Christian Barillot   David R. H
Pierre Hellier (Eds.)

Medical Image Computing and Computer-Assisted Intervention – MICCAI 2004

7th International Conference
Saint-Malo, France, September 26-29, 2004
Proceedings, Part I

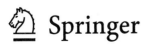 Springer

Volume Editors

Christian Barillot
IRISA-CNRS, VisAGeS Team
Campus de Beaulieu, 35042 Rennes Cedex, France
E-mail: Christian.Barillot@irisa.fr

David R. Haynor
University of Washington
Department of Radiology
Seattle, WA 98195-6004, USA
E-mail: haynor@u.washington.edu

Pierre Hellier
IRISA-INRIA, VisAGeS Team
Campus de Beaulieu, 35042 Rennes Cedex, France
E-mail: Pierre.Hellier@irisa.fr

Library of Congress Control Number: 2004111954

CR Subject Classification (1998): I.5, I.4, I.3.5-8, I.2.9-10, J.3, J.6

ISSN 0302-9743
ISBN 3-540-22976-0 Springer Berlin Heidelberg New York

Springer is a part of Springer Science+Business Media

springeronline.com

© Springer-Verlag Berlin Heidelberg 2004
Printed in Germany

Typesetting: Camera-ready by author, data conversion by PTP-Berlin, Protago-TeX-Production GmbH
Printed on acid-free paper   SPIN: 11317753   06/3142   5 4 3 2 1 0

Preface

The 7th International Conference on Medical Imaging and Computer Assisted Intervention, **MICCAI 2004**, was held in Saint-Malo, Brittany, France at the "Palais du Grand Large" conference center, September 26–29, 2004. The proposal to host **MICCAI 2004** was strongly encouraged and supported by IRISA, Rennes. IRISA is a publicly funded national research laboratory with a staff of 370, including 150 full-time research scientists or teaching research scientists and 115 postgraduate students. INRIA, the CNRS, and the University of Rennes 1 are all partners in this mixed research unit, and all three organizations were helpful in supporting **MICCAI**.

MICCAI has become a premier international conference with in-depth papers on the multidisciplinary fields of medical image computing, computer-assisted intervention and medical robotics. The conference brings together clinicians, biological scientists, computer scientists, engineers, physicists and other researchers and offers them a forum to exchange ideas in these exciting and rapidly growing fields.

The impact of **MICCAI** increases each year and the quality and quantity of submitted papers this year was very impressive. We received a record 516 full submissions (8 pages in length) and 101 short communications (2 pages) from 36 different countries and 5 continents (see figures below). All submissions were reviewed by up to 4 external reviewers from the Scientific Review Committee and a primary reviewer from the Program Committee. All reviews were then considered by the **MICCAI 2004** Program Committee, resulting in the acceptance of 235 full papers and 33 short communications. The normal mode of presentation at **MICCAI 2004** was as a poster; in addition, 46 papers were chosen for oral presentation. All of the full papers accepted are included in these proceedings in 8-page format. All of the accepted 2-page short communications are also included; they appeared at the meeting as posters. The first figure below shows the distribution of accepted contributions by topic, topics being defined from the primary keyword of the submission.

To ensure that these very selective decisions was made as fairly and justly as possible, reviewer names were not disclosed to anyone closely associated with the submissions, including, when necessary, the organizers. In addition, to avoid any unwanted pressure on reviewers, the general chair and program chair did not co-author any submissions from their groups. Each of the 13 members of the Program Committee supervised the review process for almost 50 papers. The members of the Scientific Review Committee were selected based both on a draft and on an open volunteering process and a final list of 182 reviewers was selected based on background and expertise. After recommendations were made by the reviewers and the Program Committee, a final meeting took place during two days in early May in Rennes. Because of the overall quality of the submissions and because of the limited number of slots available for presentation, about one quarter of the contributions were further discussed in order to form the final program. We are especially grateful to Nicholas Ayache, Yves Bizais,

Hervé Delingette, Randy Ellis, Guido Gerig and Wiro Niessen, who attended this meeting and helped us make the final selections. We are grateful to everyone who participated in the review process; they donated a large amount of time and effort to make these volumes possible and insure a high level of quality.

It was our great pleasure to welcome this year's **MICCAI 2004** attendees to Saint-Malo. Saint-Malo is a corsair city (a corsair was a kind of official "pirate," hired by the king) and the home city of Jacques Cartier, the discoverer of Canada and Montreal, the site of last year's **MICCAI**. The city is located on the north coast of Brittany, close to Mont Saint-Michel and to Rennes. Saint-Malo is often compared to a great vessel preparing to set out to sea, always seeking renewal and adventure. We hope that the attendees, in addition to attending the conference, took the opportunity to explore the city, the sea shore, particularly at high tide (which was unusually high at the time of the conference), and other parts of Brittany, one of France's most beautiful regions. For those unable to attend, we trust that these volumes will provide a valuable record of the state of the art in the **MICCAI 2004** disciplines.

We look forward to welcoming you to **MICCAI 2005**, to be held next year in Palm Springs, CA, USA.

September 2004   Christian Barillot, David Haynor and Pierre Hellier

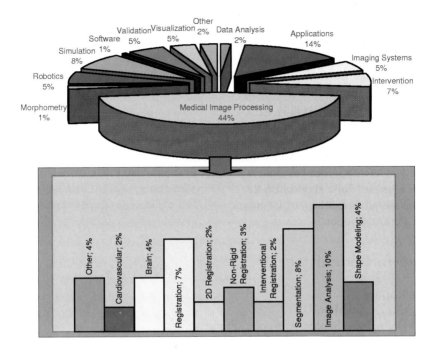

Fig. 1. View at a glance of **MICCAI 2004** contributions based on the declared primary keyword

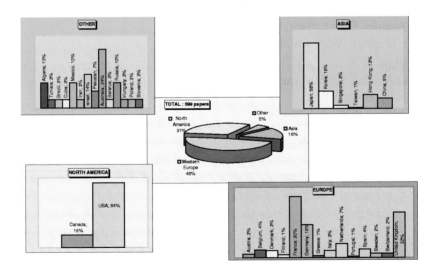

Fig. 2. Distribution of **MICCAI 2004** submissions by region

Organization

Executive Committee

Christian Barillot (General Chair), Rennes, France
David Haynor (Program Chair), Seattle, USA
Pierre Hellier (Program Co-chair), Rennes, France
James Duncan, New Haven, USA
Mads Nielsen, Copenhagen, Denmark
Terry Peters, London, Canada

Program Committee

Long Papers
Brian Davies, London, UK
Hervé Delingette, Sophia-Antipolis, France
Gabor Fichtinger, Baltimore, USA
Guido Gerig, Chapel Hill, USA
Nobuhiko Hata, Tokyo, Japan
David Hawkes, London, UK
Wiro Niessen, Utrecht, The Netherlands
Alison Noble, Oxford, UK
Gabor Szekely, Zurich, Switzerland
William (Sandy) Wells, Cambridge, USA

Short Papers
Nicholas Ayache, Sophia-Antipolis, France
Yves Bizais, Brest, France
Randy Ellis, Kingston, Canada
Steven Pizer, Chapel Hill, USA
Michael Vannier, Iowa City, USA

MICCAI Board

Alan Colchester (General Chair), Canterbury, UK
Nicholas Ayache, Sophia-Antipolis, France
Christian Barillot, Rennes, France
Takeyoshi Dohi, Tokyo, Japan
James Duncan, New Haven, USA
Terry Peters, London, Canada
Stephen Pizer, Chapel Hill, USA
Richard Robb, Rochester, USA
Russell Taylor, Baltimore, USA
Jocelyne Troccaz, Grenoble, France
Max Viergever, Utrecht, The Netherlands

Tutorial Chair

Grégoire Malandain, Sophia-Antipolis, France

Poster Coordination

Sylvain Prima, Rennes, France

Industrial Exhibition Co-chairs

Jean-Loïc Delhaye, Rennes, France
Bernard Gibaud, Rennes, France

Student Awards Coordination

Karl Heinz Höhne, Hamburg, Germany

Conference Secretariat/Management

Edith Blin-Guyot, Rennes, France
Caroline Binard, Rennes, France
Elisabeth Lebret, Rennes, France
Valérie Lecomte, Rennes, France
Nathalie Saux-Nogues, Rennes, France
Marina Surbiguet, Rennes, France

Proceedings Management

Laure Aït-Ali, Rennes, France
Arnaud Ogier, Rennes, France
Cybèle Ciofolo, Rennes, France
Valérie Lecomte, Rennes, France
Anne-Sophie Tranchant, Rennes, France
Sylvain Prima, Rennes, France
Romain Valabrègue, Rennes, France

Local Organization Committee

Christine Alami, Rennes, France
Annie Audic, Rennes, France
Yves Bizais, Brest, France
Patrick Bourguet, Rennes, France
Patrick Bouthemy, Rennes, France
Michel Carsin, Rennes, France
Pierre Darnault, Rennes, France
Gilles Edan, Rennes, France
Jean-Paul Guillois, Rennes, France
Pascal Haigron, Rennes, France
Pierre Jannin, Rennes, France
Claude Labit, Rennes, France
Jean-Jacques Levrel, Rennes, France
Eric Marchand, Rennes, France
Etienne Mémin, Rennes, France
Xavier Morandi, Rennes, France
Gérard Paget, Rennes, France
Jean-Marie Scarabin, Rennes, France

Reviewers

Purang Abolmaesumi
Faiza Admiraal-Behloul
Marco Agus
Carlos Alberola-López
Elsa Angelini
Neculai Archip
Simon R. Arridge
John Ashburner
Fred S. Azar
Christian Barillot
Pierre-Louis Bazin
Fernando Bello

Marie-Odile Berger
Margrit Betke
Isabelle Bloch
Thomas Boettger
Sylvain Bouix
Catherina R. Burghart
Darwin G. Caldwell
Bernard Cena
Francois Chaumette
Kiyoyuki Chinzei
Gary Christensen
Albert C.S. Chung

Philippe Cinquin
Jean Louis Coatrieux
Chris Cocosco
Alan Colchester
D. Louis Collins
Isabelle Corouge
Olivier Coulon
Patrick Courtney
Christos Davatzikos
Brian Davis
Benoit Dawant
Marleen De Bruijne
Michel Desvignes
Simon Dimaio
Etienne Dombre
Simon Duchesne
Ayman El-Baz
Alan Evans
Yong Fan
J. Michael Fitzpatrick
Oliver Fleig
Alejandro Frangi
Ola Friman
Robert Galloway
Andrew Gee
James Gee
Bernard Gibaud
Maryellen Giger
Daniel Glozman
Polina Golland
Miguel Angel Gonzalez Ballester
Eric Grimson
Christophe Grova
Christoph Guetter
Pascal Haigron
Steven Haker
Makoto Hashizume
Stefan Hassfeld
Peter Hastreiter
Pheng Ann Heng
Derek Hill
Karl Heinz Höhne
Robert Howe
Hiroshi Iseki
Pierre Jannin

Branislav Jaramaz
Sarang Joshi
Michael Kaus
Peter Kazanzides
Erwin Keeve
Erwan Kerrien
Charles Kervrann
Ali Khamene
Sun I. Kim
Tadashi Kitamura
Karl Krissian
Gernot Kronreif
Frithjof Kruggel
Luigi Landini
Thomas Lange
Thomas Lango
Rudy Lapeer
Rasmus Larsen
Heinz U. Lemke
Shuo Li
Jean Lienard
Alan Liu
Huafeng Liu
Jundong Liu
Marco Loog
Benoit Macq
Mahnaz Maddah
Frederik Maes
Isabelle Magnin
Sherif Makram-Ebeid
Gregoire Malandain
Armando Manduca
Jean-Francois Mangin
Marcos Martín-Fernández
Calvin Maurer Jr.
Tim McInerney
Etienne Memin
Chuck Meyer
Michael I. Miga
Xavier Morandi
Kensaku Mori
Ralph Mosges
Yoshihiro Muragaki
Toshio Nakagohri
Kyojiro Nambu

Table of Contents, Part I

LNCS 3216: MICCAI 2004 Proceedings, Part I

Brain Segmentation

Cardiovascular Segmentation

Segmentation I

Segmentation Methods

Registration II

Table of Contents, Part II

LNCS 3217: MICCAI 2004 Proceedings, Part II

Robotics

Simulation and Rendering

Interventional Imaging

Brain Imaging Applications

Cardiac and Other Applications

Short Communications

Level Set Methods in an EM Framework for Shape Classification and Estimation

Andy Tsai[1,2], William Wells[3,4], Simon K. Warfield[3,4,5], and Alan Willsky[2]

[1] Department of Medicine, Massachusetts General Hospital,
Harvard Medical School, Boston, MA, USA
[2] Department of Electrical Engineering and Computer Science,
Massachusetts Institute of Technology, Cambridge, MA, USA
[3] Department of Radiology, Brigham and Women's Hospital,
Harvard Medical School, Boston, MA, USA
[4] Computer Science and Artificial Intelligence Laboratory,
Massachusetts Institute of Technology, Cambridge, MA, USA
[5] Department of Radiology, Children's Hospital,
Harvard Medical School, Boston, MA, USA

Abstract. In this paper, we propose an Expectation-Maximization (EM) approach to separate a shape database into different shape classes, while simultaneously estimating the shape contours that best exemplify each of the different shape classes. We begin our formulation by employing the level set function as the shape descriptor. Next, for each shape class we assume that there exists an unknown underlying level set function whose zero level set describes the contour that best represents the shapes within that shape class. The level set function for each example shape is modeled as a noisy measurement of the appropriate shape class's unknown underlying level set function. Based on this measurement model and the judicious introduction of the class labels as hidden data, our EM formulation calculates the labels for shape classification and estimates the shape contours that best typify the different shape classes. This resulting iterative algorithm is computationally efficient, simple, and accurate. We demonstrate the utility and performance of this algorithm by applying it to two medical applications.

1 Introduction

Shape classification can be defined as the systematic arrangement of shapes within a database, based on some similarity criteria. It has received considerable attention in recent years with important applications to problems such as computer aided diagnosis, handwriting recognition, and industrial inspection. The various classification techniques in the literature can be broadly categorized into those based on feature matching and those based on dense matching. Dense matching algorithms are computationally expensive as they try to transform or warp one shape into another based on some energy optimization scheme. For example, Del Bimbo and Pala [3] derived a similarity measure between two shapes based on the amount of elastic deformation energy involved in matching

C. Barillot, D.R. Haynor, and P. Hellier (Eds.): MICCAI 2004, LNCS 3216, pp. 1–9, 2004.

the shapes. Cohen *et. al.,* [2] developed an explicit mapping between two shape contours based on finite element analysis. Basri *et. al.,* [1] used the sum of local deformations needed to change one shape into another as the similarity metric in comparing two shapes.

Feature matching algorithms are more popular and utilize low-dimensional feature vectors extracted from the shapes for classification. For example, Dionisio and Kim [5] classified objects based on features computed from polygonal approximations of the object. Kawata *et al.,* [8] extracted surface curvatures and ridge lines of pulmonary nodules from 3D lung CT images to discriminate between malignant and benign nodules. In Golland *et al.,* [7], skeletons are used to extract features which are then used within different linear classification methods (Fisher linear discriminant and linear Support Vectors method). Gdalyahu and Weinshall [6] constructed syntactic representation of shapes (with primitives consisting of line segments and attributes consisting of length and orientation), and used a variant of the edit matching procedure to classify silhouettes.

We consider our algorithm as a feature matching algorithm. The individual pixels associated with each shape's level set representation are the features associated with that particular shape. One might argue that the dimensionality of this feature space is too high, and is not really a feature space as it does not capture only the salient information pertinent to a shape. However, we believe that it is the over representation or redundancy within this feature space that lends simplicity to our formulation and affords us the ability to capture very subtle differences among shapes for classification. We then incorporated this high-dimensional feature vector within an EM framework to provide us with a principled approach of comparing shapes for classification.

The rest of this paper is organized as follows. Section 2 illustrates how we incorporated the level set methods into the EM framework for shape classification and estimation. In Section 3, we present experimental evaluations of our algorithm by applying our technique to two medical problems. We conclude in Section 4 with a summary of the paper and a discussion on future research.

2   Shape Classification and Estimation

Given a database of example shapes, the goal of our algorithm is two-fold: (1) to separate the example shapes into different groups of approximately the same shapes (based on some similarity measure), and (2) to estimate the shape contour for each group that best represents or typifies the shapes contained within that group. Accomplishing these two tasks of shape classification and estimation is difficult, and is the problem which we focus on in this paper.

In this shape classification and estimation problem, if the underlying shape contour of each shape class is known *a priori*, then various pattern recognition techniques in the literature can be employed to separate the shapes within the database into different groups. Similarly, if the class labels of every example in the database is known *a priori*, then the underlying contour for each shape class can be estimated by calculating the "average" shape contour within each shape class. Needless to say, it is difficult to calculate or determine either the representative shape contour of each class or the class labels of the example shapes in the database without knowledge of the other. However, we will show in this paper that it is possible to estimate both using the EM algorithm.

2.1   Shape Representation

We begin by describing our choice of the shape descriptor. Let the shape database $\mathcal{T}$ consist of a set of L *aligned* contours $\{\mathcal{C}_1, \mathcal{C}_2, ..., \mathcal{C}_L\}$.[1] We employ the signed distance function as the shape descriptors in representing each of these contours [9]. In particular, each contour is embedded as the zero level set of a signed distance function with negative distances assigned to the inside and positive distances assigned to the outside. This technique yields L level sets functions $\{Y_1, Y_2, ..., Y_L\}$, with each level set function consisting of N samples (using identical sample locations for each function).

2.2   Measurement and Probabilistic Models

For simplicity of derivation and clarity of presentation, we assume that there are only two shape classes within the database which we would like to group. It is important to realize, however, that it is straightforward to generalize our algorithm to classify more than two classes. By limiting ourselves to classify only two shape classes, we can employ the binary class label $C = \{C_1, C_2, ..., C_L\}$ to indicate which of the two shape classes each of the example shapes belong to. Specifically, each $C_l \; \forall l = 1, ..., L$ takes on the values of 0 or 1.

In our problem formulation, we postulate that there are two unknown level set functions $X = \{X_1, X_2\}$, one associated with each of the two shape classes with the property that the zero level sets of X_1 and X_2 represent the underlying shape contours of the two shape classes A and B. Importantly, there are no restrictions placed on whether X is a signed distance function. Next, we view each example shape's level set function Y_l as a noisy measurement of either X_1 or X_2. Based on this formulation, the explicit dependence of Y_l on X and C_l is given by the following measurement model:

$$Y_{l_i} = \begin{bmatrix} C_l & (1 - C_l) \end{bmatrix} \begin{bmatrix} X_{1_i} \\ X_{2_i} \end{bmatrix} + v_i \qquad \forall i = 1, ..., N \tag{1}$$

where $v \sim \mathcal{N}(0, \sigma^2 I)$ represents the measurement noise with σ as the standard deviation of the noise process.[2] This measurement model gives us the following

---

[1] Any alignment strategy that will result in the shapes having the same orientation and size can be employed.

[2] The notation I represents the identity matrix and the notation $\mathcal{N}(\mu, \Lambda)$ represents a Gaussian random vector with mean μ and variance Λ.

conditional probability of Y given C and X:

$$p(Y|X,C) = \prod_{l=1}^{L} p(Y_l|X,C_l) = \prod_{l=1}^{L} \left[C_l \quad (1-C_l) \right] \begin{bmatrix} \prod_{i=1}^{N} \frac{1}{\sqrt{2\pi}\sigma} e^{-\frac{(Y_{l_i}-X_{1_i})^2}{2\sigma^2}} \\ \prod_{i=1}^{N} \frac{1}{\sqrt{2\pi}\sigma} e^{-\frac{(Y_{l_i}-X_{2_i})^2}{2\sigma^2}} \end{bmatrix} . \quad (2)$$

Of note, this probability model bears resemblance to the stochastic framework introduced in [10] for the construction of prior shape models.

We assume that the class labels C and the level set representations of the shape contours X are statistically independent and hence

$$p(C|X) = p(C) . \quad (3)$$

Without any prior knowledge regarding the classifications of the various example shapes in the database, we set

$$p(C_l) = \begin{cases} 0.5 & \text{if } C_l = 0 \\ 0.5 & \text{if } C_l = 1 \end{cases} \qquad \forall l = 1, ..., L . \quad (4)$$

2.3   The EM Framework

The EM procedure, first introduced by Dempster *et. al.* [4] in 1977, is a powerful iterative technique suited for calculating the maximum-likelihood (ML) estimates in problems where parts of the data are missing. The missing data in our EM formulation is the class labels C. That is, if the class labels for the different shapes within the database are known, then estimating the underlying shape contour which best represents each shape class would be straightforward. The observed data in our EM formulation is Y, the collection of level set representations of the example shapes. Finally, X is the quantity to be estimated in our formulation.

The E-step. The E-step computes the following auxilliary function Q:

$$Q(X|X^{[k]}) = \left\langle \log p(Y,C|X) \big| Y, X^{[k]} \right\rangle \quad (5)$$

where $X^{[k]}$ is the estimate of X from the kth iteration, and $\langle \cdot \rangle$ represents the conditional expectation over C given Y and the current estimate $X^{[k]}$. Using Bayes' rule and our earlier simplified assumption that C and X are statistically independent, Q can be rewritten as

$$Q(X|X^{[k]}) = \left\langle \log p(Y|X,C) \big| Y, X^{[k]} \right\rangle + \left\langle \log p(C) \big| Y, X^{[k]} \right\rangle . \quad (6)$$

Since the M-step will be seen below to be a maximization of $Q(X|X^{[k]})$ over X, we can discard the second term in Eq. (6) since it does not depend on X.

Expanding the remaining term in Eq. (6), we have that[3]

$$Q(X|X^{[k]}) = -\sum_{l=1}^{L} \left[\langle C_l|Y_l, X^{[k]}\rangle \; (1 - \langle C_l|Y_l, X^{[k]}\rangle) \right] \begin{bmatrix} \sum_{i=1}^{N}(Y_{l_i} - X_{1_i})^2 \\ \sum_{i=1}^{N}(Y_{l_i} - X_{2_i})^2 \end{bmatrix}. \quad (7)$$

As evident from above, the core of the E-step is the computation of $\langle C_l|Y_l, X^{[k]}\rangle$. Using the formula for expectations, Bayes's rule, and Eqs. (2), (3), and (4), we find that

$$\langle C_l|Y_l, X^{[k]}\rangle = \frac{\prod_{i=1}^{N} e^{-\frac{(Y_{l_i}-X_{1_i}^{[k]})^2}{2\sigma^2}}}{\prod_{i=1}^{N} e^{-\frac{(Y_{l_i}-X_{1_i}^{[k]})^2}{2\sigma^2}} + \prod_{i=1}^{N} e^{-\frac{(Y_{l_i}-X_{2_i}^{[k]})^2}{2\sigma^2}}}. \quad (8)$$

This equation is equivalent to calculating the posterior shape class probabilities assuming that the underlying level set functions X_1 and X_2 are known.

The M-step. Estimates of X_1 and X_2 are obtained in the M-step of our formulation by maximizing the auxiliary function Q. In other words, the M-step calculates the $X^{[k+1]}$ such that

$$X^{[k+1]} = \arg\max_{X} Q(X|X^{[k]}). \quad (9)$$

To solve for $X^{[k+1]}$, we imposed the zero gradient condition to Eq. (7). In particular, by differentiating $Q(X|X^{[k]})$ with respect to X_{1_i} and X_{2_i} for each pixel i, and setting each resulting equation to 0, we obtain the following two expressions:

$$X_{1_i}^{[k+1]} = \frac{\sum_{l=1}^{L} \langle C_l|Y_{l_i}, X_i^{[k]}\rangle Y_{l_i}}{\sum_{l=1}^{L} \langle C_l|Y_{l_i}, X_i^{[k]}\rangle} \qquad \forall i = 1, ..., N$$

$$\qquad (10)$$

$$X_{2_i}^{[k+1]} = \frac{\sum_{l=1}^{L} \left(1-\langle C_l|Y_{l_i}, X_i^{[k]}\rangle\right) Y_{l_i}}{\sum_{l=1}^{L} \left(1-\langle C_l|Y_{l_i}, X_i^{[k]}\rangle\right)} \qquad \forall i = 1, ..., N$$

Eq. (10) is equivalent to an ML estimator of the level set functions X_1 and X_2 when the shape labels are known. Of interest, note that both X_1 and X_2 are weighted averages of distance maps from different shape examples. As a result, neither X_1 and X_2 are signed distance functions because distance functions are not closed under linear operations.

---

[3] Here, in order to take the log of $p(Y|X, C)$ in Eq. (2), we have used the fact that each C_l is a binary indicator which selects the appropriate probability distribution function.

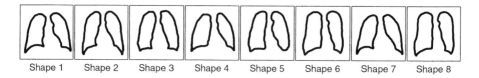

Shape 1   Shape 2   Shape 3   Shape 4   Shape 5   Shape 6   Shape 7   Shape 8

Fig. 1. Database of eight contours outlining the right and left lung fields from a collection of chest radiographs.

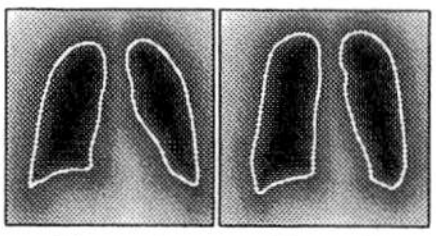

Shape	1	2	3	4	5	6	7	8
Radiologist	Nl	Nl	Dz	Nl	Dz	Dz	Nl	Dz
EM	A	A	B	A	B	B	A	B

Class A   Class B

Fig. 2. Left: Level set estimates of the two shape classes with the zero level set marked in white. Right: Comparion of chest radiograph labelings between a radiologist and our EM algorithm. The radiologist classified the chest radiographs into normal (Nl) or one with emphysema (Dz). The EM algorithm classified them into class A or class B.

3   Experimental Results

In this section, we present two medical applications to illustrate the performance of our algorithm. In both examples, we employ the alignment strategy proposed in [11] to guarantee that the example shapes in the database are all aligned to one another in terms of size and orientation. Furthermore, in these experiments, we start the iteration on the E-step, and initialize X_1 and X_2 to be the average of signed distance maps from two mutually complementary subsets of the shape database. Specifically, X_1 is set to be the average of the first four signed distance maps, and X_2 is set to be the average of the latter four signed distance maps. After convergence of our algorithm, we threshold the class labels to obtain the classification results we show in this section.

3.1   Chest Radiographs of Normal and Emphysematous Patients

Emphysema is a lung disease which involves the destruction of alveoli and its surrounding tissue. Typical findings on chest xrays of emphysema patients include hyperinflation of the lung fields and flattened diaphram. Figure 1 shows a database consisting of eight sets of contours with each set representing the outlines of the right and left lung fields from a different patient's chest radiograph. The eight patients' chest radiographs have been classified *a priori* by a radiologist as having either normal or emphysematous lung. The experiment here is two-fold: (1) to classify the eight sets of contours shown in Figure 1 into two groups based on our EM-based classifier, and (2) to compare the grouping scheme generated by our algorithm with the one from the radiologist's.

The experimental results are shown in Figure 2. The two images shown in Figure 2 represent the level set functions of the two shape classes with the zero level set of each level set function outlined in white. The white contours can be thought of as the representative shape of each shape class. The table in the figure shows that the grouping scheme generated by our EM algorithm exactly matched the one generated by the radiologist. In particular, notice that Class A corresponds to normal and Class B corresponds to diseased patients. Not surprisingly, Class B's representative shape shows the hyperinflated lung as well as the flatten diagphram typical of emphysematous patients. For this particular experiment with each shape having 300×300 pixels, it took 5 iterations to converge requiring approximiately 1.67 seconds on an Intel Xeon 4.4GHz dual processor computer.

3.2   Cerebellum of Neonates with Dandy-Walker Syndrome

Dandy-Walker Syndrome is a congenital brain malformation associated with agenesis of the cerebellum. Our task is to separate the cerebellum database shown in Figure 3 into normal cerebellums and those afflicted with Dandy-Walker Syndrome. The eight cerebellums in the database are known *a priori* to either have the disease or not. The experiment here is: (1) to classify the eight cerebellums into two different groups based on our EM-based shape classifier, and (2) to compare the results of the grouping scheme generated by our EM algorithm with the one known *a priori*.

The experimental results are shown in Figure 4. The two shapes shown in Figure 4 are the representative shapes of the two shape classes. The table in the figure shows that the grouping scheme generated by our EM algorithm matched the correct answer. In particular, notice that Class A corresponds to normal and Class B corresponds to diseased patients. Class B's representative shape shows partial agenesis of the superior aspect of the cerebellum. For this 3D experiment, each example shape's level set function is represented by $256 \times 256 \times 50$ pixels. In terms of processing time, 10 iterations were required for convergence taking approximiately 39 seconds on an Intel Xeon 4.4GHz dual processor computer.

4   Conclusions and Future Research Directions

We have outlined a novel approach for statistical shape classification and estimation based on the EM algorithm and the level set representation of shapes. The approach we have outlined is flexible as it can handle the classification of complex shapes (including those that have dimensionality greater than two and those with complex topologies) into multiple shape classes (and not just limited to two classes). The experimental results we show here are encouraging as it demonstrates low classification errors with fast processing times. We are currently exploring the use of other implicit shape representations (other than distance transforms) that will not cause any inconsistencies in the shape representation during the calculation of the M-step. We are also interested in extending this formulation to enable it to provide users with information regarding the specific differences among the different shape classes.

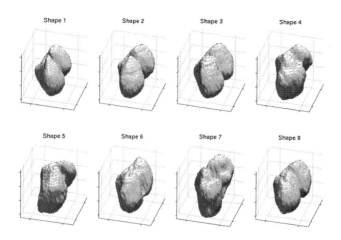

Fig. 3. Database of normal and diseased cerebellums.

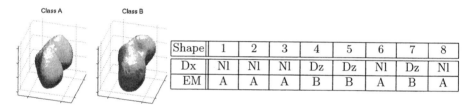

Shape	1	2	3	4	5	6	7	8
Dx	Nl	Nl	Nl	Dz	Dz	Nl	Dz	Nl
EM	A	A	A	B	B	A	B	A

Fig. 4. Left: Shape estimates of the two shape classes. Right: Comparion of labelings between the truth and our EM classifier. The diagnosis (Dx) of the cerebellums is either normal (Nl) or one with Dandy-Walker syndrome (Dz). The EM algorithm classified the cerebellums into class A or class B.

Acknowledgements. This work was supported by MGH Internal Medicine Residency Program, AFOSR grant F49620-00-1-0362, Whitaker Foundation, NIH grants R21 MH67054, R01 LM007861, P41 RR13218, NSF ERC9731748, NIH 5 P41 RR13218, and JHU EEC9731748. The authors would like to thank Drs. A. Mewes and C. Limperopoulos for their help in the segmentation of the cerebellum data set.

References

1. R. Basri, L. Costa, D. Geiger, and D. Jacobs, "Determining the similarity of deformable shapes," *IEEE Workshop: Phys Based Modeling in Comput Vis*, pp. 135-143, 1995.
2. I. Cohen, N. Ayache, and P. Sulger, "Tracking points on deformable objects using curvature information," *ECCV*, pp. 458-466, 1992.
3. A. Del Bimbo and P. Pala, "Visual image retrieval by elastic matching of user sketches," *IEEE Trans PAMI*, vol 19, pp. 121-132, 1997.

4. A. Dempster, N. Laird, and D. Rubin, "Maximum-likelihood from incomplete data via the EM algorithm," *J of Royal Statist Soc Ser B*, vol. 39, pp. 1-38, 1977.
5. C. Dionisio and H. Kim, "A supervised shape classification technique invariant under rotation and scaling," *Int'l Telecommunications Symposium*, 2002.
6. Y. Gdalyahu and D. Weinshall, "Flexible syntactic matching of curves and its application to automatic hierarchical classification of silhouettes," *IEEE Trans. on PAMI*, vol 21, pp. 1312-1328, 1999.
7. P. Golland, E. Grimson, and R. Kikinis, "Statistical shape analysis using fixed topology skeletons: corpus callosum study," *IPMI*, pp. 382-387, 1999.
8. Y. Kawata, N. Niki, H. Ohmatsu, R. Kakinuma, K. Eguchi, M. Kaneko, and N. Moriyama, "Classification of pulmonary nodules in thin-section CT images based on shape characteristics," *IEEE Trans on Nucl Sci*, vol. 45, pp. 3075-3082, 1998.
9. S. Osher and J. Sethian, "Fronts propagation with curvature dependent speed: Algorithms based on Hamilton-Jacobi formulations," *J. of Comput. Phys.*, vol. 79, pp. 12–49, 1988.
10. N. Paragios and M. Rousson, "Shape priors for level set representations," *ECCV*, June 02, Copenhagen, Denmark.
11. A. Tsai, A. Yezzi, W. Wells, C. Tempany, D. Tucker, A. Fan, E. Grimson, and A. Willsky, "A shaped-based approach to segmentation of medical imagery using level sets.," *IEEE Trans on Medical Imaging*, vol. 22, pp. 137-154, 2003.

Automatic Segmentation of Neonatal Brain MRI[*]

Marcel Prastawa[1], John Gilmore[2], Weili Lin[3], and Guido Gerig[1,2]

Department of [1]Computer Science, [2]Psychiatry, and [3]Radiology
University of North Carolina, Chapel Hill, NC 27599, USA
prastawa@cs.unc.edu

Abstract. This paper describes an automatic tissue segmentation method for neonatal MRI. The analysis and study of neonatal brain MRI is of great interest due to its potential for studying early growth patterns and morphologic change in neurodevelopmental disorders. Automatic segmentation of these images is a challenging task mainly due to the low intensity contrast and the non-uniformity of white matter intensities, where white matter can be divided into early myelination regions and non-myelinated regions. The degree of myelination is a fractional voxel property that represents regional changes of white matter as a function of age. Our method makes use of a registered probabilistic brain atlas to select training samples and to be used as a spatial prior. The method first uses graph clustering and robust estimation to estimate the initial intensity distributions. The estimates are then used together with the spatial priors to perform bias correction. Finally, the method refines the segmentation using sample pruning and non-parametric density estimation. Preliminary results show that the method is able to segment the major brain structures, identifying early myelination regions and non-myelinated regions.

1 Introduction

Magnetic resonance imaging is the preferred imaging modality for in vivo studies of brain structures of neonates. Potential applications include the analysis of normal growth patterns and the study of children at high risk for developing schizophrenia and other neurodevelopmental disorders. This typically involves the reliable and efficient processing of a large number of datasets. Therefore, automatic segmentation of the relevant structures from neonatal brain MRI is critical. This task is considerably more difficult when compared with the segmentation of brain MRI of infants and adults. This is due to a number of factors: low contrast to noise ratio, intensity inhomogeneity (bias field), and the inhomogeneity of the white matter structure. White matter is separated into myelinated

---

[*] This research is supported by the UNC Neurodevelopmental Disorders Research Center (PI Joseph Piven) HD 03110 and the NIH Conte Center MH064065. Marcel Prastawa is supported by R01 HL69808 NIH-NCI (PI E. Bullitt).

white matter and non-myelinated white matter, often with ambiguous boundaries and as a regional pattern that changes with age.

Experience shows that automatic segmentation methods for healthy adult brain MRI generally fail to properly segment neonatal brain MRI. However, the concepts and approaches for segmenting adult brains are still applicable for neonatal brains if adjusted to tackle the specific problems. Matsuzawa et al. [1] showed neonatal brain segmentation from MRI as a part of a study of early brain development. The results show that the method has difficulties dealing with tissue separation. The segmentations of one-month-old infants show mostly noise, although axial MRI slices visually leave the impression that there are intensity differences between non-myelinated white matter and gray matter. Most advanced work has been demonstrated by Warfield et al. [2,3], but subjects were mostly preterm babies presenting less complex cortical folding.

A successful concept for robust, automatic tissue segmentation of adult brains is to use the information provided by a brain atlas. The brain atlas can be used as spatial priors for segmentation [4,5]. The template-moderated segmentation proposed by Warfield et al. [6] clearly demonstrates the strength of the use of a spatial prior since regions that overlap in intensity space but are spatially disjoint can be separated. However, there is no spatial model for early myelination regions in white matter since this is an infiltrating tissue property. Cocosco et al. [7] demonstrated automatic, robust selection of training samples for different tissue categories using only regions with high atlas probabilities. Additionally, this research proposed non-parametric clustering to overcome limitations of traditional mixture Gaussian models. Brain tissue segmentation based on fractional voxel properties has been developed by Shattuck et al. [8], motivated by the need to improved tissue segmentation in the presence of pathological regional changes. Preliminary feasibility tests with our 3 Tesla neonatal MRI with the EMS method [5] were shown in Gerig et al. [9].

We have developed a new atlas based segmentation method for neonatal brain MR images. The atlas is used as a guide to determine sample locations and also defines spatial prior probabilities for tissue to improve robustness of classification. Incorporating spatial priors into the process is essential for separating different tissues that have low contrast. Our method combines the graph clustering approach by Cocosco et al. [7], the bias correction scheme by Van Leemput et al. [10], and the robust estimation algorithm by Rousseeuw et al. [11]. In contrast to most other brain segmentation schemes, our new segmentation method integrates bias correction, non-parametric classification, and brain masking into one method.

2   Method

Unlike in adult brains, white matter in neonatal brains cannot be treated as a single structure. White matter is composed of large non-myelinated regions and small regions of early myelination (mostly seen in the internal capsule and along the projection tracts towards the motor cortex). Non-myelinated white

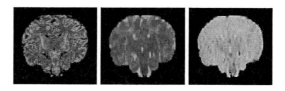

Fig. 1. Example neonatal MRI dataset with early myelination: the filtered and bias corrected Neonate-0026 dataset. From left to right: T1-weighted image, T2-weighted image, and the proton density image.

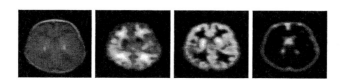

Fig. 2. The neonatal brain atlas-template created from a single subject segmentation and blurring. From left to right: T1 template image, white matter (both myelinated and non-myelinated), gray matter, and cerebrospinal fluid probabilities.

matter in infants have the inverse intensity properties as compared to adult white matter, it is dark in T1-weighted images and bright in T2-weighted images. Early myelination in white matter is shown as hyper intense regions in T1-weighted images and hypo intense regions in T2-weighted images. Fig. 1 shows an example of neonatal brain MRI in different modalities with early myelination regions.

Due to the different growth patterns across subjects and significant changes over the first few months of development, it would be difficult to obtain separate spatial models for the two different white matter classes. Therefore, we use a single spatial prior for white matter that provides the probability for every voxel to be either a myelinated white matter or non-myelinated white matter. Spatial and geometric differences between the two classes are difficult to summarize, so the identification of the different white matter classes is set to be driven by image intensities. To test our method, we have created a template atlas shown in Fig. 2. The template atlas was created from the segmentation of one dataset that was done using a semi-automatic segmentation method. The human rater first removes the skull and background using thresholding and user-supervised level set evolution. The rater then manually marks regions for each tissue type in different areas throughout the brain. From the user-selected regions, a bias field estimate is extrapolated and then used to correct the inhomogeneity. The segmentation is obtained using the k-nearest neighbor algorithm using training samples from the selected regions. The segmentation result is then edited manually to correct for possible errors. We then blur the final segmentation result to simulate the population variability. The creation of a brain atlas that sufficiently describes the true variability of the population is a significant challenge beyond the scope of this paper, but is currently in progress.

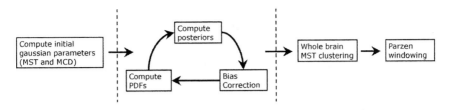

Fig. 3. Overview of the segmentation algorithm. The dashed lines show the division of the process to three major steps: initial estimation of parameters using MCD and MST clustering, bias correction, and refinement using a non-parametric segmentation method.

The segmentation process is initialized by registering the subject to the atlas using affine transformation and the mutual information image match metric [12]. The registered images are then filtered using anisotropic diffusion [13]. Since the relative ordering of the different structures are known, the clustering method using the Minimum Spanning Tree (MST) proposed by Cocosco *et al.* [7] is ideal. However, this method requires that the input images are already bias corrected and that the brain regions are identified. These tasks are not easily accomplished given the intensity properties of neonatal MRI. Our method combines the clustering method with robust estimation and bias correction using spatial probabilities. The method is composed of three major steps, as shown in Fig. 3. First, it obtains rough estimates of the intensity distributions of each tissue class. It then iteratively performs segmentation and bias correction. Finally, it refines the segmentation result using a non-parametric method.

2.1 Estimation of Initial Gaussian Parameters

The first step in the segmentation process determines the rough estimates of the intensity distributions. Here, we choose to use the Gaussian as a rough model of the intensity distributions. The parameters for the multivariate Gaussians are computed through the combination of the Minimum Covariance Determinant (MCD) estimator and MST edge breaking to the training samples.

The training samples are obtained by selecting a subset of the voxels with high probability values (ex. $\tau > 0.9$). Additionally, we use the image gradient magnitudes as a sampling constraint. The 2-norm of the image gradient magnitudes at voxel location x, $G(x) = \sqrt{|\nabla I_1(x)|^2 + \ldots + |\nabla I_n(x)|^2}$, is the measure we have chosen. Samples with $G(x)$ greater than the average $G(x)$ over the candidate white matter regions ($Pr(wm) > 0$) is removed to avoid sampling in the transition regions between myelinated and non-myelinated white matter and at white/gray matter boundaries. The removal of samples from the partial volume regions aids the clustering process (Fig. 4).

Once the samples are obtained, we compute the initial parameters for gray matter and csf using the robust mean and covariance from the MCD estimator [11]. The result of the MCD algorithm is the ellipsoid that covers at least

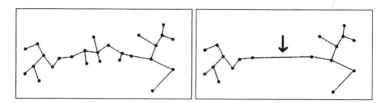

Fig. 4. Illustrations of the Minimum Spanning Trees for white matter obtained using different sampling strategies. Left: Samples with high probability values. Right: Samples with high probability values and low gradient magnitude. Choosing only samples with low gradient magnitude helps to remove samples from the transition regions between myelinated white matter and non-myelinated white matter and gray/white boundary voxels. This is crucial for clustering based on edge breaking. As seen on the right picture, breaking the longest edge marked by the arrow would give two well separated clusters.

half of the data with the smallest determinant of covariance. We then apply the graph clustering method through MST edge breaking to the white matter samples. The two white matter distributions are computed using an iterative process similar to the one described in [7]:

1. Given a threshold value T, break edges incident with node i that have length greater than $T \times A(i)$, where $A(i)$ is the average length of all edges incident on node i.
2. Determine the two largest clusters and their means using the MCD algorithm. The two clusters are sorted based on the robust mean along one of the intensity features (set the first cluster to represent early myelination).
3. Stop when the two clusters satisfy the relative ordering criterion along one of the intensity features. For example, the robust mean values for the T2 intensity feature must follow the relation: $\mu_{myel} < \mu_{gm} < \mu_{non-myel} < \mu_{csf}$
4. Otherwise, decrease the value of T and go back to step 1.

Once the two white matter clusters are identified, the robust mean and covariance of the two clusters obtained through the MCD algorithm is used as the initial Gaussian distributions for white matter. The initial Gaussian parameters are then combined with spatial priors in the next step where this initial segmentation is used to estimate the bias field.

2.2 Bias Correction

Neonatal brain MR images exhibit higher intensity variability for each tissue and low intensity contrast as compared to adult MRI. These two factors severely hamper the estimation of intensity inhomogeneity. We have experimented with a histogram based intensity inhomogeneity correction, developed by Styner *et al.* [14]. We concluded that histogram based method would often fail to obtain the optimal solution. The histogram of a neonatal brain MR dataset is generally smooth with weak maximas.

In the case of bias correction of neonatal brain MRI, the spatial context is useful to deal with the low intensity contrast. We have chosen to use the method developed by Van Leemput *et al.* [10]. The bias correction scheme uses the spatial probabilities to estimate the bias field. The bias field is estimated by fitting a polynomial to the log difference between the original image and the reconstructed homogeneous image.

2.3   Segmentation Refinement

At this stage, the images are already bias corrected and the brain regions are identified. However, the Gaussian does not seem the optimal model for the intensity distributions due to large intensity variability. Therefore, segmentation obtained using this model generally has more false positives. In order to refine the segmentation results, we apply the MST clustering method [7] to prune the samples. Instead of using probability thresholding, we simply use the previous classification labels for sample selection. The training samples obtained using this method is then used to estimate the probability density functions of each class using Parzen windowing or kernel expansion.

3   Results

We have applied the method to two cases, as shown in Fig. 5. Visual inspection shows that the major regions are properly identified, although the distinction between myelinated white matter and non-myelinated white matter is incorrect in some regions. The myelinated white matter regions are mostly distributed near the spine (central posterior). We also observed the presence of myelinated white matter around the regions associated with the sensory and motor cortex.

Quantitative validation of the segmentation results is inherently difficult due to the lack of a gold standard. The common standard, comparison with manual segmentations, does not seem to be feasible since highly convoluted structures in low-contrast, noisy data are hard to trace. In addition to that, the myelinated white matter and the non-myelinated white matter have ambiguous boundaries, which would make manual segmentation results highly variable and difficult to reproduce. This problem is solved for adult brains by offering web-based archives with simulated datasets [15] and manually segmented real datasets [1]. We are currently working on contour-based segmentation with subsequent manual interaction to provide standardize test data for validation. .

4   Discussion and Conclusion

Efficient and robust segmentation of tissue and degree of myelination would have a large impact in neonatal MRI studies, because early detection of pathology may permit early intervention and therapy. Neonatal brain MRI offers unique

---

[1] Internet Brain Segmentation Repository, http://www.cma.mgh.harvard.edu/ibsr

T1   T2   PD   Labels   3D

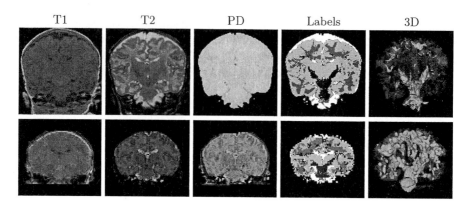

Fig. 5. The datasets and the generated segmentation results (top: high quality dataset provided by Petra Hüppi, bottom: Twin-0001A dataset). The results show that our method identifies the major brain structures, including the early myelination regions and the non-myelinated white matter regions. The classification labels are encoded as gray values, from darkest to brightest: myelinated white matter, non-myelinated white matter, gray matter, and csf. The 3D images show the segmented myelinated white matter (solid) and non-myelinated white matter (transparent).

challenges for image analysis. Standard automated segmentation methods fail as there is reduced contrast between white and gray matter in neonates. Noise is larger since non-sedated neonates need to be scanned with a high-speed MRI protocol to avoid motion artifacts. White matter is also heterogeneous, with hyper intense myelinated white matter (in T1 image) compared to non-myelinated white matter. The low contrast and visible contours in the data suggest that a boundary-based approach would be ideal as opposed to voxel-by-voxel statistical pattern recognition. Tissue segmentation by statistical pattern recognition on voxel intensities by definition lacks the concept of finding boundaries. On the other hand, the poor quality of the data and high complexity of convoluted structures presents a challenge for boundary driven segmentation methods.

We have presented an atlas-based automatic segmentation method for multi-channel neonatal MRI data. The method uses graph clustering and robust estimation to obtain good initial estimates, which are then used to segment and correct the intensity inhomogeneity inherent in the image. The segmentation is then refined through the use of a non-parametric method. Visual inspection of the results shows that the major structures are properly segmented, while the separation of myelinated and non-myelinated white matter still lacks spatial coherence in some regions. The availability of a real neonatal probabilistic brain atlas that captures the variability of the population is a critical issue for the proposed method. The creation of such an atlas requires the segmentation of a set of representative datasets and may require deformable registration for reducing the high shape variability, which make the task highly challenging.

Acknowledgements. We acknowledge Petra Hüppi for providing a high quality neonate dataset, Koen Van Leemput for providing the MATLAB code that aids the development of the bias correction software, and the ITK community (http://www.itk.org) for providing the software framework for the segmentation algorithm.

References

1. Matsuzawa, J., Matsui, M., Konishi, T., Noguchi, K., Gur, R., Bilder, W., Miyawaki, T.: Age-related volumetric changes of brain gray and white matter in healthy infants and children. Cerebral Cortex **11** (2001) 335–342
2. Warfield, S.K., Kaus, M., Jolesz, F.A., Kikinis, R.: Adaptive, template moderated, spatially varying statistical classification. Med Image Anal **4** (2000) 43–55
3. Hüppi, P., Warfield, S., Kikinis, R., Barnes, P., Zientara, G., Jolesz, F., Tsuji, M., Volpe, J.: Quantitative magnetic resonance imaging of brain development in premature and normal newborns. Ann Neurol **43** (1998) 224–235
4. Wells, W.M., Kikinis, R., Grimson, W.E.L., Jolesz, F.: Adaptive segmentation of MRI data. IEEE TMI **15** (1996) 429–442
5. Van Leemput, K., Maes, F., Vandermeulen, D., Suetens, P.: Automated model-based tissue classification of MR images of the brain. IEEE TMI **18** (1999) 897–908
6. Warfield, S., Dengler, J., Zaers, J., Guttman, C., Wells, W., Ettinger, G., Hiller, J., Kikinis, R.: Automatic identification of gray matter structures from MRI to improve the segmentation of white matter lesions. Journal of Image Guided Surgery **1** (1995) 326–338
7. Cocosco, C.A., Zijdenbos, A.P., Evans, A.C.: A fully automatic and robust brain MRI tissue classification method. Medical Image Analysis **7** (2003) 513–527
8. Shattuck, D.W., Sandor-Leahy, S.R., Schaper, K.A., Rottenberg, D.A., Leahy, R.M.: Magnetic resonance image tissue classification using a partial volume model. NeuroImage **13** (2001) 856–876
9. Gerig, G., Prastawa, M., Lin, W., Gilmore, J.: Assessing early brain development in neonates by segmentation of high-resolution 3T MRI. In: MICCAI. Number 2879 in LNCS, Springer (2003) 979–980 Short Paper.
10. Van Leemput, K., Maes, F., Vandermeulen, D., Suetens, P.: Automated model-based bias field correction of MR images of the brain. IEEE TMI **18** (1999) 885–896
11. Rousseeuw, P.J., Van Driessen, K.: A fast algorithm for the minimum covariance determinant estimator. Technometrics **41** (1999) 212–223
12. Maes, F., Collignon, A., Vandermeulen, D., Marchal, G., Suetens, P.: Multimodality image registration by maximization of mutual information. IEEE TMI **16** (1997) 187–198
13. Gerig, G., Kübler, O., Kikinis, R., Jolesz, F.: Nonlinear anisotropic filtering of MRI data. IEEE TMI **11** (1992) 221–232
14. Styner, M., Brechbuhler, C., Szekely, G., Gerig, G.: Parametric estimate of intensity inhomogeneities applied to MRI. IEEE TMI **19** (2000) 153–165
15. Collins, D.L., Zijdenbos, A.P., Kollokian, V., Sled, J.G., Kabani, N.J., Holmes, C.J., Evans, A.C.: Design and construction of a realistic digital brain phantom. IEEE TMI **17** (1998) 463–468

Segmentation of 3D Probability Density Fields by Surface Evolution: Application to Diffusion MRI

Christophe Lenglet, Mikaël Rousson, and Rachid Deriche

I.N.R.I.A. Sophia Antipolis, France
{clenglet,mrousson,der}@sophia.inria.fr

Abstract. We propose an original approach for the segmentation of three-dimensional fields of probability density functions. This presents a wide range of applications in medical images processing, in particular for diffusion magnetic resonance imaging where each voxel is assigned with a function describing the average motion of water molecules. Being able to automatically extract relevant anatomical structures of the white matter, such as the *corpus callosum*, would dramatically improve our current knowledge of the cerebral connectivity as well as allow for their statistical analysis. Our approach relies on the use of the symmetrized Kullback-Leibler distance and on the modelization of its distribution over the subsets of interest in the volume. The variational formulation of the problem yields a level-set evolution converging toward the optimal segmentation.

1 Introduction

Diffusion magnetic resonance imaging is a relatively new modality [4], [9] able to quantify the anisotropic diffusion of water molecules in highly structured biological tissues. In 1994, P. Basser [2] proposed to model the probability density function of the molecular motion $r \in \mathbb{R}^3$ by a Gaussian law whose covariance matrix is given by the diffusion tensor $\mathbf{D}$. Diffusion Tensor Imaging (DTI) then produces a volumic image containing, at each voxel, a 3×3 symmetric positive-definite tensor. The estimation of these tensors requires the acquisition of diffusion weighted images in different sampling directions together with a T2 image. Numerous algorithms have been proposed to perform a robust estimation and regularization of these tensors fields [13], [18]. Recently, Q-ball Imaging has been introduced by D. Tuch etal. [14] in order to reconstruct the Orientation Distribution Function (ODF) by the Funk-Radon transform of high b-factor diffusion weighted images acquired under the narrow pulse approximation. This ODF is the symmetric probability density function $S^2 \to \mathbb{R}$ giving the probability for a spin to diffuse in a given direction. This method provides a better angular constrast and is able to recover intra-voxel fiber crossings.

Diffusion MRI is particularly relevant to a wide range of clinical pathologies investigations such as acute brain ischemia detection [12], stroke, Alzheimer disease, schizophrenia [1] ...etc. It is also extremely useful in order to identify the

C. Barillot, D.R. Haynor, and P. Hellier (Eds.): MICCAI 2004, LNCS 3216, pp. 18–25, 2004.
© Springer-Verlag Berlin Heidelberg 2004

neural connectivity of the human brain [8], [15], [5]. As of today, diffusion MRI is the only non-invasive method that allows us to distinguish the various anatomical structures of the cerebral white matter such as the *corpus callosum*, the *arcuate fasciculus* or the *corona radiata*. These are examples of commisural, associative and projective neural pathways, the three major types of fiber bundles, respectively connecting the two hemispheres, regions of a given hemisphere or the cerebral cortex with subcortical areas. In the past, many techniques have been proposed to classify gray matter, white matter and cephalo-spinal fluid from T1-weighted MR [20] images but the literature addressing the issue of white matter internal structures segmentation is just beginning [21], [7], [17], [19].

In the following, we introduce a novel technique for the segmentation of any probability density function (*pdf*) field by examining the statistics of the distribution of the Kullback-Leibler distances between these *pdfs*. Our goal is to perform the direct segmentation of internal structures of the white matter. Zhukov et al. [21] defined an invariant anisotropy measure in order to drive the evolution of a level-set and isolate strongly anisotropic regions of the brain. The reduction of the full tensor to a single scalar gives a relatively low discrimination power to the method potentially resulting in segmentation of mixed structures. On the other side, Wiegell et al. [19], Jonasson et al. [7] and Wang et al. [16] proposed different measures of dissimilarity between full diffusion tensors: The first method uses the Frobenius norm of the difference of tensors, together with a spatial coherence term in a k-means algorithm to perform the segmentation of the thalamus nuclei. The nature of the elements to be segmented (compact, homogeneous) verify the restrictive hypothesis of the technique, which is rarely the case. The second method introduces a geometric measure of dissimilarity by computing the normalized tensor scalar product of two tensors, which can be interpreted as a measure of overlap. Finally, the third method relies on the natural distance between two Gaussian *pdfs*, given by the symmetrized Kullback-Leibler distance. The authors elegantly derive an affine invariant dissimilarity measure between diffusion tensors and apply it to the segmentation of 2D fields of *pdfs*. We generalize the existing methods to the 3D case and exploit the information provided by the statistics of the distribution of the symmetrized Kullback-Leibler (KL) distances. KL distances are taken between any *pdf* and our method is thus applicable not only to DTI but also, for example, to Q-ball data which should enable the proposed algorithm to catch even finer details. Section 2 will derive the evolution equation used to drive a 3D surface toward the optimal segmentation. Section 3 will present and discuss experimental results both on synthetic and real DTI datasets.

2   Derivation of the Level-Set Evolution

Let $p(x, r)$ be the probability density function of a random vector r of $\mathbb{R}^3$ describing the water molecules average motion at a given voxel x of a diffusion MR image $\Omega \subset \mathbb{R}^3$ and for a given diffusion time τ imposed by the parameters of the PGSE (Pulsed Gradient Spin Echo) sequence. We are interested in characterizing the global coherence of that *pdf* field and use the classical symmetrized

Kullback-Leibler distance to that end. With $p(x), q(y) \, \forall x, y \in \Omega$ two *pdfs* from $\mathbb{R}^3$ onto $\mathbb{R}^+$, their KL distance is given by

$$d(p, q) = KL(p, q) = \frac{1}{2} \int_{\mathbb{R}^3} \left(p(r) \log \frac{p(r)}{q(r)} + q(r) \log \frac{q(r)}{p(r)} \right) dr \qquad (1)$$

Assuming a partition of the data between the structure we try to segment Ω_1 and the rest of the volume Ω_2, we seek the optimal separating surface Γ between those two subsets. We denote by $\bar{p}_1$ and $\bar{p}_2$ the most representative *pdfs* over Ω_1 and Ω_2 verifying equation 5. It is then possible to model the distribution of the KL distances to $\bar{p}_1$ and $\bar{p}_2$ in their respective domains by suitable densities $p_{d,1}, p_{d,2}$. In the following, we make the assumption that $p_{d,1}, p_{d,2}$ are Gaussian of zero mean and variances σ_1^2, σ_2^2. It is indeed natural to impose the mean distance to the *pdfs* $\bar{p}_1$ and $\bar{p}_2$ to be as small as possible, while retaining an important degree of freedom by considering the variances of those distributions.

We then define the following energy in order to maximize the likelihood of these densities on their associated domain:

$$E(\Omega_i, \sigma_i^2, \bar{p}_i) = \sum_{i=1}^{2} \int_{\Omega_i} -\log p_{d,i}(d(p(x), \bar{p}_i)) dx \qquad (2)$$

where $p_{d,i} = \frac{1}{\sqrt{2\pi\sigma_i^2}} \exp \frac{-d^2(p, \bar{p}_i)}{2\sigma_i^2}$. We denote by $\phi : \Omega \to \mathbb{R}^3$ the level set distance function whose zero isosurface coincides with Γ. We define $H_\epsilon(z)$ and $\delta_\epsilon(z)$ the regularized versions of the Heaviside and Dirac functions [6] and we can now rewrite equation 2 and introduce a regularity constraint on Γ as follows:

$$\int_\Omega -\log p_{d,1}(d(p(x), \bar{p}_1)) H_\epsilon(\phi) - \log p_{d,2}(d(p(x), \bar{p}_2))(1 - H_\epsilon(\phi)) + \nu |\nabla H_\epsilon(\phi)| dx$$
$$(3)$$

The derivation of the Euler-Lagrange equations for this class of energy was studied in [11] and yields the following evolution for ϕ:

$$\phi_t(x) = \delta_\epsilon(\phi(x)) \left(\nu \operatorname{div} \frac{\nabla \phi}{|\nabla \phi|} + \frac{1}{2} \log \frac{p_{d,2}}{p_{d,1}} \right) \, \forall x \in \Omega \qquad (4)$$

Moreover, the derivation of the energy with respect to σ_i^2 and $\bar{p}_i$ provides the update formulae for these statistical parameters. It can be shown that the variance must be updated with its empirical estimation, whereas some more work is needed for the $\bar{p}_i$. We indeed have to estimate:

$$\tilde{p}_i = argmin \int_{\Omega_i} KL^2(\bar{p}_i, p(x)) dx \qquad (5)$$

For a general *pdf* $p(x)$, for instance if we consider the ODF derived from Q-ball data, the variance is easily computed as in [11] but the estimation of the $\tilde{p}_i$ might require the use of numerical approximation techniques if no closed form is available. If we now come back to the DTI case (ie. Gaussian *pdfs*), a recent paper by Wang et al. [16] nicely showed that the mean value of the tensor field is given by $\tilde{\mathbf{D}}_i = \sqrt{\mathbf{B}_i^{-1}} \left(\sqrt{\sqrt{\mathbf{B}_i} \mathbf{A}_i \sqrt{\mathbf{B}_i}} \right) \sqrt{\mathbf{B}_i^{-1}}$ where $\mathbf{A}_i = \int_{\Omega_i} \mathbf{D}(x) dx$ and $\mathbf{B}_i = \int_{\Omega_i} \mathbf{D}^{-1}(x) dx$

3   Experimental Results and Comparisons

We begin with a validation of our approach on synthetical data with limit cases where other approaches fail. Then, experiments are conducted on the extraction of the *corpus callosum* from real DTI data. Finally, we show how we can improve the robustness of our approach by introducing an anisotropy measure.

3.1   Synthetical Data

Diffusion tensor images measure the displacement of water molecules. This displacement, which characterizes different tissues, can be split into two different information: its intensity and its direction. When considering diffusion tensor images, these information are given respectively by the largest eigenvalue and the corresponding eigenvector. From this decomposition, we built one limit case where the two regions differ only with respect to the main orientation of the tensors. Moreover, to stress the algorithm, we also impose some degree of variation on the main orientation within the inside region by creating a junction as shown in Fig.1. Last, but not least, a Gaussian noise was added directly on the eigen-elements of each tensor. Initializing the surface with a bounding box, our approach is able to give the expected segmentation (Fig.1).

However, this example does not show the necessity of including a statistical model for the distance distribution of each region and the approach proposed in [16] for 2D fields of *pdf* gives a similar result. In order to show the advantages of our model, which is more general, we have generated a second test image. As shown in Fig.2, it is composed by one torus whose internal tensors are oriented according to the tangents of the central radius of the torus. Noise is also added to all the tensors of the image but with a different variance whether the tensor is inside or outside the torus. In Fig.2, we compare the results obtained using [16] and our approach, for different initializations. The first method fails to segment the torus because of the orientations high variations within each region. If we initialize with a bounding box, the surface shrinks until it disappears and if we start from a small sphere inside the torus, only a small part of the torus can be captured. Using our approach, which models the variance of the tensors, the torus is correctly extracted for the different initializations.

3.2   Real DTI Data

Data acquisition: Our dataset consists of 30 diffusion weighted images S_k : $\Omega \to \mathbb{R}$, $k = 1, ..., 30$ as well 1 image S_0 corresponding to the signal intensity in the absence of a diffusion-sensitizing gradient field. They were obtained on a GE

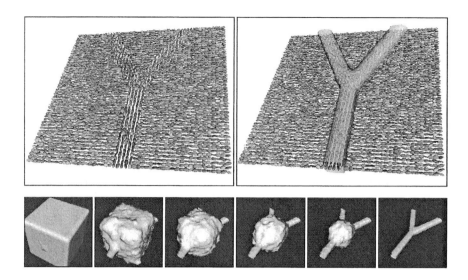

Fig. 1. Segmentation of a noisy tensor field composed by two regions with same scale but different orientations (TOP LEFT: 2D-cut of the tensor field, TOP RIGHT: same with final segmentation, BOTTOM: surface evolution).

1.5 T Signa Echospeed with standard 22 mT/m gradient field. The echoplanar images were acquired on 56 evenly spaced axial planes with a 128×128 pixels in each slice. Voxel size is 1.875 $mm \times 1.875\ mm \times 2.8\ mm$. 6 gradient directions $\mathbf{g}_k$, each with 5 different b-factors and 4 repetitions were used. Imaging parameters were: b values between 0 and 1000 $s.mm^{-2}$, $TR = 2.5\ s$, $TE = 84.4\ ms$ and a square field of view of 24 cm [10]. Those data are courtesy of CEA-SHFJ/Orsay, France[1]. References on the estimation and the regularization of diffusion tensors can be found in [13].

Experiments: The extraction of anatomical structures from DTI data is of great interest since it gives the opportunity to discriminate structures like the *corpus callosum* which is much harder to characterize using other modalities. Before any processing, the image is cropped around the element of interest to respect the assumption of bi-partitioning imposed by our model. The first experiment aims at extracting the lateral ventricles. Two small spheres are placed inside the ventricles to initialize the surface. The evolution and the final segmentation are shown in Fig.3. This result looks close to what can be expected from anatomical knowledge.

Improvements using the anisotropy: When we consider only the region terms presented in Section 2, the initialization is really important and in many cases, several seeding points have to be set manually to avoid the surface to get

---

[1] The authors would like to thank J.F. Mangin and J.B Poline for providing us with the data

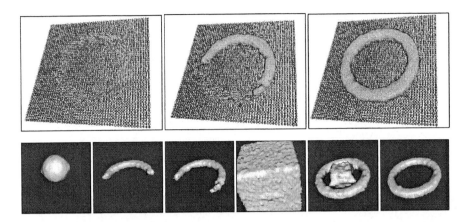

Fig. 2. Segmentation of a noisy tensor field composed by two regions with different orientations (TOP LEFT: 2D-cut of the tensor field, TOP CENTER: segmentation obtained from [16], TOP RIGHT: segmentation obtained with our method, BOTTOM: surface evolution for both of them).

stuck in a local minima. This can be overcome by introducing a global anisotropy measure. A popular one is the fractional anisotropy [3]:

$$\mathcal{A}(\mathbf{D}(x)) = \frac{\sqrt{(\lambda_1 - \lambda_2)^2 + (\lambda_2 - \lambda_3)^2 + (\lambda_1 - \lambda_3)^2}}{\sqrt{2}\sqrt{\lambda_1^2 + \lambda_2^2 + \lambda_3^2}}$$

An additional term is then defined to impose a given distribution of the anisotropy inside each region. Let $p_{a,1}$ and $p_{a,2}$ be the *pdf* of the anisotropy in Ω_1 and Ω_2, approximated by Gaussian densities. Then, according to [11] the partitioning is obtained by minimizing:

$$-\int_{\Omega} \log p_{a,1}(\mathcal{A}(\mathbf{D}(x)))H_\epsilon(\phi) + \log p_{a,2}(\mathcal{A}(\mathbf{D}(x)))(1 - H_\epsilon(\phi))dx \qquad (6)$$

This term is added to the objective function (3) defined in Section 2. Then, we obtain a new evolution equation for the level set function ϕ composed by two terms whose influence can be controlled by adjusting the weight α between zero and one:

$$\phi_t(x) = \delta_\epsilon(\phi(x)) \left(\nu \text{div}\frac{\nabla\phi}{|\nabla\phi|} + (1 - \alpha)\frac{1}{2}\log\frac{p_{d,2}}{p_{d,1}} + \alpha\frac{1}{2}\log\frac{p_{a,2}}{p_{a,1}} \right) \forall x \in \Omega \qquad (7)$$

and the statistical parameters of $p_{a,1}$ and $p_{a,2}$ are updated iteratively like in the previous part. In practice, a small weight on the anisotropy term is sufficient to avoid the surface to get stuck in a local minima. For example, the extraction of the *corpus callosum* in Fig.3 was possible thanks to this additional term by setting α to 0.3.

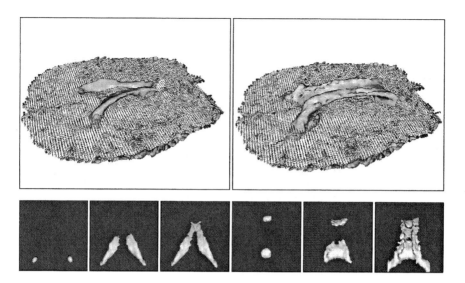

Fig. 3. Segmentation of the brain lateral ventricles (TOP LEFT) and the *corpus callosum* (TOP RIGHT) in a real diffusion tensor image, superimposed on the DTI field, BOTTOM: surface evolution for both of them).

4   Conclusion

We have presented a novel technique for the segmentation of probability density fields with a major contribution to the extraction of anatomical structures in anisotropic biological tissues such as the brain white matter. We have shown that this method performs very well on synthetic data and is able to catch fine details on real DTI thus exhibiting an adequate behavior of the Kullback-Leibler distance and of the modelization of its distribution by Gaussian densities. We are currently working on general density functions derived, for example, from Q-ball imaging to better describe the voxel-wise diffusion process.

Acknowledgements. The authors would like to thank O. Faugeras (INRIA, Sophia-Antipolis), G. Sapiro, K. Ugurbil, S. Lehericy, K. Lim (University of Minnesota), B. Vemuri and Y. Chen (University of Florida) for their valuable discussions and comments.

References

1. B.A. Ardekani, J. Nierenberg, M.J. Hoptman, D.C. Javitt, and K.O. Lim. MRI study of white matter diffusion anisotropy in schizophrenia. *NeuroReport*, 14(16):2025–2029, November 2003.
2. P.J. Basser, J. Mattiello, and D. LeBihan. MR diffusion tensor spectroscopy and imaging. *Biophysica*, (66):259–267, 1994.

3. P.J. Basser and C. Pierpaoli. Microstructural and physiological features of tissues elucidated by quantitative diffusion tensor MRI. *Journal of Magnetic Resonance,* 11:209–219, 1996.
4. D. Le Bihan, E. Breton, D. Lallemand, P. Grenier, E. Cabanis, and M. Laval-Jeantet. MR imaging of intravoxel incoherent motions: Application to diffusion and perfusion in neurologic disorders. *Radiology,* pages 401–407, 1986.
5. J.S.W. Campbell, K. Siddiqi, B.C. Vemuri, and G.B Pike. A geometric flow for white matter fibre tract reconstruction. In *IEEE International Symposium on Biomedical Imaging Conference Proceedings,* pages 505–508, July 2002.
6. T. Chan and L. Vese. An active contour model without edges. In *Scale-Space Theories in Computer Vision,* pages 141–151, 1999.
7. L. Jonasson, P. Hagmann, X. Bresson, R. Meuli, O. Cuisenaire, and J.P Thiran. White matter mapping in DT-MRI using geometric flows. In *EUROCAST,* pages 585–596, 2003.
8. C. Lenglet, R. Deriche, and O. Faugeras. Inferring white matter geometry from diffusion tensor MRI: Application to connectivity mapping. In ECCV, 4:127–140, 2004.
9. K.D. Merboldt, W. Hanicke, and J. Frahm. Self-diffusion NMR imaging using stimulated echoes. *J. Magn. Reson.,* 64:479–486, 1985.
10. C. Poupon. *Détection des faisceaux de fibres de la substance blanche pour l'étude de la connectivité anatomique cérébrale.* PhD thesis, ENST, December 1999.
11. M. Rousson and R. Deriche. A variational framework for active and adaptative segmentation of vector valued images. In *Proc. IEEE Workshop on Motion and Video Computing,* pages 56–62, Orlando, Florida, December 2002.
12. C. Sotak. The role of diffusion tensor imaging (DTI) in the evaluation of ischemic brain injury. *NMR Biomed.,* 15:561–569, 2002.
13. D. Tschumperlé and R. Deriche. Variational frameworks for DT-MRI estimation, regularization and visualization. In *Proceedings of the 9th International Conference on Computer Vision,* Nice, France, 2003.
14. D.S. Tuch, T.G. Reese, M.R. Wiegell, and V.J. Wedeen. Diffusion MRI of complex neural architecture. *Neuron,* 40:885–895, December 2003.
15. B. Vemuri, Y. Chen, M. Rao, T. McGraw, T. Mareci, and Z. Wang. Fiber tract mapping from diffusion tensor MRI. In *1st IEEE Workshop on Variational and Level Set Methods in Computer Vision,* July 2001.
16. Z. Wang and B.C. Vemuri. An affine invariant tensor dissimilarity measure and its application to tensor-valued image segmentation. In *IEEE Conference on Computer Vision and Pattern Recognition,* Washington, DC., June 2004.
17. Z. Wang and B.C. Vemuri. Tensor field segmentation using region based active contour model. In ECCV, 4:304–315, 2004.
18. Z. Wang, B.C. Vemuri, Y. Chen, and T. Mareci. Simultaneous smoothing and estimation of the tensor field from diffusion tensor MRI. In *IEEE Conference on Computer Vision and Pattern Recognition,* 1:461–466, 2003.
19. M.R. Wiegell, D.S. Tuch, H.W.B. Larson, and V.J. Wedeen. Automatic segmentation of thalamic nuclei from diffusion tensor magnetic resonance imaging. *NeuroImage,* 19:391–402, 2003.
20. Y. Zhang, M. Brady, and S. Smith. Segmentation of brain MR images through a hidden markov random field model and the expectation-maximization algorithm. *IEEE Transactions on Medical Imaging,* 20(1):45, January 2001.
21. L. Zhukov, K. Museth, D. Breen, R. Whitaker, and A.H. Barr. Level set segmentation and modeling of DT-MRI human brain data. *Journal of Electronic Imaging,* 12:125-133, 2003.

Improved EM-Based Tissue Segmentation and Partial Volume Effect Quantification in Multi-sequence Brain MRI

Guillaume Dugas-Phocion[1], Miguel Angel González Ballester[1],
Grégoire Malandain[1], Christine Lebrun[2], and Nicholas Ayache[1]

[1] Inria, Epidaure Project Team - 2004 route des Lucioles - BP 93
06902 Sophia Antipolis Cedex, France,
Guillaume.Dugas_Phocion@sophia.inria.fr,
http://www-sop.inria.fr/epidaure
[2] Pasteur Hospital, Neurology Department
30 voie romaine BP 69, 06002 Nice, France

Abstract. The Expectation Maximization algorithm is a powerful probabilistic tool for brain tissue segmentation. The framework is based on the Gaussian mixture model in MRI, and employs a probabilistic brain atlas as a prior to produce a segmentation of white matter, grey matter and cerebro-spinal fluid (CSF). However, several artifacts can alter the segmentation process. For example, CSF is not a well defined class because of the large quantity of voxels affected by the partial volume effect which alters segmentation results and volume computation. In this study, we show that ignoring vessel segmentation when handling partial volume effect can also lead to false results, more specifically to an over-estimation of the CSF variance in the intensity space. We also propose a more versatile method to improve tissue classification, without a requirement of any outlier class, so that brain tissues, especially the cerebro-spinal fluid, follows the Gaussian noise model in MRI correctly.

1 Introduction

The segmentation of pathological tissues in multi-spectral MRI is useful, for example for diagnosis purpose. The intensity signature of healthy tissues is more predictable than the one of potential lesions: having a good characterization and segmentation of healthy tissues is the first step to separate them from lesions.

For this task, the Expectation Maximization (EM) framework [1] is a popular tool. It provides a segmentation of MRI into three classes: grey matter, white matter, cerebro-spinal fluid (CSF). However, multiple artifacts affect the segmentation results. As an example, voxels at the interface between two tissues contain more than one tissue: this is called Partial Volume Effect (PVE) [2]. Furthermore, potential lesions are not handled here. Some solutions have been proposed in the literature to overcome these problems.

Lesions can be separated from healthy tissues by adding an outlier class, without any prior in the intensity space [3]. In [4], a tissue classification is performed and PVE voxels are labeled in a post-processing step. Another way to

C. Barillot, D.R. Haynor, and P. Hellier (Eds.): MICCAI 2004, LNCS 3216, pp. 26–33, 2004.

take PVE into account is to segment PVE voxels in the EM framework as a class, the parameters of which are constrained from other pure classes [5]. These PVE models have only been tested on T1 MR images though. In this study, we show that the CSF class is not well defined in the multi-spectral T2/PD MRI intensity space. Even with a PVE model such as [5], the segmentation still suffers from an over-estimation of the variance of each class, especially the CSF. We propose a method to deal with this problem, which will lead to the segmentation of vessels, in addition of other brain tissues. We validate our study on a database of T2/PD MRI of 36 multiple sclerosis patients and 9 healthy subjects, showing a significant decrease of the variance of pure classes.

2 EM-Based Segmentation of Brain Multi-spectral MR Images

Before performing any segmentation, we apply a skull-stripping technique to the images to keep brain tissues only. Many methods are available in the literature, our method is closely related to the one described in [6]. We first generate a primary EM-based segmentation that we refine with mathematical morphology. More details can be found in [7].

2.1 Basic Algorithm

MRI noise is known to follow a Rician probability density function (PDF). Since a Rician PDF, if mean value is greater than 0, can be reasonably approximated by a Gaussian PDF, it is acceptable to say that noise in multi-spectral MR images follows a Gaussian PDF. As a consequence, the segmentation is based on a Gaussian mixture model within the intensity space. Each class k is represented by the regular Gaussian parameters in the intensity space: mean μ_k and covariance matrix Σ_k. The EM algorithm consists in iterating two steps: labeling of the image – Expectation step – and estimation of the class parameters by maximizing the likelihood of the whole image – Maximization step [1].

The labeling is the computation of the probability of a tissue class given the image and the parameters. The application of Bayes' rule gives the solution to the problem, summarized in equation 1. l_j and y_j are respectively the label and the multi-spectral intensity of the voxel j; Y is the whole image and Φ is the set of parameters. $\Pi_{l_j=a}$ is the a priori probability to get the label a for the voxel j.

$$p(l_j = a|Y, \Phi^{m-1}) = \frac{p(y_j|l_j = a, \Phi^{(m-1)})\Pi_{l_j=a}}{\sum_k p(y_j|l_j = k, \Phi^{(m-1)})\Pi_{l_j=k}} \tag{1}$$

Π_{l_j} is different whether a probabilistic atlas is available or not. When no atlas is used, the prior does not depend on the position j of the voxel ($\Pi_{l_j=a} = \Pi_a$) and needs to be re-estimated at each iteration (by $\Pi_a = \sum_j p(l_j = a|Y, \Phi^{m-1})/\sum_j$) for convergence purposes. When the atlas is available, the spatially dependent prior simply needs to be normalized: $\forall j, \sum_k \Pi_{l_j=k} = 1$.

The estimators that maximize the likelihood are the MAP estimators corresponding to the mean and covariance matrix. As an approximation, we use the parameters of the last iteration $\Phi^{(m-1)}$ when computing the parameters at iteration m. Both estimators are represented within equations 2 and 3:

$$\mu_k^m = \frac{\sum_j p(l_j = k|Y, \Phi^{(m-1)})y_j}{\sum_j p(l_j = k|Y, \Phi^{(m-1)})} \tag{2}$$

$$\Sigma_k^m = \frac{\sum_j p(l_j = k|Y, \Phi^{(m-1)})(y_j - \mu_k^m)(y_j - \mu_k^m)'}{\sum_j p(l_j = k|Y, \Phi^{(m-1)})} \tag{3}$$

2.2   Results of the Basic Algorithm

This method was applied on T2/PD (TE=8/104, TR=5000, ETL=16, voxel size: 0.937*0.937*2) MR images, from an acquisition protocol concerning 36 relapsing remitting multiple sclerosis patients. Three classes were segmented: white matter, grey matter and CSF, with the corresponding atlas for each class, obtained by affinely registering the MNI probabilistic atlases [8]. It takes less than 30 seconds for 256*256*64 images on a 3Ghz PC. The results are shown in figure 1.

Visual inspection of white matter segmentation seems satisfactory. The grey matter Mahalanobis ellipse is deformed towards the CSF ellipse, mostly because of the partial volume effect, and the CSF class has a tremendously high variance, which seems quite hard to explain with these PVE voxels only, as shown next.

3   Improved Tissue Segmentation

3.1   Partial Volume Effect (PVE)

MR images have a limited resolution. Voxels at the interface between two classes, e.g. grey matter and CSF, have an intermediate intensity depending on the proportion of tissues in this voxel. Those "PVE voxels" will bias a segmentation into pure class voxel since it invalidates the Gaussian mixture model for the whole image.

Let there be two tissues a and b, their intensities y_a and y_b respectively, and α the proportion of tissue a in the considered PVE voxel. Let $N(\mu, \Sigma)$ be the Gaussian PDF with parameters μ and Σ. Both y_a and y_b follow a Gaussian PDF, respectively $N(\mu_a, \Sigma_a)$ and $N(\mu_b, \Sigma_b)$. The intensity of this voxel y_{PVE} is a random variable that can be computed using $y_{PVE} = \alpha y_a + (1 - \alpha)y_b$.

If we consider PVE voxels only, α is uniformly distributed. Separating PVE voxels from pure voxels is not trivial [2]. However, if α is fixed and known, y_{PVE} follows a Gaussian PDF with the following parameters:

$$y_{PVE} \sim N(\alpha\mu_a + (1 - \alpha)\mu_b, \alpha^2 \Sigma_a + (1 - \alpha)^2 \Sigma_b) \tag{4}$$

One solution is to emulate the partial volume effect by a fixing α to some constant values, and computing the PVE classes within the regular EM. The

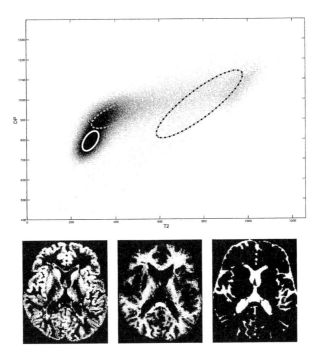

Fig. 1. Joint histogram between T2 and PD MRI, representation of tissue classes using the Mahalanobis ellipse and the corresponding classification. Three classes are segmented, corresponding to the three atlas classes (from left to right): grey matter (grey dashed), white matter (white), and CSF (black dash-dotted).

algorithm will consist in iterating three steps: labeling of all classes (including PVE classes), estimation of class parameters only for pure classes – white matter, grey matter and CSF –, and computing PVE classes parameters using equation 4. This method is interesting as it remains easy to compute and respects the original EM framework [9]. Some results are shown in figure 2.

As we can see, the grey matter class has a reasonable variance now, comparable to the one of the white matter. Indeed, adding PVE classes (between the grey matter and the CSF) allowed to decrease the variance along the T2 axis where both classes are well separate. However, the variance of the CSF remains at very high values, and the direction of the main axis shows that this problem cannot be solved solely by addressing the partial volume effect between the former segmented tissues.

3.2 Introducing a Fourth Class

As demonstrated above, the PVE does not explain the huge variance of the CSF class. A close look at the images (see figure 4.c, 4.i) shows that some dark structures (identified mainly as vessels) are also classified as CSF. Those structures

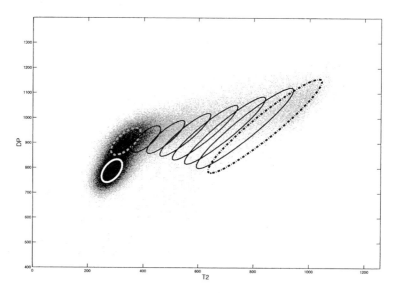

Fig. 2. Joint histogram between T2 and PD MRI, with PVE between grey-matter and CSF. 4 PVE classes were used ($\alpha \in \{0.2, 0.4, 0.6, 0.8\}$). The variance of the grey matter class has been reduced, but the CSF class is still oversized.

are not guaranteed to be labeled as outliers, if an outlier class is added as in [3]. Thus, we prefer to introduce explicitly a vessel class.

In the three class EM, vessels are classified as CSF. This CSF class has to be splitted into two classes, vessels and CSF. To achieve this, we will define an *a priori* probability for the vessels, $\pi_{l_j=\text{vessel}}$, as a fraction β of the CSF probability given by the atlas, $\Pi_{l_j=\text{CSF}}$. With this new class, the prior for CSF becomes $\pi_{l_j=\text{CSF}} = (1 - \beta)\Pi_{l_j=\text{CSF}}$.

The labeling can then be achieved into an EM framework. Since the relative ratio of vessels with respect to CSF is not known, β has to be estimated at each iteration for convergence purposes by

$$\beta = \frac{\sum_j p(l_j = \text{vessel}|Y, \Phi)}{\sum_j p(l_j = \text{vessel}|Y, \Phi) + \sum_j p(l_j = \text{CSF}|Y, \Phi)} \tag{5}$$

By introducing this fourth class, the system becomes more flexible, and still allows the adaptation of the algorithm to unforeseen tissues (e.g. with an outlier class) without loosing the information from the atlas.

The final algorithm becomes the following:

1. compute a labeling for each class (Expectation Step);
2. estimate parameters for the following classes: white matter, grey matter, CSF and vessels;
3. compute analytically PVE classes parameters using equations 4;

4. recognize the CSF class by selecting the class with highest mean on T2 axis (the CSF class has to be distinguished from the vessel class for the PVE computation with the grey matter).

Results are presented in figures 3 and 4. The CSF class only includes pure CSF (compare figure 4.i and 4.j). Its variance has decreased by a large amount, and is now comparable to grey matter and white matter class variances, which corroborates a Gaussian noise model for the MR signal.

Introducing the vessel class allows also a better recognition of PVE voxels between CSF and grey matter: Mahalanobis ellipses of PVE voxels distributions in figure 3 are now well separated.

It is important to point out that the simple usage of an outlier class may fail to separate the CSF from vessels here. Indeed, both classes have a similar number of voxels, and outlier detection assumes that the outlier class is less represented than the main class.

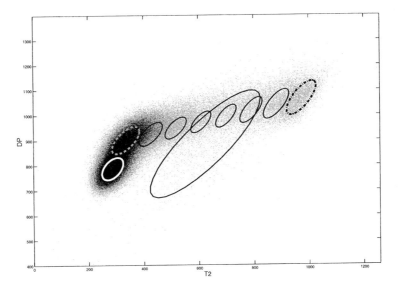

Fig. 3. Joint histogram between T2 and PD MRI, and representation of tissue classes using the Mahalanobis ellipse. As one class, which prior is a fraction of CSF atlas, is added, the CSF class does not include vessels anymore: the main three brain tissues – grey matter, white matter and CSF – follow the Gaussian noise model properly.

4 Conclusion and Future Work

Our main finding is that introducing explicitly the vessel class into the EM framework allows a significant improvement in the classification.

The system has been tested on 36 multiple sclerosis patients MRI and 9 healthy subjects, with a good estimation of the parameters, reflected by a clear

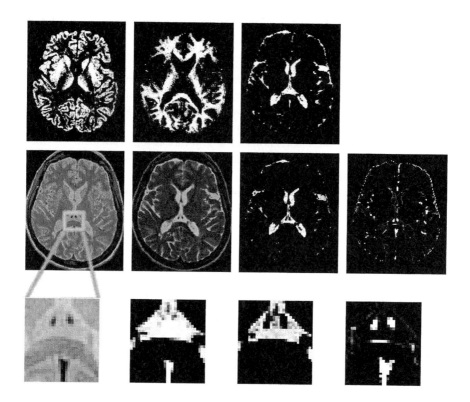

Fig. 4. Final segmentation: grey matter (a), white matter (b), CSF without vessel class (c), T2 MRI(d), Proton Density MRI (e), CSF (f), other class including vessels (g). Zoom : Proton Density (h), CSF without vessel class (i), CSF (j), other class including vessels (k).

Table 1. Estimation of T2 standard deviation for brain tissues, resulting on experiments over 36 patients and 9 healthy subjects. Notice that CSF standard deviation has been divided by 3 with the vessel class, without any intensity non-uniformity correction.

T2 std deviation	Grey matter	White matter	CSF
no PVE	68.5	32.0	160.2
PVE without vessels	49.7	33.9	167.9
PVE + vessels	46.7	34.1	58.3

PD std deviation	Grey matter	White matter	CSF
no PVE	53.3	41.8	145.2
PVE without vessels	49.9	41.2	159.6
PVE + vessels	49.7	40.4	60.5

decrease of variance for CSF class, as shown in table 1. The T2 CSF standard deviation has been divided by 3, and never exceeds 65 in all the images, although it exceeds 150 with a simple PVE model. A closer look at the final segmentation indicates that the new segmentation of CSF does not include neither vessels nor partial volume effect, that are this time correctly extracted. The whole process is still quite fast, since we simply added a few classes in the initial EM framework: it takes around 4 minutes to run the system on a 3 Ghz PC.

One application of this method may be the computation of volumes (CSF volume, or brain atrophy) since it allows a more accurate estimation of probabilities for each tissue within each voxel. Brain atrophy is indeed a good disease indicator, in Alzheimer disease or multiple sclerosis for example.

The segmentation of pathological tissues (multiple sclerosis lesions or tumors), our primary motivation, is also an interesting derived application. We argue that this may be facilitated with a good classification of healthy tissues, as the one proposed in this study. This is left as future work.

References

1. Dempster, A., Laird, N., Rubin, D.: Maximum likelihood from incomplete data via the EM algorithm. Journal of the Royal Statistical Society **39** (1977) 1–38
2. González Ballester, M.A., Zisserman, A., Brady, M.: Estimation of the partial volume effect in MRI. Medical Image Analysis **6** (2002) 389–405
3. Leemput, K.V., Maes, F., Vandermeulen, D., Colchester, A., Suetens, P.: Automated segmentation of multiple sclerosis lesions by model outlier detection. IEEE TMI **20** (2001) 677–688
4. Shattuck, D.W., Sandor-Leahy, S.R., Shaper, K.A., Rottenberg, D.A., Leahy, R.M.: Magnetic Resonance Image Tissue Classification Using a Partial Volume Model. NeuroImage **13** (2001) 856–876
5. Noe, A., Gee, J.: Efficient Partial Volume Tissue Classification in MRI Scans. In: Proc. of MICCAI. Volume 2488 of LNCS., Springer (2002) 698–705
6. Kapur, T., Grimson, W.E., Wells, W.M., Kikinis, R.: Segmentation of brain tissue from magnetic resonance images. Med Image Anal **1** (1996) 109–127
7. Dugas-Phocion, G., González Ballester, M.A., Lebrun, C., Chanalet, S., Bensa, C., Malandain, G., Ayache, N.: Hierarchical Segmentation of Multiple Sclerosis Lesions in Multi-Sequence MRI. In: International Symposium on Biomedical Imaging. (2004)
8. Collins, D., Zijdenbos, A., Kollokian, V., Sled, J., Kabani, N., Holmes, C., Evans, A.: Design and construction of a realistic digital brain phantom. IEEE TMI **17** (1998) 463–468
9. Ruan, S., Jaggi, C., Xue, J., Fadili, J., Bloyet, D.: Brain tissue classification of magnetic resonance images using partial volume modeling. IEEE Trans Med Imaging **19** (2000) 1179–1187

Cardiac Motion and Elasticity Characterization with Iterative Sequential $\mathcal{H}_\infty$ Criteria

Huafeng Liu[1,2] and Pengcheng Shi[2]

[1] State Key Laboratory of Modern Optical Instrumentation
Zhejiang University, Hangzhou, China
[2] Department of Electrical and Electronic Engineering
Hong Kong University of Science and Technology, Hong Kong
{eeliuhf, eeship}@ust.hk

Abstract. Robustness is of paramount importance in cardiac wall motion estimation and myocardial tissue elasticity characterization, especially for clinical applications. Given partial, noisy, image-derived measurements on the cardiac kinematics, we present an integrated robust estimation framework for the joint recovery of dense field cardiac motion and material parameters using iterative sequential $\mathcal{H}_\infty$ criteria. This strategy is particulary powerful for real-world problems where the types and levels of model uncertainties and data disturbances are not available *a priori*. Constructing the myocardial dynamics equations from biomechanics principles, at each time step, we rely on techniques from $\mathcal{H}_\infty$ filtering theory to first generate estimates of heart kinematics with suboptimal material parameter estimates, and then recover the elasticity property given these kinematic state estimates. These coupled iterative steps are repeated as necessary until convergence. We demonstrate the accuracy and robustness of the strategy through experiments with both synthetic data of varying noises and magnetic resonance image sequences.

1 Introduction

Regional wall function and myocardial tissue properties reveal critical information about the states of cardiac physiology and pathology. With increasingly available real-time and ECG-gated tomographic cardiac imaging data, there have been plenty image-based efforts aimed at measuring the motion and/or the material properties of the heart [3,9].

Given a set of image-derived, sparse, noisy measurements on cardiac kinematics, typical motion analysis methods need to make use of additional constraining models of mathematical or mechanical nature to obtain the dense field motion fields in some optimal senses. The underlying hypothesis is, of course, that these prior models are completely known, including their parameters, and are appropriate for the particular image data. For practical situations, especially those pathological cases, however, this assumption is rarely true. Some of the related frame-to-frame strategies can be found in a comprehensive recent review [3]. Assuming Gaussian conditions on system and data uncertainties, there are several

C. Barillot, D.R. Haynor, and P. Hellier (Eds.): MICCAI 2004, LNCS 3216, pp. 34–42, 2004.
© Springer-Verlag Berlin Heidelberg 2004

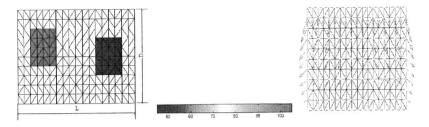

Fig. 1. Generation of the synthetic kinematic data: original configuration (left), color scale of material elasticity (middle), and displacement data at selected locations (right).

multi-frame efforts which impose the all important spatio-temporal constraints to perform motion analysis throughout the cardiac cycle [5,8,14].

The dual problem to cardiac motion recovery is the estimation of myocardial tissue elasticity based on known, image-derived kinematics observations. There have been a number of efforts on the parameter identification of the myocardium, where the basic idea is to minimize some criteria that measure the goodness of fit between the model-predicted and the data-derived mechanical responses [1,9]. More recently, an expectation-maximization (EM) strategy is proposed to estimate the composite tissue mechanical properties by using displacements reconstructed from MR tagging data [4].

We have shown that it is desirable to tackle the motion and elasticity estimation problems simultaneously, especially for disease conditions where the myocardial tissue structure and parameters undergo substantial alterations [6, 11]. By making use of the stochastic finite element and the extended Kalman filter [11], followed by a Bayesian scheme based on the maximum *a posteriori* formulation [6], these efforts were built upon a biomechanical model of the myocardium and were embedded within $\mathcal{H}_2$ filtering frameworks under known Gaussian statistics assumptions, unrealistic for real world problems. In order to relax these restrictions, we have recently proposed several $\mathcal{H}_\infty$-based robust strategies for the image-based motion recovery with fixed material model [7] and tissue elasticity estimation from known kinematics measurements [12].

In this paper, we present a robust $\mathcal{H}_\infty$ framework for the *joint* estimation of cardiac kinematics and material parameters from imaging data. It differs from the $\mathcal{H}_2$-based simultaneous estimation in: 1). no *a priori* knowledge of noise statistics is required; and 2). the min-max estimation criterion is to minimize the worst possible effects of the disturbances (model and data noises) on the signal estimation errors, which will ensure that if the disturbances are small (in energy), the estimation errors will be as small as possible (in energy), regardless the noise types. These two aspects make the $\mathcal{H}_\infty$ to be more appropriate for certain practical problems where the disturbances are unknown and non-Gaussian. In addition, our strategy is posed as an iterative sequential estimation framework which uses two separated $\mathcal{H}_\infty$ filters: one for kinematics estimation (the $\mathcal{H}_\infty$ state-filter) and one for tissue elasticity estimation (the $\mathcal{H}_\infty$ parameter-filter). At every time step, the current estimates of material parameters are used in the state-filter, and the current estimates of the kinematics are used in the

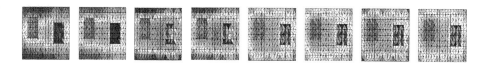

Fig. 2. Estimated elasticity distributions using the EKF [11] (the four figures on the left) and $\mathcal{H}_\infty$ (the four figures on the right) methods for noisy input data (left to right): $SNR = 20dB$ (Gaussian), $SNR = 30dB$ (Gaussian), $SNR = 20dB$ (Poisson), and $SNR = 30dB$ (Poisson).

parameter-filter. It can be thought as a generalization of the expectation maximization (EM) scheme, without the needs to know the underlying distributions.

2 Methodology

2.1 System Dynamics from Continuum Mechanics Model

For computational feasibility, our current implementation uses linear elastic material model for the myocardium. The myocardial dynamics equation, in terms of displacement field U, with a finite element representation is in the form of:

$$M\ddot{U} + C\dot{U} + KU = R \tag{1}$$

where M is the mass matrix and R the external load. The stiffness matrix K is related to the material-specific Young's modulus E and Poisson's ratio ν. In this paper, ν is fixed to 0.49 for almost incompressible material and E needs to be estimated along with the kinematics functions[1]. We also assume Rayleigh damping with $C = \alpha M + \beta K$ with fixed weighting factors α and β.

2.2 Motion Estimation: $\mathcal{H}_\infty$ State Filter

Kinematics State Space Representation. In state-space representation, Equation (1) can be rearranged by making $x(t) = (U(t), \dot{U}(t))^T$ (T denotes transpose):

$$\dot{x}(t) = A_c(\theta)x(t) + B_c w(t) \tag{2}$$

where the material parameter vector θ, the system matrices A_c and B_c, and the input term w are:

$$\theta = E, \quad A_c = \begin{bmatrix} 0 & I \\ -M^{-1}K & -M^{-1}C \end{bmatrix}, \quad B_c = \begin{bmatrix} 0 & 0 \\ 0 & M^{-1} \end{bmatrix}, \quad w(t) = \begin{bmatrix} 0 \\ R \end{bmatrix}$$

For discrete system, assuming that the input is piecewise constant over the sampling interval T between image frames, and adding the process noise $v(t)$, we arrive at the following system equation [11]:

$$x(t+1) = A(\theta)x(t) + B(\theta)w(t) + v(t) \tag{3}$$

with $A = e^{A_c T}$ and $B = A_c^{-1}(e^{A_c T} - I)B_c$.

---

[1] Here, we assume that E is spatially varying but temporally constant.

Table 1. EKF [11] and $\mathcal{H}_\infty$ estimated Young's moduli using the noise-corrupted synthetic data: each data cell represents the mean $\pm$ standard derivation for the normal (75), hard (105), and soft (45) tissues.

Method	Tissue Type	20dB(Gaussian)	30dB(Gaussian)	20dB(Poisson)	30dB(Poisson)
	Normal	61.2 ± 33.0	71.5 ± 23.9	78.0 ± 31.9	79.5 ± 23.6
EKF	Hard	95.8 ± 9.5	103.2 ± 4.5	91.9 ± 9.1	99.1 ± 6.1
	Soft	42.3 ± 18.0	47.3 ± 5.9	62.4 ± 27.8	57.3 ± 22.8
	Normal	78.8 ± 21.6	78.0 ± 17.3	77.1 ± 17.6	77.5 ± 14.1
$\mathcal{H}_\infty$	Hard	104.5 ± 6.7	104.3 ± 4.7	104.5 ± 4.7	104.8 ± 4.6
	Soft	55.0 ± 7.8	55.2 ± 7.8	55.2 ± 7.7	53.2 ± 6.3

Similarly, the system measurement equation can be expressed as:

$$y(t) = Dx(t) + e(t) \tag{4}$$

where $y(t)$ is the measurement vector, D is the measurement matrix that defines the specific input variables, and $e(t)$ is the measurement noise.

$\mathcal{H}_\infty$ **State-Filter.** Considering a system given by Equations (3) and (4), the $\mathcal{H}_\infty$ state-filtering problem is to search the optimal estimates of $x(t)$ which satisfy the following performance measure:

$$\|x(t) - \hat{x}(t)\|_Q^2 < \gamma^2 \left\{ \|v(t)\|_{W^{-1}}^2 + \|e\|_{V^{-1}}^2 + \|x(0) - \hat{x}(0)\|_{P(0)^{-1}}^2 \right\} \tag{5}$$

where the notation $\|z\|_G^2$ is defined as the square of the weighted L_2 norm of z, i.e. $\|z\|_G^2 = z^T G z$. $P(0)$, Q, W, and V are positive definite weighting matrices which are related to confidence measures and chosen by the designers to obtain desired trade-offs. $\hat{x}(0)$ is *a priori* estimate of $x(0)$, and γ is a positive constant that represents a prescribed level of noise attenuation.

The $\mathcal{H}_\infty$ estimation for the system described by Equations (3) and (4) with performance criterion (5) consists of the following iterative procedures [10]:

$$L(t) = (I - \gamma^{-2}QP(t) + D^T V^{-1} DP(t))^{-1} \tag{6}$$
$$K(t) = AP(t)L(t)D^T V^{-1} \tag{7}$$
$$\hat{x}(t+1) = A\hat{x}(t) + Bw(t) + K(t)(y(t) - D\hat{x}(t)) \tag{8}$$
$$P(t+1) = AP(t)L(t)A^T + W \tag{9}$$

It is obvious that the above $\mathcal{H}_\infty$ process has a Kalman-like structure. The only difference is that, in $\mathcal{H}_\infty$ problem, an additional condition (the Riccati matrix P is positive definite) is required for the solution to exist. It should be mentioned that directly solving Riccati equation (9) for the solution $P(t)$ is not trivial due to its nonlinearity. Instead, iterative procedure is adopted to update $R(t)$ and then $P(t)$, with $R(t)$ defined through $P(t)^{-1} = R(t)^{-1} + \gamma^{-2}Q$, and the details are omitted here.

38   H. Liu and P. Shi

Table 2. Difference between the EKF/$\mathcal{H}_\infty$ estimated displacements (from the noise-corrupted synthetic data) and the ground truth (the average displacement is 0.6).

Method	Input Data	Maximum Error	Standard Deviation
	20dB(Gaussian)	0.0246	0.0068
EKF	30dB(Gaussian)	0.0229	0.0051
	20dB(Poisson)	0.0412	0.0083
	30dB(Poisson)	0.0311	0.0057
	20dB(Gaussian)	0.0245	0.0061
$\mathcal{H}_\infty$	30dB(Gaussian)	0.0234	0.0054
	20dB(Poisson)	0.0244	0.0054
	30dB(Poisson)	0.0234	0.0054

The $\mathcal{H}_\infty$ filtering can have many solutions corresponding to different γ values. It is observed that the smaller the γ value, the smaller the estimation error. On the other hand, the Riccati equation has to have a positive definite solution, which implies that

$$[A(R(t)^{-1} + D^T V^{-1} D)^{-1} A^T + W]^{-1} - \gamma^{-2} Q > 0$$
$$\rightarrow \gamma = \xi max \left\{ eig[A(R(t)^{-1} + D^T V^{-1} D)^{-1} A^T + W] \right\}^{0.5}$$

where $max\{eig(A)\}$ denotes the maximum eigenvalue of the matrix A, and ξ is a constant larger than 1 to ensure that γ is always greater than the optimal performance level. γ value too close to the optimal performance level, i.e. $\xi \approx 1$, might actually lead to numerical instability because of matrix singularity.

2.3   Elasticity Estimation: $\mathcal{H}_\infty$ Parameter Filter

Parameter State Space Representation. In order to apply the elasticity parameter identification algorithm, the system equation (2) needs be reformulated in the form of $\dot{x}(t) = A_c(x(t))\theta + B_c$ to facilitate the process. Please note here $x(t)$ is the estimation result from the motion estimation step.

According to the finite element method, the global stiffness matrix K is assembled from the element stiffness K_e:

$$K = \sum K_e = \sum \int_{\Omega_e} B_e^T D_e B_e \, d\Omega_e \tag{10}$$

where Ω_e is the domain of an arbitrary element e, B_e is the local element strain-displacement matrix, and D_e is the element material matrix. The element stiffness matrix K_e can be stated in terms of its *unknown* Young's modulus E_e:

$$K_e = E_e \int_{\Omega_e} B_e^T D_e' B_e \, d\Omega_e = E_e K_e' \tag{11}$$

With U and $\dot{U}$ the estimation results from the $\mathcal{H}_\infty$ state-filter, we can iteratively recast KU to $G_1 E$ (and $K\dot{U}$ to $G_2 E$) [2].

---

[2] The detailed converting procedures can be found in [12]

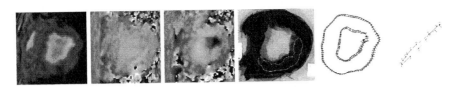

Fig. 3. From left to right: Canine MR magnitude image, x-direction, y-direction phase contrast velocity image, TTC stained postmortem myocardium with the infracted tissue highlighted, displacement constraints on the endo- and epi-cardial boundaries throughout the cardiac cycle, and blowup view of one point's trajectory.

Submitting $C = \alpha M + \beta K$, $KU = G_1 E$, and $K\dot{U} = G_2 E$ into Equation 2, we now have the following identification form of the system equation:

$$\dot{x}(t) = Fx + \mathcal{A}_c(x(t))\theta + B_c w(t) \tag{12}$$

where

$$\theta = E, \quad x(t) = \begin{bmatrix} U(t) \\ \dot{U}(t) \end{bmatrix}, \quad w(t) = \begin{bmatrix} 0 \\ R \end{bmatrix},$$

$$\mathcal{A}_c = \begin{bmatrix} 0 & 0 \\ -M^{-1}G_1 & -\beta M^{-1}G_2 \end{bmatrix}, \quad B_c = \begin{bmatrix} 0 & 0 \\ 0 & M^{-1} \end{bmatrix}, \quad F = \begin{bmatrix} 0 & I \\ 0 & -\alpha I \end{bmatrix}$$

Assuming that the elasticity parameter vector θ is temporally constant, we have the following augmented system:

$$\begin{bmatrix} \dot{x}(t) \\ \dot{\theta} \end{bmatrix} = \begin{bmatrix} Fx \\ 0 \end{bmatrix} + \begin{bmatrix} \mathcal{A}_c(x)\theta + B_c w(t) \\ 0 \end{bmatrix} + \begin{bmatrix} v_p(t) \\ 0 \end{bmatrix} \tag{13}$$

and the measurement equation is:

$$y(t) = \begin{bmatrix} D & 0 \end{bmatrix} \begin{bmatrix} x \\ \theta \end{bmatrix} + e(t) = H \begin{bmatrix} x \\ \theta \end{bmatrix} + e(t) \tag{14}$$

$\mathcal{H}_\infty$ **Parameter-Filter.** To solve the elasticity estimation problem, we introduce another cost function which seeks to achieve a guaranteed disturbance attenuation level γ_p between the unknown quantities and the parameter estimate error of the form:

$$\|\theta - \hat{\theta}\|_{Q_p}^2 < \gamma_p^2 \left\{ \|v_p\|^2 + \|e\|^2 + |\theta - \hat{\theta}(0)|_{Q_{p0}}^2 + |x(0) - \hat{x}_p(0)|_{Q_{p1}}^2 \right\} \tag{15}$$

Here, $\hat{x}_p(0)$ is the initial estimate, and Q_p, Q_{p0}, Q_{p1} are the weighting factors. Under this criterion, the $\mathcal{H}_\infty$ algorithm for the system (13) and (14) is described for $\gamma_p > \gamma^*$, with γ^* is the best-achievable disturbance attenuation level:

$$\begin{bmatrix} \dot{\hat{x}} \\ \dot{\hat{\theta}} \end{bmatrix} = \begin{bmatrix} F & \mathcal{A}_c(x) \\ 0 & 0 \end{bmatrix} \begin{bmatrix} \hat{x} \\ \hat{\theta} \end{bmatrix} + \begin{bmatrix} B_c w(t) \\ 0 \end{bmatrix} + \Sigma^{-1}H^T(y - D\hat{x}) \tag{16}$$

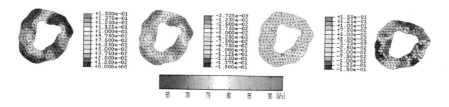

Fig. 4. From left to right: estimated radial (R) strain, circumferential (C) strain, R-C shear strain maps between end-diastole (ED) and end-systole(ES), and estimated Young's modulus distribution (the color scale is on the bottom).

where Σ satisfies the Riccati equation with initial condition $\Sigma(0) = diag(Q_{p1}, Q_{p0})$:

$$\dot{\Sigma} = -\Sigma \begin{bmatrix} F & \mathcal{A}_c(x) \\ 0 & 0 \end{bmatrix} - \begin{bmatrix} F^T & 0 \\ \mathcal{A}_c^T & 0 \end{bmatrix} \Sigma + \begin{bmatrix} D^T D & 0 \\ 0 & -\gamma_p^{-2} Q_p \end{bmatrix} - \Sigma \begin{bmatrix} I & 0 \\ 0 & 0 \end{bmatrix} \Sigma \quad (17)$$

Some of the related theoretical and practical discussions can be found in [2,12].

3   Results and Discussions

3.1   Validation with Synthetic Data

The iterative sequential $\mathcal{H}_\infty$ estimator is validated with computer-synthesized data of an object undergoing deformation in the vertical direction with fixing the bottom side. As shown in Fig. 1, the object has unit thickness, and the material properties and other parameters are taken as $E_{hard} = 105$ for the hard (red) part, $E_{normal} = 75$ for the normal (white) part, and $E_{soft} = 45$ for the soft (blue) part, D=16, L=28, Poisson's ratio $\nu = 0.49$. Under this exact model and boundary conditions, we get displacements for all nodal points, which are labelled as the ground truth data set. Then only a subset of the displacements are selected as the partial measurements on the kinematics, as shown in Fig. 1 where only displacements of the yellow points are known. Finally, different types (Gaussian and Poisson) and levels (20dB and 30dB) of noises are added to these displacements to generate the noisy data. For comparison purpose, the extended Kalman filter (EKF) framework of [11] is used to recover the displacement and elasticity modulus distribution as well.

Quantitative assessments and comparisons of the $\mathcal{H}_\infty$ and EKF results are presented in Table 1, and the recovered elasticity distributions are shown in Fig. 2. In order to validate the motion estimate results, point-by-point positional errors between the algorithm and the ground truth data are computed as shown in Table 2. Overall, the EKF results for Poisson-corrupted input data are not very satisfactory, which indicate that if the assumptions on the noise statistics are violated, it is possible that small noise errors may lead to large estimation errors for EKF. On the other hand, all the tables and figures illustrate that very similar results are obtained using the iterative sequential $\mathcal{H}_\infty$ framework for two sets of data contaminated by different types of noise, showing its desired robustness for real-world problems.

3.2   Canine Image Application

Fig. 3 demonstrates the MR phase contrast image data set. The regional volume of the postmortem injury zone is found by digitizing color photographs of the triphenyl tetrazolium chloride (TTC) stained post mortem myocardium (Fig. 3), which provides the clinical gold standard for the assessment of the image analysis results.

Myocardial boundaries and frame-to-frame boundary displacements are extracted using a unified active region model strategy [13] (as shown in Fig. 3). The estimated radial (R), circumferential (C), and R-C shear strain maps, and the material elasticity distribution are shown in Fig. 4, with initial Young's modulus set to 75000 Pascal. These maps exhibit vastly different motion and material parameters at the infarct zone from the normal tissues, and the patterns are in good agreement with the highlighted histological results of TTC stained postmortem myocardium (Fig. 3). Further, the infarct zone myocardial tissues are relatively stiffer than normal with larger Young's modulus values, which has been observed experimentally earlier.

Acknowledgments. Thanks to Dr. Albert Sinusas of Yale University for the canine experiments and the imaging data. This work is supported by HKRGC-CERG HKUST6151/03E and National Basic Research Program of China (No: 2003CB716104).

References

1. L.L. Creswell, M.J. Moulton, S.G. Wyers, J.S. Pirolo, D.S. Fishman, W.H. Perman, K.W. Myers, R.L. Actis, M.W. Vannier, B.A. Szabo, and M.K. Pasque. An experimental method for evaluating constitutive models of myocardium in *in vivo* hearts. *American Journal of Physiology*, 267:H853–H863, 1994.
2. G. Didinsky, Z. Pan, and T Basar. Parameter identification for uncertain plants using $\mathcal{H}_\infty$ methods. *Automatica*, 31(9):1227–1250, 1995.
3. A.J. Frangi, W.J. Niessen, and M.A. Viergever. Three-dimensional modeling for functional analysis of cardiac images: A review. *IEEE Transactions on Medical Imaging*, 20(1):2–25, 2001.
4. Z. Hu, D. Metaxas, and L. Axel. In-vivo strain and stress estimation of the heart left and right ventricles from mri images. *Medical Image Analysis*, 7(4):435–444, 2003.
5. W.S. Kerwin and J.L. Prince. The kriging update model and recursive space-time function estimation. *IEEE Transactions on Image Processing*, 47(11):2942–2952, 1999.
6. H. Liu and P. Shi. Simultaneous estimation of left ventricular motion and material properties with maximum a posteriori strategy. In *IEEE Computer Vision and Pattern Recognition*, pages 161–169, 2003.
7. E.W.B. Lo, H. Liu, and P. Shi. H_∞ filtering and physical modeling for robust kinematics estimation. In *IEEE International Conference on Image Processing*, volume 2, pages 169–172, 2003.

8. F.G. Meyer, R.T. Constable, A.J. Sinusas, and J.S. Duncan. Tracking myocardial deformation using spatially constrained velocities. *IEEE Transactions on Medical Imaging*, 15(4):453–465, 1996.

9. R. Muthupilla, D.J. Lomas, P.J. Rossman, J.F. Greenleaf, A. Manduca, and R.L. Ehman. Magnetic resonance elastography by direct visualization of propagating acoustic strain waves. *Science*, 269(5232):1854–1857, 1995.

10. X. Shen and L. Deng. A dynamic system approach to speech enhancement using the $\mathcal{H}_\infty$ filtering algorithm. *IEEE Transactions on Speech and Audio Processing*, 7(4):391–399, 1999.

11. P. Shi and H. Liu. Stochastic finite element framework for simultaneous estimation of cardiac kinematics functions and material parameters. *Medical Image Analysis*, 7(4):445–464, 2003.

12. P. Shi, H. Liu, and A. Sinusas. Robust filtering strategies for soft tissue Young's modulus characterization. In *IEEE International Symposium on Biomedical Imaging: Macro to Nano*, in press, 2004.

13. A.L.N. Wong, H. Liu, A. Sinusas, and P. Shi. Spatiotemporal active region model for simultaneous segmentation and motion estimation of the whole heart. In *IEEE Workshop on Variational, Geometric and Level Set Methods in Computer Vision*, pages 193–200, 2003.

14. Y. Zhu and N.J. Pelc. A spatiotemporal model of cyclic kinematics and its application to analyzing nonrigid motion with mr velocity images. *IEEE Transactions on Medical Imaging*, 18(7):557–569, 1999.

A Semi-automatic Endocardial Border Detection Method for 4D Ultrasound Data

Marijn van Stralen[1], Johan G. Bosch[1], Marco M. Voormolen[2,3], Gerard van Burken[1], Boudewijn J. Krenning[3], Charles T. Lancée[3], Nico de Jong[2,3], and Johan H.C. Reiber[1,2]

[1]Leiden University Medical Center, Radiology, Division of Image Processing C2-S, P.O. Box 9600, 2300 RC Leiden, The Netherlands
{M.van_Stralen, J.G.Bosch, G.van_Burken, J.H.C.Reiber}@lumc.nl
[2]ICIN, Interuniversity Cardiology Institute of the Netherlands, Utrecht, The Netherlands
[3]Erasmus Medical Center, Thoraxcenter, Rotterdam, The Netherlands
{M.Voormolen, B.Krenning, C.Lancee, N.deJong}@erasmusmc.nl

Abstract. We propose a semi-automatic endocardial border detection method for 3D+T cardiac ultrasound data based on pattern matching and dynamic programming, operating on 2D slices of the 3D+T data, for the estimation of LV volume, with minimal user interaction. It shows good correlations with MRI ED and ES volumes (r=0.938) and low interobserver variability (y=1.005x-16.7, r=0.943) over full-cycle volume estimations. It shows a high consistency in tracking the user-defined initial borders over space and time.

1 Introduction

For diagnosis of cardiovascular diseases, the volume and ejection fraction of the left heart chamber are important clinical parameters. 3D ultrasound offers good opportunities to visualize the whole left ventricle (LV) over the complete cardiac cycle. 3D ultrasound is non-invasive, relatively cheap, flexible in use and capable of accurate volume measurements. New, fast 3D ultrasound imaging devices are entering the market and have the potential of allowing such measurements rapidly, reliably and in a user-friendly way - provided that a suitable automated analysis is available. Manual segmentation of the large data sets is very cumbersome and suffers from inconsistencies and high variability. On the other hand, the human expert's interpretation and intervention in the detection is often essential for good results. Therefore a semi-automatic segmentation approach seems most suitable.

Some methods for segmentation of 4D echocardiographic images have been published. Angelini *et al.* [1] have reported on a wavelet-based approach for 4D echocardiographic image enhancement followed by an LV segmentation using standard snakes. Montagnat *et al.* [2] use a 2-simplex mesh and a feature detection based on a simple cylindrical gradient filter. Sanchez-Ortiz, Noble *et al.* [3] used multi-scale fuzzy clustering for a rough segmentation in 2D longitudinal slices. B-splines are used for 3D surface fitting in each time frame. These methods have not been validated successfully on a reasonable data set. The most practical approach is described by Schreckenberg [4]. It uses active surfaces that are controlled by difference-of-boxes operators applied to averages and variances of the luminance.

C. Barillot, D.R. Haynor, and P. Hellier (Eds.): MICCAI 2004, LNCS 3216, pp. 43–50, 2004.

This technique is implemented in a commercially available workstation (4D LV Analysis, TomTec, Germany). The general experience is that this technique requires much initialization and corrections and a consistent segmentation is still hard to reach.

We present a new semi-automatic endocardial border detection method for time series of 3D cardiac ultrasound data. Our method is based on pattern matching and dynamic programming techniques and combines continuity, robustness and accuracy in 2D cross sections with the spatial and temporal continuity of the 4D data. It aims at optimally using a limited amount of user interaction (capturing essential information on shape and edge patterns according to the user's interpretation of the ultrasound data) to attain a fast, consistent and precise segmentation of the left ventricle.

Although the presented method is general and suitable for any apically acquired 3D set, we performed this study on a special type of image data acquired with a new device: the Fast Rotating Ultrasound (FRU-) transducer. The transducer has been developed by the Department of Experimental Echocardiography of the Erasmus MC, the Netherlands [5,6]. It contains a linear phased array transducer that is continuously rotated around its image-axis at very high speed, up to 480 rotations per minute (rpm), while acquiring 2D images. A typical data set is generated during 10 seconds at 360 rpm and 100 frames per second (fps). The images of the left ventricle are acquired with the transducer placed in apical position. The rotation axis will approach the LV long axis in the ideal situation. The analysis assumes that the rotation axis lies within the LV lumen and inside the mitral ring.

As a consequence of the very high continuous rotation speed, the images have a curved image plane (Fig. 1a). During the acquisition, the probe rotates about 22° per image with the typical settings given above. The combination of these curved image planes, and the fact that the acquisition is not triggered by or synchronized to the ECG signal, results in an irregular distribution over the 3D+T space. A single cardiac cycle in general is not sufficient for adequate coverage of the whole 3D+T space; therefore, multiple consecutive heart cycles are merged. The cardiac phase for each image is computed offline using detected R-peaks in the ECG [7]. The total set of 2D images can be used for selection of a subset of images with a regular coverage of the 3D+T space and/or for the generation of a 4D voxel set. We perform analysis on the prior.

2   Methods

2.1   Frame Selection

To achieve adequate coverage of the whole 3D+T space, multiple consecutive cardiac cycles are merged and an optimal subset S of the total set of frames T is selected. This subset is an optimal fit of the frames on a chosen $A*P$ matrix of A equidistant rotation angles and P cardiac phases, minimizing the total deviation in rotation angle and cardiac phase. Moreover, the variation in acquisition time over the subset is minimized to limit possible motion artifacts. The constraints are translated into the following cost functions that will be minimized over the total subset S,

$$S = \arg\min_{T} \sum_{i=1}^{A} \sum_{j=1}^{P} \left(\arg\min_{b \in C_{i,j}} \left(c_{angle}(\alpha_b, i) + c_{phase}(p_b, j) + c_{time}(t_b) \right) \right), \text{ where} \qquad (1)$$

$$c_{angle}(\alpha, i) = k_1 |\alpha_{target}(i) - \alpha|; \; c_{phase}(p, j) = k_2 |p_{target}(j) - p|; \; c_{time}(t) = k_3 |t_s - t|.$$

$C_{i,j}$ is the set of candidate images for angle #i and phase #j. c_{angle} and c_{phase} describe the costs of selecting an image b with angle α_b and phase p_b for a chosen α_{target} and p_{target}. k_1, k_2 and k_3 are weighting coefficients (typically equal). Since the cost c_{time} is dependent on t_s (the average acquisition time of the subset itself), the minimization of the costs of set S is achieved in an iterative manner.

2.2   Border Detection Approach

We base our method on the knowledge that the edge patterns of the endocardial border can be complex, very different from patient to patient and even between regions within an image set. The border position need not correspond to a strong edge and may be only definable from 'circumstantial evidence' as identified by an expert observer. Rather than applying artificial, idealized edge models or templates derived from a large training set, we propose a tracking approach based on edge templates extracted from the user-defined initial borders in the patient's own images.

The method is based on these continuity assumptions (in order of strength):
1. border continuity in separate 2D slices of the left ventricle;
2. spatial continuity of shape and gray value edge patterns over the LV surface in 3D;
3. temporal and cyclic motion continuity of the endocardium.

For the FRU transducer, within the original 2D images, both spatial and temporal distances between neighboring samples are smaller than towards adjacent images in angle and phase; therefore, border continuity is supposed to be strongest here. For other devices, similar considerations apply.

The method is initialized from four manually drawn contours, taken from two roughly perpendicular views (more or less corresponding to two- and four-chamber cross sections) in two phases: end-diastole (ED) and end-systole (ES). These are used to initialize a model for the edge patterns near the 3D LV surface over time and a 3D shape model of the LV endocardial surface over the entire heart cycle. Both models are inherently 4-dimensional and can be polled at any spatial position and phase.

The actual border detection takes place in individual 2D images from the selected subset and is an extension of an approach for 2D+T sequences earlier developed by Bosch *et al.* [8]. For each image $b \in S$ (of phase p_b and angle α_b), an estimation of the border shape is derived by intersecting the 3D shape model at phase p_b by the (curved) image plane for angle α_b. The edge templates are also interpolated for the desired p_b and α_b. In the 2D image, a neighborhood of the estimated shape is resampled along lines perpendicular to the shape estimate. Using a template matching with the local edge templates, the similarity of each candidate edge point to the template is calculated. Dynamic programming is applied to find an optimal continuous border within the restrictions posed by the 3D model. In this way, the 4D surface and edge pattern models guard the (looser) spatial and temporal consistency of the detection, while the dynamic programming approach supplies a continuous and optimal

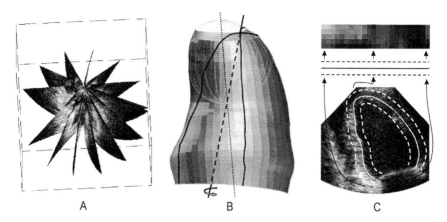

Fig. 1. (a) A sequence of seven consecutive FRU images with curved image planes. (b) 3D surface model. The LAX estimate (dotted) and the rotation axis (dashed) are shown, together with the reconstruction of the apex by spline interpolation (light gray) from two manually drawn contours (solid black). (c) The extraction of a stylized edge pattern from the image

detection locally. The set of detected contours describes the 3D endocardial surface over the whole cardiac cycle from which LV volumes, ejection fraction etc. can be computed.

The method is suitable for effective correction of the detection in other 2D images (although this was not yet used or evaluated in this study). A corrected contour will be treated as an additional manual contour and a complete new set of shape and edge pattern models will be interpolated, and all images are redetected. In this manner, corrections will cumulatively lead to a superior global solution.

2.3   3D Surface Models

As said, for two cardiac phases (ED and ES) a 3D surface model of the LV endocardium is constructed from two almost perpendicular contours. During the acquisition the rotation axis is more or less aligned with the long axis (LAX) of the left ventricle, but in practice there may be a considerable mismatch (Fig. 1b). This implies that the two image planes do not contain the true apex of the heart, and estimating the position and shape of the true apex (and the LV long axis) is a non-trivial issue. The local long axes in the 2D manually drawn contours are defined as the lines between the midpoint of the mitral valve (MV) and the 2D apex. We estimate the 3D LV long axis from the local long axes by computing the intersection of the planes perpendicular to these images through the local long axis in the image.

The endocardial surface is estimated by expressing the two contours in a cylindrical coordinate system with respect to the estimated LV long axis and applying a Kochanek spline interpolation [9] of the radial component over the angle in planes perpendicular to the long axis. This is a natural approximation of the ellipsoidal shape of the left ventricle. Since the two image planes generally do not intersect the real apex, the apical cap of the LV surface cannot be estimated simply from the two manually drawn contours, as shown in Fig. 1b. Therefore, near the 3D apex we use a spherical coordinate system oriented around the LV long axis, centered at $3/4^{th}$ of its length. The surface is estimated by a Kochanek spline interpolation of the radial component over the elevation angle for multiple rotation angles.

A contour estimate for any image at a given rotation angle and cardiac phase can be made by intersecting its curved image plane with the 3D contour models in ED and ES and then linearly interpolating between the two resulting '2D' contours over cardiac phase to get the contour estimate at the desired cardiac phase.

2.4   Edge Pattern Model

The desired edges are tracked over space and time by applying a pattern matching approach with edge templates. These edge patterns are derived from the manually drawn contours and interpolated over the (phase, angle) space.

The image is resampled clockwise along the manually drawn contour, on line segments perpendicular to this contour from the inside out. The gray values on these line segments are smoothed and subsampled to form a stylized edge pattern for this contour (Fig. 1c). A typical edge pattern for a single 2D frame is represented by 32 positions along the contour and 5 samples around each edge position.

A linear interpolation over cardiac phase is performed between the edge patterns in ED and ES. The interpolation over rotation angle is less straightforward. Since the character of the edge pattern is strongly related to the angle between the endocardial border and the ultrasound beam and the distance from the transducer, the pattern changes considerably over the rotation angle, especially when the angle between the rotation axis and LV long axis is substantial. For images with rotation angles opposite ($\bullet 180°$) to those with the manually drawn contours, the image appears nearly mirrored and the mirrored (anticlockwise) edge pattern is used. For angles in between, the edge patterns are linearly interpolated.

2.5   Contour Detection

With an edge pattern and initial contour for each image $b \in S$ (of phase p_b and angle α_b), we can now detect the individual endocardial borders. In a neighborhood of the initial contour, the image is resampled into an $N*M$ rectangular array by sampling N points along M scan lines perpendicular to the shape. From the stylized edge pattern for (p_b, α_b) an edge template for each scan line is extracted. For all nodes in the array, the sum of absolute differences with its respective edge template defines the cost of the node. We now use a straightforward dynamic programming approach [10] to find the optimal connective path through the array. A connective path contains exactly one node per line and the positions on consecutive lines cannot differ more than a predefined side step size. Dynamic programming is a well-known technique [10] that finds the optimal path (the path with the lowest sum of costs) out of all possible connective paths in an effective manner by calculating lowest cumulative costs for consecutive layers (lines) while keeping track of the partial optimal paths. Backtracking from the node with lowest cumulative cost in the last layer delivers the

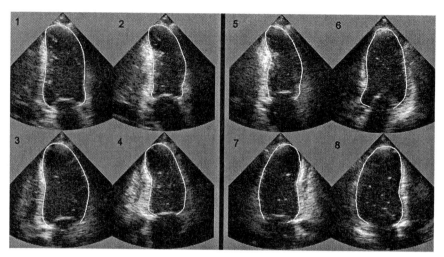

Fig. 2. Detection examples: frames at different (phase#, angle#) with contours. *Left*: 4 frames with manual contours, resp. 1: ED 2c (1,1), 2: ES 2c (6,1), 3: ED 4c (1,3), 4: ES 4c (6,3). *Right*: 4 frames with detected contours, resp. 5: frame (8,2), 6: (14,5), 7: (4,8), 8: (14,9)

overall optimal path. Smoothness constraints are enforced by applying additive costs for sidestepping during cumulative cost calculation. To limit the influence of lines with relatively poor image information, this additive penalty is calculated per line from the statistics of node costs per line with respect to overall cost statistics, such that relatively unreliable lines get higher penalties for sidestepping.

For each phase p_j, the detected contours of all angles α_i together constitute a 3D mesh that describes the endocardial surface. We observe the volume of the left ventricle over the whole cardiac cycle, by calculating the volumes inside the surface meshes of all selected heart phases.

3 Results

We performed a preliminary validation study for this method on a group of 14 subjects with different diagnoses of cardiovascular disease. MRI ED and ES volumes on these patients were determined in parallel with the 3D US study. For all patients, subsets of images were created with P=16 phases and A=10 angles. After establishing equivalent tracing conventions, two observers individually analyzed all subsets.

Reading and converting the data and the automated selection of the subset took 7 minutes per patient on average. After the drawing of the four contours, the fully automated detection of the other 156 contours took approximately 90 seconds per patient. No contour corrections were allowed afterwards. Some examples of manual and detected contours are shown in Fig. 2. From the analyses of both observers, interobserver variabilities of ED/ES volumes, EF and all other volumes were determined, as well as averages that were correlated to MRI ED and ES volumes.

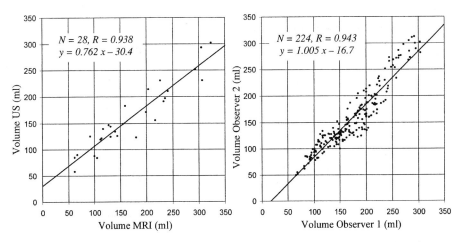

Fig. 3. (L) ED/ES volumes US vs. MRI. (R) Interobserver variability of full-cycle volumes

Results of 3DUS (average of the two observers) vs. MRI are shown in Table 1 and Fig. 3a. These show the ED and ES volumes and the corresponding correlation coefficients and regression equations.

A high correlation of r=0.938 was found between MRI and US volumes. Overall the MRI volumes were slightly higher. This has been reported in many studies and can be attributed to different tracing conventions. The differences between MRI and US volumes were not significant (paired t-test, p = 0.068). EF results showed a reasonable difference of 3.3 +/- 8.6% (regression y=0.493x + 16.6%, r=0.755).

For the interobserver variability, results are presented in Table 1 (ED and ES) and Fig. 3b (full-cycle). For ED and ES volumes only, the differences were 15.0 +/- 21.0 (av +/- SD) with a regression of y=1.013x − 17.4 (r=0.949). We found similar differences of 15.6 +/- 19.3 over all other phases (y=1.003x − 16.1, r=0.943). This difference (ED/ES vs. other phases) was not significant (unpaired t-test, p = 0.628). This implies that the detection does not introduce additional variability/errors with respect to interobserver differences from the manual contours.

Absolute differences in volumes may seem high, but this is partially due to the dilated hearts in the set and the consequent high average volumes (average MRI ED = 209 ml). The systematic differences in tracing between observers were equally reflected in the detected contours, which is encouraging.

Table 1. ED/ES volumes and correlations of 3DUS vs. MRI and Observer 1 vs. Observer 2

	ED Volume (ml)		ES Volume (ml)		Correlation	Regression
	Average	SD	Average	SD		
MRI	209	67	133	69	0.938	0.762x + 30.4
US	194	57	127	50		
Obs.1	203	56	133	48	0.949	1.013x − 17.4
Obs.2	187	63	119	52		

4 Conclusions and Future Work

We presented a new semi-automatic endocardial border detection method for 4D ultrasound data. This method offers fast and reasonably precise automated border detection with minimal user interaction and very promising results. However, one should bear in mind that this analysis is only preliminary. Methods have not yet been optimized and smaller flaws still exist. In some cases phase information was inexact, hampering the model interpolations. Also, the linear model interpolations currently disregard the complex shape and motion of the mitral valve, which is known to move nonlinearly in diastole. In addition, some distinct local misdetections were found that will be addressed in future research. Furthermore, the method was designed with advanced correction features in mind (see 2.2). These have not yet been used or tested in this analysis. It is to be expected that this will allow significantly better results with little interaction; similar improvements were found with its predecessor for the 2D+T analyses.

Despite the fact that this method is optimized for data of the FRU-transducer, the algorithm can be easily adapted to data of other image acquisition systems, for example 4D voxel sets. The detection will then be performed in 2D slices through the LV long axis.

References

1. Angelini, E.D. et al., LV Volume Quantification via Spatiotemporal Analysis of Real-Time 3D Echocardiography, IEEE Trans Medical Imaging 20 (2001), pp. 457-469, 2001
2. Montagnat, J., Delingette, H., Space and Time Shape Constrained Deformable Surfaces for 4D Medical Image Segmentation. MICCAI 2000, Springer, vol. LNCS 1935, pp. 196-205
3. Sanchez-Ortiz, G.I. et al., Automating 3D Echocardiographic Image Analysis, MICCAI 2000, Springer, LNCS 1935, pp. 687-696
4. Schreckenberg, M. et al., Automatische Objecterkennung in 3D-echokardio-graphiesequenz-en auf Basis Aktiver Oberflächenmodellen und Modellgekoppelter Merkmalsextraktion, In: Lehman, T. et al. (eds.): Bildverarbeitung für die Medizin, Springer, V087, 1998
5. Djoa, K.K. et al., A Fast Rotating Scanning Unit for Real-Time Three Dimensional Echo Data Acquisition, Ultrasound in Med. & Biol., vol 26(5), pp. 863-869, 2000
6. Voormolen, M.M. et al., A New Transducer for 3D Harmonic Imaging, Proc. Of IEEE Ultrasonics Symposium, pp. 1261-1264, 2002
7. Engelse, W.A.H., Zeelenberg, C., A Single Scan Algorithm for QRS-detection and Feature Extraction, Computers in cardiology 6, pp. 37-42, 1979
8. Bosch, J.G. et al., Overview of Automated Quantitation Techniques in 2D Echocardio-graphy, In: Reiber J.H.C. and Van der Wall, E.E. (eds.): What's New in Cardiovascular Imaging, edited by, Kluwer academic publishers, pp. 363-376, 1998
9. Kochanek, D., Bartels, R., Interpolating Splines with Local Tension, Continuity, and Bias Control, Computer Graphics, vol. 18, no. 3, pp. 33-41, 1984.
10. Sonka, M. et al., Segmentation, Ch. 5 of Image Processing, Analysis and Machine Vision, PWS Publishing, pp. 158-163, 1999

Vessel Segmentation Using a Shape Driven Flow

Delphine Nain, Anthony Yezzi, and Greg Turk

Georgia Institute of Technology, Atlanta GA 30332, USA
{delfin, turk}@cc.gatech.edu, ayezzi@ece.gatech.edu

Abstract. We present a segmentation method for vessels using an implicit deformable model with a soft shape prior. Blood vessels are challenging structures to segment due to their branching and thinning geometry as well as the decrease in image contrast from the root of the vessel to its thin branches. Using image intensity alone to deform a model for the task of segmentation often results in leakages at areas where the image information is ambiguous. To address this problem, we combine image statistics and shape information to derive a region-based active contour that segments tubular structures and penalizes leakages. We present results on synthetic and real 2D and 3D datasets.

1 Introduction

Blood vessel segmentation and visualization of blood vessels is important for clinical tasks such as diagnosis of vascular diseases, surgery planning and blood flow simulation. A number of methods have been developed for vessel segmentation, however most of those techniques do not use a shape prior, or use a strong shape prior. With strong shape priors, such as shape templates, the segmentation is constrained to a particular shape space. Since diseased vessels can have abnormal shapes, a strict shape template may result in incorrect segmentation that misses important anatomical information. However, using image intensity alone for the task of segmentation often results in leakages perpendicular to the vessel walls at areas where the image information is ambiguous. Leakages cause the segmented model to expand into areas that are not part of the vessel structure, and results in incorrect segmentation. In this paper, we introduce the notion of segmentation with a *soft* shape prior, where the segmented model is not constrained to a predefined shape space, but is penalized if it deviates strongly from a tubular structure, since those deviations have a high probability of being leaks. Our method uses a soft shape prior in addition to image statistics to deform an active contour for the task of blood vessel segmentation.

2 Related Work

Many geometric methods exist for vessel segmentation that range from using no shape priors to strong shape priors. Tubular structures can be identified by the response of derivative and Gaussian filters convolved with the image. Sato et al. use the second derivatives of a set of multiscale gaussian filters to detect

C. Barillot, D.R. Haynor, and P. Hellier (Eds.): MICCAI 2004, LNCS 3216, pp. 51–59, 2004.
© Springer-Verlag Berlin Heidelberg 2004

curvilinear structures and penalize high intensity (bumps) on the vessel walls [1]. The filter response can be used to visualize the vessels through Maximum Intensity Projections (MIP) or isosurface extraction. Since these methods rely on the intensity of the image, a noisy intensity map may result in incorrect filter response and additional shape information might be needed for a correct segmentation. Skeletons [2,3] can be used as a basis of graph analysis of vessels, and further processing is needed to extract the 3D shape of the vessel. Krissian et al. use multiscale filtering, based on a set of gaussian kernels and their derivatives to extract a skeleton of vasculature [5]. The local maxima of the filter response is used to find centerpoints and radius information in order to fit a cylindrical model to the data. The restriction of the shapes can be a limitation since diseased vessels can have cross-section that deviate from an elliptical shape.

Deformable models are a powerful technique for flexible automatic 3D segmentation. Deformable models are based on an initial contour or surface deformed by a combination of internal (shape) and external (image and user defined) forces to segment the object of interest. In particular, the addition of a shape prior as an internal force can greatly increase the robustness of deformable models when applied to the task of vessel segmentation. Snakes are parametrized models and shape templates can easily be incorporated in this framework [6, 9]. However those methods have a limitation since the surface cannot handle topological changes as easily as the level set methods and reparameterization is often necessary and complex in 3D. Level set methods represent a surface implicitly by the zero level set of a scalar-valued function. The evolution is carried out within this framework without the need for parameterization or explicit handling of topological changes [7,8]. However, since there is no explicit parameterization, incorporating a shape prior in this framework is more difficult.

To address the issue of leaks that form at the root of vessels during a fast marching segmentation, Deschamps et al. [4] freeze a percentage of the points that are closer to the starting seed (since it is assumed that they have segmented the structure of interest) while allowing the fast evolving points to evolve normally. This technique does not prevent leaks that form far away from the root of the vessels, close to the fast evolving part of the front.

Leventon et al. [10] use dimensionality reduction techniques on the distance transform of a set of previously segmented shapes to define a shape constraint within a level set framework. This technique yields good results, but requires pre-segmented data. It has also not been tested on vessel structures. Strong shape priors in combination with level set techniques for vessel segmentation was used by Lorigo et al. [11]. They evolve 1D curves in a 3D volume and then estimate the radius of the vessels locally using the inverse of principal curvature. The advantage of this technique is that it does not require pre-segmented data, however it makes a strong assumption about the shape of the vessels since they are modeled as tubes with varying width. To our knowledge, no existing level set techniques use a soft shape prior for vessel segmentation.

3   Shape Driven Flow

3.1   Region Based Flow

Our base flow deforms the curve of interest according to a smoothing term and an image term ϕ. In this paper, we use an adaptive threshold with decaying intensity from the root of the vessel (determined by the seed point of the initial contour) to the rest of the contour.

We define the following energy in the region R inside the curve C parameterized by arc-length s:

$$E(C) = -\int_R \phi d\mathbf{x} + \int_C ds \tag{1}$$

This is a region based active contour. We minimize Equation 1 by computing its first variation and solving the obtained Euler-Lagrange equation by means of gradient descent. We find the following curve evolution equation:

$$\frac{\partial C(\mathbf{x})}{dt} = (-\phi(\mathbf{x}) + \kappa(\mathbf{x}))\mathcal{N} \tag{2}$$

where ϕ is a speed determined by the underlying image, $\kappa(x)$ is the curvature of the curve at point x and $\mathcal{N}$ is the unit inward normal to the curve. We evolve this active contour using Level Set Techniques[7,8].

Image statistics alone might lead to unsatisfactory segmentations. Figure 5(a) shows an example of very noisy image data where areas of pixels close to the vessel have very similar image statistics. This results in a leak when segmented with the type of flow (2). More sophisticated algorithms can be devised based on image statistics or prior knowledge such as multiscale filter responses tuned to detect vessels [13,6,14], but these algorithms will be very specific to the type of data and image acquisition. This leakage problem can be addressed in a more general way by adding a soft shape constraint to the flow so that the algorithm penalizes obvious leaks.

3.2   Shape Filters

We would like to locally determine the shape of a contour, and particularly areas where it is widening and potentially leaking. The information from derivatives of the curve, such as curvature, is too local since widening of the contour cannot be discriminated from small noise and bumps. We propose to use a local filter at a scale larger than the derivative scale. We define a local neighborhood $B(\mathbf{x}, r)$ in the shape of a ball (disk in R^2, solid sphere in R^3) centered at the point $\mathbf{x}$ and of radius r, see Figure 1(a). For every point $\mathbf{x}$ inside and on the contour (region R), we define a filtering operation that calculates a measure ϵ_1 in the neighborhood $B(\mathbf{x}, r)$. The measure ϵ_1 is the percentage of points that fall both within the ball centered at $\mathbf{x}$ and the region R inside the contour[1]:

$$\epsilon_1(\mathbf{x}) = \int_{B(\mathbf{x},r)} \mathcal{X}(\mathbf{y})d\mathbf{y} \quad \text{where } \mathcal{X}(\mathbf{y}) = \begin{cases} 1 \text{ if } \mathbf{y} \in R \\ 0 \text{ if } \mathbf{y} \notin R \end{cases} \tag{3}$$

---

[1] If $R \to 0$, then $\epsilon_1(\mathbf{x})$ is just the curvature at $\mathbf{x}$.

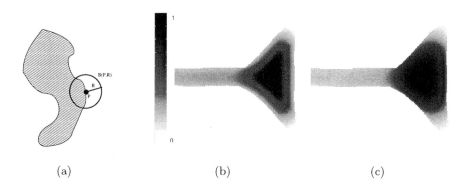

(a)   (b)   (c)

Fig. 1. (a) $\epsilon_1(\mathbf{x})$ is the intersection of the ball centered at $\mathbf{x}$ and the region R inside the contour. (b) Points inside the widening region have a higher ϵ_1 measure but most points on the contour have the same measure. (c)Contour points close to the widening of the contour have a higher ϵ_2 measure

The parameter r must be chosen by the user and be an upper bound to the expected radius of the vessels. In our simulations, the user picked the width of the largest vessel with the mouse to define r.

The filter response ϵ_1 for a synthetic shape that represents a potential leak is shown in Figure 1(b). Given a radius that is the width of the tube, the points inside the widening region will have a higher measure than the points inside the tube. We will formalize this observation in the next Section by defining an energy minimization that uses the measure ϵ_1 to penalize regions inside the contour that deviate from a tubular shape.

3.3   Curve Evolution Using Local Filters

We define such an energy as:

$$E(C) = - \int_R \phi d\mathbf{x} + \int_C ds + \alpha \int_R \epsilon_1^p(\mathbf{x}) d\mathbf{x} \qquad (4)$$

The first and second term are the same as for the region flow previously introduced. The third term is a constraint on shape. When we minimize $E(C)$, the third term will force deviations from tubular shapes to be penalized. In order to obtain a curve evolution formula, we take the first variation of Equation 4. The first variation for such an equation with nested integrals was derived in [12] and we give its solution:

$$\frac{\partial C(\mathbf{x})}{\partial t} = \left(-\phi(\mathbf{x}) + \kappa + \alpha \epsilon_2(\mathbf{x}, p) \right) \mathcal{N} \qquad (5)$$

where

$$\epsilon_2(\mathbf{x}, p) = \epsilon_1^p(\mathbf{x}) + p \int_{B(\mathbf{x},r)} \epsilon_1^{p-1}(\mathbf{y}) \mathcal{X}(\mathbf{y}) d\mathbf{y} \qquad (6)$$

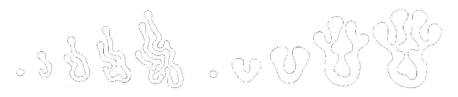

(a) Evolution in time, $p=2$, $r=20$, $\alpha=0.75$ (b) Evolution in time, $p=2$, $r=40$, $\alpha=0.75$

Fig. 2. Dilation Flow with Shape Prior

The measure ϵ_2 is again the output of a local ball filter. For a point, the response is its ϵ_1 measure plus the sum of the ϵ_1 measure of its neighbouring points that are inside the contour. For a radius r similar to the vessel width, most points on the contour have the same ϵ_1 measure since locally the same percentage of neighbors fall within the filter radius. This can be seen in Figure 1(b), on the left. To see if the contour point lies near a leak region, it is necessary to look at the ϵ_1 measure of its neighbors *inside* the contour since their measure is high for points inside widening regions. This is what ϵ_2 measures, as shown in Figure 1(c), on the right. We observe that contour points close to the widening of the contour have a higher measure than contour points on the tube [2].

Since ϵ_2 is always positive, the third part of Equation 5 is an erosion term (flow along the inward normal) that is proportional to the ϵ_2 measure. At a point with a high measure, the contour shape deviates from a tubular shape and therefore the flow is penalized. The parameter α is chosen according to the amount of penalty desired.

The filter operations are computationally expensive since at every time step, ϵ_1 is calculated for every point inside the curve and ϵ_2 is calculated for every point on the contour. As an optimization, we only recompute the filter outputs for the contour points that have moved since the previous time step and propagate the information to the neighbors that fall within the filter radius.

4   Results

It is interesting to evolve a curve using Equation 5 without an image force, to see the effect that our flow has on the evolution of a small near-circle. We chose $\phi = 1$ (a constant image term) so that without the second and third term of the equation, the curve evolution would be a simple dilation of the circle. We then ran the full curve evolution, with 2 different radii ($r = 20$, $r = 40$, $\alpha = 0.75$). As seen in Figures 2(a) and 2(b), the curve evolves keeping a "tubular" shape at all times. The width of the tube depends on the radius of the local filter.

---

[2] In our implementation, we scale both measure to lie between 0 and 1 so that all three terms in Equation 6 have similar scaling.

We now test our flow on both 2D and 3D datasets for synthetic and real data. For all flows presented, the user specified the expected biggest radius by clicking two points on the image. More investigation is needed on the effect of choosing different p, for these results we chose the parameters $p = 2$ because it is well behaved.

4.1   2D Images

In 2D,we first used our flow evolution on a synthetic model of a branching vessel. The radius was chosen to be the largest width of the vessel. We observed that the value of the chosen α influences the penalty on deviations from tubular structures. In Figure 3(a), for $\alpha > 0.65$, we observe an erosion around the branching area since points in that region have a higher measure. Figure 3(b), for $\alpha <= 0.65$, the penalty is softened and the vessel is correctly segmented. This value is used for subsequent segmentations and erosion in branching areas was not observed.

We used our flow on a noisy projection of an angiogram and compared it to the base flow without a shape constraint. We show details of the segmentation where leaks were detected. When the neck of the leak is thin, the leak disconnects from the main vessel as shown in Figure 4. This is because points on the contour near the leak region have a high ϵ_2 measure (as can be seen in Figure 1(c)) that causes the contour to erode and eventually pinch off. Once the leak pinches off, the user can then click on the disconnected contour to eliminate it, or the algorithm can detect the change of topology [15] and automatically remove the leakage. The contour points at the neck of the leak are frozen so that the leak does not re-appear while the rest of the contour evolves.

In Figure 5 we observe that the flow with a shape prior is able to prevent many leaks and produce a flow that is much better behaved than the same flow without a shape prior. We notice that without a shape prior, the flow becomes "chaotic" and leaky regions merge with vessel regions (see Figure 5(a)). The repair of such leaks with user interaction would almost amount to a manual segmentation. Figure 5(b), shows that the flow is much better behaved and produces a better segmentation for most of the image. In the left part of the image, we notice an interesting behavior of the shape-constrained flow. This part of the image

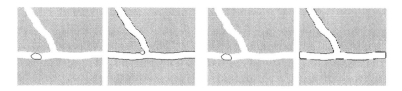

(a) A high penalty α=0.75 causes erosion around the branch.

(b) α=0.65.   Erosion   around   the branch is not observed.

Fig. 3. Flow with Shape Prior on 2D Synthetic Images

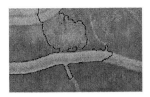

(a) Base Flow, no Shape Prior, 100 iterations

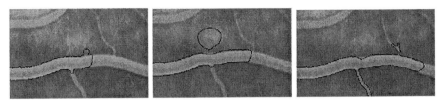

(b) Flow with Shape Prior, at t=50(left), 100(middle) and 200(right) iterations.

Fig. 4. Vessel Flow on Angiogram Images

is very noisy and image statistics are almost identical inside and outside the vessel, so the base flow without a shape prior completely leaks out of the vessel area. The flow with a shape prior also leaks into the background since the image statistics no longer discriminates between foreground and background, but the flow maintains a "vessel-like" shape and the leak is mostly contained. This is important since we do not want the leak to expand to areas of the image that are correctly segmented.

4.2   3D Images

In this section we demonstrate our flow on two 3D CT datasets of a coronary artery. In all Figures, the color on the surface represents the measure ϵ_2. We see that this measure is closely related to the thickness of a vessel.

For the first CT coronary dataset, if we use a flow based on image statistics alone, the artery "leaks" into the heart cage (Figure 6(a)). As we can see, the connecting area between the coronary and the heart has the highest measure. However, when we use the flow with the shape constraint, the leak "pinches" off

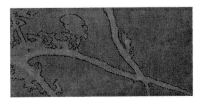
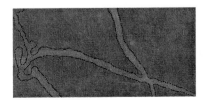

(a) Base Flow, no Shape Prior   (b) Flow with Shape Prior

Fig. 5. Vessel Flow on Angiogram Images

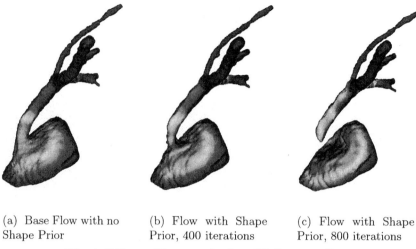

(a) Base Flow with no Shape Prior

(b) Flow with Shape Prior, 400 iterations

(c) Flow with Shape Prior, 800 iterations

Fig. 6. Different Flows on the first CT Coronary Data

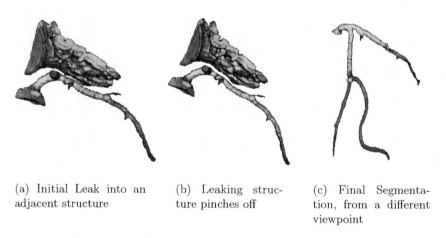

(a) Initial Leak into an adjacent structure

(b) Leaking structure pinches off

(c) Final Segmentation, from a different viewpoint

Fig. 7. Base Flow with Shape Prior on the second CT coronary dataset

from the main vessel artery (Figure 6(b) and 6(c)). The second CT coronary dataset leaks into an adjacent structure (Figure 7, left). Again, running the vessel flow separates the coronary from the leak. The user can then click on the isolated leak to remove it. The full segmentation is shown on the right.

5   Conclusion

We have presented a soft shape prior that can be combined with any other image force to deform an active contour and penalize leaks. Although the results presented are still preliminary and need to be medically validated, we found that the shape prior successfully penalizes leak regions and either disconnects the leak from the vessel, or contains the leak. We find these results encouraging since in the presence of noise, the shape driven flow is better behaved than the flow based on image statistics alone. This flow can be combined with minimal user interaction to repair leak effects that were not prevented by the algorithm.

References

1. Y. Sato, S.Nakajima, N. Shiraga, H. Atsumi, S. Yoshida, T. Koller, G. Gerig, and R. Kikinis. Three Dimensional multi-scale line filter for segmentation and visualization of curvilinear structures in medical images. Med.Imag Anal, 1998, 2, 143-168.
2. Flasque N, Desvignes M, Constans JM, Revenu M. Acquisition, segmentation and tracking of the cerebral vascular tree on 3D magnetic resonance angiography images. Med Image Anal. 2001 Sep;5(3):173-83.
3. T. Deschamps, L.D. Cohen. Fast extraction of minimal paths in 3D images and application to virtual endoscopy. Med. Image Anal, 2001 Dec; 5(4).
4. T. Deschamps, L.D. Cohen. Fast Extraction of Tubular and Tree 3D Surfaces with front propagation methods. International Conference on Pattern Recognition, 2002.
5. K. Krissian, G. Malandain, N. Ayache Model-based detection of tubular structures in 3D images. Computer Vision and Image Understanding, 80:2, pp. 130-171,2000.
6. A. Frangi, W. Niessen, K.L. Vincken, and M.A. Viergever Multiscale vessel enhancement filtering. Proc. MICCAI'98, pp.130-137, 1998.
7. S. Osher,R. Fedkiw. Level Set Methods and Dynamic Implicit Surfaces. Springer Verlag, 2002.
8. J.A Sethian. Level Set Methods and Fast Marching Methods. Cambridge University Press, 1999.
9. T. McInerney and D. Terzopoulos. T-snakes:Topology adaptive snakes. Medical Image Analysis,4(2):73-91,2000.
10. M. Leventon, E. Grimson, O. Faugeras. Statistical Shape Influence in Geodesic Active Contours. Comp. Vision and Patt. Recon. (CVPR), June 2000.
11. L. M. Lorigo, O. Faugeras, W. E. L. Grimson, R. Keriven, R. Kikinis, A. Nabavi, C.-F. Westin. Codimension-Two Geodesic Active Contours. Comp. Vision and Patt. Recon. (CVPR), June 2000.
12. G. Aubert, M. Barlaud, O. Faugeras, S. Jehan-Besson. Image Segmentation Using Active Contours: Calculus of Variations or Shape Gradients? SIAM Journal on Applied Mathematics, Volume 63, Number 6, 2003
13. Jr. Yezzi, Anthony, Andy Tsai and Alan Willsky. A Fully Global Approach to Image Segmentation via Coupled Curve Evolution Equations. Journal of Visual Communication and Image Representation, 13 (2002) 195-216.
14. A. Vasilevskiy, K. Siddiqi. Flux-Maximizing Geometric Flows. IEEE Transactions on Pattern Analysis and Machine Intelligence, 24(12), 1565-157 8, 2002.
15. X. Han, C. Xu and J.L Prince. A topology Preserving Level Set Method for Geometric Deformable Models. IEEE Transactions on PAMI, Vol 25, No. 6, pp 755-768, June 2003.

Learning Coupled Prior Shape and Appearance Models for Segmentation

Xiaolei Huang, Zhiguo Li, and Dimitris Metaxas

Center for Computational Biomedicine Imaging and Modeling,
Division of Computer and Information Sciences, Rutgers University, NJ, USA

Abstract. We present a novel framework for learning a joint shape and appearance model from a large set of un-labelled training examples in arbitrary positions and orientations. The shape and intensity spaces are unified by implicitly representing shapes as "images" in the space of distance transforms. A stochastic chord-based matching algorithm is developed to align photo-realistic training examples under a common reference frame. Then dense local deformation fields, represented using the cubic B-spline based Free Form Deformations (FFD), are recovered to register the training examples in both shape and intensity spaces. Principal Component Analysis (PCA) is applied on the FFD control lattices to capture the variations in shape as well as on registered object interior textures. We show examples where we have built coupled shape and appearance prior models for the left ventricle and whole heart in short-axis cardiac tagged MR images, and used them to delineate the heart chambers in noisy, cluttered images. We also show quantitative validation on the automatic segmentation results by comparing to expert solutions.

1 Introduction

Learning shape and appearance prior representations for an anatomical structure of interest has been central to many model-based medical image analysis algorithms. Although numerous methods have been proposed in the literature, most are hampered by the automated alignment and registration problem of training examples. In the seminal work of Active Shape and Appearance Models (ASM [3] and AAM [4]), models are built from analyzing the shape and appearance variabilities across a set of labelled training examples. Typically landmark points are carefully chosen and manually placed on all examples by experts to assure good correspondences. This assumption leads to a natural framework for alignment and statistical modeling, yet it also makes the training process time-consuming. Yang & Duncan [15] proposed a shape-appearance joint prior model for Bayesian image segmentation. They did not deal with registration of the training examples, however, and assumed the training data are already aligned.

A number of automated shape registration and model building methods have been proposed [5], [6], [7], [2]. These approaches either establish correspondences between geometric features, such as critical points of high curvature [7]; or find the "best" corresponding parametrization model by optimizing some criterion,

C. Barillot, D.R. Haynor, and P. Hellier (Eds.): MICCAI 2004, LNCS 3216, pp. 60–69, 2004.

such as minimizing accumulated Euclidean Distance [6], [2], Minimum Description Length [5], or Spline Bending Energy [2]. Both geometric feature based and explicit parameterization based registration methods are not suitable for incorporating region intensity information. In [10], the implicit shape representation using level sets is considered, and shape registration algorithms using this representation have been proposed [11,8].

Non-rigid registration is a popular approach to build statistical atlas and to model the appearance variations [14,1]. The basic idea is to establish dense correspondences between textures through non-rigid registration. However, few of the existing methods along this line are able to register training examples in arbitrary poses or to be coupled with shape registration.

In this paper, we introduce a new framework for learning statistical shape and appearance models that addresses efficiently the above limitations. This framework is an extension of our work on *MetaMorphs*, a new class of deformable models that have both shape and interior texture statistics [9], to incorporate prior information. We work in a unified shape and intensity space by implicitly representing shapes as "images" in the space of distance transforms. A novel stochastic chord-based matching algorithm efficiently aligns training examples through a similarity transformation (with rotation, translation and isotropic scaling), considering both shape and gray-level intensity information. Then the complementary local registration is performed by deforming a Free Form Deformations (FFD) control lattice to maximize mutual information between both "shape" and intensity images. we apply principal component analysis on the deformed FFD control lattices to capture variations in shape and on registered object interior textures to capture variations in intensity. This learning framework is applied to build a statistical model of the left ventricle as well as an articulated model of the whole heart in short-axis cardiac tagged MR images, then the prior models are used for automated segmentation in novel images.

2   Data Description and Algorithm Outline

2.1   Description of the Training Data

The training data are from spatial-temporal short-axis cardiac tagged MR images. A 1.5T GE MR imaging system is used to acquire the images, and an EGG-gated tagged gradient echo pulse sequence. Every 30ms, 2 sets of parallel short axis (SA) images are acquired; one with horizontal tags and one with vertical tags. These images are perpendicular to an axis through the center of the LV. A complete systole-diastole cardiac cycle is divided into 24 phases. We collected 180 images from 20 phases, discarding the beginning and ending two phases. An expert is asked to segment the epicardium (Epi), the left ventricle (LV) endocardium and the right ventricle (RV) endocardium from the images.

2.2   Learning and Segmentation Algorithm Outline

Our overall learning and segmentation framework is outlined by the flow-chart in Fig. (1). There are two major components in the framework. The procedures

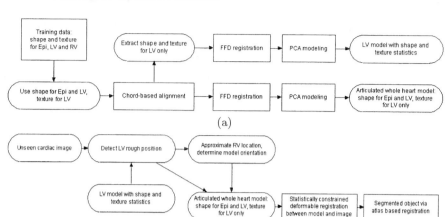

Fig. 1. (a) Learning framework. (b)Segmentation. (Rectangular boxes) Generic algorithmic steps. (Oval boxes) Specific designs for the cardiac segmentation problem.

described in the rectangular boxes are the algorithmic steps that are generic to all learning and segmentation problems. Additional procedures described in the oval boxes involve specific domain knowledge about the heart anatomy and the characteristics of the tagged MR images.

We utilize prior knowledge of the segmentation problem in devising the domain-specific procedures. First, since the images are acquired perpendicular to an axis through the center of the LV, the LV shapes appear relatively stable and near circular, and the LV interior intensities are also relatively homogeneous. Thus we learn a joint shape and texture model for the LV, which can be used for automated detection as well as segmentation. Second, for the alignment of training examples however, the LV's near-circular shape and homogeneous interior become unreliable in estimating the transformations. Thus we do the alignment based on an articulated heart model with both the epicardium (shape only) and LV endocardium (both shape and texture). Third, during segmentation in an unseen cardiac image, the LV shape and appearance model is used for automatically detecting the rough position of the heart. This position constraint and a Gabor-filter bank based method [12] are used to approximate the position of the RV. The positions of LV and RV centers determine the rough orientation of the whole heart model, which is thus transformed and further registered to the image using our statistically constrained deformable registration algorithm. The converged registration result defines the final segmentation of the heart chambers.

In the next two sections, we focus on presenting the generic algorithmic steps in our framework.

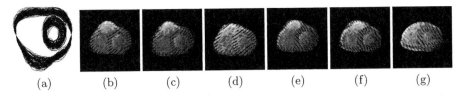

Fig. 2. Chord-based global alignment. (a) All aligned contours overlaid together. (b-g) Some examples of the globally aligned textures.

3   Learning the Shape and Appearance Statistical Model

3.1   Unified Shape and Intensity Feature Space

Within the proposed framework, we represent each shape using a Euclidean distance map. In this way, shapes are implicitly represented as "images" in the space of distance transforms where shapes correspond to the zero level set of the distance functions. The level set values in the shape embedding space is analogous to the intensity values in the intensity (appearance) space. As a result, for each training example, we have two "images" of different modalities, one representing its shape and another representing its intensity (grey-level appearance). The shape and intensity spaces are conveniently unified this way.

We use the Mutual Information criterion as the similarity measure to be optimized. Suppose A and B are two training examples. Let us denote their level set value random variables in the shape space as X_S^A and X_S^B, and their intensity random variables in the intensity space as X_I^A and X_I^B. Then the similarity between the two examples in the joint shape and intensity space can be defined using a weighted form of Mutual Information:

$$\begin{aligned}
\mathcal{M}_J(A,B) &= \mathcal{M}_S(A,B) + \alpha \mathcal{M}_I(A,B) \\
&= \mathcal{H}(X_S^A) + \mathcal{H}(X_S^B) - \mathcal{H}(X_S^A, X_S^B) + \alpha \left[\mathcal{H}(X_I^A) + \mathcal{H}(X_I^B) - \mathcal{H}(X_I^A, X_I^B) \right]
\end{aligned} \tag{1}$$

where $\mathcal{H}$ represents the differential entropy and α is a constant balancing the contributions of shape and intensity in measuring the similarity. In our experiments, we have set the values for α between $[0.2, 0.6]$. For brevity, we will use $\mathcal{M}_J$ to represent the mutual information in the joint space, $\mathcal{M}_S$ in the shape space, and $\mathcal{M}_I$ in the intensity space.

3.2   Chord-Based Global Alignment

When aligning the training examples under a common reference frame, we pursue an alignment that is "optimal" in the sense that the mutual information criterion in the joint feature space is optimized. Our solution is a novel alignment algorithm based on the correspondences between chords. Given a training example, A, suppose its un-ordered set of boundary points is $\{P_i^A = (x_i^A, y_i^A)\}, i = 1, ..., m$, a chord is a line segment joining two distinct boundary points. Our observations here are: **(i)** each of the total $\frac{1}{2}m(m-1)$ chords defines an internal, normalized reference frame for the example, in which the midpoint of the chord is the origin, the chord is aligned with the x axis, and the chord length is scaled to be of unit length 1.0; **(ii)** One pair of chord correspondences between two examples is sufficient to recover an aligning similarity transformation. So the basic idea of our algorithm is that, instead of finding correspondences between individual feature points as in most other matching algorithms, we find correspondences between chords, hence the correspondences between internal reference frames of two examples, and align the examples by aligning the best matching pair of internal reference frames.

Suppose we have an example A, as describe above, and a second example B with unordered set of boundary points $\{P_{i'}^B = (x_{i'}^B, y_{i'}^B)\}, i' = 1, ..., n$. Let us denote a chord joining two points P_i and P_j ($i \neq j$) as c_{ij}. The matching algorithm can be outlined as follows:

1. For every chord c_{ij}^A on example A,

   Find its corresponding chord $c_{i'j'}^B$ on example B as:

   $$c_{i'j'}^B = argmax_{c_{kl}^B}[\mathcal{M}_S(A_{ij}, B_{kl}(c_{kl}^B)) + \alpha\mathcal{M}_I(A_{ij}, B_{kl}(c_{kl}^B))] \qquad (2)$$

   where A_{ij} is the representation of A in its internal reference frame F_{ij}^A defined by the chord c_{ij}^A; $B_{kl}(c_{kl}^B)$ represents B in its internal reference frame F_{kl}^B defined by the chord c_{kl}^B.

2. Among all hypothesized alignments between A and B, suppose the one based on a pair of corresponding chords, c_{IJ}^A and $c_{I'J'}^B$, gives rise to the maximal mutual information in the joint shape and intensity space: $[\mathcal{M}_S(A_{IJ}, B_{I'J'}) + \alpha\mathcal{M}_I(A_{IJ}, B_{I'J'})]$, then the internal reference frames defined by this pair of chords, F_{IJ}^A and $F_{I'J'}^B$, are chosen to be the best matching reference frames.

3. Align examples A and B into a common reference frame by aligning the two reference frames F_{IJ}^A and $F_{I'J'}^B$ using a similarity transformation.

In practice, we find the chord correspondences using a stochastic algorithm based on the Chord Length Distribution (CLD) [13]. The algorithm is very efficient by considering only those chords with lengths greater than a certain percentile in the CLD of each example. On average, the computation time for aligning two examples on a $3GHz$ PC is around $15ms$ using the $85th$ percentile in our experiments. Furthermore, the algorithm can handle structures of arbitrary topology since it does not require the explicit parameterization of shapes. It is also invariant to scaling, rotation and translation, thus the training examples can be aligned robustly regardless of their initial poses. In Fig. 2, we show the aligned examples for our articulated whole heart model. Here we randomly pick one example as the atlas, and align all other examples to it.

3.3   Local Registration Using FFD and Mutual Information

After global alignment, the next step towards building a statistical model is to solve the dense correspondences problem. We proposed a nonrigid shape registration framework for establishing point correspondences in [8]. In this paper, we

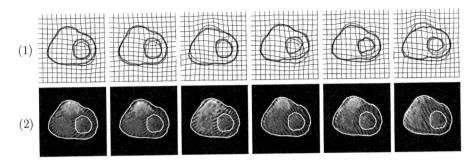

Fig. 3. Local FFD registration between training examples. (1) Each training shape (points drawn in circles) deforms to match a target mean atlas (points drawn in dots). The FFD control lattice deformations are also shown. (2) The registered textures. Note that each training texture is non-rigidly deformed based on FFD and registered to a mean texture. All textures cover a same area in the common reference frame.

extend this framework to perform nonrigid registration in the unified shape and intensity space, thus achieving simultaneous registration on both shapes and textures of the training examples. This joint registration provides additional constraints on the deformation field for the large area inside the object.

We use a space warping technique, the Free Form Deformations (FFD), to model the local deformations. The basic idea of FFD is to deform an object by manipulating a regular control lattice overlaid on its volumetric embedding space. We consider an Incremental cubic B-spline FFD in which dense registration is achieved by evolving a control lattice P according to a deformation improvement δP. Let us consider a regular lattice of control points $P_{m,n} = (P^x_{m,n}, P^y_{m,n})$; $(m,n) \in [1, M] \times [1, N]$ overlaid to a region $\Gamma_c = \{\mathbf{x}\} = \{(x,y) | 1 \leq x \leq X, 1 \leq y \leq Y\}$ that encloses a training example. Suppose the initial configuration of the control lattice is P^0, and the deforming control lattice is $P = P^0 + \delta P$. Then the incremental FFD parameters are the deformations of the control points in both x and y directions: $\boldsymbol{\Theta} = \{(\delta P^x_{m,n}, \delta P^y_{m,n})\}$. The incremental deformation of a pixel $\mathbf{x} = (x, y)$ given the deformation of the control lattice from P^0 to P, is defined in terms of a tensor product of Cubic B-spline: $\delta L(\boldsymbol{\Theta}; \mathbf{x}) = \sum_{k=0}^{3} \sum_{l=0}^{3} B_k(u) B_l(v)(\delta P_{i+k,j+l})$, where $i = \lfloor \frac{x}{X} \cdot (M-1) \rfloor + 1$, $j = \lfloor \frac{y}{Y} \cdot (N-1) \rfloor + 1$; $\delta P_{i+k,j+l}$ consists of the deformations of pixel $\mathbf{x}$'s sixteen adjacent control points; $B_k(u)$ is the kth basis function of the cubic B-spline.

To register an atlas T and a rigidly aligned training example R, we consider a sample domain Ω in the common reference frame. The mutual information criterion defined in the joint shape and intensity space can be considered to recover the deformation field $\delta L(\boldsymbol{\Theta}; \mathbf{x})$ that registers R and T:

$$\mathcal{M}_J\big(R, T(\delta L(\boldsymbol{\Theta}))\big) = \mathcal{M}_S\big(R(\Omega), T(L(\boldsymbol{\Theta}; \Omega))\big) + \alpha \mathcal{M}_I\big(R(\Omega), T(L(\boldsymbol{\Theta}; \Omega))\big) \qquad (3)$$

In the equation, $L(\boldsymbol{\Theta}; \Omega)$ represents the deformed domain of the initial sample domain Ω, i.e. $L(\boldsymbol{\Theta}; \mathbf{x}) = \mathbf{x} + \delta L(\boldsymbol{\Theta}; \mathbf{x})$, for any $\mathbf{x} \in \Omega$. A gradient descent optimization technique is used to maximize the mutual information criterion, and

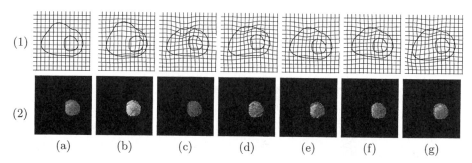

Fig. 4. PCA modeling. (1.a) The mean FFD control lattice configuration and mean shape. (1.b-c) Varying first mode of FFD deformations: -2σ reconstruction in (b) and 2σ in (c). (1.d-e) Second mode of FFD. (1.f-g) Third mode of FFD. (2.a) The mean LV texture (based on pixel-wise correspondences). (2.b-c) Varying first mode of LV texture. (2.d-e) Second mode of LV texture. (2.f-g) Third mode of LV texture.

to recover the parameters of the smooth, one-to-one registration field δL. Then dense pixel-wise correspondences can be established between each point $\mathbf{x}$ on example R, with its deformed position $\hat{L}(\mathbf{x})$ on the atlas T. The correspondences are valid on both the "shape" images and the intensity images. We show some example results using this local registration algorithm in Fig. (3).

3.4   Statistical Modeling of Shape and Appearance

After registration in the joint shape and intensity space, we apply Principal Component Analysis (PCA) on the deformed FFD control lattices to capture variations in shape. The feature vectors are the coordinates of the control points in x and y directions in the common reference frame. We also use PCA on the registered textures to capture variations in intensity. Here the feature vectors are the image pixel intensities from each registered texture. Fig. 4 illustrates the mean atlas and three primary modes of variation for both the shape deformation fields (Fig. (4).1) and intensities (Fig. (4).2). The shape model uses the articulated heart model with Epi and LV, and the texture model is for the LV interior texture only (due to tagging lines in heart walls and RV irregularity).

4   Segmentation via Statistically Constrained Registration

Given an unseen image, we perform segmentation by registering the learned prior model with the image based on both shape and texture. The mutual information criterion to be optimized is the same as Equation 3, except that here R consists of the new intensity image and a "shape" image, which is derived from the unsigned distance transform of the edge map (computed by the Canny edge detector). Another difference from the learning process is that, during optimization, instead of using directly the recovered FFD parameter increments to deform the prior model, we back-project the parameter increments to the PCA-based feature

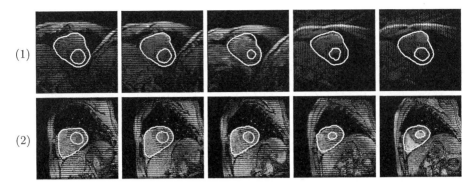

Fig. 5. Coupled prior based segmentation results on two novel tagged MR image sequences. (1) Example results from sequence 1. (2) Example results from sequence 2.

space, and magnitudes of the allowed actual parameter changes are constrained to have a 2σ upper bound. This scheme is similar to that used in AAM.

4.1 Results and Validation

Using the statistical model learned as shown in Fig. 4, we conduct automated segmentation via statistically constrained registration on two novel sequences of 4D spatial-temporal tagged MR images. Each sequence consists of 24 phases, with 16 slices (images) per phase. Since we do not use the first and last two phases in the new sequences, we have 320 images for testing from each sequence. The segmentation framework is depicted in Fig. 1.b. Example segmentation results are shown in Fig. 5. In all the experiments, following the LV detection and rough model pose estimation, the registration-based segmentation process takes less than 2 seconds to converge for each image on a $3GHz$ PC workstation.

Quantitative validation is performed by comparing the automated segmentation results with expert solutions. Denote the expert segmentation in the images as ℓ_{true}, and the results from our method as ℓ_{prior}. We define the false negative fraction (FNF) to indicate the fraction of tissue that is included in the true segmentation but missed by our method: $FNF = \frac{|\ell_{true} - \ell_{prior}|}{|\ell_{true}|}$. The false positive fraction (FPF) indicates the amount of tissue falsely identified by our method as a fraction of the total amount of tissue in the true segmentation: $FPF = \frac{|\ell_{prior} - \ell_{true}|}{|\ell_{true}|}$. And the positive fraction (TPF) describes the fraction of the total amount of tissue in the true segmentation that is overlapped with our method: $TPF = \frac{|\ell_{true} \cap \ell_{prior}|}{|\ell_{true}|}$. On the novel tagged MR sequence 1, our segmentation results produce the following average statistics: $FNF = 2.4\%, FPF = 5.1\%, TPF = 97.9\%$. On the novel sequence 2, the average statistics are: $FNF = 2.9\%, FPF = 5.5\%, TPF = 96.2\%$.

5   Discussion and Conclusions

In this paper, we have proposed a novel, generic algorithm for learning coupled prior shape and appearance models. Our main contributions in this paper are three folds. First, we work in a unified shape and intensity feature space. Second, we develop a novel stochastic chord-based matching algorithm that can efficiently align training examples in arbitrary poses, considering both shape and texture information. Third, a local registration algorithm based on FFD and mutual information performs registration both between shapes and between textures simultaneously. In our future work, we will learn a 3D coupled prior shape and texture model for the heart in tagged MR images. It is also important to explore the use of other learning techniques, such as Independent Component Analysis, in our framework.

Acknowledgements. The authors are grateful to Dr. Leon Axel for providing the MR cardiac images. We also would like to acknowledge the stimulating discussions with Dr. Nikos Paragios. Support for this research was provided by the NSF-0205671 grant.

References

1. M. Chen, T. Kanade, D. Pomerleau, and J. Schneider. 3-D deformable registration of medical images using a statistical atlas. In *MICCAI 1999*, pp. 621-630, 1999.
2. H. Chui, and A. Rangarajan. Learning an atlas from unlabeled point-sets. In *IEEE Workshop on Mathematical Methods in Biomedical Image Analysis*, 2001.
3. T. F. Cootes, C. J. Taylor, D. H. Cooper, and J. Graham. Active Shape Models - their training and application. In *Computer Vision and Image Understanding*, Vol. 61, No. 1, pp. 38-59, 1995.
4. T. F. Cootes, G. J. Edwards, and C. J. Taylor. Active Appearance Models. In *Proc. European Conf. on Computer Vision*, Vol. 2, pp. 484-498, Springer, 1998.
5. R.H. Davies, T.F. Cootes, J.C. Waterton, and C.J. Taylor. An efficient method for constructing optimal statistical shape models. In *MICCAI 2001*, pp. 57-65, 2001.
6. N. Duta, A. K. Jain, and M.-P. Dubuisson-Jolly. Learning 2D shape models. In *IEEE Conf. on Computer Vision and Pattern Recognition*, Vol. 2, pp. 8-14, 1999.
7. A. Hill, C. J. Taylor, and A.D. Brett. A framework for automatic landmark identification using a new method of non-rigid correspondences. In *IEEE Trans. on Pattern Analysis and Machine Intelligence*, Vol. 22, No. 3, pp. 241-251, 2000.
8. X. Huang, N. Paragios, and D. Metaxas. Establishing local correspondences towards compact representations of anatomical structures. In *MICCAI 2003*, LNCS 2879, pp. 926-934, 2003.
9. X. Huang, D. Metaxas, and T. Chen. MetaMorphs: deformable shape and texture models. In *IEEE Conf. on Computer Vision and Pattern Recognition*, 2004.
10. M.E. Leventon, E.L. Grimson, and O. Faugeras. Statistical shape influence in Geodesic Active Contours. In *IEEE Conf. on Computer Vision and Pattern Recognition*, Vol. 1, pp. 1316-1323, 2000.
11. N. Paragios, M. Rousson, and V. Ramesh. Matching distance functions: a shape-to-area variational approach for global-to-local registration. In *European Conf. on Computer Vision*, pages II:775–790, 2002.

12. Z. Qian, A. Montillo, D. Metaxas, and L. Axel. Segmenting cardiac MRI tagging lines using gabor filter banks. In *25th Int'l Conf. of IEEE EMBS*, 2003.
13. S. P. Smith, and A. K. Jain. Chord distribution for shape matching. In *Computer Graphics and Image Processing*, Vol. 20, pp. 259-271, 1982.
14. D. Rueckert, A.F. Frangi, and J.A. Schnabel. Automatic construction of 3D statistical deformation models using non-rigid registration. In *MICCAI 2001*, LNCS 2208, pp. 77-84, 2001.
15. J. Yang, and J.S. Duncan. 3D image segmentation of deformable objects with shape-appearance joint prior models. In *MICCAI 2003*, pp. 573-580, 2003.

A Modified Total Variation Denoising Method in the Context of 3D Ultrasound Images

Arnaud Ogier and Pierre Hellier

IRISA - INRIA**
Team Visages
35042 Rennes Cedex, France
{aogier,phellier}@irisa.fr
http://www.irisa.fr/

Abstract. Ultrasound volumes are corrupted by a multiplicative noise, the speckle, which makes high level analysis difficult. Within each resolution cell a number of elementary scatterers reflects the incident wave toward the sensor. This paper proposes a method of restoration based on variational principles adapted to ultrasound images statistics. The contribution of this paper is two-fold: we first derive a modified TV scheme to integrate the multiplicative nature of the ultrasound noise and we propose to tune the parameter λ automatically accordingly to the local noise distribution thanks to the kurtosis information. We present qualitative and quantitative results on various ultrasound volumes.

1 Introduction

Almost invasive nature, low cost and real time image formation, all of these features make ultrasound images an essential tool for medical diagnosis. This article aims at improving the use of ultrasound images so as to improve diagnosis and therapeutic treatment. However, the presence of multiplicative noise [1], called speckle, makes the interpretation of these images difficult.

This phenomenon is a common feature to all the images produced by coherent systems (SAR, laser, ultrasound, ...). For each resolution cell, it renders the spatial arrangement of the observed environment in terms of different scatterings which are not discriminated by ultrasound waves. The backscattered coherent waves with different phases undergo a constructive or a destructive interference in a random manner. Speckle statistical properties are linked to those of elementary scattering which make up the scanned area. We take into account this modeling to adjust our model based on total variation method, proposed by Rudin, Osher and Fatemi [2].

After a brief presentation of ultrasound images statistics, we will discuss briefly variational methods theory before describing our methods and comparing it to existing ones.

** This work was supported by the Council of Brittany under a contribution to the student grant.

C. Barillot, D.R. Haynor, and P. Hellier (Eds.): MICCAI 2004, LNCS 3216, pp. 70–77, 2004.

Table 1. Applications of the statistical models in ultrasonic imagery

Domain	The most adapted model(s)
cardiology	K-distribution
obstetrics and gynecology	K-distribution
abdominal	Rice, Homodyned K-distribution
Doppler	Rayleigh

2   Modeling Ultrasound Images

B-scan ultrasound images represent the back-scattering of an ultrasound beam from structures inside the body. Four models of noise are generally proposed to characterize an ultrasound image. Each noise distribution depends on two criteria, the density and the type of scatterers. Under some conditions, the classical distribution used for a random walk phenomenon is a Rayleigh distribution. It is valid only for a fully developed speckle, i.e. with a large number of incoherent scatterers. According to the number of scatterers and their space arrangement, several statistical models have been introduced. The type and distribution of scatterers is intrinsically related to the type of tissue that the ultrasound beam is passing through. Therefore this modeling is particularly adapted for restoration and segmentation purposes.

The K distribution is a generalization of the rayleigh distribution and models the presence of few diffuse scatterers. The Rician distribution is another generalization of the Rayleigh distribution and describes the presence of many coherent scatterers. The last one, introduced by Jakeman [3], the homodyned K distribution, describes the presence of few coherent scatterers.

Pragger [4] proposes to summarize these different cases (see Fig.2, left). We indicate in Tab.1 the comon application domains of these noise distribution.

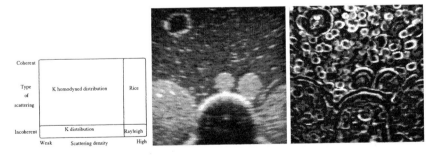

Fig. 1. Left: Distributions of noise in ultrasound images. Knowing the type and density of scatterers, appropriate distributions model the noise of ultrasound images. This illustrates the relationship between the type of noise and the type of tissue that the ultrasound beam is imaging. Middle and right: Ultrasound Image and corresponding kurtosis. The kurtosis is a relevant information to characterize edges and regions in the context of ultrasound images.

3   The Total Variation (TV) Restoration Concept

The TV anisotropic diffusion model was introduced by Rudin, Osher and Fatemi [2], and is now a popular tool for image restoration. The TV method tends to approximate the original image $u(x, y)$ by minimizing an energy.

To estimate a true signal in noise, the most frequently used methods are based on the least squares criteria which L_2 norm depends on. Rudin and Osher resort to the L_1 norm, which provides some discontinuities. Nevertheless, in practice, numerical approximation offers good results without the residual oscillations, equivalently to the Wiener filter.

In fact, Rudin and Osher propose to estimate an image u that minimizes the following energy:

$$E(u) = \int_\Omega |\nabla u| + \lambda \int_\Omega (u - u_0)^2 \tag{1}$$

where Ω is the image domain and λ is a real positive parameter. Minimizing this energy on a set of functions amounts to finding a function u_0 penalizing the oscillations. The Euler-Lagrange equation which corresponds to this energy is:

$$-\nabla u + \lambda(u - u_0) = 0,$$

For an additive noise $\sim \mathcal{N}(0, \sigma)$, this leads to the following constraints:

$$\int_\Omega u dx = \int_\Omega u_0 dx \quad \text{and} \quad \frac{1}{|\Omega|} \int_\Omega (u - u_0)^2 dx = \sigma^2. \tag{2}$$

The first constraint is satisfied thanks to TV norm translation invariance ($TV[u + c] = TV[u]$), and the corresponding gradient descent becomes:

$$\frac{\partial u}{\partial t} = div(\frac{\nabla_u}{|\nabla_u|}) + \lambda(u_0 - u), \tag{3}$$

To avoid singularities when $\nabla_u = 0$, we modify the denominator of the equation (3) as mentioned in [6], and more precisely

$$-\nabla.(\frac{\nabla_u}{\sqrt{|\nabla_u|^2 + \epsilon}}) + \lambda(u - u_0) = 0 \quad with \quad \epsilon > 0. \tag{4}$$

The steady state solution of this equation is the denoised image.

4   Application to Ultrasound Images

The purpose of this paper is to propose a modified TV restoration scheme adapted to the specific nature of ultrasound images. The afore mentioned statistics of the ultrasound images make difficult their integration in the numerical scheme directly. The contribution of this paper is two-fold: (a) we first derive a modified TV scheme to integrate the multiplicative nature of the ultrasound noise in subsection 4.1 and (b) we propose to tune the parameter λ automatically accordingly to the local noise distribution thanks to the kurtosis information in section 4.2.

Abdominal phantom

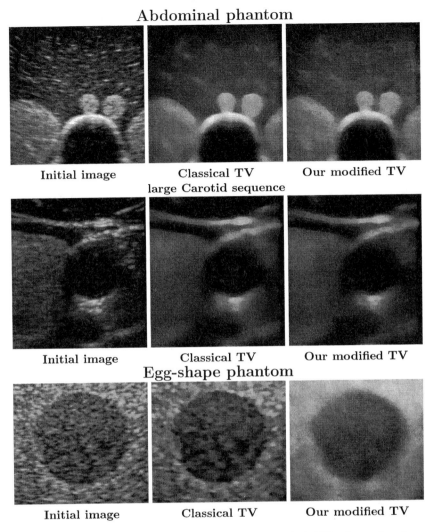

Fig. 2. Comparison of the original TV and our modified TV scheme for three ultrasound volumes. Top row: abdominal phantom, middle row: Carotid sequence and bottom row: Egg-shape phantom. Left column: original image, middle column: original TV scheme and right column: our modified TV scheme (multiplicative constraint and kurtosis-adaptive λ). Our modified TV scheme was able to smooth homogeneous regions while improving the edges of anatomical structures.

4.1   Multiplicative Noise

We take into account the multiplicative nature of the noise in the formulation of the total variation. The image u is multiplied by a noise η

$$u_0 = u\eta$$

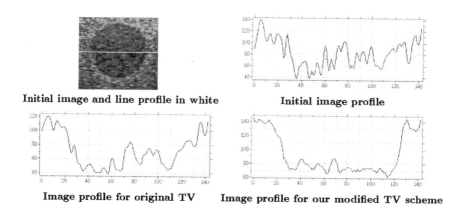

Fig. 3. Line profiles of the egg-shape phantom. Top left:image with white line for which the profile is computed. We compare image profiles of the original image, of the original TV scheme and of our modified TV scheme. We observe a reduction of the oscillation on homogeneous area and the enhancement of edges.

with the assumption of η following a normal distribution $\leadsto \mathcal{N}(0, \sigma)$. The constraints thus become:

$$\int \frac{u_0}{u} = 1, \quad \int \left(\frac{u_0}{u} - 1\right)^2 = \sigma^2.$$

A total variation denoising is applied on the image following the above constraints.

4.2   Kurtosis as a Tissue and Edge Descriptor

The kurtosis β_2 is a statistical measure corresponding to the fourth central moment. It measures the degree of steepness of the intensities distribution relative to a normal distribution. Kurtosis is defined as

$$\beta_2(x) = \frac{1}{N} \sum_{i \in V(x)} \left(\frac{x_i - \mu}{\sigma}\right)^4, \tag{5}$$

where $V(x)$ is the neighborhood of point x, N is the number of neighbors, μ is the mean gray level, σ is the standard deviation.

In the context of ultrasound images, a recent paper [5] characterizes the type of noise (Rayleigh, K, ...) according to the value of kurtosis. This value gives information about the type and density of the scatterers, consequently about the nature of the tissues. Therefore, it is a relevant information to be used for a restoration method as a region descriptor in the context of ultrasound images. In addition to this, the kurtosis is very sensitive to high transitions as any other high moment. Therefore it is a relevant information to characterize the edges of the image to be restored. Fig. 2 shows a typical kurtosis image.

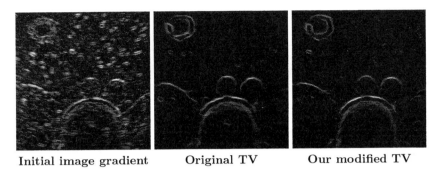

| Initial image gradient | Original TV | Our modified TV |

Fig. 4. Left: Gradient of phantom abdomen, Middle: gradient of denoised image using the original TV scheme. Right: gradient of denoised image using our modified TV scheme.

The parameter λ, which is the balance between the data term and the regularization term, can then be automatically tuned accordingly to the kurtosis in the following way:

$$\forall x \in \Omega, \lambda(x) = \frac{\beta_2^3(x)}{\max_{(\Omega)}(\beta_2^3)}$$

For a contour point, λ is maximum and the restoration scheme will preserve the contour. On the contrary, λ is minimal in homogeneous areas leading to a higher regularization.

5 Results

All the volume considered were acquired using a 3 free-hand ultrasound system. We present results on three types of images: a carotid (size $220 \times 240 \times 200$), the acquisition of a $3D$ multimodal abdominal phantom (size $531 \times 422 \times 127$) and a ultrasound phantom (egg shape, size $143 \times 125 \times 212$). The results presented here are the steady state of the restoration algorithm. Computation time on a standard PC are approximately 60 seconds, depending on the volume size.

5.1 Qualitative Assessment

The result of the denoising (Fig. 4) on the three kinds of volumes, with different number of scatterers, and thus different statistics, are visually satisfying. Indeed, for the three volumes, we obtain an piecewise smooth image with a good preservation of the structures. Our modified TV scheme seems visually better at smoothing homogeneous regions while improving the edges of anatomical structures.

5.2 Quantitative Assessment

Quantitative assessment in the context of restoration is an open problem. We here present some experiments including moments of the restored image on homogeneous areas, restored gradient images and line profiles of the images.

Table 2. Comparison of variance and mean in a 3D context on homogeneous areas.

Homogeneous area	Mean	Variance
Abdomen	50.4	289.6
Classical TV3D	53.5	66.4
TV3D, additive constraint, kurtosis based λ	53.5	66.4
TV3D, multiplicative constraint, kurtosis based λ	58.31	64.19
Carotid	54.1	74.1
Classical TV3D	67.4	36
TV3D, additive constraint, kurtosis based λ	67.4	36
TV3D, multiplicative constraint, kurtosis based λ	68.91	35.2
Egg	87.8	379.12
Classical TV3D with $\lambda = 0.1$	78.7	176.61
Classical TV3D with $\lambda = 0.01$	95.5	35
TV3D, additive constraint, kurtosis based λ	97.03	42
TV3D, multiplicative constraint, kurtosis based λ	96.18	58

Firstly, we have specified homogeneous areas -anatomically speaking - for each image sequence. Within these areas, we compute the mean and variance of image intensities. Results are presented in table 2. We compare three methods here: the original TV scheme, a first modified TV scheme (additive constraint and kurtosis-adaptive λ) and our modified TV scheme (multiplicative constraint and kurtosis-adaptive λ). We also present results with different values of parameter λ for the original TV scheme.

For the abdomen and carotid volumes, we obtain similar or better results than classical TV without tuning any parameter. Better results are obtained taking into account a multiplicative noise. The results concerning the egg volume point out the fact that the coefficient λ is critical in the classical scheme. An optimal tuning of this parameter leads to good results with the original TV scheme. For the abdominal and carotid sequence, our modified TV scheme gave better results than the original TV scheme, even for a wide range of variation for parameter λ. Based on these results, we now only compare the original TV scheme and our modified TV scheme (multiplicative constraint and kurtosis-adaptive λ). For the egg-shaped sequence, we present the profile of the image along a given line in figure 4.1. This result shows the effectiveness of our modified TV scheme since edges are enhanced and homogeneous areas are correctly smoothed.

We have also computed the image gradient. Results are presented in figure 4.2. Results show that in both restoration cases, edges are enhanced as denoted by strong image gradients. In our modified TV scheme, image gradients appear more consistent in terms of "shape".

6   Conclusion

After describing ultrasound images and fundamental concepts inherent to analysis by total variation, we propose to adapt the TV restoration scheme in two ways: we first include the constraint of a multiplicative noise and introduce a kurtosis-based parameter. In the context of ultrasound images, kurtosis is related to noise distribution and therefore to tissue properties indeed. This leads to an automatic tuning of parameter λ, which we think is useful since we experienced that the tuning of this parameter can be problematic.

Qualitative and quantitative results on various image sequences have shown the effectiveness of our modified TV scheme in smoothing homogeneous regions while enhancing edges.

References

1. J. Goodman, "Some fundamental properties of speckle," Dpt of Elec. eng, Stanford, Tech. Rep., 1976.
2. L. Rudin, S. Osher, and E. Fatemi, "Nonlinear total variation based noise removal algorithms," *Physica*,Vol 60, pages 259-268, 1992.
3. E. Jakeman and P. Pusey, "Significance of k distribution in scattering experiments," *Phys Rev Lett*, vol. 40, pp. 546–550, 1978.
4. R. W. Prager, A. H. Gee, G. M. Treece, and L. H. Berman, "Speckle detection in us images using first order statistics," Cambridge University Tech. Rep. 7, july 2001.
5. X. Hao, C. Bruce, C. Pislaru, and J. Greenleaf, "Characterization of reperfused infarcted myocardium from high-frequency intracardiac ultrasound imaging using homodyned k distribution," *IEEE Trans on Ultra., Ferro., and Freq cont.*, vol. 49, no. 11, pp. 1530–1542, 2002.
6. L. Rudin and S.Osher, "Total variation based image restoration with free local constraints," Cognitech, Tech. Rep., 1994.
7. W. H. Press, S. A. Teukolsky, W. T. Vetterling, and B. P. Flannery, *Numerical Recipes in C*, Cambridge University Press, 1995.

Correcting Nonuniformities in MRI Intensities Using Entropy Minimization Based on an Elastic Model

Ravi Bansal[1,2], Lawrence H. Staib[3], and Bradley S. Peterson[1,2]

[1] Department of Psychiatry, Columbia University, New York, NY 10032
[2] New York State Psychiatric Institute, New York, NY 10032
[3] Departments of Electrical Engineering and Diagnostic Radiology, Yale University, New Haven, CT 06512

Abstract. Nonuniformity in the pixel intensity in homogeneous regions of an observed image is modeled as a multiplicative smooth bias field. The multiplicative bias field tends to increase the entropy of the original image. Thus, the entropy of the observed image is minimized to estimate the original image. The entropy minimization should be constrained such that the estimated image is close to the observed image and the estimated bias field is smooth. To enforce these constraints, the bias field is modeled as a thin–plate deforming elastically. Mathematically, the elastic deformation is described using the partial differential equation (PDE) with the body force evaluated at each pixel. In our formulation, the body force is evaluated such that the overall entropy of the image decreases. In addition, modeling the bias field as an elastic deformation ensures that the estimated image is close to the observed image and that the bias field is smooth. This provides a mathematical formulation which is simple and devoid of weighting parameters for various constraints of interest. The performance of our proposed algorithm is evaluated using both 2D and 3D simulated and real subject brain MR images.

Keywords: Elastic Deformation, Partial Differential Equation, Expectation Maximization (EM), Entropy

1   Introduction

Magnetic resonance imaging (MRI) provides detailed information about anatomical structure. The signal-to-noise ratio (SNR) of the images is improved with the increase in the static magnetic field (B_0) strength. This improved SNR improves the image resolution and the details of the anatomical structures. However, with higher magnetic field strengths, image pixel nonuniformities, i.e. smooth variation in the intensities of the pixels of the same tissue type, tend to increase. This smooth variation of the pixel intensities within a homogeneous region makes automated image processing, such as image segmentation, visualization and derivation of computerized anatomical atlas, more difficult.

C. Barillot, D.R. Haynor, and P. Hellier (Eds.): MICCAI 2004, LNCS 3216, pp. 78–86, 2004.

There are various reasons for image nonuniformities [11], which include poor radio frequency (RF) coil uniformity, gradient–driven eddy currents, and subject anatomy both inside and outside the field of view. Some of the causes of nonuniformity, such as frequency response of the receiver and spatial sensitivity of the unloaded RF coils, can be overcome by proper calibration of the MR unit [7]. However, nonuniformities due to the geometry and the magnetic susceptibility of a subject remain [12] and require a post processing approach for correction.

The difficulty of correcting for the intensity nonuniformity stems from the fact that nonuniformities change with MRI acquisition parameters and subjects in the magnet [1]. In addition, the nonuniformities tend to change the tissue statistics such as mean and variance of the pixel intensities [1]. Thus, a robust and automatic method for correcting nonuniformities is essential for post–processing MR images. In medical image processing literature, a number of methods have been proposed [12,3,6,1,14,2,10] each with its strengths and weaknesses. Authors in [6] also proposed an entropy minimization method which optimizes a cost function that is a sum of three different terms. Thus, the estimated bias field depends upon the weights of these terms.

We propose a simple and an unifying mathematical framework where the appropriate constraints on the bias field are naturally included. The bias field forms a smooth multiplicative field, a model which has been widely used [12, 14]. The multiplicative bias field is converted into an additive field by taking the natural logarithm of the pixel intensities of the observed image. Next, the additive bias field is modeled as a thin plate deforming elastically. The elastic deformation is mathematically modeled using the partial differential equations (PDE). This model automatically incorporates the constraints that the bias field should be smooth and the estimated image should be close to the observed image. The body force in the elastic model is evaluated such that the overall entropy of the estimated image is decreased. In evaluating the body force, segmentation of the observed image into tissue classes is required which is achieved using the EM [5] algorithm which iteratively updates the mean and variance of each tissue class.

2   Methods

Image nonuniformity is usually modeled as a smooth pixelwise multiplicative bias field [12,6]. Let $(U(x, y, z))$ denote the bias field and $(T(x, y, z))$ be the pixel intensity of the original image at location (x, y, z), then the observed image pixel intensity $(S(x, y, z))$ is given as $S(x, y, z) = U(x, y, z) \cdot T(x, y, z)$.

The multiplicative bias field is converted into an additive field by taking the natural logarithm which yields $\ln S = \ln U + \ln T$. Let, $\mathbf{s}$, $\mathbf{t}$ and $\mathbf{u}$ be the random variables denoting the logarithm pixel intensities sampled from the observed image, the original image and the bias field respectively. Thus, $\mathbf{s}$ is a sum of $\mathbf{t}$ and $\mathbf{u}$. Assuming that the random variables $\mathbf{t}$ and $\mathbf{u}$ are statistically independent, the probability density function of $\mathbf{s}$ is thus obtained by convolving the probability densities of $\mathbf{t}$ and $\mathbf{u}$ [8]. Convolution operator increases entropy and hence the entropy of s is expected to be higher than the entropy of t. Hence, the original image is estimated from the observed image by reducing the entropy of the observed image. In addition, the estimation of the original image is constrained by the assumption that the bias field is smooth and that the original image is *close* to the observed image.

In our formulation, we model the logarithmic additive bias field as a thin plate deforming elastically under a body force where the body force is evaluated to minimize the entropy of the observed image. In a linear elastic model, the restoring forces are proportional to the displacement. Thus, the elastic model automatically incorporates the constraint that the estimated bias field is smooth and that the estimated image is close to the observed image. The elastic model can be modeled using elliptic partial differential equation (PDE) allowing a simple mathematical formulation which is devoid of various weighing terms. The only weights are μ and λ, the viscosity coefficients, which appear in the PDE model of the fluid dynamics. In our implementations, μ is always set to 1.0 and a variation of λ between 0.6 to 1.0 generated good results for most of the images.

The PDE governing the elastic model is given as [4]:

$$\mu \nabla^2 \vec{u} + (\lambda + \mu) \vec{\nabla}(\vec{\nabla} \cdot \vec{u}) + \vec{b}(\vec{u}) = \vec{0}, \tag{1}$$

where $\nabla^2 = \nabla^T \nabla$ is the Laplacian operator, $(\vec{\nabla} \cdot \vec{u})$ is the divergence operator, μ and λ are the elasticity constant and $\vec{u}(\vec{x}, t)$ is the field at time t and position $\vec{x}$. The PDE describing the elastic model is an elliptic boundary value problem.

The PDE in Eqn. (1), defined on a domain $\Omega = [0, 1]^3$, is a boundary value problem which is solved numerically using successive over-relaxation (SOR) method with checker board updates [9]. Zero boundary conditions of $\vec{u}(\vec{x}, t)$ for all $\vec{x} \in \partial \Omega$ and all t. Here, $\partial \Omega$ denotes the boundary of the domain Ω. Due to these boundary conditions, the bias field at $\partial \Omega$ will be zero. In our implementation we used *Forward Time Centered Space* (FTCS) [9] method for numerical estimation of the various partial derivatives in Eqn. (1).

To evaluate the body force at a pixel, the image pixels are first classified into different classes using EM [5] based maximum likelihood classification algorithm using the current estimated bias field. For the estimated classification of each pixel, body force is determined which is used to update the bias field. Using the estimated bias field, the pixel classification is again updated using the EM algorithm. This process is repeated till the estimated pixel classifications converge.

2.1   EM Based Segmentation

We assume that the image pixels can be labeled into 4 classes {*background, gray matter, white matter, fat*}. The pixel intensities in these classes are assumed to be Gaussian distributed. Thus, we need to estimate the mean and variance of the pixel intensities in each of these classes and the class to which a pixel belongs. For a given current estimate of the bias field, we estimate the class mean and variance and the pixel classification using the EM algorithm [5].

Let, $\mu = (\mu_1, \mu_2, \ldots, \mu_n)$ denote the means, $\sigma = (\sigma_1, \sigma_2, \ldots, \sigma_n)$ denote the standard deviations and $\pi = (\pi_1, \pi_2, \ldots, \pi_n)$ denote the prior probabilities of the n classes with constraint that $\sum_i \pi_i = 1$. Let, the class labels be $c_1, c_2, \cdots, c_n$ and let $z_i = (z_{1i}, z_{2i}, \ldots, z_{ni})$ be a vector of size n in $\{0,1\}$ such that $z_i = (0, 0, \ldots, 0, \underbrace{1}_{m}, 0, \ldots, 0)$ if the ith pixel belongs to mth class. That is, the vector z_i is all zero except for a 1 at the mth location if the pixel belongs to the mth class. Then given the observed image S and the estimated bias field U, the likelihood probability $P(s_i|u_i, \mu, \sigma)$ of the observed data at the ith pixel is given as:

$$P(s_i|u_i, \mu, \sigma) = \sum_{b=1}^{n} \pi_b \, p_b(s_i|u_i, \mu_b, \sigma_b) = \prod_i \left[\sum_{b=1}^{n} \pi_b \, p_b(s_i|u_i, \mu_b, \sigma_b) \right]^{z_{ai}} .$$

Then, $\quad P(c_i|s_i, u_i, \sigma, \mu) = \dfrac{P(s_i, c_i|u_i, \mu, \sigma)}{P(s_i|u_i, \mu, \sigma)} = \prod_d \left[\dfrac{\pi_a p_a(s_i|u_i, \mu_a, \sigma_a)}{\sum_{b=1}^{n} \pi_b \, p_b(s_i|u_i, \mu_b, \sigma_b)} \right]^{z_{di}} .$

Thus, for the whole image, assuming that the image pixel intensities are sampled independently, the maximum likelihood estimates of the class mean and variances using the EM algorithm are given as:

$$\mu_a = \frac{\sum_i \widehat{z_{ai}} \, (s_i - u_i)}{\sum_j \widehat{z_{aj}}}, \sigma_a^2 = \frac{\sum_i \widehat{z_{ai}} \, (s_i - u_i - \mu_a)^2}{\sum_j \widehat{z_{aj}}}, \widehat{z_{ai}} = \frac{\pi_a p_a(s_i|u_i, \mu_a, \sigma_a)}{\sum_{b=1}^{n} \pi_b \, p_b(s_i|u_i, \mu_b, \sigma_b)},$$

where $\widehat{z_{ai}}$ denotes the expected value of the ith pixel belonging to class a. Thus, the EM algorithm, in addition to estimating the class variables, also estimates a probabilistic segmentation of the image.

2.2   The Body Force

For a given estimate of the pixel classification and an estimated bias field, a body force at each pixel is estimated by minimizing the joint conditional entropy $H(C, T|S, U)$ which is a measure of uncertainty in the estimated classification and the bias field corrected image for a given observed image and the current estimated bias field. To evaluate this entropy, consider the probability distribution $p(C, T|S, U)$ which is simplified, assuming that the neighboring pixels in the observed image are statistically independent, as $p(C, T|S, U) = \prod_i p(c_i, t_i|s_i, u_i) = \prod_i P(c_i = a) p_a(t_i|s_i, u_i)$.

Thus, the joint conditional entropy is evaluated as:

$$H(C, T|S, U) = -\sum_{C,T} p(C, T|S, U) \log p(C, T|S, U)$$

$$= -\sum_i (\sum_{a, t_i} p(c_i = a, t_i|s_i, u_i) \log p(c_i = a, t_i|s_i, u_i)) = \sum_i H(c_i, t_i|s_i, u_i),$$

where the entropy $H(c_i, t_i|s_i, u_i)$ is given as:

$$H(c_i, t_i|s_i, u_i) = -\sum_a P(c_i = a) \log p(c_i = a) - \sum_{a, t_i} P(c_i = a) p_a(t_i|s_i, u_i) \log p_a(t_i|s_i, u_i).$$

Since the pixel classifications remain constant while estimating the bias field, the body force is evaluated which minimizes $H(C,T|S,U)$, i.e.,

$$\min_T H(C,T|S,U) = \min_T \sum_i H(c_i,t_i|s_i,u_i) = \min_T \sum_a H_a(t|s,u)\frac{\sum_i P(c_i = a)}{N}.$$

To evaluate the entropy functions $H_a(t|s,u)$, the probability density functions $p_a(t|s,u)$ are estimated using the Gaussian kernel based Parzen window estimate [13], i.e.,

$$p_a(t|s,u) = \frac{1}{\sum_i P(c_i = a)} \sum_i^N P(c_i = a)\frac{1}{\sigma_a\sqrt{2\pi}} \exp[-\frac{1}{2}\frac{(t - t_i)^2}{\sigma_a^2}],$$

where $t = s - u$ and $t_i = s_i - u_i$. For heuristic computation of the entropy $H_a(t|s,u)$, consider two samples of pixels $(t_i,t_j), \forall i,j$ selected at randomly from the current estimated image. The entropy terms, $H_a(t|s,u)$, are evaluated as:

$$H_a(t|s,u) = \ln(\sigma_a\sqrt{2\pi}\sum_i P_i(a)) - \frac{\sum_j P_j(a)\left\{\ln\sum_{i=1}^N P_i(a)\exp[-\frac{1}{2}\frac{(t_j-t_i)^2}{\sigma_a^2}]\right\}}{\sum_{j=1}^M P_j(a)}.$$

To evaluate $\min_T H_a(t|s,u)$, we will evaluate variation in $H_a(t|s,u)$ for small change in the bias field. Let, $\Delta\vec{u}(\vec{x},t)$ denote the small variation in the bias field at a pixel location $\vec{x}$ at time t. Also, let $h = \max_{\vec{x}}\|\Delta\vec{u}(\vec{x},t)\|$, be the maximum variation in the bias field over all pixel locations. Then the variation in the entropy for small change in the bias field is evaluated as follows:

$$\frac{dH_a(t|s,u)}{d\vec{u}(\vec{x},t)} = \mathrm{lt}_{h\to 0}\left\{\frac{H_a(t|s,u+\Delta u) - H_a(t|s,u)}{h}\right\}$$

$$= \frac{1}{\sigma_a^2\sum_{j=1}^M P_j(a)}\sum_j P_j(a)\left\{\sum_{i=1}^N W_a(i,j)(t_j - t_i)\frac{\partial}{\partial h}(t_j - t_i)\right\},$$

$$\text{where, } W_a(i,j) = \frac{P_i(a)\exp(\frac{-1}{2}(\frac{t_j(h)-t_i(h)}{\sigma_a})^2)}{\sum_k P_k(a)\exp(\frac{-1}{2}(\frac{t_j(h)-t_k(h)}{\sigma_a})^2)}.$$

To evaluate $\frac{\partial}{\partial h}(t_j - t_i)$, consider a second set of samples $(t'_i,t'_j)\forall i,j$ selected at random from the estimated image with the small variation $\Delta\vec{u}(\vec{x},t)$ in the bias field. Let $d_j = \pm$ denote increase or decrease in the pixel intensity at the pixel j in the template image and let $d_i = \pm$ be the increase or decrease at the pixel i. Also, let the image gradient at the pixel j be denoted as $\nabla T_j = (\frac{\partial t_j}{\partial x^{(1)}}\frac{\partial t_j}{\partial x^{(2)}}\frac{\partial t_j}{\partial x^{(3)}})^T$. Then the partial derivatives $\frac{\partial t_j}{\partial h}$ are defined as $\frac{\partial t_j}{\partial h} = \mathrm{lt}_{h\to 0}\left(\frac{t'_j-t_j}{h}\right) = \|\nabla T_j\|d_j$, which is the magnitude of the gradient in the deformed template image multiplied with the direction of bias field variation at the voxel j. Similarly, the partial derivative $\frac{\partial t_i}{\partial h}$ is evaluated as $\frac{\partial t_i}{\partial h} = \|\nabla T_i\|d_i$.

Let s_{ij} be the sign which between d_i and d_j, i.e., $d_i = s_{ij}d_j$. Thus, using these, we have $\frac{\partial}{\partial h}(t_j - t_i) = \frac{\partial t_j}{\partial h} - \frac{\partial t_i}{\partial h} = (\|\nabla T_j\| - s_{ij}\|\nabla T_i\|)d_j$.

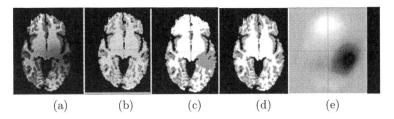

Fig. 1. Synthetic data with simulated bias field. (a) Original MRI. (b) Nonuniformity corrected. (c) Segmentation of (a). (d) Segmentation of (b). (e) Estimated bias field.

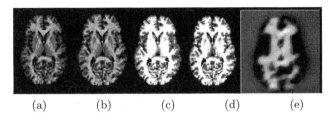

Fig. 2. Real subject 2D MR image. (a) Original MRI. (b) Nonuniformity corrected. (c) Segmentation of (a). (d) Segmentation of (b). (e) Estimated bias field.

Hence, the partial derivative of the marginal entropy can be written as:

$$\frac{dH_a(t|s,u)}{dh} = \frac{1}{\sum_j P_j(a)} \sum_j P_j(a) \underbrace{\left\{ \frac{1}{\sigma_a^2} \sum_i W_a(i,j)(t_j - t_i)\left(\|\nabla T_j\| - s_{ij}\|\nabla T_i\|\right) \right\}}_{b_j(a)} d_j.$$

Thus, we use the body force at the j pixel due to the class a is given as

$$b_j(a) = P_j(a)\left\{ \frac{1}{\sigma_a^2} \sum_i W_a(i,j)(t_j - t_i)\left(\|\nabla T_j\| - s_{ij}\|\nabla T_i\|\right) \right\}.$$

And the total body force at the pixel j is then given by the sum, $b_j = \sum_a \frac{P_i(a)}{N} b_j(a)$.

3   Results

In this section we present results of our intensity nonuniformity correction algorithm using both real and synthetic 2D and 3D MR image data.

Fig. 1 (a), shows a synthetic image with added known bias field. This synthetic image is obtained by first manually segmenting a 2D MR image into gray and white matter and then adding an off–center parabolic bias field. In this synthetic image, the gray matter pixel intensities vary from 38 to 58 and the white matter intensities vary from 46 to 57. Thus, there is a substantial overlap of pixel intensities. Fig. 1 (b) shows the image nonuniformity corrected image obtained using our proposed algorithm. In this image, the gray matter pixel intensity variation is from 46 to 58 and the white matter pixel intensity variation is from 56 to 67. Hence, in the corrected image, the variation of the pixel intensities within a class is reduced, the intensity overlap of the two classes is greatly reduced.

Fig. 1 (c) and (d) show the EM based segmentation of the images in Fig. 1 (a) and (b) respectively. Note that the segmentation is greatly improved after correcting for intensity nonuniformities. Numerically, for the image in Fig. 1 (c), the mis–classification rates of the EM algorithm are 24% and 12% for the gray matter and the white matter respectively. However, after correction, for the image in Fig. 1 (d), the mis–classification rates are 0% and 0.05% for the gray and white matter respectively.

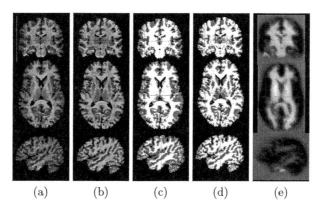

(a)   (b)   (c)   (d)   (e)

Fig. 3. Real subject 3D MRI. (1) Original MRI. (b) Nonuniformity corrected. (c) estimated segmentation of (a). (d) Estimated segmentation of (b). (e) Estimated bias field.

Fig. 2 (a) shows a real subject 2D MR image with nonuniformities. The image corrected for the nonuniformities using our algorithm is shown in Fig. 2 (b). Note that the corrected image has much better gray matter to white matter contrast. The estimated bias field is shown in Fig. 2 (e). Fig. 2 (c) and (d) show the EM based segmentation of the images in Fig. 2 (a) and (b) respectively.

Fig. 3 (a) shows three orthogonal views of a real subject 3D MR of a subject. Image obtained after correcting for intensity nonuniformities is shown in Fig. 3 (b). Fig. 3 (c) and (d) show the EM based segmentation of the images in Fig. 3 (a) and (b) respectively.

These results show that the nonuniformities in the pixel intensities can be corrected by minimizing overall entropy of the image. Also, our proposed method is robust and automated as there are no weighing parameters to be set. The estimated segmentation of the final intensity corrected image shows nonuniformity correction can lead to better post–processing of the acquired images. Also, since no underlying model of the deformation field is being assumed, the method can be used to correct any smooth bias field.

4   Discussion

We present a mathematical framework for correcting intensity nonuniformities where the bias field is modeled as a thin plate deforming elastically under a body force. The body force at each pixel is evaluated such that the overall entropy of the estimated image is reduced. The elastic deformations of the intensities is modeled using the partial differential equation (PDE), which is solved using the successive over relaxation (SOR) method.

Modeling the bias field as elastic deformations has the following advantages. First, it ensures that the estimated image is close to the original image. This is due to the fact that in the linear elastic model, the restoration forces are proportional to the amount of deformation. Second, the smoothness of the estimated bias field is ensured by the PDE modeling the elastic model. Third, the model is free of weighing parameters.

References

[1] Ahmed, M., Yamany, S., Mohamed, N., and Farag, A. (1999). A modified fuzzy C-means algorithm for MRI bias field estimation and adaptive segmentation. *MICCAI*, pages 72–81.

[2] Arnold, J., Liow, J., Schaper, K., Stern, J., Sled, J., Shattuck, D., Worth, A., Cohen, M., Leahy, R., Mazziotta, J., and Rottenberg, D. (2001). Qualitative and quantitative evaluation of six algorithms for correcting intensity nonuniformity effects. *NeuroImage*, 13:931–943.

[3] Cohen, M., DuBois, R., and Zeineh, M. (2000). Rapid and effective correction of RF inhomogeneity for high field magnetic resonance imaging. *Human Brain Mapping*, 10:204–211.

[4] Davatzikos, C. et al. (1996). A computerized method for morphological analysis of the corpus callosum. *J. Comp. Assis. Tomo.*, 20:88–97.

[5] Dempster, A. P., Laird, N. M., and Rubin, D. B. (1977). Maximum likelihood from incomplete data via EM algorithm. *J. Royal Statistical Soc., Ser. B*, 39:1–38.

[6] Mangin, J. (2000). Entropy minimization for automatic correction of intensity nonuniformity. *IEEE Workshop on Math. Methods in Bio. Image Analysis (MMBIA)*, pages 162–169.

[7] McVeigh, E., Bronskill, M., and Henkelman, R. (1986). Phase and sensitivity of receiver coils in magnetic resonance imaging. *Med. Phys.*, 13:806–814.

[8] Papoulis, A. (1991). *Probability, Random Variable, and Stochastic Processes*. McGraw–Hill, Inc., 3 edition.

[9] Press, W. H., Teukolsky, S. A., Vetterling, W. T., and Flannery, B. P. (1992). *Numerical Recipes in C. The Art of Scientific Computing*. Cambridge University Press.

[10] Prima, S., Ayache, N., Barrick, T., and Roberts, N. (2001). Maximum likelihood estimation of the bias field in mr brain images: Investigating different modelings of the imaging process. *Medical Image Computing and Computer-Assisted Intervention (MICCAI'01)*, LNCS 2208:811–819.

[11] Simmons, A., Tofts, P., Barker, G., and Arridge, S. (1994). Sources of intensity nonuniformity in spin echo images. *Magn. Reson. Med.*, 32:121–128.

[12] Sled, G., Zijdenbos, A., and Evans, A. (1998). A nonparametric method for automatic correction of intensity nonuniformity in MRI data. *IEEE Trans. of Medical Imaging*, 17(1):87–97.

[13] Viola, P. and Wells, W. M. (1995). Alignment by maximization of mutual information. *Fifth Int. Conf. on Computer Vision*, pages 16–23.

[14] Wells, W., Grimson, W., and Kikinis, R. (1996). Adaptive segmentation of MRI data. *IEEE Trans. on Medical Imaging*, 15(4):429–442.

Texture Image Analysis for Osteoporosis Detection with Morphological Tools

Sylvie Sevestre-Ghalila[1], Amel Benazza-Benyahia[2], Anne Ricordeau[3], Nedra Mellouli[3], Christine Chappard[4], and Claude Laurent Benhamou[4]

[1] Université Paris 5, Laboratoire MAP5, 45 rue des Saints Pères 75270 Paris Cédex 06, FRANCE - Université Manouba, ENSI, Laboratoire CRISTAL-GRIFT, campus de la Manouba, 2020 La Manouba, Tunisie. sevestre@math-info.univ-paris5.fr
[2] Ecole Supérieure des Communications de Tunis, URISA, Tunisia
[3] Université Paris 8, LINC, IUT de Montreuil, Montreuil, France
[4] CHR d'Orléans, France

Abstract. Osteoporosis is due to the following two phenomena: a reduction bone mass and a degradation of the microarchitecture of bone tissue. In this paper, we propose a method for extracting morphological information enabling the description of bone structure from radiological images of the calcaneus. Our main contribution relies on the fact that we provide bone descriptors close to classical 3D-morphological bone parameters. The first step of the proposed method consists in extracting the grey-scale skeleton of the microstructures contained in the underlying images. After an appropriate processing, the resulting skeleton provides discriminant features between osteoporotic patients and control patients. Statistical tests corroborate this discrimination property.

1 Introduction

Clinically, osteoporosis is a consequence of a gradual loss of calcium and collagen which induces both a dramatical bone mass decrease and, an alteration of the trabecular microarchitecture [1]. As the skeleton becomes too fragile to support the body, fractures occur frequently, especially in the wrist, spine or femur. In this context, diagnosing osteoporosis and assessing the efficacy of a treatment is a challenging issue for the health community. Since several years, various techniques have been developed in order to detect early and efficiently the apparition of this disease before fracture. The decrease of the Bone Mineral Density (BMD) is generally assessed through non-invasive methods as the dual energy X-ray absorptiometry. However, it has been recognized that in addition to BMD tests, information about the bone structure helps to determine the bone quality and hence, the probability of fractures [2]. Indeed, the bone structure consists of arches (trabeculae) that are arranged in groups according to different orientations that correspond mainly to compression/tensile stress. The analysis of such a stucture provides valuable information about the bone's mechanical strength and the alteration of its microarchitecture and hence, about the disease

C. Barillot, D.R. Haynor, and P. Hellier (Eds.): MICCAI 2004, LNCS 3216, pp. 87–94, 2004.

apparition or evolution. For instance, the bone is scanned by Magnetic Resonance Imaging (MRI) or X-rays in order to generate a textured "image" of the real bone structure. However, MRI suffers from a limited spatial resolution [3] and Computed Tomography (CT) techniques have limited applicability because of the high radiation dose. This is the reason why plane-film radiograph is preferred since it is inexpensive and requires much lower radiation doses. It is worth pointing out that the resulting 2D radiological patterns are the projection of the 3D anatomical structures on the plane film. Despite the artefacts inherent to the projection procedure, radiological trabecular patterns are assumed to reflect the anatomical one. The great irregularity (in shape, size and thickness) of the radiographic pattern and the low contrast in certain areas make difficult the interpretation of bone alteration by visual inspection. Therefore, computer-aided methods of texture analysis have been developed to assist clinicians in their diagnosis. The most challenging task consists in characterizing the bone microarchitecture by parameters automatically estimated from the images that are able to accurately detect and quantify the alterations of the bone. . In this work, we are interested in detecting osteoporosis through a texture analysis of calcaneus radiographs. Indeed, calcaneus is known to contain rich information on microarchitectural patterns and the required image acquisition system can be easily adjusted [6]. Most methods for such detection task [4]-[8] use classical approaches in texture analysis domain. Related to the approach of Gereats[9], our contribution consists in using morphological tools in order to extract characteristic features of the trabecular bone image close to classical 3D-morphological parameters. This paper is organized as follows. In Section 2, the skeletonization procedure and its composition are briefly described. In Section 3, the problem of the skeleton characterization is addressed and skeleton features are introduced. In Section 4, some experimental results are reported and commented. Finally, in Section 5, some conclusions are drawn.

2   Computing the Skeleton

2.1   Test Images

First of all, some information about image acquisition is given. Radiographic film is used for the formation of each image; the region of interest is 2.7 cm × 2.7 cm. This area only includes trabecular bone in the posterior part of the calcaneus and has a reproducible location [6]. The same X-ray clinical apparatus, with a tube voltage of 36kV, with a 18mAs exposure level with a Min-R film is employed during the acquisition procedure.The radiographs are scanned by an Agfa duoscan enabling their digital conversion. The scanning resolution amounts 100 μm so as a pixel represents an area of 105μm × 105μm. Finally, the resulting digital images $I(m, n)$ have a size of 256×256 and are coded at 8 bpp. A number of 31 images of Osteoporotic Patients (OP) with vetebral fractures and (or) with other kind of fractures and 39 images of Control Patients (CP) matched for age, are considered.

2.2   The Corresponding Skeleton

During the first stage of processing, the aim was to extract the grey-level skeleton of the microstructures contained in the underlying images. The skeleton consists of a network of arches which are located along local higher intensity regions. Its extraction was not an easy task because of the lack of a unifying approach for grey-scale image skeletonization [10,11]. In our case, a meaningful skeleton of the microarchitectures was expected preserve the microarchitecture connectivity. Therefore, we applied the skeletonization algorithm described in [12,13]. Indeed, the underlying thinning procedure is homotopic which is a crucial property for shape description applications. Furthermore, the skeletonization procedure had a very low computational cost. Figure 1.(b) provides an example of a resulting skeleton in the OP case. As can be seen, the skeleton corresponds to a very connected network of arches. The principal arches are vertical in the region of interest and originating in the subtalar joint, they correspond to the longitudinal trabeculae. The incidental arches are located in the bottom left of the region of interest originating in the inferior cortice of the calcaneus and they are associated with the transversal trabeculae.

Before characterizing the skeleton, it is necessary to determine its composition. Generally, a skeleton is viewed as the set of intersection points and the segments that connect such points. It is possible to classify the intersection pixels of the skeleton into the 2 following categories.

• The first one concerns pixels that are connected to at least 4 neighbors (according to the 8-connectivity). Since the maximum width of the skeleton amounts to 2 pixels, the pixels of this first class belong to intersection consisting of several pixels.

• The second category contains only pixels whose neighborhoods (according to the 8-connectivity) contain pixels that are not mutually 4-connected.

After determining the pixels of the first category, a label is assigned to each segment according to the segments emerging from each intersection. Indeed, at each intersection, the neighboring pixels (outside the intersection) are listed and if necessary, a new label is created for each of the listed pixels. This label is then propagated towards its nearest neighbor. It is worth noting that when the first pixel is receiving a label, two of its neighbors are potential candidates for the propagation procedure. The retained candidate is the neighbor which does not have any intersection pixel in its neighborhood. The scanning of the segment is stopped at a labeled pixel that encloses in its neighborhood an intersection pixel. The result of this classification is illustrated in the figure 1.(b). As a result, the projected portions of the trabeculae which correspond to the segments separating two adjacent multiple points can be identified.

3   Exploiting the Skeleton

The resulting grey-scale skeleton can be used to analyze the texture of the calcaneus. More precisely, we are interested here in quantifying the morphological features of the skeleton that give reliable information about the microarchitecture

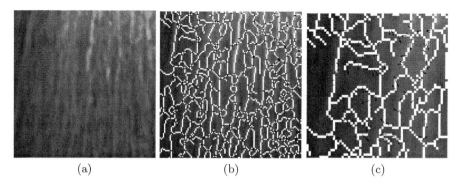

(a)   (b)   (c)

Fig. 1. Composition of skeleton: the image (b) is the pixel classification of the skeleton extrated from the image (a), the most black pixels are intersections. In the image (c) the half intra-projected distances of the left upper corner of (b) are illustrated with black arrows.

of the bone. The aim is to extract morphological features wich may be related to quantities obtained from invasive tests performed in pathological analysis.

3.1   Inter-projected Distance

An inter-projected distance is estimated as a length separating two successive intersections on a path of the skeleton, that is called a segment. The orientation of such a segment is measured with respect to the horizontal image axis. Again, for each segment, the orientation mean is defined as the average of the orientations calculated at each pixel of the underlying segment.

3.2   Intra-projected Distance

The intra-projected distances is the distances between the two lines of the maximum gradient directions around the skeleton. Hence, our objective is to determine for each segment point, the closest points to the left and the right of the segment where the absolute value of the gradient is maximum. Obviously, these points are searched along the normal to the segment [14]. The distance between the left or the right points is then computed and finally, the median value of these distances when the whole the segment is scanned could be considered as the half intra-projected distance. It is worth noting that this procedure is carried out only if the projected segment has three or more pixels, otherwise the derivative filters cannot be applied. Furthermore, the coherence between the direction of the skeleton and the direction of the detected border lines was controlled as in [14]. Among 4000 segments are generally detected in an image. With these two contraints, about 1000 intra-projected distances were estimated by using only few pixels per segment. These estimations are depicted by the black arrows in Figure 1.c.

3.3 Extracted Features

As noted by radiologists, osteoporosis tends to alterate the trabeculae that are the least required during the body motion. In the case of calcaneus, these trabeculae correspond to transversal ones [15]. Therefore, the features were separated into the two following categories :the first one is related to the transversal segments and corresponding to transversal trabeculae, the second related to the longitudinal segments corresponding to longitudinal trabeculae.

The histogram of the orientations of the segment is thresholded locally according to a sliding window. The largest value is associated with the longitudinal segments. The transversal and longitudinal projected segments do not share the same properties. To emphasize such dissymetry, the ratio between the variances of the angles and the ratio between the cardinalities of each class were evaluated. Within each class of orientation, we compute the following features :

• the mean $\bar{L}$ (resp. $\bar{l}$) of respectively the length L and the half-width l of the projected trabeculae; their variance σ_L^2 (resp. σ_l^2).
• the variance of the angles $\sigma^2(\theta)$ with respect to the local mean.
• the total number of pixels N_p belonging to the skeleton.
• the total number of ending pixels N_e of the skeleton.

4   Experimental Results

4.1   Univariate Analysis

In this part we evaluate de dispersion of each feature for CP and for OP class. The corresponding intervals mentioned in Table 1 show OP has a larger variation than CP. Althougth the OP intervals overlap the CP ones, it can be noted that for a large number of skeleton features, CP and OP are significantly different. The exceptions are N_e whatever the orientation, the mean length ($\bar{L}$) in the transverse direction, and the ratio between the values of N_p in each direction. The p-values resulting from the Wilcoxon Test show that a better discrimination between OP and CP is obtained in the longitudinal direction. More precisely, it indicates that the inter-projected and intra-projected distances take globally highest values within the CP group. Indeed, the reduction of such distances, in the OP could be imputed to a greater transparency of the bone network due to the microarchitecture deterioration. More precisely, the transparency induced by the disease is generally the result of two phenomena : a thinning effect and a perforation effect which can quantified by N_e feature.

4.2   Multivariate Analysis

In this section we are interesting to study the contribution of the morphological features combined with bone density (BMD) and Age, to discriminate between OP and CP. To visualize multidimensionality, we use the principal components analysis (PCA) approach so as to illustrate the complementary

Table 1. Statistical distributions of the considered parameters. The first table gives statistics on our features for the longitudinal direction and the second table for the transversal direction. For each direction, the associated table shows, for the length $\bar{L}$ respectively for the half-width $\bar{l}$ of the image, its interval of dispersion, its variance σ_L^2 (resp. σ_l^2), the total number of pixels N_p belonging to the skeleton and the total number of ending segments N_e of the skeleton. The third table gives global statistics of the skeleton for OP and CP as the total pixels of the skeleton N_p, the total number of intersections, the rate of the total number of pixels in longitudinal and transversal direction N_p^L/N_p^T, and the rate of the variance of the angles $\sigma^2(\theta)$ with respect to the local mean of each direction.

Longitudinal	$\bar{L}$	$\bar{l}$	σ_L	σ_l	N_p	N_e
Osteoporotic	[3.61 5.56]	[0.29 1.02]	[1.01 2.89]	[0.65 1.15]	[4078 5800]	≤ 110]
Control	[4.16 5.12]	[0.49 0.95]	[1.44 2.60]	[0.75 1.14]	[4756 5534]	[33 69]
Wilcoxon Test	$C > O$	$C > O$	$C > O$	$C > O$	$C > O$	$C > O$
(p-value)	(0.004)	(0.0056)	(0.0054)	(0.025)	(0.0018)	(0.316)
Transversal	L	l	σ_L	σ_l	N_p	N_e
Osteoporotic	[3.87 5.59]	[0.33 1.06]	[1.25 3.02]	[0.66 1.13]	[3023 4723]	[17 79]
Control	[4.20 5.33]	[0.5 0.99]	[1.53 2.81]	[0.74 1.12]	[3501 4383]	[23 64]
Wilcoxon Test	$C > O$	$C > O$	$C > O$	$C > O$	$C > O$	$C < O$
(p-value)	(0.13)	(0.035)	(0.137)	(0.056)	(0.46)	(0.13)

Global	N_p	Intersections	N_p^L/N_p^T	$\sigma_L^2(\theta)/\sigma_T^2(\theta)$
Osteoporotic	[12866 18591]	[1567 2864]	[1.01 1.56]	[0.22 5.87]
Control	[14045 16987]	[1777 2540]	[1.08 1.54]	[0.30 4.50]
Wilcoxon Test	$C < O$	$C < O$	$C > O$	$C < O$
(p-value)	(0.01)	(0.009)	(0.12)	(0.032)

information given by our features added to BMD and Age. From the analysis of the figure (2.a), we obtain three groups of features weakly correlated. The first, strongly correlated to the first factorial axis, contains length $\bar{L}$, the half-width $\bar{l}$ of the projected trabeculae, their variance for the two directions $(\bar{L}(L), \bar{L}(T), \sigma_{\bar{L}}(L), \sigma_{\bar{L}}(T), \bar{l}(L), \bar{l}(T), \sigma_l(L), \sigma_{\bar{l}}(T))$ and the number of intersections. The second, describing the second factorial axis, contains features deduced from the numbers of pixels $(N_p(L), N_p(T), N_p(L)/N_p(T))$. The last group including BMD and age is not well depicted in this first factorial plane.

The projection of our sample on the first factorial plane shows the pertinence of the first principal component ("facteur 1" in figure (2.a), to discriminate between OP and CP. We have chosen to separate the osteoporotic with vertebral fracture (black circles) from those with other fractures (darck grey circles) in addition.The discrimination between OP and CP is more striking when we limit ourselves to OP with vertebral fracture.

To classify OP and CP, logistic regression models were applied. The best models with three features were obtained as follows : one feature of first group explaining the spread of our sample was entered into the model combined with $N_e(T)$ and BMD. With $\bar{l}(T)$ as the feature of the first group, we obtained 77% well classified with 89.7% in the CP class and a very good fit with a smalle p-value ($\leq 10^{-3}$).

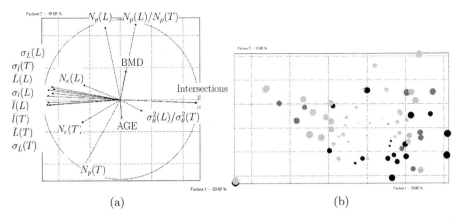

Fig. 2. The figure (a) is the correlation circle associated with the first factorial plane of the morphological features combined with bone density BMD and AGE. The figure (b) is the projection of our sample on this plane. The discs of black color give the position of OP having a vertebral fracture. The discs of dark grey color are patients having both vertebral fracture and another one fracture. Finally, the discs of light grey color give the position of CP. Bigger is the circle, higher is the proximity to the plane.

5   Conclusion and Perspectives

In this paper, we have extracted features from calcaneus radiographs that reflect the trabeculae microarchitecture of the bone. Statistical tests have indicated that the inter and intra projected distances are key-discriminant features. In fact, the results obtained are promising in the sense that :

– additional information was produced with respect to BMD and age,
– they permitted to point out well known osteoporosis symptoms related to the microarchitecture from a radiograph instead of an invasive test.

So, larger data set and more sophisticated methods should be used in order to consider more than two classes. Then it could be possible to study separately different kind of fractures.

References

1. Consensus development Conference: diagnosis, prophylaxis, and treatment of osteoporosis, *Amer. J. Med.*, vol. 94, no. 6, pp. 646-650, June 1993.
2. S.A. Goldstein, "The mechanical properties of trabecular bone: Dependence on anatomic location and function," *J. Biomech.*, vol. 20, pp. 1055-1061, 1987.
3. S. Majumdar, D. Newitt, M. Jergas, A. Gies, *et al.*, "Evaluation of technical factors affecting the quantification of trabecular bone structure using magnetic resonance imaging," *Bone*, vol. 17, pp. 417-430, 1995.
4. V. Paquet, P. Battut, H.V. Blanc D. Ferrand, "On the use of grey run lenth matrices in trabecular bone analysis," *Proc. of the Conf. on the Image Proc. and its Applic.*, pp. 445-449, 4-6 July 1995.

5. T. Lundahl, W.J. Ohley, S.M. Kay, R. Siffert, "Fractional Brownian motion: a maximum likelihood estimator and its application to image texture," *IEEE Trans. Med. Imag.*, vol. MI-5, no. 3, pp. 152-161, September 1986.

6. C.L. Benhamou, R. Harba, E. Lespessailles, E. Jacquet, D. Toulière, R. Jennane, " Fractal organisation of trabecular bone images on calcaneus radiographs," *J. Bone Mineral Res.*, vol. 9, pp. 1909-1918, 1994.

7. T.E. Southard, K.A. Southard, "Detection of simulated osteoporosis in maxillae using radiographic texture analysis," *IEEE Trans. on Biomed. Eng.*, vol. 43, no. 2, pp. 123-132, February 1996.

8. J.S. Gregory, R.M. Junold, P.E. Undrill, R.M. Aspden, "Analysis of trabecular bone structure using Fourier transforms and neural networks," *IEEE Trans. on Inf. Tech. in Biomed.*, vol. 3, no. 4, pp. 289-294, December 1999.

9. W.G.M. Geraets, "Computer-aided analysis of the radiographic trabecular pattern," *Ph. D. Thesis*, Netherlands.

10. C. Arcelli, G. Ramella, "Finding grey skeletons by iterated pixel removal," *Image and Vision Computing*, vol. 13, no. 3, pp. 159-267, April 1995.

11. S. Chen, F.Y. Shih, "Skeletonization for fuzzy degraded character images," *IEEE Trans. on Image Proc.*, vol. 5, no. 10, pp. 1481-1485, October 1996.

12. S. S. Mersal, A.M. Darwish, "A new parallel thinning algorithm for gray scale images," *IEEE Nonlinear Signal and Image Proc. Conf.*, Antalya, Turkey, June 1999.

13. S. Sevestre-Ghalila, A. Benazza-Benyahia, H. Cherif, W. Souid, "Texture analysis for osteoporosis detection with morphological tools," *Medical Imaging 2001, SPIE Conf.*, Milan Sonka, Kenneth M. Hanson Eds., vol. 4322, pp. 1534-1541, San Diego, California, USA, 17-23 February 2001.

14. C. Steger, *Unbiased extraction of curvilinear structures from 2D and 3D images*, PhD Thesis, Technical University of Munchen, 1998.

15. P. Banerji, S.G. Kabra, "The trabecular pattern of calcaneus as an index of osteoporosis" *Journal British Editorial Society of Bonne and joint Surgery* vol 65-B, no. 2, pp. 195-198, 1983.

16. T. Koller, C. Grieg, G. Szekély, D. Dettwiler, "Multiscale detection of curvilinear structures in 2D and 3D image data," *Proc. of the Fifth Internat. Conf. on Computer Vision*, pp. 864-869, 1995.

Multi-class Posterior Atlas Formation via Unbiased Kullback-Leibler Template Estimation

Peter Lorenzen[1], Brad Davis[1], Guido Gerig[1,2], Elizabeth Bullitt[1,3,4], and Sarang Joshi[1,5]

Departments of [1]Computer Science, [2]Psychiatry, [3]Surgery, [4]Radiology, and [5]Radiation Oncology,
University of North Carolina, Chapel Hill, NC 27599, USA
{lorenzen, davisb, gerig, joshi}@cs.unc,edu, bullitt@med.unc.edu

Abstract. Many medical image analysis problems that involve multimodal images lend themselves to solutions that involve class posterior density function images. This paper presents a method for large deformation exemplar class posterior density template estimation. This method generates a representative anatomical template from an arbitrary number of topologically similar multi-modal image sets using large deformation minimum Kullback-Leibler divergence registration. The template that we generate is the class posterior that requires the least amount of deformation energy to be transformed into every class posterior density (each characterizing a multi-modal image set). This method is computationally practical; computation times grows linearly with the number of image sets. Template estimation results are presented for a set of five 3D class posterior images representing structures of the human brain.

1 Introduction

Computational anatomy, the study of anatomical variation, is an active area of research in medical image analysis. An important problem in computational anatomy is the construction of an exemplar template (or atlas) from a population of medical images. This template represents the anatomical variation present in the population [1,2,3]. Understanding anatomical variability requires robust high-dimensional image registration methods where the number of parameters used to describe the mappings between images is on the order of the number of voxels describing the space of the images.

Modern imaging techniques provide an array of imaging modalities which enable the acquisition of complementary information representing an underlying anatomy. Most image registration algorithms find a mapping between two scalar images. To utilize multi-modal images of a single anatomy, we define a multi-modal image set, $\bar{I}$, as a collection of m co-registered multi-modal images, $\bar{I}(x) \in \mathbb{R}^m$. For example, $\bar{I}(x)$ might represent a CT image, a T1-weighted MR image, and a PET image of a single anatomy.

If, in traditional two-scalar image registration, the images are of different modalities, mutual information is typically used to register them. High-dimensional image registration, in the context of mutual information and other

C. Barillot, D.R. Haynor, and P. Hellier (Eds.): MICCAI 2004, LNCS 3216, pp. 95–102, 2004.
© Springer-Verlag Berlin Heidelberg 2004

dissimilarity measure frameworks, has been studied extensively. A thorough investigation of these dissimilarity measures in high-dimensional image registration is presented in [4]. A multi-modal free-form registration algorithm that matches voxel class labels, rather than image intensities, via minimizing Kullback-Leibler divergence is presented in [5,6]. This method finds correspondences between two multi-modal scalar images. A method that minimizes Kullback-Leibler divergence between expected and observed joint class histograms is presented in [7]. This technique, however, estimates class labels as a preprocessing step and is used only for rigid registration between scalar images. The method presented in this paper is more general in that registration is performed on sets of images, of arbitrary number and is not constrained by an initial class labeling. Although inter-subject high-dimensional image registration has received much attention [8, 9,10,11], to our knowledge, little attention has been given to using multi-modal image sets of subjects to estimate registration transformations.

1.1 Model-Based Multi-modal Image Set Registration

Across image sets, the number of constituent images may vary, thus registration based on an intensity similarity measure is not possible in this setting. While mutual information can be extended to multiple random variables, its extension to registration involving three or more images is problematic in that it requires maintaining an impractical number of histogram bins [12]. Given these difficulties, we move to a model-based approach where the registration is performed using underlying anatomical structures. We incorporate anatomical structures as a prior in a Bayesian framework as described in [13].

This framework is based on the assumption that human brain anatomy consists of finitely enumerable structures such as grey matter, white matter, and cerebrospinal fluid. These structures present with varying radiometric intensity values across disparate image modalities. Given a collection of multi-modal image sets representing the atlas population, we capture the underlying structures by estimating, for each image set, the class posterior densities associated with each of the structures. These class posterior densities are then used to produce the multi-class posterior atlas by estimating high-dimensional diffeomorphic registration maps relating the coordinate spaces of the densities. The Kullback-Leibler divergence is used as the distance function for the posterior densities to estimate the transformation. The use of the class posterior densities provides an image intensity independent approach to image registration.

2 Bayesian Framework

From a population of N multi-modal image sets $\{\bar{I}_i\}_{i=1}^N$, for each class c_j we first estimate the class posterior densities $p_j^i(x) = p(c_j(x)|\bar{I}_i)$ for each image set i where $c_j(x)$ is the class associated with the voxel at position $x \in \Omega \subset \mathbb{R}^3$. Again, this method is independent of the choice of the number of images comprising each image set. These class posterior densities are produced using the expectation maximization method described in [14,15]. Following [15,16], for each class c_j, the associated data likelihood, $p(\bar{I}_i(x)|c_j(x), \mu_j, \Sigma_j)$, is modeled as a normal distribution with mean, μ_j, and covariance, Σ_j. The class posteriors are computed using a new atlas developed at UNC's department of psychiatry for two year old children. This atlas is based on fourteen subjects using the same concepts as used in the construction of the Montreal Neurological Institute (MNI) International Consortium for Brain Mapping (ICBM) atlas [17].

In this paper, we focus on the construction of an exemplar template from a population of anatomical class posterior densities. We use the method developed in [18] which provides an unbiased technique for atlas construction using large deformation diffeomorphic registration.

3 Exemplar Templates

We consider the problem of estimating a template class posterior $\hat{p}$ that is the best representative for a population of N class posteriors, $\{p^i\}_{i=1}^N$, representing the N individual image sets $\{\bar{I}_i\}_{i=1}^N$. The template $\hat{p}$ is not a member of the $\{p^i\}$. To this end, we consider the problem of constructing a mapping between $\hat{p}$ and each class posterior in the set $\{p^i\}$. That is, we estimate the mappings $h_i : \Omega \to \Omega_i$ where $\Omega \subset \mathbb{R}^3$ and $\Omega_i \subset \mathbb{R}^3$ are the coordinate systems of the class posteriors $\hat{p}$ and p^i respectively. Again, Ω is independent of any of the population class posterior coordinate systems. This framework is depicted in Figure 1.

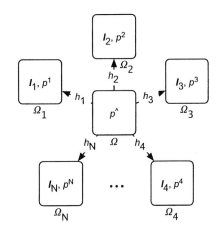

Fig. 1. Template Construction Framework

Following the template construction framework developed in [18] we seek the representative template class posterior $\hat{p}$ that requires the minimum amount of energy to deform into every population class posterior p^i. More precisely, given a transformation group $\mathcal{S}$ with associated metric $D : \mathcal{S}^2 \to \mathbb{R}$, along with a probability density dissimilarity measure $E(p, q)$, we wish to find the class posterior density $\hat{p}$ such that

$$\{\hat{h}_i, \hat{p}\} = \underset{h_i \in \mathcal{S}, p}{\operatorname{argmin}} \sum_{i=1}^N E(p^i \circ h_i, p) + D(e, h_i) \tag{1}$$

where e is the identity transformation.

In this paper we focus on the infinite dimensional group of diffeomorphisms $\mathcal{H}$ as described in [18]. We apply the theory of large deformation diffeomorphisms [9] to generate deformations h that are solutions to the Lagrangian ODEs $\frac{d}{dt}h(x,t) = v(h(x,t),t)$.

We induce a metric on the space of diffeomorphisms by using a Sobolev norm (a norm involving derivatives of a function) via a partial differential operator L on the velocity fields v. Let h be a diffeomorphism isotopic to the identity transformation e. We define the distance $D(e,h)$ as

$$D(e,h) = \min_v \int_0^1 \int_\Omega ||Lv(x,t)||^2 dx dt$$

subject to

$$h(x) = x + \int_0^1 v(h(x,t),t)dt.$$

The distance between any two diffeomorphisms is defined by

$$D(h_1,h_2) = D(e,h_1^{-1} \circ h_2).$$

The construction of h and h^{-1}, as well as the properties of D, are described in [18].

4 Large Deformation Class Posterior Template Construction

Having defined a metric on the space of diffeomorphisms, the minimum energy template estimation problem described in Equation 1 is formulated as

$$\{\hat{h}_i, \hat{p}\} = \operatorname*{argmin}_{h_i, p} \sum_{i=1}^N E(p^i \circ h_i, p) + \int_0^1 \int_\Omega ||Lv_i(x,t)||^2 dx t d$$

subject to

$$h_i(x) = x + \int_0^1 v_i(h_i(x,t),t)dt.$$

As a measure of dissimilarity between two probability density functions $p(x)$ and $q(x)$, at a spatial location x, we use the Kullback-Leibler divergence (relative entropy),

$$D_{KL}(p(x),q(x)) = \sum_{j=1}^C p_j(x) \log \frac{p_j(x)}{q_j(x)},$$

where C is the number of anatomical structure classes. From an information theoretic viewpoint [19], this dissimilarity can be interpreted as the inefficiency of assuming that an observation $q(x)$ is true when $p(x)$ is true. That is, we can use Kullback-Leibler divergence to measure how much the deformed class posteriors, $\{p^i(h_i(x))\}_{i=1}^N$, deviate from the atlas $p(x)$.

Under the Kullback-Leibler divergence measure the template estimation problem becomes

$$\hat{h}_i, \hat{p} = \underset{h_i, p}{\operatorname{argmin}} \sum_{i=1}^N \int_\Omega D_{KL}(p(x), p^i(h_i(x))) dx + \int_0^1 \int_\Omega ||Lv_i(x,t)||^2 dx dt. \quad (2)$$

This minimization problem can be simplified by noticing that for fixed transformations h_i, the $\hat{p}$ that minimizes Equation 2 is given by normalized geometric mean of the deformed class posteriors, $p^i(x)$,

$$\hat{p}_j(x) = \frac{\left(\prod_{i=1}^N p_j^i(h_i(x))\right)^{\frac{1}{N}}}{\sum_{k=1}^C \left(\prod_{i=1}^N p_k^i(h_i(x))\right)^{\frac{1}{N}}}. \quad (3)$$

Combining Equations 2 and 3 results in the following minimization problem

$$\hat{h}_i = \underset{h_i}{\operatorname{argmin}} \sum_{i=1}^N \int_\Omega D_{KL}(\hat{p}(x), p^i(h_i(x))) dx + \int_0^1 \int_\Omega ||Lv_i(x,t)||^2 dx dt. \quad (4)$$

Note that the solution to this minimization problem is independent of the ordering of the N image sets and increases linearly as image sets are added, thus, making the algorithm scalable.

5   Implementation

Following Christensen's algorithm for propagating templates described in [20], we approximate the solution to the minimization problem described in Equation 4 using an iteratively greedy method. At each iteration n, the updated transformation h_i^{n+1}, for each class posterior p^i, is computed using the update rule $h_i^{n+1} = h_i^n(x + \epsilon v_i^n(x))$. The fields h_i^n and v_i^n are the current estimated transformations and the velocity for the ith class posterior, and ϵ is the time step size. That is, each final transformation h_i is built form the composition of n transformations.

The velocity v_i^n for each iteration n is computed as follows. First, compute the updated template estimate (i.e. the normalized geometric mean)

$$\hat{p}_j^n(x) = \frac{\left(\prod_{i=1}^N p_j^i(h_i^n(x))\right)^{\frac{1}{N}}}{\sum_{k=1}^C \left(\prod_{i=1}^N p_k^i(h_i^n(x))\right)^{\frac{1}{N}}}$$

for each class component j. Next, following the second order approximation to

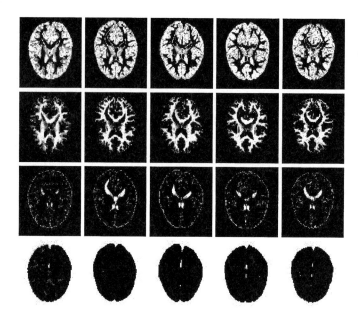

Fig. 2. Five class posteriors each with three classes and a background class. These images clearly show the large inter-subject variability, especially in the ventricular system.

Kullback-Leibler divergence described in [13] define the body force functions

$$F_i^n(x) = \sum_{k=1}^{C} \left[\frac{p_k^i(h_i(x))}{\hat{p}_k(x)} - 2 \right] \nabla p_k^i \Big|_{h_i(x)}^T .$$

This is the variation of the class posterior dissimilarity term in Equation 4 with respect to the transformation h_i. The velocity field v_i^n is computed at each iteration by applying the inverse of the differential operator L to the body force function, that is, $v_i^n(x) = L^{-1}F_i^n(x)$, where $L = \alpha\nabla^2 + \beta\nabla \cdot \nabla + \gamma$ is the Navier-Stokes operator. This computation is performed in the Fourier domain [21].

6   Results

To evaluate the performance of this method we applied the algorithm to a set of five class posterior densities that were derived from a population of T1-weighted, T2-weighted, and proton density 3D MR images of brains of health two year old children using an expectation maximization segmentation method [15,16]. As a preprocessing step, these images were aligned using affine registration. An axial slice from each derived class posterior density is shown in Figure 2. There is noticeable variation between these anatomies, especially in the ventricular region.

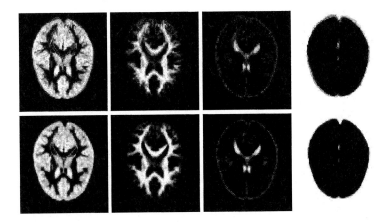

Fig. 3. Template Construction. The top row shows the normalized geometric mean class posterior density following an affine registration of all five subjects. The bottom row represents the estimated template after the final iteration of the algorithm.

Figure 3 shows the normalized geometric mean of the five class posterior densities following the affine registration and the final estimate of the template. The normalized geometric mean is blurry since it is an "average" of the varying individual neuroanatomies. Ghosting is evident around the lateral ventricles and near the boundary of the brain. In the final estimate of the template these variations have been accommodated by the high-dimensional registration.

Acknowledgments. The authors would like to thank Matthieu Jomier for producing the class posterior densities and Dr. Mark Foskey for insightful discussions. This work was supported by NIBIB-NIH grant R01 EB000219, DOD Prostate Cancer Research Program DAMD17-03-1-0134, NIMH grant MH064580 Longitudinal MRI Study of Brain Development in Fragile X, and the NDRC.

References

1. Miller, M., Banerjee, A., Christensen, G., Joshi, S., Khaneja, N., Grenander, U., Matejic, L.: Statistical methods in computational anatomy. Statistical Methods in Medical Research **6** (1997) 267–299
2. Grenander, U., Miller, M.: Computational anatomy: an emerging discipline. Quarterly of Applied Mathematics **56** (1998) 617–694
3. Thompson, P., Woods, R., Mega, M., Toga, A.: Mathmatical/computational challenges in creating deformable and probabilistic atlases of the human brain. Human Brain Mapping **9** (2000) 81–92
4. Hermosillo, G.: Variational Methods for Multimodal Image Matching. PhD thesis, Universite de Nice - Sophia Antipolis (2002)
5. D'Agostino, E., Maes, F., Vandermeulen, D., Suetens, P.: A viscous fluid model for multimodal non-rigid image registration using mutual information. Medical Image Analysis (MedIA) **7** (2003) 565–575

6. D'Agostino, E., Maes, F., Vandermeulen, D., Suetens, P.: An information theoretic approach for non-rigid image registration using voxel class probabilities. In: International Workshop on Biomedical Image Registration (WBIR). Volume 2717 of Lecture Notes in Computer Science (LNCS)., Springer-Verlag (2003) 122–131

7. Chan, H.M., Chung, A.C.S., Yu, S.C.H., Norbash, A., Wells W.M. III, Multi-modal image registration by minimizing Kullback-Leibler distance between expected and observed joint class histograms. Proceedings of the IEEE Computer Vision and Pattern Recognition (CVPR) **2** (2003) 570–576

8. Rueckert, D., Hayes, C., Studholme, C., Summers, P., Leach, M., Hawkes, D.J.: Non-rigid registration of breast mr images using mutual information. In: Proceedings of Medical Image Computing and Computer-Assisted Intervention (MICCAI). Lecture Notes in Computer Science (LNCS), Springer-Verlag (1998) 1144–1152

9. Miller, M.I., Joshi, S.C.: Large deformation fluid diffeomorphism for landmark and image matching. In: Brain Warping. Academic Press, San Diego (1999) 115–131

10. Gaens, T., Maes, F., Vandermeulen, D., Suetens, P.: Non-rigid multimodal image registration using mutual information. In: Proceedings of Medical Image Computing and Computer-Assisted Intervention (MICCAI). Lecture Notes in Computer Science (LNCS), Springer-Verlag (1998) 1099–1106

11. Studholme, C., Hill, D.L.G., Hawkes, D.J.: An overlap invariant entropy measure of 3d medical image alignment. Pattern Recognition (1998) 71–86

12. Bhatia, K.K., Hajnal, J.V., Puri, B.K., Edwards, A.D., Rueckert, D.: Consistent groupwise non-rigid registration for atlas construction. In: Proceedings of IEEE International Symposium on Biomedical Imaging (ISBI), IEEE (2004) 908–911

13. Lorenzen, P., Joshi, S.: High-dimensional multi-modal image registration. In: International Workshop on Biomedical Image Registration (WBIR). Volume 2717 of Lecture Notes in Computer Science (LNCS)., Springer-Verlag (2003) 234–243

14. Moon, N., van Leemput, K., Gerig, G.: Automatic brain and tumor segmentation. In: Medical Image Computing and Computer-Assisted Intervention (MICCAI). Volume 2489 of Lecture Notes in Computer Science (LNCS)., Tokyo, Springer-Verlag (2002) 372–379

15. van Leemput, K., Maes, F., Vandermeulen, D., Suetens, P.: Automated model-based tissue classification of mr images of the brain. IEEE Transactions on Medical Imaging (TMI) **18** (1999) 897–908

16. van Leemput, K., Maes, F., Vandermeulen, D., Suetens, P.: Automated model-based bias field correctionof mr images of the brain. IEEE Transactions on Medical Imaging (TMI) **18** (1999) 885–896

17. Cocosco, C., Kollokian, V., Kwan, R.S., Evans, A.: Brainweb: Online interface to a 3d mri simulated brain database. In: NeuroImage (Proceedings of 3-rd International Conference on Functional Mapping of the Human Brain). Volume 5., Copenhagen (1997) S425

18. Davis, B., Lorenzen, P., Joshi, S.: Large deformation minimum mean squared error template estimation for computation anatomy. In: Proceedings of IEEE International Symposium on Biomedical Imaging (ISBI), IEEE (2004) 173–176

19. Cover, T., Thomas, J.: Elements of Information Theory. John Wiley & Sons, Inc., New York (1991)

20. Christensen, G., Rabbit, R., Miller, M.: Deformable templates using large deformation kinematics. Transactions on Image Processing **5(10)** (1996) 1435–1447

21. Joshi, S., Lorenzen, P., Gerig, G., Bullitt, E.: Structural and radiometric asymmetry in brain images. Medical Image Analysis (MedIA) **7** (2003) 155–170

Dual Front Evolution Model and Its Application in Medical Imaging

Hua Li[1,2*], Abderr Elmoataz[3], Jalal Fadili[1], and Su Ruan[4]

[1] GREYC-ENSICAEN, CNRS UMR 6072, 6 Bd. Maréchal Juin, 14050 Caen, France
[2] Dept. of Elec. & Infor. Eng., Huazhong Univ. of Sci. & Tech., Wuhan, P.R.China
[3] LUSAC, Site Universitaire, BP78, 50130 Cherbourg-Octeville, France
[4] Equipe Image, L.A.M.(EA2075), IUT de Troyes, 10026 Troyes, France
{hua.li,abderr.elmoataz,j.fadili,su.ruan}@greyc.ismra.fr

Abstract. This paper presents a curve evolution model for 3D slice-by-slice image segmentation and its application in medical imaging. It is an iterative process based on the dual front evolution and the morphological dilatation to iteratively deform the initial contour towards the segmentation result. The dual front evolution model is proposed to form the new boundary by the contact position of two (or more) curves evolving in opposite directions. The fast sweeping evolution scheme is introduced for the contour evolution and the velocities for the propagation of the different curves are defined in accordance with the region-based characteristics. This model can achieve the global energy minimum and solves the disadvantages of classical level set evolution methods. Experimental results are given to illustrate the robustness of the method and its performance in precise region boundary localization and medical imaging.

1 Introduction

In computer vision literatures, various methods dealing with object segmentation and feature extraction are discussed [1]. Among them, active contour models [2] have emerged as a powerful tool for semi-automatic object segmentation. In recent years, many approaches have been proposed to improve the robustness and stability of active contour models [3].

Based on the Mumford-Shah minimal partition functional [4], Chan and Vese [5] proposed a new active contour model without a stopping edge-function to detect objects whose boundary are not necessarily defined by a gradient. The authors formulated this functional in terms of the level set formalism. Later, they generalized this process to treat multiple regions, and applied it to medical imaging [6]. The similar works were also proposed by Yezzi and Tsai [7,8]. Furthermore, under suitable assumptions, Chan and Vese's model [5] simply reduces to the k-means algorithm with a nonlinear diffusion preprocessing step. Then, Gibou and Fedkiw developed a hybrid numerical technique [9] that draws on

---

* This research work is financial supported by GRAVIR (Groupe Régional d'Action pour la Valorisation Industrielle de la Recherche) of Basse-Normandie, France.

C. Barillot, D.R. Haynor, and P. Hellier (Eds.): MICCAI 2004, LNCS 3216, pp. 103–110, 2004.

the speed and simplicity of k-means procedures and the robustness of level set algorithms. In [10], Xu proposed a graph cuts-based active contours approach, which combines active contour model and the optimization tool of graph cuts, for object segmentation. In his method, the graph-cuts optimization is used to iteratively deform the contour to achieve the segmentation result.

All the above interesting active contour models are implemented based on level set method [11]. However, the level set method has the disadvantage of a heavy computation requirement even using the narrow band evolution. The fast marching method [12] is extremely faster than level set evolution. But within this method, the front only can move strictly positive or negative, it often exceeds the true boundary.

Recently, some improved fast marching methods were proposed for image segmentation. Cohen [13] proposed a global minimal path approach, based on fast marching method, for their active contour models. It is a global energy minimization method with complexity $O(NlogN)$, where N is the number of grids. Another interesting region-growing approach was the multi-label fast marching evolution proposed by Sifakis [14] for motion analysis in video processing. An automatic stopping criterion was guaranteed due to the multiple contours marching towards the boundaries from opposite sides. Deschamps [15] also proposed an improved fast marching method in his dissertation. In these methods, the speed functions are derived from the local image information (not just gradients). The use of region's statistical information to differentiate the different front speeds has a bigger potential than the traditional speed function, which is only decided by the edge function.

In this paper, a dual front evolution model is proposed to iteratively drive the initial contour towards the segmentation result, and the fast sweeping evolution scheme is introduced in its evolution. Furthermore, the velocities for the propagation of the different contours are defined according to the region-based characteristics. A 2D slice-by-slice process for segmenting 3D image is also introduced. Our approach is simple and fast with complexity $O(N)$, in which N is the number of grid points. It can easily extract the close and smooth boundary of the desired object. It is efficient and reliable, and requires very limited user intervention. Experimental results are given to illustrate the robustness of the method against noise and its performance in precise region boundary localization and medical imaging.

2   Description of Dual Front Evolution Model

Within the minimal path theory proposed by Cohen and coauthors [13], the surface of minimal action $U_0(p)$ is defined as the minimal energy integrated along a path between a starting point p_0 and any point p, and is shown in the following Equation (1):

$$U_0(p) = \inf_{A_{p_0,p}} \{ \int_\Omega \widetilde{P}(L(s))ds \} = \inf_{A_{p_0,p}} \{E(L)\} \tag{1}$$

Where $A_{p_0,p}$ is the set of all paths between p_0 and p. $L(s)$ represents a curve on a 2D image. Ω is its domain of definition. $E(L)$ represents the energy along the curve L, and $\widetilde{P}$ is the integral potential. Given the minimal action surface U_0 to p_0 and U_1 to p_1, the minimal geodesic between p_0 and p_1 is exactly the set of points p_g that satisfy

$$U_0(p_g) + U_1(p_g) = \inf_p \{U_0(p) + U_1(p)\} \tag{2}$$

The minimal path between p_0 and any point p in the image can be easily deduced from the action map U by solving the following Eikonal Equation (3):

$$|\nabla U| = \widetilde{P} \qquad \text{with} \qquad U(p_0) = 0 \tag{3}$$

Now, considering all the points satisfying $U_0(p) = U_1(p)$ and the above Equation (2), at these points, the front starting from p_0 to compute U_0 first meets the front starting from p_1 to compute U_1 and the propagation stops. These points are the global minimum energy points between point p_0 and p_1. Without loss of generality, Let X be a set of continuous points in the image, U_X is the minimal action with potential $\widetilde{P}$ and starting points $\{p, p \in X\}$. Clearly, $U_X = min_{p \in X} U_p$. Considering all the points satisfying $U_{X_i}(p) = U_{X_j}(p)$ and $U_{X_i}(p_g) + U_{X_j}(p_g) = \inf_p \{U_{X_i}(p) + U_{X_j}(p)\}$, these points are the global minimum energy points in the region enclosed by X_i and X_j.

Therefore, we proposed the dual front evolution model to extract the region's boundary by finding all the points where different minimal actions U are equal to any others. The besic concept of this model was introduced in [16]. In this paper, a futher detailed algorithm description is shown in Appendix. In this algorithm, the size of the narrow band can be specified by the user for a given segmentation, or a class of images. We use the morphological dilatation operator to obtain the narrow band because the iteration step size can be controlled easily by adjusting the size of the structure element and the dilatation times.

The front evolution scheme in our dual front evolution method is an extension of fast sweeping method because of its low complexity. The fast sweeping method [17] was presented by Zhao for computing the numerical solution of Eikonal equations on a rectangular grid. and gives the same result as the fast marching method but with lower complexity $O(N)$. Since the low computational cost of the fast sweeping method is maintained, the complexity of our dual front evolution method is still $O(N)$, where N is the number of grid points.

3   3D Image Segmentation Approach

For segmenting the 3D image, we proposed a 2D slice-by-slice process [18]. In this paper, we tested more synthetic images and 3D medical images to prove the validity of this 3D algorithm. The segmentation process includes two steps: the boundary mapping between the connective slices and the 2D boundary tracking. The flowchart in Figure 1 shows the sequence of all steps we undertake to obtain the segmentation result of 3D medical image.

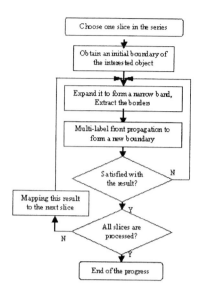

Fig. 1. Flowchart depicting the sequence of steps to segment 3D image

In medical image series, the statistics information of the corresponding regions generally change very slowly from one slice to the next, which means that the segmented region's statistics information in one slice is a good estimate of the corresponding region in the next consecutive un-segmented slice. This information is very helpful to guide the boundary tracking process. Here, we calculate the mean values u_{in}, u_{out} and the variances σ_{in}, σ_{out} of the regions inside and outside the segmented boundary in the previous slice. In the boundary tracking process of the current slice, let l_{in} and l_{out} be the labels of the inner and outer borders of the dilated narrow band from the mapped boundary. The propagation speeds for the labeled points (x, y) are decided by the following Equations:

$$
\begin{cases}
F_{in}(x, y) = \exp(\frac{|\overline{I}(x,y)-u_{in}|^2}{2\sigma_{in}^2}) + f(\nabla I(x, y)) & \text{if } L(x, y) = l_{in} \\
F_{out}(x, y) = \exp(\frac{|\overline{I}(x,y)-u_{out}|^2}{2\sigma_{out}^2}) + f(\nabla I(x, y)) & \text{if } L(x, y) = l_{out}
\end{cases}
\tag{4}
$$

$$
f(\nabla I(x, y)) = \frac{1}{1 + \alpha|\nabla I(x, y)|}
\tag{5}
$$

where $\overline{I}(x, y)$ is the average value of the image intensity in a window of size 3×3 centered at the examined point. $|\nabla I(x, y)|$ is the image local gradient, and α is a constant.

In this 2D slice-by-slice segmentation process, the mapped boundary from the previous slice provides a good initialization of the boundary tracking process in current slice. In the boundary tracking process, the result of every dual front evolution step provides the initialization for the next dual front evolution. The speed function decided by the region's statistical information together with the

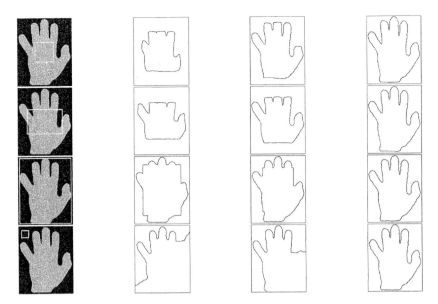

Fig. 2. The segmentation result on a hand image with different initialization

gradient information ensures an appreciate evolution. The dual front evolution method ensures an automatic evolution stopping criterion for every front propagation. The boundary tracking process stops automatically when the change between the current formed boundary and that of the previous iteration is lower than a pre-specified threshold. The total complexity of our 3D image segmentation approach is $O(M \times N)$, in which M is the number of 2D slices and N is the number of pixels in one slice.

4   Experimental Results

One very attractive feature associated with our method is that it automatically proceeds in the correct direction without relying upon additional inflationary terms commonly employed by many active contour algorithms. We illustrate this in Figure 2 with a noisy synthetic image of a hand. An initial contour completely contained within the interested object will flow outward towards the boundary (shown in the first row). An initial contour partially inside and partially outside the interested object will flow in both directions towards the boundary (shown in the second row). An initial contour encircling the interested object will flow inward towards the boundary (shown in the third row). And finally, an initial contour situated outside the interested object will flow outward towards and wrap around the boundary (shown in the last row). In Figure 2, the first column shows the initializing contour with the original image. The second and the third column show two intermediate steps of the algorithm. The last column shows the final segmentation curve.

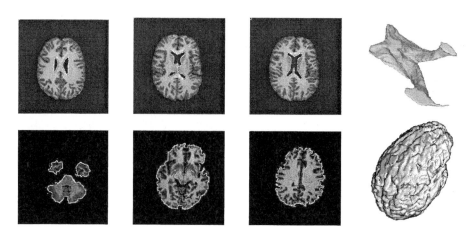

Fig. 3. The segmentation result on 3D MRI brain data

In [7], the authors also test their method on a similar hand image, but when the initial contour was outside the object, in addition to the curves that outline the boundary of the hand, there exist extraneous curves around the four corners of the image which do not correspond to image edges. This is due to the fact that their algorithm was trapped in a local minimum—a common problem faced by all algorithms which rely on gradient descent methods for minimization. However, in our experimental results on the similar image with similar initial contour, there are no extraneous curves around the corners of the image which do not correspond to image edges.

We tested our approach on two 3D medical images based on the approach described in Section 3. In the first row of Figure 3, the first three panels are the segmentation results on three different slices. The last panel is the 3D surface modeling of the segmented ventricle. In the second row of Figure 3, the first three panels are the segmentation results on three different slices. The last panel is the 3D surface modeling of the segmented brain. The segmentation results show the validaty of our method.

5   Conclusions

In this paper, a novel level set-based framework for image segmentation is presented. The dual front evolution model has been introduced to iteratively deform the initial contour towards the segmentation result and the fast sweeping scheme is introduced for the contour evolution. Our approach can detect contours with or without gradients, and provide a more global result by avoiding the disadvantage of local minima of many active contour models. Several segmentation results illustrate that this new framework is a fast, precise technique for un-supervised segmentation or labeling.

In this paper, we have demonstrated the feasibility of incorporating region information into the evolution equations for the dual front evolution model. Moreover, future extensions of our work can be focused on the combined use of several pattern features, such as texture, gradient vector value, and color information. This can be performed using the same general framework by incorporating these distinct features into the velocity field definition. However, much more work is needed in order to test on large data sets and to improve the current algorithm.

Finally, we would like to mention that this segmentation framework using the dual front evolution model has potential applications in other image analysis domains. Examples include object tracking problems in video sequences and so on.

References

1. Munoz, X., et al.: Strategies for image segmentation combining region and boundary informa-tion. Pattern Recognition Letters **24** (2003) 375–392
2. Kass, M., Witkin, A., Terzopoulos, D.: Snakes: Active contour models. International Journal of Computer Vision **1** (1988) 321–332
3. Suri, J., Liu, K., et al.: Shape recovery algorithms using level sets in 2D/3D medical imagery: A state of the art review. IEEE Trans. on Infor. Tech. in Biomedicine **6** (2002) 8–28
4. Mumford, D., Shah, J.: Optimal approximation by piecewise smooth functions and associated variational problems. Commun. Pure Appl. Math. **42** (1989) 577–685
5. Chan, T., Vese, L.: Active contours without edges. IEEE Trans. on Image Processing **10** (2001) 266–277
6. Chan, T., Vese, L.: A multiphase level set framework for image segmentation using the mumford and shah model. International Journal of Computer Vision **50** (2002) 271–293
7. Tsai, A., Yezzi, A., Willsky, A.: Curve evolution implementation of the mumford-shah functional for image segmentation, denoising, interpolation, and magnification. IEEE Trans. on Image Processing **10** (2001) 1169–1186
8. Yezzi, A., Tsai, A., Willsky, A.: A fully global approach to image segmentation via coupled curve evolution equations. Journal of Visual Communication and Image Representation **13** (2002) 195–216
9. Gibou, F., Fedkiw, R.: A fast hybrid k-means level set algorithm for segmentation. International Journal of Computer Vision (2003)
10. Xu, N., Bansal, R., Ahuja, N.: Object segmentation using graph cuts based active contours. In: Proceedings of IEEE International Conference on Computer Vision and Pattern Recognition(CVPR). Volume 2. (2003) 46–53
11. Osher, S., Sethian, J.: Fronts propagating with curvature dependent speed: algorithms based on the Hamilton-Jacobi formulation. Journal of Computational Physics **79** (1988) 12–49
12. Sethian, J.: Fast marching methods. SIAM Review **41** (1999)
13. Cohen, L., Kimmel, R.: Global minimum for active contour models: A minimal path ap-proach. In: IEEE International Conference on CVPR (CVPR'96). (1996)
14. Sifakis, E., Tziritas, G.: Moving object localization using a multi-label fast marching algorithm. Signal Processing: Image Communication **16** (2001) 963–976
15. Deschamps, T.: Curve and Shape Extraction with Minimal Path and Level-Sets Techniques:Applications to 3D Medical Imaging. PhD thesis, UNIVERSITE de PARIS-DAUPHINE (2001)

16. Li, H., Elmoataz, A., Fadili, J., Ruan, S.: A multi-label front propagation approach for object segmentation. In: International Conference of Pattern Recognition (ICPR2004), Combridge, UK (2004)
17. Zhao, H.: Fast sweeping method for Eikonal equation I: Distance function. http://www.math.uci.edu/ zhao (2002)
18. Li, H., Elmoataz, A., Fadili, J., Ruan, S.: 3D medical image segmentation approach based on multi-label front propagation. In: International Conference of Image Processing(ICIP2004), Singapore (2004)

Appendix:
The Description of the Dual Front Evolution Scheme

Initialization:
Label map L: The initial separating contours are $B_1, \ldots, B_k$, labeling $B_i (1 \leq i \leq k)$ as a label l_i, other rest points are labeled as -1.
Action map U: For any point p of the initial contours, set $U(p) = 0$; for other points, set $U(p) = \infty$.

Input:
Original image A need to be segmented, the size of A is $I \times J$
Initial Label map L
Initial Action map U

Marching Forward Loop:
For each point $x(i, j)$ in image A, calculating its new label and new action value by the ordering $i = 1 \to I$, $j = 1 \to J$ as following:
- The new label of x is the label of the point having the smallest U value among point x and its 4-connexity neighbors.

$$x_{min} = \{x | u(x) = min(u_{i,j}, u_{i-1,j}, u_{i+1,j}, u_{i,j-1}, u_{i,j+1}\} \qquad l_{i,j}^{new} = l(x_{min})$$

- The new speed of point x for Eikonal equation $|\nabla u(x)| = P(l(x))$ is:

$$h_{i,j}^{new} = P(l_{i,j}^{new})$$

- Finding the two minimum U in the 4-connexity neighbors of point x:

$$a = u_{x_{min}} = min(u_{i-1,j}, u_{i+1,j}) \qquad b = u_{y_{min}} = min(u_{i,j-1}, u_{i,j+1})$$

- Calculating the new U from the current value of its 4-connexity neighbors:

$$\overline{u}_{i,j} = \begin{cases} min(a, b) + h_{i,j}^{new} & \text{if } |a - b| \geq h_{i,j}^{new} \\ a + b + \frac{\sqrt{2(h_{i,j}^{new})^2 - (a-b)^2}}{2} & \text{if } |a - b| \leq h_{i,j}^{new} \end{cases}$$

- Updating $u_{i,j}$ to be the smaller one of $\overline{u}_{i,j}$ and its current value:

$$u_{i,j}^{new} = min(u_{i,j}, \overline{u})$$

Repeat the above computation for calculating the new label and new distance value of all the points in image A by the alternating ordering according the following alternating order $i = I \to 1$, $j = 1 \to J$; $i = I \to 1$, $j = J \to 1$; $i = 1 \to I$, $j = J \to 1$; $i = 1 \to I$, $j = 1 \to J$.

Output:
The label map L represents the final segmentation into k regions R_k.

Topology Smoothing for Segmentation and Surface Reconstruction

Pierre-Louis Bazin and Dzung L. Pham

Johns Hopkins University, Baltimore, USA,
pbazin1@jhmi.edu,
http://medic.rad.jhmi.edu/

Abstract. We propose a new method for removing topological defects in surfaces and volumes segmented from medical images. Unlike current topology correction approaches, we define a smoothing operator that acts solely on the image volume and can be integrated into segmentation procedures. The method is based on an analysis of the scalar field underlying the isosurface of interest, and performs only local changes. No assumptions are required on the structure to segment, or on the desired topology. We show that segmentation algorithms that incorporate toplogical smoothing produce results with fewer topological defects.

1   Introduction

Topological considerations are a central element in the problem of reconstructing the geometric surface of an anatomic tissue from medical images. Most of these objects have a very simple topology, usually the topology of a sphere. For instance, cortical surfaces despite their intricate geometry, are typically assumed to be topologically spherical. However, surfaces obtained from unconstrained image segmentation are generally not consistent with the anatomical topology: isosurfaces extracted from the segmented volumes often produce large numbers of topological handles due to small errors in the original segmentation.

Mainly for the purpose of cortical reconstruction, recent works have addressed the problem of correcting the defects on the volume or the surface obtained [13,4,12] until spherical topology is reached. These methods act on geometric information alone by placing cuts and filling holes in the surface (or a binary representation of the surface) with little regard to whether this is reflected in the actual data. Alternatively, other strategies start from a topologically correct surface model and then deform it with topology-preserving transformations to perform the segmentation [8,15]. The main drawback of this approach is that finding an initial surface close enough to converge to the desired object becomes a problem with complex geometric shapes.

In this paper, we propose a "topology smoothing" algorithm that locally regularizes surface topology. The technique removes small topological defects while keeping major structures unchanged. No requirements are made on the surface to start from, or on the correct topology to obtain. We also show how the algorithm can be incorporated into a tissue classficiation algorithm to improve the topological consistency of segmentation results. Because it does not impose a hard constraint on the segmentation, it allows deviations from topological regularity where it is deemed appropriate. If a hard topological

C. Barillot, D.R. Haynor, and P. Hellier (Eds.): MICCAI 2004, LNCS 3216, pp. 111–118, 2004.
© Springer-Verlag Berlin Heidelberg 2004

constraint is desired, then the previously described topology correction approaches [13, 4,12] can still be used. Because the topology has already been regularized, fewer cuts and merges will be required.

This paper is organized as follows. We first analyze the link between image segmentation and surface topology, and design a smoothing algorithm from the analysis (Sec.2). That algorithm is then integrated into any tissue classification technique based on fuzzy clustering (Sec.3). It is validated on cortical segmentation and reconstruction examples (Sec.3.3).

2 Smoothing the Topology of Scalar Fields

2.1 Duality Between Scalar Fields and Surfaces

The topology of surfaces is characterized globally by its Euler Number. This measure, however, does not account for the type or extent of local topology changes. Let us consider a surface as the zero level set of a 3D scalar field (for instance, the field of distances to the surface). The surface is in turn recovered from the field as an isosurface (using marching cubes [7,9]). It follows that the surface and the scalar field are two complementary descriptions.

We should expect changes in the surface topology to reflect changes in the field, and vice versa. Indeed, if random noise is added to the scalar field, many small-scale topology changes will occur in the surface. This is the main problem of surface reconstruction from medical images, where some of the noise is propagated into the segmentation, and introduces many topological defects. Smoothing the field smooths the geometry of the associated surface, and should also "smooth" its topology, i.e. remove those topology defects.

2.2 Critical Points and Topological Variations

In scalar fields, topology changes occur only at critical points [6,14]. These points are locally the singular points of the implicit isosurfaces, an extension of the non-simple points of binary images[1,3,5]. They have been classified in [14] as *regular, flat, minimal, maximal* and *saddle* points, either *local* or *extended*. At any non-regular point, or non-regular region made of extended non-regular points, topology changes for the isosurface can occur when the isovalue used to construct the surface is equal to the value at that point.

If a field has many non-regular points, its topology is likely to be complicated, and to change drastically if the isovalue is modified. It results in a "topological noise", as the topology of the isosurface is unstable for small changes in the isovalue. Following this idea, a field with mostly regular points will be "topologically smooth", i.e. its topology will change only at a small number of isovalues. It is our goal here to produce such smooth topologies: segmented tissues should have a regular topology, wherever the segmentation threshold is.

2.3   Classification of Topological Types

To identify critical points, let us consider a point X with value $f(X)$. We define as *positive*, *negative* and *equal* neighbors the points Y in a neighborhood of X with respectively $f(Y) > f(X)$, $f(Y) < f(X)$ and $f(Y) = f(X)$. With an appropriate neighborhood, the number of positive, negative and equal regions determines the type of the point. We will refer to this type as the *topological type* of the point[1]. Appropriate neighborhoods here are the smallest possible regions around X with connected neighbors Y [14]. In a discrete field, it is the 6, 18 or 26 neighbors of a voxel in a cubic 3D volume, with the connectivity rules usual to volume or surface extraction from digital images[13,5] (however, the connectivity rules don't affect much the smoothing presented here).

Table 1. Topological types and neighbors: N_p, N_n, N_e are the numbers of positive, negative and equal regions in the neighborhood of X, $\langle \cdot \rangle$, $\langle \cdot \rangle^+$, $\langle \cdot \rangle^-$ are the mean values over the complete neighborhood, the positive regions or the negative regions, respectively.

Topological type	Minimum	Maximum	Regular	Saddle	Flat
Conditions	$N_p = 1,$ $N_n = 0$	$N_p = 0,$ $N_n = 1$	$N_p = 1,$ $N_n = 1$ Local: $N_e = 0$, Extended: $N_e > 0$	$N_p > 1$ or $N_n > 1$	$N_p = 0,$ $N_n = 0$
Topological neighbor $f^T(X)$	$\langle f(Y) \rangle^+$	$\langle f(Y) \rangle^-$	$\langle f(Y) \rangle$	$\langle f(Y) \rangle^+_{(\text{join})}$ $\langle f(Y) \rangle^-_{(\text{split})}$	$f(X)$

Table 1 lists all the possible types, both in 2D and 3D, and the necessary conditions to discriminate between them. This classification is sufficient to detect all topological changes [14]: surfaces appearing and disappearing at maxima and minima, and joining at saddles. The topological type of points will change if and only if its value goes above or below the closest values of its neighbors. Depending on the topological type, we define *topological neighbor* $f^T(X)$ for the value of X, as listed in Table 1.

For a minimum, a maximum or a saddle point, replacing $f(X)$ with the topological neighbor will force its topological type to change. Saddle points can be affected in two ways: either we lower the value to its negative neighbors value, or raise it to its positive neighbors value. For the underlying surface, it corresponds to "split" or "join" operations. Both choices are valid, so we have to select the most appropriate (usually, the closest value). Flat points are just kept unchanged. Regular points are those we want to reinforce. If a point is regular but close to its above or below neighbors, it will change its topological type with a small perturbation. So to ameliorate the regularity of the point, we place it at a central value.

---

[1] Rigorously, it is the geometric type of the field itself seen as an hyper-surface; we abuse of the topology term to avoid confusing the geometries of the isosurface of interest and of the associated field.

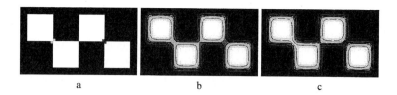

Fig. 1. Effects of smoothing: a) original field image, b) result of geometric smoothing, c) result of topological smoothing. The original image is an artificial field for an isocontour halfway between black (0) and white (1). The 0.25, 0.5 and 0.75 isocontours are displayed for b) and c), with decreasing thickness. Topological smoothing differs from geometric smoothing on saddle regions: likely junctions (left) or cuts (right) are strengthened, undetermined regions are not affected (middle).

2.4   The Topology Smoothing Algorithm

If we replace the original values of the scalar field with the topological neighbors, we are not guaranteed to reach a simpler topology. Due to the change of neighbors, some regular points become critical: we then have to iterate the operation to reach a stable regularity. We perform the following relaxation:

$$f(X) \leftarrow f(X) + \mu \frac{w_0[f_0(X) - f(X)] + w_T[f^T(X) - f(X)]}{w_0 + w_T}$$

where $f_0(X)$ is the original value of the scalar field, w_0 and w_T the relative weights of the original and the topological value, and μ the update parameter. w_0, w_T, μ are all in $[0, 1]$. This algorithm minimizes the following energy function:

$$E = \sum_X \left(w_0 \| f(X) - f_0(X) \|^2 + w_T \| f(X) - f^T(X) \| \right).$$

We have to keep in mind that $f^T(X)$ varies whenever $f(X)$ reaches a new topological type: this is why we have to compute an iterative solution rather than a direct solution, that would not account for topology transitions. A low update factor ($\mu = 0.5$ is enough) will also reduce oscillations due to simultaneous topological changes of several neighboring points.

Example: Geometric vs. Topological Smoothing. The algorithm can be used on any scalar field, but only makes sense for fields associated to an isosurface (in 3D) or an isocontour (in 2D). The toy example of Fig. 1 illustrates the effects of topological smoothing on critical points. Compared to traditional geometric smoothing (i.e. using the average value of the neighborhood instead of $f^T(X)$; anisotropic or robust smoothing are not considered here for simplicity), topologic smoothing will increase the junctions or the cuts at saddles, depending on initial conditions.

Fig.2 presents a more relevant comparison: a membership function representing gray matter obtained from the segmentation of a noisy 2D phantom is processed with the topological and geometric smoothing algorithms. Geometric smoothing has been previously observed to simplify the topology of extracted isosurfaces[16]. Our analysis confirms

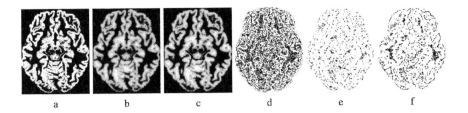

Fig. 2. Example on a a segmented phantom: a) original segmented gray matter, b) geometric smoothing, c) topological smoothing. d,e,f) display the critical (black) and extended critical (gray) points for the three images.

that observation: averaging the field over its neighbors are likely to reinforce regular points and remove critical points. However, geometric smoothing makes no distinction between small topological changes (removing the noise) and large ones (affecting the ideal object topology). Topological smoothing will transform the image in a more hierarchical way, preserving and compacting the main topology information, while removing noise-related critical points. The amount of corrected topology is driven by the smoothing factor w_T; even large critical regions will disappear with repeated iterations, if the factor w_T is high enough.

3   Topology Smoothing in Tissue Classification

In this section, we show how topological regularization can be incorporated into a segmentation algorithm. Tissue classification techniques often produce on membership or probability functions that represent the likelihood each pixel of the image belongs to a particular tissue class. This function can then used to build an isosurface, e.g. taking the 0.5 isovalue. Topological regularization of this function will therefore improve the topological properties of surfaces derived from the function.

3.1   Topology-Smoothing Segmentation

We use a Robust Fuzzy C-means (RFCM) algorithm [11] as the basis for tissue classification. This algorithm imposes a spatial penalty on the standard fuzzy C-means algorithm to improve robustness to noise. The following embedding of topological smoothing applies similarly to expectation-maximization algorithms that perform Gaussian clustering [10]. We integrate the smoothing as an additional step in RFCM:

1. compute the RFCM membership functions $u_{j,k}$:

$$u_{j,k} = \frac{\left(\|y_j - v_k\|^2 + \beta \sum_{l \in N_j} \sum_{m \neq k} u_{l,m}^{*q} \right)^{1/q-1}}{\sum_k \left(\|y_j - v_k\|^2 + \beta \sum_{l \in N_j} \sum_{m \neq k} u_{l,m}^{*q} \right)^{1/q-1}},$$

2. relax the membership functions $u^*_{j,k}$ toward the topological neighbors $u^T_{j,k}$:

$$u^*_{j,k} = u^*_{j,k} + \mu \frac{w_0[u_{j,k} - u^*_{j,k}] + w_T[u^T_{j,k} - u^*_{j,k}]}{w_0 + w_T}$$

3. compute the RFCM class mean values $v_k = \frac{\sum_j u^{*q}_{j,k} y_j}{\sum_j u^{*q}_{j,k}}$.

The membership functions are the topologically smoothed $u^*_{j,k}$, but the algorithm is still very similar to the original RFCM algorithm (steps 1 and 3 only). The convergence of the topological smoothing is fast, usually around 20 iterations. The smoothing step only adds one tuning parameter to the algorithm, w_T (we set $\mu = 0.5$, $w_0 = 1$ in all cases). Its usual scope is from 0.1 to 1.

A constraint of segmentation algorithms (FCM or EM-based) is that the membership functions all add to one. When the smoothing is introduced, that property is verified if and only if $\sum_k u^T_{j,k} = 1$. To meet this constraint, the values $u^T_{j,k}$ are reprojected using $u^T_{j,k} = u^T_{j,k} / \sum_k u^T_{j,k}$. In practice the projection is small, and no significant change has been observed in the result.

3.2   Over-Smoothing Correction

An issue that must be addresssed with topological smoothing is the flattening of membership values over small regions. As the smoothing computes a mean of the region, it will lower maxima on thin, elongated regions and spread boundaries between low and high regions. To counteract this effect, we enforce changes only at topologically relevant regions. We used the following property: as long as the corrected value $u^c_{j,k}$ stays between the closest inferior and superior values $u^{inf}_{j,k}$, $u^{sup}_{j,k}$ of $u^*_{j,k}$, the topological type of the point is preserved. We apply the following correction:

$$u^c_{j,k} = \min[\max[(u^*_{j,k} + w_c u_{j,k})/(1 + w_c), u^{inf}_{j,k}], u^{sup}_{j,k}]$$

This correction step will guarantee that the smoothed field has values as close to the original data as possible, but with a simplified topology. The parameter w_c is not critical, and is set in practice to 0.25. We also considered using a robust weighted mean for computing $u^T_{j,k}$ as an alternative, with similar results.

3.3   Experimental Evaluation

The algorithm has been validated on a simulated MR image from the Brainweb database [2], with 3% and 5% noise. The segmentation was performed using the FCM, RFCM, topology-smoothing RFCM (T-RFCM), topology-smoothing with correction (TC-RFCM) algorithms, both with $w_T = 1$. The RFCM parameter has been set to near optimal values, from [11].

We report in Table 2 the misclassification rate (ratio of misclassified pixels over the volume), the RMS error on the membership functions, the ratio of critical points in the volume, the number of handles detected in a connectivity graph (from [13]) for the segmented volume of white matter, and the Euler number of the extracted surface.

Table 2. Error measures and Topological numbers from Simulated MR results

	FCM		RFCM		T-RFCM		TC-RFCM	
noise	3 %	5 %	3 %	5 %	3 %	5 %	3 %	5 %
Misclassification rate (%)	3.988	6.587	3.755	4.947	4.483	5.654	4.057	5.230
Average RMS error	0.131	0.173	0.119	0.139	0.136	0.156	0.126	0.147
Critical points (%)	60.63	63.84	49.96	48.74	33.31	34.62	36.34	37.61
Detected handles	286	956	129	90	76	48	74	65
Euler number	-950	-2750	-408	-290	-268	-184	-304	-240

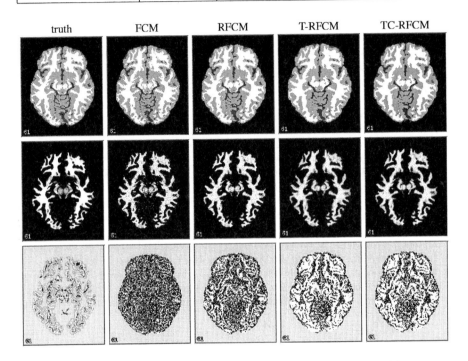

truth   FCM   RFCM   T-RFCM   TC-RFCM

Fig. 3. Results on the simulated MR image with 5% noise, for the different algorithms: segmentation (top), white matter membership (middle) and corresponding critical points (bottom).

The results show that the topology smoothing is efficient, removing about a third of the critical points and half of the handles. With the correction step, the segmentation errors remain very close to those of RFCM, and are comparable if not better to those of FCM. The membership functions are very similar to RFCM memberships (see Fig.3), free of noise, slightly smoother. The number of critical points is greatly reduced, and they are moved away from the boundaries. The topology is simplified (less handles) and even stabilized (fewer variations with different isovalues) from the smoothing. A posterior correction to reach spherical topology will need to impose fewer modifications of the segmentation, improving accuracy.

4   Discussion

Although many image processing algorithms employ regularization or smoothing to improve robustness to noise, they do not consider how the the topology of the data is affected. We have proposed a smoothing algorithm that directly addresses the topology of scalar fields, and have embedded it into a standard segmentation technique. It makes no assumption on the nature of the object, uses all the information from the image, and avoids hard constraints. Experiments for cortical reconstruction have demonstrated that it imposes minor changes in the overall segmentation, while effectively removing many topology defects. Although our embedding within the segmentation algorithm is currently suboptimal, it should be possible to incorporate topological regularity as a penalty or prior probability function more formally into the optimization.

References

1. G. Bertrand. Simple points, topological numbers and geodesic neighborhood in cubic grids. *Pattern Recognition Letters*, 15(10):1003–1011, 1994.
2. D. L. Collins, *et al.* Design and construction of a realistic digital brain phantom. *IEEE Trans. Med. Img.*, 17(3), 1998.
3. M. Couprie, F. Bezerra, and G. Bertrand. Topological operators for grayscale image processing. *J. Electronic Imaging*, 10(4):1003–1015, 2001.
4. X. Han, C. Xu, U. Braga-Neto, and J. L. Prince. Topology correction in brain cortex segmentation using a multiscale, graph-based algorithm. *IEEE Trans. Med. Img.*, 21(2):109–121, 2002.
5. X. Han, C. Xu, and J. L. Prince. A topology preserving level set method for geometric deformable models. *IEEE Trans. Pat. Analysis and Mach. Intelligence*, 25(6):755–768, 2003.
6. J. C. Hart. Morse theory for implicit surface modeling. In H.-C. Hege and K. Polthier, editors, *Mathematical Visualization*, pp 257–268. Springer-Verlag, Oct. 1998.
7. W. E. Lorensen and H. E. Cline. Marching cubes: A high resolution 3d surface construction algorithm. In *Proc. SIGGRAPH'87*, volume 21, pp 163–169, 1987.
8. J.-F. Mangin, V. Frouin, I. Bloch, J. Regis, and J. Lopez-Krahe. From 3d magnetic resonance images to structural representations of the cortex topography using topology preserving deformations. *J. Mathematical Imaging and Vision*, 5:297–318, 1995.
9. G. M. Nielson. On marching cubes. *IEEE Trans. Visualization and Computer Graphics*, 9(3):283–297, 2003.
10. D. Pham, C. Xu, and J. Prince. Current methods in medical image segmentation. In *Annual Review of Biomedical Engineering*, volume 2 of *Annual Reviews*, pp 315–337. 2000.
11. D. L. Pham. Spatial models for fuzzy clustering. *Computer Vision and Image Understanding*, 84:285–297, 2001.
12. F. Segonne, E. Grimson, and B. Fischl. Topological correction of subcortical segmentation. In *Proc. MICCAI'03*, Montreal, november 2003.
13. D. W. Shattuck and R. M. Leahy. Automated graph-based analysis and correction of cortical volume topology. *IEEE Trans. Med. Img.*, 20(11), 2001.
14. G. H. Weber, G. Scheuermann, and B. Hamann. Detecting critical regions in scalar fields. In *Proc. EUROGRAPHICS - IEEE TCVG Symposium on Visualization*, Grenoble, may 2003.
15. C. Xu, D. L. Pham, and J. L. Prince. *SPIE Handbook on Medical Imaging - Vol. 2*, chapter Medical Image Segmentation Using Deformable Models, pp 129–174. SPIE Press, 2000.
16. C. Xu, D. L. Pham, M. E. Rettmann, D. N. Yu, and J. L. Prince. Reconstruction of the human cerebral cortex from magnetic resonance images. *IEEE Trans. Med. Img.*, 18(6), 1999.

Simultaneous Boundary and Partial Volume Estimation in Medical Images

Dzung L. Pham and Pierre-Louis Bazin

Laboratory of Medical Image Computing, Johns Hopkins University, Baltimore, MD 21224

Abstract. Partial volume effects are present in nearly all medical imaging data. These artifacts blur the boundaries between different regions, making accurate delineation of anatomical structures difficult. In this paper, we propose a method for unsupervised estimation of partial volume fractions in single-channel image data. Unlike previous methods, the proposed algorithm simultaneously estimates partial volume fractions, the means of the different tissue classes, as well as the the locations of tissue boundaries within the image. The latter allows the partial volume fractions to be constrained to represent pure or nearly pure tissue except along tissue boundaries. We demonstrate the application of the algorithm on simulated and real magnetic resonance images.

1 Introduction

Segmentation of three-dimensional volumetric images is an important goal in many medical imaging applications such as in the localization of pathology, quantification, and computer integrated surgery. Because of the finite resolution of imaging devices, however, nearly all images suffer from partial volume effects. These artifacts result when different tissue classes in the image contribute to a single voxel, thereby causing boundaries to be blurred and ambiguously defined. As a result, standard voxel-based segmentation techniques that do not address partial volume effects often fail to capture fine details that may be present in the original image. In many applications, this preservation of fine details can be critical in the quantification and analysis of anatomical structures and pathology.

In tissue classification methods, the most common approach to dealing with partial volume effects is to obtain a soft or fuzzy segmentation. Rather than exclusively classifying a voxel as belonging to a particular class, soft segmentation methods allow for a continuous grade of membership within different classes. These memberships can be computed using fuzzy clustering [1,2] or probabilistic classification alorithms [3,4]. This approach, however, does not explicitly model partial volume effects and can therefore be susceptible to certain artifacts in the resulting segmentation [5]. Rather than measure the partial volume content, some methods have attempted to segment out partial volume voxels as separate classes [6]. Recent work has focused on directly estimating partial volume fractions in multi-channel [7,8,9] and single-channel images [5,10,11]. Because of the ill-posed nature of the problem, a fundamental difficulty in most of these partial volume estimation methods has been how to incorporate appropriate prior information into the estimation framework.

C. Barillot, D.R. Haynor, and P. Hellier (Eds.): MICCAI 2004, LNCS 3216, pp. 119–126, 2004.
© Springer-Verlag Berlin Heidelberg 2004

In this paper, we incorporate boundary information into the estimation procedure. Tissue boundaries within the image play a key role in partial volume effects because they, in fact, define where partial voluming will occur. Knowledge of the boundary locations allows us to constrain the partial volume fractions to be smooth and to represent pure tissue away from boundaries. The overall framework for estimating partial volume fractions and boundaries is based on an approximation of the Mumford-Shah functional. This leads to an iterative algorithm for estimation of the partial volume fractions, mean intensities of the tissue classes, and the boundaries. A multigrid algorithm is used to solve the discretized partial differential equation in the boundary estimation. This paper builds upon our previous work presented in [12,5].

2   Background

In [13] and [14], segmentation of two-dimensional magnetic resonance (MR) images was performed based on the minimization of the following energy functional with respect to the segmentation f, and the boundary field b:

$$\int\int_{\Omega} \alpha(y-f)^2 + \beta(1-b)^2|\nabla f|^2 + \gamma(\rho|\nabla b|^2 + \frac{1}{\rho}s^2)dxdy \tag{1}$$

The above equation closely resembles the well-studied Mumford-Shah functional [13], except it uses a continuously-valued boundary function rather than a binary one. In this equation, Ω is the domain of the image, y is the image data, and α, β, γ, and ρ are weighting parameters controlling the balance of each term. The estimated image f is an approximation of y and not a true segmentation or tissue classification. It will be piecewise smooth, as dictated by the second term that penalizes the gradient of f where the boundary field is small. The boundary field at each pixel possesses a value between zero and one and will be large where f is discontinuous. The third term penalizes both the existence of boundaries, as well as the gradient of the boundary field. The effectiveness of equation (1) stems from the fact that the f is smoothed within but not across boundaries, and because the boundary field itself is constrained to be smooth.

3   Energy Formulation

In this section, it is shown how the edge-adaptive properties of (1) can be incorporated into a partial volume estimation algorithm. Three major modifications of (1) are made. First, the approximate image f is replaced with a partial volume image representation:

$$f_j = \sum_{k=1}^{C} s_{jk}c_k$$

where s_{jk} is the partial volume fraction at voxel j for class k, and c_k is the representative tissue class intensity for class k. The summation over classes on s_{jk} is restricted to be equal to one and we will refer to c_k as the class mean. Second, instead of penalizing the gradient of the partial volume fractions, we employ a penalty function that constrains the partial volumes to be pure or nearly pure away from boundaries. Third, the boundary field is allowed to exist between voxel locations on a complementary grid and is decomposed into its directional components. For notational simplicity in the equations that follow, we focus on the single channel two-dimensional case, but the generalization to three dimensions and multiple channels is straightforward.

We propose to minimize the following energy functional with respect to the partial volume fractions s, the mean intensities c, and the boundary field b:

$$E = \alpha \sum_{j \in \Omega} \left\| y_j - \sum_{k=1}^{K} s_{jk} c_k \right\|^2 \tag{2}$$

$$+ \frac{\beta}{2} \sum_{j \in \Omega} \sum_{k=1}^{K} \sum_{m \neq k} \left(\sum_{l \in N_j^{(x)}} (1 - b_{j|l}^{(x)})^2 s_{jk} s_{lm} + \sum_{l \in N_j^{(y)}} (1 - b_{j|l}^{(y)})^2 s_{jk} s_{lm} \right)$$

$$+ \frac{\gamma}{2} \sum_{j \in \Omega_x} \left(\frac{1}{\rho} (b_j^{(x)})^2 + \rho \sum_{l \in N_j} (b_j^{(x)} - b_l^{(x)})^2 \right) + \frac{\gamma}{2} \sum_{j \in \Omega_y} \left(\frac{1}{\rho} (b_j^{(y)})^2 + \rho \sum_{l \in N_j} (b_j^{(y)} - b_l^{(y)})^2 \right)$$

Although Eq. 2 may appear complicated, it can be broken down into fairly simple parts. The first term follows the standard linear assumption used in most partial volume estimation methods.

The second line of Eq. 2 is based on the smoothness penalty on partial volume fractions proposed in [5]. This penalty is similar to the Potts model used in Markov random field theory and enforces two constraints: 1) the partial volume should be similar to its neighbors; 2) the partial volume should be close to zero or one. The main difference is that the penalty is now modulated by horizontal and vertical boundary fields, $b^{(x)}$ and $b^{(y)}$. Thus, the penalty function is relaxed at voxels near boundaries. We use the notation $N_j^{(x)}$ and $N_j^{(y)}$ to denote the set of horizontal and vertical neighbors of j, and $b_{j|l}$ to denote the boundary value between pixel locations j and l.

The third line of Eq. 2 consists of penalty functions on the horizontal and vertical boundary fields to ensure that they are also smooth. This penalty function is the same as the boundary penalty functions utilized in [15] except that the boundary field has been decomposed into separate horizontal and vertical components. The complementary horizontal and vertical grids of the boundary fields are denoted Ω_x and Ω_y, respectively. It is possible to also consider diagonal boundaries at the cost of greater computational expense. The parameters α, β, γ, and ρ control the relative balance of each term. For the boundary field, γ controls the magnitude of each field while ρ controls the overall smoothness. Figure 1 shows the boundary fields estimated from a synthetic image with some additive noise. The estimated partial volumes are used to construct a hard classification by assigning each pixel to the class with the greatest partial volume contribution, as shown in Figure 1(b). Figures 1(c)-(d) shows the horizontal and vertical boundary fields estimated on the complimentary grid. By increasing ρ, it is possible to diffuse the boundary field to a greater extent, as shown in Figure 1(e). Note that the diffusion is symmetric.

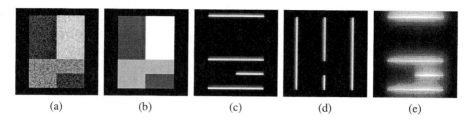

$$(a) \qquad (b) \qquad (c) \qquad (d) \qquad (e)$$

Fig. 1. Illustration of boundary fields: (a) input image, (b) classification result, (c) horizontal boundary field, (d) vertical boundary field, (e) horizontal boundary field with increased ρ parameter.

4 Algorithm

To minimize the energy function, a coordinate descent method is employed. The algorithm iteratively seeks a zero gradient condition of (2). For single-channel images, we employ the simplifying assumption that only two classes can contribute to a single voxel. To improve readability, we present the equations for b_j on the standard grid. It is straightforward to modify the equations such that the neighborhoods are decomposed to consider horizontal and vertical boundaries. The basic computations are the same.

If a and b denote the two contributing classes to a voxel j, the estimator for the partial volume fraction is derived by taking the first derivative of (2) with respect to s_{ja} and setting it to zero. This yields

$$s_{ja} = \frac{(c_b - y_j)(c_b - c_a) + \beta(1 - b_j)^2 \sum_{i \in N_j}\left(\sum_{m \neq b} s_{lm} - \sum_{m \neq a} s_{lm}\right)}{(c_b - c_a)^2} \qquad (3)$$

Values of s_{ja} are restricted to lie between zero and one and we sort the mean intensities such that $c_b > c_a$. The value of s_{jb} is computed as $1 - s_{ja}$.

A necessary condition on b_j for (2) to be minimized is

$$\sum_{l \in N_j}\sum_{k=1}^{K}\sum_{m \neq k} s_{jk}s_{lm} = \left(\sum_{l \in N_j}\sum_{k=1}^{K}\sum_{m \neq k} s_{jk}s_{lm} + \frac{\gamma}{\rho\beta}\right)b_j + \frac{\gamma\rho}{\beta}\nabla^2 b_j \qquad (4)$$

Equation (4) is a difference equation with spatially varying coefficients. A multigrid algorithm is employed to efficiently determine a solution [2].

The class means are computed iteratively using the following equation:

$$c_k = \frac{\sum_{j \in \Omega} s_{jk}\left(y_j - \sum_{l \neq k} s_{jl}c_l\right)}{\sum_{j \in \Omega} s_{jk}^2}. \qquad (5)$$

Our algorithm can be summarized as follows:

1. Obtain the initial class means.
2. Estimate the spread coefficients using the following procedure:
   a) Compute (3) for $\binom{K}{2}$ combinations of a and b.

    b) Select partial volume configuration with minimal energy.
    c) Repeat 3(a) & 3(b) for all voxels in the image.
3. Estimate the boundary field using (4).
4. Estimate the class means (5).
5. Repeat 2-4 until convergence.

Convergence is assumed to be achieved when the maximum change over all spread coefficients between iterations is less than 0.01. To improve stability of the algorithm, we employ a simple relaxation procedure that weights the current estimate with the previous estimate. This relaxation is eventually removed as iterations are increased and the algorithm nears convergence.

5   Gain Field Correction for MR Images

MR images can suffer from signal inhomogeneities, causing smooth intensity variations over the image space. This effect is usually represented by a multiplicative gain field [3]. This can be modeled by placing an additional variable, g_j, within the first term of (2:

$$\sum_{j \in \Omega} \|y_j - g_j \sum_{k=1}^{K} s_{jk} c_k\|^2$$

We model the gain field as a 2D polynomial function of low degree (degree 3 or 4 usually provides enough flexibility):

$$g_j = \sum_{n,m=1}^{N,M} v_{n,m} P_{n,m}(j),$$

where $P_{n,m}$ is a polynomial basis function of degree n in the horizontal and m in the vertical directions. We choose Chebyshev polynomials for their numerical stability and their properties for function approximation [16].

    The optimal polynomial coefficients $v_{n,m}$ are the solution of the least-squares equation:

$$\sum_{j \in \Omega} \|y_j - \sum_{n,m=1}^{N,M} v_{n,m} P_{n,m}(j) \sum_{k=1}^{C} s_{jk} c_k\|^2 = 0$$

In matrix notations, we can rewrite the above equation as $(Y - S \cdot P \cdot V)^T (Y - S \cdot P \cdot V) = 0$, with vectors $Y = [y_j], V = [v_{n,m}]$ and matrices $P = [P_{n,m}(j)]$ and S is a diagonal matrix with central elements $\sum_{k=1}^{C} s_{jk} c_k$. The solution is given by:

$$V = (P^T C P)^{-1} P^T Y. \qquad (6)$$

To reduce the computational burden of estimating for all unknown variables simultaneously, we solve the gain field in an initialization step using the simplified model described in [5]. This model does not use a spatial prior and assumes that the contributing tissue classes for a voxel are the classes whose centroids bound the intensity value of that voxel.

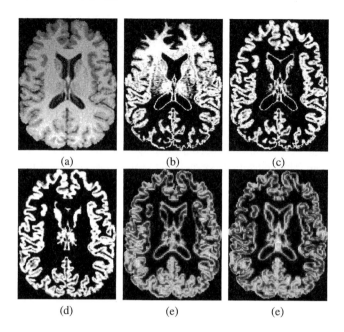

Fig. 2. (a) Actual MR image with simulated inhomogeneity, (b) fuzzy c-means gray matter segmentation, (c) enhance fuzzy c-means result, (d) partial volume result, (e)-(f) horizontal and vertical boundary fields.

6   Results

Figure 2 compares the results of the partial volume estimation algorithm with the standard fuzzy c-means algorithm, and an enhanced fuzzy clustering algorithm that incorporates gain field and noise correction [17]. Figure 2(a) is a slice from a real MR image data set. A gain field has been artificially applied to the image to increase the difficulty of the segmentation. The standard fuzzy c-means algorithm yields rather poor results, while the partial volume and enhanced fuzzy clustering algorithm provide reasonable results. The partial volume result has a reduced rim artifact around the ventricle but possesses thicker gray matter. The boundary fields illustrate that most of the structure within the boundary field is not purely horizontal or vertical. For this example, the following parameter settings were used: $\alpha = 1$, $\beta = 100$, $\gamma = 100$, and $\rho = 1$. The relaxation weight was initially set to 0.25 and incremented by 0.25 until equal to one. A third degree polynomial was used to the model the inhomogeneity field.

Figure 3 shows the results of our algorithm when applied to the Brainweb phantom from McGill University [18]. The image was simulated with 5% noise and 40% inhomogeneity. The results of the algorithm very closesly follow the true partial volume fractions used to generate the synthetic image. The estimated fractions are mostly free from the effects of the noise. In addition, the estimated gain field captures the darkening of intensities seen at the bottom of the image. For this example, the following parameter settings were used: $\alpha = 1$, $\beta = 150$, $\gamma = 100$, $\rho = 1$, 3rd degree polynomial for the inhomogeneity field..

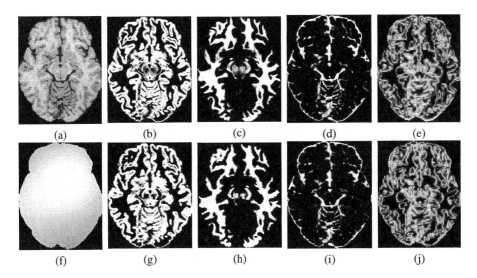

Fig. 3. Brainweb phantom image: (a) T_1-weighted image, (b)-(d) true gray matter, white matter, and cerebrospinal fluid partial volumes, field, (e) horizontal boundary field, (f) estimated gain field, (g)-(i) estimated partial volume fractions, (j) vertical boundary field.

7 Discussion

We have proposed a new approach for partial volume estimation that simultaneously computing a boundary field. The boundary field allows the partial volume fractions to be smooth and represent pure tissue at pixels that are away from the boundaries. A subtle benefit of this approach is that in our previous approach [5], a prior probability function on the tissue class means was required to stabilize the estimation. This is no longer needed because the boundary field allows the segmentation to be essentially binary or "hard" everywhere except at boundaries, thereby making it more stable. We have found that convergence is still rather slow however. Execution times for two-dimensional images were on the order of a couple of minutes on Pentium IV 3.0 GHz, with most of the time devoted to the solution of the boundary fields. Although the multigrid solution is efficient, hundreds of iterations are usually required for the overall algorithm to converge. In future work, we plan to investigate improving the convergence properties of the algorithm and perform further validation of its performance. We have found that gray matter in brain images is perhaps overestimated. This can be corrected by using separate variances for different class configurations, similar to mixture model approaches.

References

1. R.C. Herndon, J.L. Lancaster, J.N. Giedd, and P.T. Fox. Quantification of white matter and gray matter volumes using T1 parametric images using fuzzy classifiers. *J. Magnetic Resonance Imaging*, 6:425–435, 1996.
2. D.L. Pham and J.L. Prince. Adaptive fuzzy segmentation of magnetic resonance. *IEEE Trans. Med. Imag.*, 18:737–752, 1999.

3. W.M. Wells, W.E.L. Grimson, R. Kikins, and F.A. Jolesz. Adaptive segmentation of MRI data. *IEEE Trans. Med. Imag.*, 15:429–442, 1996.

4. K.V. Leemput, F. Maes, D. Vandermulen, and P. Seutens. Automated model-based tissue classification of MR images of the brain. *IEEE Trans. Med. Imag.*, 18(10):897–908, 1999.

5. D.L. Pham and J.l. Prince. Unsupervised partial volume estimation in single-channel image data. In *Proceedings of the IEEE Workshop on Mathematical Methods in Biomedical Image Analysis*, pages 170–177, Hilton Head, SC, June 11-12 2000.

6. P. Santago and H.D. Gage. Quantification of MR brain images by mixture density and partial volume modeling. *IEEE Trans. Medical Imaging*, 12:566–574, 1993.

7. H.S. Choi, D.R. Haynor, and Y. Kim. Partial volume tissue classification of multichannel magnetic resonance images— a mixel model. *IEEE Trans. Medical Imaging*, 10:395–407, 1991.

8. H. Soltanian-Zadeh, J.P. Windham, D.J. Peck, and A.E. Yagle. Optimal transformation for correcting partial volume averaging effects in magnetic resonance imaging. *IEEE Trans. Nucl. Sci.*, 11:302–318, 1992.

9. D.H. Laidlaw, K.W. Fleischer, and A.H. Barr. Partial-volume bayesian classification of material mixtures in MR volume data using voxel histograms. *IEEE Trans. Med. Imag.*, 17:98–107, 1998.

10. D.W. Shattuck, S.R. Sandor-Leahy, K.A. Schaper, D.A. Rottenberg, and R.M. Leahy. Magnetic resonance image tissue classification using a partial volume model. *Neuroimage*, 13:856–876, 2001.

11. K. Van leemput, F. Maes, D. Vandermeulen, and P. Suetens. A unifying framework for partial volume segmentation of brain mr images. *IEEE Trans. Med. Imag.*, 22:105 – 119, 2003.

12. D.L. Pham. Unsupervised tissue classification in medical images using edge-adaptive clustering. In *Proceedings of the 25th International Conference of the IEEE Engineering in Medicine and Biology Society*, Cancun, Mexico, Sept. 17-21 2003.

13. H.H. Pien and J.M. Gauch. Variational segmentation of multi-channel MRI images. In *Proceedings of the 1994 IEEE International Conference on Image Processing*, volume 3, pages 508–512, 1994.

14. J. Kaufhold, M. Schneider, A.S. Willsky, and W.C. Karl. A statistical method for efficient segmentation of MR imagery. *Internation Journal of Pattern Recognition and Artificial Intelligence*, 11(8):1213–1231, 1997.

15. J.M. Gauch J. Shah, H.H. Pien. Recovery of surfaces with discontinuities by fusing shaing and range data within a variational framework. *IEEE Trans. on Image Processing*, 5(8):1243–1251, 1996.

16. Philip J. Davis. *Interpolation and Approximation.* Dover, 1975.

17. D.L. Pham. Robust fuzzy segmentation of magnetic resonance images. In *Proceedings of the 14th IEEE Symposium on Computer-Based Medical Systems*, pages 127–131, Bethesda, MD, July 26-27 2001.

18. D.L. Collins, A.P. Zijdenbos, V. Kollokian, J.G. Sled, N.J. Kabani, et al. Design and construction of a realistic digital brain phantom. *IEEE Trans. Med. Imag.*, 17:463–468, 1998.

Local Watershed Operators for Image Segmentation

Hüseyin Tek and Hüseyin Can Aras

Imaging and Visualization, Siemens Corporate Research, Inc.
755 College Road East, Princeton NJ 08540, USA

Abstract. In this paper, we propose local watershed operators for the segmentation of medical structures. Watershed transform is a powerful technique to partition an image into many regions while retaining edge information very well. Most watershed algorithms have been designed to operate on the whole or cropped image, making them very slow for large data sets. In this paper, we propose a computationally efficient local implementation of watersheds. In addition, we show that this local computation of watershed regions can be used as an operator in other segmentation techniques such as seeded region growing, region competition or markers-based watershed segmentation. We illustrate the efficiency and accuracy of the proposed technique on several MRA and CTA data.

1 Introduction

Recent technological advances in imaging acquisition devices increase the spatial resolution of image data significantly. For example, new multi-detector CT machines can produce images with sizes as large as 512x512x1000. Thus, segmentation algorithms for these data sets need to operate locally in order to be computationally efficient since there is limited amount of time and memory available. While cropping data via user defined region of interest may be a solution for well localized pathologies, the user selected regions can still be very large in many applications, e.g. vascular segmentation or bone removal in CTA. Alternatively, images can be thresholded to reduce the area, where the segmentation and visualization algorithms need to operate, however, usually at the expense of removing anatomically important structures from the data.

We focus on the watershed-based segmentation of medical images in this paper. In medical image analysis, accurate detection of object boundaries are extremely important for quantification reasons, thus, making edge-based algorithms popular. While advances in edge detection algorithms increase the accuracy and performance of edge detectors, they are still not robust enough for many practical applications because edge grouping and linking (especially in 3D) is still quite a difficult problem. Unlike edge detectors, watershed transforms [8,5] produce closed contours and give good performance at junctions and places, where the object boundaries are diffused. Unfortunately, most watershed transforms are designed to operate on the whole image, which becomes a computational problem for large data sets.

C. Barillot, D.R. Haynor, and P. Hellier (Eds.): MICCAI 2004, LNCS 3216, pp. 127–134, 2004.
© Springer-Verlag Berlin Heidelberg 2004

In this paper, we propose a local implementation of watershed transform. Stoev and Strasser [7] also attempted to compute watersheds locally, which is discussed in Section 2. Our algorithm is based on filling operations from a user selected point. In the proposed algorithm, for each region to be filled accurately, its immediate two outer layers must be represented and filled at the same time. This *three layer* representation makes a user selected region (or catchment basin) [1] and its watershed lines to be computed correctly and locally. While the proposed algorithm can be used for the local computation of traditional watershed transform, it can also be used as an operator in segmentation algorithms. Specifically, instead of using pixel-based growth in many locally operating segmentation algorithms, regions can be used via the proposed local watershed operators. The incorporation of regions into the local segmentation algorithms allows much more accurate localization of object boundaries especially when boundaries are diffused. In the paper, we illustrate our ideas on two different segmentation algorithms namely, seeded region growing [1] and region competetition [10,6]. Several examples will be presented to illustrate the effectiveness of the proposed algorithm.

2   Watershed Transforms: Overview

Watershed segmentation [8,5] is a morphological gradient-based technique, which can be intuitively described as follows: View the gradient image as a height map, and gradually "immerse it in water", with water leaking through the minimum gradient points, rising uniformly and globally across the image. Place a "dam" when two distinct bodies of water (catchment basins) meet and continue the process until water has reached all the points of the image. The dams provide the final segmentation. This can be interpreted in the image domain as the growth of seeds placed on the minima of the image gradient height map at a time proportional to their height that finally converges on the crest lines of the gradient map. This is a powerful approach especially where local gradients cannot be defined, *e.g.* diffused edges. Since most structures contain several catchment basins on them, a typical watershed segmentation produces a large number of regions for even simple images, which is known as the *over-segmentation* problem. Many regions can be effectively reduced via nonlinear smoothing filtering [9,2]. The rest of them can be grouped together via region-growing techniques [8] or using marker methods [8,4].

Recently, Stoev and Strasser [7] proposed a technique for local computation of watersheds via simulating the rain-falling process. While this algorithm may work well on certain images, it cannot fill every basin correctly. Specifically, errors occur at places where basins have necks, or protrusions, *i.e.* water may not flow into the correct basin during the raindrop tracking process, Figure 1. Our implementation of this algorithm has proved the existence of this problem and the basins extracted from this algorithm appear *blocky* due to missed protrusions and necks in basins. In fact, Vincent and Soille [8] also discussed the errors that arise in tracking the path of a raindrop in digital image domain.

---

[1] Region and basin terms are interchangeably used throughout of this paper.

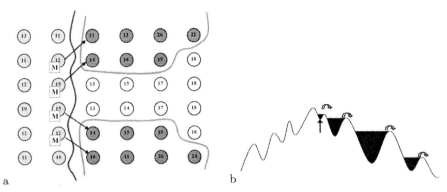

Fig. 1. (a) Breadth-First Problem: Water cannot flow through narrow regions in the breath-first type basin-filling algorithm since flooding on the dam (at the maxima) is stopped. Arrows show the pixels, which cause maxima to stop (b) Depth-First Problem: Whenever water reaches a dam, it starts filling the neighboring region from its minimum. The same process is applied to all neighboring regions iteratively, resulting in exploring too many regions if the minima of neighboring regions are in monotonocally decreasing order.

3   Local Watershed Operators

In this paper, we propose a new algorithm for computing watershed transform of an image *locally*. It is based on filling a region from a user selected point. The main goal is to fill a basin and compute its boundaries correctly and locally. This goal is satisfied via filling the main region and its immediate neighboring regions *simultaneously*. This *three-layer basin filling* algorithm, is based on the following two filling techniques.

Breadth-First Basin Filling: The first and most obvious approach of basin extraction is based on filling it with water and building dams at its ridges. First, the minimum of a user-selected region is computationally determined with gradient descent algorithm. Then, the region is filled with water starting from the minimum. When the water level reaches the ridges (watershed lines), dams (called maxima in our representation) are constructed to stop the water flowing into the neighboring regions. When a region is surrounded by dams, the filling process terminates. Second, the minimum of a neighboring region is determined from the dams (maxima points), again with a gradient descent algorithm. The same filling and construction of dams approach is recursively applied to fill the neighboring basins. Once the neighboring regions are filled, they can be checked for merging to the main region via segmentation criteria.

We have implemented the above algorithm. The filling process is implemented via region growing type operators, *i.e.* pixels visit eight-neighborhood, and bucket-based queueing for computational efficiency. Queueing is necessary for simulating the water rise. Specifically, we start from the minimum point and visit its eight neighbors and put them into buckets based on their height function. Then, the pixel with the minimum value is removed from the bucket for further growing. First, we check if any neighbor of this pixel has a lower

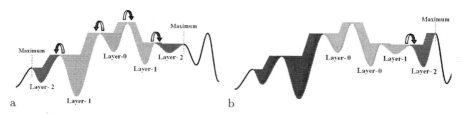

Fig. 2. The three-layer representation of basins during flooding (a) and the update of the layers after merging and continued flooding (b).

intensity value. If there is such a pixel, it means that we are in the vicinity of a watershed line and we mark that point as maximum, and its neighbors are not inserted into buckets. This growth process continues until no more pixels are left in the buckets, *i.e.* the basin is filled and surrounded by maxima points. As illustrated in Figure 1a, this filling process prevents passing through narrow regions, necks or protrusions, thus, basins cannot be correctly determined. The neck problem in this algorithm may be solved by using differential operators, such as second order derivatives, however, they are sensitive to noise and filter sizes. Our goal is to have a robust basin filling algorithm with no higher order gradient computations.

Depth-First Basin Filling: The above algorithm builds dams wherever it sees a lower height during the filling process. The next possible approach for computing local watershed transform is based on filling the neighboring regions whenever water flows into them instead of building dams. Specifically, when a pixel visits a neighboring pixel with a lower intensity, the minimum of the neighboring region is computed and water level is reduced to its minimum. The filling process continues from the new minimum until the user selected basin is filled, Figure 1b. During this process, the pixels where water from different basins are visited more than once are marked as *watershed-pixels* [2] as in [8]. The algorithm works very well if the selected basin is surrounded by regions with higher minima. However, when a region neighbors several regions with lower minima, which in turn also neighbors other regions with lower minima, the algorithm will fill considerably a large number of regions. In our experiments, we have observed that the algorithm can easily explore more than half of an image. Thus, this algorithm cannot be used where the local growth process is extremely important.

Three-Layer Basin Filling Algorithm: We now present a *three-layer basin filling* watershed algorithm, which combines the two approaches mentioned above. In this algorithm, the user selected region of interest is assigned to *layer-zero* and its immediate neighboring layers are marked as *layer-one* while the immediate neighbors of layer-one regions are marked as *layer-two*, Figure 2.

It is already shown that a basin and its watershed lines can be correctly computed if its neighboring regions are filled simultaneously, *i.e.* they reach the ridges at the same time. It is enough to start (or continue) the filling process

---

[2] Watershed-pixels are equidistant to two or more regions and are important in watershed implemetations. Watershed line is a more general term for describing ridges.

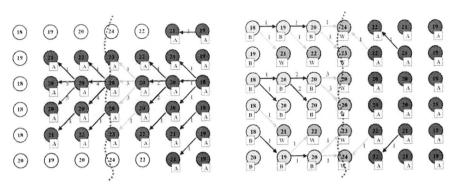

Fig. 3. The partitioning of plateau (level 20) between two basins A and B seperated by dashed line: Some pixels next to plateau are marked as watershed-pixels(W) incorrectly. They are corrected by using the source information. The propogation of distance is indicated by arrows.

right before the lowest level ridge they share. Then, the filling algorithm simulates region competition between these two regions and correctly constructs all watershed lines the regions share. This property is used in our algorithm between layer-zero vs. layer-one, and layer-one vs. layer-two regions. In other words, layer-zero and layer-one regions initialize the neighboring regions whenever they reach to the first watershed line that they share with their neighbors, thus allowing simultaneous filling and correct determination of watershed lines between these layers. On the other hand, layer-two regions build dams wherever they see new regions. Thus, it is possible that layer-two basins cannot be fully filled due to the neck problem. The three-layer filling process stops when layer-zero and all layer-one regions are completely filled, *i.e.* all watershed lines have been formed.

Watershed algorithms apply special processes when water reaches plateau, a local flat region. A plateau does not introduce any problems if it is totally inside a basin. However, when it is located between two or more basins, extra care must be taken to partition the plateau between the regions correctly. Like traditional watershed algorithms, the distance transform [3] is used in our algorithm to partition the plateaus between regions. Specifically, assume that a pixel P_i visits its neighboring pixel P_j, then the distance value at P_j is defined as

$$dist(P_j) = \begin{cases} 1 & \text{if} \quad g(P_i) < g(P_j) \\ min(dist(P_j), dist(P_i) + 1) & \text{else if} \quad g(P_i) = g(P_j) \end{cases} \quad (1)$$

where $g(P)$ is the height function at P. The above equation uses a simple distance metric. More accurate distance metrics, such as Euclidean can be used as well, however, at the expense of more computational time.

The distance transform allows the correct partitioning of plateaus between two regions. However, when a layer-zero (or layer-one) initializes a region from a plateau, a special case occurs, as in Figure 3. In the figure, region A propagates on the plateau (level 20) until it detects a new region B, *i.e.* it sees an empty lower level (level 18). During the propagation, all plateau points and the pixels next to the plateau are marked as region A. When water is initialized from B, it corrects the pixels at the plateau via distance transform. However, pixels next to the plateau are marked as watershed-pixels because collision from regions A and B are marked at these pixels. Specifically, region B visits these pixels but it cannot change their region labels because it brings a distance value of one as region A does. This error is corrected when the pixels from watershed-pixels are selected from the bucket. Specifically, if their sources are different, then they were correctly marked as watershed pixels; otherwise their correct regional labels are assigned to them and water starts rising from them.

Once the layer-zero and layer-one regions are filled correctly, *i.e.* no pixels exist in the buckets, the filling process terminates. Now, region merging can be applied between the layer-one basins and the layer-zero basin. When a layer-one region is merged to the layer-zero basin via some merging criterion, e.g. thresholding, it is also marked as layer-zero and the regional information of layer-zero is updated accordingly, Figure 2. In addition, all the neighboring layer-two regions of the merged layer-one region are updated to layer-one status. After merging, the filling process is restarted from the minimum point of the previous level-two regions' maxima list. This may cause some parts of layer-two regions to be processed again, but it is important to lower the water level to the place where the first maximum was marked. The lowering of water level to the first maximum point allows the algorithm to initialize the neighbors of the previous level-two regions(converted to layer-one after merging) as the new level-two regions, thus, avoiding the neck problem, Figure 1. The filling process continues until there are no more pixels left in the buckets, *i.e.* all new layer-one regions are also filled. The algorithm continues by merging, updating and flooding until a user-defined convergence criterion or a combination of several criteria are satisfied.

In this section, we proposed a new method for computing watershed transforms locally and correctly. The new algorithm consists of filling and merging processes. We call them watershed operators. Similarly, a deletion operator can be easily defined. We believe that these watershed operators, namely filling, merging and deleting can be used as basis for the segmentation processes, which will be described in the next section.

4   Medical Image Segmentation via Watershed Operators

In most local segmentation algorithms, the growing/deleting operations are done on pixels. However, we propose that regions can be used instead of pixels. Specifically, we illustrate the ideas on seeded region growing [1] and region competition algorithms [10,6].

Combined with morphological operations, seeded region growing can be considered as one of the most practical segmentation algorithms in medical image applications due to its simple implementation and near real-time execution. Typically, from a user selected point, pixels are added to the growing region until a threshold criterion is no longer satisfied. This method works well if the regions are rather well isolated and a good threshold value is determined. However, region growing algorithms cannot localize edges, especially when boundaries are

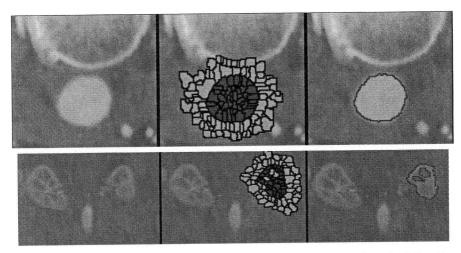

Fig. 4. Results of seeded region growing: The segmented region is red while other explored regions are green and watershed lines are black. (Top) Segmentation of aorta from CTA in orthogonal view. Seed point is given by the user (or from vessel centerline model) inside the aorta. (Bottom) Partial segmentation of a kidney from MRA. Again, user enters the seed point on the part of kidney.

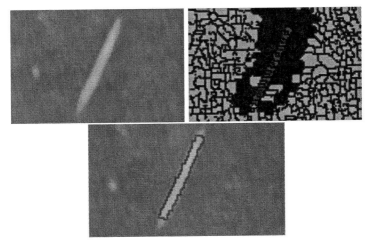

Fig. 5. Result of region competition: One seed is given in the vessel, one seed is given in the background. Red represents segmented vessel. Green represents the background regions. Blue represents the regions, which are first taken by the vessel, but then lost to background after competition.

diffused. In this paper, we propose that region growing can be implemented via watershed operators. Instead of pixels, basins are added to the growing region. We have implemented this algorithm and the threshold is determined from a bleeding criterion. Specifically, the bleeding criterion monitors the size of the growing region and the histogram of the segmented region. If a newly added basin changes the histogram and the number of pixels in the segmentation significantly, bleeding occurs and this stops the propagation. The main advantage of this algorithm is its ability to better localize edges even in the case of diffused edges. Figure 4 presents the segmentation of vessels and parts of the kidney by this algorithm.

The second example of applying watershed operators for image segmentation is the region competition [10]. In general, region competition works well, but it cannot guarantee detecting the boundaries at the edge point since it is rather difficult to incorporate edge information to this process, and it requires advanced deformable model evolution [6]. We have implemented a rather simpler version of region competition via watershed operators. Specifically, in our implementation, the growing regions compete for basins via watershed operators, namely, filling, merging and deleting, and produce well localized boundaries. The result of this region competition algorithm is also illustrated in Figure 5.

5   Conclusion

In this paper, we presented a three-layer basin filling algorithm for computing watershed transforms locally and accurately. We expect that the proposed algorithm will be important in the semi-automatic segmentation of medical structures in large data sets, *e.g.* CTA data obtained from multi-detector CT machines. In addition, we proposed that these watershed operators can be efficiently used in segmentation algorithms.

References

1. R. Adams and L. Bischof. Seeded region growing. *PAMI*, 16(6):641–647, 1994.
2. E. B. Dam and M. Nielsen. Nonlinear diffusion schemes for interactive watershed segmentation. In *MICCAI*, pages 596 – 603, 2000.
3. P. Danielsson. Euclidean distance mapping. *Computer Graphics and Image Processing*, 14:227–248, 1980.
4. R. J. Lapeer, A. C. Tan, and R. Aldridge. Active watersheds: Combining 3D watershed segmentation and active contours to extract abdominal organs from MR images. In *MICCAI*, pages 596 – 603, 2002.
5. L. Najman and M. Schmitt. Watersheds of a continuous function. *Signal Processing*, 38(1):99–112, 1994.
6. T. B. Sebastian, H. Tek, J. J. Crisco, S. W. Wolfe, and B. B. Kimia. Segmentation of carpal bones from 3d CT images using skeletally coupled deformable models. *Medical Image Analysis*, 7(1):21–45, 2003.
7. S. L. Stoev and W. Strasser. Extracting regions of interest applying a local watershed transformation. In *IEEE Visualization*, 2000.
8. L. Vincent and P. Souille. Watersheds in digital spaces: an efficient algoritm based on immersion simulations. *PAMI*, 13(6):583–598, 1991.
9. J. Weickert. Review of nonlinear diffusion filtering. In *First International Conference, Scale-Space*, pages 3–28, Utrecht, The Netherlands, 1997. Springer.
10. S. C. Zhu and A. L. Yuille. Region competition: Unifying Snakes, Region growing, and Bayes/MDL for multiband Image Segmentation. *PAMI*, 18(9):884–900, 1996.

Medical Image Segmentation Based on Mutual Information Maximization

Jaume Rigau, Miquel Feixas, Mateu Sbert, Anton Bardera, and Imma Boada

Institut d'Informatica i Aplicacions, Universitat de Girona, Spain
{jaume.rigau,miquel.feixas,mateu.sbert,anton.bardera,imma.boada}@udg.es

Abstract. In this paper we propose a two-step mutual information-based algorithm for medical image segmentation. In the first step, the image is structured into homogeneous regions, by maximizing the mutual information gain of the channel going from the histogram bins to the regions of the partitioned image. In the second step, the intensity bins of the histogram are clustered by minimizing the mutual information loss of the reversed channel. Thus, the compression of the channel variables is guided by the preservation of the information on the other. An important application of this algorithm is to preprocess the images for multimodal image registration. In particular, for a low number of histogram bins, an outstanding robustness in the registration process is obtained by using as input the previously segmented images.

1 Introduction

In image processing, grouping parts of an image into units that are homogeneous with respect to one or more features results in a segmented image. Thus, we expect that segmentation subdivides an image into constituent regions or objects, a significant step towards image understanding. The segmentation problem is very important in clinical practice, mainly for diagnosis and therapy planning.

In this paper we introduce a new algorithm for medical image segmentation based on mutual information (MI) optimization of the information channel between the histogram bins and the regions of the partitioned image. The first step of the algorithm partitions an image into relatively homogeneous regions using a binary space partition (BSP). The second step clusters the histogram bins from the previously partitioned image. This algorithm provides us with a global segmentation method without any human interaction. Our approach has similar characteristics to the agglomerative information bottleneck method [6] applied to document clustering.

An important application of the previous algorithm is to use the segmented images in the registration process. This allows for an extremely robust and very fast registration. Multimodal image registration is a fundamental task in medical image processing since it is a necessary step towards the integration of information from different images of the same or different subjects. Results obtained from different image modalities show good behavior of our segmentation algorithm and resulting segmented images perform well in medical image registration using mutual information-based measures.

C. Barillot, D.R. Haynor, and P. Hellier (Eds.): MICCAI 2004, LNCS 3216, pp. 135–142, 2004.

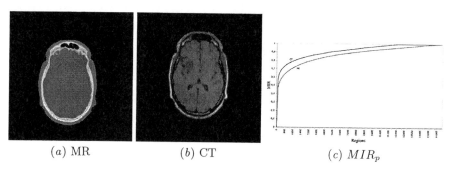

(a) MR   (b) CT   (c) MIR_p

Fig. 1. Test images: (a) MR and (b) CT. The two plots in (c) show the MIR_p with respect to the number of regions for (a) and (b).

2 Information Theoretic Tools

Some of the most basic information theoretic concepts [3] are presented here. The *Shannon entropy* $H(X)$ of a discrete random variable X with values in the set $\mathcal{X} = \{x_1, \ldots, x_n\}$ is defined as $H(X) = -\sum_{i=1}^{n} p_i \log p_i$, where $n = |\mathcal{X}|$ and $p_i = Pr[X = x_i]$. Shannon entropy expresses the average information or uncertainty of a random variable. If the logarithms are taken in base 2, entropy is expressed in bits. If we consider another random variable Y with probability distribution q, corresponding to values in the set $\mathcal{Y} = \{y_1, \ldots, y_m\}$, the *conditional entropy* is defined as $H(X|Y) = -\sum_{j=1}^{m} \sum_{i=1}^{n} p_{ij} \log p_{i|j}$ and the *joint entropy* is defined as $H(X,Y) = -\sum_{i=1}^{n} \sum_{j=1}^{m} p_{ij} \log p_{ij}$, where $m = |\mathcal{Y}|$, $p_{ij} = Pr[X = x_i, Y = y_j]$ is the joint probability, and $p_{i|j} = Pr[X = x_i|Y = y_j]$ is the conditional probability. Conditional entropy can be thought of in terms of an *information channel* whose input is the random variable X and whose output is the random variable Y. $H(X|Y)$ corresponds to the uncertainty in the information channel input X from the point of view of receiver Y, and vice versa for $H(Y|X)$. In general, $H(X|Y) \neq H(Y|X)$ and $H(X) \geq H(X|Y) \geq 0$.

The *mutual information* between X and Y is defined as

$$I(X,Y) = \sum_{i=1}^{n} \sum_{j=1}^{m} p_{ij} \log \frac{p_{ij}}{p_i q_j}. \tag{1}$$

It can also be expressed as $I(X,Y) = H(X) - H(X|Y) = H(Y) - H(Y|X)$ and is a measure of the *shared information* between X and Y.

A fundamental result of information theory is the *data processing inequality* which can be expressed in the following way: if $X \to Y \to Z$ is a Markov chain, i.e., $p(x, y, z) = p(x)p(y|x)p(z|y)$, then

$$I(X,Y) \geq I(X,Z). \tag{2}$$

This result demonstrates that no processing of Y, deterministic or random, can increase the information that Y contains about X.

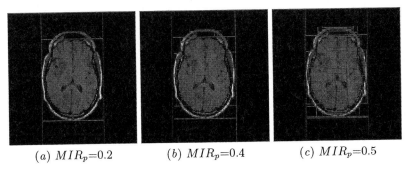

(a) MIR_p=0.2   (b) MIR_p=0.4   (c) MIR_p=0.5

Fig. 2. Partition of the MR image of Fig.1.a with three different MIR_p.

3   Two-Step Segmentation Algorithm

In this section, we present a general purpose global two-step segmentation algorithm that can be applied to different medical image modalities.

Given an image with N pixels and an intensity histogram with n_i pixels in bin i, we define a discrete information channel $X \to Y$ where X represents the bins of the histogram, with marginal probability distribution $\{p_i\} = \{\frac{n_i}{N}\}$, and Y the pixel-to-pixel image partition, with uniform distribution $\{q_j\} = \{\frac{1}{N}\}$. The conditional probability distribution $\{p_{j|i}\}$ of this channel is given by the transition probability from bin i of the histogram to pixel j of the image, and vice versa for $\{p_{i|j}\}$. This channel fulfills that $I(X,Y) = H(X)$ since, given a pixel, there is no uncertainty about the corresponding bin of the histogram. From the data processing inequality (2), any clustering or quantization over X or Y, respectively represented by $\widehat{X}$ and $\widehat{Y}$, will reduce $I(X,Y)$. Thus, $I(X,Y) \geq I(X,\widehat{Y})$ and $I(X,Y) \geq I(\widehat{X},Y)$.

3.1   Image Partitioning

The first step of the algorithm is a greedy top-down procedure which partitions an image in quasi-homogeneous regions. Our splitting strategy takes the full image as the unique initial partition and progressively subdivides it with vertical or horizontal lines (BSP) chosen according to the maximum MI gain for each partitioning step. Note that other strategies, as a quad-tree, could be used, obtaining a varied polygonal subdivision. This partitioning process is represented over the channel $X \longrightarrow \widehat{Y}$. Note that this channel varies at each partition step because the number of regions is increased and, consequently, the marginal probabilities of $\widehat{Y}$ and the conditional probabilities of $\widehat{Y}$ over X also change. Similar algorithms were introduced in the context of pattern recognition [5], learning [4], and DNA segmentation [1].

The partitioning algorithm can be represented by a binary tree [5] where each node corresponds to an image region. At each partitioning step, the tree acquires information from the original image such that each internal node i

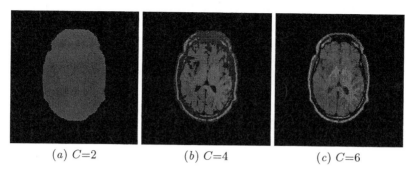

(a) $C=2$ (b) $C=4$ (c) $C=6$

Fig. 3. MR image segmentations obtained respectively from the partitioned images of Fig.2, indicating the number of colors C chosen in each case. The efficiency coefficients α are, respectively, 0.25, 0.22, and 0.22.

contains the mutual information I_i gained with its corresponding splitting. The total $I(X,\widehat{Y})$ captured by the tree can be obtained adding up the MI available at the internal nodes of the tree weighted by the relative area $q_i = \frac{N_i}{N}$ of the region i, i.e., the relative number of pixels corresponding to each node. Thus, the total MI acquired in the process is given by $I(X,\widehat{Y}) = \sum_{i=1}^{T} \frac{N_i}{N} I_i$, where T is the number of internal nodes. It is important to stress that this process of extracting information enables us to decide locally which is the best partition. This partitioning algorithm can be stopped using different criteria: the ratio $MIR_p = \frac{I(X,\widehat{Y})}{I(X,Y)}$ of mutual information gain, a predefined number of regions R, or the error probability [3,5]. The partitioning procedure can also be visualized from equation $H(X) = I(X,\widehat{Y}) + H(X|\widehat{Y})$, where the acquisition of information increases $I(X,\widehat{Y})$ and decreases $H(X|\widehat{Y})$, producing a reduction of uncertainty due to the progressive homogenization of the resulting regions. Observe that the maximum MI that can be achieved is $H(X)$.

Figure 1 shows the two test images used in our experiments. The two plots in Fig. 1.c indicate the behavior of MIR_p with respect to the number of partitions. Both plots show the concavity of the MI function. It can be clearly appreciated that a big gain of MI is obtained with a low number of partitions. Thus, for instance, 50% of MI is obtained with less than 0.5% of the maximum number of partitions. Observe that in the CT image less partitions are needed to extract the same MIR_p than in the MR image. Figure 2 presents the results of partitioning the MR test image. We show the partitioned images corresponding to three different MIR_p. Observe that the first partitioned image (Fig. 2.a) only separates the brain structure from the background.

3.2   Histogram Quantization

The second step of the algorithm is a greedy bottom-up segmentation procedure which takes as input the previously obtained partition and results in a histogram clustering based on the minimization of the loss of MI.

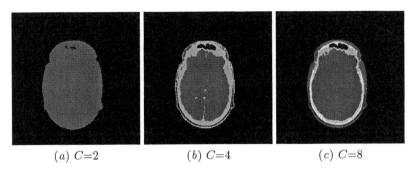

(a) C=2   (b) C=4   (c) C=8

Fig. 4. CT image segmentations obtained from a partition of Fig.1.b (with MIR_p=0.5), indicating the number of colors. The coefficients α are, respectively, $0.21, 0.24$, and 0.23.

The basic idea underlying our quantization process is to capture the maximum information of the image with the minimum number of colors (histogram bins). The clustering of the histogram is obtained efficiently by merging two neighbor bins so that the loss of MI is minimum. The stopping criterion is given by the ratio $MIR_q = \frac{I(\widehat{X},\widehat{Y})}{I(X,\widehat{Y})}$, a predefined number of bins C, or the error probability P_e [3,5]. Our clustering process is represented over the channel $\widehat{Y} \longrightarrow \widehat{X}$. Note that this channel changes at each clustering step because the number of bins is reduced. At the end of the quantization process, the following inequality is fulfilled: $I(X,Y) \geq I(X,\widehat{Y}) \geq I(\widehat{X},\widehat{Y})$.

In our experiments, the quality of the segmentation is measured by the coefficient of efficiency $\alpha = \frac{I(\widehat{X},\widehat{Y})}{H(\widehat{X},\widehat{Y})}$ [2]. In Fig. 3 we show three MR segmented images obtained from the corresponding partitions of Fig.2 with the indicated number of colors. Also, Fig. 4 shows three CT segmented images (2, 4, and 8 colors) built from a partition with MIR_p=0.5. Graphs plotting α versus the number of bins are presented in Fig. 5, showing a similar behavior in the two cases. These graphs correspond to a sequence of partitioned images of the MR and CT images of Fig. 1. It is important to observe from Fig. 5 that the images with a high number of partitions (with MIR_p from 0.6 to 1) have a decreasing efficiency, while the images with a low number of partitions (from 0.1 to 0.4) present a maximum of efficiency for a low number of bins. Observe also that MR and CT plots in Fig. 5 show a relatively stable α value for a partitioned image with MIR_p=0.5. In all performed experiments, an interesting pattern has been found. For each image, all MIR curves cross at a common point (see Fig. 5). This can be interpreted as an intrinsic property of the image. The number of bins at the crossing point might correspond inversely to the segmentation complexity of the image. For instance, in the plots (a) and (b) of Fig. 5, we have values 6 and 9 respectively, which reflects the higher complexity of the MR image.

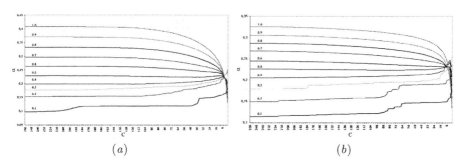

(a) (b)

Fig. 5. Plots of α corresponding to a sequence of partitioned images (with MIR_p from 0.1 to 1.0) for the (a) MR (Fig. 1.a) and (b) CT (Fig.1.b) images.

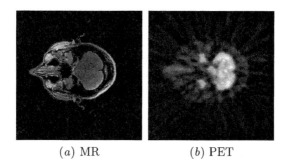

(a) MR (b) PET

Fig. 6. Test images: (a) MR and (b) PET.

4   Application to Image Registration

In this section, segmented images obtained with the MI-based segmentation algorithm are applied to medical rigid registration. The registration measure criterion used is the normalized MI (NMI) introduced by Studholme et al.[7]:

$$NMI(X,Y) = \frac{H(X) + H(Y)}{H(X,Y)} = 1 + \frac{I(X,Y)}{H(X,Y)}. \tag{3}$$

Experiments on MR-CT and MR-PET images are presented, showing a high robustness of NMI for a low number of histogram bins. The robustness of NMI has been evaluated in terms of the partial image overlap. This has been done using the parameter AFA (Area of Function Attraction) introduced by Čapek et al.[8] This parameter evaluates the range of convergence of a registration measure to its global maximum, counting the number of pixels, i.e. x-y translations in image space, from which the global maximum is reached by applying a maximum gradient method. The higher the AFA, the wider the attraction basin of the measure is.

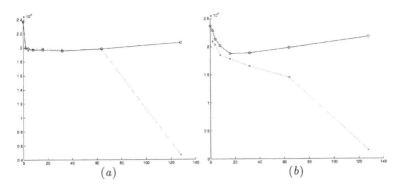

Fig. 7. AFA values obtained from the registration of (a) MR-CT (Fig. 1) and (b) MR-PET (Fig. 6) images using uniform (dotted line) and MI-based (solid line) quantizations. The x-axis represents the size of the bins.

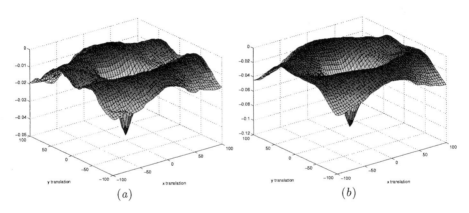

Fig. 8. Attraction basins of NMI obtained with 4 bins for the MR-PET (Fig. 6) registration with (a) uniform and (b) MI-based quantizations.

The robustness of NMI is analyzed with respect to the uniform quantization of the histogram and the quantization given by the MI-based segmentation algorithm. In Fig. 7, we show the AFA values obtained from the registration of the MR-CT pair of Fig. 1 and the MR-PET of Fig. 6, where the bin size is given by the successive powers of 2, going from 1 to 128. In these experiments, we have quantized only the MR image, partitioned with MIR_p=0.5, although similar results are obtained by quantizing both images. Figure 8 shows the attraction basins of NMI obtained with only 4 bins (bin size = 64) for the MR-PET images with a uniform quantization (Fig. 8.a) and a MI-based quantization (Fig. 8.b). Note the smoothness of the basin obtained with the MI-based segmentation. From these results, we can observe that the use of the segmented images provides us with a high robustness. For a high number of bins, the uniform quantization has a positive effect since it basically reduces the noise of the images. On the other hand, a negative effect is obtained when a very coarse quantization is applied without an information preservation criterion. In contrast, while the MI-based segmentation does not improve the uniform quantization for a high number of bins, it presents a remarkable improvement for a very coarse quantization. This is basically due to the fact that the segmentation is guided by an information optimization criterion.

5   Conclusions

We have presented in this paper a general purpose two-step mutual information-based algorithm for medical image segmentation, based on the information channel between the image intensity histogram and the regions of the partitioned image. We have applied this algorithm to preprocess the images for multimodal image registration. Our experiments show that, using as input the segmented images, an outstanding robustness is achieved in the registration process for a low number of histogram bins. In the future we will compare our segmentation algorithm against other state-of-the-art methods, and analyze two open problems: the optimal partition and the optimal number of clusters.

References

1. Pedro Bernaola, José L. Oliver, and Ramón Román. Decomposition of DNA sequence complexity. *Physical Review Letters*, 83(16):3336–3339, October 1999.
2. Torsten Butz, Olivier Cuisenaire, and Jean-Philippe Thiran. Multi-modal medical image registration: from information theory to optimization objective. In *Proceeding of 14th International Conference on Digital Signal Processing (DSP'02)*, July 2002.
3. Thomas M. Cover and Joy A. Thomas. *Elements of Information Theory*. Wiley Series in Telecommunications, 1991.
4. Sanjeev R. Kulkarni, Gábor Lugosi, and Santosh S. Venkatesh. Learning pattern classification – a survey. *IEEE Transactions on Information Theory*, 44(6):2178–2206, 1998.
5. Ishwar K. Sethi and G.P.R. Sarvarayudu. Hierarchical classifier design using mutual information. *IEEE Transactions on Pattern Analysis and Machine Intelligence*, 4(4):441–445, July 1982.
6. Noam Slonim and Naftali Tishby. Agglomerative information bottleneck. In *Proceedings of NIPS-12 (Neural Information Processing Systems)*, pages 617–623. MIT Press, 2000.
7. Colin Studholme. *Measures of 3D Medical Image Alignment*. PhD thesis, University of London, London, UK, August 1997.
8. Martin Čapek, Lukas Mrož, and Rainer Wegenkittl. Robust and fast medical registration of 3D-multi-modality data sets. In *Proceedings of the International Federation for Medical and Biological Engineering*, volume 1, pages 515–518, June 2001.

Adaptive Segmentation of Multi-modal 3D Data Using Robust Level Set Techniques

Aly Farag and Hossam Hassan

Computer Vision and Image Processing Laboratory
University of Louisville, Louisville, KY 40292.
{hossam,farag}@cvip.uofl.edu
http://www.cvip.louisville.edu

Abstract. A new 3D segmentation method based on the level set technique is proposed. The main contribution is a robust evolutionary model which requires no fine tuning of parameters. A closed 3D surface propagates from an initial position towards the desired region boundaries through an iterative evolution of a specific 4D implicit function. Information about the regions is involved by estimating, at each iteration, parameters of probability density functions. The method can be applied to different kinds of data, e.g for segmenting anatomical structures in 3D magnetic resonance images and angiography. Experimental results of these two types of data are discussed.

1 Introduction

Both surgical planning and navigation benefit from image segmentation. Also the 3D segmentation of anatomical structures is very important for medical visualization and diagnostics. The segmentation process is still a challenging problem because of image noise and inhomogeneities. Therefore this process can not depend only on image information but also has to exploit the prior knowledge of shapes and other properties of the structures to be segmented.

In many cases, the 3D segmentation is performed using deformable models. The mathematical foundation of such models represents the confluence of physics and geometry [1]. The latter represents an object shape and the former puts constraints on how the shape may vary over space and time. Deformable models have had great successes in imaging and computer graphics. In particular in [2], the deformable models recover the object's structure using some properties of its shape. The model evolves iteratively towards the steady state of energy minimization. But the disadvantage of this method is that the initial contour should be close to the final one. The model faces also problems with topological changes of a complex structure.

Level set techniques of segmentation overcome problems of the classical deformable models [3,4,5]. A curve in 2D or a surface in 3D evolves in such a way as to cover a complex shape or structure. Its initialization is either manual or automatic and it need not to be close to the desired solution. But these methods depend on a big number of parameters to be tuned for the success of the process.

C. Barillot, D.R. Haynor, and P. Hellier (Eds.): MICCAI 2004, LNCS 3216, pp. 143–150, 2004.
© Springer-Verlag Berlin Heidelberg 2004

In [6], a more efficient 3D segmentation technique was proposed. In this approach, surface evolution is controlled by current probabilistic region information. Probability density functions for the object and the background are estimated using the Stochastic Expectation Maximization algorithm (SEM). The level set model designed is based on these density functions. But this method can work only for bimodal images, and this may be too restrictive for many applications.

Also in [7,8], new segmentation methods were proposed using level set techniques. The former provided results for segmenting thin structure while the latter gave results for some real and synthetic images.

In this paper, a novel and robust segmentation based on the level set technique is proposed. A statistical model of regions is explicitly embedded into partial differential equations describing the evolution of the level sets. The probability density function for each region is modelled by a Gaussian with adaptive parameters. These parameters and the prior probability of each region are automatically re-estimated at each iteration of the process. The level set model designed depends on these density functions. The region information over the image is also taken into account.

Initialization of level set functions is very important for success of this segmentation process. An automatic seed initialization is used to accelerate the process and make it less sensitive to noise. The chosen initialization needs an accurate estimate of the parameters for each class. The SEM algorithm is used to give initial estimates of class parameters. During the level sets evolution, these parameters are iteratively re-estimated in order to obtain more accurate segmentation. Our work differs from that in [6] due to its suitability for multi-modal images and due to adaptive estimation of the probability density functions. Our experiments in 3D segmentation of MR images and angiography demonstrate the accuracy of the algorithm.

The paper is organized as follows. Section 2 considers the proposed level set formalism. Section 3 explains in brief the estimation of probability densities of image signals. The proposed evolutionary surface model is presented in Section 4. Experiments with simulated and real 3D images are discussed in Section 5.

2   Surface Modelling by Level Sets

Within the level set formalism [9], the evolving surface is a propagating front embedded as the zero level of a 4D scalar function $\phi(x,t)$. This hypersurface is usually defined as the signed distance function positive inside, negative outside, and zero on the boundary of a region. The continuous change of ϕ can be described by the partial differential equation:

$$\frac{\partial \phi(x,t)}{\partial t} + F|\nabla \phi(x,t)| = 0, \tag{1}$$

where F is a scalar velocity function depending on the local geometric properties (local curvature) of the front and on the external parameters related to the input data e.g, image gradient. The hypersurface ϕ deforms iteratively according to F, and the position of the 3D front is given at each iteration step by the equation $\phi(x, t) = 0$. Practically, instead of Eq. 1, the value $\phi(x, t_{n+1})$ at step $n + 1$ is computed from $\phi(x, t_n)$ at step n by the relation:

$$\phi(x, t_{n+1}) = \phi(x, t_n) - \triangle t \cdot F |\nabla \phi(x, t_n)|, \tag{2}$$

The design of the velocity function F plays the major role in the evolutionary process. Among several formulations proposed in [10,11], we have chosen the following formulation:

$$F = \nu - \epsilon k, \tag{3}$$

where $\nu = 1$ or -1 for the contracting or expanding front, respectively, ϵ is a smoothing coefficient always small with respect to 1, and k is the local curvature of the front defined in the 3D case as follows:

$$k = ((\phi_{xx} + \phi_{yy})\phi_z^2 + (\phi_{xx} + \phi_{zz})\phi_y^2$$
$$+(\phi_{zz} + \phi_{yy})\phi_x^2 - 2\phi_x\phi_y\phi_{xy} - 2\phi_x\phi_z\phi_{xz}$$
$$-2\phi_z\phi_y\phi_{zy})/(2(\phi_x^2 + \phi_y^2 + \phi_z^2)^{3/2}), \tag{4}$$

The latter parameter acts as a regularization term.

With this representation a single level set either contracts until vanishing or expands to cover all the space. To stop the evolution at the edge, F can be multiplied by a value which is a function of the image gradient[12]. But if the edge is missed, the surface can not come back. So to depend only on the edge is not sufficient for accurate segmentation and other information from the image should be used.

The segmentation partitions the image into regions each belonging to a certain class. In our approach a separate level set function is defined for each class and automatic seed initialization is used. Given parameters of each class, the volume is initially divided into equal non-overlapped sub-volumes. For each sub-volume, the average gray level is used to specify the most probable class with the initial parameters estimated by the SEM. Such initialization differs from that in [13] where only the distance to the class mean is used. Then a signed distance level set function for the associated class is initialized. Therefore selection of the class parameters is very important for the successful segmentation. The probability density functions of classes are embedded into the velocity term of each level set equation. The parameters of each one of these density functions are re-estimated at each iteration. The automatic seed initialization produces initially non-overlapped level set functions. The competition between level sets based on the probability density functions stops the evolution of each level set at the boundary of its class region.

3   Estimation of Intensity Probability Density Functions

A segmented image I consists of homogeneous regions characterized by statistical properties related to a visual consistency. The inter-region transitions are assumed to be smooth. Let $\Omega \in R^p$ be open and bounded p-dimensional volume. Let $I : \Omega \to R$ be the observed p-dimensional image data. We assume that the number of classes K is known. Let $p_i(I)$ be the intensity probability density function of class i. Each density function must represent the region information to discriminate between two different regions. In our experience Gaussian models show satisfactory results in medical image segmentation. In this work we also use such density functions and associate the mean μ_i, variance σ_i^2, and prior probability π_i with each class i. The priors satisfy the obvious condition:

$$\sum_{i=1}^{K} \pi_i = 1. \tag{5}$$

In accord to the estimation method in [14], the model parameters are updated at each iteration as follows:

$$\mu_i = \frac{\int_\Omega H_\alpha(\phi_i)I(x)dx}{\int_\Omega H_\alpha(\phi_i)dx}. \tag{6}$$

$$\sigma_i^2 = \frac{\int_\Omega H_\alpha(\phi_i)(\mu_i - I(x))^2 dx}{\int_\Omega H_\alpha(\phi_i)dx}. \tag{7}$$

We propose the following equation to estimate the prior probability by counting the number of pixels in each region and divide it by the total number of pixels:

$$\pi_i = \frac{\int_\Omega H_\alpha(\phi_i)dx}{\sum_{i=1}^{K} \int_\Omega H_\alpha(\phi_i)dx}. \tag{8}$$

Here, $H_\alpha(z)$ is the Heaviside step function defined in [15] as a smoothed differentiable version of the unit step function. The function $H_\alpha(z)$ changes smoothly at the boundary of the region. By the above equations, the model parameters are estimated based on the region information.

4   Evolutionary Surface Model

The term $(\nu = \pm 1)$ in Eq. 3 specifies the direction of the front propagation. Several approaches were developed to make all fronts either contracting or expanding (see, e.g., [16]) in order to evolve in both directions and avoid overlaps between the regions.The problem can be reformulated as classification of each point at the evolving front. If the point belongs to the associated class, the front expands otherwise it contracts.

4.1   PDE System

The classification decision is based on Bayes' decision [17] at point x as follows:

$$i^*(x) = \arg \max_{i=1,..,K} (\pi_i p_i(I(x))). \tag{9}$$

The term (ν) for each point x is replaced by the function $\nu_i(x)$ so the velocity function is defined as:

$$F_i(x) = \nu_i(x) - \epsilon \cdot k(x), \ \forall \ i = 1..K. \tag{10}$$

where

$$\nu_i(x) = \begin{cases} -1 \text{ if } i = i^*(x) \\ 1 \qquad \text{otherwise} \end{cases} \tag{11}$$

If the pixel x belongs to the front of the class $i = i^*(x)$ associated to the level set function, the front will expand, otherwise it will contract. Now, we put the Eq. 1 in the general form using the derivative of the Heaviside step function $(\delta_\alpha(z))$ [13] as follows :

$$\frac{\partial \phi_i(x,t)}{\partial t} = \delta_\alpha(\phi_i(x,t))(\epsilon \cdot k(x) - \nu_i(x))|\nabla \phi_i(x)|. \tag{12}$$

The function $\delta_\alpha(z)$ selects the narrow band points around the front. Solution of the PDEs requires numerical processing at each point of the image or volume which is a time consuming process. Actually we are interested only in the changes of the front, so that the solution is important at the points near the front. Such narrow band points are selected in Eq. 12. Points outside the narrow band are given large positive or large negative values to be excluded from processing in order to accelerate the iterations.

5   Experimental Results

5.1   Brain MR Images

We have four classes: (i)bones, (ii)gray matter (GM), (iii)white matter (WM), and (iv)cerebral spinal fluid (CSF). Applying the automatic seed initialization directly may result in miss-classifying some pixels that share the gray level range of the brain as shown in Fig. 1. That may lead to segment the eye as a brain for example. Therefore gray levels only are not sufficient for accurate segmentation. To solve this problem, the level sets for the classes have the automatic seed initialization except the (GM) class is initialized manually inside the volume as small balloons. But such initialization yields a lower prior probability of the (GM) growing region than it should have in Eq. 8 comparing to the other two classes. To avoid this problem, we compute the prior probabilities for all the classes by Eq. 8 but for the (GM) prior use the condition of Eq. 5: $\pi_2 = 1 - \pi_1 - \pi_3 - \pi_4$ and Eq. 8 is modified as follows:

$$\pi_i = \frac{\int_\Omega H_\alpha(\phi_i)dx}{\int_\Omega dx}, \ \forall \ i = 1, 3, 4. \tag{13}$$

After these modifications, the initial balloons (Fig. 1-right image) will evolve to cover the GM region without overlapping other regions. We only show results for WM/GM regions that represent the brain.

Table 1. Classification accuracy at different noise and inhomogeneity levels.

Noise and Inhomogeneity	Bones	GM	WM	CSF
0%–0%	99.8%	98.1%	99.1%	98.5%
3%–20%	97.9%	97.5%	98.3%	97.2%
9%–40%	97.3%	97.2%	96.4%	95.4%

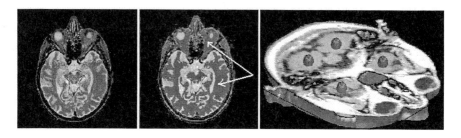

Fig. 1. $T2$ weighted MR image (left), showing that some areas outside the brain may have the same range of gray levels of the GM(the areas marked by the arrows) (middle), and the initialization of level set function of the GM inside the volume (right).

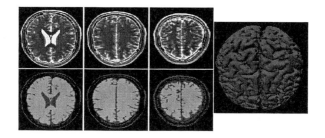

Fig. 2. Brain segmentation (light gray areas in the bottom images) and its 3D view to the right.

Simulated T2-weighted MR 3D image data sets of the size $181 \times 217 \times 174$ are downloaded from the web sight $http://www.bic.mni.mcgill.ca/brainweb/$. These data sets have different noise and inhomogeneity levels. Table 5.1 shows the accuracy of the approach for each region. Figure 2 shows results of the segmented brain and its 3D view.

5.2   Magnetic Resonance Angiography

Magnetic Resonance Angiography(MRA) is based on amplification of signals from blood vessels and suppression of signals from other tissues. The blood vessels appear as lighter spots in the image. Traditional segmentation needs an extra post-processing to remove the non-blood-vessel areas from the final region maps [18,19]. In our approach, the data set has three classes, namely, CSF with bones, GM with WM, and blood vessels (BV) combined with the fat around

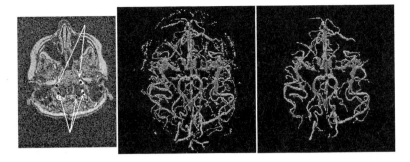

Fig. 3. MRA slice with the cross-sections of the initialized BV level set functions (black circles) (left), visualization of the segmented $512 \times 512 \times 93$ data set using traditional techniques in [18] with fat(middle), and the visualization of our results(right).

the brain which has practically the same range of the gray levels as the blood vessels. Once again, the level set function for the BV class is initialized manually as balloons inside the vessels that have the largest cross sectional area as shown in Fig. 3-left image, and the prior probabilities are estimated as in previous section (with the obvious changes of the class indices). As a result, the fat does not appear in the final segmentation results. Data sets were collected using a Picker 1.5T Edge MRI scanner. It consists of 512x512x93 axial slices with slice thickness 1 mm, TR = 27 ms, TE = 6 ms. The proposed segmentation approach is tested on 20 data sets.

6   Conclusions and Future Research

We developed a simple and fast statistical evolutionary model based on the level set techniques. The model does not need fine tuning of weighting parameters, but the number of classes (regions) has to be known. Each class is assigned with a level set function, and the SEM algorithm provides initial estimates of parameters of the Gaussian model of each class. These estimates permit us to initialize the level sets near to the optimal solution in order to reduce considerably the number of iterations. The Gaussian models of each class are re-estimated at each iteration.

Experiments with real and simulated 3D images confirm that the proposed method is robust and accurate. We expect it may fail on the images where simple Gaussian models cannot discriminate between the regions which makes a limitation. In future work we are going to use more general parametric types of probability distributions which can be estimated with the level sets evolution.

References

1. S. Osher and N. Paragios, *Geometric Level Set Methods in Imaging, Vision, and Graphics,* Springer, 2003.
2. D. Terzopoulos, "Regularization of inverse visual problems involving discontinuities," *IEEE Tr. on PAMI,* 8(2):413–424, 1986.
3. V. Caselles, R. Kimmel, and G. Sapiro., "Geodesic active contours," *IJCV,* 22:61–79, 1997.
4. H-K. Zaho, T. Chan, B. Merriman, and S. Osher, "A variational level set approach to multiphase motion," *J. of Computational Physics,* 127:179–195, 1996.
5. R. Goldenberg, R. Kimmel, E. Rivlin, and M. Rudzsky, "Cortex Segmentation: A Fast Variational Geometric Approach," *IEEE Tr. on Medical Imaging,* Vol. 21, No. 2, pp. 1544–1551, December 2002.
6. C. Baillard, and C. Barillot, "Robust 3D segmentation of anatomical structures with level sets," *MICCAI* LNCS 1935, Pages 236–245, Pittsburgh, Pennsylvania, October 2000.
7. M. Holtzman-Gazit, D. Goldsher, and R. Kimmel. "Hierachical Segmentation of Thin Structures in Volumetric Medical Images ," *MICCAI,* Montreal, Canada, November 16–18, 2003.
8. T.Kadir, and M. Brady. "Unsupervised Non-parametric Region Segmentation Using Level Sets,"*ICCV,* Niece, France, October 11-17, 2003.
9. J.A. Sethian, *Level Set Methods and Fast Marching Methods,* Combridge University Press, USA, 1999.
10. J. Gomes and O. Faugeras, "Reconciling distance functions and Level-Sets,", *Technical Report 3666,*INRIA, April 1999.
11. N. Paragios and R. Deriche., "Unifying boundary and region-based information for geodesic active tracking," *CVPR,* Vol. 2, pp 300–305, Fort Collins, Colorado, jun. 1999.
12. R. Malladi, J. Sethian, and B. Vemuri. "Shape modeling with front propagation: A level set approach," *IEEE Tr. on PAMI,* 17(2):158–175, febreuary, 1995.
13. C. Samson, L. Blanc-Féraud, G. Aubert, and J. Zerubia. "Multiphase Evolution and Variational Image Classification," *Technical Report 3662,* INRIA, France, 1999.
14. T. Chan and L. Vese. "A multiphase level set framework for image segmentation using the mumford and shah model.," *International Journal of Computer Vision,* 50(3):271–293,2002.
15. T. Chan, B.Sandberg, and L. Vese."Active Contours without Edges for Vector Valued Images," *Journal of Visual Communications and Image Representations,* 2:130–141, 2000.
16. X. Zeng, L.H. Staib, R.T. Schultz, H. Tagare, L. Win, and J.S. Duncan. "A new approach to 3D sulcal ribbon finding from MR images," *MICCAI,* pages 148–157, sep. 1999.
17. R. Duda, P. Hart, and D. Stork. "Pattern Classification ," *John Wiley and Sons Inc.,* 2001.
18. M.Sabry, A. Farag, S. Hushek, and T. Moriarity. "Statistical-Based Approach for Extracting 3D Blood Vessels from TOF-MRA Data,"*MICCAI,* Montreal, Canada, November 16–18, 2003.
19. H. Hassan, A. Farag. "MRA Data Segmentation Using Level Sets,"*in Proc IEEE International Conference on Image Processing,* Barcelona, Spain, Sep. 14–17, 2003.

Coupling Statistical Segmentation and PCA Shape Modeling

Kilian M. Pohl[1], Simon K. Warfield[2], Ron Kikinis[2], W. Eric L. Grimson[1], and
William M. Wells[2]

[1] Computer Science and Artificial Intelligence Lab, http://www.csail.mit.edu,
Massachusetts Institute of Technology, Cambridge MA, USA.,
{kpohl,welg}@csail.mit.edu
[2] Surgical Planning Laboratory, http://www.spl.harvard.edu, Harvard Medical School
and Brigham and Women's Hospital, 75 Francis St., Boston, MA 02115 USA,
{warfield,kikinis,sw}@bwh.harvard.edu

Abstract. This paper presents a novel segmentation approach featuring shape
constraints of multiple structures. A framework is developed combining statistical
shape modeling with a maximum a posteriori segmentation problem. The shape is
characterized by signed distance maps and its modes of variations are generated
through principle component analysis. To solve the maximum a posteriori segmentation problem a robust Expectation Maximization implementation is used.
The Expectation Maximization segmenter generates a label map, calculates image
intensity inhomogeneities, and considers shape constraints for each structure of
interest. Our approach enables high quality segmentations of structures with weak
image boundaries which is demonstrated by automatically segmenting 32 brain
MRIs into right and left thalami.

1 Introduction

For many age or disease related brain studies large quantities of Magnetic Reasoning Images (MRI) have to be accurately segmented into anatomical regions. Achieving
high quality brain MRI segmentation is quite challenging for automatic methods so
researchers often have to rely on labor intensive, manual delineation. The task is challenging because some structures have very similar intensity characteristics, such as substructures in the cortical gray matter, while others have only weakly visible boundaries
(e.g. thalamus). Recent methods using enhanced anatomical knowledge have greatly
improved the quality of automatically generated results. We briefly summarize methods
that incorporate shape constraints into the segmentation process. A promising approach
[1,2,3] is based on level set functions. It characterizes shape based signed distance maps
in combination with the Principle Component Analysis (PCA) [4] . Generally, PCA
finds the largest modes of variation among the signed distance maps. Besides level sets,
deformable model methods have used many different shape representations, such as
spherical harmonics [5], point based models [4], skeleton or medial representations [6],
and finite element models [7].

The novel approach presented in this paper is most closely related to work by Tsai and
Leventon [1,2]. While PCA based segmentation methods are very robust they are also

C. Barillot, D.R. Haynor, and P. Hellier (Eds.): MICCAI 2004, LNCS 3216, pp. 151–159, 2004.
© Springer-Verlag Berlin Heidelberg 2004

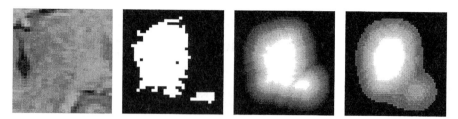

Fig. 1. Example of a left thalamus and corresponding segmentation, related signed distance map, and structure's mean where the voxel's brightness corresponds to the value in the distance map.

constraint in the degrees of freedom of the shape variations allowed. We therefore couple the PCA based shape modeling with a maximum a posteriori estimation problem which will be solved through an Expectation Maximization (EM) implementation developed by Pohl et al. [8]. This allows the system to accommodate shapes that differ some what from those modeled by the PCA. Additionally, the method can segment multiple objects and estimate intensity inhomogeneities in the image.

2   Method

This section discusses the integration of shape constraints into an EM segmentation algorithm. First, the shape variations across subjects are captured through PCA [9]. Afterwards, the shape constraints are added to the parameter space of an EM-based segmentation algorithm [8].

2.1   Shape Representation

Various shape representations have been explored in medical imaging. For our work, we chose signed distance maps due to their robustness. The structure's shape variations are captured by PCA. To apply PCA to the training data we first align all training sets using the affine registration method developed by Warfield [10]. Then, each data set i is transferred into structure specific signed distance maps $\mathcal{D}_a^{(i)}$, where a represents the structure of interest (see also Figure 1). In these distance maps positive values are assigned to voxels within the boundary of the object, while negative values indicate voxels outside the object. By taking the average over all these distance maps $\mathcal{D}_a^{(i)}$ we define the mean distance map $\overline{\mathcal{D}}_a := \frac{1}{n} \sum_i \mathcal{D}_a^{(i)}$ and the mean corrected signed distance maps $\tilde{\mathcal{D}}_a^{(i)} := \mathcal{D}_a^{(i)} - \overline{\mathcal{D}}_a$. The input for PCA is the vector $\tilde{\mathcal{D}}^{(i)} := (\tilde{\mathcal{D}}_1^{(i)^T}, \cdots, \tilde{\mathcal{D}}_N^{(i)^T})^T$ defined by the mean corrected signed distance maps of the N structures of interests. Therefore, PCA is applied to all structures at once. This analysis defines the shape constraints of the entire image which is represented by the eigenvector or modes of variation matrix U, eigenvalue matrix Λ, and $\overline{\mathcal{D}} := (\overline{\mathcal{D}}_1^T, \cdots, \overline{\mathcal{D}}_N^T)^T$ (see also Figure 2). To reduce the computational complexity for the EM implementation, U and Λ will only be defined by the first K eigenvectors and eigenvalues, where K represents 99 % of the eigenvalues' energy.

The shapes in a specific brain image will be captured by the expansion coefficients of the eigenvector representation which we call shape parameters $\mathcal{S} = (\mathcal{S}_1, \cdots, \mathcal{S}_K)$.

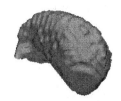 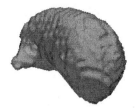

Fig. 2. These are the results of PCA applied to a training set of manually segmented thalami. As clearly visible from the images the first mode of variation, i.e. the deformation along the eigenvector with the largest eigenvalue, defines the size of the structure.

S relates to the distance maps by $\mathcal{D}_S = \overline{\mathcal{D}} + U \cdot S$. We will refer to the shape parameter generated distance map of a specific structure a as $\mathcal{D}_{S,a} = \overline{\mathcal{D}}_a + U_a \cdot S$, where U_a are just the entries in U that refer to structure a.

The probability distribution over the shape parameters $p(S)$ is now defined by the Gaussian distribution

$$p(S) = \frac{1}{\sqrt{(2\pi)^K |\Lambda|}} \exp\left(-\frac{1}{2} S^T \Lambda^{-1} S\right)$$

where K is the dimension of eigenvalue matrix Λ.

2.2   Estimating Intensity Inhomogeneities and Shape

The algorithm proposed in this chapter is based on an EM-based segmentation algorithm by Pohl et al. [8] which uses probability atlases to define the spatial distribution of structures . Expanding this approach, we will not only approximate the maximum a posteriori estimate (MAP) of the image intensity inhomogeneities $\mathcal{B}$ but also the MAP estimate of the shape parameters S. In this framework the MAP estimates of the parameter space, i.e. $\mathcal{B}$ and S, depend on the partition of the image in anatomical regions $\mathcal{T}$ (the hidden data), the log intensities of the input image $\mathcal{I}$ (the observed data), and previous estimations of the inhomogeneities $\mathcal{B}'$ as well as the shape parameter S'. Therefore, our approach tries to solve the following problem:

$$(\mathcal{B}'', S'') = \arg\max_{\mathcal{B}, S} Q(\mathcal{B}, S | \mathcal{B}', S') = \arg\max_{\mathcal{B}, S} E_{\mathcal{T} | \mathcal{I}, \mathcal{B}', S'}(\log p(\mathcal{B}, S | \mathcal{T}, \mathcal{I}))$$

$$= \arg\max_{\mathcal{B}, S} E_{\mathcal{T} | \mathcal{I}, \mathcal{B}', S'}(\log p(\mathcal{I} | \mathcal{T}, S, \mathcal{B}) + \log p(S | \mathcal{T}, \mathcal{B}) + \log p(\mathcal{B} | \mathcal{T}))$$

$$= \arg\max_{\mathcal{B}, S} E_{\mathcal{T} | \mathcal{I}, \mathcal{B}', S'}(\log p(\mathcal{I} | \mathcal{T}, \mathcal{B}) + \log p(S | \mathcal{T}, \mathcal{B}) + \log p(\mathcal{B} | \mathcal{T}))$$

$$(1)$$

where $E_{\mathcal{T} | \mathcal{I}, \mathcal{B}', S'}(\log p(\mathcal{B}, S | \mathcal{T}, \mathcal{I})) := \sum_{\mathcal{T}} p(\mathcal{T} | \mathcal{I}, \mathcal{B}', S') \cdot \log p(\mathcal{B}, S | \mathcal{T}, \mathcal{I})$ and we assume independence of S in $p(\mathcal{I} | \mathcal{T}, S, \mathcal{B})$. If we further assume independence between $\mathcal{B}$ and S, and $\mathcal{B}$ and $\mathcal{T}$ than the maximization problem can be simplified to :[1]

$$\mathcal{B}'' = \arg\max_{\mathcal{B}} E_{\mathcal{T} | \mathcal{I}, \mathcal{B}', S'}(\log p(\mathcal{I} | \mathcal{T}, \mathcal{B})) + \log p(\mathcal{B}) \qquad (2)$$

$$S'' = \arg\max_{S} E_{\mathcal{T} | \mathcal{I}, \mathcal{B}', S'}(\log p(S | \mathcal{T})) \qquad (3)$$

---

[1] $p(S | \mathcal{T}, \mathcal{B}) = \frac{p(S, \mathcal{T}, \mathcal{B})}{p(\mathcal{T}, \mathcal{B})} = \frac{p(S, \mathcal{T}) p(\mathcal{B})}{p(\mathcal{T}) p(\mathcal{B})} = p(S | \mathcal{T})$ and $p(\mathcal{B} | \mathcal{T}) = p(\mathcal{B})$.

To solve these two equations the EM algorithm iterates between the Expectation Step (E-Step) and the Maximization Step (M-Step). The E-Step first updates $\mathcal{B}'$ and $\mathcal{S}'$ with $\mathcal{B}''$ and $\mathcal{S}''$. Then it calculates the expected value of the two functions based on $\mathcal{B}'$ and $\mathcal{S}'$. The M-Step approximates separately the MAP estimates $\mathcal{B}''$ and $\mathcal{S}''$ based on the results of the E-Step. For a general overview of EM we refer the reader to [11].

In the remainder of this section we will first discuss the two MAP estimation problems separately and then integrate these two MAP estimation problems into the EM framework.

Estimating the Intensity Inhomogeneities

To find the MAP estimate of $\mathcal{B}$ we assume statistical independence of the voxel location x for $\mathcal{B}$ and $\mathcal{I}$. Therefore, Equation (2) simplifies to:

$$0 = \frac{\partial}{\partial \mathcal{B}_x} \left(E_{\mathcal{T}|\mathcal{I},\mathcal{B}',\mathcal{S}'} \left(\log p(\mathcal{I}_x|\mathcal{B}_x, \mathcal{T}_x) \right) \right) + \frac{\frac{\partial}{\partial \mathcal{B}_x} p(\mathcal{B})}{p(\mathcal{B})} \tag{4}$$

The conditional intensity distribution is modeled by a Gaussian distribution:

$$p(\mathcal{I}_x|\mathcal{T}_x = e_a, \mathcal{B}_x) := \frac{1}{\sqrt{(2 \cdot \pi)^n |\sigma_a|}} e^{-\frac{1}{2}(\mathcal{I}_x - \mathcal{B}_x - \mu_a)^T \cdot \sigma_a^{-1} \cdot (\mathcal{I}_x - \mathcal{B}_x - \mu_a)} \overset{2}{}$$

where n is the number of input channels, and (μ_a, σ_a) define the intensity distribution of structure a. '$\overset{x}{=}$' refers to footnote x for further explanation. Let's define

$$A_x(a) := \frac{\partial}{\partial \mathcal{B}_x} p(\mathcal{I}_x|\mathcal{T}_x = e_a, \mathcal{B}_x) = \sigma_a^{-1} \cdot (\mathcal{I}_x - \mathcal{B}_x - \mu_a)$$

and the weights $\mathcal{W}_x(a) := E_{\mathcal{T}|\mathcal{I},\mathcal{B}',\mathcal{S}'}(\mathcal{T}_x(a))$ so that Equation (4) turns into

$$0 = \frac{\partial}{\partial \mathcal{B}_x} \left(E_{\mathcal{T}|\mathcal{I},\mathcal{B}',\mathcal{S}'} \left(\log p(\mathcal{I}_x|\mathcal{T}_x, \mathcal{B}_x) \right) \right) + \frac{\frac{\partial}{\partial \mathcal{B}_x} p(\mathcal{B})}{p(\mathcal{B})}$$

$$= E_{\mathcal{T}|\mathcal{I},\mathcal{B}',\mathcal{S}'}(\mathcal{T}_x) \cdot \frac{\partial}{\partial \mathcal{B}_x} \log p(\mathcal{I}_x|\mathcal{T}_x, \mathcal{B}_x) + \frac{\frac{\partial}{\partial \mathcal{B}_x} p(\mathcal{B})}{p(\mathcal{B})} = \mathcal{W}_x^T \cdot A_x + \frac{\frac{\partial}{\partial \mathcal{B}_x} p(\mathcal{B})}{p(\mathcal{B})}$$

As Wells shows [12] the above problem can be approximated by a low pass filter H applied to the weighted residual $\bar{R}$: $\mathcal{B} \approx H\bar{R}$. Now, we will explicitly define the weights $\mathcal{W}_x(a) := E_{\mathcal{T}|\mathcal{I},\mathcal{B}',\mathcal{S}'}(\mathcal{T}_x(a))$:

$$\mathcal{W}_x(a) := E_{\mathcal{T}|\mathcal{I},\mathcal{B}',\mathcal{S}'}(\mathcal{T}_x(a)) \overset{3}{=} E_{\mathcal{T}_x|\mathcal{I}_x,\mathcal{B}'_x,\mathcal{S}'}(\mathcal{T}_x(a))$$

$$= 0 \cdot p(\mathcal{T}_x(a) = 0|\mathcal{I}_x, \mathcal{B}'_x, \mathcal{S}') + 1 \cdot p(\mathcal{T}_x(a) = 1|\mathcal{I}_x, \mathcal{B}'_x, \mathcal{S}') \tag{5}$$

$$= p(\mathcal{T}_x(a) = 1|\mathcal{I}_x, \mathcal{B}'_x, \mathcal{S}') \overset{4}{=} \frac{p(\mathcal{I}_x|\mathcal{T}_x(a) = 1, \mathcal{B}'_x) \cdot p(\mathcal{T}_x(a) = 1|\mathcal{S}')}{p(\mathcal{I}_x|\mathcal{B}'_x, \mathcal{S}')}$$

We will model $p(\mathcal{T}_x(a) = 1|\mathcal{S})$ as a measure of agreement among the shape $\mathcal{S}$ an the label map $\mathcal{T}$. This is achieved by transforming the distance maps $\mathcal{D}_\mathcal{S}$ produced by $\mathcal{S}$ into binary maps through $\mathcal{H}$:

---

[2] e_a has a 1 at position a and 0 otherwise

[3] Bayes' rule: $\sum_{\mathcal{T}(i,a_j)} p(\mathcal{T}(1,a_1), \cdots, \mathcal{T}(n,a_m)|\mathcal{I}, \mathcal{B}') \cdot \mathcal{T}_x(a) = p(\mathcal{T}_x(a) = 1|\mathcal{I}, \mathcal{B}')$

[4] Based on previous independence assumption

$$\mathcal{H}_S(x,a) := \begin{cases} 1 & , \text{if } \mathcal{D}_{S,a}(x) \geq 0 \\ 0 & , \text{if } \mathcal{D}_{S,a}(x) < 0 \end{cases}$$

where $\mathcal{H}_S(x,a)$ is the Heaviside function for structure a. $p(\mathcal{T}|S)$ penalizes any disagreement between $\mathcal{T}_x$ and $\mathcal{H}_S(x) = (\mathcal{H}_S(x,1), \cdots, \mathcal{H}_S(x,N))^T$:

$$p(\mathcal{T}|S) := \frac{1}{Z} e^{-\frac{1}{2}\sum_x d(\mathcal{T}_x, \mathcal{H}_S(x)) + \log(f(\mathcal{T}_x))}$$

where d is a correlation metric between $\mathcal{T}_x$ and $\mathcal{H}_S(x)$. Here $d(v_1, v_2) := (v_1 - v_2)^T (v_1 - v_2)$, which means d is zero when v_1 and v_2 agree, and 1 or greater when they disagree. $f(\mathcal{T}_x)$ represents a prior probability on $\mathcal{T}_x$ defined by a probability atlas [8]. We therefore can ignore f in the normalizing function Z with m being the number of voxels in the image

$$Z := \sum_{\mathcal{T}'} e^{\sum_x -\frac{1}{2}d(\mathcal{T}_x', \mathcal{H}_S(x))} = \prod_x \sum_{\mathcal{T}_x} e^{-\frac{1}{2}d(\mathcal{T}_x, \mathcal{H}_S(x))}$$

$$\overset{5}{=} \prod_x (1 + (N-1) \cdot e^{-1}) = (1 + (N-1) \cdot e^{-1})^m$$

If $p(\mathcal{T}_x|S) := (1 + (N-1) \cdot e^{-1})^{-1} \cdot e^{-\frac{1}{2}d(\mathcal{T}_x, \mathcal{H}_S(x))} \cdot f(\mathcal{T}_x)$ defines the local conditional probability than

$$p(\mathcal{T}|S) := (1 + (N-1) \cdot e^{-1})^{-m} \cdot e^{\sum_x -\frac{1}{2}d(\mathcal{T}_x, \mathcal{H}_S(x)) + \log(f(\mathcal{T}_x))} = \prod_x p(\mathcal{T}_x|S)$$

Estimating the Shape Parameters S

As mentioned in Section 2.1 statistical independence among the coefficients of $S = (S_1, \cdots, S_N)^T$ is assumed. Therefore, Equation (3) is solved for each component of S:

$$0 = \frac{\partial}{\partial S_i} E_{\mathcal{T}|\mathcal{I}, \mathcal{B}', S'} (\log p(S|\mathcal{T})) = \frac{\partial}{\partial S_i} E_{\mathcal{T}|\mathcal{I}, \mathcal{B}', S'} (\log p(\mathcal{T}|S) + \log p(S))$$

$$= \left(\sum_x \frac{\partial}{\partial S_i} (E_{\mathcal{T}_x|\mathcal{I}_x, \mathcal{B}_x', S'} (\log p(\mathcal{T}_x|S))) \right) + \log \frac{\partial}{\partial S_i} p(S) \tag{6}$$

$$= \sum_x E_{\mathcal{T}_x|\mathcal{I}_x, \mathcal{B}_x', S'} (\mathcal{T}_x)^T \frac{\partial}{\partial S_i} \log p(\mathcal{T}_x|S) - \Lambda_i^{-1} S_i$$

where $\frac{\partial}{\partial S_i} \log p(\mathcal{T}_x|S)$

$$= \frac{\partial}{\partial S_i} - \frac{1}{2}(\mathcal{T}_x - \mathcal{H}_S(x))^2 = \frac{\partial \mathcal{H}_S(x)}{\partial S_i}$$

$$\cdot (\mathcal{T}_x - \mathcal{H}_S(x)) \overset{6}{=} (\delta(\mathcal{D}_S(x))^T U_i(x)) \cdot (\mathcal{T}_x - \mathcal{H}_S(x))$$

$^5 \sum_{\mathcal{T}_x} e^{-\frac{1}{2}d(\mathcal{T}_x, \mathcal{H}_S(x))} = |\mathcal{H}_S(x)|^2 e^{-\frac{1}{2}(|\mathcal{H}_S(x)|^2 - 1)} + (N - |\mathcal{H}_S(x)|^2) e^{-\frac{1}{2}(|\mathcal{H}_S(x)|^2 + 1)}$. If we assume each voxel is part of only one shape then $|\mathcal{H}_S(x)| = 1$ and $\sum_{\mathcal{T}_x} e^{-\frac{1}{2}d(\mathcal{T}_x, \mathcal{H}_S(x))} = 1 + (N-1)e^{-1}$

is zero unless $\mathcal{T}_x(a) \neq \mathcal{H}_\mathcal{S}(a)$ for a structure a and voxel x is located at the border of the shape of a. Thus, if Ω is the set of voxels at the boundaries of $\mathcal{H}_\mathcal{S}$ Equation (6) simplifies to :

$$
\begin{aligned}
0 &= \left(\textstyle\sum_{x \in \Omega} E_{\mathcal{T}_x | \mathcal{I}_x, \mathcal{B}'_x, \mathcal{S}'}(\mathcal{T}_x)^T \cdot \left(\delta^0 (\mathcal{D}_\mathcal{S}(x))^T U_i(x)\right) \cdot (\mathcal{T}_x - \mathcal{H}_\mathcal{S}(x))\right) - \Lambda_i^{-1} \mathcal{S}_i \\
&= \left(\textstyle\sum_{x \in \Omega} W_x^T \cdot \left(\delta^0 (\mathcal{D}_\mathcal{S}(x))^T U_i(x)\right) \cdot (\mathcal{T}_x - \mathcal{H}_\mathcal{S}(x))\right) - \Lambda_i^{-1} \mathcal{S}_i \\
\Rightarrow \mathcal{S}_i &= \Lambda_i \cdot \textstyle\sum_{x \in \Omega} \left(\delta^0 (\mathcal{D}_\mathcal{S}(x))^T U_i(x)\right) \cdot W_x^T (\mathcal{T}_x - \mathcal{H}_\mathcal{S}(x))
\end{aligned}
$$

From the above equation the updated shape parameter $\mathcal{S}_i$ is defined by the weighted sum of its eigenvector values located at borders and scaled by the ith eigenvalue. In other words, the eigenvector values $U_i(x)$ defines the 'direction of change' for parameter $\mathcal{S}_i$ and the $W_x^T(\mathcal{T}_x - \mathcal{H}_\mathcal{S}(x))$ control the 'speed of change'.

2.3 The Shape Constraint EM Algorithm

The EM Algorithm is now defined by the E-Step who generates the structure posterior probabilities W, called *weights*, based on the constraints imposed by shape, intensity, image inhomogeneities, and location (see Equation (5))

$$
W_x(a) = \frac{p(\mathcal{I}_x | \mathcal{T}_x(a)=1, \mathcal{B}'_x) p(\mathcal{T}_x(a)=1 | \mathcal{S}')}{p(\mathcal{I}_x | \mathcal{B}'_x, \mathcal{S}')} = \frac{p(\mathcal{I}_x | \mathcal{T}_x(a)=1, \mathcal{B}'_x) p(\mathcal{T}_x(a)=1 | \mathcal{S}')}{\sum_{a'} p(\mathcal{I}_x | \mathcal{T}_x(a)=1, \mathcal{B}'_x) p(\mathcal{T}_x(a)=1 | \mathcal{S}')}
$$

The M-Step calculates the image inhomogeneities $\mathcal{B}$ and shape parameters $\mathcal{S}$ based on the newly updated weights W. $\mathcal{B} = H \cdot \bar{R}$ is approximated by a simple low pass filter H and the weighted residuum $\bar{R}_x = \sum_a W_x(a) \sigma_a^{-1}(\mathcal{I}_x - \mu_a)$ (see also [12]).

Table 1. Summary over 32 cases of the Dice comparison between the results of EM implementations and expert segmentations. The minimum and maximum list the worst and best Dice measure over all cases. As clearly by the numbers the new approach of this paper, EM-Shape, outperformed the other two methods

DICE Measure over 32 cases

Method	Mean	Variance	Minimum	Maximum
EM-Rigid	0.755	0.0221	0.449	0.883
EM-NonRigid	0.715	0.0149	0.34	0.883
EM-Shape	0.82	0.0117	0.625	0.909

---

[6] $\frac{\partial \mathcal{H}_\mathcal{S}(x,a)}{\partial \mathcal{S}_i} = \delta(\mathcal{D}_{\mathcal{S},a}(x)) \cdot \frac{\partial \mathcal{D}_{\mathcal{S},a}(x)}{\partial \mathcal{S}_i} = \delta(\mathcal{D}_{\mathcal{S},a}(x)) \cdot U_{a,i}(x)$ where δ is the Dirac's delta function and the Eigenvector matrix U_a was defined in Section 2.1

[7] where δ^0 is the null function with $\delta^0(0) = 1$, $\delta^0(x) = 0$ for $x \neq 0$, and $\delta^0(X) := (\delta^0(X(1)), \cdots, \delta^0(X(n)))^T$ for a vector X

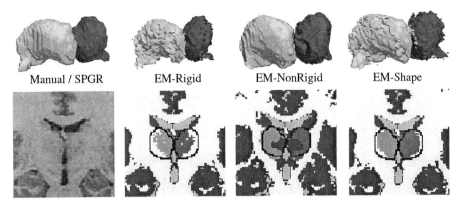

Manual / SPGR   EM-Rigid   EM-NonRigid   EM-Shape

Fig. 3. Segmentation results from different EM implementation. As clearly visible in the 2D images the shape constraint approach (EM-Shape) is closest to the expert's segmentation indicated by the black lines. EM-Shape was also the only method who properly captured the hypothalamus (see 3D models), while EM-NonRigid is too smooth and EM-Rigid underestimated the structure.

The shape parameters $\mathcal{S} = (\mathcal{S}_1, \cdots, \mathcal{S}_N)^T$ are updated in the M-Step by:

$$\mathcal{S}_i = \Lambda_i \cdot \sum_{x \in \Omega} \left(\delta^0(\mathcal{D}_\mathcal{S}(x))^T U_i(x) \right) \cdot \mathcal{W}_x^T (\mathcal{T}_x - \mathcal{H}_\mathcal{S}(x))$$

The EM algorithm iterates between E- and M-Step until the cost function $Q((\mathcal{B},\mathcal{S}),(\mathcal{B}',\mathcal{S}'))$ of Equation (1) converges to a local maximum, which is guaranteed by the EM framework if the iteration sequence has an upper bound [11].

3   Validation

We validate our approach by segmenting 32 test cases into white matter, grey matter, cortical spinal fluid, and the left and right thalamus. The study uses segmentations from one expert which are restricted to the right and left thalamus, which this study regards as gold standard. To introduce no bias into the segmentation approach we only generated shape atlases for those two structures (see also Section 2.1). The shape atlases are produced for each test case by applying PCA to the remaining 31 cases. From the analysis we use the first five modes of variations, which corresponds to 99% of the eigenvalues' energy. Furthermore, we manually calibrate the EM segmentations by comparing one automatic segmentation result to an expert's segmentation. Especially for structures like the thalamus, where borders are not clearly visible, large variations of the experts' opinion about structure's boundary exist. Therefore, this manual calibration is essential so that automatically generated results meet the experts' expectations. To measure the robustness of the method (EM-Shape) we compare the automatic with the expert segmentations using the volume overlap measure Dice [13]. We then compare the experts segmentations to the results of two different EM implementations. The first algorithm (EM-Rigid) uses rigid alignment of atlas information and no shape constraints. The second implementation (EM-NonRigid) also does not incorporate shape constraints but uses non-rigid registration for the initial alignment and models neighborhood relationships through Markov Random Field approximation [8].

Generally, EM-Shape outperformed the other two method (see also Table 1). It had the highest mean average value of agreement, the lowest variance, the highest minimum Dice measure over all cases, and the highest maximum dice measure. Of the three methods, EM-Shape relies the least on the initial registration of the atlas to the patient. The new shape constraints allow a better adjustment of the EM parameters to the specific brain images during the segmentation process. It can capture subtle difference in the shape as the hypothalamus which is underrepresented in both EM-Rigid and EM-NonRigid (see 3D images in Figure 3).

The EM-NonRigid heavily relies on the initial non-rigid registration. Even though it produced excellent results for the superior temporal gyrus [14], it performed worse on the thalamus, because the initial alignment process cannot detect the thalamus' weakly visible boundaries. It produces very smooth segmentations due to the Mean Field approximation which models neighborhood dependencies within an image. On the downside, it also smoothed over subtle differences within small gyri and the thalamus, which are better captured by EM-Shape and EM-Rigid.

4   Discussion

A novel shape constraint segmentation approach has been presented. Embedded in an EM segmentation framework, the algorithm deals with multiple brain structures as well as estimates the intensity inhomogeneities. It generates high quality segmentations of structures with weakly visible boundaries. The approach is not restricted to the modes of variations presented in the shape model but models patient specific abnormalities. Furthermore, we have documented its robustness by segmenting 30 different cases and comparing them to other EM-like methods as well as manual segmentations. In the future we would like to include more complex conditional probabilities that better model the dependencies between label maps and the shape of the object. We also would like to couple pose and labeling of the objects because their solution depend on each other.

Acknowledgments. This investigation was supported by a research grant from the Whitaker Foundation, by NIH grants (R21 MH67054, R01 LM007861, P41 RR13218, P01 CA67165) and by NSF ERC 8810-27499. We would like to thank Katherine Long, Florent Segonne, Lilla Zollei, Polina Golland, Samson Timoner, and Monica Vantoch for their valuable contributions to this paper.

References

1. M.E. Leventon, W.E.L. Grimson, O.D. Faugeras, "Statistical shape influence in geodesic active contours," in *CVPR*, pp. 1316 – 1323, 2000.
2. A. Tsai, A. Yezzi, W. Wells III, C. Tempany, D. Tucker, A. Fan, W. Grimson, A. Willsky, "A shape-based approach to the segmentation of medical imagery using level sets," *IEEE Transaction on Medical Imaging*, vol. 22, no. 2, pp. 137 – 154, 2003.
3. R. D. M. Rousson, N. Paragios, "Active shape models from a level set perspective," Tech. Rep. 4984, Institut National de Recherche en Informatique et en Automatique, Sophia-Antipolis, 2003. ftp://ftp.inria.fr/INRIA/publication/publi-pdf/RR/RR-4984.pdf.
4. T.F. Cootes, A. Hill, C.J. Taylor, J. Haslam, "The use of active shape models for locating structures in medical imaging," *Imaging and Vision Computing*, vol. 12, no. 6, pp. 335–366, 1994.

5. A. Kelemen, G. Szekely, G. Gerig, "Elastic model-based segmentation of 3-d neuroradiolog-ical data sets medical imaging," *IEEE Transactions on Medical Imaging*, vol. 18, pp. 828 – 839, 1999.
6. Stephen M. Pizer and Guido Gerig and Sarang Joshi and Stephen R. Aylward, "Multiscale medial shape-based analysis of image objects," in *Proceedings of the IEEE, Special Issue on: Emerging Medical Imaging Technology*, vol. 91, pp. 670 – 679, 2003.
7. Xenophon Papdemetris and Albert J. Sinusas and Donald P. Dione and R. Todd Constable and James S. Duncan, "Estimation of 3-d left ventricular deformation form medical images using biomechanical models," *IEEE Transactions on Medical Imaging*, vol. 21, pp. 786 – 800, 2002.
8. Kilian M. Pohl, Sylvain Bouix, Ron Kikinis, W. Eric L. Grimson, "Anatomical guided segmen-tation with non-stationary tissue class distributions in an expectation-maximization frame-work," in *ISBI*, pp. 81–84, 2004.
9. T.F. Cootes, G.J. Edwards, C.J. Taylor, "Active appearance model," in *ECCV*, vol. 2, pp. 484–498, 1998.
10. S. K. Warfield, J. Rexilius, P. S. Huppi, T. E. Inder, E. G. Miller, W. M. Wells, G. P. Zientara, F. A. Jolesz, R. Kikinis, "A binary entropy measure to assess nonrigid registration algorithm," in *MICCAI*, pp. 266–274, Oct. 2001.
11. Geoffrey J. McLachlan, Thriyambakam Krishnan, *The EM Algorithm and Extensions*. John Wiley and Sons, Inc., 1997.
12. W.M. Wells III, W.E.L Grimson, R. Kikinis, F.A Jolesz, "Adaptive segmentation of MRI data," *IEEE Transactions on Medical Imaging*, vol. 15, pp. 429–442, 1996.
13. L.R.Dice, "Measure of the amount of ecological association between species," *Ecology*, vol. 26, pp. 297–302, 1945.
14. K. M. Pohl and W. M. Wells and A. Guimond and K. Kasai and M. E. Shenton and R. Kikinis and W. E. L. Grimson and S. K. Warfield, "Incorporating non-rigid registration into expectation maximization algorithm to segment MR images," in *MICCAI*, pp. 564–572, 2002.

Image Segmentation Adapted for Clinical Settings by Combining Pattern Classification and Level Sets

S. Li, T. Fevens, and A. Krzyżak

Computer Science Department, Concordia University, Montréal, Québec, Canada
{shuo_li, fevens, krzyzak}@cs.concordia.ca

Abstract. An efficient clinical image segmentation framework is proposed by combining a pattern classifier, hierarchical and coupled level sets. The framework has two stages: training and segmentation. During training, first, representative images are segmented using hierarchical level set. Then the results are used to train a pattern classifier. During segmentation, first the image is classified by the trained classifier, and then coupled level set functions are used to further segment to get correct boundaries. The classifier provides an initial contour which is close to correct boundary for coupled level sets. This speeds up the convergence of coupled level sets. A hybrid coupled level set method which combines minimal variance functional and Laplacian edge detector is proposed. Experimental results show that by the proposed framework, we achieve accurate boundaries, with much faster convergence. This robust autonomous framework works efficiently in a clinical setting where there are limited types of medical images.

Keywords: Segmentation, variational level set, support vector machine, variational methods, energy minimization, Bayesian decision.

1 Introduction

Image segmentation has always been a critical component in medical imagery since it assists in medical diagnoses. It is more challenging compared to other imaging fields. This is primarily due to the large variability in topologies, complexity of medical structures, several kinds of artifacts and restrictive scanning methods. This is especially true for volumetric medical images where a large amount of data is coupled with complicated 3D medical structures.

One of latest techniques in segmentation is based on the class of deformable models, referred as "level set" or "geodesic active contours/surfaces." The application of the level set in medical image segmentation became extremely popular because of its ability to capture the topology of shapes in medical imagery. There are some related works that have been proposed mainly for two-dimensional segmentation. Codimension-two geodesic active contours were used in [10] for the segmentation of tubular structures. The fast marching algorithm [11] and level set method were used in [7] and [14], while Region competition, introduced in [17], was used in [2]. In [2] and[15], Chan and Vese proposed a method using the Mumford-Shah model for both

C. Barillot, D.R. Haynor, and P. Hellier (Eds.): MICCAI 2004, LNCS 3216, pp. 160–167, 2004.
© Springer-Verlag Berlin Heidelberg 2004

two dimensional and volumetric segmentation. Later a hierarchical scheme was used to extend this method to segment multiple regions [14]. Very recently Michal et al [6] proposed a hierarchical volumetric segmentation which combines Chan and Vese method and geodesic active contour [1] with edge alignment for volumetric segmentation. To apply level set methods to real time applications, LeFohn [8] has translated level set techniques to graphic cards and run in nearly real time.

Although efficient, level sets are not suitable for clinical segmentation due to several reasons: (1) high computational cost; (2) complicated parameter settings; (3) sensitivity to the placement of initial contours. With regard to the latter, as will be shown in experimental results, the running time of level set method heavily relies on the position and size of initial curves and complexity of objects. Moreover for some cases, coupled level set do not converge for some initial curves. This paper reports the efforts to overcome the above problems by combining pattern classifier and level sets as a continuation of work reported in [9]. The approach takes the strength of classifier, hierarchical and coupled level set segmentation. In this framework, clinical segmentation is divided into three steps. First, sample images or representative slices of volumetric images are segmented by the hierarchical level set segmentation method. The hierarchical method allows the detection of multiple objects in an image while limiting the complexity of the computation. Then these results are used to train the pattern classifier. We choose support vector machine (SVM) which is widely used in pattern recognition. Therefore the segmentation problem is expressed as a classification problem temporarily. Since medical images usually contain a large amount of redundant information for classification, to accelerate the segmentation by SVM, an information reduction scheme [9] is used. Although SVM training takes some time, once the SVM is trained, we can use it to segment the image whenever we want. Finally, coupled level sets are used to represent multiple objects. The evolution of these level set curves will give a final fine segmentation. A hybrid coupled level sets segmentation algorithm combining Samson's algorithm [12], optimal edge integrator [7] and geodesic active contour model is also proposed. Although the second stage only gives a coarse result, it helps the coupled level set curves by finding good initial curves. Therefore it takes much less time for the coupled curves to converge. By above framework, with the help of SVM, we naturally combined hierarchical and coupled level set to achieve a fast and robust autonomous medical image segmentation framework for clinical setting. An error analysis model is also proposed to analyze and compare hierarchical and coupled level sets.

2   Segmentation Methods: Variational Approach

Minimal Variance Functional. Due to its simplicity and efficiency, minimal variance is widely used in variational level set methods [2, 12 and 15]. In our framework, two minimal variance based level set methods will be combined. A brief introduction is given below. To focus our discussion, regularity terms will be ignored. In [2], Chan and Vese proposed a variational level set approach based on minimal variance and

Mumford-Shah functional described as following. Given a two-dimensional gray level image, $I(x,y): \Omega \rightarrow R^+$.

$$E(C, c_1, c_2) = \iint_{\Omega_c} (I - c_1)^2 dxdy + \iint_{\Omega \backslash \Omega_c} (I - c_2)^2 dxdy \ , \tag{1}$$

where C is the active contour which separates the image into interior and exterior parts respectively. And c_1 and c_2 are the means of interior and exterior parts of C.

Samon [12] proposed a similar minimal variance functional for coupled level sets. Assume there are K regions; the proposed method used K level set functions ϕ_i ($i \in [1,k]$) to represent each of them as

$$E_{coupled}(\phi_1, \ldots, \phi_k) = \sum_{i=1}^{K} e_i \int_{\Omega} H_\alpha(\phi_i)(I - c_i)^2 / \sigma_i^2 dxdy \ , \forall i, \alpha_i \in \mathbb{R}., \tag{2}$$

where H_α is the Heaviside function, c_i and σ_i are mean and covariance of positive areas in level set function ϕ_i.

Hierarchical versus coupled. Level set methods naturally divide an image into two regions. Therefore it is very efficient at extracting one object in an image consisting of several disconnected pieces. In order to extract multiple objects, people normally use hierarchical methods [5, 12] or coupled level set methods [15, 16, 17]. Although straightforward and fast, hierarchical segmentations simply assume a single mean inside and outside of zero level. So for multiple objects detection, it tends to be less accurate than coupled level sets. As a result the boundaries may not be optimal. A detailed error analysis is performed and shown in section 2. Coupled level set on the other hand uses one level set function to represent each object. But it is not only slow but it also suffered from the problem of placement of initial curve, a common problem that exists in numerical minimization when functions are non-convex the numerical results may depend on the choice of the initial curves [6, 15].

Error Analysis with Bayes model. Although hierarchical level set segmentation is widely used in segmentation, the accuracy of the obtained boundaries is unknown. In the following, a Bayes model is proposed to analysis the results. A simulation on energy minimization for hierarchical and coupled level set is performed and compared. In this simulation, data is randomly generated with given means and covariance. We use Bayes decision to calculate the correct decision boundary and benchmark with the decision boundary calculated by the energy minimization. The error measurements are defined in eq. 3. The correct decision boundary is calculated using Bayesian decision approach.

Fig. 1(a) shows that when there are two classes in the image, energy minimization is able to get perfect decision boundary which is almost the same as Bayesian decision boundary. However when there are more than two classes, hierarchical scheme will introduce more error as shown in Fig. 1(b). Moreover the energy curve in Fig. 1(b) is not very sharp around the global minima which means that numerical algorithm may not converge to global minimum. Fig. 2 shows energy surface of eq. 3. The error is much lower than with hierarchical level sets. From above we can conclude that coupled level sets tend to find more accurate decision boundaries than those for hierarchical level sets when there are more than two classes in the image.

1. $E_c(w_1, w_2) = \int_0^{w1}(I - \mu_{left})dx + \int_{w1}^{w2}(I - \mu_{middle})dx + \int_{w2}^{max}(I - \mu_{right})dx$.

$E_h(w) = \int_0^w (I - \mu_{left})dx + \int_w^{max}(I - \mu_{right})dx$, w_i are decision boundaries. \hfill (3)

2. Normalized energy $E(x) = E(x)/N$ where N is the total number of pixels.

3. e_1 = misclassed pixels/total pixels;

   e_2 = misclassed pixels/pixels of two classes

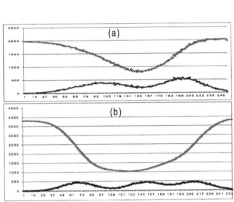

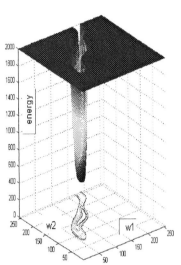

Fig. 1. Energy minimization and Bayesian boundary. Top curve: energy curve E_n or E_c. Bottom curve: histogram of the image. (a) Two regions case: first decision boundary by hierarchical energy minimization ($e_1 = 0.0020$; $e_2 = 0.0020$). (b) Three regions case: first decision boundary calculated by hierarchical energy minimization ($e_1 = 0.0607$; $e_2 = 0.0911$).

Fig. 2. Energy minimization and Bayesian boundary using energy function $E_c (e_1 = 0.0207$; $e_2 = 0.0411)$.

3 Proposed Framework

The proposed framework has two stages: a training stage and a segmentation stage. In the training stage, first, representative images are segmented using hierarchical level set region detection. Then the results are used to train a SVM classifier. In segmentation stage, first images are classified by the trained SVM, and then coupled level set functions are used to further segment the images to get accurate boundaries.

Hierarchical region detection. First hierarchical level set described in section 2.1 is used to detect hierarchically how many regions inside of representative images. The energy function we use is shown in eq. 1. Level set formula is given in [2].

Optimal SVM training and segmentation. Due to the fact that level set normally takes long time to segment the image, to adapt it to clinical applications, recently researchers [9, 4] are working on initializing a level set segmentation with an approximated segmentation from another method to get a more time-efficient method. In [4], Chen *et al.* initialize level set with marching cube method. In [9], Li *et al.* initialize level set with a trained SVM in volumetric image and clinical images. In current application, we adapt the SVM based initialization proposed in [11, 12].

The results obtained from hierarchical region detection are input into SVM. A window based feature extraction is used to extract features from the regions segmented by hierarchical level set segmentation. The SVM classifier we use is modified from [3]. To accelerate the segmentation by SVM, an information reduction is used [9]. For segmentation we only need to compute 3% of the total pixels since rest of the 97% are the repetition of the 3%.

Hybrid Coupled Level Sets Segmentation. SVM classification naturally provides a novel initial contour for coupled level sets. We use one level set function to represent one region. Since boundary segmented by SVM is close to the correct boundary, a hybrid coupled level sets segmentation algorithm combining Samson's algorithm [12], optimal edge integrator [7] and geodesic active contour model are proposed as shown in eq. 4. A similar functional is used in [1] for a single level set function.

$$E = -\gamma_1 E_{Edge} + \gamma_2 E_{Coupled} + \gamma_3 E_{GAC} , \tag{4}$$

where γ_i are constants and geodesic active contour (E_{GAC}) is defined as $E_{GAC} = \iint g(S) dS$ where $g(S)$ is an inverse edge indicator function. As suggested in [1], we use $g(S) = \alpha^2/(\alpha^2 + |\nabla I|^2)$, where α is a constant. E_{Edge} is the functional proposed in [7] where Kimmel shows that the Laplacian edge detector ΔI provides optimal edge integration with regard to a very natural geometric functional as shown in eq. 5.

$$E_{Edge}(S) = \int \int_S \langle \nabla I, \mathbf{n} \rangle da - \int \int_{\Omega_s} K_I |\nabla I| dxdy , \tag{5}$$

where S is the evolving contour, K_I is the mean curvature of level sets, $\mathbf{n}$ is the unit vector to the curve and da is the surface area element.

Eq.6 shows the level set function we use. In eq.6, $\phi: \Omega \to R^+$ is Lipschitz continuous function, δ_a is the direct delta function, $I_{\xi\xi} = \Delta I - K_I|\nabla I|$ and β is a constant.

$$\frac{\phi_i^{t+1} - \phi_i^t}{\Delta t \cdot \delta_\alpha(\phi_i^t)} = \left[\gamma_3 div\left(g\frac{\nabla\phi_i}{|\nabla\phi_i|} \right) - \gamma_2 e_i \frac{(u_0 - c_i)^2}{\sigma^2} - \beta \frac{\left(\sum_{i=1}^{K} H_\alpha(\phi_i) - 1 \right)^2}{(u_0 - c_i)^2} - \gamma_1 I_{\xi\xi} \right] . \tag{6}$$

Confidence map. To measure the confidence of the segmentation, a confidence measurement is proposed: $\psi(x,y) = max(H_\alpha(\phi_i)/\Sigma|H_\alpha(\phi_i)|)$. The larger the value of $\psi(x,y)$, the higher the confidence of the data segmented.

4 Experiments

First, some experiments were done to show the final results and computational time of the level set in terms of the number of iterations to convergence could heavily rely on position and size of initial curve and complexity of the object. The level set algorithm is described in section 3.1. Then different two-dimensional and volumetric images are used to test the framework we proposed.

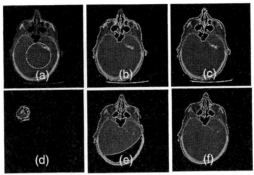

Fig. 3. Challenging nose. (a) Iteration 0. (b) Iteration 150. (c) Iteration 350. (d) Iteration 0. (e) Iteration 600. (f) Iteration 1200.

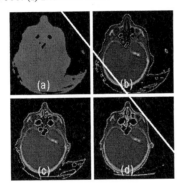

Fig. 4. Comparison of level set (b, c, and d) and SVM based segmentation (a). (a) SVM based. (b) Iteration 0. (c) Iteration 5. (d) Iteration 15.

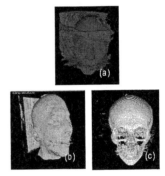

Fig. 5. Volumetric segmentation results. (a) Volumetric segmentation by SVM. (b) Volumetric segmentation by hierarchical level set. (c) Internal part (skull) rendering.

As can be seen from Figs. 3 (a) to (c), the majority of the objects are segmented in the first 150 iterations while it takes another 200 iterations to segment only the nose. It is very difficult for the user to set appropriate stopping conditions, since from iteration 150 to iteration 350, each iteration only causes a few pixel changes. Therefore a too relaxed stopping term will not able to stop the iterations while a strict stopping condition will stop the iteration before it is correctly segmented. The images here are obtained from CT head volumetric data set of Stanford. Figs. 3(d) to (f) show those iterations when different size and position of the initial curve are used. To segment the same image, the iteration used varies a lot when different positions and sizes of initial curves are used. It becomes even worse when complicated structure encountered. Fig. 4 shows the comparison between the level set and SVM based segmentation. As shown in Fig.4(c) the boundary find by SVM is not very accurate. Comparison of Fig. 3(c) and Fig. 4(d) shows that SVM is able to greatly accelerate level set segmentation. Previously 350 iterations are needed while 15 iterations are sufficient now. Figs. 5 and 6 show another two volumetric segmentation results. Fig. 7 gives results of coupled level sets and confidence map (fig. 7(d)). The brightness in the image indicates the confidence of the segmentation. The brighter the data, the more confident the segmentation is. Confidence map shows, as expected, that the boundary parts have lower confidence.

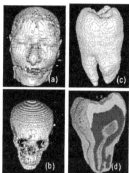

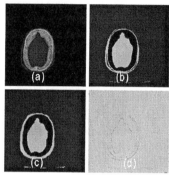

Fig. 6. Volumetric segmentation of another CT head and tooth. (a) The external part of the head. (b) Internal part of the head. (c) External part of tooth. (d) Internal part of the tooth.

Fig. 7. Coupled level sets. (a) Original image. (b) Iteration 0. (c) Iteration 20. (d) Confidence map calculated.

5   Conclusion

In this paper, we first propose a Bayesian model to analyze the error in hierarchal level set and coupled level sets. The error analysis shows that coupled level sets are able to converge to more accurate boundaries even thought it takes much longer time to converge. Based on that analysis, an image processing approach adapted to the clinical setting is proposed and implemented. With the aid of techniques from the field of pattern recognition, we naturally combined hierarchical with coupled level set to achieve a fast and robust autonomous image segmentation framework for clinical initialization where the complicated setting for level sets can be transparent to user. The framework is not only able to achieve fast segmentation, but is also able to give more accurate boundary. To help the clinical physician to evaluate the segmentation results, a confidence map is computed. Two dimensional and volumetric images were used to test the framework. The experimental results are very promising. This framework works efficiently in a clinical setting where a specialist works with limited types of medical images. The classifiers need to be trained only once with representative images or slices segmented by hierarchical level set. The clinical physician just needs to indicate the classifier the image type. As a continuation of the work in this paper, we are currently implementing a real time segmentation system for selected types of clinical images.

References

1. V. Casseles, R. Kimmel, and G. Sapiro. Geodesic active contours. *International Journal of Computer Vision*, 22(1):61-79, 1997.
2. T. Chan and L. Vese. Active contour model without edges. *IEEE Trans. Image Processing*, vol. 24, 10(2):266-277, 2001.
3. C.-C. Chang and C.-J. Lin. Training nu-support vector classifiers: theory and algorithms. *Neural Computation* 13(9):2119-2147, 2001.
4. T. Chen and D. N. Metaxas. Gibbs prior models, marching cubes, and deformable models: a hybrid framework for 3D medical image segmentation, *Proc. MICCAI*, 703-710. 2003.
5. T. Deschamps. Curve and shape extraction with minimal path and level set techniques. Applications to 3D medical imaging. PHD thesis. University of Paris Daphine, 2001.
6. M. Holtzman-Gazit, D. Goldsher, and R. Kimmel. Hierarchical segmentation of thin structure in volumetric medical images. In *Proc. MICCAI*, 562-569, 2003.
7. R. Kimmel and A. M. Bruckstein. Regularized laplacian zero crossings as optimal edge integrators. *International Journal of Computer Vision,* 53(3):225-243, 2003.
8. A.E. Lefohn, J.E. Cates, and R.T. Whitaker. Interactive, GPU-Based Level Sets for 3D Segmentation, in *Proc. MICCAI*, 564-572. 2003.
9. S. Li, T. Fevens, and A. Krzyżak. An SVM based framework for autonomous volumetric medical image segmentation using hierarchical and coupled level sets. *Proc. of Computer Aided Radiology and Surgery(CARS)*, 2004.
10. L. M. Lorigo, O. Faugeras, W. Grimson, R. Keriven, R. Kikinis, C.F. Westin, and Ayra Nabavi. Codimention-two geodesic active contours for the segmentation of tubular structures. *Proc. of Computer vision and pattern recognition*, 2000.
11. S. Osher and J. Sethian. Fronts propagating with curvature-dependent speed: algorithms based on Hamiltons–Jacobi formulations. *J. Comput. Phys.*, 79(1):12–49, 1988.
12. C. Samson, L. Blanc-Feraud, G. Aubert, and J. Zerubia. A level set model for image classification. *International Journal of Computer Vision,* 40(3):187–197, 2000.
13. A. Tsai, A. Yezzi, and A. S. Willsky. Curve evolution implementation of the Mumford-Shah functional for image segmentation, denoising, interpolation, and magnification. *IEEE Trans. Image Processing,* 10:1169 -1186, 2001.
14. A. Vasilevskiy and K. Siddiqi. Flux maximizing geometric flow. *IEEE Trans. Pattern Anal. Machine Intel.* , 24(12):1565-1578, December 2002.
15. L. Vese and T. Chan. A Multiphase Level Set Framework for Image Segmentation Using the Mumford and Shah Model. *Intern. Journal of Computer Vision*, 50(3):271-293, 2002.
16. X. Zeng, L. H. Staib, R. T. Schultz, and J. S. Duncan. Segmentation and measurement of the cortex from 3-D MR images using coupled surfaces propagation. *IEEE Trans. Med. Imag.*, 18: 927–937, Sept. 1999.
17. H. K. Zhao, T. Chan, B. Merriman, and S. Osher. A variational level set approach to multiphase motion. *J. Comput. Phys.*, 127:179-195. 1996.
18. S. Zhu and A. Yuille. Region competition: Unifying snakes, region growing, energy/Bayes/MDL for multi-band image segmentation. *IEEE Trans. Pattern Anal. Machine Intel.*, 19(9): 884-900, 1996.

Shape Particle Filtering for Image Segmentation

Marleen de Bruijne and Mads Nielsen

IT University of Copenhagen, Denmark

Abstract. Deformable template models are valuable tools in medical image segmentation. Current methods elegantly incorporate global shape and appearance, but can not cope with localized appearance variations and rely on an assumption of Gaussian gray value distribution. Furthermore, initialization near the optimal solution is required.

We propose a maximum likelihood shape inference that is based on pixel classification, so that local and non-linear intensity variations are dealt with naturally, while a global shape model ensures a consistent segmentation. Optimization by stochastic sampling removes the need for accurate initialization.

The method is demonstrated on three different medical image segmentation problems: vertebra segmentation in spine radiographs, lung field segmentation in thorax X rays, and delineation of the myocardium of the left ventricle in MRI slices. Accurate results were obtained in all tasks.

1 Introduction

Statistical models of global object appearance are widely used for image segmentation [7, 13,12], and form powerful tools especially in the case of missing or locally ambiguous boundary evidence.

However, entirely global models can be too constrained to adhere to new images adequately. Intensity variations occurring at random locations within an object, such as for example calcification or lesions, can not be captured in a global appearance model and will impair the model fit. To keep model complexity within bounds usually a simple linear model of appearance is applied and thus results are unreliable if the image gray values are not Gaussian distributed. Linear models of object appearance were shown to fail in many medical image segmentation tasks [18,9,4,14]. Another drawback of current deformable model approaches it that they require initialization near the final solution, and thus need manual intervention [9,16] or automatic object recognition [5,20].

Suggested solutions for region segmentation of images with a non-linear appearance are based on non-linear filtering or normalization of the images before applying the appearance model [4,14]. This overcomes some of the problems related to non-Gaussian distributed gray values, but the application to different types of distributions is still rather limited. In edge-based segmentation, non-linear appearance has been modeled as a mixture of Gaussians [5], or by using non-parametric classifiers to discriminate between object and background pixels [18] or between boundary and non-boundary pixels [9]. The classifier-based approaches can cope with arbitrary gray value distributions but can not directly be extended to a region appearance model due to the computational complexity and the amount of data needed.

C. Barillot, D.R. Haynor, and P. Hellier (Eds.): MICCAI 2004, LNCS 3216, pp. 168–175, 2004.

On the other hand, performance of pixel classification methods was shown to improve by adding global information, for instance in the form of spatially varying priors obtained from digital atlases [19]. These methods rely on the (rigid or elastic) matching of an atlas to the image, and therefore requires the image appearance to be fairly consistent in the entire image.

We propose a shape model inference on the basis of pixel classification. Localized intensity variations are thus dealt with naturally, while the global shape model ensures a consistent segmentation. By applying a non-parametric classifier we will be able to cope with arbitrary gray value distributions. We show that the maximum likelihood solution can be found using iterated likelihood weighing, which can be implemented using a particle filtering scheme such as are often used in object tracking (see for instance [11]). This makes the segmentation result relatively independent of the initialization, guarantees convergence provided that enough samples are used, and allows for straightforward extension to multi-modal shape models or multiple solutions.

2   Maximum Likelihood Shape Inference

Several different schemes for efficient optimization of shape models or combined models of shape and appearance have been proposed, usually resulting in a local maximum likelihood or maximum a posteriori (MAP) estimate. In this work, we will estimate the maximum likelihood rather than the MAP solution, since the latter has an inherent bias towards the local mode of the prior.

In the following we will prove that a maximum likelihood estimate of the shape may be obtained through an iterated likelihood weighing that may simply be implemented by a particle filtering scheme. We will show global convergence to the global maximum.

Theorem 1 (Maximum likelihood convergence). *The maximum of $P(I|S)^t P(S)$ converges to the maximum of $P(I|S)$ for any $P(S)|\forall S, P(S) > 0$, and $S \in \mathcal{B}$, where $\mathcal{B}$ is a separable Banach space endowed with a weak (or strong) topology.*

Proof. Let us define

$$f_t(S) = (P(I|S)^t P(S))^{1/t}$$

Since $f_t(S)$ is just a monotonic transformation of $P(I|S)^t P(S)$ it has the same properties of extrema, and we may examine f_t instead. Since f_t converges to $P(I|S)$ uniformly (remember $P(S) > 0$), it also Γ-converges to $P(I|S)$ ([3] page 35, Theorem 2.1.8). Since Γ-convergence is obtained,

$$\lim_{t \to \infty} \arg\max_S f_t(S) = \arg\max_S P(I|S)$$

([3] page 34, Theorem 2.1.7)

Hence we have proved that the maximum likelihood shape may be obtained as the maximum of $P(I|S)^t P(S)$ as t approaches infinity. Let us define

$$L_t(S) = \frac{P(I|S)^t P(S)}{Z_t}$$

where $Z_t = \int P(I|S)^t P(S) dS$. As t tends to infinity $L_t(S) \rightarrow \sum_i a_i \delta(S_i)$, where δ is the Dirac delta functional, a_i are positive constants summing to 1, and S_i is the shapes taking the global maximum value $P(I|S)$. Especially in the case where $P(I|S)$ has a unique maximum, Z_t tends to a single $\delta(S_0)$, where S_0 is the maximum likelihood estimate.

Hence we have shown that samples of $L_t(S)$ with probability 1 tends to the maximum likelihood estimate of S.

Notice that the above arguments could have been made simpler if S belongs to a normed space with a strong topology (like R^N). However, the above results are valid for shapes defined as points in Kendall's shape space, closed curves, surfaces in 3D, functions of bounded variation on the real plane, etc. That is, any shape representation living in a Banach space (a complete normed linear space) equipped with a weak or strong topology.

2.1   Shape Particle Filtering

As shown, iterated likelihood weighing of a shape distribution leads to the maximum likelihood shape solution. We will implement this using a particle filtering scheme [10]. It must be noted, that the argumentation in the previous section holds in the continuous domain; in a discretized shape space and within a finite evolution time the maximum likelihood solution may not be reached. However, using a sufficiently dense sampling of the shape distribution and a sufficiently slow evolution, the algorithm will converge.

We will use a shape model derived from hand annotated examples for $P(S)$, and estimate the likelihood $P(I|S)$ using pixel classification. Within this framework, any kind of shape model, any set of local image descriptors and any classifier can be used.

Shape Model. The object shape and shape variation are described using a point distribution model (PDM) [8]. Shapes are defined by the coordinates of a set of landmark points which correspond between different shape instances. Each shape can be approximated by a linear combination of the mean shape and several modes of shape variation which describe a joint displacement of all landmarks. The modes of variation are given by the principal components of a collection of aligned example shapes. Usually only a small number of components is needed to capture most of the variation in the training set.

Image term. Each shape has associated with it a labeling that divides the image pixels into two or more classes, for example inside and outside an object. A pixel classifier is trained to distinguish between pixels of different classes on the basis of local image descriptors. We have chosen a general scheme in which pixels are described by the outputs of a set of Gaussian derivative filters at multiple scales, and a k-NN classifier is used for probability estimation.

We use a moderated k-NN classifier by which the posterior probability of a pixel with feature vector $\mathbf{x}$ belonging to class ω is given by

$$P(\omega|\mathbf{x}) = \frac{k_\omega + 1}{k + m},$$

where k_ω among the k nearest neighbors belong to class ω, and m is the number of classes [1]. The moderation with respect to a standard k-NN classifier with $P(\omega|\mathbf{x}) = k_\omega/k$ ensures that probabilities are always nonzero for finite k, thus avoiding a 'veto-effect' if probabilities of separate pixels are multiplied.

Pixel intensities are assumed to be conditionally independent on the class label, and the likelihood of a shape template is thus given by the product of separate pixel likelihoods. Particle weights are then defined as

$$w_i = \exp\left[\frac{c}{n} \sum_{j=1}^{n} \log P(\mathbf{x}_j|\omega_{s_i})\right], \tag{1}$$

where c is a constant which controls the randomness of the sampling process, n is the number of pixels in the template, and $P(\mathbf{x}_j|\omega_{s_i})$ is the likelihood term for the observed pixel feature vector $\mathbf{x}_j$ given the implied label ω_{s_i}.

Particle Filtering. A random set of N shape hypotheses — 'particles' — s_i is sampled from the prior shape-and-pose model. Each hypothesis has an associated image labeling, which is compared to the label probability map as obtained from the initial pixel classification. Particles are weighed by their likelihood term and a new set of N hypotheses is generated from the current set by random sampling proportionally to these weights. In this way, particles representing unlikely shapes vanish while successful particles multiply. After a small random perturbation of duplicate particles, the process of importance resampling is repeated. The initial sparse sampling eventually evolves into a δ-peak at the maximum likelihood solution.

In practice, the solution may be approximated by the strongest local mode of the particle distribution before the process has converged. The local modes can be efficiently obtained using the mean shift algorithm [6].

3   Experiments

Cross-validation experiments are performed on spine and thorax radiographs and on short-axis cardiac MRI slices. Examples of each of these image types, with the desired segmentation, are given in Fig. 1(a-b).

The spine data set contains 91 lateral spine radiographs of both healthy and fractured vertebrae, in which the vertebrae L1 through L4 are delineated manually. Image sizes are ca. 210×505 pixels. Shape models are constructed by equidistant sampling along the contours of each of the vertebrae. A set of cross-validation experiments is performed in which each time the method is trained on 84 images and tested on the remaining 7.

The lung data set contains 30 digitized posterior-anterior chest radiographs of size 512×512, taken from the publicly available JSRT (Japanese Society of Radiological Technology) database [15]. Both lung fields have been delineated manually by two observers. Shape models are constructed by equidistant sampling of each lung, starting from the outer and lower corner. The left and right lungs are modeled independently. Leave-one-out experiments are performed.

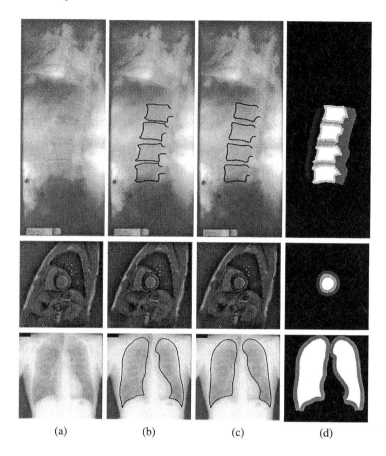

(a)   (b)   (c)   (d)

Fig. 1. Example images from each data set. Top row: spine X ray; middle row: cardiac MRI; bottom row: thorax X ray. (a) Normalized image; (b) Manual segmentation; (c) Automatic segmentation using shape particle filtering; (d) Label template used.

The cardiac data set was made publicly available by M.B. Stegmann [17] and consists of 14 short-axis, end-diastolic cardiac MRI slices of size 256×256 with manually placed landmarks on the epicardial and endocardial contours. Leave-one-out experiments are performed.

All images have been normalized to zero mean and unit variance prior to processing, using a global normalization for the X rays, and for the MR images a Gaussian local normalization according to $\bar{L} = (L - L_\sigma)/\sqrt{(L^2)_\sigma - (L_\sigma)^2}$, where L_σ is the image L convolved with a Gaussian kernel of width σ (σ=16 pixels).

3.1 Settings

The parameter settings used for pixel classification were the same for all experiments: Features include the original image and the derivatives up to the third order computed

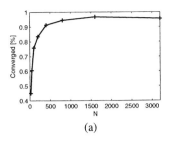

	N	mean	stdev	max
Spine	1600	1.4	0.4	3.1
Cardiac	1000	1.1	0.3	1.9
Left lung	2000	4.4	2.0	12
Right lung	2000	3.8	1.5	9.8
Left lung, 2nd observer		3.6	3.8	23
Right lung 2nd observer		3.0	1.7	8.4

(a)   (b)

Fig. 2. (a) Percentage of spine segmentations converged with an average error below 2 mm, as a function of the number of particles in the distribution N. (b) Average point-to-contour segmentation errors in pixels.

at a scale of 1, 2, 4, and 8 pixels, resulting in a 41 dimensional feature space. The set of samples is normalized to unit variance for each feature, and k-NN classification is performed with an approximate k-NN classifier [2] with k=25.

For each task, class templates have been defined from the manually drawn contours. For lung and heart segmentation, this is simply the interior of the contour, and a border on the outside. In the spine data one can, on the basis of the shape alone, make a distinction between parts of the image with a different appearance, without requiring additional annotation. We have defined a template with five separate image regions: anterior background, posterior background, inter vertebral space, vertebra boundary and vertebra interior (see Fig. 1(d)).

Apart from N, the number of shape particles used in the process, all particle filtering parameters are equal in all experiments. The noise added to duplicates in the particle filtering process is of standard deviation $\sigma_d = 0.05\,\sigma$, with σ the standard deviation of the prior shape model. Iteration stops if the change in the maximum local mode of the shape distribution, computed using mean shift filtering with a kernel of size $0.05\,\sigma$, becomes negligibly small. The constant c, determining the speed of convergence according to Eq. 1, is set to 50.

3.2   Results

Examples of segmentations obtained are given in Fig. 1(c). Segmentation accuracy is evaluated by the mean point-to-contour distance with respect to the manual outlines Fig. 2(a) shows performance of vertebra segmentation for particle distributions of varying size. Results for a fixed number of particles and for all three data sets are listed in Fig. 2(b). In the case of vertebra segmentation, where the model describes only a part of the entire spine, a shape instance shifted one or more vertebra heights upwards or downwards with respect to the manual segmentation can also represent accurate vertebra segmentations. We allow the model to shift one vertebra and report the errors of the three overlapping vertebrae.

4 Discussion and Conclusion

The obtained accuracy of vertebra segmentation is close to the maximum accuracy that can be expected with the given shape model, and results are likely to improve if higher resolution images, a higher dimensional shape model, and more training images are used. Nevertheless, the results are competitive with results described in the literature. Zamora et al. reported success rates of 50% with average errors below 6.4 mm in active shape model (ASM) segmentation of lumbar vertebrae in spine radiographs [20]. Smyth et al. performed ASM segmentation of vertebrae in dual energy X ray absorptiometry (DXA) images [16] and obtained success rates of 94 – 98%, with errors in the order of 1 mm for healthy vertebra and success rates of 85 – 98% with errors in the order of 2 mm for fractured vertebrae. Scott et al. reported successful convergence of a modified active appearance model (AAM) in 92% of DXA scans of healthy spines with an average error of ca. 1.5 mm [14].

Segmentation of cardiac MRI is a task where linear AAMs have been shown to perform well. Stegmann et al. [17] reported point-to-contour errors of basic AAM of 1.18 (max 2.43), on the same data set. If a border of background appearance was added to the model, which usually improves segmentation performance, the mean error increased to 1.73. The mean errors obtained using shape particle filtering, with a border around the template, are comparable to those of the basic AAM (1.1 ± 0.3, max 1.9). Without a border we obtained similar errors (1.2 ± 0.3, max 2.1), which indicates that our method is less sensitive than AAM to the large variation in intensity of tissue surrounding the left ventricle, even though these different tissues end up in the same class of 'background tissue'.

The errors for lung field segmentation are a little larger than those of the other two tasks, but inter observer variation is also large in these images. It must be noted that the placement of landmarks, equidistantly along the contour with only one specific corresponding point, is far from optimal in this case and an optimization of landmark positioning will likely improve segmentation results.

The use of a large number of hypotheses makes segmentation by shape particle filtering robust to local maxima and independent of initialization. An additional advantage of particle filters, not employed in this work, is their ability to represent multiple solutions simultaneously. This could for instance be used to segment the entire spine with only a partial spine model. Furthermore, possible multimodal shape distributions would be dealt with naturally.

To conclude, we propose a robust and general method for the segmentation of images with localized or non-linear gray value variations.

Acknowledgements. The authors would like to thank L. Tánko and C. Christiansen of the Center for Clinical and Basic Research (CCBR A/S), Denmark, J.C. Nilsson and B.A. Grønning of the Danish Research Center for Magnetic Resonance (DCRMR), M.B. Stegmann of the Technical University of Denmark and B. van Ginneken and M. Loog of the Image Sciences Institute, Utrecht, The Netherlands, for providing the data sets and manual segmentations used in this study.

References

1. F.M. Alkoot and J. Kittler. Moderating k-NN classifiers. *Pattern Analysis & Applications*, 5(3):326–332, 2002.
2. S. Arya, D.M. Mount, N.S. Netanyahu, R. Silverman, and A.Y. Wu. An optimal algorithm for approximate nearest neighbor searching. *Journal of the ACM*, (45):891–923, 1998.
3. Gilles Aubert and Pierre Kornprobst. *Mathematical problems in image processing*, volume 147 of *Applied Mathematical Sciences*. Springer Verlag, 2002.
4. H.G. Bosch, S.C. Mitchell, B.P.F. Lelieveldt, F. Nijland, O. Kamp, M. Sonka, and J.H.C. Reiber. Active appearance-motion models for endocardial contour detection in time sequences of echocardiograms. In *Med Imaging: Image Process*, volume 4322 of *Proc of SPIE*. SPIE Press, 2001.
5. M. Brejl and M. Sonka. Object localization and border detection criteria design in edge-based image segmentation: automated learning from examples. *IEEE Trans Med Imaging*, 19(10):973–985, 2000.
6. D. Comaniciu and P. Meer. Mean shift: A robust approach toward feature space analysis. *IEEE TPAMI*, 24(5):603–619, 2002.
7. T.F. Cootes, G.J. Edwards, and C.J. Taylor. Active appearance models. *IEEE TPAMI*, 23(6):681–684, 2001.
8. T.F. Cootes, C.J. Taylor, D.H. Cooper, and J. Graham. Active shape models – their training and application. *Comput Vis Image Underst*, 61(1):38–59, 1995.
9. M. de Bruijne, B. van Ginneken, M.A. Viergever, and W.J. Niessen. Adapting active shape models for 3D segmentation of tubular structures in medical images. In *IPMI*, volume 2732 of *LNCS*, pages 136–147. Springer, 2003.
10. A. Doucet, N. de Freitas, and N. Gordon, editors. *Sequential Monte Carlo methods in practice*. Springer-Verlag, New York, 2001.
11. M. Isard and A. Blake. CONDENSATION – conditional density propagation for visual tracking. *Int J Comput Vis*, 29(1):5–28, 1998.
12. A.K. Jain, Y. Zhong, and M.P. Dubuisson-Jolly. Deformable template models: A review. *Signal Processing*, 71(2):109–129, 1998.
13. S. Sclaroff and J. Isidoro. Active blobs: region-based, deformable appearance models. *Comput Vis Image Underst*, 89(2-3):197–225, 2003.
14. I.M. Scott, T.F. Cootes, and C.J. Taylor. Improving appearance model matching using local image structure. In *IPMI*, volume 2732 of *LNCS*, pages 258–269. Springer, 2003.
15. J. Shiraishi, S. Katsuragawa, J. Ikezoe, T. Matsumoto, T. Kobayashi, K. Komatsu, M. Matsui, H. Fujita, Y. Kodera, , and K. Doi. Development of a digital image database for chest radiographs with and without a lung nodule: Receiver operating character- istic analysis of radiologists' detection of pulmonary nodules. *Am J Roentgenol*, 174:71–74, 2000.
16. P.P. Smyth, C.J. Taylor, and J.E. Adams. Vertebral shape: Automatic measurement with active shape models. *Radiology*, 211(2):571–578, 1999.
17. M.B. Stegmann, R. Fisker, and B.K. Ersbøll. Extending and applying active appearance models for automated, high precision segmentation in different image modalities. In *Proceedings of the 12th Scandinavian Conference on Image Analysis*, 2001.
18. B. van Ginneken, A.F. Frangi, J.J. Staal, B.M. ter Haar Romeny, and M.A. Viergever. Active shape model segmentation with optimal features. *IEEE Trans Med Imaging*, 21(8):924–933, 2002.
19. S.K. Warfield, M. Kaus, F.A. Jolesz, and R. Kikinis. Adaptive, template moderated, spatially varying statistical classification. *Med Image Anal*, 4:43–55, 2000.
20. G. Zamora, H. Sari-Sarrafa, and R. Long. Hierarchical segmentation of vertebrae from x-ray images. In *Med Imaging: Image Process*, volume 5032 of *Proc of SPIE*, pages 631–642. SPIE Press, 2003.

Profile Scale-Spaces for Multiscale Image Match

Sean Ho* and Guido Gerig

Department of Computer Science
University of North Carolina, Chapel Hill, NC 27599, USA
seanho@cs.unc.edu

Abstract. We present a novel statistical image-match model for use in Bayesian segmentation, a multiscale extension of image profile models akin to those in Active Shape Models. A spherical-harmonic based 3D shape representation provides a mapping of the object boundary to the sphere S^2, and a scale-space for profiles on the sphere defines a scale-space on the object. A key feature is that profiles are not blurred across the object boundary, but only along the boundary. This profile scale-space is sampled in a coarse-to-fine fashion to produce features for the statistical image-match model. A framework for model-building and segmentation has been built, and testing and validation are in progress with a dataset of 70 segmented images of the caudate nucleus.

1 Why Are Anatomical Objects So Hard to Segment?

Model-based segmentation has come a long way since Kass and Witkin's original snakes [1], but segmentation of anatomical structures from real-world 3D medical images still presents some difficult challenges for automatic methods. Bayesian model-based segmentation balances a geometry prior, guided by a model of the expected object shape, against an image match likelihood, guided by a model of the expected image appearance around the object. Much has been done on the shape representation and prior; here we will focus on the image match model.

In many objects, a simple gradient-magnitude based image-match model is insufficient. The profile of the image across the object boundary can vary significantly from one portion of the boundary to another. Some portions of the boundary might not even have a visible contrast, in which case the shape prior is needed to define the contour. In real-world medical images, the contrast-to-noise ratio is often low, and models need to be robust to image noise.

In our study, one of the applications we focus on is the caudate nucleus in the human brain. From a partnership with our Psychiatry department, we have access to over 70 high-resolution MRIs (T1-weighted, 1x1x1mm) with high-quality manual expert segmentations of both left and right caudates. The manual raters, having spent much effort on developing a reliable protocol for manual segmentation, indicate some of the challenges in caudate segmentation, which motivate a multiscale statistical image-match model for automatic methods.

---

* Supported by NIH-NIBIB P01 EB002779.

Portions of the boundary of the caudate can be localized with standard edge detection at appropriate scales. However, there are also nearby false edges which may be misleading. In addition, where the caudate borders the nucleus accumbens, there is no contrast at the boundary; the manual raters use a combination of shape prior and external landmarks to define the boundary. Figure 1 shows the challenge.

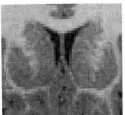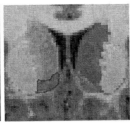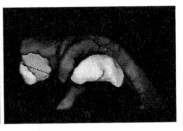

Fig. 1. Coronal slice of the caudate: original T1-weighted MRI (left), and segmented (middle). Right and left caudate are shown shaded in green and red; left and right putamen are sketched in yellow, laterally exterior to the caudates. Nucleus accumbens is sketched in red outline. Note the lack of contrast at the boundary between the caudate and the nucleus accumbens, and the fine-scale cell bridges between the caudate and the putamen. At right is a 3D view of the caudate and putamen relative to the ventricles.

Another "trouble-spot" for the caudate is where it borders the putamen; there are "fingers" of cell bridges which span the gap between the two. The scale of the object structure relative to the scale of the image noise may swamp single-scale image-match models with the noise.

Many other segmentation tasks in medical images present challenges similar to the caudate; in automatic segmentation methods, this motivates image-match models which are statistically trained and multiscale. This paper focuses on the image match likelihood model, not on the shape prior; the shape prior we use is from the statistical spherical harmonics shape model [2].

2   Related Work

There are various image match models in use by current model-based segmentation methods, but relatively few which incorporate scale.

Perhaps the simplest image match model is simply to optimize for high gradient magnitude of the image. This is often used by both classical mesh-based snakes [1] and implicit (geodesic) snakes [3]. The gradient magnitude is usually computed at a fixed, global scale. Region-competition snakes use global probability distributions of "inside" intensities vs. "outside" intensities to drive the image match [4]. van Ginneken et al [5] perform a local inside/outside classification using not just the raw greylevels but a high-dimensional n-jet feature vector, which incorporates multiple scales. Leventon et al [6] train a global profile model that relates intensity values to signed distances from the boundary, incorporating more information than a simple inside/outside classifier, but without treating the scale issue.

Cootes and Taylor's seminal Active Shape Model (ASM) work [7] samples the image along 1D profiles around boundary points, normal to the boundary, using correspondence given by the Point Distribution Model (PDM). Probability distributions are trained for each profile independently. Multi-resolution ASMs [8] use a Gaussian image pyramid in the original image coordinate system. The "hedgehog" model in the 3D spherical harmonic segmentation framework [2] can be seen as a variant of ASMs, and uses a training population linked with correspondence from that geometric model. Profiles have also been used in 2D cardiac MR images [9]. Fenster et al [10] use coarse-scale profiles to summarize sectors of the object boundary.

A different approach is taken by Cootes and Taylor's Active Appearance Models [11], which perform a global Principal Components Analysis on intensities across the whole object after registration. The global PCA is particularly well-suited for capturing global illumination changes in their face recognition applications.

Image features at the boundary may appear at various scales, which motivates a multiscale approach. However, traditional multiscale approaches blur in Euclidean space, which may blur across the object boundary. In the spirit of Canny [12], we wish to construct multiscale features where the blurring is *along* the boundary and not *across* the boundary. Our approach is to construct a *scale-space* on the image profiles, similar to classical scale-spaces [13,14] but on a curved non-Euclidean space. We then sample the profile scale-space after the fashion of Laplacian image pyramids [15], to obtain multiscale features upon which Gaussian models are trained using the training population.

3   Method

We first describe the process of sampling image profiles across the boundary of the object, in Section 3.1. A scale-space on those profiles is defined in Section 3.2, blurred only along the object boundary, and not across the boundary. Finally, Section 3.3 shows the sampling of the profile scale-space to obtain multiscale features for the statistical model.

3.1   Extracting Image Profiles of the Object

The shape representation we use is based on 3D spherical harmonics [2], and provides a diffeomorphic mapping from each object to the unit sphere S^2. There are many ways to parameterize the objects [16]; our method would work naturally with other parameterizations.

A uniform sampling of the object boundary is obtained from a sampling of the sphere S^2. At each point on the object boundary, the image is sampled evenly along a straight line normal to the boundary, producing an image profile. The first image in Figure 2 shows 512 profiles taken around one caudate from our training set. The 1D ordering of the profiles represents a certain traversal of the 2D surface of the object; adjacent profiles in this visualization are not necessarily adjacent on the surface.

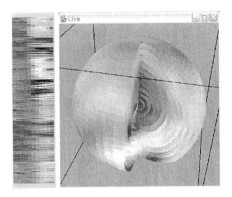

Fig. 2. Intensity profiles from the boundary of a single caudate. At left is a linear visualization of the profiles; the left half is inside the caudate, and the right half is outside. At right is an "onionskin" visualization of the profiles mapped onto concentric spheres. Each sphere represents sampled intensities at a fixed distance away from the boundary, from -5mm to +5mm, with 1mm spacing.

The right image in Figure 2 shows a different visualization of the same profiles. We use the diffeomorphic mapping of the object to the sphere S^2 to map each level of the profiles to a sphere. The outermost sphere represents intensities sampled from an "onionskin" +5mm outside the object boundary. Each profile is 11 samples long, so there are 11 concentric spheres in the visualization. The uniform grey matter interior of the caudate can be seen on the interior spheres.

3.2   Profile Scale-Space

To extend the classical single-scale profile models to a multiscale framework, we define a scale-space on the profiles sampled on the boundary. The "onionskin" visualization in Figure 2 shows the profiles mapped onto spheres. The intensities at each onionskin level can be mapped onto the sphere S^2, where a scale-space can be more easily constructed. Each onionskin level is blurred separately, so the blurring stays within each onionskin without blurring across onionskin levels.

The scale-space on S^2 is defined via the orthonormal spherical harmonic basis on $L^2(S^2)$. Note that this is separate from the use of spherical harmonics in the shape representation. Let $f \in L^2(S^2)$ be a scalar-valued function on the sphere; e.g. the sampled intensities from a single onionskin about the object. The spherical harmonics $\{Y_l^m\}$ form a complete orthonormal basis of $L^2(S^2)$, so the function f has a *Fourier expansion* in spherical harmonics:

$$f(\theta, \phi) = \sum_{l=0}^{\infty} \sum_{m=-l}^{l} c_l^m Y_l^m(\theta, \phi), \tag{1}$$

where c_l^m are the complex coefficients of the spherical harmonics:

$$c_l^m = \int_{\phi=0}^{2\pi} \int_{\theta=0}^{\pi} f(\theta, \phi) Y_l^m(\theta, \phi) \sin\theta \, d\theta \, d\phi. \tag{2}$$

We make use of the well-known fact that the spherical harmonics are eigenfunctions of the Laplace operator on S^2, with eigenvalues $l(l+1)$; i.e. $\triangle_{S^2} Y_l^m + l(l+1)Y_l^m = 0$, where the Laplace operator on S^2 is

$$\triangle_{S^2} = \frac{\partial^2}{\partial\theta^2} + \frac{\cos\theta}{\sin\theta}\frac{\partial}{\partial\theta} + \frac{1}{\sin^2\theta}\frac{\partial^2}{\partial\phi^2} \tag{3}$$

We define the *scale-space* of f on S^2 to be $\Phi(f) : S^2 \times R^+ \to R$ given by:

$$\Phi(f)(\theta, \phi; \sigma) = \sum_{l=0}^{\infty} \sum_{m=-l}^{l} e^{-l(l+1)\sigma} c_l^m Y_l^m(\theta, \phi). \tag{4}$$

This is the solution to the diffusion equation, $\frac{\partial \Phi(f)}{\partial \sigma} = \triangle_{S^2}\Phi(f)$.

The scale-space on the sphere defines a scale-space on the image profiles, via the diffeomorphic mapping provided by the shape representation. If the diffeomorphism were an isometry, the Laplacian on S^2 would map to the Laplace-Beltrami operator on the surface of the object, and our scale-space would be equivalent to Laplace-Beltrami blurring on the object surface. In general, such an isometry is impossible to obtain, but we have an approximation, since the mapping provided by the spherical harmonic shape representation preserves area exactly and approximately preserves angles. The scale-space on image profiles is constructed using a spherical harmonic basis for the image intensities on each "onionskin", analogous to the use of the spherical harmonic basis for the (x, y, z) coordinates of the boundary.

3.3   Multiscale Features and Statistical Model

With a scale-space defined on the image profiles about the object boundary, we sample features from the scale-space in a coarse-to-fine fashion, and build a statistical model on the multiscale tree of features. The coarse-to-fine sampling follows the recursive triangular subdivision of the sphere. In our implementation, we use 512 samples at the finest σ scale, down to 8 samples at the coarsest scale, with a total of four scale levels. A schematic of the sampling scheme is illustrated in the left image in Figure 3. The node at the top of the tree represents a single coarse-scale profile summarizing an eighth of the boundary.

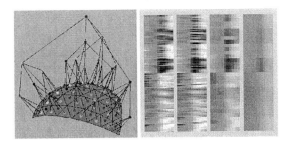

Fig. 3. At left, a visualization of the coarse-to-fine sampling of the profile scale-space. Distance away from the grey sphere indicates coarser scale in the scale-space. At right, average profiles across the training population, at four scales, fine to coarse.

These blurred profiles are calculated for each object in the training population. The right image in Figure 3 shows the mean profiles at multiple scales, where the mean is taken at corresponding locations over the training population. Correspondence is established via the spherical harmonic parametrization [2]. Again, in this visualization, the ordering of the profiles from top to bottom represents a traversal of the object boundary; this blurring is not the same as a simple y-axis blur.

Finally, the features used to build the statistical model are scale residuals: differences between each profile at scale (each node in the tree in Figure 3) and its parent profile (parent in the tree, at coarser scale). The eight profiles at the coarsest scale are included unchanged as features. This is analogous to the classical Laplacian image pyramid [15] in Euclidean space. Each scale-residual profile is then modelled with a Gaussian. With profiles 11 samples long, we have (512+128+32+8) Gaussian models, each 11-dimensional. The local Mahalanobis distances are summed to produce a global goodness-of-fit. This model is similar to the single-scale profile model in Active Shape Models, which would have 512 Gaussians, each 11-dimensional, and in contrast with Active Appearance Models, which would have a single very high dimensional Gaussian.

4   Ongoing/Future Work

4.1   Segmentation

We have implemented a self-contained framework in Mathematica for building this model and using it for segmentation. The shape representation and prior is from Brechbühler and Kelemen, et al [2]. The Bayesian segmentation is just an optimization of the posterior, the product of the shape prior and the image-match likelihood. We use Mathematica's built-in *NMinimize* non-linear optimization routines. The dimension of the search space is only 18; we search over the 12 main eigenmodes of shape variation, and let translation and rotation be unconstrained. Test segmentations, initialized at the mean shape and pose, have been run on a couple test images, with promising results.

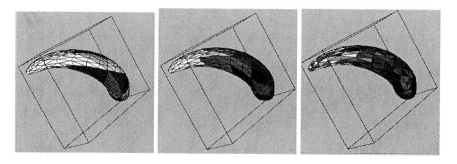

Fig. 4. Local image match goodness-of-fit textured onto deformable caudate segmentation, at initialization (after 1 iteration). White represents worse fit, dark represents better fit. The image match is computed at multiple scales; three scales are shown from coarse to fine.

4.2   Validation

Validation is in progress on the new image match model, as well as its use in segmentation. It is anticipated that due to increased robustness to noise and better modelling of population variability, our new multiscale profile model will yield segmentations closer to the manual expert than those from the single-scale profile model. We have access to a large database of over 70 segmented images, as well as intra- and inter-rater reliability figures for the manual raters. Evaluation of specificity/compactness and generalizability of the profile model itself is also planned.

5   Conclusions

We present a new multiscale statistical image profile model for use in Bayesian segmentation. The complex image appearance of anatomical structures in noisy medical images motivates a multiscale approach to modelling image profiles. We make use of the spherical harmonic shape representation to map the boundary profiles onto the sphere, where we define a scale-space which blurs image intensities along the object boundary, but not across the boundary. From the continuous scale-space, profiles are sampled at various locations and scales, and scale residuals akin to the Laplacian image pyramid are used as features in the statistical model. We have built the model and run preliminary segmentation tests; in-depth validation is in progress.

Acknowledgments. The caudate images and expert manual segmentations are funded by NIH RO1 MH61696 and NIMH MH 64580 (PI: Joe Piven). Manual segmentations are by Michael Graves, with protocol development by Rachel Gimpel and Heather Cody Hazlett. Image processing, including Figure 1, by Rachel Gimpel. The formalism for a scale-space on S^2 arose from discussions with Remco Duits at the Technical University of Eindhoven.

References

1. M. Kass, A. Witkin, and D. Terzopoulos, "Snakes: Active shape models," *International Journal of Computer Vision*, vol. 1, pp. 321–331, 1987.
2. András Kelemen, Gábor Székely, and Guido Gerig, "Elastic model-based segmentation of 3d neuroradiological data sets," *IEEE Transactions on Medical Imaging (TMI)*, vol. 18, pp. 828–839, October 1999.
3. H. Tek and B.B. Kimia, "Volumetric segmentation of medical images by threedimensional bubbles," *Computer Vision and Image Understanding (CVIU)*, vol. 65, no. 2, pp. 246–258, 1997.
4. S. Zhu and A. Yuille, "Region competition: Unifying snakes, region growing, and Bayes/MDL for multi-band image segmentation," in *International Conference on Computer Vision (ICCV)*, 1995, pp. 416–423.
5. Bram van Ginneken, Alejandro F. Frangi, Joes J. Staal, Bart M. ter Haar Romeny, and Max A. Viergever, "A non-linear gray-level appearance model improves active shape model segmentation," in *Proc. of IEEE Workshop on Mathematical Methods in Biomedical Image Analysis (MMBIA)* 2001, 2001.
6. M. Leventon, O. Faugeraus, and W. Grimson, "Level set based segmentation with intensity and curvature priors," in *Workshop on Mathematical Methods in Biomedical Image Analysis Proceedings (MMBIA)*, June 2000, pp. 4–11.
7. Timothy F. Cootes, A. Hill, Christopher J. Taylor, and J. Haslam, "The use of active shape models for locating structures in medical images," in *Information Processing in Medical Imaging (IPMI)*, 1993, pp. 33–47.
8. T. Cootes, C. Taylor, and A. Lanitis, "Active shape models: Evaluation of a multiresolution method for improving image search," 1994.
9. Nicolae Duta, Anil K. Jain, and Marie-Pierre Dubuisson-Jolly, "Learning-based object detection in cardiac MR images," in *International Conference on Computer Vision (ICCV)*, 1999, pp. 1210–1216.
10. Samuel D. Fenster and John R. Kender, "Sectored snakes: Evaluating learned-energy segmentations," *IEEE Transactions on Pattern Analysis and Machine Intelligence*, vol. 23, no. 9, pp. 1028–1034, 2001.
11. Timothy F. Cootes, Gareth J. Edwards, and Christopher J. Taylor, "Active appearance models," *IEEE Transactions on Pattern Analysis and Machine Intelligence (PAMI)*, vol. 23, no. 6, pp. 681–685, 2001.
12. J.F. Canny, "A computational approach to edge detection," *IEEE Trans on Pattern Analysis and Machine Intelligence (PAMI)*, vol. 8, no. 6, pp. 679–697, November 1986.
13. J. J. Koenderink, "The structure of images," *Biological Cybernetics*, vol. 50, pp. 363–370, 1984.
14. L. M. J. Florack, B. M. ter Haar Romeny, J. J. Koenderink, and M. A. Viergever, "The Gaussian scale-space paradigm and the multiscale local jet," *International Journal of Computer Vision (IJCV)*, vol. 18, no. 1, pp. 61–75, April 1996.
15. Peter J. Burt and Edward H. Adelson, "The laplacian pyramid as a compact image code," *IEEE Transactions on Communications*, vol. COM-31,4, pp. 532–540, 1983.
16. Martin A. Styner, Kumar T. Rajamani, Kutz-Peter Nolte, Gabriel Zsemlye, Gabor Szekely, Chris J. Taylor, and Rhodri H. Davies, "Evaluation of 3d correspondence methods for model building," in *Information Processing in Medical Imaging (IPMI)*, 2003.

Classification Improvement by Segmentation Refinement: Application to Contrast-Enhanced MR-Mammography

Christine Tanner[1], Michael Khazen[2], Preminda Kessar[2], Martin O. Leach[2], and David J. Hawkes[1]

[1] Imaging Sciences, Guy's Hospital, King's College London, UK
[2] Clin. MR Section, Inst. of Cancer Research & Royal Marsden NHS Trust, Sutton, UK
christine.tanner@kcl.ac.uk

Abstract. In this study we investigated whether automatic refinement of manually segmented MR breast lesions improves the discrimination of benign and malignant breast lesions. A constrained maximum a-posteriori scheme was employed to extract the most probable lesion for a user-provided coarse manual segmentation. Standard shape, texture and contrast enhancement features were derived from both the manual and the refined segmentations for 10 benign and 16 malignant lesions and their discrimination ability was compared. The refined segmentations were more consistent than the manual segmentations from a radiologist and a non-expert. The automatic refinement was robust to inaccuracies of the manual segmentation. Classification accuracy improved on average from 69% to 82% after segmentation refinement.

1 Introduction

The development of computer aided diagnostic systems for MR mammography relies on the collection of ground truth information of the breast lesion's image position and extent. Currently, a radiologist's segmentation is the accepted gold standard for this definition. Manual segmentation is, however, very labour-intensive and prone to inaccuracies. The workload of radiologists often prohibit building large annotated databases.

While humans can rapidly perceive image objects, the exact definition of the object boundary is time consuming, especially for contrast-enhanced image sequences. Fully automatic segmentation, on the other hand, has proven more difficult than expected. We therefore aim to develop a semi-automatic method that reduces the segmentation workload significantly, that is also applicable for weakly enhancing structures and that can readily be applied to registered images.

A few automatic and semi-automatic segmentation algorithms have been proposed for the extraction of breast lesion from dynamic contrast-enhance MR images. Lucas-Quesada et al. [1] recommended segmentation of MR breast lesions by manually thresholding the similarity map, generated from the normalized cross-correlation between the time-intensity plot of each voxel and a reference plot derived from a small user defined region of interest (ROI). This method compared favourably to a multispectral analysis method, where 20 to 30 manually selected lesion voxels were used to generate a lesion cluster in the 2D pre- to post-contrast intensities space by means of the k-nearest

C. Barillot, D.R. Haynor, and P. Hellier (Eds.): MICCAI 2004, LNCS 3216, pp. 184–191, 2004.
© Springer-Verlag Berlin Heidelberg 2004

neighbour algorithm. Note that the multispectral analysis method may have been disadvantaged by exploiting only limited data from the temporal domain, while the temporal correlation method was dependent on a single reference enhancement curve. Jacobs et al. [2] employed a k-means related clustering algorithm for extracting 4D feature vectors of adipose, glandular and lesion tissue from T1- and T2-weighted images and 3D fat-suppressed T1-weighted pre- and post-contrast images. Lesion classification was based on the angular separation from the adipose feature vector. Adipose and glandular reference feature vectors were provided by the user. Extraction of lesion outlines was not attempted. Fischer et al. [3] clustered the intensity enhancement profiles employing self-organizing Kohonen maps. The cluster results were shown to the user for interrogation of the dynamic sequences. No segmentation was attempted.

Our segmentation refinement method aims to extract the most probable lesion object of the contrast-enhanced MR image sequence from the data provided by the manual segmentation and prior knowledge about the segmentation process. The problem was posed as a two-class classification problem where the training data were provided by the manual segmentation. The segmentation decision was based on a constrained *maximum a-posteriori probability* (MAP) estimation in order to account for the imbalanced number of lesion and background voxels. The class conditional probability density functions were directly estimated from the temporal domain of the data samples. Sparsely sampled distributions were avoided by reducing the temporal dimensions with principle component analysis.

In the spatial domain, we observed that regions of non-enhancing tissue (like small heterogeneities, necrotic centres or fatty regions) were generally included in the manually segmented lesions. A MAP estimation solely based on the temporal domain would therefore lead to misclassifications. Instead, we rearranged the MAP estimation such that the ratio of prior class probabilities can be viewed as a threshold for the *likelihood ratio*. The segmentation process was then modelled by extract the biggest connected and filled lesion object for a given thresholded likelihood ratio map. The lesion candidate with the highest average a-posteriori probability that changed in size by less than a given limit was then selected as the most probable lesion. No assumptions were made about the edge strength or the shape or the enhancement profile of the lesion to avoid removing valuable information for the discrimination of benign and malignant lesions.

The aim of this study was two-fold. Firstly to assess the robustness and consistency of the segmentation refinement in comparison to the manual segmentations from an expert and a non-expert. Secondly, we compared the classification accuracy based on the segmentation refinement to that based on manual segmentation.

2   Materials

For this initial work we selected 18 patients from the symptomatic database of the UK multi-centre study of MRI screening in women at genetic risk of breast cancer (MARIBS) where patient motion was small enough allow interpretation of the images. The patients had in total 10 benign and 16 malignant histologically proven lesions. The images came from three centres of the MARIBS study and were all acquired according to the agreed protocol (3D gradient echo sequence on a 1.5T MR system with TR=12ms, TE=5ms, flip angle=35°, field of view of 340mm, 1.33x1.33x2.5mm³ voxel size, coronal slice orientation, 90s acquisition time, 0.2mmol Gd-DTPA, see [4]).

The lesions were manually segmented by an experienced radiologist and a non-expert. The radiologist segmented the lesions by defining contours on the coronal slices of a selected post- to pre-contrast difference image. The radiologist had access to previous radiological reports to ensure that the correct lesion was segmented. Views of all original and all difference images of the dynamic sequence were provided. The non-expert segmented the lesions by employing region growing techniques from ANALYZE (Biomechanical Imaging Resource, Mayo Foundation, Rochester, MN, USA) with manual corrections if necessary. Generally, the same intensity threshold was applied to all slices while the seed voxel was moved. No information about the lesion location was provided to the non-expert. Eight missed lesions were segmented after comparison with the radiologist's segmentations. All manual segmentations were conducted without knowledge of the pathological results.

3   Methods

3.1   Data-Preprocessing

The image data was preprocessed by subtracting the mean of the two pre-contrast images from each post-contrast image. The sequence of subtracted images was then normalized to zero mean and unit variance for each 3D lesion ROI.

Many of the multispectral segmentation algorithms assume that the intensity distributions of the separate objects can be approximated with multivariate Gaussian distributions. There is, however, no reason to expect that the temporal data of MR mammograms conform to this assumption. Therefore we performed density estimations with Gaussian kernels and a bandwidth selected according to [5]. We reduced the dimensionality of the preprocessed data by principle component analysis to reduce sparseness.

3.2   Segmentation

The segmentation refinement aimed to extract the most probable connected lesion object of a 3D region of interest (ROI) for a given manual segmentation. The ROI was defined as the rectangular box extending the manual segmentation by 7mm in each direction. The problem was posed as a two-class classification problem where the training data was provided by the manual segmentation. The segmentation decision was based on the *maximum a-posteriori probability* (MAP) estimation in order to account for the unequal number of lesion and background voxels within the ROI.

Assuming equally likely image features x and taking the prior class probability $P(C_k)$ for class C_k into account, the most probable segmentation refinement is given by maximizing the a-posteriori probabilities, i.e. $argmax_k P(C_k|x) = P(x|C_k)P(C_k)$ where $P(x|C_k)$ was estimated from the manual segmentation. For a two class problem the discrimination function $y(x)$ can be written as

$$y(x) = \frac{P(x|C_1)}{P(x|C_2)} \quad \text{with} \quad x \in \begin{cases} C_1 & \text{if } y(x) > \theta \\ C_2 & \text{otherwise} \end{cases} \quad \text{where} \quad \theta = \frac{P(C_2)}{P(C_1)}. \quad (1)$$

Equation (1) emphasizes that the ratio of the prior probabilities act as a threshold (θ) on the *likelihood ratio*. Instead of estimating θ from the number of lesion and background voxels in the manual segmentation, we propose to use θ for implicitly incorporating prior knowledge about the segmentation process.

Assuming that one connected lesion was manually segmented per ROI we firstly extracted for a given threshold θ the biggest connected object. Thereafter we applied morphological closing and hole filling operations to model the observation that manually segmented lesions generally include non-enhancing regions. A set of lesion candidates was then generated by varying the threshold θ. Assuming that the manual segmentation is similar in size to the actual lesion object, we selected all candidates that had a volume change of less than a certain percentage compared to the manual segmentation. Of this subset we finally choose the object with the maximum average a-posteriori probability for the whole lesion. We tested ten threshold variations, namely **MAP**: $\theta = V(C_2)/V(C_1)$ with volume $V(C_k)$ estimated from input segmentation, **Tp**: connected filled lesion that changed volume by less than $p\%$ while maximizing the average posterior probability, tested for $p \in \{0, 10, 20, 30, 40, 50, 60\}$, **Tmax**: lesion with maximal average posteriori probability and **ML**: maximum likelihood decision $\theta = 0$.

Coarse input segmentations were simulated by approximating the manual segmentation by an ellipse on each 2D slice. The sensitivity to the size of the initial segmentation was assessed by changing the size of these ellipses by $s\%$ for all cases or by randomly selecting a size change $s\%$, with $s \in \{-33, -20, 0, 25, 50\}$.

Segmentations were compared by means of the overlap measure $O = V(A \cap B) / V(A \cup B)$ where A and B are two segmented lesion regions; $A \cap B$ ($A \cup B$) are the intersection (union) of region A and B; and $V(C)$ is the volume of region C.

3.3   Feature Extraction

The size of our dataset limits the number of feature candidates that can reasonably be assessed. We therefore restricted ourselves to the 10 least correlated features of 27 previously reported 3D features used in this context [6,7,8]. These were selected by hierarchical clustering the feature vectors derived from the radiologist's segmentation according to their correlation. The 10 selected features were the following: *Irregularity* was determined by $irr = 1 - V_{in}/V$ where V_{in} is the volume within the effective radius $(3V/(4\pi))^{1/3}$. *Eccentricity* was determined by $ecc = \sqrt{a^2 - b^2}/a$ where $2a$ ($2b$) was the longest (shortest) axis, of the ellipsoid approximating the lesion shape. *Rectangularity* was defined as $rec = V/V_{rec}$ where V_{rec} is the volume of the smallest enclosing rectangular box. *Entropy of Radial Length Distribution* was calculated as $erl = \sum_{n=1}^{20} P_n log(P_n)$, where P_n is the probability that a surface vertex has an Euclidean Distance to the lesion's centre of gravity that lies within the nth increment of the distribution. *Peripheral-Central* and *Adjacent-Peripheral Ratio* were derived from partitioning the lesion and its immediate surrounding into 4 equally sized regions (central, middle, peripheral, adjacent) with boundaries kept in similar shape as the lesion itself. The ratios were given by $pcr = MITR(peripheral)/MITR(central)$ and $apr = MITR(adjacent)/MITR(peripheral)$ where $MITR$ is the maximum intensity time ratio as defined in [4]. *Slope Factor* m was derived from non-linearly fitting the general saturation equation $I_a/((T_{1/2}/t)^m + 1)$ to the average intensity difference

$I_t - I_0$ of the lesion where I_t is the intensity at time t after contrast infusion and I_0 is the pre-contrast intensity. *Texture parameters* were derived from the average *Spatial Gray-Level Dependence* matrix (one voxel distance, average of 9 directions) of the first post-contrast image intensities with values scaled from 1 to 40. *Spatial Correlation* is defined as $cor = \sum\sum (i - \mu_x)(j - \mu_y)P(i,j)/(\sigma_x\sigma_y)$ where $\mu_x = \sum iP_x(i)$, $\mu_y = \sum jP_y(j)$, $\sigma_x^2 = \sum(i - \mu_x)^2 P_x(i)$, $\sigma_y^2 = \sum(j - \mu_x)^2 P_x(j)$. *Angular Second Moment* is given by $asm = \sum\sum [P(i,j)]^2$. *Difference Average* was calculated by $dia = \sum\sum kP_{x-y}(k)$.

3.4   Classification

Single features were combined using stepwise linear discriminate analysis. The ability of combined features to discriminate between benign and malignant lesions was quantified by receiver operating characteristics (ROC) analysis. The ROC curve is defined by the fraction of false positives (1-specificity) to the fraction of true positives (sensitivity) for various thresholds on the decision criterion. The classification performance was summarized by the area under the ROC curve (A_{ROC}) for leave-one-out tests on a per-lesion basis. The statistical significance of the difference between ROC curves was tested using the ROCKIT program from Metz et al. [9].

4   Results

4.1   Data Preprocessing

The background (lesion) distributions of the original data were statistically significantly different (Lilliefors test, 5% level) from Gaussian normal distributions in 100% (67%) of all cases. The first two principle components of the preprocessed enhancement curves describe on average 98% of the variation in the data (range [91,100]%). The background (lesion) distributions of these two component were statistically significantly different from Gaussian normal distributions in 98% (69%) of all cases.

4.2   Segmentation

Fig. 1 illustrates for two neighbouring example slices the 3D segmentation refinement. It can be observed that the MAP refinement (contours in row 2) of the initial coarse segmentation (row 1) underestimated the extent of the lesion when compared with the radiologist's segmentation (row 6). The ML refinement (row 5) overestimated the lesion. The T0 (row 3) and Tmax (row 4) refinements produced almost identical results that are reasonable improvements to the radiologist's segmentation.

The average lesion size was statistically significantly bigger (paired t-test, P<0.001) for the radiologist's segmentation than for the non-expert (4.11ml vs 2.77ml). The average overlap between the two manual segmentations improved statistically significantly (paired t-test, P<0.01) after T0 refinement for all scenarios (from 59% to [64,68]%).

Fig. 2 shows how thresholding the likelihood ratio and changing the size of the initial segmentations affected the overlap measure O. Applying a threshold to keep

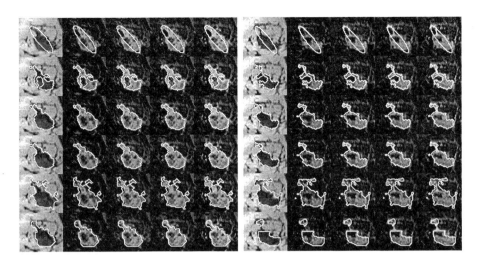

Fig. 1. Two example slices showing each (left to right) mean pre-contrast image and difference images after subtracting the mean pre-contrast image from 1st, 2nd, 3rd or 4th post-contrast image. Overlayed contours show (top to bottom) initial segmentation (E-20%), refinements of E-20% by MAP, T0, Tmax or ML criterion (see section 3.2); and radiologist's segmentation.

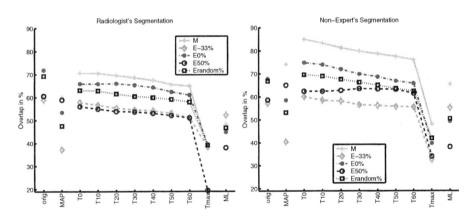

Fig. 2. Average overlap of refined and manual segmentation for (left) radiologist's and (right) non-expert's segmentation. Values along x-axis represent initial overlap (orig) and overlap after refinement with 10 threshold variations (MAP, T0-60, Tmax, ML) described in 3.2. Refinement was tested for manual segmentation (M) or for ellipsoidal approximations of manual segmentation that either all changed in size by $s\%$ (E$s\%$) or that randomly changed in size (Erandom%).

volume changes to a minimum (T0) provided on average the biggest overlap of all refinement strategies apart from input scenario E50%. Refinements of the ellipsoidal approximations (E$s\%$) produced generally smaller mean overlaps than refinements of the manual segmentations (M). The maximal possible average overlap when thresholding the likelihood ratio was 73% and 86% for the two manual segmentations. Optimal thresholding of the temporal correlation maps (created with respect to the most enhancing 5x5 ROI within the lesion) resulted in a maximal mean O of 60% for both manual segmentations.

4.3   Classification

We compared the classification performance of features derived from manually segmented lesion to that from refined segmentations. A combination of 3 refinement strategies (MAP, T0, ML) and 5 initial segmentations (M, E-33%, E0%, E50%, Erandom%) was tested (see section 3.2). Tp ($p > 0$) and Tmax refinements were not assessed because their overlaps were either very similar to T0 or were very small. The assessment was based on the area under the ROC curve (A_{ROC}) created from leave-one-out tests.

The best feature extracted from the radiologist's segmentation was *Texture Correlation* with an A_{ROC} of 0.57. After segmentation refinement, the best feature changed to *Peripheral-Central Ratio* (*pcr*) with average A_{ROC} values of 0.40, 0.66, 0.74 for MAP, T0 and ML, respectively. The best feature for the non-expert's segmentation was already *pcr* (A_{ROC}=0.69) and remained so after refinement (mean A_{ROC} 0.42, 0.71, 0.82 for MAP, T0 and ML). The *pcr* mean values of benign and malignant lesions were statistically significantly different (pooled t-test, 5% level) in 90% of all input scenarios after T0 and ML refinement.

To avoid overfitting the data, we combined not more than two features during stepwise linear discriminate analysis. This resulted in A_{ROC} of 0.57 and 0.70 for features extracted from the radiologist's and the non-expert's segmentation, respectively. Classification based on the refined segmentations provided A_{ROC} values between 0.57 and 0.89, of which none was statistically significantly worse (ROCKIT, 5% level) than the results of the manual segmentation. The best results were achieved with the ML refinement strategy. It produced in all cases the highest A_{ROC} (mean 0.80, range [0.69,0.89]). For half of the initial segmentations it was statistical significantly better at the 5% level than the manual segmentations. The second best results were produced by T0 with A_{ROC} values between 0.53 to 0.76 (mean 0.70). MAP was on average not better than the manual segmentation (mean 0.64, range [0.52,0.77]).

5   Conclusion

We have shown that the refinement of manual segmentations based on thresholding the likelihood ratio map can significantly improve the discrimination of benign and malignant breast lesions from contrast-enhanced MR images. Simplification of the lesion delineation by 2D ellipses and change of lesion size before refinement did not lead to inferior classification results. The consistent classification success of the maximum-likelihood refinement strategy was surprising, given its low overlap measures and apparent overestimation of the lesions extent, and requires further investigations.

The overlap between a manual segmentation and its refinement was on average significantly higher for the non-expert. This is likely due to region growing being more similar to the refinement technique than manual outlining. Classification results improved to a similar level for both manual segmentations after segmentation refinement.

Thresholding optimized for maximal overlap provided higher results for the likelihood map than for the temporal correlation map. This could be because the probabilistic approach removed the dependency on a single reference enhancement curve.

Computerized segmentation methods are generally evaluated against radiologist's manual segmentations. It is, however important to assess the effects of the segmentation on the ultimate goal, in this case the ability to discriminate benign and malignant MR breast lesion. To our knowledge, such a study has not been published, apart from evaluating the enhancement characteristics of region subsampling methods [10,11].

Classification of MR breast lesion based on step-wise linear discriminant analysis of extracted features from lesion segmentations has been reported previously [6,7,8]. These studies achieved classification accuracies of 72%, 79% (without leave-one-out tests) and 87%, respectively, when combining two features. Our classification results were on the lower end when based on features from the manual segmentations (69%) but improved to 78% and 85% after maximum-likelihood segmentation refinement. In future work, we will study how much segmentation refinement and registration improves classification for a large dataset.

Acknowledgements. CT acknowledges funding from EPSRC (MIAS-IRC). The image data were provided by MARIBS [4]. This study and MK are supported by the MRC (G9600413).

References

1. F. A. Lucas-Quesada et al., "Segmentation Strategies for Breast Tumors from Dynamic MR Images," *J Magn Reson Imaging*, vol. 6, p. 753, 1996.
2. M. A. Jacobs et al., "Benign and Malignant Breast Lesions: Diagnosis with Multiparametric MR Imaging," *Radiology*, vol. 229, p. 225, 2003.
3. H. Fischer et al., "Local Elastic Matching and Pattern Recognition in MR Mammography," *Int J Imaging Syst Technol*, vol. 10, p. 199, 1999.
4. J. Brown et al., "Magnetic Resonance Imaging Screening in Women at Genetic Risk of Breast Cancer: Imaging and Analysis Protocol for the UK Multicentre Study," *Magn Reson Imaging*, vol. 18, p. 765, 2000.
5. B. W. Silverman, *Density Estimation for Statistics and Data Analysis*. Chapman Hall, 1986.
6. S. Sinha et al., "Multifeature Analysis of Gd-Enhanced MR Images of Breast Lesions," *J Magn Reson Imaging*, vol. 7, p. 1016, 1998.
7. K. G. A. Gilhuijs et al., "Computerized Analysis of Breast Lesions in Three Dimensions using Dynamic Magnetic-Resonance Imaging," *Med Phys*, vol. 1, p. 1647, 1998.
8. L. I. Sonoda, *Classification of Lesions in Magnetic Resonance Images of the Breast*. PhD thesis, King's College London, 2003.
9. C. E. Metz et al., "Maximum Likelihood Estimation of Receiver Operating Characteristics Curves from Continuously-Distributed Data," *Statistics in Medicine*, vol. 17, p. 1033, 1998.
10. S. Mussurakis et al., "Primary Breast Abnormalities: Selective Pixel Sampling on Dynamic Gadolinium-Enhanced MR Images," *Radiology*, vol. 206, p. 465, 1998.
11. G. P. Liney, P. Gibbs, C. Hayes, M. O. Leach, and L. W. Turnbull, "Dynamic Contrast-Enhanced MRI in the Differentiation of Breast Tumors: User-Defined Versus Semi-automated Regions-of-Interest Analysis," *J Magn Reson Imaging*, vol. 10, p. 945, 1999.

Landmark-Driven, Atlas-Based Segmentation of Mouse Brain Tissue Images Containing Gene Expression Data

Ioannis A. Kakadiaris[1], Musodiq Bello[1], Shiva Arunachalam[1], Wei Kang[1], Tao Ju[2], Joe Warren[2], James Carson[3], Wah Chiu[3], Christina Thaller[3], and Gregor Eichele[4]

[1] Visual Computing Lab, Dept. of Computer Science, Univ. of Houston, Houston TX, USA
[2] Dept. of Computer Science, Rice University, Houston TX, USA
[3] Verna and Marrs McLean Dept. of Biochemistry, Baylor College of Medicine, Houston TX, USA
[4] Max Planck Institute of Experimental Endocrinology, Hannover, Germany

Abstract. To better understand the development and function of the mammalian brain, researchers have begun to systematically collect a large number of gene expression patterns throughout the mouse brain using technology recently developed for this task. Associating specific gene activity with specific functional locations in the brain anatomy results in a greater understanding of the role of the gene's products. To perform such an association for a large amount of data, reliable automated methods that characterize the distribution of gene expression in relation to a standard anatomical model are required. In this paper, we present an anatomical landmark detection method that has been incorporated into an atlas-based segmentation. The addition of this technique significantly increases the accuracy of automated atlas-deformation. The resulting large-scale annotation will help scientists interpret gene expression patterns more rapidly and accurately.

1 Introduction

With the successful efforts in mammalian genome sequencing, biologists are increasingly interested in understanding the function of different gene products at the molecular level. One strategy towards this end is high-throughput *in situ* hybridization (HITISH) [1]. Using HITISH, the spatial distribution of gene expression patterns (where genes are actively transcribed) can be generated throughout an entire organ or organism for thousands of genes each year. By relating a gene's activity to specific functional populations of cells, one gains insight into the function of that gene's products. In addition, genes that express in the same set of cell populations are likely to be related in function. For these reasons, accurately characterizing the location of gene expression in relation to the underlying anatomical morphology is prerequisite to the interpretation of HITISH results. Such a characterization must become both rapid and accurate in order to handle the vast amount of data generated by HITISH. A major computational challenge is to develop efficient algorithms that can accomplish this task with little or no human intervention.

HITISH is currently being applied to both the mouse brain and the mouse embryo [2,3]. For our algorithm development, we initially focus on the postnatal mouse brain. The postnatal mouse brain is small, accessible, and contains hundreds of functional subregions, making it a particularly good specimen choice for HITISH. To date, several

C. Barillot, D.R. Haynor, and P. Hellier (Eds.): MICCAI 2004, LNCS 3216, pp. 192–199, 2004.

steps in the computational process of gene expression localization have already been developed: (1) an image filter that identifies the location of cells and the amount of gene expression in each cell [4]; (2) a deformable atlas of the mouse brain anatomy [5] built using subdivision meshes [6] that, when deformed to accurately overlay the anatomy of the HITISH image data collected, segments the major anatomical regions of the image and serves as a standard coordinate system onto which cellular gene expression information is attached; and (3) global deformation of the atlas using affine transformation to account for rotation and translation, and local deformation based on iterated least-squares to account for shape variation [5]. However, the accuracy of the local fitting, and thus the segmentation and interior coordinate system, is limited by its reliance on only tissue boundary detection. Thus, manual deformation of the internal regions of the atlas must still be performed (Fig. 1(a)). In this paper, we present a method that detects anatomical landmarks in tissue images using texture features. This method has been incorporated into the atlas deformation procedure and substantially improves the segmentation and fitting of the atlas' internal boundaries.

The challenges in segmentation are due to the nature of the images. Each individual mouse brain is inherently slightly different from every other one in structure, although the main anatomical features are the same. In spite of the extreme precision employed in carrying out the HITISH process, sectioning induces local distortion upon tissue slices. Also, due to the nature of gene expression patterns, different genes are not expressed equally in different anatomical regions, making it difficult to construct a consistent model of each landmark in all images.

The rest of the paper is organized as follows: Section 2 presents our method in detail including acquisition of the training data for our experiments, locating each landmark in an image, and utilizing the information about the location of the landmark to improve the mesh fitting. Section 3 presents our results and the validation techniques used.

2   Methods

2.1   Experimental Data

In situ hybridization to label cells expressing a gene of interest was performed on 20μm-thick serially sliced cross-sections of the postnatal day 7 (P7) C57BL/6 mouse brain, which were then imaged with a light microscope at 3.3μm per pixel resolution [2]. This resulted in approximately 400 2D images per brain, with each image being 2000 x 3500 pixels in size. For each gene, 11 images were selected that best matched a set of 11 previously defined standard sagittal sections (i.e., levels), to provide a consistent and global representation of the expression patterns. For this work, we selected 100 images of level 9 sagittal sections expressing different genes.[1] We marked the ground truth coordinates for seven selected anatomical landmarks (Fig. 1b) in each of the 100 images. The images were sorted into four categories (Q_1, Q_2, Q_3, Q_4) based on the average signal strength of gene expression in the images.

---

[1] The complete data set is available at www.geneatlas.org and currently consists of 1207 images across 11 sagittal levels.

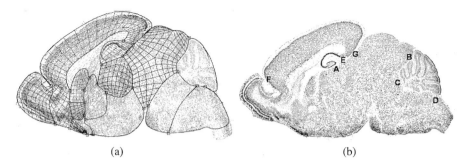

(a)   (b)

Fig. 1. (a) *Sca1* gene expression image overlaid with a subdivision mesh manually fitted by neuroanatomists. (b) A typical mouse brain image showing the expression of the *Camk2g* gene as revealed by *in situ* hybridization with the seven landmarks under consideration marked as follows: A - Dentate gyrus; B - Intersection of midbrain and cerebellum; C - Intersection of pons and cerebellum; D - Intersection of medulla and cerebellum on the outer boundary; E - Tip of the corpus callosum; F - Intersection of the cortex and olfactory bulb on the outer boundary; and G - Intersection of the cortex and the midbrain on the outer boundary.

2.2   Landmark Localization

To locate the desired landmarks in a given gene expression image, first we designed a template for the landmarks and selected their neighborhoods. We then extracted several features before selecting an optimal set of features. Based on a selected training set of images and the selected set of features, classifiers were constructed to distinguish each landmark from its neighborhood. These steps are further elaborated below.

Template Design: We designed a template that sufficiently includes the features of interest in a landmark, and that can be used to distinguish it from its neighbors (Fig. 2(a)). We allowed the rectangular template to have multiple regions so that different textures may be extracted from different areas around the landmark. The dimension (21x11 pixels) was chosen based on examining the area around the landmarks in several images.

Neighborhood Definition: For each landmark, we selected adjacent windows that do not include the landmark and that are different enough to be considered as typical examples of what the landmark is not (i.e., 'out-class'). For example, for landmark A we selected same-sized windows for the out-class, to the immediate right, above, and below the in-class window (Figs. 2(b-i)).

Feature Extraction: To be able to classify each landmark, features based on the statistics of local histograms were extracted as follows:

1. Convolve the original image (I_0) with two Gaussian kernels of width 5 (with $\sigma = 1$, 2) resulting in two smoothed images (I_1, I_2).

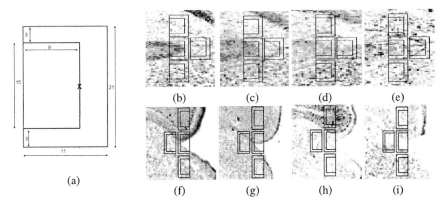

Fig. 2. (a) Landmark template. Selected neighborhood for landmark A in (b) Q_1 (c) Q_2 (d) Q_3, and (e) Q_4 image categories. (f-i) Selected neighborhoods for landmark D.

2. Convolve the three images (I_0, I_1, I_2) with two appropriate edge detector filters (e.g., 45° & 135° for landmark A, 135° & 180° for landmark E). This results in six filtered images. The choice of kernel is guided by the landmark edge orientation.

3. When the template is appropriately placed on the image, the image region under the inner part of the template is divided into overlapping 5x5 windows two pixels apart, and then into overlapping 9x9 windows. The outer part of the template is divided into three windows. The local histogram for each sub-window is obtained and the mean, standard deviation, and skewness are computed. The resulting feature vector with 414 elements (three features in 23 windows in six images) is labeled '1' ('in-class'). Similar features are extracted from the 'out-class' neighbors and labeled '-1'.

Selecting the Optimal Feature Set: It is expected that not all the features extracted will contribute equally to the classification. Using discriminant analysis with F-Test and Wilk's lambda, we ranked the features in order of discriminant power and performed a forward selection process [7]. For example, for landmark A, zero misclassification was obtained consistently with 164 features (out of 414) and these were selected as the optimal feature set.

Selecting the Training Set: Based on methods suggested in [8], we selected an optimal training set of images as follows (let N be the total number of images):

1. Select the first image and extract the optimal features for the in- and out-classes based on the ground truth.

2. Classify the ground truth in the remaining $N - 1$ images based on the single-image training set.

3. Repeat for all N images. The image that gives the smallest number of misclassifications when used as training to classify all the other $N - 1$ images is selected as the first training image.

4. For the remaining $N - 1$ images, form a new training set by adding each in turn to the first image. The two are used to classify the remaining $N - 2$ images and the pair that gives the least misclassification becomes the best two images.

5. Repeat the steps above adding one image in turn until zero misclassification is achieved (or until misclassification reduces below a threshold).

A classifier is needed to distinguish features of the landmark from that of neighboring regions. We used the k-Nearest Neighbor (KNN) [9] classifier in selecting the best training set because of its ability to classify even with a one-member training set. Figure 3(a) depicts the number of misclassifications as the number of images in the training set increases. The categories with low gene expression signals required more images to be included in the training set to reduce the misclassification to zero. However, in all categories, the misclassification is sufficiently low when half of the images are included. The best result was obtained by combining the optimal training images from categories Q_1, Q_2, and Q_3. Out of 100 images, 54 images formed this optimal set.

Estimating Classifier Parameters: We considered various classifiers including KNN [9], Support Vector Machines (SVM) [10], and Adaboost [11]. The best results were obtained for SVM. The Radial Basis Function (RBF) kernel [12] was used in the SVM and optimal values for the kernel parameters (C and γ) were obtained by cross validation. The training data was divided into four sets, with one set used as training data to classify the remaining three, in turn, using values of C between 2^{-5} and 2^{25} and γ between 2^{-15} and 2^3 as suggested in [13]. The results were sorted in descending order of misclassifications and the C and γ pair that gave the least misclassification across the four sets was chosen as the optimal. For the 24 images in the Q_1 category, the optimal values are $C = 2$ and $\gamma = 0.0078125$ for landmark A.

Locating Landmark Position: Given an approximate location of the desired landmark in the image (obtained after affine and local fitting as described in Sec. 1) and a given radius, a search is conducted in a square region around the approximate location. Rather than extracting features for all the pixels in the search area, features are extracted for every third pixel initially to expedite the process without making the search too coarse. A pixel-by-pixel search is then conducted around the area with the highest decision values (from SVM). This is possible because the decision values were found to be monotonically increasing towards the expected ground truth in all the images tested.

2.3 Integration into Mesh Fitting Process

To incorporate the knowledge of the landmarks into the mesh fitting framework [5], we set up a quadratic energy function $E^k(x)$ of the form: $E^k(x) = E_f^k(x) + E_d^k(x)$, where $E_f^k(x)$ measures the fit of the mesh at subdivision level k to the image and $E_d^k(x)$ measures the energy used in deforming the mesh. The fitting term $E_f^k(x)$ is formulated as: $E_f^k(x) = \alpha B^k(x) + \beta L^k(x)$, where $B^k(x)$ is the fitting error of the boundary of the mesh to the outer boundary of the image. $L^k(x)$ is the fitting error of the mesh to the landmarks defined as: $\sum_j (l_j - p_j(x))^2$, where $p_j(x)$ is the vertex of the mesh associated with landmark l_j. The formulation of $B^k(x)$ and the deformation energy term $E_d^k(x)$ are the same as in [5]. The minimizer of $E^k(x)$ is then computed using a linear solver such as conjugate gradients.

3   Results

After incorporating the feature-driven landmark localization algorithm into the mesh-fitting framework, the fitting of internal region boundaries was substantially improved. Figures 3(b,c) depict the performance for different image categories. For each landmark, the distance to the ground truth before and after incorporating the feature-driven algorithm was compared (Fig. 4). It was observed that the distance from the ground truth is reduced in 89%, 68%, and 76% of the images for landmarks A, E, and F respectively. In cases where the initial fitting is very far from the ground truth, the result of fitting is similarly poor.

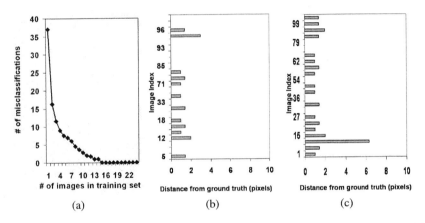

(a)   (b)   (c)

Fig. 3. (a) Number of misclassifications of landmark A and its neighbors as the number of training images increases for image category Q_1. Localization error for landmark A in image categories (b) Q_1, and (c) Q_2.

Different landmarks are more accurately detected in some images than others. As summarized in Table 1, at least three landmarks were found within a 4x4 neighborhood of the ground truth in 87% of the images. In 58% of the images, at least four landmarks were detected within a 3x3 neighborhood of the actual ground truth, and the number increases to 76% in a 5x5 neighborhood. Considering the inter-observer variability in locating the ground truth for the landmarks, detection errors within a 3x3 neighborhood are deemed acceptable. Figure 5 illustrates typical improvements after incorporating the feature-driven algorithm.

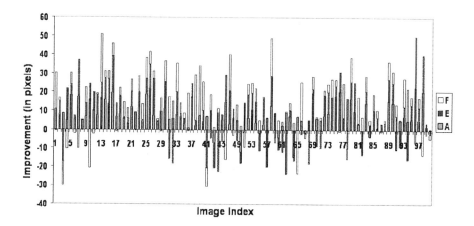

Fig. 4. Difference in distance to the ground truth in landmarks A, E and F after incorporating the feature-driven algorithm. A positive value indicates improvement. The cases where no improvement is observed are mainly due to the fact that the initial fitting would place the search window too far from the location of the landmark.

Table 1. Summary of results when fitting all the landmarks simultaneously.

No. of Landmarks	1x1 window	2x2 window	3x3 window	4x4 window	5x5 window
1	93	100	100	100	100
2	62	91	94	96	97
3	27	59	78	87	89
4	9	33	58	68	76
5	1	10	28	47	62
6	0	3	9	16	25
7	0	0	0	0	3

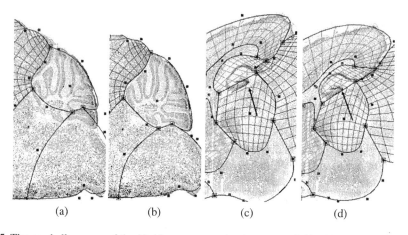

(a)   (b)   (c)   (d)

Fig. 5. The cerebellum area of the *Ntrk3* gene expression image overlaid with the mesh fitted (a) without, and (b) with the feature-driven algorithm. The area around the dentate gyrus for the *Calb1* image fitted (c) without, and (d) with our algorithm.

4   Conclusion

In fitting a deformable atlas to mouse brain images, the accuracy is greatly improved when internal region boundaries are used for aiding the fitting process. In biological images such as sagittal sections of the mouse brain, there is a lot of variation in shape and appearance making it difficult to use traditional methods (e.g., snakes, active shape and appearance models) for segmentation of internal region boundaries. We have selected a feature-based approach that extracts information about the texture of specific landmarks (distinguishing anatomical features) in the image and locates those landmarks in any new image. The locations of the detected landmarks are then incorporated into an energy-minimization framework to fit the standard mesh to the given image. Incorporating the internal landmarks has substantially improved the segmentation results.

Acknowledgements: This work was supported in part by a training fellowship (to Musodiq Bello) from the W.M. Keck Foundation to the Gulf Coast Consortia through the Keck Center for Computational and Structural Biology.

References

1. Herzig, U., Cadenas, C., Sieckmann, F., Sierralta, W., Thaller, C., Visel, A., Eichele, G.: Development of high-throughput tools to unravel the complexity of gene expression patterns in the mammalian brain. In Bock, G., Goode, J., eds.: Complexity in Biological Information Processing. Novartis Foundation Symposium 239. John Wiley & Sons, Chicester (2001) 129–149
2. Carson, J., Thaller, C., Eichele, G.: A transcriptome atlas of the mouse brain at cellular resolution. Current Opinion in Neurobiology **12** (2002) 562–5
3. Visel, A., Thaller, C., Eichele, G.: Genepaint.org: an atlas of gene expression patterns in the mouse embryo. Nucleic Acids Research **32** (2004) D552–556
4. Carson, J.: Quantitative annotation and analysis of gene expression patterns with an atlas of the mouse brain. PhD thesis, Baylor College of Medicine (2004)
5. Ju, T., Warren, J., Eichele, G., Thaller, C., Chiu, W., Carson, J.: A geometric database for gene expression data. In Kobbelt, L., Schröder, P., Hoppe, H., eds.: Eurographics Symposium on Geometry Processing, Aachen, Germany (2003) 166–176
6. Warren, J., Weimer, H.: Subdivision Methods for Geometric Design: A Constructive Approach. Morgan Kaufmann Publishers, San Francisco, CA (2002)
7. Jain, A.K., Duin, R.P.W., Mao, J.: Statistical pattern recognition: A review. IEEE Transactions on Pattern Analysis and Machine Intelligence **22** (2000) 4–37
8. Plutowski, M., White, H.: Selecting concise training sets from clean data. IEEE Transactions on Neural Networks **4** (1993) 305–318
9. Duda, R.O., Hart, P.E., Stork, D.G.: Pattern Classification. John Wiley & Sons Inc. (2001)
10. Vapnik, V.N.: The Nature of Statistical Learning. Springer (1998)
11. Freund, Y., Schapire, R.E.: An introduction to boosting. Journal of Japanese Society for Artificial Intelligence **14** (1999) 771–780
12. Schölkopf, B., Smola, A.: Learning with Kernels. MIT Press, Cambridge, MA (2002)
13. Hsu, C., Chang, C., Lin, C.: A practical guide to support vector classification. Technical report, National Taiwan University, Taipei 106, Taiwan (2003)

On Normalized Convolution to Measure Curvature Features for Automatic Polyp Detection

C. van Wijk[1], R.Truyen[2], R. E. van Gelder[3], L.J. van Vliet[1], and F.M. Vos[1,3]

[1] Quantitative Imaging Group, Delft University of Technology
Lorentzweg 1, 2628 CJ Delft, The Netherlands
{vanwijk,lucas,frans}@ph.tn.tudelft.nl
[2] MIMIT AD Group, Philips Medical Systems Nederland B.V.
P.O. Box 10000, 5680 DA Best, The Netherlands
{roel.truyen}@philips.com
[3] Department of Radiology, Academic Medical Centre Amsterdam
P.O. Box 22700, 1100 DE Amsterdam, The Netherlands
{r.e.vangelder, f.m.vos}@amc.uva.nl

Abstract. Early removal of polyps has proven to decrease the incidence of colon cancer. We aim to increase the sensitivity of the screening by automatic detection of polyps. It requires accurate measurement of the colon wall curvature. This paper describes a new method which computes the curvatures using space-variant derivative operators in a strip along the edge of the colon. It optimizes the trade-off between noise reduction and mixing of adjacent image structures. The derivative operators incorporate an applicability function for regularization and interpret the strips as confidence measure; certain inside and uncertain outside. To that purpose the technique of normalized convolution is utilized and adapted to allow a local Taylor expansion of the image signal. A special scheme to compute the confidence values is also presented.

1 Introduction

The colorectal polyp is an important precursor to colon cancer [10,13]. This benign lesion typically protrudes from the colon wall as a small, sloped mound (see Figure 1). Fortunately, the long pre-malignant stadium (5-10 years) enables efficient prevention by a timely removal. Virtual colonoscopy is a procedure to inspect the colon based on 3D CT images. However, current visualization techniques are still too time consuming for large scale use. Additionally, significant polyps are sometimes missed. Therefore many authors have suggested methods of automatic polyp detection [8,5,4,6].

Accurate curvature measurement is essential for any polyp detection scheme. Yoshida reported a method based on the implicit function theorem, computing

C. Barillot, D.R. Haynor, and P. Hellier (Eds.): MICCAI 2004, LNCS 3216, pp. 200–208, 2004.
© Springer-Verlag Berlin Heidelberg 2004

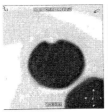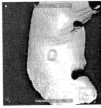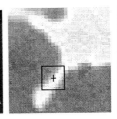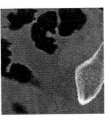

Fig. 1. From left to right: First two pictures: Cross-sectional view of small polyp and endoluminal view of same polyp. The last two pictures show a thin fold with overlay of a 7x7 kernel and tissue and folded structures

the radius of curvature directly from the first and second order derivatives. These derivatives were computed by employing isotropic Gaussian derivative kernels at scale σ [15][1]. Summers advocates a local B-spline fit through the triangulated surface voxels from which the radius of curvature is calculated [11]. Unfortunately a local model obtained from only surface voxels (without using grey value information) tends to become rather noisy. We have seen this happening in the computation of surface normals from triangulated meshes [9].

Noisy data asks for a certain amount of regularization, whereas thin colonic structures require a very small filter kernel. Violating the first requirement yields a noisy result (stochastic error) whereas violating the second causes a substantial bias in the derivatives (systematic error). Both errors hamper the curvature measurement. Finding a trade-off between the conflicting requirements is very difficult due to the presence of small folded structures on the colon wall as well as the presence of other structures in the tissue (see Figure 1).

In this paper we present a novel method to adapt the size and shape of the filter kernels to the local image data. The method avoids the systematical error due to mixing of nearby image structures and is optimized for noise reduction. However, using irregular shaped filter kernels requires a space-variant normalization of the derivative filters. Therefore we present an intuitive framework for deriving normalized differential convolution of arbitrary order (Section 2.1). In section 2.2 we present a scheme to compute space-variant kernels from the local image structure. The performance of the new method is assessed on both simulated data as well as CT data.

2   Methods

Derivatives in 3D images can be computed by convolution with derivatives of Gaussian kernels. In order to adapt the Gaussian (derivative) kernels to the local geometry they are multiplied with a confidence function which is extracted from

---

[1] Unfortunately no information on the scale at which the derivatives are computed is given.

the local image structure. This additional weighting requires re-normalization as well as a (re-)orthogonalization. The technique which takes care of both is normalized convolution ([7,14,3,2]).

For the detection of polyps the resulting image derivatives can be combined into principal curvatures, κ_1 and κ_2 (Thirion and Gourdon [12]). Based on the principal curvatures a number of polyp detectors can be constructed. Yoshida [15] uses primarily the shape index and curvedness. The shape index is given by $SI = \frac{1}{2} - \frac{1}{\pi} atan(\frac{\kappa_1 + \kappa_2}{\kappa_1 - \kappa_2})$ and the curvedness is given by $CV = \sqrt{\frac{k_1^2 + k_2^2}{2}}$.

2.1 A Least Squares Approach to Normalized Convolution

The following assumes a 2D image (extension to 3D image space is straightforward). Consider a local neighbourhood of $N \times N$ pixels f_i that is modeled by a Taylor expansion around the center of the local neighborhood (indicated by 0):

$$f_i = I(0) + x_i I_x(0) + y_i I_y(0) + \frac{x_i^2 I_{xx}(0)}{2!} + \frac{y_i^2 I_{yy}(0)}{2!} + \frac{2x_i y_i I_{xy}(0)}{2!} + R(i) \quad (1)$$

in which I indicates the 'true', underlying image function and i is a linear index. Using terms up to the second order and substituting $\eta_1 = I(0)$, $\eta_2 = I_x(0)$, ..., Equation 1 is rewritten as:

$$\begin{bmatrix} f_1 \\ ... \\ f_{N^2} \end{bmatrix} \approx \begin{bmatrix} 1 & x_1 & y_1 & 0.5\,x_1^2 & 0.5\,y_1^2 & x_1 y_1 \\ ... & ... & ... & ... & ... & ... \\ 1 & x_{N^2} & y_{N^2} & 0.5\,x_{N^2}^2 & 0.5\,y_{N^2}^2 & x_{N^2} y_{N^2} \end{bmatrix} \begin{bmatrix} \eta_1 \\ ... \\ \eta_6 \end{bmatrix} \quad (2)$$

The local neighbourhood can be depicted as a point in an N^2-dimensional space spanned by the orthonormal basis $\{\mathbf{e}_i\}$. A new set of basis vectors $\mathbf{b}_j = \{\mathbf{1}, \mathbf{x}, \mathbf{y}, \frac{\mathbf{xx}}{2}, \frac{\mathbf{yy}}{2}, \mathbf{xy}\}$ are the basis functions of the Taylor expansion (i.e. the columns of the matrix in Equation 2). Thus, $\{\eta_1, \eta_2, \eta_3, \eta_4, \eta_5, \eta_6\}$ are the coordinates of the signal on the new basis and directly yield the first and second order derivatives. It can be stated that:

$$f_e^i \approx \mathbf{B}\eta_b^j \quad (3)$$

Equation 3 merely rewrites Equation 2, implying that the signal f on basis $\mathbf{e}_i$ is approximated by the so-called basis tensor $\mathbf{B}$ times the coordinates of f on basis $\mathbf{b}_j$, (η_b^j). It must be emphasized that, in general, the basis functions can be freely selected and need not be orthonormal. Our basis was merely chosen to comply with the Taylor expansion. The objective now is to find the new coordinates η_b^j by minimizing the error $\epsilon = \|f - \mathbf{B}\eta\| = (f - \mathbf{B}\eta)^2$. The result is the general least squares solution to 3:

$$(\mathbf{B}^T\mathbf{B})^{-1}\mathbf{B}^T f_e^i = \eta_b^j \quad (4)$$

with $(\mathbf{B}^T\mathbf{B})^{-1}\mathbf{B}^T$ the pseudo-inverse of $\mathbf{B}$.

To reduce the influence of points further away from the neighborhood center we multiply the set of equations in eq. 2 by a (rotation invariant) matrix $\hat{\mathbf{A}}$, with $\mathbf{A} = \hat{\mathbf{A}}^T\hat{\mathbf{A}}$. The $N^2 \times N^2$ diagonal matrix $\mathbf{A}$ contains the spatial weights and is called the applicability function[2].

$$\hat{\mathbf{A}}f_e^i = \hat{\mathbf{A}}\mathbf{B}\eta_b^j. \tag{5}$$

Multiplication with $\hat{\mathbf{A}}$ is allowed as long as it does not yield a singular system of equations. Similarly, each equation in (2) can be multiplied again by other weights. It is now clear how confidence levels assigned to each neighbor can be incorporated. The result is a double weighted least squares solution:

$$(\mathbf{B}^T\mathbf{ACB})^{-1}\mathbf{B}^T\mathbf{AC}f_e^i = \eta_b^j \tag{6}$$

with the diagonal matrix $\mathbf{C} = \hat{\mathbf{C}}^T\hat{\mathbf{C}}$ holding the confidence value of each neighbor.

2.2   Local Confidence Values

The framework presented in the previous section accommodates normalized space variant-kernels. The confidence values which are inserted into this regularization are computed locally and will adapt the kernel to the local image structure. The goal is to assign high confidence to voxels on the image structure under consideration and a low confidence to neighboring structures. Such structures might be neighboring folds, changes in tissue structures, the opposite side of a fold, etc. We propose the following scheme to compute the confidence values.

1. Segment the air to find the air-tissue interface. Usually this is achieved by simple thresholding. We use a dynamic threshold [1] to allow for a correct segmentation of geometries affected by partial volume effects.
2. Compute for all voxels the distance to the air-tissue interface. We perform two distance transforms. One to compute the distance to air. From this we subtract a second distance transform, the distance to tissue. This operation results in positive values for air and negative values for tissue. On the colon wall the values of the distance transform are zero.
3. Compute the gradient of the distance transform which will act as a normal vector field. We will use these normals to distinct between different structures.

Steps 1 to 3 can be computed for the entire image at once. In contrast the following step is a local one to be incorporated in the convolution process. To distinguish between different geometries one can remark that the surface normal of the structure under consideration will differ from that of the direct neighboring structures.

---

[2] We use a Gaussian weighting $A = e^{-\frac{x^2}{2\sigma^2}}$ such that the scale at which the least squares solution is obtained is identical to the scale at which isotropic Gaussian derivatives are computed.

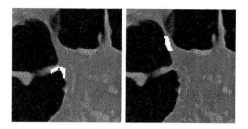

Fig. 2. Constructed confidence values for a neighborhood of 13^2 pixels. The neighborhood center is indicated by the black dot.

4. Assign neighboring voxels to belong to the current structure by taking the inner product of the normal at the neighborhood center with the normal of a neighbor. A threshold on this value (e.g. ¿0) classifies the neighbor and sets it's confidence value to zero or one.

An example of a region selected by the above scheme is given in Figure 2 . Note that the confidence values are weighted with the applicability function in the regularization process.

3   Results

The performance of the space-variant filtering is assessed on both simulated objects as well as CT data. Two test images were created to test the computation of radii of curvature with both the isotropic method as well as the new method. The first image, displayed in Figure 3a, is a 3D cylinder (only cross-section shown) which was constructed using the error function with a σ of 2. The cylinder has a radius of 18 pixels. Gaussian noise was added to the images. The standard deviation of the noise was 4% of the contrast (intensity difference between air and tissue). The second test image contains two 3D cylinders, their centers separated by 40 pixels. The image was constructed by multiplying two separate cylinder images after which noise was added.

Figure 3 shows that noise affects the derivative computation at small scales (a and b). Increasing the (isotropic) scale of the operator improves the results (c), but adjacent structures inside the footprint of the filter spoil the final result (d).

The isotropic Gaussian derivative filtering fails to return the correct curvatures. In this paper we propose to improve the curvature measurement by introducing space variant kernels. The performance is compared to the isotropic method in Figure 4a. The result of the isotropic method are repeated on the left cylinder. The results obtained with the proposed method are plotted on the right cylinder. It is clear that in the region where the two cylinders are close together the new method outperforms the method using isotropic kernels.

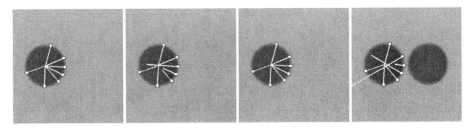

Fig. 3. Trade-off between noise suppression and resolution. On several positions on the edge the normal direction (line direction) and radius of curvature (line length) are plotted. From left to right: (a) noise free image, small scale $\sigma = 1$. (b) Gaussian noise added, $\sigma = 1$. (c) computation at larger scale suppresses the noise, $\sigma = 3$. At larger scale ($\sigma = 3$) incorrect curvature and gradient direction are obtained close to neighboring structures (d).

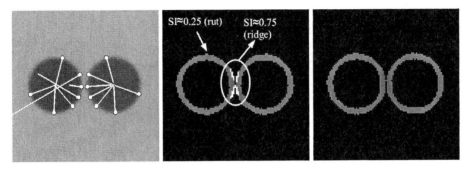

Fig. 4. Radius of curvature (left) and shape index (middle,right) computed on two cylinders (Only a cross section of the cylinders is shown). On several positions on the edge the gradient (line direction) and radius of curvature (line length) are plotted. Left cylinder: isotropic method. The gradient direction is obtained using isotropic Gaussian kernels ($\sigma = 3$). Right cylinder: both gradient direction and radius of curvature are obtained with space variant kernels ($\sigma = 3$).
The middle image shows the classification by shape index computed by the isotropic method. The isotropic method classifies large part of the cylinders to a ridge like structure. The new method (right) using space variant kernels classifies all voxels correctly.

The new method does not suffer from the systematic error introduced when using isotropic filters. The cost is a small increase in a stochastic error due to the fact that the incorporation of confidence levels into the filtering in effect reduces the number of voxels used to suppress noise. However, the specific choice of confidence levels based on the local structure allows to discard just those voxels which would have introduced a systematic error. In other words our method optimizes the trade-off between noise reduction and preservation of image structure.

The shape index is computed from the principal curvatures and is often used to select polyp candidates by means of thresholding. Applying such classification to the image in Figure 4a yield Figure 4b. The isotropic method will result in

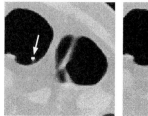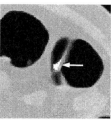

Fig. 5. One slice from the 3D Ct dataset. Voxels labelled as belonging to polyps (white). The new method finds the polyp (left). The isotropic method fails to find the polyp and selects a false positive. The results were obtained by filtering with $\sigma = 3$.

Table 1. Detection results. The isotropic method detects 3 false positives. The space variant method detection the true positive and one (small) false positive. The results were obtained by filtering with $\sigma = 3$.

id	method	cluster size	label
1	isotropic	9	false positive
2	isotropic	28	false positive
3	isotropic	86	false positive
4	space-variant	31	true positive
5	space-variant	3	false positive

a classification of a large part of the cylinder to a ridge-like structure. The new method correctly classifies all the voxels to a rut-like structure (8c).

To demonstrate the performance of the method on CT data, a scheme similar to [8] is applied. Yoshida et al. use the the shape index and curvedness to select the set of polyp candidates. In [8] thresholds were presented for the shape index (between 0.9 and 1.0) and for curvedness ($0.05\,mm^{-1}$ and $0.25\,mm^{-1}$). We applied the same scheme using hysteresis thresholding [8] to investigate the performance with respect to the candidate selection step. Initial test results on a few patients show promising results. The power of the method is clearly demonstrated in Figure 5 and Table 1 which are obtained by applying the method to a small dataset ($200 \times 200 \times 100$ voxels) containing one polyp (approx. 4 mm). The new method detects the polyp and finds one false positive. The isotropic method detects three false positives and misses the true positive.

From the demonstration of our method both on simulated data as well as CT data we feel confident that space-variant kernels will yield fewer false positives. Especially for small polyps the new method is likely to increase the sensitivity. However, we are aware that the performance of the operator can only be assessed by statistical validation on a large number of datasets. This is the focus of future work.

4   Conclusions

The measurement of curvature in CT data for the detection of polyps is difficult due to the highly folded colon. Therefore noise suppression with larger isotropic filters is not possible. We have shown that with a specific formulation of normalized convolution using a local Taylor expansion space-variant kernels can be used. In addition we have shown that space-variant kernels can be constructed which discards just those voxels belonging to neighboring image geometries. Thereby the derivative filtering optimizes the trade-off between noise suppression and preservation of local image structure.

The assessment of the method by simulated images shows that the space-variant filtering outperforms isotropic filtering. Also, on CT data the new method seems to indicate a higher sensitivity and higher specificity. However, the authors do realize an investigation on more data is needed to be conclusive on the overall improvement of polyp detection.

References

1. J. Bernsen: Dynamic Thresholding of grey level images. In ICPRA'86: Proc. Int. Conf. on Pattern Recognition, pp 1251–1255, Berlin, Germany, 1986
2. G. Farnebäck: A Unified Framework for Bases, Frames, Subspace Bases, and Subspace Frames. SCIA 1999, pages 341–349, Kangerlussuaq, Greenland, 1999.
3. Gunnar Farnebäck. Spatial Domain Methods for Orientation and Velocity Estimation. PhD Thesis, Linköping University, Sweden, 1999.
4. S.B. Goturk et al.: A statistical 3-d pattern processing method for computer-aided detection of polyps in ct colonography. IEEE Trans. on Med. Imag. 20:1251–1260, 2001
5. A. K. Jerebko et al.: Multiple neural network classification scheme for detection of colonic polyps in ct colonography data sets. Acad. Radiol., 10:154–160, 2003
6. G. Kiss et al.: Computer-aided diagnosis in virtual colonography via combination of surface normal and sphere fitting methods. European Radiology, 12:77–88, 2002
7. H. Knutsson and C.-F. Westin: Normalized Convolution - a technique for filtering incomplete and uncertain data. SCIA, 2:997–1006, 1993
8. J. Nappi and H. Yoshida: Automated detection of polyps with ct colonography: evaluation of volumetric features for reduction of false-positive findings. Acad. Radiol., 9:386–397, 2002
9. M. Persoon, I.W.O. Serlie, F. Post, R. Truyen and F. M. Vos: Visualization of noisy and biased volume data using first and second order derivative techniques. IEEE Visualization 2003 (Proc. Conf. Seattle, WA), pages 379–385, 2003
10. J.D. Potter, M.L. Slattery and R. M. Bostick. Colon cancer: a review of the epidemiology. Epidemiol. Rev., 15:499–545, 1993
11. R. M. Summers, C. F. Beaulieu, L. M. Pusanik, J. D. Malley, R. Brooke, J. D. Glazer and S. Napel: Automated polyp detector for ct colonography: Feasibility Study. Radiology, 216:284–290, 2000
12. J.P. Thirion and A. Gourdon. Computing the Differential Characteristics of Isointensity Surfaces. Computer Vision and Image Understanding, 61(2):190–202, 1995

13. B. Vogelstein, E. R. Fearon and S. R. Hamilton: Genetic alterations during colorectal-tumour development. N.Eng.J.Med., 319:525–532, 1998
14. C-.F. Westin A Tensor Framework for Multidimensional Signal Processing. PhD Thesis, Linköping University, Sweden, 1994.
15. H. Yoshida: Three-dimensional computer-aided diagnosis scheme for detection of colonic polyps. IEEE Transactions on Medical Imaging, 20:1261–1274, 2001

Implicit Active Shape Models for 3D Segmentation in MR Imaging

Mikaël Rousson[1], Nikos Paragios[2], and Rachid Deriche[1]

[1] I.N.R.I.A. Sophia Antipolis, France
{Mikael.Rousson,Rachid.Deriche}@sophia.inria.fr
[2] Ecole Nationale des Ponts et Chaussées, Paris, France
Nikos.Paragios@cermics.enpc.fr

Abstract. Extraction of structures of interest in medical images is often an arduous task because of noisy or incomplete data. However, hand-segmented data are often available and most of the structures to be extracted have a similar shape from one subject to an other. Then, the possibility of modeling a family of shapes and restricting the new structure to be extracted within this class is of particular interest. This approach is commonly implemented using active shape models [2] and the definition of the image term is the most challenging component of such an approach. In parallel, level set methods [8] define a powerful optimization framework, that can be used to recover objects of interest by the propagation of curves or surfaces. They can support complex topologies, considered in higher dimensions, are implicit, intrinsic and parameter free. In this paper we re-visit active shape models and introduce a level set variant of them. Such an approach can account for prior shape knowledge quite efficiently as well as use data/image terms of various form and complexity. Promising results on the extraction of brain ventricles in MR images demonstrate the potential of our approach.

1 Introduction

Object extraction is one of the first steps in medical imaging. Further analysis will highly depend on the quality of the segmented structures. However, medical images often suffer from noise, occlusions and incomplete data. Therefore, regularization constraints and prior knowledge are usually of good use. In this paper, we address this application with objective to recover a structure of particular geometric form.

B-splines deformable models as well as point distribution models are mathematical formulations introduced to the snake framework [4] to account for shape consistency. Active shape models [2] were a major breakthrough in object extraction and image segmentation. Such a framework consists of two stages; (i) the modeling and (ii) the segmentation phase.

During modeling the objective is to recover a compact representation for the geometric form of the structure of interest. Using a set of registered training examples, one can either represent prior knowledge using simple or more

C. Barillot, D.R. Haynor, and P. Hellier (Eds.): MICCAI 2004, LNCS 3216, pp. 209–216, 2004.

complicated density functions. Gaussian distribution [2], mixture models [1] or non-parametric function [3] were considered in the past.

The segmentation/object extraction stage aims at recovering a geometric structure in the image plane that accounts for the desired image characteristics while being in the family of shapes generated by the model . To this end, a mechanism for recovering the most probable object location in the image was considered. Then, one can iterate and move closer to the target by updating the position of the model such that it gets closer to the desired image characteristics.

Level set representations [8] is an established technique for tracking moving interfaces in imaging, vision and graphics [7]. One can see numerous advantages for considering a level set variant of the active shape model. Such a formulation could account for various forms (boundary or regional) of data/image terms of various nature (edges, intensity properties, texture, motion, etc.), an important limitation of the active shape model. Furthermore, one can maintain the implicit and intrinsic property of the level set method as well as the ability to account for topological changes while being able to introduce prior shape knowledge, a task partially addressed up to now [6,12,10].

In this paper we propose a level set variant of active shape models that consists of various terms. Quite critical is the term that refers to the prior knowledge with objective to constrain the evolving surface to belong to a compact family of shapes - the one recovered through the training set. Such a term couples two unknown variables; (i) the evolving contour, (ii) the optimal projection parameters of this contour to the model space and imposes the active shape model behavior on the process. Furthermore, various image-driven terms - a major advantage/characteristics of the method - could be considered to guide the evolving contour towards the desired image characteristics.

The most closely related work with our approach, the active shape model can be found in [2]. In [6,12,10] substantial efforts to integrate prior knowledge within level set representations were considered. Worth mentioning is [6, 12] where modeling of prior knowledge is done in a consistent active shape model manner. Contrary to [6], where two optimization processes alternate, we propose a variational integration of data and prior terms. Moreover, the evolving surface is not restricted within the modeled space like in [12], but only attracted to this space, allowing more flexibility.

The reminder of the paper is organized as follows: in Section 2 we briefly introduce the level set representations, while in Section 3 we address the construction of the prior model in the space of level set functions. The main contribution of the paper, the level set variant of the active shape model is presented in Section 4, while in Section 5 we demonstrate the efficiency and the flexibility of our approach through the integration of a region-based data term for 3D segmentation in MR images.

2   Level Set Representations

Level set representations [8] are a useful mathematical formulation for implementing efficiently curve/surface propagation. One can also consider the level set space as an optimization framework Let $\phi : \Omega \times \mathcal{R}^+ \to \mathcal{R}^+$ be a Lipschitz function with the following properties,

$$\phi((x,y);t) = \begin{cases} 0 & , (x,y) \in \mathcal{C}(t) \\ +\mathcal{D}((x,y), \mathcal{C}(t)) > 0 & , (x,y) \in \mathcal{C}_{in}(t) \\ -\mathcal{D}((x,y), \mathcal{C}(t)) < 0 & , (x,y) \in \mathcal{C}_{out}(t) = [\Omega - \mathcal{C}_{in}(t)] \end{cases}$$

where $(x,y) = p$, $\mathcal{C}_{in}(t)$ is the area enclosed by the curve $\mathcal{C}$, $\mathcal{D}((x,y), \mathcal{C}(t))$ the minimum Euclidean distance between the pixel (x,y) and $\mathcal{C}(t)$ at time t.

Let us also introduce the approximations of Dirac and Heaviside distributions as defined in [10]. Then one can define terms along $\mathcal{C}$ as well as interior and exterior to the curve using the Dirac and Heaviside functions:

$$(x,y) \in \Omega : \{\lim_{\alpha \to 0+} [\delta_\alpha(\phi(x,y)] = 1\} = \mathcal{C}$$
$$(x,y) \in \Omega : \{\lim_{\alpha \to 0+} [H_\alpha(\phi(x,y))] = 1\} = \mathcal{C}_{in}$$

Such terms will be used later to introduce the active shape prior term as well as data/image-driven terms that guides the contour ($\mathcal{C}$) towards the object of interest. The extension to higher dimensions is straightforward and in the following parts, we use this representation for an an evolving surface ($\mathcal{S}$) in $\mathcal{R}^3$.

3 Modeling Prior Knowledge in the Level Set Space

Learning the distribution of geometric/image structures is a common problem in computer vision with applications to segmentation, tracking, recognition, etc. It is clear that the selection of the representation is important. Given the selected optimization framework, level set functions is a natural selection to account for prior knowledge with numerous earlier described advantages. Let us consider a training set $\mathcal{C}_i$ of N registered curves or surfaces. Then, a distance transform can be used to represent $\mathcal{C}_i$ as a level set function ϕ_i.

The next step is the construction of the shape model, using the aligned contours. In order to create an invariant representation, one should first normalize the training set ϕ_i. Subtraction of the mean (that can be recovered by averaging ϕ_i's) is a common selection to this end. However, a simple averaging over the training will not give a istance function. To overcome this limitation, we consider a more rigorous approach [10], seeking to estimate the distance function (ϕ_M) that minimizes:

$$E(\phi_M) = \sum_{i=1}^{n} \int_\Omega (\phi_i - \phi_M)^2 d\Omega, \quad \text{SUBJECT TO} : |\nabla \phi_M|^2 = 1$$

One can optimize such a term though a gradient descent method:

$$\frac{d}{dt} \phi_M = \sum_{i=1}^{n} (\phi_i - \phi_M)$$

while ϕ_M is projected to the space of distance functions following [11]. The two steps alternate until the system reaches a steady-state solution. Then, we consider the modeling approach introduced in [6,12]. Once the samples ϕ_i centered

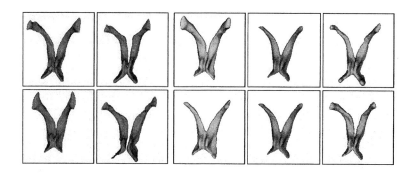

Fig. 1. LEFT: Some surfaces of the Training Set (segmented lateral brain ventricles of several patients), RIGHT: Model with the most important shape of variations [principal two modes after rigid alignment (blue:mean, red: $+\sigma$, green:$-\sigma$)].

with respect to $\phi_{\mathcal{M}}$, $[\psi_i = \phi_i - \phi_{\mathcal{M}}]$, the most important modes of variations can be recovered through Principal Component Analysis:

$$\phi = \phi_{\mathcal{M}} + \sum_{j=1}^{m} \lambda_j \, U_j$$

where m is the number of retained modes of variation, U_j are these modes (eigenvectors), and λ_j are linear weight factors within the allowable range defined by the eigenvalues.

An example of such an analysis is shown in [fig. (1)] for the 3D modeling of lateral brain ventricles. The model was built using 8 surfaces from different subjects. This example includes a difficult issue for classical parametric approaches because of different surface topologies within the training set. For example, the fourth surface in [fig. (1)] shows a separation between left and right ventricles. Our approach can deal naturally with this type of data. The obtained model gives a compact representation of the shape family: the first two modes of variation represent the major part of the class (80%), while the third one (9%) accounts for non-symetric properties of the ventricles that can be observed in some of the training samples. Moreover, the implicit representation of the surfaces make the modeling phase entirely automatic.

4   Introducing Prior Knowledge in the Level Set Space

Let us now consider an interface represented by a level-set function $\phi(\mathbf{x})$ as described in Section 2 (where $\mathbf{x}$ is in $\mathcal{R}^2$ or $\mathcal{R}^3$). We would like to evolve it while respecting some shape properties $\phi_{\mathcal{P}}(\mathbf{x})$ modulo a transformation $\mathcal{A}$ belonging to a predefined family. Assuming a rigid transformation $\mathcal{A}(\mathbf{x}) = \mathbf{R}\mathbf{x} + \mathbf{T}$, the evolving interface and the transformation should satisfy the conditions:

$$\begin{cases} \mathbf{x} \to \mathcal{A}(\mathbf{x}) \\ \phi(\mathbf{x}) \approx \phi_{\mathcal{P}}(\mathcal{A}(\mathbf{x})), & \forall \mathbf{x} \in \Omega \end{cases}$$

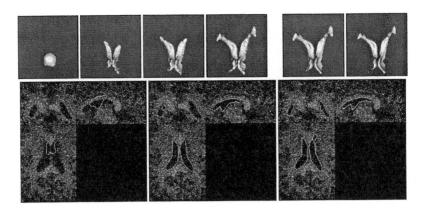

Fig. 2. Segmentation of lateral brain ventricles with Shape Prior ($b = 0.3$) of a noisy MR image. TOP LEFT: surface evolution, TOP RIGHT: projected surface in the learning space and ground-truth surface (from the training set), BOTTOM: surface cut (green) and its projection in the learning space (red) during surface evolution.

In that case, the optimal transformation $\mathcal{A}$ should minimize:

$$E(\phi, \mathcal{A}) = \int_{\Omega} \rho(\phi, \phi_{\mathcal{P}}(\mathcal{A})) d\Omega$$

where ρ is a dissimilarity measure. For the sake of simplicity, we will use the sum of squared differences. Scale variation can be added to the rigid transformation $\mathcal{A}$, leading to a similarity one $\mathcal{A}(\mathbf{x}) = \mathcal{S}\mathbf{R}\mathbf{x} + \mathbf{T}$ (for 3D images, we obtain 7 parameters: $\mathcal{S}$, $\mathbf{R}(\theta_1, \theta_2, \theta_3)$, $\mathcal{T} = (\mathcal{T}_x, \mathcal{T}_y, \mathcal{T}_z)^T$). In that case, the objective function should be slightly modified (refer to [10] for further details). Furthermore, one can assume that estimating and imposing the prior within the vicinity of the zero-crossing of the level set representation is more meaningful. Within distance transforms, shape information is better captured when close to the origin of the transformation. The prior can be thus rewritten:

$$E(\phi, \mathcal{A}) = \int_{\Omega} \delta_{\epsilon}(\phi) \left(\mathcal{S}\phi - \phi_{\mathcal{P}}(\mathcal{A})\right)^2 d\Omega \quad \text{where } \epsilon \gg \alpha$$

During the model construction, we have analyzed the principal modes of variation within the training set. Including this information, the ideal transformation will map each value of current representation to the "best" level set representation belonging to the class of the training shapes. If a shape representation $\phi_{\mathcal{P}}$ belongs to this class, then it can be derived from the principal modes:

$$\phi_{\mathcal{P}} = \phi_{\mathcal{M}} + \sum_{j=1}^{m} \lambda_j U_j$$

Hence, we define a new objective function by introducing the modes weights $\lambda = (\lambda_1, \ldots, \lambda_m)$ as additional free parameters:

$$E(\phi, \mathcal{A}, \lambda) = \int_{\Omega} \delta_{\epsilon}(\phi) \left(\mathcal{S}\phi - \left(\phi_{\mathcal{M}}(\mathcal{A}) + \sum_{j=1}^{m} \lambda_j U_j(\mathcal{A})\right)\right)^2 d\Omega$$

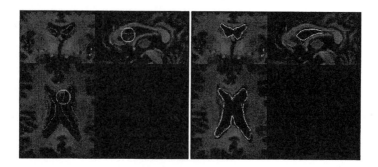

Fig. 3. Segmentation of lateral brain ventricles with Shape Prior ($b = 0.3$) in an MR image which was not used during the learning phase: surface cut (green) and its projection in the learning space (red) at initialization (LEFT) and after convergence (RIGHT).

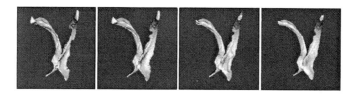

Fig. 4. Segmentation of lateral brain ventricles varying the influence of the shape prior term. From left to right, the shape prior weight b is 0, 0.3, 0.4, 0.5.

In order to minimize the above functional with respect to the evolving level set representation, the global linear transformation and the modes weights λ_j, we use the calculus of variations. The equation of evolution for ϕ is given by the calculus of its variations:

$$\frac{d}{dt}\phi = -2\delta_\epsilon(\phi)\mathcal{S}(\mathcal{S}\phi - \phi_\mathcal{M}(\mathcal{A})) - \frac{d}{d\phi}\delta_\epsilon(\phi)(\mathcal{S}\phi - \phi_\mathcal{M}(\mathcal{A}))^2$$

The differentiation with respect to the modes weights gives us a close form of the optimal parameters by solving the linear system $\bar{U}\lambda = b$ with:

$$\begin{cases} \bar{U}(i,j) = \int_\Omega \delta_\epsilon(\phi)U_i(\mathcal{A})U_j(\mathcal{A}) \\ b(i) = \int_\Omega \delta_\epsilon(\phi)(\mathcal{S}\phi - \phi_\mathcal{M}(\mathcal{A}))U_i(\mathcal{A}) \end{cases}$$

where $\bar{U}$ is a $m \times m$ positive definite matrix. Finally, the minimization of the energy with respect to the pose parameters is done by considering the gradient of each parameter:

$$\begin{cases} \frac{d}{dt}\mathcal{S} = 2\int_\Omega \delta_\epsilon(\phi)(\mathcal{S}\phi - \phi_\mathcal{P}(\mathcal{A}))(-\phi + \nabla\phi_\mathcal{P}(\mathcal{A}) \cdot \frac{\partial}{\partial\mathcal{S}}\mathcal{A})d\Omega \\ \frac{d}{dt}a_i = 2\int_\Omega \delta_\epsilon(\phi)(\mathcal{S}\phi - \phi_\mathcal{P}(\mathcal{A}))(\nabla\phi_\mathcal{P}(\mathcal{A}) \cdot \frac{\partial}{\partial a_i}\mathcal{A})d\Omega \quad \text{with } a_i \in \{\theta_1, \theta_2, \theta_3, \mathcal{T}_x, \mathcal{T}_y, \mathcal{T}_z\} \end{cases}$$

5   Active Shapes, Level Sets, and Object Extraction

In this section, we integrate the proposed level set variant of the active shape model to the Geodesic Active Region model [9], that on top of salient features uses global region statistics.

5.1   Geodesic Active Region

Introducing global region properties is a common technique to improve segmentation performance. To this end, one can assume a two-class partition problem where the object and the background follow different intensity distribution. Let $p_{\mathcal{C}_{in}}$ and $p_{\Omega-\mathcal{C}_{in}}$ be the densities of $I(\mathbf{x})$ in $\mathcal{C}_{in}$ and $\Omega - \mathcal{C}_{in}$. Then according to the Geodesic Active Region model [9] one can recover the object through the optimization of the following function:

$$E(\phi, p_{\mathcal{C}_{in}}, p_{\Omega-\mathcal{C}_{in}}) = (1-a) \int_\Omega \delta_\alpha(\phi) g(|\nabla I|) |\nabla \phi| d\Omega$$
$$-a \int_\Omega [H_\alpha(\phi) \log(p_{\mathcal{C}_{in}}(I)) + (1 - H_\alpha(\phi)) \log(p_{\Omega-\mathcal{C}_{in}}(I))] d\Omega$$

One can consider either parametric approximation [9] or a non-parametric density [5] functions to describe intensity properties. In both cases the new term will result in a local balloon force that moves the contour in the direction that maximizes the posterior segmentation probability as shown in [9].

5.2   Object Extraction

The Geodesic Active Region module is used jointly with the shape prior constraint. This data-specific information make the contour evolve toward the object of interest while keeping a global shape consistant with the prior shape family. For this purpose a variational formulation incorporating two terms is used:

$$E(\phi, \mathcal{A}, \lambda) = b E_{shape}(\phi, \mathcal{A}, \lambda) + (1 - b) E_{data}(\phi)$$

where E_{shape} is the shape prior and E_{data} is the Geodesic Active Region module.

This framework has been tested on the extraction of the lateral brain ventricles. [Fig. (2)] show the robustness to noise brought by the prior shape knowledge (the image is one of the training images but with additional Riccian noise). In [fig. (3)], we show the ability of our approach to extract objects from new images (not used for building the model). The active shape model is able to approximate the surface with a similar one from the modeled class while the object extraction allows small local variations with respect to the model. Finally, in [fig. (4)], we show the influence of the shape prior term by changing its weight. While prior knowledge improves the quality of the object extraction, overweighting shape prior will make object details to be missed. The possibility of tuning this parameter is an important advantage of our approach compared to [12].

6   Conclusion

We have proposed a level set variant of active shape models to deal with object extraction in medical MR images. Our approach exhibits numerous advantages. It can deal with noisy, incomplete and occluded data because of its active shape nature. It is intrinsic, implicit parameter and topology free, a natural property of the level set space. Examples on the brain ventricles extraction demonstrate the potential of our method. The nature of the sub-space of plausible solutions is a limitation of the proposed framework. Quite often the projection to this space does not correspond to a level set distance function. To account for this limitation, we currently explore prior modeling directly on the Euclidean space, and then conversion to the implicit space during the object extraction.

References

1. T. Cootes and C. Taylor. Mixture model for representing shape variation. *Image and Vision Computing*, 17:567–574, 1999.
2. T. Cootes, C. Taylor, D. Cooper, and J. Graham. Active shape models-their training and application. *Computer Vision and Image Understanding*, 61(1):38–59, 1995.
3. D. Cremers, T. Kohlberger, and C. Schn orr. Nonlinear Shape Statistics in Mumford-Shah Based Segmentation. In *ECCV*, volume 2, pages 93–108, 2002.
4. M. Kass, A. Witkin, and D. Terzopoulos. Snakes: Active contour models. In *First International Conference on Computer Vision*, pages 259–268, London, June 1987.
5. J. Kim, J. Fisher, A. Yezzi, M. Cetin, and A. Willsky. Nonparametric methods for image segmentation using information theory and curve evolution. In *IEEE Internation Conference on Image Processing*, pages 797–800, Sept. 2002.
6. M. Leventon, E. Grimson, and O. Faugeras. Statistical Shape Influence in Geodesic Active Controus. In *IEEE CVPR*, pages I:316–322, 2000.
7. S. Osher and N. Paragios, editors. *Geometric Level Set Methods in Imaging, Vision and Graphics*. Springer Verlag, 2003.
8. S. Osher and J. Sethian. Fronts propagating with curvature dependent speed: algorithms based on the Hamilton–Jacobi formulation. *Journal of Computational Physics*, 79:12–49, 1988.
9. N. Paragios and R. Deriche. Geodesic active regions and level set methods for supervised texture segmentation. *The International Journal of Computer Vision*, 46(3):223, 2002.
10. M. Rousson and N. Paragios. Shape priors for level set representations. In A. Heyden, G. Sparr, M. Nielsen, and P. Johansen, editors, *Proceedings of the 7th European Conference on Computer Vision*, volume 2, pages 78–92, Copenhagen, Denmark, May 2002. Springer–Verlag.
11. M. Sussman, P. Smereka, and S. Osher. A Level Set Method for Computing Solutions to Incomprenissible Two-Phase Flow. *Journal of Computational Physics*, 114:146–159, 1994.
12. A. Tsai, A. Yezzi, et al. Model-based curve evolution technique for image segmentation. In *IEEE Conference on Computer Vision and Pattern Recognition*, volume 1, pages 463–468, Dec. 2001.

Construction of 3D Dynamic Statistical Deformable Models for Complex Topological Shapes

Paramate Horkaew and Guang-Zhong Yang

Royal Society/Wolfson Foundation MIC Laboratory,
Department of Computing,
Imperial College of Science, Technology and Medicine, London, SW7 2BZ, UK
{phorkaew, g.z.yang}@imperial.ac.uk
http://vip.doc.imperial.ac.uk

Abstract. This paper describes the construction of 3D dynamic statistical deformable models for complex topological shapes. It significantly extents the existing framework in that surfaces with higher genus can be effectively modeled. Criteria based on surface conformality and minimum description length is used to simultaneously identify the intrinsic global correspondence of the training data. The proposed method requires neither surface partitioning nor artificial grids on the parameterization manifold. The strength of the method is demonstrated by building a statistical model of the complex anatomical structure of the left side of human heart that includes the left ventricle, left atrium, aortic outflow tract, and pulmonary veins. The analysis of variance and leave-one-out-cross-validation indicate that the derived model not only captures physiologically plausible modes of variation but also is robust and concise, thus greatly enhancing its potential clinical value.

1 Introduction

With the increasing popularity of the Active Shape and Appearance Models [1, 2], 3D shape modeling and segmentation based on these techniques are gaining significant clinical interest. In essence, the technique recovers the underlying shape by exploiting a priori knowledge about the plausible variations of anatomical structures captured by the Point Distribution Model (PDM). The practical quality of a PDM relies on the definition of correspondence across a set of segmented samples. Brett and Taylor [3] generated correspondences using ICP while a diffeomorphism between the shapes was maintained by harmonic map. Davies *et al.* [4] solved this problem by manipulating global parameterization subject to the Minimum Description Length (MDL) criterion. For time varying 3D objects, identification of dense correspondence within the training set is a significant challenge. Landmark techniques based on anatomical features has been proven to be problematic for 3D shapes that undergo large deformation over time. To resolve this difficulty, Horkaew and Yang recently proposed a harmonic embedding technique for establishing optimal global correspondence for a set of

C. Barillot, D.R. Haynor, and P. Hellier (Eds.): MICCAI 2004, LNCS 3216, pp. 217–224, 2004.

dynamic surfaces whose topological realization is homeomorphic to a compact 2D manifold with boundary [5]. Its application to left ventricular modeling has demonstrated its compactness and ability for capturing principal modes of variation that are biologically meaningful.

One of the key challenges of 3D statistical shape modeling is the parameterization of surfaces with generic topologies. For high genus shapes, most of the current techniques [6,7,8] have limited their investigation to surface remeshing, texture mapping and metamorphosis between a pair of objects. The method recently proposed by Praun *et al.* [9], suggests a parameterization algorithm based on heuristic legal checks to avoid path intersection for a group of surfaces. Although being able to create a valid set of smooth surface partitions, the resultant meshes are not necessarily statistically optimal. This is also true for other approaches [10,11]. The alternatives of using level set embedded in higher dimension manifold or volumetric registration, on the other hand, are less compact and do not explicitly guarantee the topology of the final result [12,13].

General anatomical structures can have shapes with higher genuses. A normal human heart as shown in Figure 1, for example, consists of four chambers, each topologically equivalent to a sphere with different numbers of boundaries corresponding to valvular and vascular orifices. The left and right ventricles are connected with the atria at mitral and tricuspid valves. When all the valvular structures and inflow/outflow tracts are considered, the shape to be modeled becomes highly complex even in its static form. The purpose of this paper is to extend the harmonic embedding techniques proposed by Horkaew and Yang for anatomical structures with complex topology. One possible extension to the technique is to use surface subdivision such that each surface patch can be harmonically embedded on its own. This, however, requires the identification of geometrical landmarks for separating the overall structure into physiologically independent but topologically simple substructures. The network of partitioning curves implies the initial boundary correspondence and surface subdivision. For dynamic shapes, the treatment of surface continuity and correspondence across boundaries with this approach, however, is challenging. In this paper, a more effective embedding scheme that incorporates multiple boundaries associated with high genus objects is proposed. Whilst ensuring the generative PDM is geometrically and statistically optimal, the method also has the following features:

– *No surface partitioning prior to parameterization is required while maintaining the conformal structure and multi-resolution properties for the surface.*
– *No artificial structure is introduced to the parameterization domain, i.e., the correspondence is implicit to ensure flexibility in mathematical treatment and reduce shape artifacts.*

We demonstrate in this paper how the proposed method can be used for modeling the entire left side of the heart including Left Atrium (LA), Left Ventricle (LV), major Pulmonary Veins (PV) and the Left Ventricular Outflow Tract (LVOT).

2   Material and Methods

2.1   Surface Parameterization

One of the key steps for the proposed statistical shape modeling scheme is the parameterization of a generic surface with its equivalent topological domain. The base domain used in this study is a unit sphere. Since the underlying anatomy of LV and LA across subjects is consistent, the vertices correspond to the boundary orifices are mapped onto given locations of the base domain before surface parameterization. For LV and LA, the mitral annulus was parameterized onto a contour connecting the unit spheres used for mapping the LA and LV, as shown in Figure 1(c). Without loss of generality, the mitral annulus was always parameterized onto a contour centered by the north pole so as to ensure that no singularity was introduced by mapping infinitesimal area of the surface to infinity. During the subsequent analysis the G^1 continuity across the mitral valve boundary was maintained by conformal parameterization.

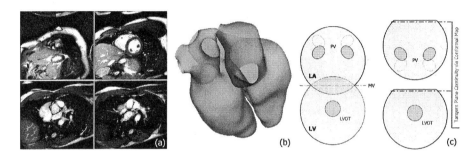

Fig. 1. Short axis MR images covering 4 chambers of the heart from the apex to the atria during diastole (a) and its corresponding 3D surface reconstruction (b). (c) The configuration used for surface parameterization of the LV and LA used for this study

The remaining internal vertices were then uniformly distributed on each sphere by using Tutte's mapping [14]. With the introduction of boundary contours as shown in Figure 1(c), the trimmed sphere is no longer convex and mesh folding is inevitable. To alleviate this problem, the vertices were first mapped to a stereographic complex domain followed by iterative mesh untangling and smoothing [15]. The technique was based on maximizing the minimum area of simplicial elements in a local sub-mesh such that

$$\hat{\mathbf{x}} = \max_{\mathbf{x}} \left(\min_{1 \leq i \leq N} \left| \mathbf{x}_i^1 - \mathbf{x}\,\mathbf{x}_i^2 - \mathbf{x} \right| \right) \tag{1}$$

In the above equation, the ith triangle in the local submesh is defined by the positions of the free vertex $\mathbf{x}$ and the positions of the two other vertices $\mathbf{x}_i^1$ and $\mathbf{x}_i^2$, and $\hat{\mathbf{x}}$ is the new optimal position of the free vertex. In this study, Polak-Ribiere's conjugate gradient optimization was adopted. This unfolding scheme results in topologically valid mesh that can be spatially degenerated. A variant of constrained Laplacian smoothing was subsequently applied to enhance mesh quality. The algorithm relocates the free vertex to the geometric center of the immediate neighboring vertices, only if the quality of the local submesh was improved according to the quality metric given by [16],

$$\alpha(T_x) = (I)2\sqrt{3}\frac{\|(\mathbf{x}_2 - \mathbf{x}_0) \times (\mathbf{x}_1 - \mathbf{x}_0)\|}{\|\mathbf{x}_2 - \mathbf{x}_0\|^2 + \|\mathbf{x}_0 - \mathbf{x}_1\|^2 + \|\mathbf{x}_1 - \mathbf{x}_2\|^2} \tag{2}$$

$$I = \begin{cases} +1 \text{ , if } (\mathbf{x}_2 - \mathbf{x}_0) \times (\mathbf{x}_1 - \mathbf{x}_0) \cdot N_x > 0 \\ -1 \text{ , otherwise} \end{cases}$$

Where T_x is a triangle defined by three vertices $\mathbf{x}_0$, $\mathbf{x}_1$ and $\mathbf{x}_2$ and the surface normal vector N_x is evaluated at the center of the triangle. The function I captures the inversion of the element to prevent mesh folding.

2.2   Variational Approach to Conformal Surface Embedding

The mesh obtained above generally has a good quality but its parameterization may not preserve the local geometric property. The purpose of conformal embedding at this stage is to reparameterize the LV and LA surfaces M to their respective topologically equivalent unit spheres S with corresponding boundaries. A variational approach to piecewise linear *Harmonic Maps* was used [17]. The advantage of the variational approach over the leastsquare ones [5,10] is that the convex constraints on the manifolds may be relaxed, provided that the initial parameterization is already of valid topology. Let $(M, m) \in \mathbf{R}^3$ and $(S, s) \in \mathbf{R}^3$ be two diffeomorphic Riemannian manifolds and $\Phi : (M, m) \to (S, s)$ is a conformal map, which minimizes metric dispersion. This metric can be represented as a sum of potential energy in a configuration of springs, each of which is placed along an edge of the triangulation. For this approach, we define linear Laplacian operator $\triangle_{PL} : C^{PL} \to C^{PL}$ on function Φ to be

$$\triangle_{PL}\,\Phi = \sum_{\{i,j\}\in M} \kappa_{ij}\,(\Phi(i) - \Phi(j)) \tag{3}$$

where $\Phi = (\phi_x, \phi_y, \phi_z)$ is a harmonic map from the surface mesh M to a unit sphere S and κ is a spring constant, defined as a summation of cotangent weighting coefficients of its subtended angles of a given edge (i, j). Since map Φ is harmonics if it only has a normal component $(\triangle\Phi)^\perp$ and its tangent component $\triangle\Phi$ is zero, therefore at critical point we have $\triangle\Phi \to (\triangle\Phi)^\perp$. In this case, Φ can be solved by iteratively displacing internal free vertices in the steepest gradient direction, *i.e.*,

$$\delta\Phi \;=\; -D\Phi \times \delta t \tag{4}$$

$$D\Phi(i) = \triangle\Phi(i) - (\triangle\Phi(i))^\perp \text{ and } (\triangle\Phi(i))^\perp = \langle\triangle\Phi(i), \mathbf{n}(\Phi(i))\rangle\mathbf{n}(\Phi(i))$$

where $\langle,\rangle$ is inner product in $\mathbf{R}^3$ and $\mathbf{n}(\mathbf{p})$ is a normal vector on S at point $\mathbf{p}$. For a sufficiently small step size δt, the resultant parameterization is guaranteed to converge to the conformal approximation. Finally, Deluanay triangulation was used to remesh the conformal domain with equilateral triangles to ensure that the final mesh is topologically correct, angle-preserving, and not degenerated. It is worth noting here that the conformal property used here also ensures the shape consistency, *i.e.*, the G^1 continuity from LV to LA across the mitral annulus.

2.3 Identifying Optimal Correspondence

The next step of building the statistical shape model is to establish optimum point correspondence within the training set. With the proposed framework, we formulate the correspondence problem as that of defining a set of dense vector fields, by which each surface in the training set is deformed. These vector fields are interpolated with radial basis splines whose control points are constrained around the defined boundaries. It is worth noting that by doing so, no artificial grids were imposed on the parameterization process. To reduce the computational cost, a k-d tree was used for sampling a deformed surface point on the parametric domain. Similar to previous studies, MDL was employed as the optimization criterion for the derived statistical model. It is well known that the MDL function is highly non-linear and can have multiple local minima, the optimization is therefore carried out in a hierarchical manner. At the coarsest parameterization level, the correspondence vector fields were deformed such that they minimized the Euclidean distances between a pair of surfaces. At the subsequent levels L, a set of 4^{L-1} spline control points and corresponding vector values were recursively inserted into the domain, with their positions determined by maximizing the multi-site geodesic distances on an individual surface. The parameterization was optimized subject to the MDL of the entire training set on a per-surface basis. The ordering, by which each sample was optimized, was randomly permutated before each iteration [18]. Conjugate gradient method was used to identify the optimal deformation fields and finally, Principal Component Analysis (PCA) was applied to capture the mean shape and principal modes of variation.

2.4 Data Acquisition and Validation

Four healthy subjects, (mean age = 27, range 25-29 years) were studied in supine position with a Siemens Sonanta 1.5T (40mT/m, 200mT/m/ms). A breath-hold retrospectively ECG-gated trueFISP cine sequence (TE = 1.63ms, TR = 3.26ms) was used. The effective temporal resolution was 22-30ms and multiple parallel short axis images were acquired in two multislice groups, one to cover from the valvular plane to the apex of the LV with 10mm increments, and the other from the aortic arch to the valvular plane in 5mm increments, due to the geometrical complexity of the LA. The in-plane and through-plane image resolution used was 1.2mm x 1.2mm and 7mm, respectively. The image segmentation scheme follows the method used in [5] for depicting the cardiac borders. For the LV, the mitral and aortic valve planes were manually defined along with the left ventricular in-flow and out-flow tracts. Similarly, the planes cutting through the pulmonary veins were also specified, giving a total of five boundary contours including the mitral annulus. A total of thirty-four shapes of the LV and LA were used for building the dynamic statistical shape model.

3   Results

Figs. 2(a) shows an example of the initial Tutte's mapping of the LA projected onto a stereographic plane. It is evident that significant mesh folding is introduced particularly around the pulmonary veins. The resultant parameterization of the unfolded mesh after applying the proposed mesh smoothing and conformal parameterization are illustrated in Figs. 2 (b) and (c), respectively. A total of 10 control points, excluding those on the boundaries, as shown in Figs. 2(d) were used to interpolate correspondence vector fields to establish the optimal set of control points. It is worth noting that these vector fields were bounded on the manifold and determined by the MDL objective.

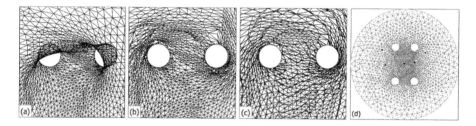

Fig. 2. The stereographic projection of the zoom up around the boundaries of the parameterized LA surfaces showing the initial state (a), after applying mesh untangling and smoothing (b) and conformal maps (c) and positions of the control points (d)

Fig. 3 demonstrates the principal modes of variation captured by the derived optimal PDM. An animation of the first three modes corresponds to contraction, radial twisting and shortening (http://vip.doc.ic.ac.uk/~gzy/osdm/). The compactness of a model is measured by using the total variance captured by the principal modes. The generalization ability is assessed by using leave-one-out reconstruction, *i.e.*, the PDM was built by using both LV and LA surfaces from all but one subject and then fitted to the excluded samples. The accuracy of the reconstruction is measured as the residue of the fitted model to the actual data. The process is repeated by excluding each of the remaining subjects in turn. The averaged residue over the samples is then computed.

Fig. 4 shows the quantitative comparison of these measurements for the model obtained by sampling on the conformal map, and that obtained by minimizing Euclidean distance between a pair of surfaces, *i.e.*, parameterization given at the first level of recursion, and the optimal model proposed in this paper. It can be observed from the graphs that the optimal model is 67% and 25%, respectively, more compact than the conformal and minimized Euclidean models.

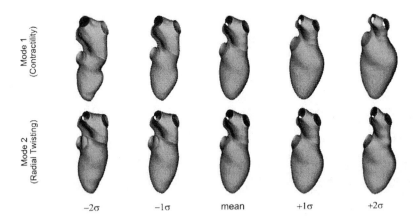

Fig. 3. The variation captured by the first two modes of variations. The shape parameters were varied by $\pm 2\sigma$, seen within the training set. They corresponds to contraction and radial twisting

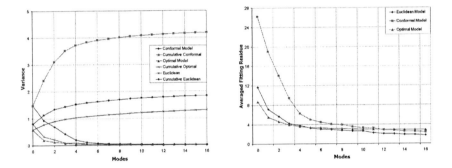

Fig. 4. Quantitative comparison of these measurements among the conformal, minimizing Euclidean distance, and the proposed optimal models, showing analysis of variances (left) and leave-one-out fitting residue (right)

Further analysis of the model shows that the averaged fitting residue of generated PDMs to the actual data by taking into account other modes of variation, the optimal model gives consistently less residue than that of the other methods.

4 Discussions and Conclusion

Conformal surface embedding is an essential step towards optimal statistical deformable surface modeling for dynamic structures. We have shown that the basic concept described in [5] can be extended to shapes with complex topology, thus enhancing its practical clinical value. The proposed method produces a PDM that is significantly more compact than the one obtained from the conformal and minimized Euclidean techniques. It must be pointed out, however, that the method proposed above applies only to a sub-class of all mathematically plausible shapes and is not suitable for shapes such as *n-torus*. From our experience, however, the restriction imposed on our framework is realistic for modeling cardiovascular and other visceral structures.

References

1. T.F. Cootes, C.J. Taylor, D.H. Cooper and J. Graham: Active Shape Models - Their Training and Application, CVIU, 61(1) (1995) 38-59.
2. T.F. Cootes, G.J. Edwards, and C. J. Taylor: Active Appearance Models, ECCV, 2 (1998) 484-498.
3. A.D. Brett and C.J. Taylor: Construction of 3D Shape Models of Femoral Articular Cartilage Using Harmonic Maps, MICCAI (2000) 1205-1214.
4. R.H. Davies, C.J. Twining, T.F Coots J.C. Waterton and C.J. Taylor: A Minimum Description Length Approach to Statistical Shape Modelling, IPMI (2001) 50-63.
5. P. Horkaew and G. Z. Yang: Optimal Deformable Surface Models for 3D Medical Image Analysis, IPMI (2003) 13-24.
6. M. S. Floater: Parametrization and Smooth Approximation of Surface Triangulations, CAGD, 14 (1997) 231-250.
7. S. Haker *et al.*: Conformal Surface Parameterization for Texture Mapping, IEEE Trans. Visualization and Computer Graphics, 6(2) (2000) 181-189.
8. B. Lévy and J. Mallet: Non-distorted Texture Mapping for Sheared Triangulated Meshes, SIGGRAPH (1998) 343-352.
9. E. Praun, W. Sweldens and P. Schroder: Consistent Mesh Parameterizations, SIGGRAPH (2001) 179-184.
10. M. Eck *et al.*: Multiresolution Analysis of Arbitrary Meshes, SIGGRAPH, (1995) 173-182.
11. O. Sorkine, D. Cohen-Or, R. Goldenthal and D. Lischinski: Bounded-distortion Piecewise Mesh Parameterization, IEEE Visualization (2002) 355-362.
12. A. Tsai *et al.*: Coupled Multi-Shape Model and Mutual Information for Medical Image Segmentation, IPMI (2003) 185-197.
13. A.F. Frangi, D. Rueckert, J.A. Schnabel, and W.J. Niessen: Automatic Construction of Multiple-object Three-dimensional Statistical Shape Models: Application to Cardiac Modeling, IEEE Trans. Med. Imag., 21, (2002) 1151-66.
14. W. T. Tutte: Convex Representations of Graphs, London Math. Soc., III Ser. 10 (1960) 304-320.
15. L. Freitag and P. Plassmann: Local Optimization-based Simplicial Mesh Untangling and Improvement. Intl. J. of Num. Meth. in Engr., 49 (2000) 109-125.
16. S.A. Canann, J.R. Tristano and M.L. Staten: An Approach to Combined Laplacian and Optimization-Based Smoothing for Triangular, Quadrilateral and Quad-Dominant Meshes, 7th Int. Meshing Roundtable, (1994) 479-494.
17. X. Gu, Y. Wang, T.F. Chan, P. Thompson and S. Yau: Genus Zero Surface Conformal Mapping and Its Application Surface Mapping, IPMI (2003) 172-184.
18. R.H. Davies, C.J. Twinig, P.J. Allen, T.F Coots and C.J. Taylor: Shape Discrimination in the Hippocampus using an MDL Model, IPMI (2003) 38-50.

Shape Representation via Best Orthogonal Basis Selection

Ashraf Mohamed[1,2] and Christos Davatzikos[1,2]

[1] CISST NSF Engineering Research Center,
Department of Computer Science, Johns Hopkins University
http://cisstweb.cs.jhu.edu/
[2] Section for Biomedical Image Analysis, Department of Radiology,
University of Pennsylvania School of Medicine
http://oasis.rad.upenn.edu/sbia/
{ashraf,christos}@rad.upenn.edu

Abstract. We formulate the problem of finding a statistical representation of shape as a best basis selection problem in which the goal is to choose the basis for optimal shape representation from a very large library of bases. In this work, our emphasis is on applying this basis selection framework using the wavelet packets library to estimate the probability density function of a class of shapes from a limited number of training samples. Wavelet packets offer a large number of complete orthonormal bases which can be searched for the basis that optimally allows the analysis of shape details at different scales. The estimated statistical shape distribution is capable of generalizing to shape examples not encountered during training, while still being specific to the modeled class of shapes. Using contours from two-dimensional MRI images of the corpus callosum, we demonstrate the ability of this approach to approximate the probability distribution of the modeled shapes, even with a few training samples.

1 Introduction

The statistical study of anatomical shape variability in medical images allows for the morphometric characterization of differences between normal and diseased poplulations [1,2,3],the detection of shape changes due to growth or disease progression [4,5], the construction of models capable of automatically segmenting and labelling structures in images [6,7], and the estimation of missing shape features from obsereved ones [8].

A space of high dimensionality is typically needed to represent shapes in medical images faithfully. With the limited availability of training samples, the statistical shape modeling and analysis task becomes infeasible in the original high dimensional space. This problem has traditionally been approached by applying dimensionality reduction methods, such as principal component analysis (PCA), to yield a compact shape representation (shape descriptor) with a small number of parameters that can estimated easily from the training samples. However, with the limited availability of training samples, PCA becomes sensitive

C. Barillot, D.R. Haynor, and P. Hellier (Eds.): MICCAI 2004, LNCS 3216, pp. 225–233, 2004.

to noise and data outliers, and it allows only a small number of degrees of freedom for the shape descriptor, which makes it unable to generalize to valid shape
instances not encountered during training.

In this work, we propose the of use of the best orthogonal basis selection
framework of Coifman and Wickerhauser [9] to decide a multi-resolution shape
representation that is optimal according to an application-dependent criterion.
Multi-resolution analysis offers a shape representation with a large number of
degrees of freedom by analyzing shape at different scales independently [10]. For
example, wavelet packets (WPs) – of which the discrete wavelet transform is a
special case – offers a large library of complete orthonormal bases, each of which
capable of linearly mapping shape onto a different multi-resolution feature space.
This library can be searched for the optimal basis according to a criterion that
depends on the shape analysis task at hand. We demonstrate the use of this basis
selection framework for approximating the probability density function (pdf) of
a class of shapes by minimizing the entropy of WP coefficients [11]. This yields
wavelet coefficients that are as decorrelated as possible, and therefore, coupled
with a Gaussian assumption, allows the expression of the pdf as the product of
lower dimensional pdfs that can be estimated more accurately from the limited
available training samples. Such estimates of shape pdfs are useful for computing
the likelihood of shapes in classification problems, and can consitute a shape prior
to be used in generative models for shape segmentation and estimation tasks.

The rest of the paper is organized in four sections. In Section 2, we explain
our shape representation and review the use of PCA for shape modeling and
analysis. In Section 3, we present the details of our approach with a brief overview
of wavelet packets and best basis selection. In Section 4, using contours of two-
dimensional (2D) corpora callosa extracted from MRI images, we demonstrate
the ability of our approach to approximate the pdf of the modeled shapes even
with a few training samples. In Section 5, we explain how our approach is readily
extendable to 3D images and we present an outlook for future work.

2   Shape Descriptors Using PCA

A continuous shape instance in $\Re^d$ may be represented by a map from a d_r
dimensional reference space to the shape space, $\psi : \Re^{d_r} \to \Re^d$. For example, in
case of 3D shapes, $d = d_r = 3$ with ψ defined for each shape instance as the
deformation map that registers this instance to a reference template [3]. For the
sake of simplicity, we will restrict our discussion to shapes represented by a closed
2D contour which therefore, may be defined by $\psi : [0, 1) \to \Re^2$ $(d_r = 1, d = 2)$,
with values in $[0, 1)$ being the normalized distance along the contour.

Assume that n_s examples are available from $\mathcal{C}$, the class of shapes of interest. Also, assume that Procrustes alignment was performed on the shapes
to remove effects of translation, rotation, and scaling [6]. A uniform sampling
of the interval $[0, 1)$ with n_p points $(n_p = 2^{K_o}$, and K_o a positive integer) is
achieved by piece-wise constant speed reparameterization of the original contours obtained via manual or automatic landmark selection. Let the coordi-

nates $\{(x_i, y_i)\}_{i=1}^{n_p}$, of the resulting points around the contour be concatenated into a vector $\mathbf{x} = [x_1, .., x_{n_p}, y_1, .., y_{n_p}]^T \in \Re^n$ $(n = 2n_p)$. Therefore, the set $\mathcal{T} = \{\mathbf{x}_1, \mathbf{x}_2, \cdots, \mathbf{x}_{n_s}\}$, may be regarded as n_s independent realizations of a random vector $\mathbf{X}$ with an unknown pdf, $f_{\mathbf{X}}$.

For anatomical shapes, $n_s \ll n$ which makes shape analysis impractical or even infeasible in the original n-dimensional space. However, if $\mathcal{C}$ has an intrinsic dimensionality $m \ll n$ (e.g., due to correlations between the shape point coordinates), the analysis may be performed in a low-dimensional subspace $\mathcal{Q}$ of $\Re^n$, which we hope to include $\mathcal{C}$. To analyze data in $\mathcal{Q}$, a map $\mathcal{V} : \Re^n \to \mathcal{Q}$ must be defined. In this work, we restrict our attention to linear maps which can be defined by an invertible real $n \times n$ matrix $\mathbf{A}$, whose columns are basis vectors spanning $\Re^n$. Let $\mathbf{X} = \mathbf{AV}$. The map $\mathcal{V}$ is decided by choosing $\mathbf{A}^*$ as the optimal basis matrix according to some criterion that measures the efficiency of the basis with respect to $\mathcal{T}$, followed by selecting a collection $\{\mathbf{a}_i^*\}_{i=1}^r$ from among its columns.

Applying PCA to $\mathcal{T}$, yields the matrix $\mathbf{A}_{pca}^*$ whose columns are the eigenvectors of the sample covariance matrix of $\mathbf{X}$. The matrix $\mathbf{A}_{pca}^*$ is the rotation satisfying a number of optimality criteria including attaining the minimum of $h_{\mathbf{X}}$, the entropy function of the coefficients $\mathbf{V} = \mathbf{A}^T\mathbf{X}$ defined by [12]:

$$h_{\mathbf{X}}(\mathbf{A}) = \sum_{i=1}^n \hat{\sigma}_i^2(\mathbf{A}) \log \hat{\sigma}_i^2(\mathbf{A}), \tag{1}$$

with $\hat{\sigma}_i^2(\mathbf{A}) = \mathrm{E}[v_i^2]/\sum_{j=1}^n \mathrm{E}[v_j^2]$, and v_i's being components of $\mathbf{V}$. The maximum number of degrees of freedom (dof) of the shape descriptor $\mathbf{V}$ is $n_s - 1$ which is the number of eigenvectors of the sample covariance matrix with non-zero eigenvalues. These eigenvectors span the linear space in which the training samples lie. Therefore, if $m < n_s - 1$, $\mathbf{V}$ will be unable to represent legal shapes outside the linear subspace spanned by the training samples.

3   Methods

The abovementioned drawbacks of PCA may be addressed in the best basis selection (BBS) framework described in detail in [9,12]. In this context of shape analysis, the goal of BBS is to find the optimal representation of $\mathbf{X}$ in terms of the columns of $\mathbf{A}$ which are selected from the components of a library $\mathcal{L}$ of overcomplete bases ($|\mathcal{L}| > n$). The choice of the library $\mathcal{L}$ and the optimization criterion are task dependent. For example, for shape classification, $\mathcal{L}$ may be designed to test one or more hypothesis of local shape differences between two poplulations, while the optimization criterion would encourage the representation of shape in terms of the basis that provides the best clustering [13]. In general, $\mathbf{A}$ need not have n columns or constitute a complete basis. However, this will be the case in our work here.

We now direct our attention to the task of estimating $f_{\mathbf{X}}$ given $\mathcal{T}$. We assume that $\mathcal{L}$ is formed of orthonormal bases, such as the wavelet packets (WP) library [11], briefly explained in Section 3.1. Any complete minimal basis from this library will correspond to a rotation matrix $\mathbf{A}_S$. Such a basis can be partitioned into N groups of basis vectors, with each group spanning a subspace $\mathcal{S}_l$, and the subspaces $\{\mathcal{S}_l\}_{l=1}^N$ mutually orthogonal. The partitioning is decided so that the subspaces $\{\mathcal{S}_l\}_{l=1}^N$ will correspond to shape features that can be analyzed independently of the others. One obvious, example would be localized shape details, and global shape characteristics. Defining $\mathbf{x}_p^l = \mathrm{Proj}(\mathbf{x}, \mathcal{S}_l)$, we can write

$$f_{\mathbf{X}}(\mathbf{x}) = \prod_{l=1}^N f_{\mathbf{X}_p^l}(\mathbf{x}_p^l). \tag{2}$$

If each of the subspaces in $\{\mathcal{S}_l\}_{l=1}^N$, is of low dimensionality, then the independence assumption has effectively decomposed the pdf into the product of marginal pdfs that can be estimated more accurately from the limited samples. Moreover, it improves the generalization ability of the estimated pdf over that of PCA since the shape descriptor can have up to $n_s - 1$ dof from each subspace $\mathcal{S}_l$ compared to a total of $n_s - 1$ dof in PCA. On the other hand, high correlation between $\mathbf{x}_p^l$ implied by the training samples, may betray the invalidity of this assumption, and therefore suggests that the improved generalization ability of the estimated $f_{\mathbf{X}}$ comes at the expense of its low specificity (i.e., the estimated $f_{\mathbf{X}}(\mathbf{x})$ may include invalid shapes). Therefore, we select the optimal basis $\mathbf{A}_S$ according to an information cost that, coupled with a Gaussian assumption on $f_{\mathbf{X}}$, supports independence of shape projections on the subsapces $\{\mathcal{S}_i\}_{i=1}^N$. This criterion is explained in Section 3.2.

3.1   The Wavelet Packet Bases Library

Wavelet packets (WPs) form a family of orthonormal bases for discrete functions in $L^2(\Re)$ [9]. Dyadic multi-resolution analysis of a signal may be performed by defining wavelet analysis functions $\{W_k\}_{k=0}^\infty$ associated with an exact quadrature mirror filter pair, $h(i)$ and $g(i)$, as:

$$\begin{aligned} W_{2i}(z) &= \sqrt{2}\sum h(k)W_i(2z - k) \\ W_{2i+1}(z) &= \sqrt{2}\sum g(k)W_i(2z - k) \end{aligned} \tag{3}$$

The functions $W_0(z)$ and $W_1(z)$ correspond to the mother wavelet and the scaling function respectively.

A wavelet packet basis (WPB) of $L^2(\Re)$ is any orthonormal basis selected from the functions $W_{k,i,j} \equiv 2^{k/2}W_i(2^k t - j)$ [9]. For an analyzed signal of length 2^{K_o}, each $W_{k,i,j}$ is identified by the indices

- $k = 0, \cdots, K$: the scale parameter, where K is the maximum scale ($K \le K_o$),
- $i = 0, \cdots, 2^k - 1$: the frequency index at scale k, and
- $j = 0, \ldots, 2^{K_o-k} - 1$: the translation index at scale k.

The library of WPs may be organized into a binary tree with each level representing the projection of the signal of the parent node onto two subspaces corresponding to its low frequency component and high frequency details. If each wavelet packet $W_{k,i,j}$ is represented by a $2^{K_o} \times 1$ vector, we can define

$$\mathbf{W}_{k,i} = [W_{k,i,0}|\cdots|W_{k,i,2^{K_o-k}-1}] \tag{4}$$

to be the collection of WPs for all translations at node (k,i) of the tree. If a collection $\{\mathbf{W}_{k,i}\}$ corresponds to to a disjoint cover of the frequency domain, then it forms an orthonormal basis [9]. The discrete wavelet transform constitutes one of these basis. Every such basis will correspond to the leaves of a full binary wavelet packet tree (WPT). There are 2^{2^K} such bases for a binary tree of K levels. This flexibility can be exploited to select the most efficient representation of a signal according to some information cost.

3.2   Best Basis Selection (BBS) for Estimating 2D Shape pdf

The shape vector $\mathbf{X}$, may be decomposed into two signals written as column vectors $\mathbf{X}^1 = [x_1, \cdots, x_{n_p}]^T$ and $\mathbf{X}^2 = [y_1, \cdots, y_{n_p}]^T$, with $\mathbf{X} = [\mathbf{X}^{1^T} \mathbf{X}^{2^T}]^T$. We elect to use the same WPB for both signals. Any set $\{\mathbf{W}_{k,i}\}$ forming a WPB of $\Re^{n_p}$ may be written in the form an $n_p \times n_p$ basis matrix $\mathbf{B}$. The matrix $\mathbf{A}_{wpt} = \mathrm{diag}(\mathbf{B}, \mathbf{B})$ forms a basis for $\Re^n$, and the shape descriptor is $\mathbf{V} = \mathbf{A}_{wpt}^T \mathbf{X} = [\mathbf{V}^{1^T} \mathbf{V}^{2^T}]^T$ with $\mathbf{V}^1 = \mathbf{B}^T \mathbf{X}^1$ and $\mathbf{V}^2 = \mathbf{B}^T \mathbf{X}^2$.

The goal of the BBS algorithm is to find the matrix $\mathbf{A}_{wpt}^*$ attaining the minimum of an information cost functional $\mathcal{M}_{\mathbf{X}}(\mathbf{A})$ that measures the efficiency of the basis $\mathbf{A}_{wpt}$ in representing $\mathbf{X}$. Defining the function $\mathcal{M}$, as a map from real sequences $\{v_i\}$ to $\Re$, we can now define $\mathcal{M}_{\mathbf{X}}(\mathbf{A}) \equiv \mathcal{M}(\{v_i\})$, with v_i's the components of $\mathbf{V} = \mathbf{A}^T \mathbf{X}$. Coifman and Wickerhauser [9] proposed a fast BBS algorithm suitable for searching the WP library when $\mathcal{M}$ is additive, (i.e., $\mathcal{M}(0) = 0$ and $\mathcal{M}(\{v_i\}) = \sum_i \mathcal{M}(v_i)$). Here, we use $\mathcal{M}_{\mathbf{X}}(\mathbf{A}_{wpt}) = h_{\mathbf{X}^1}(\mathbf{B}) + h_{\mathbf{X}^2}(\mathbf{B})$, where $h_{\mathbf{X}^1}(B)$ and $h_{\mathbf{X}^2}(B)$ are defined analogous to equation (1). It can be shown that since $h_{\mathbf{X}^l}$ is an additive information cost for $l = 1, 2$ [11], so will $\mathcal{M}$ be. This choice of $\mathcal{M}$ will provide the optimal WPB, $\mathbf{B}^*$, and therefore $\mathbf{A}_{wpt}^*$, that produces $\mathbf{V}^1$ and $\mathbf{V}^2$, each composed of a set of coefficients that are as decorrelated as possible. This basis is called the Joint Best Basis (JBB) [11].

The shape descriptor $\mathbf{V}$ may be decomposed into a collection $\{\mathbf{v}_{k,i}\}$ of WP coefficients with $\mathbf{v}_{k,i} \equiv [(\mathbf{W}_{k,i}^{*T} \mathbf{x}^1)^T (\mathbf{W}_{k,i}^{*T} \mathbf{x}^2)^T]^T$ for the set $\{\mathbf{W}_{k,i}^*\}$ which forms the optimal basis $\mathbf{B}^*$. Here, we assume that each $\mathbf{v}_{k,i}$ is independent of $\mathbf{v}_{u,v}$ for all $(k,i) \neq (u,v)$. With this choice, it can be seen that each $\mathbf{W}_{k,i}^{*T}$ describes one of the subspaces $\mathcal{S}_l$ mentioned above. In the work presented here, each coefficients vector $\mathbf{v}_{k,i}$ is assumed to follow a Gaussian distribution and PCA is applied to estimate this distribution [13].

4   Experimental Results

We compare the estimated shape pdfs generated by PCA basis (PCAB), JBB, and the approach in [10] which will be referred to as WT basis (WTB). We

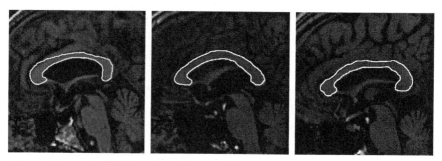

Fig. 1. Example MRI images with manually outlined corpus callosum contours.

use a dataset composed of 100 manually-outlined corpora callosa contours in midsaggital MR images of normal subjects. Landmarks were manually selected by an expert and the contours were then reparametrized by piece-wise constant speed parameterization. We used $n_p = 512$, and therefore $K_o = 9$. Example contours from the dataset are shown in Figure 1. More details about the datasets can be found in [10]. For wavelet analysis, we used the Daubechies wavelet with 6 vanishing moments and $K = 5$ (5 levels of wavelet decomposition).

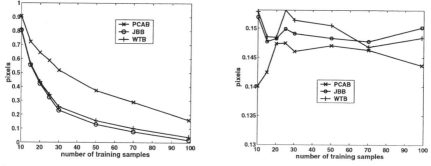

Fig. 2. Average generalization (left) and specificity (right) errors for the estimated $f_{\mathbf{X}}$ by JBB, WTB, and PCAB.

Ideally, an estimated $f_{\mathbf{X}}$ may be evaluated by comparing it with the actual pdf responsible for generating the analyzed shapes. For naturally occuring shapes, the latter, is however, not known. Therefore, we adopt the measures of generalization and specificity used in [14]. We do not address the issue of compactness here since our goal is to increase the number of degrees of freedom over that of PCA. PCA will always produce a more compact representation than WTB or JBB for any percentage of the total variance obsereved in the training samples. Constructing a more compact shape descriptor may be a achieved via wavelet shrinkage or the approach in [13] and is subject to future investigations.

We introduce the maximum absolute distance (MAD) across all corresponding points in two shapes as a measure the similarity between them. Cross validation via the leave-one-out method is used for measuring the generalization

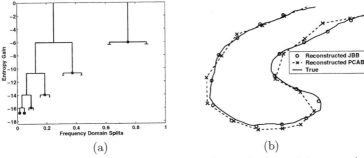

Fig. 3. (a) The JBB tree compared to the WTB tree for 25 training samples. Circles denote the terminal nodes of the WTB. The length of each branch in the tree indicates the amount of entropy reduction achieved by splitting a node into its two children. (b) Zoom-in to the reconstruction of a corpus callosum contour using PCAB and the JBB tree in (a).

ability of an the estimated $f_{\mathbf{X}}$. The generalization error for the left-out sample is defined as the MAD between this sample and its best possible reconstruction using the model. Since each of the tested models is composed orthonormal vectors, the best-possible reconstruction of a shape is found by projecting it on the model's basis vectors, followed by restricting the coefficients of the basis to be within three standard deviations from the mean as estimated from the training samples. The average generalization error of a model can then be computed over the complete set of trials which involve leaving-out a different sample each time.

To evaluate the specificity, a shape is randomly generated according to the estimated pdf, and MAD is computed between this shape and all available samples, whether used for estimating $f_{\mathbf{X}}$ or not. The minimum MAD is recorded as the specificity error. The average specificity error is then computed for 1000 randomly generated shapes.

The average generalization and specificity errors for varying number of training samples are shown in Figure 2. JBB and WTB estimates of $f_{\mathbf{X}}$ have better generalization ability than that of PCAB. On the other hand, the specificity error is higher for both JBB and WTB compared to PCAB. The increase in the specificity error of JBB over that of PCA is maximum of 9% (with 10 training samples). JBB has better specificity than WTB for 50 training samples or less.

In Figure 3.a, the WPT of JBB for 25 training samples is compared to that of the WTB. The structure of the two trees are similar, although not identical. Some bands in the WTB are split into their two children in the JBB because the coefficients of the children offer a lower entropy. JBB has a total of 10 nodes giving rise to a maximum of 240 dof while WTB has 6 nodes, which gives rise to a maximum of 144 dof. On the other hand PCAB has a maximum of 24 dof.

To qualitatively evaluate the generalization ability of the JBB prior in this case, in Figure 3.b reconstructions of a corpus callosum contour (not used in training) is shown for PCAB and JBB. The JBB reconstruction follows the original contour closely, while the PCAB contour shows some significant differences.

5   Discussion and Future Work

We presented the problem of finding a shape descriptor as a BBS problem in which the goal is to select the optimal basis for shape representation from a very large library of bases. Within this framework of BBS, we demonstrated the use of the WP library for estimating the pdf of shapes of 2D corpus callosa contours. The independence assumption between the wavelet coefficients at different nodes of the selected WPT allows the expression the pdf as a product of lower dimensional pdfs which can easily be estimated from the training samples. This assumption reveals similarities between our approach and that of Staib and Duncan [15], although ours enjoys the advantages of wavelet analysis over Fourier analysis. The assumption is also equivalent to imposing a block diagonal prior on the structure on the covariance matrix of $\mathbf{V} = \mathbf{A}_S^T \mathbf{X}$ [10]. This observation connects our approach to that in [7] and the references therein, which have the effect of imposing some form of a structure on the covariance matrix of $\mathbf{X}$. A key difference is that transforming shapes using $\mathbf{A}_S$ allows the shape description in a basis for which prior knowledge about shape (e.g., independence between local and global shape) has direct a implication on the covariance structure that is not a result of an ad hoc physical or general smoothness model.

As pointed out in the body of this work, with the use of other orthogonal basis libraries and selection criteria, many shape analysis applications can benefit from the approach presented here. With the availability of deformation fields mapping shape to a standard template, the extension of this work to 3D and 4D shapes is straight forward. Usually, such deformation fields are readily avaialable as a product of an image warping procedure, which is essential for establishing automatic correspondence between shapes in 3D and 4D images. The application of this approach for 3D shapes is currently underway. Also, we plan to investigate other approaches for the grouping of basis vectors rather than using the nodes of the WPT, and approaches to achieve more compact descriptors.

Acknowledgments. The authors would like to thank Xiaodong Tao for providing the repraremetrized corpus callosum data. WavPack library was used for programing and creating some figures in this work. This work was supported in part by the National Science Foundation under Engineering Research Center grant EEC9731478, and by the National Institutes of Health grant R01NS42645.

References

1. P. Golland, W. E. L. Grimson, M. E. Shenton, and R. Kikinis. Deformation analysis for shape based classification. In *Proc. of IPMI'2001*, LNCS 2082, pages 517–530, 2001.
2. P. Yushkevich, S. Joshi, S. M. Pizer, J. G. Csernansky, and L. E. Wang. Feature selection for shape-based classficiation of biological objects. In *Proc. of IPMI'2003*, LNCS 2732, pages 114–125, 2003.

3. J. G. Csernansky, S. Joshi, L. Wang, J. W. Haller, M. Gado, J. P. Miller, U. Grenander, and M. I. Miller. Hippocampal morphometry in schizophrenia by high dimensional brain mapping. In *Proc. Natl. Acad. Sci.*, 95:11406–11411, Sept. 1998.

4. P. R. Andersen, F. L. Bookstein, K. Conradsen, B. K. Ersbøll, J. L. Marsh, and S. Kreiborg. Surface-bounded growth modeling applied to human mandibles. *IEEE Trans. Med. Imag.*, 19(11):1053–1063, Nov. 2000.

5. C. Davatzikos, A. Genc, D. Xu, and S. M. Resnik. Voxel-based morphometry using the ravens maps: Mehods and validation using simulation of longitudinal atrophy. *Neuroimage*, 14:1361–1369, Dec. 2001.

6. T. F. Cootes, C. J. Taylor, D. H. Cooper, and J. Graham. Active shape models – their training and application. *Computer Vision and Image Understanding*, 61(1):38–59, 1995.

7. Y. Wang and L. H. Staib. Boundary finding with prior shape and smoothness models. *IEEE Trans. PAMI*, 22(7):738–743, July 2000.

8. A. Mohamed, S. K. Kyriacou, and C. Davatzikos. A statistical approach for estimating brain tumor induced deformation. *Proc. of the IEEE MMBIA Workshop*, pages 52–59, December 2001.

9. R. R. Coifman and M. V. Wickerhauser. Entropy-based algorithms for best basis selection. *IEEE Trans. on Inf. Theory*, 38(2), March 1992.

10. C. Davatzikos, X. Tao, and D. Shen. Hierarchical active shape models using the wavelet transform. *IEEE Trans. on Med. Imag.*, 22(3):414–423, March 2003.

11. M. V. Wickerhauser. Fast approximate factor analysis. In *Curves and Surfaces in Computer Vision and Graphics II*, In *SPIE Proc.*, 1610:23–32, Boston, 1991.

12. N. Saito. Image approximation and modeling via least statistically dependent basis. *Pattern Recognition*, 34:1765–1784, 2001.

13. F. G. Meyer and J. Chinrungrueng. Analysis of event-related FMRI data using best clustering basis. *IEEE Trans. on Med. Imag.*, 22(8):933–939, Aug. 2003.

14. M. A. Styner, K. T. Rajamani, L. R. Nolte, G. Zsemlye, Gábor Székely, C. J. Taylor, and R. H. Davies. Evaluation of 3d correspondence methods for model building. In *Proceedings of IPMI'2003*, 2003.

15. L. H. Staib and J. S. Duncan. Boundary finding with parametrically deformable models. *IEEE Trans. on PAMI*, 14(11):1061–1075, Nov. 1992.

Robust Generalized Total Least Squares Iterative Closest Point Registration

Raúl San José Estépar[1], Anders Brun[1,2], and Carl-Fredrik Westin[1]

[1] Laboratory of Mathematics in Imaging, Brigham and Women's Hospital,
Harvard Medical School, Boston, MA, USA
{rjosest,anders,westin}@bwh.harvard.edu
[2] Department of Biomedical Engineering, Linköping University, Sweden.

Abstract. This paper investigates the use of a total least squares approach in a generalization of the iterative closest point (ICP) algorithm for shape registration. A new Generalized Total Least Squares (GTLS) formulation of the minimization process is presented opposed to the traditional Least Squares (LS) technique. Accounting for uncertainty both in the target and in the source models will lead to a more robust estimation of the transformation. Robustness against outliers is guaranteed by an iterative scheme to update the noise covariances. Experimental results show that this generalization is superior to the least squares counterpart.

1 Introduction

The iterative closest point (ICP) algorithm [1] has been extensively used as optimization technique for rigid model based registration based on features extracted from medical datasets. ICP is an iterative descent procedure which seeks to minimize the sum of the squared distances between all points in a source and their closest points in a target model. As stated by Besl and McKay [1], ICP cannot deal with outliers and unequal uncertainty among points.

When there is a known correspondence between the points in the source and the target, the rigid transformation between those sets can be solved in a least squares sense with a closed form solution [2]. From a statistical point of view, least squares methods assume that the points are observed with isotropic, identical and independent Gaussian noise. A more general approach would be to assume that both the source and the target have noise that can be neither isotropic nor identical. This kind of model leads to a Generalized Total Least Squares (GTLS) problem. Kanatani et al. [3] have introduced a total least squares solution to the problem of rotations of correspondent points.

This paper introduces a novel total least squares generalization of ICP. This generalization will allow us to consider anisotropic noise both in the target shape and the source shape. Moreover, an iterative technique is presented that allows us to estimate the optimal set of covariance matrices so the effect of outlier points is minimized. An evaluation study is carried out to show the superiority of the proposed method compared to the standard ICP.

C. Barillot, D.R. Haynor, and P. Hellier (Eds.): MICCAI 2004, LNCS 3216, pp. 234–241, 2004.

1.1 Iterative Closest Points

Let $\mathcal{P}$ be the data shape (source shape) and $\mathcal{X}$ the model shape (target shape) to be registered with. The data shape is decomposed in point set form, if not already available in that form. The model shape could originally be given in any representation but for our purpose we will assume that is also decomposed in a point set. Thus, let N_P, N_X be the number of points in the shapes. P and X are respectively defined by the N_P-tuple $\mathcal{P} = \{\mathbf{p}_1, \mathbf{p}_2, \cdots, \mathbf{p}_{N_P}\}$ and the N_X-tuple $\mathcal{X} = \{\mathbf{x}_1, \mathbf{x}_2, \cdots, \mathbf{x}_{N_X}\}$. There is not a preestablished correspondence between the points $\mathbf{p}_j$ and $\mathbf{x}_j$.

ICP finds the rigid body transformation[1], rotation $\mathbf{R}$ and translation $\mathbf{t}$ that aligns the source with the target by minimizing the distance metric

$$J(\mathbf{R}, \mathbf{t}) = \sum_{i=1}^{N_P} \|\mathbf{y}_i - \mathbf{R}\mathbf{p}_i - \mathbf{t}\|^2, \qquad \text{where} \quad \mathbf{y}_i = \mathcal{C}(\mathbf{R}\mathbf{p}_i + \mathbf{t}, \mathcal{X}) \qquad (1)$$

is a point on the surface of the target model $\mathcal{X}$ that corresponds to the point $\mathbf{p}_i$. Given that *a priori* correspondence between source points and target points does not exist, an iterative search is needed in order to solve the problem. At each iteration, a correspondence is established by means of the *correspondence operator* $\mathcal{C}$. Then, the transformation that minimizes a mean square metric is computed. The data points are transformed using the computed transformation and the process is repeated until a minimum error threshold is achieved or a maximum number of iterations is reached. The correspondence operator is typically the *closest point* operator: $\mathcal{C}_{cp}(\mathbf{a}, \mathcal{X}) = \arg\min_{\mathbf{x} \in \mathcal{X}} \|\mathbf{x} - \mathbf{a}\|$.

One of the main drawbacks of ICP is that unequal uncertainty among points is not considered in the process. Several authors have tried to *partially* take into account unequal uncertainty by using a weighted least squares minimization [4, 5,6]. This approach, although effective and intuitively correct, is not optimal due to isotropic assumptions.

2 Method

Real problems present data with noise both in the source and in the target. Moreover, the noise is typically anisotropic, i.e. certain directions are prone to being more inaccurate than others. These facts lead us to introduce a generalized total least squares approach to the aforementioned registration problem.

2.1 GTLS Registration of Corresponding 3-D Point Sets

Let us assume that the target points and the source points are corrupted with additive noise: $\mathbf{x}_i = \bar{\mathbf{x}}_i + \Delta\mathbf{x}_i$ and $\mathbf{p}_i = \bar{\mathbf{p}}_i + \Delta\mathbf{p}_i$, where $\Delta\mathbf{x}_i$ and $\Delta\mathbf{p}_i$ are independent random variables with zero mean and known covariance matrices

---

[1] The method can also handle affine transformations by looking for the solution in a linear affine subspace

$V[\mathbf{x}_i] = E[\Delta\mathbf{x}_i\Delta\mathbf{x}_i^T]$ and $V[\mathbf{p}_i] = E[\Delta\mathbf{p}_i\Delta\mathbf{p}_i^T]$. The relation between the free noise data is given by the rigid transformation model

$$\bar{\mathbf{x}}_i = \mathbf{R}\bar{\mathbf{p}}_i + \mathbf{t}, \qquad i = 1, \cdots, N_P. \tag{2}$$

Our problem is to find an estimator of the rotation matrix, $\hat{\mathbf{R}}$, and the translation term, $\hat{\mathbf{t}}$ from the noisy data $\{\mathbf{x}_i\}$ and $\{\mathbf{p}_i\}$.

The Gauss-Markov theorem states that the linear minimum variance unbiased estimator when the noise is correlated is given by the minimization of the *Mahalanobis* distance

$$J(\mathbf{R}, \mathbf{t}) = \sum_{i=1}^{N_P}(\mathbf{p}_i - \bar{\mathbf{p}}_i)^T V[\mathbf{p}_i]^{-1}(\mathbf{p}_i - \bar{\mathbf{p}}_i) + \sum_{i=1}^{N}(\mathbf{x}_i - \bar{\mathbf{x}}_i)^T V[\mathbf{x}_i]^{-1}(\mathbf{x}_i - \bar{\mathbf{x}}_i), \tag{3}$$

subject to the model constraint (2). This problem can be seen as a Generalized Total Least Squares problem [7] from the matrix algebra point of view. The main difficulty of this problem is that we are looking for the solution in the group of rotations $SO(3)$. To find a feasible implementation, we have decoupled the problem over the minimization variable. Thus, we will independently minimize the rotation variable and the translation variable. An iterative approach will seek the optimal solution in both spaces.

Rotation term. Let us restrict our data model to be

$$\bar{\mathbf{x}}_i = \mathbf{R}\bar{\mathbf{p}}_i, \qquad i = 1, \cdots, N_P. \tag{4}$$

The minimization of the functional J in eq. (3) subject to (4) has been previously addressed by Ohta and Kanatani [3]. The authors show that the values of $\hat{\mathbf{x}}_i$ and $\hat{\mathbf{p}}_i$ that minimize (3) can be solved analytically using Lagrange multipliers and considering $\mathbf{R}$ fixed. From this solution, the resulting minimum is minimized with respect to $\mathbf{R}$. The problem reduces to

$$J_R(\mathbf{R}) = \sum_{i=1}^{N_P}(\mathbf{x}_i - \mathbf{R}\mathbf{p}_i)^T\mathbf{W}_i^{\mathbf{R}}(\mathbf{x}_i - \mathbf{R}\mathbf{p}_i) \qquad \hat{\mathbf{R}} = \arg\min_{\mathbf{R}\in SO(3)} J_R, \tag{5}$$

where $\mathbf{W}_i^{\mathbf{R}} = (\mathbf{R}V[\mathbf{p}_i]\mathbf{R}^T + V[\mathbf{x}_i])^{-1}$. The same authors proposed an optimization scheme based on quaternions using the renormalization technique of Kanatani [8]. The implementation of this optimization method has been proven to be robust and stable.

Translation term. In this case, the data model is merely

$$\bar{\mathbf{x}}_i = \bar{\mathbf{p}}_i + \mathbf{t}, \qquad i = 1, \cdots, N_P. \tag{6}$$

Following the same approach as in [3], we have solved the values of $\hat{\mathbf{x}}_i$ and $\hat{\mathbf{p}}_i$ that minimize (3) considering $\mathbf{t}$ fixed. Again, minimizing that result with respect to $\mathbf{t}$, we can write

$$J_t(\mathbf{t}) = \sum_{i=1}^{N_P} (\mathbf{x}_i - \mathbf{p}_i - \mathbf{t})^T \mathbf{W}_i^{\mathbf{t}} (\mathbf{x}_i - \mathbf{p}_i - \mathbf{t}), \qquad \hat{\mathbf{t}} = \arg\min_{\mathbf{t} \in R^3} J_t \qquad (7)$$

where $\mathbf{W}_i^{\mathbf{t}} = (V[\mathbf{p}_i] + V[\mathbf{x}_i])^{-1}$. $\hat{\mathbf{t}}$ can be analytically obtained by equating the gradient to zero and solving for $\mathbf{t}$. The solution is given by

$$\hat{\mathbf{t}} = (\sum_{i=1}^{N_P} \mathbf{W}_i^{\mathbf{t}})^{-1} \sum_{i=1}^{N_P} \mathbf{W}_i^{\mathbf{t}} (\mathbf{x}_i - \mathbf{p}_i). \qquad (8)$$

Note that setting the covariance matrices to the identity, the solutions $\hat{\mathbf{R}}$ and $\hat{\mathbf{t}}$ reduce to the least squares ones.

Robustness. A total least squares approach has the flexibility of encoding the uncertainty information of the observed data points in the covariance matrices. In point correspondence problems we can identify two sources of noise: extrinsic noise due to sensor errors and intrinsic noise due to incorrect matches. The extrinsic noise is problem dependent and we try to model it by means of the covariance matrices. The intrinsic noise has paramount importance as recognized by Haralick et al. [9]. Outliers make ordinary LS estimators the estimator of least virtue. We have enforced the robustness of the correspondence problem by an iterative algorithm that looks for the optimal set of covariance matrices. At the same time, the iterative approach will allow us to look for the solution in both parameter spaces, rotation and translation.

Our aim is to make the outlier points having a noise covariance higher than initially expected by adding an isotropic part. The covariance matrix can be written as the sum of two terms

$$V[\mathbf{x}_i] = V_{ex}[\mathbf{x}_i] + \sigma_{x_i}^2 \mathbf{I}_3 \qquad V[\mathbf{p}_i] = V_{ex}[\mathbf{p}_i] + \sigma_{p_i}^2 \mathbf{I}_3. \qquad (9)$$

An iterative scheme will look for the optimal set of $\sigma_{x_i}^2$ and $\sigma_{p_i}^2$ such that the outliers are identified.

The robust corresponding points algorithm can be summarized as follows:

1. Set initial variable: $\hat{\mathbf{t}} = [0, 0, 0]^T$, $V[\mathbf{x_i}] = V_{ex}[\mathbf{x_i}] + \mathbf{I}$, $V[\mathbf{p_i}] = V_{ex}[\mathbf{p_i}] + \mathbf{I}$.
2. Estimate $\hat{\mathbf{R}}$ as described in [3] using $\{\mathbf{x}'_i = \mathbf{x_i} - \hat{\mathbf{t}}\}$ and $\{\mathbf{p_i}\}$.
3. Rotate source points with estimated $\hat{\mathbf{R}}$: $\{\mathbf{p}'_i = \hat{\mathbf{R}}\mathbf{p}_i\}$.
4. Estimate $\hat{\mathbf{t}}$ using eq. (8) with points $\{\mathbf{x_i}\}$ and $\{\mathbf{p}'_i\}$.
5. Update covariance matrix before next iteration
   a) $\{\mathbf{p}'_i = \hat{\mathbf{R}}\mathbf{p}_i + \hat{\mathbf{t}}\}$.
   b) Transform source covariance matrix: $V_{ex}[\mathbf{p_i}] = \hat{\mathbf{R}} V_{ex}[\mathbf{p_i}] \hat{\mathbf{R}}^T$.
   c) $\sigma_{x_i}^2 = \begin{cases} \|\mathbf{p}'_i - \mathbf{x}_i\|^2 / 2 & \text{if} \quad \text{Tr}[V_{ex}[\mathbf{x}_i]] < 3\|\mathbf{p}'_i - \mathbf{x}_i\|^2 / 2, \\ 0 & \text{otherwise}, \end{cases}$

   $\sigma_{p_i}^2 = \begin{cases} \|\mathbf{p}'_i - \mathbf{x}_i\|^2 / 2 & \text{if} \quad \text{Tr}[V_{ex}[\mathbf{p}_i]] < 3\|\mathbf{p}'_i - \mathbf{x}_i\|^2 / 2, \\ 0 & \text{otherwise}. \end{cases}$
6. Check for convergence, if not go to step 2.

2.2   Generalized Total Least Squares ICP: GTLS-ICP

The iterative closest points problem defined in section 1.1 can be solved using the minimization method presented in the previous section. In this case, the correspondence between the data points, $\{\mathbf{p}_i\}$, and the model points, $\{\mathbf{x}_i\}$, is not known. For each point, we know the covariance matrix of the noise, $V_{ex}[\mathbf{p_i}]$ and $V_{ex}[\mathbf{x_i}]$ respectively. The functional (1) can be rewritten as

$$J(\mathbf{R},\mathbf{t}) = \sum_{i=1}^{N_P}(\mathbf{p}_i - \bar{\mathbf{p}}_i)^T V[\mathbf{p}_i]^{-1}(\mathbf{p}_i - \bar{\mathbf{p}}_i) + \sum_{i=1}^{N_X}(\mathbf{y}_i - \bar{\mathbf{y}}_i)^T V[\mathbf{y}_i]^{-1}(\mathbf{y}_i - \bar{\mathbf{y}}_i). \quad (10)$$

where $\mathbf{y}_i$ is the result of the closest point operator. An iterative closest point approach will start by assuming a matching between data and model points. From this matching, the transformation that minimizes the function (10) will be solved by using the previous algorithm. In the initial iterations, it is dangerous to minimize J using the initial covariances, V_{ex}, since the dominant noise will be due to the uncertainty of the matching. Sharp et al. [10] have shown that the noise due to the closest point correspondence operator can be modeled as an isotropic Gaussian noise with variance equal to the distance between the data point and the closest point in the model. This noise model can be introduced to update the covariance matrices globally for each iteration. Thus, the algorithm will initially look for the solution in the least squares sense and the closer the data points and model points get, the more the algorithm will rely on the provided noise covariances, V_{ex}.

The *GTLS-ICP* algorithm can be summarized as follows:

1. Set the initial transformation: $\hat{\mathbf{R}} = \mathbf{I}_3,\ \hat{\mathbf{t}} = [0,0,0]^T$.
2. Transform data points: $\{\mathbf{p}'_i = \hat{\mathbf{R}}\mathbf{p}_i + \hat{\mathbf{t}}\}$.
3. Find closest points: $\{\mathbf{y}_i = \mathcal{C}_{cp}(\mathbf{p}'_i, \mathcal{X})\}$.
4. Noise level estimation due to $\mathcal{C}_{cp}$: $\sigma^2 = \frac{1}{N_P}\sum_{i=1}^{N_P}\|\mathbf{y}_i - \mathbf{p}'_i\|^2$.
5. Update model covariance matrices: $V[\mathbf{y}_i] = V_{ex}[\mathbf{y}_i] + \sigma^2\mathbf{I}_3$.
6. Solve corresponding points registration between $\{\mathbf{y}_i\}$ and $\{\mathbf{p}_i\} \rightarrow \hat{\mathbf{R}}$ and $\hat{\mathbf{t}}$.
7. Check for convergence, if not go to step 2.

3   Experiments

3.1   Methodology

The reliability of our algorithm has been tested by random noise simulations. A hip model has been used as the model shape. Points have been randomly sampled from that mesh and transformed with a known rotation matrix $\mathbf{R}$, and translation vector $\mathbf{t}$ (see Fig. 1).

Noise has been independently added to the mesh and the transformed points. The noise between points is independent but not identically distributed with a known covariance matrix. Noise has been generated according to two distributions: Normal and Tukey's *slash* distribution. The slash distribution can be

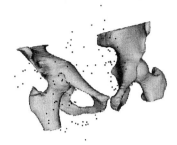

Fig. 1. Hip and random sampled points after transformation used for the evaluation of the algorithm.

Table 1. Eigenvalues of noise covariance matrices for each class. The degree of anisotropy decreases with the the number of the class

Cov. class	λ_1	λ_2	λ_3	Cov. class	λ_1	λ_2	λ_3	Cov. class	λ_1	λ_2	λ_3
1	1.00	0.00	0.00	6	0.67	0.17	0.17	11	0.44	0.33	0.22
2	0.80	0.20	0.00	7	0.57	0.29	0.14	12	0.40	0.40	0.20
3	0.67	0.33	0.00	8	0.50	0.38	0.12	13	0.40	0.30	0.30
4	0.57	0.43	0.00	9	0.44	0.44	0.11	14	0.36	0.36	0.27
5	0.50	0.50	0.00	10	0.50	0.25	0.25	15	0.33	0.33	0.33

obtained as a Gaussian random variable with zero mean and a given covariance divided by a uniform random variable over the interval $[0, 1]$. The slash distribution has been used to model outliers due to its broad tails. 15 different classes of noise have been simulated depending on the covariance. Table 1 shows the eigenvalues of the different noise covariance matrices. The first five classes correspond to the case of noise confined onto a plane.

A distance metric on rotation matrices can be defined as the minimal angle of rotation needed, around some axis, to transform one rotation into another. This can be calculated using quaternions of the relative rotation error $\mathbf{R}_e = \hat{\mathbf{R}}\mathbf{R}^T$. The quaternion representation of $\mathbf{R}_e$ is $\mathbf{q}_e = [q_0, q_1, q_2, q_3]^T$. The error vector is defined as $\Delta\Omega = \Delta\Omega\mathbf{l}_r$, where $\Delta\Omega = \arccos(2q_0)$ is the angle of the rotation error $\mathbf{R}_e$ and $\mathbf{l}_r = [q_1, q_2, q_3]^T / \sin(\frac{\Delta\Omega}{2})$ is the axis of rotation. The variance of the error is given by $V[\Delta\Omega] = E\{\Delta\Omega\Delta\Omega^T\}$.

The two statistics that we have used to assess the rotation error have been the mean rotation error E_Ω and the standard deviation S_Ω defined as

$$E_\Omega = \|E\{\Delta\Omega\}\|, \qquad S_\Omega = \sqrt{\text{Tr}[V[\Delta\Omega]]}. \qquad (11)$$

Regarding the translation, we have used the mean translation error E_t and the standard deviation S_t defined as

$$E_t = \|E\{\mathbf{t} - \hat{\mathbf{t}}\}\|, \qquad S_t = \sqrt{\text{Tr}[E\{(\mathbf{t} - \hat{\mathbf{t}})(\mathbf{t} - \hat{\mathbf{t}})^T\}]}. \qquad (12)$$

To estimate the error statistics, 100 independent realizations have been carried out for each anisotropic noise class and variance. We have compared our method

Rotation Error (degrees)

E_Ω S_Ω

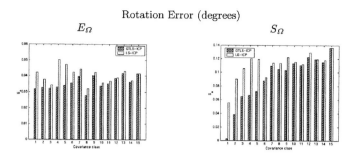

Fig. 2. Evaluation of the rotation error and translation error for different covariance matrices and Gaussian noise. Dark bar: GTLS-ICP. Light bar: LS-ICP

Rotation Error (degrees)

E_Ω S_Ω

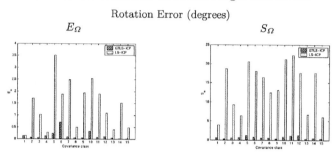

Fig. 3. Evaluation of the rotation error and translation error for different covariance matrices and slash noise. Dark bar: GTLS-ICP. Light bar: LS-ICP.

(GTLS-ICP) with the standard least squares ICP (LS-ICP) using Horn method [2] to minimize the functional at each iteration.

3.2   Results

The GTLS-ICP algorithm has been tested by randomly sampling 150 points from the mesh. A rotation of 30° around the axis $[1,1,1]^T$ and a translation $[1,1,1]^T$ have been applied. Noise has been added to the mesh and to the sampled points after the transformation.

Figure 2 shows the rotation error statistics for Gaussian noise. From these results we can see that, as long as rotations are involved, the mean error is similar for both methods; however the standard deviation of our solution is significantly smaller for anisotropic noise classes. The more isotropic the noise becomes, our solution tends to the standard least squares as expected. The translation error follows a similar tendency, our method shows a lower S_t when the noise distributes in an anisotropic way.

Figure 3 shows the error statistics for slash noise. Slash noise has been only added to the sampled points, while the mesh has been corrupted with Gaussian noise. The results clearly shows the stability and robustness of our method. It is fair to say that a preprocessing for outliers rejection may improve the results for

LS-ICP. However, our method seamlessly incorporates the rejection of outliers by setting up the covariance matrices adequately.

4 Conclusions

A generalization of the iterative closest points algorithm has been presented using a generalized total least squares framework. The main contributions of this work are: 1) noise is modeled both in the target shape and the source shape (total least squares), 2) anisotropic noise can be taken into account in the estimation of the transformation (generalized total least squares) and 3) outlier rejection is intrinsically handled by iterative estimation of the optimal isotropic noise variance of the covariance matrices. We believe that registration techniques that use ICP, or some of its variants, as optimization process will directly benefit of the generalized approach introduced in this paper, yielding a more robust estimation.

Acknowledgments. This work has been funded by CIMIT and NIH grant P41 RR 13218.

References

1. Paul J. Besl and Neil D. McKay. A method for registration of 3-D shapes. *IEEE Transaction on Pattern Analysis and Machine Intelligence*, 14(2):239–256, 1992.
2. B. K. P. Horn. Closed-form solution of absolute orientation using unit quaternions. *Journal of the Optical Society of America*, 4(4):629–642, 1987.
3. N. Ohta and K. Kanatani. Optimal estimation of three-dimensional rotation and reliability evaluation. *IEEE Transactions on Information and Systems*, E81-D(11):1247–1252, 1998.
4. Zhengyou Y. Zhang. Iterative point matching for registration of free-form curves and surfaces. *International Journal of Computer Vision*, 13(2):119–152, Oct 1994.
5. Calvin R. Maurer, Georges B. Aboutanos, Benoit M. Dawant, Robert J. Maciunas, and J. Michael Fitzpatrick. Registration of 3-D images using weighted geometrical features. *IEEE Transaction on Medical Imaging*, 15(6):836 – 849, Dec 1996.
6. Chitra Dorai, John Weng, and Anil K. Jain. Optimal registration of objects view using range data. *IEEE Transaction on Pattern Analysis and Machine Intelligence*, 19(10):1131 – 1138, Dec 1997.
7. S. van Huffel and J. Vandewalle. Analysis and properties of the generalized total least squares problem $AX \approx B$, when some or all columns are subject to error. *SIAM Journal on Matrix Analysis and Applications*, 10(3):294 – 315, 1989.
8. K. Kanatani. *Statistical Optimization for Geometric Computation: Theory and Practice*. Elsevier, 1996.
9. Robert M. Haralick, Hyonam Joo, Chung-Nan Lee, Xinhua Zhuang, Vinay G. Vaidya, and Man Bae Kim. Pose estimation from corresponding point data. *IEEE Transactions on Systems, Man. and Cybernetics*, 19(6):1426 – 1446, Nov 1989.
10. Gregory C. Sharp, Sang W. Lee, and David K. Wehe. ICP registration using invariant features. *IEEE Transaction on Pattern Analysis and Machine Intelligence*, 24(1):90–102, Jan 2002.

Robust Inter-slice Intensity Normalization Using Histogram Scale-Space Analysis

Julien Dauguet[1,2,3], Jean-François Mangin[1], Thierry Delzescaux[1], and Vincent Frouin[1]

[1] Service Hospitalier Frédéric Joliot, CEA, Orsay, France
[2] INRIA, Epidaure Project, Sophia Antipolis, France
[3] Ecole Centrale Paris, Laboratoire de Mathématiques Appliquées aux Systèmes,
Châtenay-Malabry, France

Abstract. This paper presents a robust method to correct for intensity differences across a series of aligned stained histological slices. The method is made up of two steps. First, for each slice, a scale-space analysis of the histogram provides a set of alternative interpretations in terms of tissue classes. Each of these interpretations can lead to a different classification of the related slice. A simple heuristics selects for each slice the most plausible interpretation. Then, an iterative procedure refines the interpretation selections across the series in order to maximize a score measuring the spatial consistency of the classifications across contiguous slices. Results are presented for a series of 121 baboon slices.

1   Introduction

Histological data often present large and discontinuous changes of intensities between slices. The sectioning process, indeed, does not assure a perfect constant thickness for all the slices. The staining intensity is sensitive to these variations of thickness, and is also sensitive to the concentration of the solution and the incubation time. Finally, the acquisition of the slices on the scanner can accentuate these differences.

The design of postprocessing procedures overcoming these intensity inhomogeneities is complex for several reasons:

- the number of homogenous tissues and their relative sizes vary from one slice to another;
- the intensity distributions may present high discontinuities from one block of contiguous slices to another : actually, the brain after extration is usually divided into small blocks mainly for a more homogeneous fixation;
- the relative contrasts between the intensity ranges corresponding to the different tissue classes can be radically different from one slice to another;
- large spatial inhomogeneities can occur inside some slices, which disturbs the classification of the different types of tissues, especially in case of low contrast.

A previous attempt to overcome this kind of problems led to match the intensity distribution of contiguous slices using a strategy based on a 1D linear registration of histograms [3]. This approach was successful for a dataset including two tissue classes only and presenting a good contrast. However, we observed some failures of the same approach for datasets corrupted by the various artifacts mentioned above. Some of these failures

C. Barillot, D.R. Haynor, and P. Hellier (Eds.): MICCAI 2004, LNCS 3216, pp. 242–249, 2004.

resulted from local maxima of the similarity measure used to register the histograms. In the worst cases, the global maximum of this similarity measure did not correspond to the targeted registration.

We present in this paper a different strategy which aims at increasing the robustness of the intensity restoration process. Some of the difficulties of the linear-registration based approach could be overcome using some non linear normalization [6], in order to get the possibility to deal with more than two classes. Such an approach, however, may still be sensitive to minimization problems. Therefore, rather than performing a blind registration between histograms, our new strategy detects the ranges of intensities corresponding to the different tissues before matching the histograms. For the sake of robustness, an iterative algorithm updates these detections until achieving consistent tissue classifications across contiguous slices. This new strategy is applied on a set of 121 realigned histological slices of a baboon brain acquired with a resolution of 0.16mm in the sectioning incidence (coronal) and an inter-slice distance of 0.72mm. The slices have been stained with a general marker which created a contrast between gray and white matter (Nissl staining), and a more specific marker of the basal ganglia and thalamus (Acetylcholinesterase histochemistry) which produces a very intense staining. The set has been realigned following a method described in [1].

2   Method

The method described in this paper is made up of two steps. First, for each slice, a multi-scale histogram analysis is performed. This analysis provides several possible interpretations of the histogram shape in terms of underlying tissue classes. Each interpretation can be used to compute a classification of the corresponding slice. A simple heuristics selects for each slice the most likely interpretation according to *a priori* knowledge about the acquisition process. The second step leads to question the spatial consistency of the resulting classifications across contiguous slices in order to detect some failures of this heuristics. This second step is based on an iterative process. For each slice, a simple score is used to rank the set of histogram interpretations according to consistency with the interpretations selected for the neighboring slices. If the current selected interpretation is not the best one, an update is applied. Several loops on the set of slices are performed until convergence of the process.

2.1   Histogram Scale-Space Analysis

Because of the various artifacts mentioned in the introduction, few *a priori* knowledge on the shapes of the histograms can be used to analyse them automatically. The main one lies in the relative positions of the tissues: the marker of the basal ganglia is darker than grey matter, which is darker than white matter. Another interesting property is true for most of the slices: the contrast between basal ganglia and grey matter is higher than the contrast between grey and white matters. Otherwise, the distributions of intensities of each of the tissues vary largely across slices. In the worst cases, one given tissue can correspond to several histogram modes (several maxima), induced by some variability in the staining process or by intra-slice spatial inhomogeneities. The fact that one class of tissue can be represented by several neighboring histogram modes leads to develop

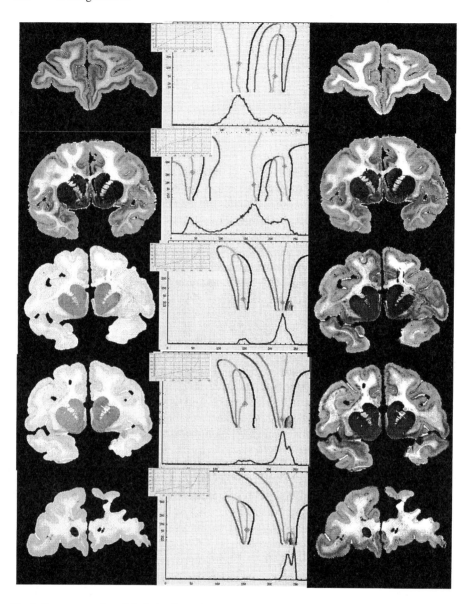

Fig. 1. Some examples of the behaviour of the heuristics analysing successfully most of the slices of the dataset. **left:** raw slice, **middle:** The scale-space trajectories of the extrema used to interpret the histogram. Cyan (respectively violet) color corresponds to the second derivative minima (resp. maxima). Green and dark blue colors correspond to first derivative extrema. Diamond shapes mark the drift velocity minima corresponding to the scale of the detected modes. The polynomial normalizing the slice intensity is superimposed. **right:** normalized slice.

a multiscale strategy. Smoothing the histogram, indeed, is supposed to mix together the modes corresponding to the same tissue before merging the different classes.

Linear scale-space analysis is an appealing multiscale approach when dealing with 1D signals because of the simplicity of the extrema behavior induced by the causality property [7,2]. This scale-space can be computed by applying the heat equation to the signal, which corresponds to smoothing it with a Gaussian kernel with increasing width. The extrema of the initial signal can be tracked throughout the scales until their extinction, which occurs when one maximum and one minimum get in touch with each other at a bifurcation point. For a 1D signal, the number of maxima always decreases with scale until reaching a stage where only one maximum remains. Since extrema of the histogram and of its first derivatives often have direct semantic interpretations, they allow the analysis of the histogram shape relative to the underlying tissue classes.

In simple cases, smoothing the histogram until only three maxima survive is sufficient to detect the modes corresponding to the three classes of tissues. The general situation, however, requires a better heuristics. For instance, the slices which do not cross the basal ganglia lead to only two classes of tissues, which has to be inferred. More difficult cases occur when the contrast between grey and white matter is very low. In such cases the two related histogram modes merge very early in the scale-space, while several maxima induced by the basal ganglia may still exist. In the worst cases, this contrast is so low that the part of the histogram corresponding to grey and white matter includes only one maximum (see Fig. 1). It has been shown elsewhere, however, that such situations can be overcome through the use of the second derivative minima [5]. This larger set of extrema, which is related to the histogram curvature, embeds more information about the various classes of tissues making up the slice.

Hence, each second derivative minimum is supposed to mark a mode of the histogram. Moreover, the location of this minimum along the intensity axis provides an estimation of the average intensity of this mode. This location, however, varies with the scale. The mode represented by this minimum, indeed, varies also with scale. Intuitively, a minimum may stand for an artifactual mode at low scales, and represent a tissue of interest at higher scales after several artifactual modes have been merged together by the smoothing. During this merging process, the location of the minimum along the intensity axis varies rapidly from the average intensity of the artifactual mode to the average intensity of the tissue of interest. In fact, most of the extrema trajectories in scale-space alternate such periods of high horizontal drift velocity with periods of stability which could be related to scale ranges where they are catched by some underlying mode. Therefore, our method associates a different mode to each local minimum of the horizontal drift velocity along the trajectory of second derivative minima [5].

In order to sort these modes in decreasing order of interest, two features are used: the extinction scale of the second derivative minimum trajectory they belong to, and an evaluation of the number of slice's pixels they stand for. This evaluation is the integral of the histogram in the range defined by the locations at the mode's scale of the second derivative minimum and the closest first derivative minimum [5]. First derivative minima correspond in fact to the largest slope points of the histogram's hills. Hence, this integral corresponds approximately to half the volume of the mode in terms of slice's pixels. Several interpretations of the histogram shape can be derived from the modes at the top of the hierarchy. The interpretation systematicaly selected as the most plausible one results from the following heuristics:

1. Compute the scale-space until only one second derivative minimum survives;

2. Detect the highest drift velocity minimum along the trajectory of this minimum, which stands for a mode GW representing the sum of grey and white matter;
3. Detect the second derivative minimum trajectory with the highest extinction scale located on the right of the first derivative minimum associated to the left slope of GW;
4. Detect the next drift velocity minimum along the first trajectory and the highest one along the second trajectory. The minimum on the left stands for a mode G representing grey matter, the one on the right stands for a mode W representing white matter;
5. Detect the second derivative minimum with the highest extinction scale located on the left of the intensity range explored previously. The highest mode M is associated to the marker of the basal ganglia if its volume is more than 100 pixels.

The Figure 1 gives a few examples of the behaviour of this heuristics. For each slice, alternative interpretations are also derived from the scale-space of the histogram, to deal with potential failures of this heuristics. They correspond for instance to associating the modes G and W respectively to the leftmost and to the rightmost two biggest modes. Here is the list of the different alternative interpretations taken into account for the results presented in this paper:

1. The biggest mode can stand for either "G" or "W" modes (extreme or pathological slices);
2. The two biggest modes stand for "G and W modes";
3. The three biggest modes stand for "M, G and W modes" or "M, G and X modes", where the mode X does not lead to a class of tissue;
4. The four biggest modes stand for "M, X, G and W modes".

It should be noted that this list of interpretations does not explore all the combinatorial possibilities and results from a tuning to some events found in our data.

Each interpretation can be simply converted into a classification of the respective slice: the histogram is split into classes by thresholds defined as the middle points between the estimated mode's averages. These classifications may include one, two or three classes.

2.2 Classification Spatial Consistency

The second step of the process detects the failure of the main heuristics, using for each slice a score based on the consistency between the slice's classification and the two classifications of the contiguous slices. This score is based on the number of voxels which belong to the same class in two contiguous slices. For each slice, the score obtained by the heuristics interpretation is compared to the scores obtained by the other interpretations. The interpretation with the best score is selected (see Fig; 2). This process is iterated until convergence, which occured in two or three iterations in our experiments, thanks to the robust behaviour of the heuristics.

During a final stage, we correct the intensity of each slice by estimating the best polynom matching the detected classes of tissues with template values selected by the user. The degree of this polynom (1, 2, or 3) depends on the number of tissues found in the slice. Three-degree polynoms are replaced by a linear interpolation on the $[0, m]$

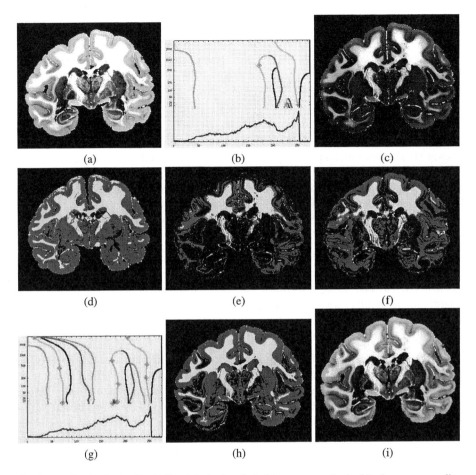

Fig. 2. An histological stained slice (a), its heuristic histogram analysis (b), the corresponding normalisation. The classification of the previous slice (d), of the current slice following the heuristics (e) and of the next slice (f). Alternative histogram analysis with 4 biggest mode detected (M,X,G,W) (g), the best classification according to the consistency with the neighboring slices (h) and the final corrected slice (i).

segment, where m stands for the position of the marker maximum, to avoid polynom "rebunds" problems.

3   Results and Discussion

We present in figure 3 a slice orthogonal to the sectioning incidence, first before any processing, second after intensity normalization using only the heuristics, and finally after the whole process. The iterative step has converged after two iterations. The final histogram interpretation selected by the whole process stems from the heuristics for about 85% of the slices. For the final intensity normalization, we set the average intensity of the white matter to 230, the intensity of the grey matter to 160 and finally 80 for the marker. As far as computing time is concerned, a complete normalization of the whole volume 500*440*121 with 2 iterations on a Pentium IV 1.8GHz takes about 10 minutes. The result is globally satisfying. In fact, the remaining problems (imperfections in the marker regions) stem mainly from intra-slice spatial inhomogeneities that were not taken into account by the process described in this paper, or from pathological sections.

The Figure 1 provides an insight into the variability of the histogram shapes to be analysed. The first and the second raws show simple histograms with two or three modes. The third row shows an example of low contrast where the white matter mode does not lead to any maximum in the histogram but is recovered via the curvature-related second derivative minimum. The fourth row shows a successful estimation of the average intensity of the marker at high scale while this class of tissues is split into a lot of modes at lower scales. The fifth row shows the detection of the marker mode in a limit case where it is made up of a few hundred pixels, namely for a slice located at the beginning of basal ganglia.

The figure 2 describes the behaviour of the second step of the method for a slice leading to a failure of the heuristics. The competition between the alternative interpretations of the histogram leads to the selection of the (M,X,G,W) hypothesis. In fact none of the interpretations is fully satisfying in terms of classification, because of a large spatial inhomogeneity inside the slice. Therefore, our algorithm can only select the interpretation leading to the best 3D consistency.

This kind of situations calls for applying some intra-slice bias correction procedure somewhere into the restoration process. The very low grey/white contrast of some of our slices, however, prevented us to perform such a correction systematically before intensity normalization. Indeed, the risk of mixing definitively the range of intensities corresponding to grey and white matter is too high. To prevent such problems to occur, we plan to address the bias correction process through a two stage procedure performed on a slice by slice basis. An initial correction will be performed before intensity normalization using a highly regularized correction field preventing any mixing between grey and white matter. A final correction will be performed with more degrees of freedom for the field after interpretation of the histogram. This interpretation, indeed, yields an estimation of the contrast between grey and white matter, which can be used to perform a slice by slice tuning of the bias field regularization. First experiments using an entropy minimization approach are promising but beyond the scope of this paper [4].

While our method includes some *ad hoc* tuning to some of our dataset features (the heuristics and the set of alternative interpretations), the strategy is generic and could be adapted easily to other kinds of dataset. Thanks to the iterative correction process, indeed, no strong robustness is required for the initial heuristics. The main requirement to assure a good behaviour of the whole process is that the set of alternative histogram interpretations is rich enough to cover all the possible cases. In our opinion, with a reasonable intra-slice bias, the hypothesis that each tissue class leads to one of the biggest scale-space mode should give the possibility to build a small successful set of alternative interpretations for various kinds of data. Compared to a blind registration procedure prone to local maxima of the similarity measure [3], our point of view assumes that each of these potential local maxima corresponds to a different matching of the histograms modes. Hence our method selects first the most frequent matching with a template histogram shape provided by the

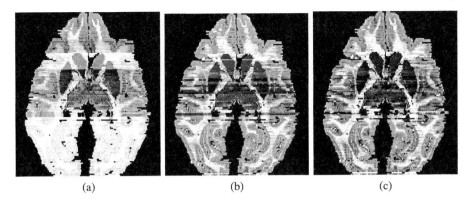

(a)   (b)   (c)

Fig. 3. An axial view of the histological volume : before intensity correction (a), after the heuristic strategy (b) and after the spatial consistency checking (c).

heuristics and iteratively propagates this choice throughout the series of slices in order to achieve 3D spatial consistency of the resulting classification.

4   Conclusion

We have presented in this paper a generic strategy to perform robust histogram normalization throughout a series of registered images. This method can deal with variations of the number of tissue classes throughout the series and provides a 3D consistent classification of the data. While the approach described in the paper requires an heuristics providing an initial correct classification of most of the slices, the framework may be extended to complex situations where no such heuristics is available. The iterative step indeed could consists in a global stochastic minimization of the sum of scores evaluating spatial consistency of the classification of contiguous slices.

References

1. T. Delzescaux, J. Dauguet, F. Condé, R. Maroy, and V. Frouin. Using 3D non rigid FFD-based method to register post mortem 3D histological data and in vivo MRI of a baboon brain. In *MICCAI, Montréal, LNCS 2879, Springer Verlag*, pages 965–966, 2003.
2. J.J. Koenderink. The structure of images. *Biol. Cybernetics*, 50:363–370, 1984.
3. Grégoire Malandain and Eric Bardinet. Intensity compensation within series of images. In *MICCAI*, volume 2879 of *LNCS*, pages 41–49, Montréal, Canada, 2003. Springer Verlag.
4. J.-F. Mangin. Entropy minimization for automatic correction of intensity nonuniformity. In *IEEE Work. MMBIA*, pages 162–169, Hilton Head Island, South Carolina, 2000. IEEE Press.
5. J.-F. Mangin, O. Coulon, and V. Frouin. Robust brain segmentation using histogram scale-space analysis and mathematical morphology. In *Proc. 1st MICCAI*, LNCS-1496, pages 1230–1241, MIT, Boston, Oct. 1998. Springer Verlag.
6. S. Prima, N. Ayache, A. Janke, S. Francis, D. Arnold, and L. Collins. Statistical Analysis of Longitudinal MRI Data: Application for detection of Disease Activity in MS. In *MICCAI*, pages 363–371, 2002.
7. A.P. Witkin. Scale-space filtering. In *In* International Joint Conference on Artificial Intelligence, pages 1019–1023, 1983.

Quantification of Delayed Enhancement MR Images

Engin Dikici[1], Thomas O'Donnell[1], Randolph Setser[2], and Richard D. White[2]

[1] Siemens Corp Research 755 College Rd East Princeton, NJ 08540
[2] Cleveland Clinic Foundation 9500 Euclid Ave Cleveland, OH 44195

Abstract. Delayed Enhancement MR is an imaging technique by which non-viable (dead) myocardial tissues appear with increased signal intensity. The extent of non-viable tissue in the left ventricle (LV) of the heart is a direct indicator of patient survival rate. In this paper we propose a two-stage method for quantifying the extent of non-viable tissue. First, we segment the myocardium in the DEMR images. Then, we classify the myocardial pixels as corresponding to viable or non-viable tissue. Segmentation of the myocardium is challenging because we cannot reliably predict its intensity characteristics. Worse, it may be impossible to distinguish the infracted tissues from the ventricular blood pool. Therefore, we make use of MR Cine images acquired in the same session (in which the myocardium has a more predictable appearance) in order to create a prior model of the myocardial borders. Using image features in the DEMR images and this prior we are able to segment the myocardium consistently. In the second stage of processing, we employ a Support Vector Machine to distinguish viable from non-viable pixels based on training from an expert.

1 Introduction

Delayed enhancement magnetic resonance (DEMR) is an image acquisition technique applied typically to the left ventricle (LV), or the main pumping chamber of the heart, whereby non-viable tissue may be identified. Tissues that are non-viable will *not* benefit from interventions such as coronary by-pass or stent placement, etc. These actions serve to increase blood flow to a region, and while helpful for damaged regions provide no advantages once a tissue is necrotic. Therefore, we seek to distinguish non-viable heart tissue from healthy or damaged tissue so that unnecessary invasive procedures may be avoided and patients whose condition might improve from revascularization are identified.

Delayed Enhancement Magnetic Resonance (DEMR) is an image acquisition technique applied almost exclusively to the Left Ventricle (LV) whereby non-viable tissues may be discriminated. Typically in DEMR, a paramagnetic contrast agent (Gd-DTPA) is administered and the patient imaged after 20-30 minutes using a standard inversion recovery MR protocol. Non-viable cardiac tissues appear with increased signal intensity (see Figure 1a). It should be noted that during this 20-30 minute waiting period other MR protocols are generally acquired, specifically Cine MR, a time series over the cardiac cycle. Compared to DEMR, in Cine MR the LV myocardium appears with much more uniform texture (see Figure 1b) with which contraction of the myocardium can be visualized.

C. Barillot, D.R. Haynor, and P. Hellier (Eds.): MICCAI 2004, LNCS 3216, pp. 250–257, 2004.
© Springer-Verlag Berlin Heidelberg 2004

The goal of our work is to automatically quantify the degree to which the left ventricle of an individual is non-viable in short axis DEMR images. This quantification is a two-step process. First, the left ventricle borders are segmented. Following this, tissues belonging to the left ventricle are classified.

Segmentation of the LV in DEMR images is challenging since we cannot reliably predict its intensity characteristics. Compared to segmentation of Cine MR images, in which assumptions may be made about the relative intensities of air, blood, and muscle, little can be said of the DEMR myocardium. Worse, non-viable tissues may have intensities that render it indistinguishable from the blood pool. Thus, radiologists in analyzing DEMR images often refer to a "corresponding" Cine image in which the heart wall is visible. By "corresponding" we mean a Cine image that has the most similar slice plane with respect to the heart and closest trigger time in the cardiac cycle. Note that slice planes may not be identical due to patient motion or respiratory artifacts; and, the ECG time of the DEMR may not exactly match the temporal sampling of the Cine with respect to the ECG.

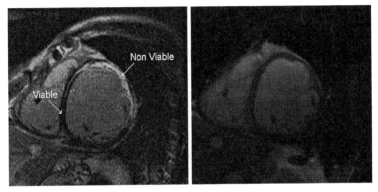

Fig. 1a. DEMR image showing viable and non-viable myocardium. Fig. 1b An MR Cine acquisition at approximately the same slice position and phase in the cardiac cycle.

In determining the myocardial border in the LV we take an approach similar to that taken by radiologists who look back and forth between the DEMR and corresponding Cine to infer the heart wall. We perform an automatic segmentation on a corresponding Cine image using the technique by Jolly [2]. While this cine segmentation is generally quite good, we make it available to the user for editing (the only manual portion of our procedure). This Cine segmentation is then employed as a prior in the segmentation of the LV in the DEMR image.

Once the LV borders in the DEMR image are identified, classification of the myocardial pixels is performed using a Support Vector Machine (SVM), a supervised machine learning technique in which the computer is taught to recognize a phenomenon given a series of examples. The SVM is trained using ground truth provided by experts at Cleveland Clinic.

2 Related Work

Very little has been published on automated techniques for classifying non-viable tissues in DEMR and none, to our knowledge, on segmenting myocardial borders in these images.

The classification techniques in the literature have typically relied on either visual inspection of images [6], which precludes quantitation, or manual delineation of the non-viable region [7,10], which can be time prohibitive. Semi-automatic segmentation techniques, based on the signal intensity characteristics of viable myocardium, have been used extensively in previous studies [8]. Some of these studies have defined a threshold for non-viable pixels as >2*std dev of the signal intensity of remote, viable myocardium (which was defined manually) [8]; other studies have used 3*std dev as the threshold [9]. More recently, Kolipaka et al. have validated these thresholding techniques [3], demonstrating good agreement with manually thresholded images. Furthermore, this study showed that alternate thresholding methods, based on the histogram of signal intensities in the LV blood pool or the histogram of LV myocardium (including non-viable tissue) were too inconsistent for routine clinical implementation.

This work differs from our previous work [1] in that we include the segmentation of the myocardium; and, our feature space for the classification of non-viable tissues has changed. We have reduced the number of features used in the SVM as we found three of the features (e.g., thickness of the myocardium) to provide redundant information for the task. With regard to general classification using SVM, El-Naqa's work on mammogram analysis is the closest to our work [12].

To perform our segmentation of the myocardial borders we employ non-rigid registration between the DEMR and Cine images (to approximate the location of the LV in the DEMR) and between different Cine images (to interpolate the image characteristics where there is no data). Noble et. al., successfully employed Cine to Cine non-rigid registration to segment the LV in a method similar to ours [5]. They do not segment DEMR images, however, and direct Cine to DEMR registrations can only provide approximate deformation fields since the image characteristics differ so significantly.

3 Methods

Let $\overline{C}_{n,m}$ represent a $n \times m$ matrix of Cine images with n adjacent slice positions and m consecutive phases equally spaced in time. Let $\overline{V}_n$ represent the set of n DEMR images with n adjacent slice positions. For a $V_i \in \overline{V}_n$, let the corresponding cine image be $C_{i,k} \in \overline{C}_{n,m}$ such that

$$k = \left\lfloor \frac{t_{V_i} - t_{C_{i,1}}}{t_{C_{i,m}} - t_{C_{i,1}}} \right\rfloor m$$

where t represents the ECG trigger time of the image. We apply a myocardial border detection algorithm to $C_{i,k}$ which employs a region segmentation combined with an active contour formulation [2]. The result, which may be manually edited, is $S_{C_{i,k}}(r)$, the segmentation of the corresponding Cine image. Adjacent to the corresponding cine image $C_{i,k}$ is $C_{i,k+1}$ such that

$$t_{C_{i,k}} \leq t_{V_i} \leq t_{C_{i,k+1}}$$

3.1 Determination of Segmentation Prior

We register $C_{i,k}$ and $C_{i,k+1}$ using a non-rigid variational approach [4]. The resulting deformation field, $U(\vec{x})$, such that

$$C_{i,k}(\vec{x}) \mapsto C_{i,k+1}(U(\vec{x}))$$

is linearly interpolated

$$U'(\vec{x}) = \frac{(t_{V_i} - t_{C_{i,1}})}{(t_{C_{i,m}} - t_{C_{i,1}})} U(\vec{x})$$

to calculate the deformation field at t_{V_i}. This deformation field is then applied to $S_{C_{i,k}}(r)$

$$S_{prior}(r) = U'(S_{C_{i,k}}(r))$$

to arrive at our segmentation prior, i.e., the segmentation of the cine acquisition interpolated to time t_{V_i}.

3.2 Localization of the LV in the DEMR Image

The center of the bloodpool in V_i is computed by registering $C_{i,k}$ with V_i resulting in the deformation field $D(\vec{x})$ such that

$$C_{i,k}(\vec{x}) \mapsto V_i(D(\vec{x}))$$

The segmentation $S_{C_{i,k}}(r)$ is then deformed by $D(\vec{x})$ to arrive at

$$S_{center}(r) = D(S_{C_{i,k}}(r))$$

The centroid of S_{center}

$$\vec{x}_{center} = \int_{S_{center}} S_{center}(r)dr$$

is the position from which we start our search of the LV in V_i. Note that the deformation field is too imprecise for any other inferences.

3.3 Determination of the LV Borders in the DEMR Image

We deform the prior model, S_{prior}, to fit to the DEMR image V_i to maximize the probability that the resulting S_{V_i} is the correct segmentation of V_i. In the fitting process, we apply an affine registration with five parameters: translation in the x and y dimensions $\vec{\tau}$, shearing parameters s_q and s_m, and a scaling parameter ω. The translation is bound by the distance of 10 pixels but is allowed to change without penalty. Also, the shearing is bound by ±60 degrees and ±%20 scaling again without any penalty.

The scale bound, ω', is based on the change in the size of the LV from slice level i to an adjacent slice level, $i+1$ or $i-1$. The slice level with the maximal change is selected in the case of $i \neq 1, m$. We make the assumption that the change in scale due to motion artifacts, through-plane motion, etc., will not be greater than ω'.

3.3.1 Computation of Scale Bound ω'

For brevity we will assume the adjacent slice is $i+1$. We register $C_{i,k}$ with $C_{i+1,k}$ resulting in the deformation field $F(\vec{x})$ such that $C_{i,k}(\vec{x}) \mapsto C_{i+1,k}(F(\vec{x}))$

We then calculate the average of the deformation between the endo and epi contours of $S_{C_{i,k}}(r)$

$$\vec{g} = \oint_{S_{C_{i,k\,epi}}} F(\vec{x})dr - \oint_{S_{C_{i,k\,endo}}} F(\vec{x})dr$$

The scale bound, ω', is then the norm of $\vec{g}$, $\omega' = \|\vec{g}\|_2$

3.3.2 Penalty upon Scaling

Unlike translation, $\vec{\tau}$, a penalty is incurred on scaling. This penalty is a coefficient in our energy formulation that is maximized (to be described in Section 3.3.3). The penalty varies from 1 (no penalty) to e^{-1} (maximal penalty resulting from a scaling equal to the scale bound ω') and is bell shaped.

In our implementation the scale ω is iteratively increased by 1.5% from a value of 1 to ω' (similarly decreased to $-\omega'$) with the total energy formulation is evaluated at each step. Thus, at iteration γ, the scale ω is $\omega = (1.015)^\gamma$.

The penalty for a scale ω is based on the ratio of the iteration number, γ, and the iteration number corresponding to the maximal number of iterations, γ' where $\omega' = (1.015)^{\gamma'}$. Specifically, $e^{\frac{\gamma}{\gamma'}}$; which may be rewritten as $e^{\frac{\log_{1.015}\omega}{\log_{1.015}\omega'}}$.

3.3.3 Energy Maximization

The energy formulation that is maximized by affine registration procedure is expressed as

$$S_{V_i}(r) = ArgMax_{\vec{\tau},q,m,\omega}\{(e^{\log \omega'})\{W_1 \int_{S_{V_i}} E_1(\omega s_q s_m S'_{V_{i\,epi}}(r)+\vec{\tau})dr +$$

$$W_2 \int_{S_{V_i}} E_2(\omega s_q s_m S'_{V_{i\,endo}}(r)+\vec{\tau})dr + W_3 \oint_{\omega s_q s_m S'_{V_{i\,endo}}(r)+\vec{\tau}} E_3(x)dr\}\}$$

where $E_1(\vec{x})$ and $E_2(\vec{x})$ are the inner and outer edge images created by applying a steering filter and detecting directional dark to bright edges and bright to dark edges respectively. Our steering filter is a modified Sobel Filter that adapts its convolution kernel by using the relative location of the convolved pixel with respect to $\vec{x}_{center}$.

$E_3(\vec{x})$ is the "bloodpoolness"image created by making an estimation of bloodpool's mean intensity via the intensities of the central pixels as calculated during the localization procedure.

3.4 Classification

We employ an SVM to perform the classification of myocardial pixels once the borders have been detected. We prefer this approach over automatic thresholding since the distribution of gray levels in the myocardium is not strictly a bimodal distribution of non-viable (bright) and viable (dark) pixels. This is due to partial voluming effects and the degree of damage.

For our kernel function of the SVM we use a Gaussian radial basis function of the form:

$$k(\overline{\phi}(\vec{x}),\overline{\phi}(\vec{x}')) = e^{-\|\overline{\phi}(x)-\overline{\phi}(x')\|^2/2\sigma^2}$$

where $\overline{\phi}$ is the vector of features. It may be shown that kernels of this form (following Mercer's conditions [11]) have corresponding optimization problems that are convex, thus lacking local minima.

To determine σ in our kernel as well as K, a compromise between maximizing the margin and minimizing the number of training set errors, we employed the "leave-one-out strategy". For more details see [1]

The following three features make up $\overline{\phi}$: The first feature, ϕ_1, is the intensity of a pixel, I_p,relative to the average myocardial intensity, $\overline{I}_M = \dfrac{\sum\limits_{p\in M} I_p}{\sum\limits_{p\in M} 1}$ thus $\phi_1 = \dfrac{I_p}{I_M}$.

The second of these features is the standard deviation $\phi_2 = std(I_r)$ of the relative pixel intensities with respect to its next neighbors. The final feature ϕ_3 is related to the image as a whole and not to a single pixel. We call this feature myocardial contrast and it is defined as $\phi_3 = \dfrac{\overline{I_M}}{\overline{I}}$ i.e., the ratio of the mean myocardial intensity

$\overline{I_M}$ and the mean image intensity $\overline{I}$ of the image.

3.5 Image Acquisition Parameters

Forty-five patients with known multi-vessel chronic ischemic heart disease underwent DEMR (Sonata, Siemens Medical Solutions, Erlangen, Germany) using an IR Turbo-FLASH sequence (FOV 300-360mm2, TE 4ms, TR 8ms, flip angle 30 deg, TI 190-470ms), approximately 20 minutes after intravenous 0.2mmol/kg Gd-DTPA injection, with (n=9) or without (n=31) phase sensitive reconstruction. TrueFISP cine images (FOV 260-360mm, TE 1.5msec, TR 25-43msec, 49-65o) were also acquired. For both types of imaging, 3 representative short-axis slices (thickness 6-10mm) were acquired at the base, mid-ventricle and apex of the left ventricle during repetitive 10-15 second breath-holds.

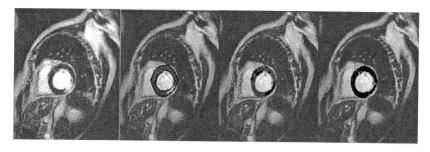

Fig. 2. Left to Right: A DEMR image. Our automatic segmentation. Our classification of non-viable tissues (black indicated non-viability). Agreement with the expert (black pixels indicate agreement; white pixels indicate disagreement).

4   Results

Our 45 patients were broken down in to training (31 patients) and testing (14 patients) groups. For the training group the myocardial borders were manually drawn and the pixels classified as viable or non-viable by an expert. Appropriate SVM parameters were found to be $\sigma = 0.01$ and $K = 20$. For the testing group, segmentations and classifications were obtained automatically. For each of the 42 (14 test patients with 3 slices levels each) DEMR images, the myocardial borders on the corresponding Cine images were automatically segmented and an expert oversaw any additional editing.

To evaluate the segmentation results, the expert delineated the ground truth myocardial borders on the DEMR images using the Argus package from Siemens. Using this ground truth we found our technique's contour pixel location error to be 1.54 pixels on average with the standard deviation of 0.39 pixels over the 42 images.

The 42 DEMR image slices segmented above were then classified using the SVM. Our classification module achieved to 88.39% accuracy rate with a standard deviation of 6.15%, sensitivity of %81.34 and specificity of 92.28%. Figure 2 shows the results on one set.

5 Conclusions

We have presented preliminary results on the automatic segmentation and classification of non-viable tissue in DEMR images. In future work we hope to include affine transformations of the segmentation priors as well as a degree of local deformation.

References

1. O'Donnell Thomas, Ning Xu, Randolf Setser, Richard D. White. Semi-Automatic Segmentation of Non-Viable Cardiac Tissue Using Cine and Delayed Enhancement Magnetic Resonance Images. *SPIE Medical Imaging 2003 Physiology and Function: Methods, Systems, and Applications*, pp 242 – 251.
2. M. –P. Jolly, N. Duta, and G. Funka-Lea. Segmentation of the Left Ventricle in Cardiac MR Images. *Proc. ICCV,* Vancouver, Canada, 2001.
3. Kolipaka A, Chatzimavroudis GP, White RD, O'Donnell TP, and Setser RM. Segmentation of Non-Viable Myocardium in Delayed Enhancement Magnetic Resonance Images. ISMRM, Toronto, CA, 2003.
4. Christophe Chefd'Hotel, Gerardo Hermosillo, and Olivier Faugeras. A Variational Approach to Multi-Modal Image Matching *IEEE Workshop on Variational and Level Set Methods (VLSM'01),* p.21, July 13-13, 2001.
5. Nicholas M.I. Noble, Derek L.G. Hill, Marcel Breeuwer, Julia A. Schnabel, David J. Hawkes, Frans A. Gerritsen, and Reza Razavi. Myocardial Delineation via Registration in a Polar Coordinate System. *MICCAI (1) 2002:* 651-658.
6. Choi, K. M., Kim, R. J. et. al.,. (2001). Transmural Extent of Acute Myocardial Infarction Predicts Long-Term Improvement in Contractile Function. *Circulation* 104: 1101-1107.
7. Setser RM, Bexell DG, et al. Quantitative Assessment of Myocardial Scar in Delayed Enhancement Magnetic Resonance Imaging. *J Magn Reson Imaging 2003* 18: 434-41.
8. R. J. Kim, D. S. Fieno, et. Al.,. Relationship of MRI delayed contrast enhancement to irreversible injury, infarct age, and contractile function. *Circulation* 1999; 100: 1992-2002.
9. Fieno DS, Kim RJ,et.al.,. Contrast enhanced MRI of myocardium at risk: distinction between reversible and irreversible injury throughout infarct healing. 2000;36:1985-1991.
10. Sandstede JJW, et. al.(2000). Analysis of First-Pass and Delayed Contrast-Enhancement Patterns of Dysfunctional Myocardium on MR Imaging: Use in the Prediction of Myocardial Viability. (Monographie)
11. Cristianini N, Shawe-Taylor J. An Introduction to Support Vector Machines and other kernel-based learning methods. Cambridge University Press 2000.
12. El-Naqa I,, Yongyi Yang, Miles N. Wernick, Nikolas P. Galatsanos, and Robert Nishikawa, "Support Vector Machine Learning for Detection of Microcalcififcations in Mammograms", IEEE ICIP, Rochester, NY, September 2002

Statistical Shape Modelling of the Levator Ani with Thickness Variation

Su-Lin Lee[1,2], Paramate Horkaew[1], Ara Darzi[2], and Guang-Zhong Yang[1,2]

[1] Royal Society/Wolfson Foundation Medical Image Computing Laboratory
[2] Department of Surgical Oncology and Technology
Imperial College London, London, UK
{su-lin.lee, paramate.horkaew, a.darzi, g.z.yang}@imperial.ac.uk

Abstract. The levator ani is vulnerable to injury during childbirth and effective surgical intervention requires full knowledge of the morphology and mechanical properties of the muscle structure. The shape of the levator ani and regional thickening during different levels of physiological loading can provide an indication of pelvic floor dysfunction. This paper describes a coupled approach for shape and thickness statistical modelling based on harmonic embedding for volumetric analysis of the levator ani. With harmonic embedding, the dynamic information extracted by the statistical modelling captures shape and thickness variation of the levator ani across different subjects and during varying levels of stress. With this study, we demonstrate that the derived model is compact and physiologically meaningful, demonstrating the practical value of the technique.

1 Introduction

The pelvic floor is a complex structure composed of a diaphragm of striated muscle covered by fascia. The levator ani is the part of the pelvic floor for visceral support and for drawing the anal canal upwards and forwards. It is highly susceptible to injuries during natural childbirth, which can lead to problems with urination and defecation [1]. Defective pelvic organ support is one of the most common problems in women. Among them, over 20% require a second operation. The management of pelvic floor disorders in women is traditionally divided between gynaecologists, urologists and colorectal surgeons. The modern surgical approach to the problem is to perform all necessary repairs during one single operation to avoid the usual territorial subdivision and patient re-operation. This requires an accurate preoperative identification of all prolapsed organs and their mechanical properties.

Magnetic Resonance Imaging (MRI) in both closed and open access scanners has been used to assess any injuries of the levator. Open access (interventional) scanners are becoming popular as the subject sits in an anatomically natural position, where the pelvic floor muscles can optimally exert its full function [2]. Dynamic information can also be acquired by using fast acquisition protocols with which each image can be acquired in less than 2 seconds. Full 3D acquisition of the entire levator ani volume during straining has so far proven to be difficult due to the prolonged imaging time required to recover the fine structural details of the levators. Diagnosis has usually

C. Barillot, D.R. Haynor, and P. Hellier (Eds.): MICCAI 2004, LNCS 3216, pp. 258–265, 2004.
© Springer-Verlag Berlin Heidelberg 2004

been made based on distances to specific landmarks in a single image slice – typically mid-sagittal or mid-coronal [3].

Hoyte *et al* [4] used 3D reconstructions of the levator ani to observe the differences between symptomatic and asymptomatic subjects. Similar work in the reconstruction of the entire levator ani has been accomplished in other research institutions [5] to compare the levators of symptomatic and asymptomatic subjects. The scans have been limited to levators at rest due to the time constraint for which a subject can maintain a certain dynamic position. Previous work at this institution has investigated the shape variation of the levator ani by using statistical shape modelling of the surface of the levators with harmonic embedding [6]. The training set consisted of levators at rest, maximal contraction and maximal squeeze down with 3D MR data sets acquired using a fast spin echo gradient recalled echo protocol. As the surface of the levator is topologically equivalent to a compact 2D manifold with boundary, the model was constructed based on original work by Horkaew and Yang [7].

Existing research has shown that the strain distribution of the levator ani during different levels of physiological loading plays an important part in assessing its mechanical function. To this end, Hoyte *et al* have recently extended their work to study the thickness of the levator ani [8]. They have shown that colour thickness mapping of the levator ani can be used for the swift evaluation of a large number of levators. In their study, levators of symptomatic and asymptomatic subjects at rest were manually segmented and then divided into four quadrants. It was found that the right anterior quadrant was thicker in asymptomatic subjects although the significance of this has not yet been determined. This is an indirect way of assessing the strain distribution during stress, and thickness mapping may be performed in a number of ways. The direction along which the thickness is determined may be the direction to a corresponding control point on the opposite surface, the direction to the closest point on the opposite surface or the surface or vertex normal. For more detailed analysis, it is possible to adopt previous work in shape and volume modelling in medical image computing. For example, medial representations [9] can be used to model the thickness of the levator ani. This consists of a set of medial atoms that contain two vectors of equal length, each originating from the atom. A mesh of medial atoms could be used to represent the thickness of a sheet muscle such as the levator ani.

The purpose of this paper is to extend our previous work on optimal statistical shape modelling for volumetric analysis of the levator ani. With harmonic embedding, it provides an effective framework for combining shape with tensor distribution for optimal statistical modelling. We demonstrate that for sheet muscles such as the levator ani, the method can capture meaningful dynamic shape and thickening variations.

2 Method

2.1 Data Acquisition

For assessing shape and volumetric variations across subjects and during different levels of physiological loading, two training data sets were acquired for this study. The first was built from transverse images acquired from a 1.5T Siemens Sonata closed access scanner. A fast turbo-spin echo non-zone selective protocol was used to acquire T_2 weighted images (TR=1500ms, TE=130ms, slice thickness = 3mm) of the pelvic floor at rest, with the subjects in a supine position. Acquisition time was approximately 5 minutes with 32 slices obtained from each subject with image size 256x168 pixels and spatial resolution of 1x1 mm. Ten subjects were scanned with this protocol. The second set was built from coronal slices from a 0.5T GE iMR open access scanner. A fast turbo spin echo protocol was used to acquire T_2 weighted images (TR=4900ms, TE=102ms, slice thickness = 5mm) of the pelvic floor with the subjects in both sitting and squatting positions. A total of 15 slices were acquired for each subject and the acquisition time was approximately 8 minutes. Whilst a subject is in the squatting position, the shape of the levator ani changed due to the weight bearing down on the levators, and four subjects were scanned with this protocol. All subjects scanned were nulliparous females.

2.1 Harmonic Shape Embedding

Similar to our previous study, the levators were manually segmented from the MR images. Each volume was automatically separated into the top and bottom surfaces [10] by determining the points of highest curvature. Each surface was then triangulated, scaled and aligned by using the Iterative Closest Points algorithm [11]. Shape embedding was performed by using the technique previously developed [7], where triangulated and aligned surfaces are harmonically mapped to a unit quadrilateral based domain. A B-spline surface patch was constructed from each mesh by reparameterising the harmonic embedding over uniform knots. The surfaces are reparameterised over the unit base domain with the parameterization defined by a piecewise bilinear map.

2.2 Incorporating Thickness Variation

After harmonic shape embedding, the associated muscle thickness $d(p)$ was measured at each control point p by using its minimum distance to the corresponding surface [12]. By using the bottom surface of the levator as the base domain, the surface tangents to the control points on the top surface give a local linear approximation of the top surface. Therefore, the shortest distance between p and the plane Tp gives a local thickness measure. That is,

$$d(p) = \min dist(p, Tp) \tag{1}$$

To achieve a combined statistical shape and volume modelling, the dimensionality of the original problem of shape modelling needs to be extended to include d described above. For this study, the Minimum Description Length (MDL) criterion was used to determine the optimal control points that can yield the most compact description of the shape and thickness variations. In this case, the corresponding objective function can be written as:

$$F = \sum_m \left(-\sum_s \ln P\left(\left\{ \begin{matrix} x \\ y \\ z \\ d \end{matrix} \right\}_s^{T} \middle|^m \middle| \sigma_m \right) + L(\sigma_m) \right) \tag{2}$$

where $\left\{ x, y, z, d \right\}^T \Big|_s^m$ is the projection of the sth shape and thickness into the mth axis of the model whose variance is σ_m^2. We assume in this study that the distributions of the coordinates and d are of Gaussian and the model parameters are uniformly distributed. In this case, the log likelihood and length of the model parameters are:

$$\ln P\left(x_s^m \mid \sigma_m \right) = \ln \Delta + \frac{1}{2}\ln\left(2\pi\sigma_m^{\,2}\right) - \frac{1}{2}\left(\left\{ \begin{matrix} x \\ y \\ z \\ d \end{matrix} \right\}_s \middle|^m \middle/ \sigma_m \right)^2 \tag{3}$$

$$L(\sigma_m) = 1 + \ln\left(\frac{\sigma_{max} - \sigma_{min}}{\delta} \right) + \left| \ln \delta \right|$$

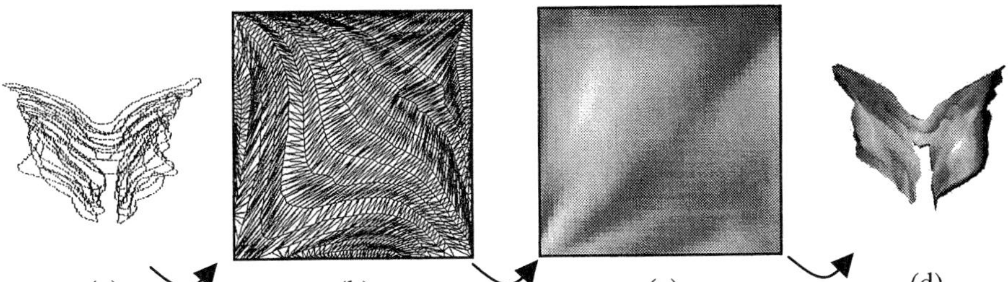

(a)   (b)   (c)   (d)

Fig. 1. (a) A segmented levator ani volume whose bottom surface has been made into a (b) harmonic map and shown here (c) with corresponding thickness map and (d) the thickness map displayed on the bottom surface of the levator ani.

The optimisation was performed by using Polak-Ribiere's conjugate gradient optimisation algorithm [13]. At each iteration, the coordinates of each control point were moved in the harmonic embedded space and the associated thickness was recalculated in the original re-projected 3D shape space by following the local thickness measure described above. Figure 1 schematically summarises the overall computational steps involved in the proposed algorithm, showing the harmonic embedded space used for determining the optimal control points for capturing both shape and thickness variations, and the final modelling results before and after re-mapping the thickness distribution to the 3D model of the levator ani.

3   Results

Figure 2 illustrates two example cross sections of the pelvic floor acquired by using the closed and open access scanners respectively, where the structure associated with the levator ani is indicated by the arrows. They generally provide enough resolution for the manual segmentation of the levators. The corresponding training sets used in the study are shown in (c) and (d) where local muscle thickness is mapped by using a colour scale ranging from cool to warm colours[1]. Warmer shades indicate a thicker part of the levator and the maximum scale used is 10 mm.

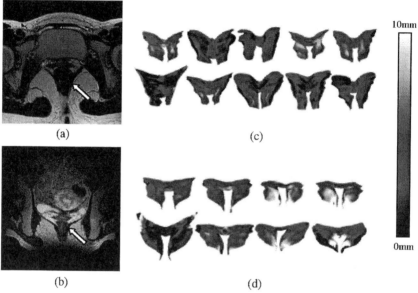

Fig. 2. Example magnetic resonance images from (a) the closed access scanner and (b) the open access scanner and their respective training sets with thickness representation as shown on the scale to the right: (c) the ten subjects and (d) the four subjects in two positions. The levator ani in (a) and (b) is indicated by the white arrows.

The corresponding results by using the proposed combined shape and thickness modelling after principal components analysis is shown in Figure 3. The purpose of the first training set is to depict detailed morphological variations across different subjects by using relatively high SNR images. It is evident from the modelling results that the first mode of variation of the proposed modelling scheme captures the thickness variation in the anterior part of the levator along with a change in position of the levator arms while the second mode shows a slight change in the right section of the levator in both shape and thickness. In the second set showing the dynamic information of the levators during stress, the first mode displays a change in the shape of the levator arms and a change in height of the posterior of the levator and the second mode shows a shape and thickness variation in the anterior of the levator ani. These modes correspond to the shape and thickness change in the levator during

---

[1] A colour version of this paper can be found at http://www.doc.ic.ac.uk/~gzy/PFM

squeezing where the levator is under stress. In this case, the levator arms flatten out, the posterior plate of the levator changes angle and it is expected that the thickness shifts accordingly. In both sets, the third mode of variation shows little variation in both shape and thickness.

Figure 4 shows a comparison of the accumulative variance of the statistical models from the parameterization based on shape information only and the parameterization based on both shape and thickness information combined, the proposed modelling technique. As expected, the compactness of the combined technique is less than that of the shape only model due to the increased information dimensionality in the optimization.

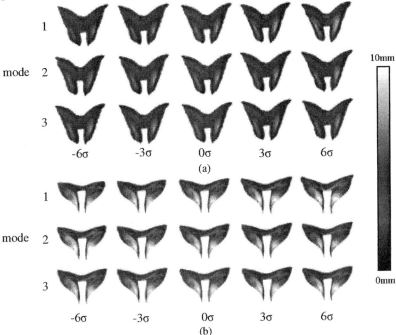

Fig. 3. Principal components analysis showing the first three modes of variation of the levator ani shapes and corresponding thicknesses of the training set built from images acquired in (a) the closed access scanner to assess shape and thickness variation across subjects at rest, and (b) the open access scanner to assess shape and thickness variation during stress. The thickness color map used can be seen on the right.

4 Conclusion

In conclusion, we have described the use of a statistical shape model that includes both surface and thickness information of the levator ani. The objective function used to select the parameterisation of the shape model was based on the MDL criterion. The work extends our previous research on optimal statistical shape modelling for volumetric analysis of the levator ani. With harmonic embedding, it provides an

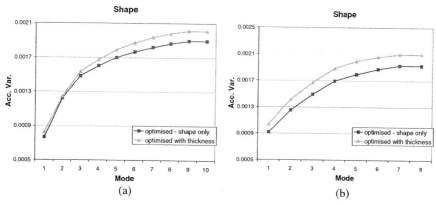

Fig. 4. Accumulative variance of the shape from the training sets built from images acquired in (a) the closed access scanner and (b) the open access scanner.

effective framework for combining shape with tensor distribution, and is particularly suited for modelling sheet muscles such as the levator ani. Principal component analysis of the derived model has shown meaningful shape and thickening variation of the levator ani, demonstrating the practical value of the technique.

Acknowledgements. The authors would like to thank W. Caspersz at St Mary's Hospital and S. Masood, L. Crowe and D. Firmin at the Royal Brompton Hospital for their assistance in MR data acquisition.

References

1. Healy, J.C., Halligan, S., Reznek, R.H., Watson, S., Phillips, R.K., Armstrong, P. Patterns of Prolapse in Women with Symptoms of Pelvic Floor Weakness: Assessment with MR Imaging. Radiology, Vol. 203. (1997) 77-81.
2. Law, P.A., Danin, J.C., Lamb, G.M., Regan, L., Darzi, A., Gedroyc, W.M. Dynamic Imaging of the Pelvic Floor Using an Open-Configuration Magnetic Resonance Scanner. Journal of Magnetic Resonance Imaging, Vol. 13. (2001) 923-929.
3. Fielding, J.R., Hoyte, L., Schierlitz, L. MR Imaging of Pelvic Floor Relaxation. Journal of Women's Imaging, Vol. 2. (2000) 82-87.
4. Hoyte, L., Schierlitz, L., Zou, K., Flesh, G., Fielding, J.R. Two- and 3-dimensional MRI comparison of levator ani structure, volume, and integrity in women with stress incontinence and prolapse. American Journal of Obstetrics and Gynecology, Vol. 185. (2001) 11-19.
5. Duchinela, K., Ryhammer, A., Nagel, L.L., Djurhuus, J.C., Constantinou, C.E. MRI of the Aging Female Pelvic Floor; A 3D Perspective of its Principal Organization. International Continence Society Congress, Seoul. (2001)
6. Lee, S-L., Horkaew, P., Darzi, A., Yang, G-Z. Optimal Scan Planning with Statistical Shape Modelling of the Levator Ani. MICCAI (2003). 714-721.
7. Horkaew, P., Yang, G-Z. Optimal Deformable Surface Models for 3D Medical Image Analysis. IPMI (2003).

8. Hoyte, L., Jakab, M., Warfield, S., Paquette, R., Flesh, G., Zou, K., Fielding, J. Comparison of Levator Ani Thickness in Symptomatic and Asymptomatic Women Using MR-Based 3D Color Mapping. American Urogynecologic Society Scientific Meeting (2003).
9. Pizer, S.M., Gerig, G., Joshi, S., Aylward, S.R. Multiscale Medial Shape-Based Analysis of Image Objects. Proceedings of the IEEE, Vol. 91, No. 10. (2003) 1670-1679.
10. Kanai, T., Suzuki, H., Kimura, F. Three-dimensional geometric metamorphosis based on harmonic maps. The Visual Computer, Vol. 14. (1998) 166-176.
11. Besl, P.J., McKay, N.D. A Method for Registration of 3-D Shapes. IEEE Transactions on Pattern Analysis and Machine Intelligence, Vol. 14. (1992) 239-256.
12. Hoppe, H., DeRose, T., Duchamp, T., McDonald, T., Stuetzle, W. Surface Reconstruction from Unorganized Points. ACM SIGGRAPH (1992) 71-78.
13. Press, W.H., Teukolsky, S.A., Vetterling, W.T., Flannery, B.P. Numerical Recipes in C, 2nd edn. Cambridge University Press (1996) ISBN 0-521-43108-5.

Characterizing the Shape of Anatomical Structures with Poisson's Equation

Haissam Haidar[1,2], Sylvain Bouix[2,3], James Levitt[2,3], Chandley Dickey[2,3], Robert W. McCarley[3], Martha E. Shenton[2,3], and Janet S. Soul[1,2]

[1] Department of Neurology, Children's Hospital and Harvard Medical School, Boston, MA.
{haissam, sylvain}@bwh.harvard.edu,
[2] Surgical Planning Laboratory, Department of Radiology, Brigham and Women's Hospital and Harvard Medical School, Boston, MA.
Janet.Soul@childrens.harvard.edu
[3] Clinical Neuroscience Division, Laboratory of Neuroscience, Boston VA Health Care System, Brockton Division, Department of Psychiatry, Harvard Medical School, Boston, MA.
{james_levitt, chandlee_dickey, robert_mccarley, martha_shenton}@hms.harvard.edu,

Abstract. This paper presents a novel approach to analyze the shape of anatomical structures. Our methodology is rooted in classical physics and in particular Poisson's equation, a fundamental partial differential equation [1]. The solution to this equation and more specifically its equipotential surfaces display properties that are useful for shape analysis. We demonstrate the solution of this equation on synthetic and medical images. We present a numerical algorithm to calculate the length of streamlines formed by the gradient field of the solution to this equation for 3D objects. We used the length of streamlines of equipotential surfaces to introduce a new function to characterize the shape of objects. A preliminary study on the shape of the caudate nucleus in Schizotypal Personality Disorder (SPD) illustrates the power of our method.

1 Introduction

Shape analysis methods play a key role in the study of medical images. They enable us to go beyond simple volumetric measures to provide a more intuitive idea of the changes an anatomical structure undergoes. There are mainly three classes of shape analysis methods. The first class relies on a feature vector, such as spherical harmonics or invariant moments [2, 3], as a representation of shape and tries to discriminate between classes of shapes using clustering methods such as principal component analysis. These methods are usually numerically stable and relevant statistics can be computed from them. However, their interpretation is often difficult and they rarely provide an intuitive description of the shape. The second class of methods is based on a surface boundary representation of the object and the study of the mechanical deformations required to transform one object into another [4, 5]. This popular technique is very intuitive, but relies on registration methods which are difficult to implement and not always reliable. Calculating significant statistics from the deformation also poses a challenge. The third class makes use of medial representa

C. Barillot, D.R. Haynor, and P. Hellier (Eds.): MICCAI 2004, LNCS 3216, pp. 266–273, 2004.
© Springer-Verlag Berlin Heidelberg 2004

tions which provide insightful information about the symmetry of the object. Unfortunately, the medial models still need to be registered with each other before any statistics can be derived [6-8]. In clinical studies, different classes of methods are often combined in order to obtain intuitive and statistically significant results, see for example [9].

In this paper, we propose a novel shape analysis method based on Poisson's equation with a Dirichlet boundary condition. This equation, most known in electrostatics, has very interesting properties for the study of shape. Most notably, its solution is always smooth, has one sink point and can be made independent of the scale of the original object. Our approach is to extract one scalar value and use this number to compare different classes of objects.

Section 2 provides details on Poisson's equation and how it can be used for shape analysis. Section 3 illustrates and validates the method on synthetic objects and finally Section 4 presents a preliminary case study of the caudate in Schizotypal Personality Disorder.

2   Methods

2.1   Poisson's Equation

Poisson's equation is fundamental to mathematical physics and has been widely used over a range of phenomena. Examples include electrostatic fields, gravitational fields, thermo-dynamic flows and other applications. Mathematically, Poisson's equation is a second-order elliptic partial differential equation defined as:

$$\Delta u = -1 \tag{1}$$

Poisson's equation is independent of the coordinate system and characterizes the entire domain (volume in 3D) not only its boundary. Functions u satisfying Poisson's equation are called potential functions. These functions have many mathematical properties related to the underlying geometry of the structure. Among the properties are the following:

1. The shape of the potential function is correlated to the geometry of the structure. This correlation gives a mathematical meaning to the medical concept of anatomical sublayers.
2. In the special case of Dirichlet conditions on the outer surface of a closed homogeneous domain, the potential function converges smoothly to a single sink point. Moreover, a unique streamline can be drawn from each point of the boundary to the sink point by following the gradient field of the potential function.
3. The pattern of streamlines is independent of the value of the potential on the boundary and is closely related to the shape of the domain.

The length of each streamline can be calculated by summing the Euclidean distances between neighboring points along the streamline. For example, in electrostatics, this length is called the 'electric displacement'.

In Figure 1, we illustrate the solution of Poisson's equation for simple two dimensional domains, a circle (Figure 1a) and a square (Figure 1b). In both examples, the initial conditions on the boundary were set to u = 100. The solution represents a lay-ered set of equipotential curves making a smooth transition from the outer contour to the center. The equipotential curves for a circle are simply smaller circles. However, the equipotential curves inside a square smoothly change shape as they approach the sink point. This change is illustrated in Figure 1a where two streamlines connect the sink point to two equipotential points inside the circle. Figure 1b shows similar streamlines inside the square. Inside a circle the 'electric displacement' along an equipotential curve is constant. Inside a square, this displacement varies due to the shape of the boundary. Note however, that the variation of displacement decreases from one equipotential level to another while moving towards the sink point. We used this concept of displacement as the basis of our approach to apply Poisson's equation for the analysis of shape of anatomical structures.

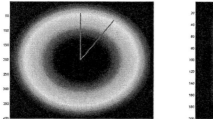 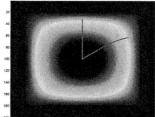

Fig. 1. a) potential function inside a circle with streamlines of two equipotential points. b) po-tential function inside a square with streamlines of two equipotential points.

2.2 Calculating the Displacement

Since there are many standard numerical methods for solving Poisson's equation (1), we will not discuss in this work the numerical solution of Poisson's equation for 3D MRI. We refer the reader to [10] for details on numerical solutions of standard partial differential equations. We will focus instead on the computation of the displacement for each point in the given domain.

Because all streamlines converge to one unique sink point, P_s, we can design a downwinding algorithm to calculate the displacement at a voxel P_0 by summation of the Euclidean distances between consecutive voxels along the streamline connecting P_0 to P_s.

First, P_s is found by solving the following equation:

$$\|\text{grad}(u)\| = 0 \tag{2}$$

The displacement D at a voxel P_0 is then defined as:

$$D(P_0) = \Sigma L_i \tag{3}$$

L_i is the Euclidean distance between consecutive voxels P_i and P_{i+1} on the streamline connecting P_0 to the sink point. Depending on the direction of the gradient field at voxel P_i, L_i can have one of the following values:

$h_1, h_2, h_3, (h_1^2 + h_2^2)^{1/2}, (h_1^2 + h_3^2)^{1/2}, (h_2^2 + h_3^2)^{1/2}$ or $(h_1^2 + h_2^2 + h_3^2)^{1/2}$;
h_1 is the voxel width, h_2 the voxel height and h_3 the slice thickness.

The direction of the gradient is assessed using a simple transformation from a Cartesian to a spherical coordinate system. The azimuth θ and the elevation φ of the gradient are calculated at P_i and used to determine L_i. The coordinates of the following voxel on the streamline, P_{i+1}, can be computed using;

$$\begin{cases} x_{i+1} = x_i + L_i.\sin\varphi_i\cos\theta_i \; ; \\ y_{i+1} = y_i + L_i.\sin\varphi_i\sin\theta_i \; ; \\ z_{i+1} = z_i + L_i.\sin\theta_i \end{cases} \qquad (4)$$

L_i is added to the current $D(P_0)$ using (3), the procedure is then repeated at P_{i+1} until the sink point P_s is reached. Figure 2 presents the displacement maps of a circle and square.

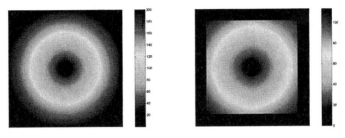

Fig. 2. Displacement map of a circle (left) and a square (right).

2.3 Analysis of Shape Using Poisson's Equation

Earlier, we demonstrated that the dynamics of change of the equipotential surfaces inside the domain while approaching the center is related to the domain geometry. To evaluate this process we first define the normalized drop of potential E at an equipotential surface S_i as:

$$E = (U_0 - U_i)/(U_0 - U_s); \qquad (5)$$

U_0, U_s and U_i are the potentials on the boundary, at the sink point and on the current equipotential surface respectively. E characterizes the amount of energy needed to transform the surface boundary into the current equipotential surface.

We then introduce v, the coefficient of variance of the displacement along the current equipotential surface S_i:

$$v(E) = \text{stdev}(D(S_i))/\text{mean}(D(S_i)) \qquad (6)$$

Function $v(E)$, which we call the "shape characteristic", displays some very interesting properties:
1. It is independent of the potential on the outer boundary.
2. It is independent of the overall volume and defined exclusively by the shape.
3. A given value v corresponds to a known drop of potential E.

4. The slope of $v(E)$ dramatically decreases on a well-determined interval for each specific shape. We call the 'critical point' the point $P_c(E_c, v_c)$ where the curvature of $v(E)$ changes sign. This point characterizes the shape in a unique way.

Thus, the shape of a structure can be represented, through the "shape characteristic", by one unique point $P_c(E_c, v_c)$ independent of both the initial conditions on the outer boundary and the volume of the structure. This point defines the amount of energy, needed for the structure to lose its initial shape and to deform into a new one comparable to a sphere.

3   Experiments on Synthetic Data

In addition to the 2D examples given in Section 2, we created two simple phantoms with different shapes to test our algorithm. The first phantom is a single 3D tube, the second is a tubular tree. Poisson's equation was solved, and then the displacement map was calculated. Figure 3 shows the resulting potential functions and displacement maps for a cross section of both objects.

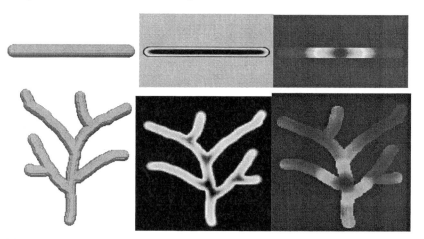

Fig. 3. Potential functions and (middle) and displacement maps (right) for two simple synthetic objects

A graph of the shape characteristic function, $v(E)$, is shown in Figure 4. Notice v is 0 for the circle as expected. For the other phantoms, v is a monotically decreasing function, i.e., as the equipotential surface approaches the sink point, the shape characteristic approaches zero.

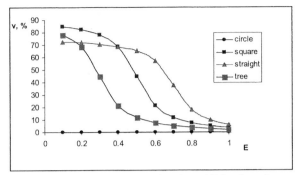

Fig. 4. Shape characteristic ν as a function of E for four phantoms.

4   Shape Analysis of the Caudate Nucleus

The caudate nucleus is an essential part in the "cognitive" circuitry connecting the frontal lobe to subcortical structures of the brain. Pathology in any of the core components of this circuitry may result in neurological disease such as schizophrenia[11, 12] and schizotypal personality disorder (SPD) . Previous studies have shown volumetric and shape differences of the caudate between normal controls and SPD subjects [13, 14]. In this paper we propose to validate our methodology by applying our shape analysis method to the data used in [13, 14] and verify the previously observed shape differences.

4.1   Methods

Fifteen right-handed male subjects with Schizotypal Personality Disorder (SPD) with no previous neuroleptic exposure and fourteen normal comparisons subjects (NC), underwent MRI scanning. Subjects were group matched for parental socioeconomic status, handedness and gender. MRI images were acquired with a 1.5T GE scanner, using a SPoiled Gradient Recalled (SPGR) sequence yielding to a (256x256x124) volume with (0.9375x0.9375x1.5mm) voxel dimensions. The scans were acquired coronally. The caudates were drawn manually and separated by an Anterior/Posterior boundary. Details of the segmentation procedure can be found in [14].

We applied our novel method to the entire caudate to investigate any difference in shape between normal controls and SPD subjects. Poisson's equation was solved for each left and right caudate. Afterwards, the displacement maps were calculated using the algorithm presented in Section 2. An example caudate nucleus and its corresponding potential function and displacement map are shown in Figure 5. The function ν was then computed for each structure. We used E_c = 30% as 'critical' value to calculate the corresponding v_c. We applied a Mann-Whitney non-parametric test to compare the values of v_c between the two groups. Figure 6 presents a plot graph of v_c for our data set.

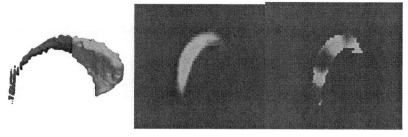

Fig. 5. 3D rendering of the caudate nucleus (left), sagittal cross section displaying the potential function (middle) and displacement map (right).

4.2   Results and Discussion

Our test revealed a statistically significant difference in the head of the right caudate for the value v_c ($p< 0.03$) between NC and SPD. No significant group differences ($p< 0.167$) in the head of the left Caudate were found.

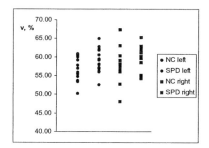

Fig. 6. Plot of the 'critical' value v_c ($E_c=0.3$) of the caudate for 14 SPD and 15 controls.

Previous analysis of the same data set revealed a group difference in volume on both sides and a shape difference on the right side using the "shape index" measure[13, 14]. We are glad to report that our method confirms the results previously published.

5   Conclusion

We have developed a novel method for shape analysis of anatomical structures. Our method is based on using the solution of Poisson's equation to assess the dynamics of change of shape of the equipotential surfaces inside the structure. We have developed an algorithm for calculating the displacement maps defined by the length of the streamlines generated by the gradient field of the potential function. We used these maps to introduce a new function, called 'shape characteristic', which characterizes in a unique way the shape of a structure. Our method was validated on synthetic 2D and 3D and on real medical data. Our results on the shape of the caudate nucleus in SPD correlate nicely with the literature. This suggests that our method can be used as a powerful tool to correlate shape of anatomical structures with different factors such as aging or diseases. The "shape characteristic" is one of many tools one can build based on Poisson's equation. In future work, we propose to design more intuitive shape analysis techniques based on this equation and its solutions.

Acknowledgements. We gratefully acknowledge the support of the National Institute of Health (K02 MH 01110 and R01 MH 50747 to MES, R01 MH 40799 to RWM), the Department of Veterans Affairs Merit Awards (MES, RWM), Career Development Award (CCD) and the United Cerebral Palsy Foundation (JSS).

References

1. Farlow, S.J., *Partial Differential Equations for Scientists and Engineers.* 1993: Dover.
2. Mangin, J.-F., et al. *3d Moment Invariant Based Morphometry.* in *MICCAI.* 2003. Montreal: Springer-Verlag.
3. Brechbuhler, C., G. Gerig, and O. Kubler, *Parametrization of Closed Surfaces for 3D Shape Description.* CVGIP: Image Understanding, 1995. **61**: p. 154-170.
4. Bookstein, F.L., *Shape and the Information in Medical Images.* Computer Vision and Image Understanding, 1997. **66**(2): p. 97-118.
5. Csernansky, J.G., et al., *Hippocampal Morphometry in Schizophrenia via High Dimensional Brain Mapping.* Proc. Natl. Acad. Sci., 1998. **95**: p. 11406-11411.
6. Styner, M. and G. Gerig, *Medial Models Incorporating Object Variability for 3D Shape Analysis,* in *IPMI'2001.* 2001. p. 502--516.
7. Styner, M., et al., *Statistical Shape Analysis of Neuroanatomical Structures based on Medial Models.* Medical Image Analysis, 2003. **7**(3): p. 207-220.
8. Bouix, S., et al. *Hippocampal Shape Analysis Using Medial Surfaces.* in *MICCAI.* 2001. Utrecht: Springer-Verlag.
9. Styner, M., J.A. Lieberman, and G. Gerig. *Boundary and Medial Shape Analysi of the Hippocampus in Schizophrenia.* in *MICCAI.* 2003. Montreal: Springer-Verlag.
10. Lapidus, L. and G.F. Pinder, *Numerical solutions of partial differential equations in science and engineering.* 1982: Wiley-Interscience.
11. Keshavan, M.S., et al., *Decreased Caudate Volume in neuroleptic-naive psychotic patients.* American Journal of Psychiatry, 1998. **155**(774-778).
12. Corson, P.W., et al., *Caudate size in first-episode neuroleptic-naive schizophrenic patients measured using an artificial neural network.* Biological Psychiatry, 1999. **46**: p. 712-720.
13. Levitt, J., et al., *Shape of Caudate Nucleus and Its Cognitive Correlates in Neuroleptic-Naive Schizotypal Personality Disorder.* Biological Psychiatry, 2004. **55**: p. 177-184.
14. Levitt, J.J., et al., *MRI Study of Caudate Nucleus Volume and Its Cognitive Correlates in Neuroleptic-Naive Patients With Schizotypal Personality Disorder.* American Journal of Psychiatry, 2002. **159**: p. 1190-1197.

Automatic Optimization of Segmentation Algorithms Through Simultaneous Truth and Performance Level Estimation (STAPLE)

Mahnaz Maddah, Kelly H. Zou, William M. Wells, Ron Kikinis, and
Simon K. Warfield

Computational Radiology Laboratory, Surgical Planning Laboratory, Brigham and Women's
Hospital, Harvard Medical School, Boston MA 02115, USA.
{mmaddah, zou, sw, kikinis, warfield}@bwh.harvard.edu
http://spl.bwh.harvard.edu

Abstract. The performance of automatic segmentation algorithms often depends critically upon a number of parameters intrinsic to the algorithm. Appropriate setting of these parameters is a pre-requisite for successful segmentation, and yet may be difficult for users to achieve. We propose here a novel algorithm for the automatic selection of optimal parameters for medical image segmentation. Our algorithm makes use of STAPLE (Simultaneous Truth and Performance Level Estimation), a previously described and validated algorithm for automatically identifying a reference standard by which to assess segmentation generators. We execute a set of independent automated segmentation algorithms with initial parameter settings, on a set of images from any clinical application under consideration, estimate a reference standard from the segmentation results using STAPLE, and then identify the parameter settings for each algorithm that maximizes the quality of the segmentation generator result with respect to the reference standard. The process of estimating a reference standard and estimating the optimal parameter settings is iterated to convergence.

1 Introduction

The analysis of medical images is a critical process, enabling applications ranging from fundamental neuroscience, to objective evaluation of interventions and drug treatments, to monitoring, navigation and assessment of image guided therapy. Segmentation is the key process by which raw image acquisitions are interpreted. Interactive segmentation is fraught with intra-rater and inter-rater variability which limits its accuracy, while also being costly and time-consuming. Automatic segmentation holds out the potential of dramatically increased precision, and reduction in time and expense. However, the performance of automatic segmentation algorithms often depends critically upon a number of parameters intrinsic to the algorithm. Such parameters may control assumptions regarding tissue intensity characteristics, spatial homogeneity constraints, boundary smoothness or curvature characteristics or other prior information. Appropriate setting of these parameters by users is often a prerequisite for successful segmentation, and yet may be difficult for users to achieve

C. Barillot, D.R. Haynor, and P. Hellier (Eds.): MICCAI 2004, LNCS 3216, pp. 274–282, 2004.

due to the potentially nonlinear effects and interactions between different parameter settings which are challenging for human operators to optimize over. Furthermore, the selection of parameters based on a synthetic phantom may not be appropriate for clinical applications since the normal and pathological appearance of subjects from any particular clinical population may be quite different from that readily captured in a phantom.

To overcome these problems, we present here an approach to estimate the true segmentation from several automatic or semi-automatic segmentation algorithms and optimize their free parameters for a category of medical images. The ground-truth estimation is done by an Expectation-Maximization algorithm, called STAPLE (Simultaneous Truth and Performance Level Estimation), presented in [1]. In that work, a collection of expert-segmented images was given to STAPLE and a probabilistic estimate of the true segmentation was computed along with the performance level measurement of each expert. The idea here is to employ this method in order to obtain the optimal values for the parameters of different automated segmentation algorithms and to evaluate their performance compared with the estimated true segmentation. This is significantly important in medical application such as neuroscience and surgical planning, since the users often face difficulty to find good parameter settings and yet their results are utilized for the research studies and disease therapies.

The paper is organized as follows: In Section 2, we outline our evaluation and parameter optimization methodology. The ground-truth estimation, the optimization algorithm, and the assessment metric used in this study are described in this section. The optimization and evaluation of the four algorithms for brain tissue segmentation as well as the obtained results are presented in Section 3, and finally the conclusion and further work are brought in Section 4.

2 Methods

The proposed method is an iterative process with two main stages: ground-truth estimation and parameter setting which can be performed on a specific case or a collection of subjects:

a) Optimization on One Subject:

To find the best parameters for each subject, we first need to estimate a ground truth and performance level on a training dataset segmented using the algorithms under study. In this stage, the segmented images from different algorithms are given to STAPLE which computes simultaneously a probabilistic estimate of the true segmentation and a measure of the performance level represented by each segmentation algorithm. Then, we optimize the performance of each algorithm with respect to the estimated ground truth. Given a set of algorithms with optimized parameters, we recompute the ground truth and re-optimize the parameters until the ground truth estimate converges. At the end of this stage we have the optimized segmentation algorithms, an estimated true segmentation, and the levels of performance for each algorithm on one experimental data.

b) Optimization on a Collection of Subjects:

The goal of this step would be to expand the capability of the approach to optimize parameters of each algorithm across N training subjects, for $N > 1$. This is achieved by changing the quality measure to be the mean of the performance level across all cases. Each optimization step is performed based on the impact of the parameter across the N cases rather than just one case. This would give us optimized parameters for a set of subjects, finding a tradeoff in settings across all of the subjects. It might do worse than possible if we optimized just for one case, but on average leads to a better result over all the subjects.

In fact, our approach is technically an instance of a generalized expectation maximization algorithm, where we have extra parameters (the segmentation algorithm parameters) for which no closed form maximization exists and so an approximate local maximization strategy is used.

2.1 STAPLE

STAPLE takes a collection of segmentations of an image, and constructs a probabilistic estimate of the true segmentation and a measure of the performance level of each segmentation generator [1]. This algorithm is an instance of the Expectation-Maximization (EM) in which the segmentation decision at each voxel is directly observable, the hidden true segmentation is a binary variable for each voxel, and the performance level, achieved by each segmentation method is represented by sensitivity and specificity parameters [1]. At each EM iteration, first, the hidden true segmentation variables are replaced with their conditional probabilities and are estimated given the input segmentation and a previous estimate of the performance level. In the second step, the performance parameters are updated. This process is iterated until the convergence is reached. STAPLE is also capable of considering several types of spatial constrains, including a statistical atlas of prior probabilities for the distribution of the structure of interest which we make use of it in our approach.

2.2 Performance Metric

The "ideal" performance point represents true positive rate (*TP*) of 1 and false positive rate (*FP*) of 0. With the *TP* and *FP* obtained by comparing each segmentation with the estimated ground truth, a performance metric can be defined based on the weighted Euclidean distance from this point:

$$Performance = 1 - \sqrt{w^2 (1 - TP)^2 + (1 - w)^2 FP^2} \qquad (1)$$

The weighting factor, w, is set equal to the foreground prevalence. When the foreground occupies a small portion of the image (small w), *TP* is very sensitive to the number of foreground errors, while *FP* is relatively insensitive to the errors in the background. Weighting the errors makes the overall error almost equally sensitive to the errors in the foreground and background.

2.3 Optimization Method

Numerous optimization algorithms exist in the literature and each might be invoked in our application provided that it is able to find the global optimum and can be applied to discrete optimization problems.

Here, we make use of simultaneous perturbation stochastic approximation (SPSA) method [2]. It requires only two objective function measurements per iteration regardless of the dimension of the optimization problem. These measurements are made by simultaneously varying in a proper random fashion of all the parameters. The random shift of parameters is controlled by a set of SPSA algorithm coefficients which must be set for each algorithm under-optimization. The error function here, is 1–*Performance* computed for each segmentation from equation (1). Note that the behavior of the error in terms of the parameter should be known in order to correctly set the acceptable range of parameters.

3 Experiments and Results

We have applied our method to the problem of tissue segmentation of human's brain, which has received continues attention in medical image analysis, focusing on white mat classification.

3.1 Human Brain Tissue Segmentation Algorithms

We considered four algorithms including two research segmentation algorithms and two well-known packages which are briefly described in the following:

SPM – SPM uses a modified maximum likelihood "mixture model" algorithm for its segmentation, in which each voxel is assigned a probability of belonging to each of the given clusters [3]. Assuming a normal distribution for the intensity of the voxels belonging to each cluster, the distribution parameters are computed. These parameters are then combined with a given priority map to update the membership probabilities. The smoothing parameter applied to affine registration is considered as the parameter to be optmimally set.

FSL – The segmentation algorithm in this package is based on a hidden Markov random field (HMRF) model [4]. It starts with an initial estimation step to obtain initial tissue parameters and classification, followed by a three-step EM process which updates the class labels, tissue parameters and bias field iteratively. During the teratn MRF-MAP (maximum a posteriori) approach is used to estimate class labels, mp is applied to estimate the bias field, and the tissue parameters are estimated by maximum likelihood (ML). We used the MRF neighborhood beta value as the controlling parameter for optimization.

k-NN Classification – The k-Nearest Neighbor (k-NN) classification rule is a technique for nonparametric supervised pattern classification. Given a training data set consisting of N prototype patterns and the corresponding correct classification of each prototype into one of C classes, a pattern of unknown class, is classified as class C if most of the closest prototype patterns are from class C. The algorithm we used is a fast implementation of this basic idea[5]. The number of training data patterns, their position and K, the number of nearest neighbors to consider, are the controlling factors of this method which the latter, K is considered here as the parameter to be optimized.

EM – This method is an adaptive segmentation, which uses an Expectation Maximization (EM) algorithm [6]. It simultaneously labels and estimates the intensity inhmogeneities artifacts in the image. It uses an iterated moving average low-pass filter in bias field estimation which its width is considered as the parameter for our study. We set the number of EM iteration steps to 10 according to [6].

3.2 Training and Test Data

We applied the approach on five sets of T1-weighted MR brain images with resolution of 0.9375×0.9375×1.3 mm³, each consists of 124 slices. The images were first filtered by a multi-directional flux-diffusion filter, implemented in 3D Slicer [7]. Next, the non-brain tissues are removed from the images by brain extraction tool (BET) in the FSL package which uses a deformable model to fit the brain's surface [8]. The average of the semi-automatic segmentation of 82 cases was used as the atlas for STAPLE.

3.3 Optimization Results

In Table I, the optimization results for each of the four algorithms are shown. In the first step (iteration 0), each algorithm has been run with the default value of its parameter. With the estimated ground-truth in Iteration i, each algorithm goes through the optimization loop and the obtained optimal values are set for the next ground-truth estimation (iteration $i+1$). The iteration stops when the parameters converge. Once the optimized parameters are found for one case randomly selected from the pool of datasets, we use these values as the initial parameter setting for optimizing on a collection of datasets. The k-NN algorithm is an exception to this, as discussed later. The sensitivity (p) and specificity (q) obtained from STAPLE, are given in Table I as the performance measures.

EM – As seen in Table I, this algorithm gains a high performance score from STAPLE. The error rate versus its parameter, *i.e.* the width of the low-pass filter for bias field estimation in pixels, is shown in Fig. 1(a) for one of the cases under study. The minimum error corresponds to relatively large value of 90 which reflects the low RF coil artifact in the image. A similar trend was observed for other cases.

Table 1. The sensitivity (p) and specificity (q) of each segmentation algorithms are given for the iterations of optimization process. In Iteration 0, STAPLE runs given the four segmentations extracted by each method with the corresponding initial parameters. The new parameters are obtained with respect to the estimated ground-truth in iteration 0. In Iteration 1, the STAPLE runs with the obtained parameters and a new ground-truth and (p,q) pairs are estimated. No changes in parameters occurs in the next optimization, so we stop. Note that for optimization on five cases, the mean and the standard deviation of (p,q)'s over all cases are given in the Table.

Alg.		Optimization on one case		Optimization on five cases	
		Iter. 0	Iter. 1	Iter. 0	Iter. 1
SPM	Window Len.	8	12	12	10
	p	0.6866	0.6843	0.5912±0.1085	0.6014±0.0999
	q	0.9996	0.9995	0.9943±0.0073	0.9966±0.0062
FSL	MRF β	0.3	0.2	0.2	0.1
	p	0.9017	0.9135	0.8149±0.1664	0.8498±0.1892
	q	0.9990	0.9983	0.9960±0.0068	0.9955±0.0063
k-NN	K	9	6	15	12
	p	0.9983	0.9554	0.9497±0.0480	0.9574±0.0482
	q	0.9937	0.9988	0.9986±0.0020	0.9987±0.0020
EM	Filter Width	31	90	90	90
	p	0.9000	0.9899	0.9890±0.0164	0.9857±0.0191
	q	1.0000	0.9990	0.9955±0.0043	0.9951±0.0052

k-**NN** – This algorithm also gets a good performance score. However the resulting optimum K, number of neighbors to be considered, is smaller than its default value 9 which is inconsistent with the fact that the error rate in *k*-NN method is inversely proportional to K. This can be investigated by looking at Fig. 1(b) in which the error vs. the parameter K is illustrated. Although, the graph shows a minimum at K = 6 (which might be due to excluding specific prototypes), the error is very sensitive to the choice of K in that region. A better parameter setting is to set K>12 to avoid the transition region (Note that the upper limits for K is the smallest number of prototypes, selected by the user for each tissue class). In order to prevent the optimization algorithm from stopping in such unwanted minima, one can define the optimization goal as a combination of the error and the error sensitivity to the parameter.

FSL – The optimum value for MRF neighborhood beta is obtained to be 0.2 when considering one subject and 0.1 for our collection of subjects. As seen in Fig. 1(c), the error rate is a well-behaved function of the parameter, however contrary to EM and *k*-NN methods, the error rate increases as the optimization algorithm proceeds. This is due to the fact that the estimated ground-truth converges to EM and *k*-NN results, and therefore the difference between the segmentation by FSL and the estimated ground-truth increases more and more.

SPM – This algorithm underestimates the white matter tissue compared to the prevailing algorithms (EM and *k*-NN), and thus, a low performance level is assigned to it by STAPLE. Furthermore, the selected parameter is not able to push the segmentation results to the estimated ground-truth, though the improvement is apparent in Fig.2 (e). The algorithm gets even lower performance level in the second run, as can be observed in Fig. 1(d).

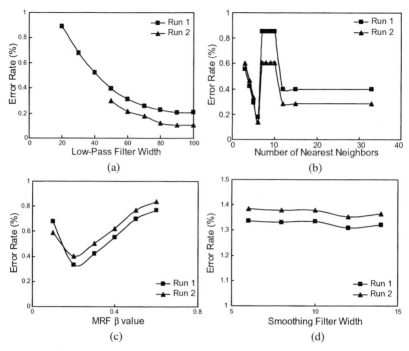

Fig. 1. The error rates versus the parameter for (a) EM (b) k-NN (c) FSL and (d) SPM algorithms after the first and second ground-truth estimations. The overall error rate obtained for EM and k-NN algorithms decreases as the estimated ground-truth approaches the results of these two algorithms.

The effect of parameter adjustment can be observed in Fig.2, where the segmentations with the default and optimized parameters are illustrated.

4   Conclusion and Further Work

In this paper, we presented a novel approach for the automatic selection of optimal parameters for segmentation. This algorithm is an iterative process with two main stages: ground-truth estimation and parameter setting. Two widely-used packages, SPM and FSL, and two research algorithms, k-NN and EM were considered for the optmization. We applied these algorithms on a set of 3D MR images of brain to segment the white matter tissue. The optimal parameters were obtained first for a single case and then for a collection of five cases. The process of estimating a ground-truth and estimating the optimal parameter settings converges in a few iterations. The proposed approach was shown to provide improved segnmentation results compared with algorithms with default parameter setting.

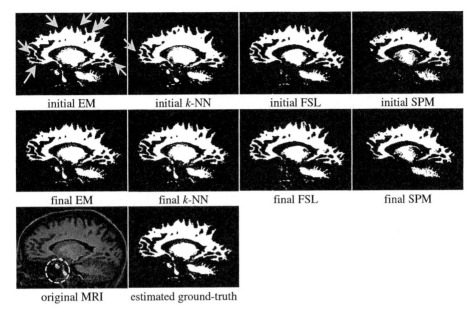

| initial EM | initial *k*-NN | initial FSL | initial SPM |

| final EM | final *k*-NN | final FSL | final SPM |

original MRI   estimated ground-truth

Fig. 2. The optimized segmentations are improved as compared to the initial segmentations. White matter segmentations obtained from different algorithms before and after optimization along with the original MR image and the final estimated ground truth. Some of the errors in the initial segmentation corrected by the proposed algorithm are highlighted by arrows.

Further work is under way to apply this approach to more medical images, to segmentation of other structures. Removing the artifacts in the images such as that highlighted in Fig. 2 with a circle, is another important step to improve the final ground-truth estimation.

Acknowledgement. This investigation was supported by a research grant from the Whitaker Foundation, and by NIH grants R21 MH67054, R01 LM007861, P41 RR13218, P01 CA67165.

References

1. Warfield, S. K., Zou, K. H., Wells, W. M.: Validation of Image Segmentation and Expert Quality with an Expectation-Maximization Algorithm. MICCAI 2002: 5th International Conference, Tokyo, Japan, September 25-28, Proceedings, Part I. (2002) 298 – 306.
2. Spall, J. C.: Stochastic Approximation and Simulated Annealing. Encyclopedia of Electrical and Electronics Engineering, Wiley, New York, Vol. 20, (1999) 529–542.
3. Ashburner, J.: Computational Neuroanatomy. PhD Thesis, University College London (2000). Available at http://www.fil.ion.ucl.ac.uk/spm.

4. Zhang, Y., Brady, M., and Smith S.: Segmentation of Brain MR Images Through a Hidden Markov Random Field Model and the Expectation-Maximization Algorithm. IEEE Trans. Medical Imaging, Vol. 20, No. 1, (2001) 45-57.
5. Warfield, S. K.: Fast k-NN Classification for Multichannel Image Data. Pattern Recognition Lett., Vol. 17, No. 7 (1996) 713-721.
6. Wells, W.M., Grimson, W.E.L., Kikinis, R., Jolesz, F.A.: Adaptive Segmentation of MRI data. IEEE Trans. Medical Imaging. Vol. 15, (1996) 429-442.
7. Krissian, K.: Flux-Based Anisotropic Diffusion: Application to Enhancement of 3D Angiogram. IEEE Trans. Medical Imaging, Vol. 22, No. 11 (2002)1440-1442.
8. Smith, S.: Fast Robust Automated Brain Extraction. Human Brain Mapping, Vol.17, No. 3, (2002) 143-155.

Multi-feature Intensity Inhomogeneity Correction in MR Images

Uroš Vovk, Franjo Pernuš, and Boštjan Likar

Faculty of Electrical Engineering, Tržaška 25, 1000 Ljubljana, Slovenia
{uros.vovk, franjo.pernus, bostjan.likar}@fe.uni-lj.si

Abstract. In MRI, image intensity inhomogeneity is an adverse phenomenon that increases inter-tissue overlapping and hampers quantitative analysis. This study provides a powerful fully automated intensity inhomogeneity correction method that makes no a prior assumptions on the image intensity distribution and is able to correct intensity inhomogeneity with high dynamics. Besides using intensity features, as in most of the existing methods, spatial image features are also incorporated into the correction algorithm. A force is computed in each image point so that distribution of multiple features will shrink in the direction of intensity feature. Extensive regularization of those forces produces smooth inhomogeneity correction estimate, which is gradually improved in an iterative correction framework. The method was tested on simulated and real MR images for which gold standard segmentations were available. The results showed that the method was successful on uniform as well as on low and highly dynamic intensity uniformity images.

1 Introduction

Image intensity inhomogeneity, also referred to as bias field, intensity nonuniformity or shading, is perceived as a smooth intensity variation across the image. In MRI, intensity inhomogeneity may be caused by a number of factors, such as poor radio frequency coil uniformity, static field inhomogeneity, radio frequency penetration, gradient-driven eddy currents, and overall patient anatomy and position [1, 2]. The problem is especially cumbersome because inhomogeneity depends on the measured object and therefore cannot be eliminated or reduced by scanner calibration. A common solution is to conduct retrospective inhomogeneity correction, which is a necessary pre-processing step in many automatic image analysis tasks, e.g. in segmentation or registration, and especially if quantitative analysis is the final goal.

The most intuitive approach for intensity inhomogeneity correction is image smoothing or homomorphic filtering [3, 4, 5]. These methods are based on the assumption that intensity inhomogeneity is a low frequency signal which can be suppressed by high pass filters. However, since the imaged objects themselves usually contain low frequencies, filtering methods often fail to produce meaningful correction. Iterative optimisation that maximises the frequency content of the distribution of tissue intensity has been proposed in [6]. Dawant *et al.* [7] manually selected some points inside white matter and estimated the bias field by fitting splines to the intensities of these points. Styner *et al.* [8] modelled each tissue simply by its

C. Barillot, D.R. Haynor, and P. Hellier (Eds.): MICCAI 2004, LNCS 3216, pp. 283–290, 2004.
© Springer-Verlag Berlin Heidelberg 2004

mean intensity value. A parametric bias field is fitted to the image in an iterative process, which requires initialisation in a form of class means and special masks that have to be defined for each type of images. Information minimisation technique [9] has proved to be very robust and accurate approach in which bias field is modelled by polynomials and applied to acquired image in an optimisation process. The method based on fuzzy C-means [10] minimises the sum of class membership function and the first and second order regularisation terms that ensure the smooth bias field. Ahmed *et al.* [11] used a fuzzy C-means algorithm and combined bias field with adaptive segmentation. Other segmentation-based methods use expectation-maximisation algorithm to compute the bias field from the residue image by either spatial filtering [12] or by weighted least-squares fit of the polynomial bias model [13]. These methods interleave classification and bias field estimation [12] and also the estimation of class-conditional intensity distribution [13] but require initialisation, which is not trivial and practical. Besides, the assumption on normality of intensity distribution of individual tissues may often not be valid, especially when correcting pathological data.

In this paper we propose a novel fully automated bias correction method that makes no assumption on the distribution of image intensities and provide non-parametric correction. As most of the existing methods, the method is based on intensity features but also additional spatial image features are incorporated to improve bias correction and to make it more dynamic.

2 Method

Corruption of intensity homogeneity in MR imaging is a multiplicative phenomenon that is most commonly described by the following model,

$$u(x) = v(x)s(x) + n(x), \tag{1}$$

in which the acquired image $u(x)$ is a combination of the uncorrupted image $v(x)$, corrupted by the multiplicative bias field $s(x)$, and statistically independent noise $n(x)$. The problem of correction of intensity inhomogeneity is to estimate $v(x)$, given the acquired image $u(x)$.

The proposed method can be outlined in four steps:

S1. Calculate probability distribution $p(.)$ of image features
S2. Estimate the forces that will shrink $p(.)$ in the direction of intensity feature
S3. Estimate the bias correction field
S4. Perform partial correction and stop if predefined number of iterations is reached. Otherwise go to S1.

The above steps are described in more detail in the following sections.

2.1 Probability Distribution Calculation

Probability distribution of image features $p(i,d)$ is determined by binning the intensities (i) and the corresponding second spatial derivatives (d) into a discrete two-dimensional feature space. Second derivatives are obtained by convoluting the original image by the Laplacian operator, which was implemented as a 3×3 kernel and applied separately for each slice.

The purpose of using additional image features in a form of second derivatives is to additionally separate tissue clusters in the feature space [14]. This is especially important when image intensities are not enough discriminating features, i.e. when intensity distributions of distinct tissues overlap significantly. This adverse and unfortunately quite frequent phenomenon in MRI is the main source of error in segmentation and inhomogeneity correction methods.

2.2 Force Estimation

In order to obtain an estimation of forces F_x for each image point x that will shrink the probability distribution $p(i,d)$ of an image $u(x)$ in the direction of intensity feature i, we first define a global energy, say E, as a measure of probability distribution dispersion. For this purpose we use the Shannon entropy H,

$$E = H(u(x)) = -\sum_{i,d} p(i,d)\log p(i,d).$$ (2)

The entropy H is usually computed as above by summation of the uncertainties $\log p(i,d)$ in the feature space domain but since we are seeking a contribution of each image point x to the global entropy we will compute the entropy alternatively by summation of the uncertainties over the image domain x of a size X,

$$E = H(u(x)) = -\frac{1}{X}\sum_x \log p(i(x),d(x)).$$ (3)

We can now derive point energy, say E_x, which is the contribution of each image point x to the global energy E,

$$E_x = -\frac{1}{X}\log p(i(x),d(x)).$$ (4)

E_x is, therefore, a contribution of image point x to the dispersion of probability distribution $p(i,d)$. Corresponding point force F_x that will shrink the probability distribution $p(i,d)$ in the direction of intensity feature i can, thus, be obtained by deriving the point energy E_x over the intensities and changing the sign to plus,

$$F_x = \frac{1}{X}\frac{\partial}{\partial i}\left(\log p(i(x),d(x))\right).$$ (5)

Forces F_x are computed by a Sobel operator in the feature space for all feature pairs (i,d) and then mapped to the points with corresponding features in the image space. The obtained forces can be viewed upon as votes for point intensity changes that would result in less disperse probability distribution.

2.3 Bias Correction Estimation

To control the speed of the iterative bias correction and to make it independent of the shape of feature probability distributions, point forces F_x are first normalized in magnitude. The normalized forces are then regularized in the image domain by a sufficiently wide Gaussian kernel g. This yields smooth field of normalized forces that is used to derive an estimation of multiplicative bias correction field $s^{-1}(x)$,

$$s^{-1}(x) = 1 + \left(f \frac{F_x}{\mu(|F_x|)} \right) * g, \qquad (6)$$

where $\mu(|F_x|)$ denotes mean of absolute force, f a predefined magnitude of forces, and $*$ a convolution. A degree of smoothness of bias correction field $s^{-1}(x)$ is determined by the standard deviation σ_g of the Gaussian kernel g.

2.4 Partial Correction

Partial bias correction is performed in each iteration, say n^{th}, by applying bias correction field $s^{-1}(x)$ to the input image $u_n(x)$ so that mean intensity (brightness) and standard deviation (contrast) of the input image are preserved,

$$u_{n+1}(x) \Leftarrow u_\sigma(x) + \mu(u_0(x)) - \mu(u_\sigma(x)), \quad u_\sigma(x) = u_n(x)s^{-1}(x) \frac{\sigma(u_0(x))}{\sigma(u_n(x)s^{-1}(x))}. \qquad (7)$$

The size of partial correction depends on the predefined force magnitude f and the standard deviation σ_g that controls the regularization step, i.e. the smoothness of the bias correction field.

3 Results

Removal of background in MRI images is essential in nearly all methods because background represents air voxels that are not corrupted by the multiplicative bias field and would therefore hamper inhomogeneity correction of the neighbouring tissue voxels. To mask out dark air voxels we remove all voxels with intensities smaller than the predefined intensity threshold, which is the simplest and most commonly used approach [9, 6, 13].

To demonstrate and evaluate the performance of proposed method, we applied it to several simulated and real magnetic resonance images of the human brain.

In the first set of images, variations of digital brain phantom acquired from Brainweb-MRI Simulator [15] were considered: six pairs of volumes with 3% Gaussian noise, including T1-, T2- and PD-modalities, normal and Multiple Sclerosis (MS) lesion cases. Each pair comprised shading free volume and its corrupted version with 40% intensity inhomogeneity. The resolutions were 181×217×181 voxels, sized 1×1×1mm³.

In the second set of images, extra bias fields with higher degree of dynamics were added to the images from the first set. Bias fields were generated by cubic B-spline interpolation between equally spaced nodes at every 50 voxels in each direction. Node values (multiplication factors) were randomly distributed on the interval between 0.8 and 1.2.

Third set consisted of six volumes, three of a normal volunteer (256×256×25 voxels 8bit) and three of a tumour patient (256×256×20 voxels, 8bit, slice thickness of 5mm, in plane resolution of 1×1mm). White and grey matter manual segmentations were available [16].

Volumes of the second set were used to show the capability of our method to successfully cope with bias fields, which have high degree of dynamics. Changing the size of the regularization kernel has a direct impact on the estimated fields. Reducing kernel size makes the fields more locally flexible, but looses a part of its regularization functionality. The effect of regularization kernel size on the shape of reconstructed bias field is shown in Fig. 1. Image (a) indicates the position of the bias field profiles shown on the images (b) and (c). Solid lines indicate generated bias field and broken lines the corresponding reconstruction after inhomogeneity correction. Standard deviations of the regularization kernels were set to 30 mm in case (b) and to 90 mm in case (c). In the first case high correlation between applied and reconstructed bias fields was found, while the in second case the correlation was poor due to too high regularization.

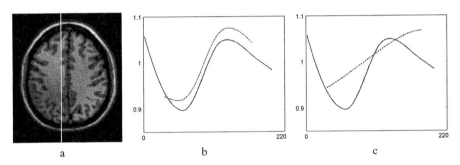

Fig. 1. Image (a) shows the profile position, (b) and (c) the applied (solid curve) and reconstructed bias field (broken curve) for the regularization of 30 and 90 mm, respectively

Quantitative evaluation was performed by computing the coefficient of joint variations (*cjv*) [9] between grey (GM) and white matter (WM) of the brain, which were segmented in all three sets of images. *Cjv* is computed from standard deviations (σ) and mean values (μ) of the voxel intensities belonging to the two matters,

$$cjv(GM,WM) = \frac{\sigma(GM) + \sigma(WM)}{|\mu(GM) - \mu(WM)|}. \tag{8}$$

The measure is independent of the changes in contrast and brightness and measures the intensity inhomogeneity in the sense of minimizing the intensity overlapping between two tissues.

In Table 1 the results of inhomogeneity correction in the first set of images are given. The four columns describe the volume properties (modality, bias field and pathology) and starting, final and ideal *cjv* values. The method successfully corrected the first six volumes and did not induce any artefacts into the second half of the inhomogeneity free volumes.

Table 1. Coefficient of joint variations of grey and white matter for the first dataset

Volume	$cjv_{start}[\%]$	$cjv_{end}[\%]$	$cjv_{ideal}[\%]$
T1 40%	69.3	51.7	51.6
T2 40%	106.4	83.4	83.2
PD 40%	163.0	62.8	64.9
T1 40% MS lesions	68.0	51.0	50.9
T2 40% MS lesions	123.8	74.5	74.9
PD 40% MS lesions	195.6	64.9	66.9
T1 0%	51.6	51.9	51.6
T2 0%	83.2	83.4	83.2
PD 0%	64.9	65.5	64.9
T1 0% MS lesions	50.9	51.2	50.9
T2 0% MS lesions	74.9	75.0	74.9
PD 0% MS lesions	66.9	67.7	66.9

Table 2. Coefficient of joint variations of grey and white matter for the second dataset

Volume (df – dynamic field)	$cjv_{start}[\%]$	$cjv_{end}[\%]$	$cjv_{ideal}[\%]$
T1 40% × df	86.8	51.7	51.6
T2 40% × df	107.7	84.5	83.2
PD 40% × df	228.5	64.7	64.9
T1 40% MS lesions × df	84.8	51.0	50.9
T2 40% MS lesions × df	128.1	75.8	74.9
PD 40% MS lesions × df	276.3	66.6	66.9
T1 0% × df	78.5	51.9	51.6
T2 0% × df	93.1	84.7	83.2
PD 0% × df	125.6	67.2	64.9
T1 0% MS lesions × df	76.6	51.2	50.9
T2 0% MS lesions × df	98.7	76.6	74.9
PD 0% MS lesions × df	141.8	69.4	66.9

The results of inhomogeneity correction in the second set of images are given in Table 2. The proposed method successfully corrected the inhomogeneities with high dynamics. Final *cjv* values did not match the ideal ones as perfectly as in the first set, because the induced bias fields could not be exactly reconstructed by Gaussian convolution. Parameters were fixed for all experiments with $f = 0.02$, $\sigma_g = 30$ mm, number of iterations was 30. Size of the histogram was 256 (*i*) by 400 (*d*) bins.

Table 3 shows the results on real MR volumes of the third set. The volumes without intensity inhomogeneity were not known so that the extent of the achieved correction cannot be determined. The Last column states relative change of *cjv* value, where it can be seen that improvement was achieved in all volumes.

Table 3. Coefficient of joint variations of grey and white matter for the real volumes

Volume	$cjv_{start}[\%]$	$cjv_{end}[\%]$	$cjv_{change}[\%]$
T1 normal	138.0	132.6	-3.9
T2 normal	90.7	89.0	-1.9
PD normal	77.8	70.4	-9.6
T1 tumour	175.7	169.4	-3.6
T2 tumour	169.3	159.6	-5.7
PD tumour	133.8	117.3	-12.4

4 Conclusion

The proposed fully automated bias correction method makes no assumption on the distribution of image intensities and provides non-parametric correction. No *a priori* knowledge such as digital brain atlases or reference points is needed. Spatial image features are incorporated in addition to commonly used intensity features, which give the method enough information to successfully correct even highly dynamic bias fields.

The method performed well on all tested images. The second set of images with artificially generated dynamic bias fields showed a possible advantage over many other methods that incorporate more rigid correction models. The performance of the proposed method depends on the overlap between the probability distributions of image features, which should be small. The proposed correction framework, however, enables straightforward incorporation of additional image features that could yield additional discriminative power and improve the correction performance on the images of poor quality.

Acknowledgement. This work has been supported by the Slovenian Ministry of Education, Science and Sport under grant P2-0232.

References

1. Condon, B. R., Patterson, J., Wyper, D., Jenkins, A.,Hadley, D. M.: Image non-uniformity in magnetic resonance imaging: its magnitude and methods for its correction. The British Journal of Radiology 60 (1987) 83-87
2. Simmons, A., Tofts, P. S., Barker, G. J.,Arridge, S. R.: Sources of intensity nonuniformity in spin echo images at 1.5 T. Magn Reson Med 32 (1994) 121-128
3. Johnson, B., Atkins, M. S., Mackiewich, B.,Anderson, M.: Segmentation of multiple sclerosis lesions in intensity corrected multispectral MRI. IEEE transaction on medical imaging 15 (1996) 154-169
4. Koivula, A., Alakuijala, J.,Tervonen, O.: Image feature based automatic correction of low-frequency spatial intensity variations in MR images. Magn Reson Imaging 15 (1997) 1167-1175
5. Haselgrove, J.,Prammer, M.: An algorithm for compensating of surface-coil images for sensitivity of the surface coil. Magnetic Resonance Imaging 4 (1986) 469-472

6. Sled, J. G., Zijdenbos, A. P.,Evans, A. C.: A nonparametric method for automatic correction of intensity nonuniformity in MRI data. IEEE Trans Med Imaging 17 (1998) 87-97

7. Dawant, B. M., Zijdenbos, A. P.,Margolin, R. A.: Correction o fintensity variations in MR images for computer-aided tissues classification. IEEE Trans Med Imaging 12 (1993) 770-781

8. Styner, M., Brechbuhler, C., Szekely, G.,Gerig, G.: Parametric estimate of intensity inhomogeneities applied to MRI. IEEE Trans Med Imaging 19 (2000) 153-165

9. Likar, B., Viergever, M. A.,Pernuš, F.: Retrospective correction of MR intensity inhomogeneity by information minimization. IEEE Trans Med Imaging 20 (2001) 1398-1410

10. Pham, D. L.,Prince, J. L.: Adaptive fuzzy segmentation of magnetic resonance images. IEEE Trans Med Imaging 18 (1999) 737-752

11. Ahmed, M. N., Yamany, S. M., Mohamed, N., Farag, A. A.,Moriarty, T.: A modified fuzzy C-means algorithm for bias field estimation and segmentation of MRI data. IEEE Trans Med Imaging 21 (2002) 193-199

12. Wells III, W. M., Grimson, W. E. L.,Jolezs, F. A.: Adaptive segmentation of MRI data. IEEE Trans Med Imaging 15 (1996) 429-442

13. Van Leemput, K., Maes, F., Vandermeulen, D.,Suetens, P.: Automated model-based bias field correction of MR images of the brain. IEEE Trans Med Imaging 18 (1999) 885-896

14. Derganc, J., Likar, B., Pernuš, F.: Nonparametric segmentation of multispectral MR images incorporating spatial and intensity information. In: Sonka, M., Fitzpatrick, J.M. (eds.): Proceedings of SPIE Medical Imaging 2002: Image processing, Vol. 4684. SPIE Press, San Diego USA (2002) 391-400

15. Cocosco, C. A., Kollokian, V., S, K. R. K.,Evans, A. C.: BrainWeb: Online Interface to a 3D MRI Simulated Brain Database. NeuroImage 5 (1997) 425-425

16. Velthuizen, R. P., Clarke, L. P., Phuphanich, S., Hall, L. O., Bensaid, A. M., Arrington, J. A., Greenberg, H. M.,Silbiger, M. L.: Unsupervised measurement of brain tumor volume on MR images. J Magn Reson Imaging 5 (1995) 594-605

Using a Maximum Uncertainty LDA-Based Approach to Classify and Analyse MR Brain Images

Carlos E. Thomaz[1], James P. Boardman[2], Derek L.G. Hill[3], Jo V. Hajnal[2],
David D. Edwards[4], Mary A. Rutherford[2], Duncan F. Gillies[1], and Daniel Rueckert[1]

[1] Department of Computing, Imperial College, London, UK
cet@doc.ic.ac.uk
[2] Imaging Sciences Department, Imperial College, London, UK
[3] Division of Imaging Sciences, King's College, London, UK
[4] Division of Paediatrics, Obstetrics and Gynaecology, Imperial College, London, UK

Abstract. Multivariate statistical learning techniques that analyse all voxels simultaneously have been used to classify and describe MR brain images. Most of these techniques have overcome the difficulty of dealing with the inherent high dimensionality of 3D brain image data by using pre-processed segmented images or a number of specific features. However, an intuitive way of mapping the classification results back into the original image domain for further interpretation remains challenging. In this paper, we introduce the idea of using Principal Components Analysis (PCA) plus the maximum uncertainty Linear Discriminant Analysis (LDA) based approach to classify and analyse magnetic resonance (MR) images of the brain. It avoids the computation costs inherent in commonly used optimisation processes, resulting in a simple and efficient implementation for the maximisation and interpretation of the Fisher's classification results. In order to demonstrate the effectiveness of the approach, we have used two MR brain data sets. The first contains images of 17 schizophrenic patients and 5 controls, and the second is composed of brain images of 12 preterm infants at term equivalent age and 12 term controls. The results indicate that the two-stage linear classifier not only makes clear the statistical differences between the control and patient samples, but also provides a simple method of analysing the results for further medical research.

1 Introduction

Multivariate pattern recognition methods have been used to classify and describe morphological and anatomical structures of MR brain images [5, 8, 17]. Most of these approaches analyse all voxels simultaneously, and are based on statistical learning techniques applied to either segmented images or a number of features pre-selected from specific image decomposition approaches. Although such pre-processing strategies have overcome the difficulty of dealing with the inherent high dimensionality of 3D brain image data, an intuitive way of mapping the classification results back into the original image domain for further interpretation has remained an issue.

C. Barillot, D.R. Haynor, and P. Hellier (Eds.): MICCAI 2004, LNCS 3216, pp. 291–300, 2004.
© Springer-Verlag Berlin Heidelberg 2004

In this paper, we describe a new framework for classifying and analysing MR brain images. It is essentially a linear two-stage dimensionality reduction classifier. First the MR brain images from the original vector space are projected to a lower dimensional space using the well-known PCA and then a maximum uncertainty LDA-based approach is applied next to find the best linear discriminant features on that PCA subspace. The proposed LDA method is based on the maximum entropy co-variance selection method developed to improve quadratic classification performance on limited sample size problems [15].

In order to demonstrate the effectiveness of the approach, we have used two MR brain data sets. The first contains images of 17 schizophrenic patients and 5 controls; and the second is composed of brain images of 12 preterm infants at term equivalent age (mean post-menstrual age [PMA] at birth 29 weeks, mean PMA at MR image acquisition 41 weeks), and 12 term born controls (mean PMA at birth 40.57 weeks, mean time of image acquisition day 4 of postnatal life). The results indicate that the two-stage linear classifier not only makes clear the statistical differences between the control and patient samples, but also provides a simple method of analysing the results for further medical research.

2 Principal Component Analysis (PCA)

Principal Component Analysis has been used successfully as an intermediate dimensionality reduction step in several image recognition problems. It is a feature extraction procedure concerned with explaining the covariance structure of a set of variables through a small number of linear combinations of these variables. In other words, PCA generates a set of orthonomal basis vectors, known as principal components (or most expressive features [12]), that minimizes the mean square reconstruction error and describes major variations in the whole training set considered [4]. For this representation to have good generalisation ability and make sense in classification problems, we assume implicitly that the distributions of each class are separated by their corresponding mean differences.

However, there is always the question of how many principal components to retain in order to reduce the dimensionality of the original training sample. Although there is no definitive answer to this question for general classifiers, Yang and Yang [16] have proved recently that the number of principal components to retain for a best LDA performance should be equal to the rank of the total covariance matrix composed of all the training patterns.

3 Linear Discriminant Analysis (LDA)

The primary purpose of the Linear Discriminant Analysis is to separate samples of distinct groups by maximising their between-class separability while minimising their within-class variability.

Let the between-class scatter matrix S_b and within-class scatter matrix S_w be defined as

$$S_b = \sum_{i=1}^{g} N_i(\overline{x}_i - \overline{x})(\overline{x}_i - \overline{x})^T \quad \text{and} \quad S_w = \sum_{i=1}^{g}\sum_{j=1}^{N_i}(x_{i,j} - \overline{x}_i)(x_{i,j} - \overline{x}_i)^T , \tag{1}$$

where $x_{i,j}$ is the n-dimensional pattern j from class π_i, N_i is the number of training patterns from class π_i, and g is the total number of classes or groups. The vector $\overline{x}_i$ and matrix S_i are respectively the unbiased sample mean and sample covariance matrix of class π_i [4]. The grand mean vector $\overline{x}$ is given by

$$\overline{x} = \frac{1}{N}\sum_{i=1}^{g} N_i\overline{x}_i = \frac{1}{N}\sum_{i=1}^{g}\sum_{j=1}^{N_i} x_{i,j} , \tag{2}$$

where N is the total number of samples, that is, $N = N_1 + N_2 + \cdots + N_g$. It is important to note that the within-class scatter matrix S_w defined in (1) is essentially the standard pooled covariance matrix multiplied by the scalar $(N - g)$, that is

$$S_w = \sum_{i=1}^{g}(N_i - 1)S_i = (N - g)S_p . \tag{3}$$

The main objective of LDA is to find a projection matrix P_{lda} that maximizes the ratio of the determinant of the between-class scatter matrix to the determinant of the within-class scatter matrix (Fisher's criterion), that is

$$P_{lda} = \arg\max_{P} \frac{|P^T S_b P|}{|P^T S_w P|} . \tag{4}$$

It has been proved [4] that if S_w is a non-singular matrix then the Fisher's criterion is maximised when the column vectors of the projection matrix P_{lda} are the eigenvectors of $S_w^{-1}S_b$ with at most $g-1$ nonzero corresponding eigenvalues. This is the standard LDA procedure.

However, the performance of the standard LDA can be seriously degraded if there are only a limited number of total training observations N compared to the dimension of the feature space n. Since the within-class scatter matrix S_w is a function of $(N - g)$ or less linearly independent vectors, its rank is $(N - g)$ or less. Therefore, S_w is a singular matrix if N is less than $(n + g)$, or, analogously, might be unstable if N is not at least five to ten times $(n + g)$ [7].

4 The Maximum Uncertainty LDA-Based Approach

In order to avoid the singularity and instability critical issues of the within-class scatter matrix S_w when LDA is applied in limited sample and high dimensional problems, we have proposed a new LDA approach based on a straightforward stabilisation method for the S_w matrix [14].

4.1 Related Methods

In the past, a number of researchers [1, 2, 9, 10] have proposed a modification in LDA that makes the problem mathematically feasible and increases the LDA stability when the within-class scatter matrix S_w has small or zero eigenvalues.

The idea is to replace the pooled covariance matrix S_p of the scatter matrix S_w (equation (3)) with a ridge-like covariance estimate of the form

$$\widehat{S}_p(k) = S_p + kI ,\tag{5}$$

where I is the n by n identity matrix and $k \geq 0$. However, a combination of S_p and a multiple of the identity matrix I as described in equation (5) expands all the S_p eigenvalues, independently of whether these eigenvalues are either null, small, or even large [14].

Other researchers have imposed regularisation methods to overcome the singularity and instability in sample based covariance estimation, especially to improve the Bayes Plug-in classification performance [3, 6, 13]. According to these regularisation methods, the ill posed or poorly estimated S_p could be replaced with a convex combination matrix $\widehat{S}_p(\gamma)$ of the form

$$\widehat{S}_p(\gamma) = (1-\gamma)S_p + (\gamma)\overline{\lambda}I ,\tag{6}$$

where the shrinkage parameter γ takes on values $0 \leq \gamma \leq 1$ and could be selected to maximise the leave-one-out classification accuracy. The identity matrix multiplier would be given by the average eigenvalue $\overline{\lambda}$ of S_p calculated as

$$\overline{\lambda} = \frac{1}{n}\sum_{j=1}^{n}\lambda_j = \frac{tr(S_p)}{n} ,\tag{7}$$

where the notation "tr" denotes the trace of a matrix.

The regularisation idea described in equation (6) has the effect of decreasing the larger eigenvalues and increasing the smaller ones, thereby counteracting the biasing inherent in sample-based estimation of eigenvalues [3]. However, such approach would be computationally expensive to be used in practice because it requires the calculation of the eigenvalues and eigenvectors of an n by n matrix for each training observation of all the classes in order to find the best mixing parameter γ.

4.2 The Proposed Method

The proposed method considers the issue of stabilising the S_p estimate with a multiple of the identity matrix by selecting the largest dispersions regarding the S_p average eigenvalue.

Since the estimation errors of the non-dominant or small eigenvalues are much greater than those of the dominant or large eigenvalues [4], we have used the following selection algorithm [14] to expand only the smaller and consequently less reliable eigenvalues of S_p, and keep most of its larger eigenvalues unchanged:

i. Find the Φ eigenvectors and Λ eigenvalues of S_p, where $S_p = S_w/[N-g]$;

ii. Calculate the S_p average eigenvalue $\overline{\lambda}$ using equation (7);

iii. Form a new matrix of eigenvalues based on the following largest dispersion values

$$\Lambda^* = diag[\max(\lambda_1,\overline{\lambda}),\max(\lambda_2,\overline{\lambda}),...,\max(\lambda_n,\overline{\lambda})]\,;\tag{8a}$$

iv. Form the modified within-class scatter matrix

$$S_w^* = S_p^*(N-g) = (\Phi\Lambda^*\Phi^T)(N-g)\,.\tag{8b}$$

The proposed LDA is constructed by replacing S_w with $S_w^{\cdot\cdot}$ in the Fisher's criterion formula described in equation (4). It is a straightforward method that overcomes both the singularity and instability of the within-class scatter matrix S_w when LDA is applied in small sample and high dimensional problems. It also avoids the computational costs inherent to the aforementioned shrinkage processes.

5 Experimental Results

In order to demonstrate the effectiveness of the approach, we have used two MR brain data sets. The first contains images of 17 schizophrenic patients and 5 controls and the second is composed of brain images of 12 preterm infants at term equivalent age and 12 term controls.

Before registration, the MR brain images of each subject in the schizophrenia dataset have been stripped of extra-cranial tissue [18]. All MR images are then registered to the MNI brainweb atlas using the non-rigid registration described in [11]. Finally, the registered images have been resampled with a voxel size of 1x1x1 mm³. After registration and resampling the schizophrenia dataset consists of 181x217x181 = 7,109,137 voxels. An analogous procedure has been adopted for the infant images consisting of 256x256x114 = 7,471,104 voxels.

Throughout all the experiments, we have used for the schizophrenia analysis a total of 13 training examples, i.e. all the 5 controls and 8 schizophrenia patients randomly selected. The remaining 9 schizophrenia subjects have been used for classification testing. The infant training and test sets have been composed of 8 and 4 images respectively. For instance, the PCA schizophrenia transformation matrix is composed of 7,109,137 (= number of voxels) rows and 12 (= total of training samples − 1) columns, where each column corresponds to a principal component. The LDA transformation matrix is composed of 12 rows and 1 (= number of groups − 1) column. Using these PCA plus LDA transformation matrices, every original image composed of 7,109,137 voxels has been reduced to a one-dimension vector on the final (or most discriminant [12]) feature space.

Figures 1 and 2 show the projected schizophrenia and infant data on the most expressive and discriminant features. White circles and squares represent the training sample of the controls and schizophrenia (or infant) examples used. The black circles and squares describe the corresponding subjects selected for testing. As can be seen, although the two and three most expressive features explain more than 50% of the total sample variance, the classification superiority of the two-stage dimensionality reduction technique based on a maximum uncertainty LDA approach is clear in both applications.

Another result revealed by these experiments is related to the linear discriminant feature found by the maximum uncertainty approach. In fact, this one-dimensional vector corresponds to a hyper-plane on the original space which direction describes statistically the most discriminant differences between the controls and the patients images used for training. A procedure of moving along this most discriminant feature and mapping back into the image domain might provide an intuitive interpretation of the results.

Figures 3 and 4 show respectively the schizophrenia and infant five points chosen from left to right on the most discriminant feature space and projected back into the image domain using the corresponding transpose of the LDA and PCA linear transformations previously computed. In Figure 3, although the differences are very subtle, the visual analysis of the example sagittal, axial, and coronal slices suggests that the regions of the normal brains are slightly better represented than the ones observed on the schizophrenia images. In looking at the preterm analysis illustrated in Figure 4, there is enlargement of the lateral ventricular system in the preterm infants at term equivalent age compared to the term control group. This is a common finding at term equivalent age among infants who have been born prematurely [19,20].

6 Conclusion

In this paper, we introduced the idea of using PCA plus the maximum uncertainty LDA-based approach to classify and analyse MR brain images. It avoids the computation costs inherent in the commonly used optimisation processes, resulting in a simple and efficient implementation for the maximisation and interpretation of the Fisher's criterion.

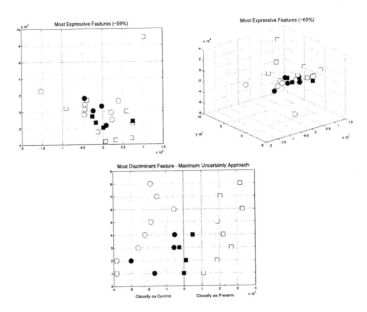

Fig. 1. Schizophrenia sample data projected on the most expressive and discriminant[*] features.

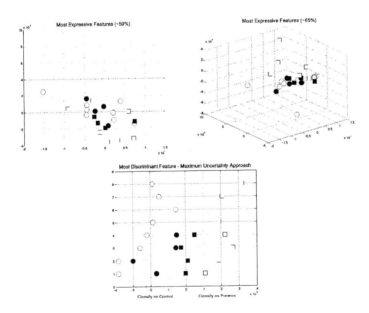

Fig. 2. Infant sample data projected on the most expressive and discriminant[*] features.

---

[*] The vertical value of each point is illustrative only and represents its corresponding index in the sample set.

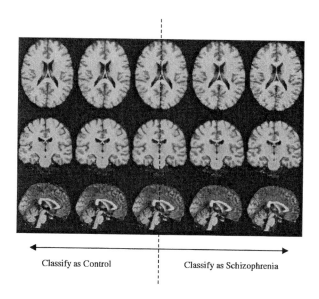

Fig. 3. Visual analysis of the schizophrenia most discriminant feature.

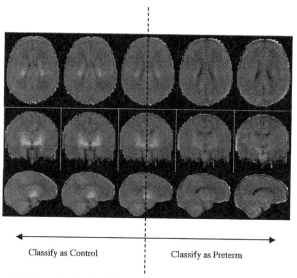

Fig. 4. Visual analysis of the preterm most discriminant feature.

The two-stage dimensionality reduction technique is a straightforward approach that considers the issue of stabilising the ill posed or poorly estimated within-class scatter matrix with a multiple of the identity matrix. Although the experiments carried out were based on small MR data sets, we believe that such recent multivariate statistical advances for targeting limited sample and high dimensional problems can provide a new framework of characterising and analysing the high complexity of MR brain images.

Acknowledgments. This work is part of the UK EPSRC e-science project "Information eXtraction from Images" (IXI). Also, the first author was partially supported by the Brazilian Government Agency CAPES under Grant 1168/99-1.

References

1. N.A. Campbell, "Shrunken estimator in discriminant and canonical variate analysis", *Applied Statistics*, vol. 29, pp. 5-14, 1980.
2. P.J. Di Pillo, "Biased Discriminant Analysis: Evaluation of the optimum probability of misclassification", *Comm. in Statistics-Theory and Methods*, vol. A8, no. 14, pp. 1447-1457, 1979.
3. J.H. Friedman, "Reguralized Discriminant Analysis", *JASA*, vol. 84, no. 405, pp. 165-175, 1989.
4. K. Fukunaga, *Introduction to Statistical Pattern Recognition*, 2nd ed. Academic Press, 1990.
5. P. Golland, W. Grimson, M. Shenton, and R. Kikinis, "Small Sample Size Learning for Shape Analysis of Anatomical Structures", In Proc. *MICCAI*, pp. 72-82, 2000.
6. T. Greene and W.S. Rayens, "Covariance pooling and stabilization for classification", *Computational Statistics & Data Analysis*, vol. 11, pp. 17-42, 1991.
7. A. K. Jain and B. Chandrasekaran, "Dimensionality and Sample Size Considerations in Pattern Recognition Practice", *Handbook of Statistics*, vol. 2, pp. 835-855, 1982.
8. Z. Lao, D. Shen, Z. Xue, B. Karacali, S. Resnick, and C. Davatzikos, "Morphological classification of brains via high-dimensional shape transformations and machine learning methods", *NeuroImage*, vol. 21, pp. 46-57, 2004.
9. R. Peck and J. Van Ness, "The use of shrinkage estimators in linear discriminant analysis", *IEEE PAMI*, vol. 4, no. 5, pp. 531-537, September 1982.
10. W.S. Rayens, "A Role for Covariance Stabilization in the Construction of the Classical Mixture Surface", *Journal of Chemometrics*, vol. 4, pp. 159-169, 1990.
11. D. Rueckert, A. F. Frangi, and J. A. Schnabel, "Automatic Construction of 3-D Statistical Deformation Models of the Brain Using Nonrigid Registration", *IEEE Transactions on Medical Imaging*, vol. 22, no. 8, pp. 1014-1025, 2003.
12. D. L. Swets and J. J. Weng, "Using Discriminant Eigenfeatures for Image Retrieval", *IEEE PAMI*, vol. 18, no. 8, pp. 831-836, 1996.
13. S. Tadjudin, "Classification of High Dimensional Data With Limited Training Samples", PhD thesis, Purdue University, West Lafayette, Indiana, 1998.
14. C. E. Thomaz and D. F. Gillies, "A Maximum Uncertainty LDA-based approach for Limited Sample Size problems - with application to Face Recognition", *Technical Report TR-2004-01*, Department of Computing, Imperial College, London, UK, January 2004.
15. C. E. Thomaz, D. F. Gillies and R. Q. Feitosa. "A New Covariance Estimate for Bayesian Classifiers in Biometric Recognition", *IEEE CSVT*, vol. 14, no. 2, pp. 214-223, February 2004.
16. J. Yang and J. Yang, "Why can LDA be performed in PCA transformed space? ", *Pattern Recognition*, vol. 36, pp. 563-566, 2003.

17. P. Yushkevich, S. Joshi, S.M. Pizer, J.G. Csernansky and L.E. Wang. "Feature Selection for Shape-Based Classification of Biological Objects", *Information Processing in Medical Imaging,* 2003.
18. S. Smith, "Fast robust automated brain extraction",*Human Brain Mapping,*17(3):143-155, 2002.
19. L. R. Ment et al. "The etiology and outcome of cerebral ventriculomegaly at term in very low birth weight preterm infants", *Pediatrics* 104, 243-248, 1999.
20. J. P. Boardman et al. "An evaluation of deformation-based morphometry applied to the developing human brain and detection of volumetric changes associated with preterm birth", In Proc. *MICCAI,* Lecture Notes in Computer Science (2878), 697-704, 2003.

Data Driven Brain Tumor Segmentation in MRI Using Probabilistic Reasoning over Space and Time

Jeffrey Solomon[1,3], John A. Butman[2], and Arun Sood[1]

[1] Center for Image Analysis, George Mason University,
{jsolomon,jbutmana}@cc.nih.gov
asood@cs.gmu.edu
[2]Diagnostic Radiology Department, Clinical Center, National Institutes of Health,
[3] Medical Numerics Inc.

Abstract. A semi-automated method for brain tumor segmentation and volume tracking has been developed. This method uses a pipeline approach to process MRI images. The pipeline process involves the following steps: 1) automatic alignment of initial and subsequent MRI scans for a given patient, 2) automatic de-skulling of all brain images, 3) automatic segmentation of the brain tumors using probabilistic reasoning over space and time with a semi-automatic correction of segmentation results on the first time point only and, 4) brain tumor tracking, providing a report of tumor volume change. To validate the procedure, we evaluated contrast enhanced MRI images from five brain tumor patients, each scanned at three times, several months apart. This data was processed and estimated tumor volume results show good agreement with manual tracing of 3D lesions over time.

1 Introduction

The best accepted measure of brain tumor viability is interval change in tumor size and decisions on efficacy of clinical treatments in a given patient and in clinical trials are most commonly based on this measure. Commonly used measurement methods to assess changes in lesion or tumor size over time include (1) greatest diameter [1], (2) greatest diameter multiplied by greatest perpendicular diameter [2], (3) manual lesion tracing, [3] (4) computer-based automated techniques to segment the lesion and calculate volume [4].

The one and two dimensional measures are accurate only when lesions are spherical or elliptical in nature. While this assumption is often invalid, these techniques are used in clinical situations because of their simplicity [3]. However, the use of such measurements on serial studies can be problematic as it is difficult to define precisely the same location for measurement of subsequent studies. As stated by Sorenson [3] and others, 3D segmentation techniques can improve lesion measurement accuracy relative to 1D and 2D methods. Although manual 3D techniques are more accurate, they are not commonly used clinically largely due to limitations of time involvement and inter-rater variability. As medical imaging devices provide higher spatial resolution, more image slices are created for each study. This requires processing of a significant number of images to determine lesion

C. Barillot, D.R. Haynor, and P. Hellier (Eds.): MICCAI 2004, LNCS 3216, pp. 301–309, 2004.

volume. There is a need to develop automated techniques that can detect lesions (e.g. tumors) in medical images and track their progression in size, shape and intensity.

An interesting class of intensity based 3D segmentation techniques uses Bayesian analysis for tissue classification. These methods assume that the image histogram can be modeled as a sum of Gaussian distributions, known as a Gaussian mixture model. The probability distribution for this model is:

$$P(x_j) = \sum_{i=1}^{k} P(C_i)P(x_j \mid C_i) \qquad (1)$$

where $P(x_j)$ is the probability of pixel j having intensity x_j, $P(C_i)$ is the probability of class C_i in the image, k is the number of classes and $P(x_j|C_i)$ is the probability of obtaining pixel intensity x_j given that the tissue class is C_i. Using the approaches of others [5], $P(x_j|C_i)$ is assumed to follow a Gaussian probability distribution for each tissue type, C_i, in the brain. Bayes' Rule states that the probability of pixel j being in tissue class C_i given its intensity x_j is given by:

$$P(C_i \mid x_j) = \frac{P(x_j \mid C_i)P(C_i)}{P(x_j)} \qquad (2)$$

The expectation-maximization (E-M) algorithm has been used to iteratively estimate the parameters of the Gaussians in the mixture model in order to classify various tissue classes [5]. To segment and track the progression of diseased tissue, e.g. multiple sclerosis lesions or brain tumors, in MR images of the brain, segmentation is performed independently on each 3D image of the 4D time series (three spatial dimensions plus time). Temporal information does not influence the segmentation.

Since there is some relation between images at different times, temporal information has the potential to improve segmentation of lesions in MR images. Perhaps, the simplest temporal technique is image differencing as explored in a paper by Hajnal et al [6]. This difference image only represents change in intensity not shape. If a lesion does not change much over time, it will not be detected by this system.

Detecting change by estimating the displacement field was proposed by Rey et al [7]. This automatic method performed well on the task of lesion detection but did not perform as well with segmentation accuracy. Gerig et al explored the use of pixel-based temporal analysis in lesion detection [8]. In this work, rigid registration and global intensity normalization (to account for global pixel intensity differences across scanning sessions) were performed on a series of MR images of patients with multiple sclerosis. This method was shown to be sensitive to registration accuracy producing false positives. In order to reduce the number of false positives resulting from registration errors, a spatio-temporal model was developed [9]. While this technique has some limitations, the work is significant in the author's realization that methods exclusively concentrating on the spatial or temporal aspects cannot be expected to provide optimal results.

It is hypothesized that using both temporal and spatial properties of the 4D image set will improve the automatic segmentation of lesions in the time series compared with techniques that independently detect lesions from one scan to the next or focus only on areas of change. Solomon and Sood [10] have demonstrated positive results comparing the E-M algorithm with a combined E-M+HMM (Hidden Markov Model) approach which incorporates probabilistic reasoning over space and time to segment

4D lesions in MR images. This work was validated on simulated data generated with Gaussian mixture model.

This paper describes the validation of this technique on sample data from 5 patients whose brain tumor volume was assessed both by manual tracings and by automated 4D segmentation. In addition, a practical pipeline approach to the automatic processing of the 4D MRI data sets was developed that minimizes user interaction.

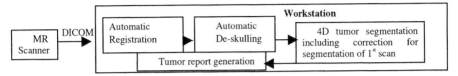

Fig. 1. MR images are sent from the scanner to a workstation via the DICOM protocol. The MR images are automatically registered using FLIRT. Next the brains are automatically skull stripped. The 4D data is segmented using probabilistic reasoning over space and time via the E-M+HMM method. As part of this technique, the segmentation of the 1st time point is manually corrected by removing tissue incorrectly classified as tumor by the E-M algorithm (e.g. enhancing vasculature). The remaining volumes in the time series are segmented automatically without user interaction. Finally a report is generated presenting the tumor volumes over time.

2 Methods

A pipeline approach was used to pre-process the series of MR images for each patient.

2.1 Registration Engine

A software program termed the "registration engine" was used to automatically align all MR images in the time series for each patient. This engine automatically searches for new DICOM formatted images on the workstation. If a new data set exists, the engine determines if a previous study exists for this patient. If not, the data set is saved as a reference scan for that patient. If a previous scan does exists, its reference is automatically retrieved and registered via the FLIRT [11] linear registration program with a 6 parameter rigid registration using correlation as the cost function and sinc interpolation to minimize effects of resampling the image data. The results of the registration are stored for further processing.

2.2 Automatic De-skulling

Once all desired images are registered, a process known as de-skulling is performed to exclude all extracranial tissue (e.g. scalp fat, head and neck musculature, bone marrow) from the MR image and minimize the number of tissue classes for further segmentation. The normal intracranial contents include predominantly brain tissue (gray and white matter), cerebrospinal fluid (CSF), and vasculature. In the pathologic cases, brain tumor serves as an additional tissue class. Automated programs have been developed for de-skulling, but do not behave as well on data with pathology, such as the brain tumors in this study, as they do on normal brains. In addition to a change in morphology due to the tumors, these images are acquired with contrast agents making vessels appear hyper-intense. These vessels create bridges between tissues in the brain and the skull, thus making the automated delineation of the brain more difficult. We have used a template based approach to automatically de-skull brain MRIs in this group. This process is accomplished by registering the first time point in the MR series for a given patient to the MNI template brain. The transformation matrix derived from this 12-parameter affine registration [11] was saved using the MEDx software package (Medical Numerics, Inc. Sterling, VA). The matrix is inverted and applied to a previously de-skulled brain mask image, available from the SPM99 software package (http://www.fil.ion.ucl.ac.uk/spm/) which shares the same coordinate system as the MNI template. The pixel values in the brain mask image represent probability of brain tissue. This image was thresholded such that all voxels above a 60% probability of brain tissue were set to 1. This transformed brain mask is multiplied by all registered MR images in the time series, resulting in de-skulled time series of data ready for tumor segmentation.

2.3   4-D Lesion Segmentation Using Probabilistic Reasoning over Space and Time

Segmentation of aligned de-skulled images is performed using probabilistic reasoning in space (via the expectation-maximization) algorithm and time (using the hidden Markov model). Initialized by a K-means clustering, the E-M algorithm is applied to each volume in the time series. This results in estimates of the Gaussian parameters for the pixel distributions of all tissue classes (including tumor) for each volume. This information is used by a hidden Markov model which makes use of previous and subsequent scans to estimate the classification of a voxel in the image.

Change over time is modeled as a series of snapshots, each describing the state of the world at a particular time with a set of random variables (some observable and some not). If we assume that the entire state is determined by a single discrete unobservable random variable, we have a hidden Markov model (HMM).

If we consider the state of each voxel in our 4D medical image data to be lesion status, with possible values of lesion and non-lesion, then the problem of segmenting and tracking lesions over time can be modeled as a HMM. The state of the system (lesion/non-lesion), represented in this model as X_t, is not observable. What is observable is the pixel intensity value. This "evidence" variable will be represented as E_t. We will also make a 1st order Markov assumption (the current state can be determined completely from the previous state). The equation below represents this 1st order Markov state to state "Transition model".

$$P(\overline{X}_t \mid \overline{X}_{t-1}) = P(\overline{X}_t \mid \overline{X}_{0:t-1}) \qquad \text{Transition Model} \qquad (3)$$

The evidence variable E_t is dependent on only the current state. This dependence is known as the Sensor Model.

$$P(E_t \mid \overline{X}_t) = P(E_t \mid \overline{X}_{0:t-1}) \qquad \text{Sensor Model} \qquad (4)$$

Each voxel in the 4D image will independently follow the HMM.

In a process known as *filtering*, one computes the posterior distribution over the current state given all evidence to date $P(X_t \mid E_{1:t})$. In our case, if the state X_t equals lesion or non-lesion and E_t is equal to the pixel's intensity, then $P(X_t|E_{1:t})$ provides the tissue classification given the pixel's intensity value. It can be shown that there is a recursive formula to express this posterior distribution:

$$P(\overline{X}_{t+1} \mid E_{1:t+1}) = \alpha P(E_{t+1} \mid \overline{X}_{t+1}) \sum_{x_t} P(\overline{X}_{t+1} \mid \overline{X}_t) P(\overline{X}_t \mid E_{1:t}) \tag{5}$$

The current state is projected forward from t to $t+1$ then updated using new evidence E_{t+1}. Another process known as *smoothing* is used to compute past states given evidence up to the present. In other words, you may re-estimate the state at time points 1-4 given that you have estimates up to time point 5. This will theoretically improve the estimates of these states by using more information gathered. The following expression represents the probability of state X_k ($1 <= k < t$), given all evidence acquired so far.

$$P(\overline{X}_k \mid E_{1:t}) = \alpha P(\overline{X}_k \mid E_{1:k}) P(E_{k+1:t} \mid \overline{X}_k) \tag{6}$$

The right side of this equation contains a normalization constant, α, the familiar filtering expression from equation (5) and a backward expression, $P(E_{k+1:t}|X_k)$. This backward expression is given by the recursion:

$$P(E_{k+1:t} \mid \overline{X}_k) = \sum P(E_{k+1} \mid \overline{X}_{k+1}) P(E_{k+2:t} \mid \overline{X}_{k+1}) P(\overline{X}_{k+1} \mid \overline{X}_k) \tag{7}$$

The sensor model used is given below:

$$P(E_t \mid X_t(0)) = A_l (1/\sqrt{2\pi}\sigma_l) \exp(-(x-\mu_l)^2/2\sigma_l^2) \tag{8}$$

$$P(E_t \mid X_t(1)) = \sum_i A_i \sqrt{2\pi}\sigma_i \exp(-(x-\mu_i)^2/2\sigma_i^2) \tag{9}$$

where the probability at time t of having a pixel value equal to E_t given that this pixel represents lesion (state $X_t(0)$) is the Gaussian of the lesion tissue class l. The probability of having the pixel value E_t given that the pixel does not represent lesion (state $X_t(1)$)is the sum of the other Gaussians in the mixture model. There is a coefficient, α, used to sum the probabilities to 1 as seen in the equation below.

$$\alpha \sum_{i=0}^{1} P(E_t \mid X_t(i)) = 1 \tag{10}$$

A transition model was developed that is dependent on the distance from the lesion border and growth of the lesion. Exponential lesion growth is a simple model often employed [12] and is used here. The likelihood of a transition from lesion to non-lesion or vice versa is greater when the voxel is close to the lesion border (margin). This new model is shown below in equation (11).

$$T = P(\overline{X}_t \mid \overline{X}_{t-1}) = \begin{pmatrix} 1-\exp(-dist/C) & \exp(-dist/C) \\ \exp(-dist/C) & 1-\exp(-dist/C) \end{pmatrix} \tag{11}$$

The coefficient, C is a constant, and *dist* represents the distance from the border of the lesion. This distance is modified to take into account exponential lesion growth as follows:

$$dist_{t+1} = dist_t + \exp(\gamma * \Delta t) \tag{12}$$

for voxels inside the lesion, and

$$dist_{t+1} = |\exp(\gamma * \Delta t) - dist_t| \tag{13}$$

for voxels outside of the lesion. The term Δt represents the time between scans and γ represents the rate of exponential growth. This transition model is therefore unique for each voxel in the image and varies with each volume in the time series.

The choice of γ, the rate of exponential lesion growth, is initially estimated based on results of the E-M algorithm on successive image scans in the time series.

Theoretically, there is a separate γ for each point on the lesion border, allowing for modeling of lesion growth that is anisotropic. The transition model described here requires an estimate of the lesion border on the first scan in the series. This estimate was performed by running the E-M algorithm on the first time point and using the manual tracings to limit false positive results. This semi-automated correction is only performed on the first image of the temporal series.

2.4 Report Generation

The output of the 4D lesion segmentation process is a series of probabilistic images where voxel intensity represents the probability of being tumor. For classification purposes, any voxel whose probability was above 0.5 was labeled as tumor. A total volume of voxels assigned as tumor is computed. An html report is displayed showing tumor volume estimates over time.

2.5 Ground Truth Data

The 5 patients in the study each had 3 MRI scans with near isotropic voxel sizes (0.9375mm x 0.9375mm x 1.0mm). To validate the method, the tumors were manually traced at each time point, using MEDx software. The volumes based on these tracings were computed. Binary image masks were generated from these tracings for the validation process. In addition, the tracings of the tumor in the first scan were used in the correction step for the 4D tumor segmentation technique described in section 2.3.

3 Results

Scans from 5 patients were processed as described in the Methods section. Resulting tumor volumes taken from the generated report were compared with tumor volumes recording during the ground truth creation. Figure 2 shows the correlation between the tumor volumes calculated by the automatic 4D method and manual tracing. The correlation is strong with an R^2 value of 0.89.

In order to determine if the automated method classified as tumor the same voxels as the manual tracing, the Dice similarity coefficient (DSC) was used. The mean DSC value for all time point 2 and 3 measures was 0.71. Table 1 shows these values for the second and third time points in all 5 cases. Time point 1 was left out because the tumor volume estimated from the automated technique is based in part on the manual tracings for time point 1 as described in the methods section.

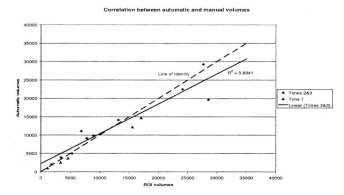

Fig. 2. Comparison of tumor volumes (# voxels) measured by 4D E-M+HMM to that measured by manual tracing. Identical measurements fall on the dashed line. The coefficient of determination, R^2 for the two methods was 0.89 (Correlation was performed for time points two and three as these were obtained without any manual interaction).

Table 1. Dice similarity coefficients for Time points 2 and 3. These measures show the amount of overlap between the automated 4D tumor volume and the manual tracing.

	DSC Time 2	DSC Time 3
Patient 1	0.82	0.84
Patient 2	0.75	0.77
Patient 3	0.70	0.64
Patient 4	0.79	0.75
Patient 5	0.62	0.45

The low DSC for patient 5 is attributed to the manual tracing of the irregularly shaped tumor.

Figure 3 below illustrates one section of the tumor from the MRI of Patient 3. Figure 3A illustrates an enhancing brainstem tumor which is relatively hyperintense and shares signal characteristics with the nearby cavernous sinuses. Figure 3B shows the voxels classified as tumor in white with the black outline representing manual tracing (for validation purposes). Despite the irregularity of the tumor, as well as iso-intensity with the cavernous sinus, the 4D E-M+HMM algorithm reliably classifies the enhancing portion of the tumor and segments it from the cavernous sinuses.

4 Discussion

This paper discusses an automated pipeline process for segmenting and tracking brain tumor lesions from MRI data requiring minimal user interaction. A 4D segmentation algorithm that makes use of probabilistic reasoning over space and time (E-M+HMM) has been tested on 5 patients. Previous work validated this technique on simulated

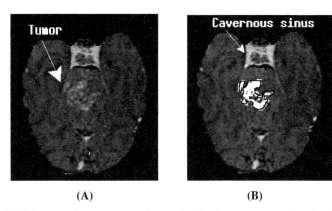

(A)   **(B)**

Fig. 3. A) MRI image of a tumor at time point 2 after pre-processing but before tumor segmentation. The tumor shares signal intensity with the vessels of the cavernous sinus. B) Automatic segmentation of the tumor via 4D E-M+HMM (in white) matches the enhancing tumor. The black contour represents manual tracing for validation purposes. Note that the cavernous sinus is not identified as tumor.

images demonstrating that this 4D method yields better segmentation accuracy for the current scan than independently segmenting with the E-M algorithm alone [10]. The proposed segmentation technique also has advantages over change detection techniques. By making use of both spatial and temporal information, our technique will detect tumors even if they are not changing significantly. While our technique is dependent on proper alignment across time points, it is not dependent on intensity normalization since the E-M algorithm is applied for each time point in the series. In addition, changes in tissue distribution (e.g. tumor less or more enhancing) are handled. This automated tumor segmentation process produces a report containing tumor volume change, providing estimates of tumor progression which can be incorporated into treatment planning.

One can certainly ask to what degree temporal information improves segmentation as compared to simply performing E-M at each time point. We could not perform the direct comparison as the E-M alone fails to segment brain tumors in any individual data sets without some form of manual interaction. This is because there are spatially distinct regions in the brain (notably blood vessels) which share signal characteristics with the brain tumor so that E-M classifies both tissue types into the same class. Manually excluding this data on the first data set allows the HMM to propagate this information forward and perform subsequent segmentation in a fully automated way. This is perhaps the most important advantage of applying the HMM in conjunction with the E-M algorithm.

Correlation of brain tumor volumes with manual tracings was strong. However, a degree of mismatch in overlapping areas was caused primarily by difficulty in manual tracing of the tumor boundaries. The tumors are quite irregular, making the manual segmentation task difficult. Future work will include validation on additional patients as well as evaluating how estimates and models of the growth rate of the tumors affect the segmentation results obtained from the HMM model. By estimating the rate of growth for each point on the tumor boundary, it may be possible to predict tumor location at times in the future. This might have further application in treatment planning. Another future goal is to include the Markov Random Field as a prior probability of the segmentation, modeling spatial correlation among neighborhood voxels in the 4D segmentation algorithm.

Automated tumor segmentation has the potential to play an important role in medical imaging, both in the management of individual patients and in the conduct of clinical trials where changes in tumor volume is a primary endpoint.

References

1. R. Therasse, S. Arbuck, E.A. Eisenhauer et al, "New Guidelines to Evaluate the Response to Treatment in Solid Tumors", *Journal of the National Cancer Institute,* Vol 92, pp. 205-216, 2000
2. A.B. Miller, B. Hoogstraten, M. Staquet et al, "Reporting Results of Cancer Treatment" *Cancer,* 47, pp. 207-214, 1981.
3. G. Sorensen, S. Patel, C. Harmath, et al, "Comparison of Diameter and Perimeter Methods for Tumor Volume Calculation", *Journal of Clinical Oncology*, Vol 19, Issue 2, pp.551-557, 2001.
4. S.M. Haney, P.M. Thompson, T.F. Cloughesy, et al, "Tracking Tumor Growth Rates in Patients with Malignant Gliomas: A Test of Two Algorithms", *Am J Neuroradiology*, 22:73-82, January 2001.
5. K. Van Leemput, F. Maes, D. Vandermeulen, et al, "Automatic segmentation of brain tissues and MR bias field correction using a digital brain atlas" *Proceedings of Medical Image Computing and Computer-Assisted Intervention – MICCAI'98*, volume 1496 of Lecture Notes in Computer Science, pages 1222-1229, Springer, 1998.
6. S. Hajnal, W. Oatridge, B. Young, "Detection of Subtle Brain Changes Using Subvoxel Registration and Subtraction of Serial MR Images", *Journal of Computer Assisted Tomography*, 19(5) pp.677-691, 1995.
7. D. Rey, G. Subsol, H. Delingette, et al, "Automatic Detection and Segmentation of Evolving Processes in 3D Medical Images: Applications to Multiple Sclerosis", *Medical Image Analysis*, 6, pp. 163-179, 2002.
8. G. Gerig, D. Welti, C. Guttmann, et al, "Exploring the discrimination power of the time domain for segmentation and characterization of active lesion in serial MR data", *Medical Image Analysis*, 4, pp.31-42, 2000.
9. D. Welti, G. Gerig, E.W. Radu, et al, "Spatio-temporal Segmentation of Active Multiple Sclerosis Lesions in Serial MRI Data", *IPMI, LNCS 2082*, pp. 438-445, 2001.
10. J. Solomon, A. Sood, *"4-D Lesion Detection using Expectation-Maximization and Hidden Markov Model"*, Proceedings of the IEEE International Symposium on Biomedical Imaging. (ISBI), pp 125-128. April, 2004.
11. M. Jenkinson, S. Smith, "A global optimisation method for robust affine registration of brain images", *Medical Image Analysis*, 5(2), pp.143-156, 2001.
12. K. Swanson, C. Bridge, J. Murray et al, "Virtual and real brain tumors: using mathematical modeling to quantify glioma growth and invasion", *Journal of the Neurological Sciences*, 216 pp. 1-10, 2003.

Atlas-Based Segmentation Using Level Sets and Fuzzy Labels

Cybèle Ciofolo

IRISA / CNRS**
Team Visages
35042 Rennes Cedex, France
Cybele.Ciofolo@irisa.fr

Abstract. We propose to segment volumetric structures with an atlas-based level set method. The classical formulation of the level set evolution force presents a stopping criterion, a directional term and a regularization term. Fuzzy labels registered from an atlas provide useful information allowing to automatically tune the respective influence of the different terms according to the desired application. This is done with a fuzzy decision system based on simple rules corresponding to an expert knowledge. Two applications are presented in details in the context of 3D brain MRI: the segmentation of white matter with the tuning of the regularization term, and the segmentation of the right hemisphere. Experimental results on the MNI Brainweb dataset and on a database of real MRI volumes are presented and discussed.

1 Introduction

Segmentation of anatomical structures is a critical task in medical image processing, with a large spectrum of applications that ranges from visualisation to diagnosis. For example, to obtain useful quantitative information for the study of evolutive brain diseases like multiple sclerosis, an accurate segmentation of the white matter is needed.

In such a task, the main difficulties are the non-homogeneous intensities within the same class of tissue, as well as the high complexity and large variability of the anatomical structures. Among the various surface evolution methods that have been proposed in this framework, the non-parametric ones [3,8,7] showed abilities to deal with this difficulties. In particular, the level set formalism [6] provides an efficient implementation for these approaches, with the following advantages: (i) efficient numerical schemes are available, (ii) topological changes are allowed, and (iii) extension of the method to higher dimensions is easy.

However, segmentation results on anatomical areas with very high positive or negative curvatures, such as sulci or ventricle horns in brain, sometimes show inaccuracies due to the regularization term involved in the evolution force. These areas generally correspond to interfaces between different classes of tissues.

** This work was supported by the CNRS and the Council of Brittany

C. Barillot, D.R. Haynor, and P. Hellier (Eds.): MICCAI 2004, LNCS 3216, pp. 310–317, 2004.
© Springer-Verlag Berlin Heidelberg 2004

Therefore, an expert can easily locate them and select an appropriate processing. In this context, the fuzzy labels of tissue classes provided by an atlas and registered toward the processed volume are useful. However, this example can be generalized to the combination of any set of fuzzy labels and expert knowledge in order to strongly constrain the segmentation task according to the desired medical application.

Following previous work [4], we propose to integrate atlas knowledge into a level set segmentation framework [1] via a fuzzy decision system. We first focus on white matter segmentation. Fuzzy label maps adapted to any MRI volumes are created by registration and used to automatically choose the weight on curvature in the level set evolution force. Then we propose another example of level set evolution constrained to only one hemisphere with fuzzy labels.

The next section of this paper presents our methods with atlas-based preprocessing and integration of the fuzzy decision in the level set formalism. Section 3 shows our results on the MNI Brainweb dataset and on a real MRI volume database, and our conclusions and perspectives are presented in section 4.

2   Method

In this section, we focus on the automatic processing set up to segment (i) the white matter with a curvature constrain tuned by fuzzy labels and (ii) the right hemisphere of the brain.

2.1   A Fully Automatic Processing

In order to achieve the segmentation of brain structures of interest in MRI volumes coming from any acquisition system, we included the segmentation algorithm in a fully automatic succession of operations. These operations are the same for each processed MRI volume. First, a brain mask and the fuzzy maps corresponding to the application are created from the data available in the MNI Brainweb dataset [5]. Then, the segmentation is performed with a level set algorithm including a fuzzy decision module. The following sections present these steps for one processed volume.

2.2   Atlas-Based Preprocessing

Atlas Description
The atlas we use is the MNI Brainweb dataset, which provides MRI volumes of a brain and the associated fuzzy maps. For each tissue class, the fuzzy map is a volume where each voxel has an intensity value that is proportional to its membership to this class. To segment the white matter, we use the fuzzy maps associated to the white matter, the grey matter and the cerebro-spinal fluid (CSF), as presented in the next paragraphs. For the right hemisphere application, we use only the brain tissues labeled with right laterality.

Creation of a Brain Mask

To create an adjusted brain mask for the processed volume from the MNI Brain-web dataset, we use an affine registration algorithm (12 parameters that maximize the mutual information are computed). The grey matter, white matter and internal CSF volumes of the MNI phantom were previously combined to obtain a brain segmentation. The white matter and grey matter volumes were binary versions of the corresponding fuzzy maps, and the internal CSF was segmented with the level set algorithm described in section [1]. We then use a morphological dilation on the registration result to get a mask including the whole brain of the processed volume.

Creation of the Fuzzy Label Maps

To perform the segmentation of the white matter as precisely as possible, the evolution of the contour is constrained at the following high curvature areas:
- the interface between the grey matter and the white matter,
- the interface between the white matter and the CSF.
Concerning the segmentation of the right hemisphere, we need the distance to this hemisphere.

The fuzzy maps of the Brainweb MNI dataset are thus affinely registered to provide fuzzy maps that are adapted to the current volume.

2.3   Integration in a Level Set Segmentation Framework

To perform the segmentation of brain structures, the mask obtained as described in 2.2 is applied on the processed volume, and the masked data is processed with a level set algorithm.

General Formulation of the Level Set Evolution Force

In [1], the authors proposed the following region-based evolution force:

$$F = g(P_T)(\rho \kappa - \nu), \tag{1}$$

where ν is a constant module force, which sign leads the current interface toward the desired contour; κ is the local curvature of the interface; ρ is the weight on curvature; g is a decreasing function; and P_T is the probability of transition between the inside and the outside of the structure to be segmented. It is computed according to a preliminary classification of tissues, as described in [1]. The role of the term $g(P_T)$ is thus to stop the evolution of the contour at the desired location.

In previous work [4], we showed how to improve the impact of $g(P_T)$ with fuzzy logic. In this paper, we focus on the other parameters so that they are automatically tuned according to the application, as presented in the next paragraphs.

Application to White Matter Segmentation: Design of ρ

The role of ρ is to regularize the contour. However, this regularization should be adapted to any part of complex volumes like the white matter. In details, it should allow the contour to propagate in very narrow protusions as the gyri.

However, in areas corresponding to "holes" in the structure, as the ventricles, the contour should strongly contract to match the edges of the holes.

To this end, the value of ρ is locally derived from the fuzzy label maps with a fuzzy decision system. This system is drawn from fuzzy control [2] and chooses appropriate weights on curvature according to a small set of rules corresponding to an expert knowledge. It is designed with the following characteristics.

The *inputs* are the local proportion between the grey matter and the white matter (noted GM/WM), and between the CSF and the white matter (noted CSF/WM). They correspond respectively to the membership of the current voxel to the interface between the grey matter and the white matter, and to the interface between the CSF and the white matter. There are two *outputs* of the fuzzy decision system, noted $\rho+$ and $\rho-$, which represent the weight on curvature, respectively on positive and negative curvature areas. High values of $\rho+$ and $\rho-$ respectively encourage contraction and expansion.

We use five states modeled with gaussian-like functions to represent the memberships of the fuzzy variables GM/WM, CSF/WM, $\rho+$ and $\rho-$. It is a common choice in the field of fuzzy control, which provides a partition of the universe of the fuzzy variables that is accurate enough. Our preliminary experiments showed that there was no significant change in the results with the inclusion of an offset in the design of the membership functions. Consequently, they are distributed uniformly on the universe of the variables.

Table 1. Fuzzy rules for weight on positive curvature ($\rho+$) and negative curvature ($\rho-$). VL: very low; L: low; M: medium; H: high; VH: very high

	VL GM/WM	L GM/WM	M GM/WM	H GM/WM	VH GM/WM
VL CSF/WM	VL $\rho+$ / VH $\rho-$		VL $\rho+$		M $\rho+$
L CSF/WM		M $\rho+$	H $\rho-$	H $\rho+$	
M CSF/WM		H $\rho+$ / H $\rho-$	L $\rho-$		
H CSF/WM				VH $\rho+$	
VH CSF/WM			VL $\rho-$		VH $\rho+$ / VL $\rho-$

The fuzzy *decision rules* are presented in Tab. 1. They were designed according to the following principles. In areas with a high positive local curvature, as gyri, the contour should expand even if the structure is very thin. This corresponds to lower the curvature constraint in regions where the proportion of white matter is large (VL $\rho+$, VH $\rho-$). On the contrary, in areas with a high negative curvature, as sulci, or in the neigbouring of ventricles, the contour should strongly contract, in order not to cross regions where the proportion of white matter is low. As this is a common problem in white matter segmentation, we take it into account by giving the priority to the proportion of CSF in the design of the rules associated to $\rho+$. This explains how Tab. 1 does not appear as a symmetric matrix.

The associative tables between input and output fuzzy variables are computed at the beginning of the algorithm in order not to lower the speed of evolution of the level set with intermediate calculations.

Let us note that with fuzzy decision, only a few rules are needed to compute $\rho+$ and $\rho-$ [2]. Thus, most of the boxes of Tab. 1 are empty, which consequently decreases the complexity of the fuzzy system. This is one of the major advantages of fuzzy logic, which avoids the use of manually-tuned parameters, and directly translates the knowledge of an expert from words to numerical decision.

Application to Right Hemisphere Segmentation: Modification of the Evolution Force According to Fuzzy Labels

This application requires a simpler system than the segmentation of white matter. As a distance map to the right hemisphere is available, the propagation of the contour can be constrained in order to minimize this distance. In details, the ν and $g(P_T)$ terms of the propagation force are modified until the distance is small enough (a few voxels) to use the original evolution force proposed in [1]:

- the sign of ν is chosen so that the contour propagates toward the right hemisphere,
- if the distance is large enough, $g(P_T)$ is set to 1 in order to increase the evolution speed.

3   Results

3.1   White Matter Segmentation with Fuzzy Regularization

Results on the MNI Brainweb Dataset

The experiments were run on the MNI Brainweb dataset [5]. After the application of a brain mask created with the combined segmentations of the white matter, grey matter and CSF, we tested the segmentation algorithm on the white matter by comparing the results with the version presented in [1], which did not involve fuzzy labels.

Let us stress that the image quality of these volumes is very good. Consequently the sulci were correctly segmented with any version of the algorithm. However, as shown on Fig. 1, the contraction of the contour was not strong enough in the occipital part of the ventricles region with the previous version, and this effect was corrected by the introduction of fuzzy labels.

The overlapping rate between our segmentation results and the MNI white matter volume was improved from 97.7 % to 98.3 % with the introduction of fuzzy labels, and the computation time was the same with both versions of the method.

Results on 18 Real MRI Volumes

The experiments were run on a database of 18 MRI volumes (size $256 \times 256 \times 176$). It was acquired on a GE 1.5T system with a sagittal orientation. The patients were all male, 35 ± 10 year old, healthy and right-handed persons. Let us stress

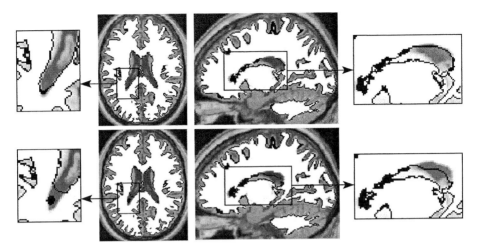

Fig. 1. White matter segmentation: the black contour shows the result with fuzzy labels (first row) and without fuzzy labels (second row), the white area corresponds to the true white matter.

that for each segmentation, we used exactly the same set of parameters for the 18 volumes.

To create adapted initial volumes, we used the registered version of the MNI brain mask that was obtained as described in 2.2, and perform a morphological erosion, as we know that the white matter is located inside the brain. The obtained volume is thus a full volume, with no hole corresponding to the location of the ventricles.

As for the previous set of experiments, we compared the segmentation results with and without the fuzzy labels. As the initial contour does not present any hole around the ventricles, its evolution in this area corresponds to a strong contraction and requires to increase the constraint on curvature. Fig. 2 shows how the introduction of fuzzy labels improved the final segmentation result. Moreover the computation time was increased by only 5 % with the introduction of fuzzy labels.

For comparison, we also tested the white matter segmentation with a gradient-based level set, with the same set of parameters. The gradient-based method failed to follow the white matter borders in the areas that are too far from the initialization volume, on the MNI volume as well as on the 18 volumes database.

3.2 Right Hemisphere Segmentation

The experiments were run on the same database as the white matter segmentation. The level set algorithm was initialized with a parallelepipedic box located inside the brain.

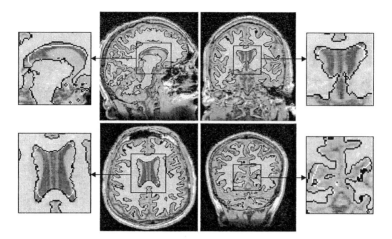

Fig. 2. White matter segmentation: the black contour shows the result with fuzzy labels and the white contour without fuzzy labels. The final contour matches the edges of ventricles and sulci with the use of fuzzy labels.

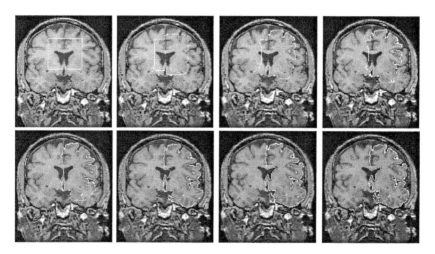

Fig. 3. Brain segmentation constrained to the right hemisphere

As soon as the contour begins to evolve, it is attracted to the right hemisphere because of the distance constraint. The evolution is shown on Fig. 3, and the priority given to the distance constraint can be observed in the ventricles area. The contour is attracted to the right hemisphere before segmenting the ventricle. It finally converges at the desired location.

This shows that the level set evolution can be constrained relatively to a given set of fuzzy labels in order to focus on any anatomical structure.

4   Conclusion and Future Work

We presented an automatic method for the segmentation of volumetric structures. Fuzzy labels coming from an atlas were used to constrain the propagation of a level set contour. Two examples of label-constrained evolution forces were described: one designed for the segmentation of the white matter, the other one dedicated to the right hemisphere segmentation. In all the cases, fuzzy logic avoided the introduction of weighting parameters to balance the respective influence of the terms involved in the evolution force.

Experimental results showed that the combined fuzzy logic and level set methods were at least as robust as the original algorithm. The quality of results was improved for white matter segmentation both on the MNI Brainweb dataset and on a database of 18 volumes. Concerning the right hemisphere segmentation, the evolving contour converged rapidly to the desired structure.

This last set of experiments provides a lot of perspectives. We demonstrated that fuzzy labels could constrain the level set evolution in specific areas, while improving the accuracy of the segmentation. A variety of medical applications could thus take advantage of this technique to quantitatively assess the evolution of anatomical structures, such as lesions. Moreover, the use of several contours propagating in competition, for example one for each hemisphere, could lead to very precise segmentation results in the region of convergence.

References

1. Baillard, C., Barillot, C.: Robust 3D Segmentation of Anatomical Structures with Level Sets. Proceedings of MICCAI (2000), 236–245
2. Bouchon-Meunier, B.: La logique floue et ses applications. Addison-Wesley (1995)
3. Caselles, V., Kimmel, R., Sapiro, G.: Geodesic Active Contours. Int. Journal of Computer Vision, Vol 22 (1997) **1** 61–79
4. Ciofolo, C., Barillot, C., Hellier, P.: Combining Fuzzy Logic and Level Set Methods for 3D MRI Brain Segmentation. Proceedings of the IEEE International Symposium on Biomedical Imaging (2004)
5. Collins, D. L., Zijdenbos, A.P., Kollokian, V., Sled, J.G., Kabani, N.J., Holmes, C.J., Evans, A.C.: Multimodality Imaging - Design and Construction of a Realistic Digital Brain Phantom. IEEE Transactions on Medical Imaging, Vol 17 **3** (1998) 463–468
6. Osher, S., Sethian, J.A.: Fronts Propagating with Curvature Dependant Speed: Algorithms Based on Hamilton-Jacobi Formulation. Journal of Computational Physics, Vol 79 (1998) 12–49
7. Paragios, N.: A Variational Approach for the Segmentation of the Left Ventricle. Int. Journal of Computer Vision, Vol 50 (2002) **3** 345–362
8. Yezzi Jr., A., Tsai, A., Willsky, A. A Statistical Approach to Snakes for Bimodal and Trimodal Imagery. Proceedings of the IEEE Conference on Computer Vision (1999)

Multi-phase Three-Dimensional Level Set Segmentation of Brain MRI

Elsa D. Angelini[1], Ting Song[2], Brett D. Mensh[3], and Andrew Laine[2]

[1] Ecole Nationale Supérieure des Télécommunications, Département Traitement du Signal et des Images, 46 rue Barrault, 75013 Paris, France.
elsa.angelini@enst.fr
[2] Columbia University, Heffner Biomedical Imaging Laboratory,
Department of Biomedical Engineering, 1210 Amsterdam Avenue,
New York, NY 10027, USA.
{ts2060, laine}@columbia.edu
[3] Columbia University, Department of Biological Phsychiatry, College of Physicians and Surgeons, Columbia University, New York, NY, 10032, USA.
bm189@columbia.edu

Abstract. This paper presents the implementation and quantitative evaluation of a four-phase three-dimensional active contour implemented with a level set framework for automated segmentation of cortical structures on brain T1 MRI images. The segmentation algorithm performed an optimal partitioning of three-dimensional data based on homogeneity measures that naturally evolves to the extraction of different tissue types in the brain. Random seed initialization was used to speed up numerical computation and avoid the need for *a priori* information. A simple post-processing, based on morphological operators, was applied to correct for segmentation artifacts. The segmentation method was tested on ten MRI brain data sets and quantitative evaluation was performed by comparison to manually labeled data, Computation of false positive and false negative assignments of voxels for white matter, gray matter and cerebrospinal fluid were performed. Results reported high accuracy of the segmentation methods, demonstrating the efficiency and flexibility of the multi-phase level set segmentation framework to perform the challenging task of automatically extracting cortical brain tissue volume contours.

1 Introduction

This paper presents the implementation and quantitative evaluation of a four-phase three-dimensional active contour implemented within a level set framework for automated segmentation of cortical brain structure on T1 magnetic resonance images (MRI). A level set implementation of surface propagation offers the advantage of easy initialization, computational efficiency, and the ability to capture deep sulcal folds. In recent years, several works have focused on using level set methods for MRI brain segmentation. Zeng *et al.*[1] proposed a segmentation method of the cortex from 3-D MR images using coupled level set surface propagation, assuming a constant thickness range of the cortical mantle. By evolving two embedded surfaces simultaneously, each

C. Barillot, D.R. Haynor, and P. Hellier (Eds.): MICCAI 2004, LNCS 3216, pp. 318–326, 2004.

driven by its own image-derived information and within a certain distance range from each other, a segmentation of the cortical gray matter was achieved. Recently, Yang *et al.* [2] proposed a new method for three-dimensional MRI segmentation based on the combination of joint-prior shape appearance models within a level set deformable model. This method was motivated by the observation that the shapes and gray levels variations in an image had some consistent relations. Building a maximum *a-posteriori* shape-appearance prior model provided some configurations and context information to assist the segmentation process. The model was formulated in a level set framework rather than using landmark points for parametric shape description. Goldenerg *et al.*[3] formulated their 3D MR image segmentation problem as a geometric variational problem for propagation of two coupled bounding surfaces, similar to Zeng *et al.*[1] . The authors put forward an efficient numerical scheme for the implementation of a geodesic active surface model, where a surface evolution was performed.

In this work, we have implemented the multi-phase level set framework first proposed by Chan and Vese [4]. This framework simultaneously deforms coupled level set functions without any prior models or shape constraints. A global partition of the image data results in 2^N homogenous areas for N level set curves, solely based on average gray values measures.

2   Method

2.1 Active Contours Without Edges

A new energy functional for homogeneity-based segmentation derived from the work of Mumford and Shah was proposed by Chan and Vese [5]. Let us assume that a given image, u_0 is formed by two regions of approximate piecewise constant intensities, of distinct values u_0^i and u_0^o . Let us denote the boundary between the two regions by C_0 . Given an initial curve C defined on the image, the following "fitting energy" can be minimized to segment the two regions:

$$F_1(C) + F_2(C) = \int_{inside(C)} |u_0 - c_1|^2 \, dx + \int_{outside(C)} |u_0 - c_2|^2 \, dx . \qquad (1)$$

The parameters c_1, c_2 correspond to the mean values of the image inside and outside the curve C . The curve C_0 that corresponds to the boundary of the object minimizes this energy functional:

$$\inf_C \{F_1(C) + F_2(C)\} = 0 = F_1(C_0) + F_2(C_0) \qquad (2)$$

As a special case of the Mumford-Shah functional, Chan and Vese proposed an active contour model derived from this energy functional with the addition of two regularizing terms to constrain the length of C and the area inside C :

$$E = \mu\left(length(C)\right) + \upsilon\left(area\left(inside\,C\right)\right) + \lambda_1 \int_{inside(C)} |u_0 - c_1|^2 \, dx + \lambda_2 \int_{inside(C)} |u_0 - c_2|^2 \, dx \qquad (3)$$

where $\mu \geq 0$, $\upsilon \geq 0$, $\lambda_1, \lambda_2 > 0$ are fixed parameters.

This energy functional can be extended to the segmentation of multiple homogeneous objects in the image by using several curves $\{C_1, C_2, ..., C_i\}$. In the case of two curves we use the following fitting energy.

$$E = \begin{aligned} &\lambda_1 \int_{\substack{inside\,C_1 \\ inside\,C_2}} |u_0 - c_{11}| dx + \lambda_2 \int_{\substack{inside\,C_1 \\ outside\,C_2}} |u_0 - c_{10}| dx + \lambda_3 \int_{\substack{outside\,C_1 \\ inside\,C_2}} |u_0 - c_{01}| dx + \lambda_4 \int_{\substack{outside\,C_1 \\ outside\,C_2}} |u_0 - c_{00}| dx + \\ &\mu_1 length(C_1) + \mu_2 length(C_2) + v_1 area(inside\,C_1) + v_2 area(inside\,C_2) \end{aligned}$$

Minimization of this energy functional deforms simultaneously two curves and identifies four homogeneous areas defined by the intersection of the two curves as illustrated in Fig. 1.

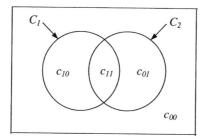

Fig. 1. Partitioning of an image into four areas with two curves C_1, C_2.

2.2 Level Set Formulations of Minimization Problems

Minimization of the functional in Equation (3) is performed with a level set implementation. The level set framework, introduced by Osher and Sethian [6], provides an effective implicit representation for evolving curves and surfaces, which has found many applications, as it allows topological changes, such as merging and breaking.

In this framework, a given curve C (being now the boundary of an open set $\omega \in \Omega$) is represented implicitly, as the zero level set of a scalar Lipschitz function, called the level set function, negative inside ω, positive outside ω and zero on the contour. Given the curve C embedded in a level set function ϕ, its associated Heaviside function H and Dirac function δ are defined respectively as described in [4]. Using these functions, the different components of the functional in Equation (3), parameterized with the contour curve C, can be reformulated with the level function ϕ as described in [4].

Detection of multiple objects is performed via the introduction of multiple level set functions $\{\phi_1, \phi_2\}$ and the computation of mean data values in areas of constant values is defined via the combination of their Heaviside functions $\{H(\phi_1), H(\phi_2)\}$. In this study we implemented the segmentation functional with two level set functions generating four phases defined with mean values defined as:

$$c_{11}(\phi_1,\phi_2) = \frac{\int_\Omega u_0(x)H(\phi_1)H(\phi_2)d\Omega}{\int_\Omega H(\phi_1)H(\phi_2)d\Omega} \ , \ c_{10}(\phi_1,\phi_2) = \frac{\int_\Omega u_0(x)H(\phi_1)\big(1-H(\phi_2)\big)d\Omega}{\int_\Omega H(\phi_1)\big(1-H(\phi_2)\big)d\Omega} \ ,(4)$$

$$c_{01}(\phi_1,\phi_2) = \frac{\int_\Omega u_0(x)\big(1-H(\phi_1)\big)H(\phi_2)d\Omega}{\int_\Omega \big(1-H(\phi_1)\big)H(\phi_2)d\Omega} \ , c_{00}(\phi_1,\phi_2) = \frac{\int_\Omega u_0(x)\big(1-H(\phi_1)\big)\big(1-H(\phi_2)\big)d\Omega}{\int_\Omega \big(1-H(\phi_1)\big)\big(1-H(\phi_2)\big)d\Omega}$$

The Euler-Lagrange systems for the two level set functions are defined as:

$$\frac{\partial\phi_1}{\partial t} = \delta(\phi_1)\left\{\begin{aligned}&\mu div\left(\frac{\nabla\phi_1}{|\nabla\phi_1|}\right) - \upsilon + \lambda_1\left(u_0 - c_{11}\right)^2 H\left(\phi_2\right) + \lambda_2\left(u_0 - c_{10}\right)^2\left(1 - H\left(\phi_2\right)\right)\\&-\lambda_3\left(u_0 - c_{01}\right)^2 H\left(\phi_2\right) - \lambda_4\left(u_0 - c_{00}\right)^2\left(1 - H\left(\phi_2\right)\right)\end{aligned}\right\}$$

$$\frac{\partial\phi_2}{\partial t} = \delta(\phi_2)\left\{\begin{aligned}&\mu div\left(\frac{\nabla\phi_2}{|\nabla\phi_2|}\right) - \upsilon + \lambda_1\left(u_0 - c_{11}\right)^2 H\left(\phi_1\right) - \lambda_2\left(u_0 - c_{10}\right)^2 H\left(\phi_1\right)\\&+\lambda_3\left(u_0 - c_{01}\right)^2\left(1 - H\left(\phi_1\right)\right) - \lambda_4\left(u_0 - c_{00}\right)^2\left(1 - H\left(\phi_1\right)\right)\end{aligned}\right\} \quad (5)$$

In our implementation we kept the Heaviside function negative inside the contour. This explains the modification of the signs of the homogeneity terms compared to the original paper by Vese [4]. The level set algorithm was implemented with a semi-implicit scheme proposed by Chan and Vese [5] but extended to three dimensions. This implicit scheme provides unconditional stability for any temporal and spatial discretization parameters.

In our implementation, the segmentation was initialized with two level set functions defined as the distance function from two sets of initial curves. The initial curves were defined as 64 cylinders centered at regularly spaced seed locations across the entire data volume and slightly shifted from each other, as illustrated in Fig. 2.

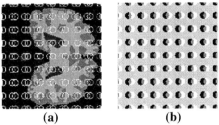

(a)   **(b)**

Fig. 2. Initialization of the level set segmentation. (a) Original MRI slice with two sets of cylinders. (b) Corresponding partitioning of the image domain into 4 phases defined by the overlap of the two level set functions.

Note that such initialization does not use any *a priori* information on the location of tissues or on the anatomy of the brain and does not require manual input by a user.

2.3 Post Processing with Morphological Operators

Initial experiments on clinical data showed potential misclassification of pixels located at the interface between two structures. This type of error is due to the fact that the segmentation method performs a global segmentation of the data and does not apply any constraints on the size or the shape of the tissues segmented so that misclassification of pixels might cancel each other in the homogeneity measure. To correct for these errors we designed a simple post-processing scheme that adjusted interface pixel assignments. After the level set segmentation was completed, WM, GM and CSF structures, corresponding to separate phases, were saved as binary volumes. These volumes were then used as masks applied to the original data to compute the mean μ and variance σ of the underlying tissue. First, the GM mask was dilated, to correct for any under segmentation of thin structures. According to the statistics of the segmented GM, two threshold values were set as $\mu \pm 3\sigma$. Contour pixel with gray values inside this interval were kept within the GM phase, while pixels with gray values outside the interval were removed from the phase and assigned to the adjacent WM phase. This process was iterated until no new points were added in the GM phase. A similar process was then applied to the CSF phase with dilation of the binary mask and comparison to the GM with threshold values of $\mu \pm 4\sigma$ using the CSF statistics.

Finally, a 3-D connectivity algorithm was performed to correct for spurious isolated pixels in the three phases. This simple post-processing approach provided very robust performance on the ten clinical MRI cases segmented in this study, described next.

3   Experiments and Results

We applied our segmentation to ten T1-weighted MRI data sets acquired on healthy young volunteers. The MRI data sets were of size (256×256×73) with a 3mm slice thickness and 0.86mm in-plane resolution. These data sets had been previously labeled via a labor-intensive (40 hours per brain) manual method in which expert raters with extensive training in neuroanatomy choose histogram thresholds on locally hand-drawn regions of interest. This labeled data was used as ground truth for evaluation of the segmentation accuracy.

MRI data sets were pre-processed to remove all non-brain tissue by using the corresponding manually labeled data sets as binary masks. Before segmenting the data sets, we evaluated the homogeneity of the three main tissues targeted for segmentation: WM, GM and CSF again using the labeled data for masking each region. Results showed very stable estimates of mean and variance values for each tissue type across the entire volumetric data set, confirming our assumption that a homogeneity-based segmentation method could be applied to these MRI data sets to extract the three main tissue types. A Gaussian fit was performed on the histogram of the entire gray level distribution of the three brain tissues for each case. We observed that the three tissue types have well separated average values suggesting that the assumption of homogeneity and separability of gray scale values is valid for each patient and each tissue type. The agreement between the volume histograms and the fitted Gaussian distribution was calculated with a chi-squared test. Results for the different tissues did not show a systematic agreement between the data and the Gaussian fit, at level 0.05, except for the gray matter. Therefore, despite reasonable agreement between the data and the fitted Gaussian distribution, we need further investigation before being able to introduce additional constraints based on *a priori* Gaussian statistics to the method as proposed for example by Baillard *et al.*[7] .

As detailed in [8], we used a phantom MRI to tune the parameters of the segmentation method set to:

$$\lambda_1 = \lambda_2 = \lambda_3 = \lambda_4 = 0.01, \upsilon = 0, \quad \mu = 4.10^{-8} \times \text{Volume\_size} / \text{Diagonal\_distance}$$

$$\Delta t = 10^4, \Delta x = \Delta y = \Delta z = 1.$$

The diagonal distance was defined as the diagonal within the data volume. Setting the constant speed term υ to zero eliminates the use of a constant inflating force on the model.

3.1   Quantitative Assessment of Segmentation Performance

We present in Fig. 3 a selected slice and a three-dimensional rendering of the white matter and CSF cortical structures from a MRI clinical case segmented for this study. Visual rendering of the cortical structures confirmed the overall high performance of the multi-phase segmentation method to extract homogenous objects that correspond to distinct anatomical tissues. The segmentation method was able to handle multiple challenges without any *a priori* information or shape constraints that include the extraction of highly-convoluted white matter surfaces, the extraction of separate ventricular structures for the CSF, and handling of different volume sizes of the three structures in a simultaneous segmentation scheme.

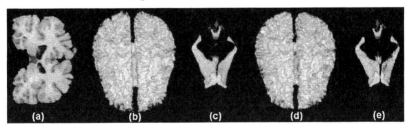

Fig. 3. Rendering of WM and CSF segmented structures. (a) MRI slice. (b-c) Structures from manual labeling. (d-e) Structures from level set segmentation.

Segmentation errors were measured using a recent methodology proposed by Udupa [9] for comparison of segmentation method performance. Accuracy of the object contours obtained with the proposed level set segmentation method was evaluated by comparing the results to our ground truth segmentation of each object, using manually labeled contours. The overlap and difference between the two contours was measured via counting of true positive (*TP*), false positive (*FP*) and false negative (*FN*) voxels. These quantities are reported as volume fractions (*VF*) of the true delineated object volume in Table 1, for the three clinical cases.

Table 1. Error measurements for segmentation of clinical MRI cases.

Case	FNVF (%)			FPVF (%)			TPVF (%)		
	GM	WM	CSF	GM	WM	CSF	GM	WM	CSF
1	4.2	8.5	21.9	8.1	4.8	4.8	95.8	91.5	78.1
2	6.5	5.1	28.5	5.0	8.9	6.1	93.5	94.9	71.5
3	4.5	6.3	27.5	5.9	5.2	7.8	95.5	93.7	72.5
4	8.6	4.1	32.7	4.5	9.2	16.2	91.3	95.9	63.7
5	5.4	4.3	35.7	3.9	6.8	1.0	94.6	95.7	64.3
6	5.5	18.9	26.5	17.3	0.6	0.5	99.5	81.1	73.5
7	6.9	4.1	20.6	4.0	7.9	11.3	93.1	95.9	79.4
8	8.3	4.6	33.8	6.4	9.3	0.005	91.7	95.4	66.2
9	8.9	2.9	37.3	2.9	11.2	0.7	91.1	97.1	62.7
10	11.0	3.8	48.7	3.9	13.5	5.3	89.0	96.2	51.3
Average	7.0	6.3	31.3	6.2	7.7	5.4	93.5	93.7	68.3

Significantly high FNVF errors were observed for the CSF, corresponding to under-segmentation of the ventricles, whose pixels were assigned to white matter. Very low resolution at the ventricle borders can explain in part this result. On the other hand, labeling of the MRI data for the ventricle can also bear some error as localizations of its borders is difficult even for an expert performing manual tracing. Indeed, Kikinis *et a.l* [10] reported a variation in volumetric measurements of manual observers in the order of 15% for WM, GM and CSF.

We also compared our error measurements to results reported by Zeng *et al.*[1] and Niessen *et al.*[11]. In Zeng *et al.*[1], the authors tested their algorithm for the segmentation of frontal lobes on seven high-resolution MRI datasets from a randomly chosen subset of young autistic and control adult subjects. They ran a coupled-surfaces level set algorithm to isolate the brain tissue and segment the cortex. The average TP and FP volume fractions for the cortical gray matter in the frontal lobe were 86.7% and 20.8% (compared to 93.5% and 6.2% obtained using the present methods on whole brain). In Niessen *et al.*[11], a 'hyperstack' segmentation method, based on multiscale pixel classification, was tested for 3D brain MRI segmentation. A supervised segmentation framework with manual post-editing was applied to a probabilistic brain phantom for estimation of segmentation error. First, a binary segmentation of the brain phantom was performed to evaluate the minimal segmentation error due to partial volume effects. The study reported a volume fraction of misclassified pixels (FP+FN) around 20% for WM, GM and CSF. 'Hyperstack' segmentation was applied with and without a probabilistic framework. Optimal (FP+FN) volume fraction errors were obtained with the probabilistic version reporting: 10% for WM, 21% for GM, and 25% for CSF.

4 Conclusion

This paper presented a novel clinical application and quantitative evaluation of a recently introduced multiphase level-set segmentation algorithm using T1-weighted brain MRIs. The segmentation algorithm performed an optimal partitioning of a three-dimensional data set based on homogeneity measures that naturally evolves to the extraction of different tissue types in the brain. Experimental studies including ten MRI brain data sets showed that the optimal partitioning successfully identified regions that accurately matched WM, GM and CSF areas. This suggests that by combining the segmentation results with fiducial anatomical seed points, the method could accurately extract individual tissue types from these tissues. Random seed initialization was used to speed up the numerical calculation and avoid convergence to local minima. This random initialization also ensured robustness of the method to variation of user expertise, biased or erroneous *a priori* input information, and initial settings influenced by variation in image quality. Future work will include incorporation of available co-registered FLAIR and T2-weighted MRI data to improve the segmentation performance for the CSF, running the algorithm on vectorial-type data.

References

[1] X. Zeng, L. H. Staib, R. T. Schultz, and J. S. Duncan, "Segmentation and measurement of the cortex from 3-D MR images using coupled-surfaces propagation," *IEEE Transactions on Medical Imaging*, vol. 18, pp. 927-937, 1999.

[2] J. Yang and J. S. Duncan, "3D Image segmentation of deformable objects with shape-appearance joint prior models," MICCAI, Montreal, Canada, pp. 573-580, 2003.

[3] R. Goldenberg, R. Kimmel, E. Rivlin, and M. Rudzsky, "Cortex segmentation - a fast variational geometric approach," IEEE Workshop on Variational and Level Set Methods in Computer Vision, pp. 127-133, 2001.

[4] L. A. Vese and T. F. Chan, "A multiphase level set framework for image segmentation using the Mumford and Shah model," University of California, Los Angeles, CA, USA, Computational and Applied Mathematics Report 01-25, 2001.

[5] T. F. Chan and L. A. Vese, "Active contours without edges," *IEEE Transactions on Image Processing*, vol. 10, pp. 266 - 277, 2001.

[6] S. Osher and J. A. Sethian, "Fronts propagating with curvature-dependent speed: algorithms based on Hamilton-Jacobi formulation.," *Journal of computational physics*, vol. 79, pp. 12-49, 1988.

[7] C. Baillard, C. Barillot, and P. Bouthemy, "Robust Adaptive Segmentation of 3D Medical Images with Level Sets," INRIA, Rennes, France, Research Report Nov. 2000.

[8] E. Angelini, T. Song, B. D. Mensh, and A. Laine, "Segmentation and quantitative evaluation of brain MRI data with a multiphase three-dimensional implicit deformable model," SPIE International Symposium Medical Imaging, San Diego, CA, USA, 2004.

[9] J. Udupa, V. LeBlanc, H. Schmidt, C. Imielinska, P. Saha, G. Grevera, Y. Zhuge, P. Molholt, Y. Jin, and L. Currie, "A methodology for evaluating image segmentation algorithm," SPIE Conference on Medical Imaging, San Diego CA, USA, pp. 266-277, 2002.

[10] R. Kikinis, M. E. Shenton, G. Gerig, J. Martin, M. Anderson, D. Metcalf, C. R. Guttmann, R. W. McCarley, W. Lorensen, H. Cline, and F. A. Jolesz, "Routine quantitative analysis of brain and cerebrospinal fluid spaces with MR imaging," *Journal of Magnetic Resonance Imaging*, vol. 2, pp. 619-629, 1992.

[11] W. J. Niessen, K. L. Vincken, J. Weickert, and M. A. Viergever, "Three-dimensional MR brain segmentation," International Conference on Computer Vision, pp. 53-58, 1998.

[12] B. Fischl, D. H. Salat, E. Busa, M. Albert, M. Dieterich, C. Haselgrove, A. v. d. Kouwe, R. Killiany, D. Kennedy, S. Klaveness, A. Montillo, N. Makris, B. Rosen, and A. M. Dale, "Whole brain segmentation: automated labeling of neuroanatomical structures in the human brain," *Neuron*, vol. 33, pp. 341-355, 2002.

[13] W. A. Barrett, L. J. Reese, and E. N. Mortensen, "Intelligent segmentation tools," IEEE International Symposium on Biomedical Imaging, 2002. Proceedings, Washington D.C., USA2002.

Effects of Anatomical Asymmetry in Spatial Priors on Model-Based Segmentation of the Brain MRI: A Validation Study

Siddarth Srivastava, Frederik Maes, Dirk Vandermeulen, Wim Van Paesschen, Patrick Dupont, and Paul Suetens

Katholieke Universiteit Leuven, Faculties of Medicine and Engineering, Medical Image Computing (Radiology - ESAT/PSI), University Hospital Gasthuisberg, Herestraat 49, B-3000 Leuven, Belgium.
Siddharth.Srivastava@uz.kuleuven.ac.be

Abstract. This paper examines the effect of bilateral anatomical asymmetry of spatial priors on the final tissue classification based on maximum-likelihood (ML) estimates of model parameters, in a model-based intensity driven brain tissue segmentation algorithm from (possibly multispectral) MR images. The asymmetry inherent in the spatial priors is enforced on the segmentation routine by laterally flipping the priors during the initialization stage. The influence of asymmetry on the final classification is examined by making the priors subject-specific using non-rigid warping, by reducing the strength of the prior information, and by a combination of both. Our results, both qualitative and quantitative, indicate that reducing the prior strength alone does not have any significant impact on the segmentation performance, but when used in conjunction with the subject-specific priors, helps to remove the misclassifications due to the influence of the asymmetric priors.

1 Introduction

A normal human brain has systematic bilateral asymmetry, exhibited, most notably, in the frontal and the occipital regions. This effect is referred to as the *brain torque*. For a normal population, the right frontal lobe is larger than the left, the left occipital lobe is larger than the right ([8] and references therein). This normal inter-hemispheric morphological variability is reflected in all databases that are built upon a large representative population study. An example of such a database is the digital brain atlas provided with SPM99 [6] (figure 1) which contains spatially varying probability maps for gray matter (GM), white matter (WM) and cerebro-spinal fluid (CSF), obtained by averaging deterministic classifications of respective tissue classes from a large normal population, aligned to a standard reference space by affine transformations [2]. The asymmetry inherent in the normal brains, hence, is reflected in the inter-hemispheric asymmetry of the priors. This atlas has wide applications in the field of automated brain tissue segmentation, wherein it is used as a first estimate of the classification, and to spatially constrain the classification [3]. The use of the priors

C. Barillot, D.R. Haynor, and P. Hellier (Eds.): MICCAI 2004, LNCS 3216, pp. 327–334, 2004.

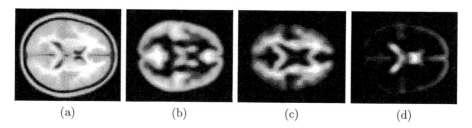

Fig. 1. Digital Brain Atlas as provided by SPM99 [6]. (a) Normal T1 brain template, (b)-(d): apriori spatial probability maps for gray matter, white matter and csf respectively

in their usual form, however tends to introduce a spatial bias in the derived classifications, of a nature similar to the asymmetry content in the priors. Furthermore, asymmetry studies and anatomical lateralization over and above the normal morphogenic incongruity of the human brain are strong indicators of widespread and local neurodegenerative disorders. Typically, in such computational neuroscience methodologies, it is the segmentation map which is under examination. This fact, combined with the ubiquity of the automated segmentation methodologies using a brain atlas as spatial *a-priori* information merits a study examining the influence that the asymmetric priors have on the final results, and devise ways to attenuate or ideally, obliterate their influence. Such a study will ensure that the morphological findings are intrinsic to the data under examination, and not an artifact of the intermediate processing steps.

2   Materials and Methods

We use high-resolution simulated 3D T1 weighted brain MR images provided by Brainweb [1]. All the data sets have 1 mm isotropic voxel dimensions. The intensity homogeneity was chosen to be 20% to engage the bias correction component of the segmentation scheme. The experiments were performed for noise levels $\sigma = \{3, 5, 7, 9\}\%$. Corresponding to these data sets were anatomical deterministic ground truths G per tissue class, which were used as a reference to which we compare the segmentation maps produced by each segmentation methodology. We use the spatial priors P^o in their original orientation, as provided in the standard distribution of SPM99 [6]. We also derive a new set of priors P^f by flipping P^o bilaterally in the native space. This is done to transfer the intrinsic bilateral asymmetry in the spatial priors to the opposite side. Because of the flipping in the native space of the atlas, no re-alignment of P^f to P^o was performed.

2.1   Standard Segmentation

The standard segmentation strategy under examination is the method presented in [3], which parameterizes the tissue-specific intensity distribution as a gaussian, resulting in a mixture model for the entire data set. We denote this strategy by

$\mathcal{U}$. At the core is the classical Expectation-Maximization (EM) loop which is initialized by model parameter estimates from P^o or P^f . The standard processing methodology involves reformating the spatial priors for each tissue class, to the space of the study subject, which has already been aligned to a standard reference space by a 12 parameter affine transformation using maximization of mutual information [4] as an image similarity measure. The realigned spatial priors are then used to initialize the EM loop, and also to spatially constrain the tissue classification during the search for ML estimates of model parameters. The results of the segmentation, however, differ, depending on whether the classification has been initialized by P^o or P^f. The effect is clearly visible in figure 2, which shows an axial slice of the GM classification map obtained by initialization and constraining the classification by P^o, and by P^f respectively, and the absolute difference between the two classifications.

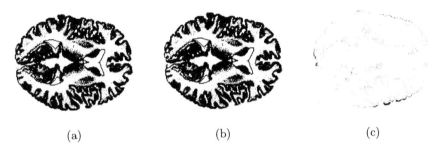

(a)   (b)   (c)

Fig. 2. (a) Probabilistic GM classification obtained by model-based tissue classification initialized with P^o, (b) probabilistic GM classification obtained on initialization with P^f, (c) absolute difference of (a) and (b), showing a systematic misclassification on the outer periphery of the cortex, predominantly at the frontal and contralateral occipital lobe. The colormap is inverted (high(dark) to low(bright)).

2.2   Segmentation with Subject Specific Priors

An affine mapping of the priors P^o or Pf to the study subject ensures global anatomical correspondence between the subject and the prior. Local morphological variability in the brain of the subject to be segmented is not taken into account by this methodology. A more optimal way of providing the EM segmentation routine with initial estimates would be to normalize the priors to the study subject by using a high-dimensional non-rigid registration technique [7]. Warping the priors to the subject brings the priors in better anatomical correspondence with the subject, resulting in a more accurate initialization, which is likely to improve the overall segmentation. Starting from the initial affine alignment of the spatial priors to the study subject, a set of deformation fields were estimated from the T1 weighted template provided with SPM99 [6], using the non-rigid registration tool of SPM99 [6], with default parameter settings. These deformation fields were then applied to the priors, enhancing the local anatomical correspondence. The deformed priors were then provided to the segmentation routine as initial estimates and for successive spatial constraints. We denote this strategy by $\mathcal{W}$.

2.3   Segmentation with Reduced Priors

In [5] it is argued that it is not convenient to initialize the segmentation with actual *a-priori* probabilities because the empirical frequencies in the atlas tissue maps encode a wide variation in population, and are different from the anatomical variation in the study subject. As proposed in [5] we moderate the priors by a small factor before initialization and subsequent processing steps. If $p_t(r)$ denotes the a-priori probability of voxel r being of the tissue type t, then the prior is modified into

$$q_t(r) = \alpha p_t(r) + (1 - \alpha)\frac{1}{K} \tag{1}$$

where K is the number of classes under consideration, and $\alpha \in [0,1]$ is the weighing parameter that serves to reduce the influence of the spatial priors on classification. We have applied this prior reduction strategy to each of the segmentation strategies mentioned in sections 2.1 and 2.2, for values of $\alpha = \{0.3, 0.5, 0.7, 0.9, 1.0\}$, where $\alpha = 1.0$ refers to unmodified spatial priors. In cases where reduced priors were used in combination with $\mathcal{W}$ (section 2.2), the reduction was applied after the non-rigid registration.

2.4   Segmentation Performance Index

Each segmentation methodology yields a classification map for each of the tissue classes, which we denote by $\mathcal{C}$. The free parameters for our experiments are the segmentation methodologies $\mathcal{M} \in \{\mathcal{U}, \mathcal{W}\}$ representing the affine and warped priors respectively, orientations $k \in \{o, f\}$ of the priors P^o and P^f respectively and the reduction fraction $\alpha \in \{0.3, 0.5, 0.7, 0.9, 1.0\}$ for the priors, and the noise content of the data $\sigma \in \{3, 5, 7, 9\}\%$. For ease of reference, a segmentation for a particular tissue class performed on data with a particular noise content σ, with methodology $\mathcal{M}$, and initialization performed with priors in orientation k will be denoted by $\mathcal{C}_\alpha^{k,\mathcal{M}}$. Based on this notation, we have, for a particular orientation k of the prior, and for a particular noise level, 10 possible segmentations for each tissue class. Since the basic objective of the work is to check for the effects of asymmetry of the priors on the segmentation, our hypothesis is that a segmentation $\mathcal{C}_\alpha^{k,\mathcal{M}}$ is immune to the asymmetry effects if it agrees well with its corresponding ground truth G, and also if $\mathcal{C}_\alpha^{o,\mathcal{M}}$ and $\mathcal{C}_\alpha^{f,\mathcal{M}}$ agree well with each other. We use the Dice Similarity Coefficient (DSC) described in [9] as a measure of agreement between the segmentations for a particular tissue class using different methodologies. This similarity index is defined as $DSC(\mathcal{C}_1, \mathcal{C}_2) = \frac{2V(\mathcal{C}_1 \cap \mathcal{C}_2)}{V(\mathcal{C}_1) + V(\mathcal{C}_2)}$, where $V(\mathcal{C})$ is the volume of the classification map $\mathcal{C}$, defined, in our case, as the total number of voxels classified in a classification map (all voxels with non-zero probability). This measure is used to evaluate a ratio of twice the number of commonly classified voxels, to the number of all the voxels classified in C_1 and C_2, without taking into account the probability of the classification. This makes the measure more stringent as compared to discretizing both the volumes by deterministic assignment (hard segmentation) [3], and more responsive to spatial misclassifications even with a small membership probability. The value of this DSC lies between 0 and 1, and serves as a performance index increasing from 0 to 1, indicating an excellent agreement for $DSC > 0.7$ [7]. For ease of reference, we define $s_\alpha^{k,\mathcal{M}} = \mathrm{DSC}(C_\alpha^{k,\mathcal{M}}, G)$ and $s_\alpha^{\mathcal{M}} = \mathrm{DSC}(C_\alpha^{o,\mathcal{M}}, C_\alpha^{f,\mathcal{M}})$, where G refers to the ground truth corresponding to the classification map C.

3 Results

We have studied the segmentation performance based on DSC, on simulated Brainweb data [1]. Since most of the systematic errors occur in the GM (figure 2(c)), we present results only for the GM, for noise content of 5% and 7%. This is the noise content from moderate to extreme that is typically present in most of the high resolution acquisitions that are used. Table 1 shows the DSC based performance index for GM, and its variations across methodologies and noise level. Figure 3 shows the GM segmentations for all methodologies (for $\alpha = 1.0$ and $\alpha = 0.7$), for $\sigma = 5\%$, allowing visual inspection of the improvement in segmentation for each methodology.

Table 1. Similarity index (DSC) for GM, for all methodologies. The results are shown for noise levels $\sigma = 5\%$ and $\sigma = 7\%$. The left-most column shows the segmentation methodology, standard ($\mathcal{U}$) or warped ($\mathcal{W}$), along with the reduction fraction α.

$\sigma \Longrightarrow$	$\sigma = 5\%$			$\sigma = 7\%$		
$(\mathcal{M}, \alpha) \Downarrow$	$s_\alpha^{o,\mathcal{M}}$	$s_\alpha^{f,\mathcal{M}}$	$s_\alpha^{\mathcal{M}}$	$s_\alpha^{o,\mathcal{M}}$	$s_\alpha^{f,\mathcal{M}}$	$s_\alpha^{\mathcal{M}}$
$(\mathcal{U}, 1.0)$	0.725612	0.722171	0.986609	0.709364	0.708018	0.992829
$(\mathcal{W}, 1.0)$	0.730665	0.730551	0.992660	0.713761	0.712719	0.994128
$(\mathcal{U}, 0.3)$	0.722913	0.714043	0.980580	0.709440	0.708352	0.993268
$(\mathcal{U}, 0.5)$	0.721188	0.714287	0.981220	0.708900	0.708214	0.993152
$(\mathcal{U}, 0.7)$	0.721942	0.713215	0.980316	0.708662	0.708607	0.993026
$(\mathcal{U}, 0.9)$	0.722741	0.715180	0.981435	0.708951	0.709029	0.992880
$(\mathcal{W}, 0.3)$	0.730177	0.729552	0.993097	0.713373	0.712819	0.994267
$(\mathcal{W}, 0.5)$	0.730270	0.729546	0.992827	0.713594	0.712928	0.994203
$(\mathcal{W}, 0.7)$	0.731153	0.729602	0.992718	0.713463	0.712810	0.994210
$(\mathcal{W}, 0.9)$	0.730947	0.729415	0.992680	0.713562	0.712726	0.994411

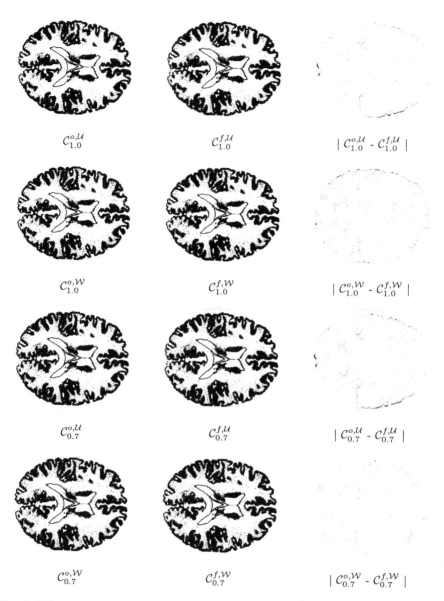

Fig. 3. Column-wise: segmentations initialized with P^o, P^f, and their absolute differences respectively. Methods vary row-wise, as designated by the corresponding labels. The noise level for the data is $\sigma = 5\%$

4   Discussion

Table 1 gives a global overview of segmentation performance of various methodologies, and their ability to make the segmentation maps indifferent to the spatial asymmetry content in the prior probability maps. We observe a small improvement, with respect to the similarity index, between the affine-transformed, and non-rigidly deformed prior based initialization strategy, with un-modified ($\alpha = 1.0$) priors. Upon inclusion of the reduction strategy (section 2.3) in the standard segmentation procedure $\mathcal{U}$ there is a drop in the DSC measure, and it remains less than the performance of $\mathcal{U}$ for $\alpha = 1.0$. The use of $\mathcal{W}$, however, performs better than $\mathcal{U}$ for all values of α, and performs better than ($\mathcal{W}$,1.0) (table 1) for $0.7 \leq \alpha \leq 0.9$. This holds true for all noise ranges $\sigma \in \{3, 5, 7, 9\}\%$. Within a particular methodology, there seems to be a very minimal dependence of α upon the DSC based comparison with the ground truth. This does not agree well with the findings reported in [5]. The differences could be because of the fact that we calculate volumes in DSC metric as voxel counts in the posterior probability maps, and not as voxel counts in hard segmented classification maps. Since the basic objective of this work is to make the segmentations immune to the anatomical asymmetry in the priors, a successful strategy will be one that gives high values of performance index s_α^k, indicating that the segmentations of the same study subject, obtained by initializations with P^o and P^f respectively agree well with each other, while at the same time are in good agreement with their respective ground truths. Table 1 demonstrates that some improvement is gained in s_α^k by changing the normalization strategy from affine-only to non-rigid. Further, there is a slight improvement, for the non-rigid normalization, for values of $0.3 \leq \alpha < 1.0$, in comparison to the values for ($\mathcal{U}$,1.0) and ($\mathcal{W}$, 1.0). It should be mentioned here that the similarity across segmentations, as demonstrated under column labeled s_α^k in table 1 is high even without any modification to the segmentation methodology. Since the misclassifications due to asymmetry represent a small fraction of connected voxels at anatomically specific locations, a removal of this effect lends a very small fraction to the performance index as an improvement, making small changes in performance very significant. Residual errors ($1.0 - DSC$) in the most optimal segmentation (figure 3, bottom row) can be attributed to the remaining misclassified voxels spread over the entire segmentation map, while segmentation errors due to the misclassified voxels at the outer edge of the cortex are completely removed.

5   Conclusion

This paper investigates the effect of anatomical bilateral asymmetry in the spatial prior probability maps used to initialize, and spatially guide intensity based segmentation, on the resulting classifications. The premise for the experiments performed was that the same study-subject brain, segmented under laterally flipped conditions (P^o or P^f) should result in the same segmentation, and should also agree well with the corresponding anatomical ground truth. To this end, we have used the volume similarity as the performance index, and compared gray matter segmentations obtained after initialization of the classification method with P^o and P^f respectively. Since the effects of asymmetry are more visible in the gray matter segmentation maps, we have presented results only for the gray matter. Our results indicate that anatomical asymmetry in the prior probability maps influence the segmentation by severely misclassifying small but significant regions of the brain, especially at the outer surface of the cortex. Such an effect might get swamped in volumetric studies, but is of significance in studies where topological and geometrical properties of the cortex are under examination. Further, the use of non-rigid registration improves the segmentation performance, as compared to the usual affine-only spatial correspondence, and also helps to remove the effects of asymmetry from the final GM classification map. Reducing the prior strength alone does not result in any significant improvement of the segmentation. Further, visual analysis of figure 3 (bottom row) shows that the reduced prior strategy, when used in conjunction with the non-rigid registration, serves to remove the effect of the spatial prior asymmetry from the classification.

Acknowledgements. This work was funded by grant KU Leuven A99-005. The authors would like the acknowledge the contribution of Kristof Baete and Natalie Nelissen.

References

1. C.A. Cocosco, V. Kollokian, R.K.-S. Kwan, and A.C. Evans. Brainweb: Online interface to a 3d mri simulated brain database. *NeuroImage*, 5(4):S425, 1997. part 2/4.
2. A.C. Evans, D.L. Collins, S.R. Mills, E.D. Brown, R.L. Kelly, and T.M. Peters. 3d statistical neuroanatomical models from 305 mri volumes. *Proc. IEEE Nuclear Science Symposium and Medical Imaging Conference*, pages pp 1813–1817, 1993.
3. K. Van Leemput, F. Maes, D. Vandermeulen, and P. Suetens. Automated model based tissue classification of MR images of the brain. *IEEE Transactions on Medical Imaging*, 18(10):pp 897–908, 1999.
4. F. Maes, A. Collignon, D. Vandermeulen, and P. Suetens. Multimodality image registration by maximization of mutual information. *IEEE Transactions on Medical Imaging*, 16(2):pp 187–198, 1997.
5. J.L. Marroquin, B.C. Vemuri, S. Botello, F. Calderon, and A. Fernandez-Bouzas. An accurate and efficient bayesian method for automatic segmentation of brain MRI. *IEEE Transactions on Medical Imaging*, 21(8):pp 934–945, 2002.
6. Wellcome Department of Cognitive Neurology. Statistical Parametric Mapping (SPM). http://www.fil.ion.ucl.ac.uk/spm/.
7. Killian M. Pohl, William M. Wells, Alexandre Guimond, Kiyoto Kasai, Martha E. Shenton, Ron Kikinis, W. Eric L. Grimson, and Simon K. Warfield. Incorporating non-rigid registration into expectation maximization algorithm to segment mr images. *MICCAI*, LNCS 2488:pp 564–571, 2002.
8. S. Prima, S. Ourselin, and N. Ayache. Computation of the mid-saggital plane in 3d brain images. *IEEE Transactions on Medical Imaging*, 21(2):pp 122–138, 2002.
9. A.P. Zijdenbos, B.M. Dawant, R.A. Margolin, and A.C. Palmer. Morphometric analysis of white matter lesions in MR images: Methods and validation. *IEEE Transactions on Medical Imaging*, 13(4):pp 716–724, 1994.

How Accurate Is Brain Volumetry?

A Methodological Evaluation

Horst K. Hahn[1], Benoît Jolly[1], Miriam Lee[1], Daniel Krastel[2], Jan Rexilius[1],
Johann Drexl[1], Mathias Schlüter[1], Burckhard Terwey[2], and Heinz-Otto Peitgen[1]

[1] MeVis – Center for Medical Diagnostic Systems and Visualization,
Universitätsallee 29, 28359 Bremen, Germany, hahn@mevis.de
[2] Center for Magnetic Resonance Imaging, St.-Jürgen Str., Bremen, Germany

Abstract. We evaluate the accuracy and precision of different techniques for measuring brain volumes based on MRI. We compare two established software packages that offer an automated image analysis, EMS and SIENAX, and a third method, which we present. The latter is based on the Interactive Watershed Transform and a model based histogram analysis. All methods are evaluated with respect to noise, image inhomogeneity, and resolution as well as inter-examination and inter-scanner characteristics on 66 phantom and volunteer images. Furthermore, we evaluate the N3 nonuniformity correction for improving robustness and reproducibility. Despite the conceptual similarity of SIENAX and EMS, important differences are revealed. Finally, the volumetric accuracy of the methods is investigated using the ground truth of the BrainWeb phantom.

1 Introduction

Various indications exist for brain volume measurements. Major fields of application are diagnosis, disease monitoring, and evaluation of potential treatments in Multiple Sclerosis (MS) [1,2,3] and neurodegenerative diseases, most importantly Alzheimer's disease (AD) [4,5]. Rudick *et al.* propose the brain parenchymal fraction (BPF), which they define as the ratio of brain parenchymal volume to the total volume within the brain surface contour, as a marker for destructive pathologic processes in relapsing MS patients [1]. De Stefano *et al.* found substantial cortical gray matter (GM) volume loss in MS. They propose that neocortical GM pathology may occur early in the course of both relapsing-remitting and primary progressive forms of the disease and contribute significantly to neurologic impairment [2]. In addition to a process that is secondary to white matter (WM) inflammation, they also assume an independent neurodegenerative process, which mainly affects GM and raises the need for robust measures to independently quantify WM and GM volumes.

Fox *et al.* report a mean brain atrophy progression of approximately one percent (12.3 ml) per year in the AD group compared to less than 0.1 percent (0.3 ml) in the control group [4]. I. e., the relative precision of brain volume measurements must be approximately 0.5 percent in order to significantly measure atrophy within one year. Brunetti *et al.* conclude that GM and WM atrophy quantification could complement neuropsychological tests for the assessment of disease severity in AD, possibly having an impact on therapeutic decisions [5].

C. Barillot, D.R. Haynor, and P. Hellier (Eds.): MICCAI 2004, LNCS 3216, pp. 335–342, 2004.
© Springer-Verlag Berlin Heidelberg 2004

In addition to global measurements, a regional analysis is important, for example to derive separate volumes for brain lobes, deep gray matter, hippocampus, cerebellum, etc. Fox *et al.* visualize regional atrophy by the differences between aligned and normalized serial scans, while computing tissue loss that takes into account partial volume effects (PVE) by the integral of the change over the whole brain [4]. Andreasen *et al.* derive volume measurements for twelve standardized regions based on the Talairach coordinate system [6].

In this paper, we concentrate on whole brain characteristics, for total brain volume (TBV=WM+GM), BPF (=TBV/(TBV+CSF)), as well as GM and WM volumes. These measures are expected to remain important parameters in clinical imaging and within clinical trials [1,2,5]. Our objectives are:

1. To evaluate the accuracy and precision of different methodologies for whole brain volumetry on a software phantom with known ground truth and on real MRI data. We aim toward contributing to a methodological comparison that we find poorly developed for image analysis in general and for brain volumetry in particular.
2. To investigate the importance of image nonuniformity, noise, and resolution in brain volumetry and the possibility of improving results using nonuniformity correction.
3. To propose a novel technique which is simple, fast, robust, and accurate. Robustness will be assessed with respect to nonuniformity, noise, and resolution, while the major criterion is reproducibility in terms of inter-examination (scan-rescan) and also inter-scanner characteristics.

2   Material and Methods

For the evaluation of brain volumetry, we used phantom, volunteer, and patient data. The phantom data was obtained from the BrainWeb database [7] at different noise (3%, 5%, 7%, 9%) and nonuniformity levels (0%, 20%, 40%) as well as axial resolutions (1 mm, 3 mm, 5 mm; cf. Fig. 5). The in-plane resolution of the phantom is $(1.0\,\text{mm})^2$ throughout. The exact volumetric ground truth is known a-priori and provided on the web site; the values for GM and WM are 902.9 ml and 680.8 ml, respectively, if glial matter (6.0 ml) is counted as WM; TBV sums up to 1583.7 ml.

To evaluate scan-rescan reproducibility, we used data from three healthy volunteers (subjects 1–3), which have been scanned each five times on the same day with independent repositioning and head rotation. Two of the subjects have also been repeatedly scanned twice on two different scanners on another day, such that inter-scanner characteristics are available. The two devices and acquisition protocols were: (A) Siemens Magnetom Symphony, T1 MPR 3D, TR = 1900 ms, TE = 4.15 ms, TI = 1100 ms, and (B) an older Siemens Magnetom Vision Plus, T1 MPR 3D, TR = 9.7 ms, TE = 4.0 ms, TI = 300 ms. We used an isotropic resolution of $(1.0\,\text{mm})^3$ for all volunteer images with an acquisition time of approximately nine minutes. Inter-examination images were acquired on scanner A for subjects 1 (M, 39 y) and 2 (F, 34 y) and on scanner B for subject 3 (F, 27 y). To limit scan times, we resampled the image data from subject 3 (all five independent acquisitions) at four different axial resolutions using a three-lobed Lanczos filter (1.8 mm, 3.0 mm, 4.8 mm, 7.2 mm).

Various techniques exist to address brain volumetry based on MRI. We have evaluated two of them, which have reached a certain popularity, namely the software packages

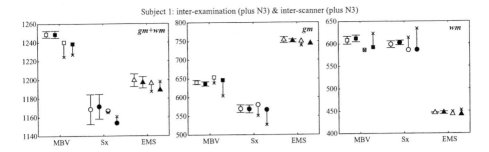

Fig. 1. Inter-examination and inter-scanner characteristics (subject 1) of total brain (***gm+wm***), GM, and WM volumes (mean and SD) for three methods: MBV ('square'), SIENAX (Sx, 'circle'), and EMS ('triangle'). The filled symbols represent the results after N3 nonuniformity correction. Error bars correspond to single SD. The candle plots show inter-scanner differences ('cross' for scanner B), while each symbol represents the mean of two independent acquisitions.

SIENAX [8] and EMS [9]. Both are well documented and available on the internet for research purposes [8,9]. Furthermore, we have evaluated a novel method that builds upon the image analysis platform MeVisLab [10], referred to as MeVisLab Brain Volumetry (MBV). We briefly describe the concepts of the three methods.

SIENAX is a fully automated command-line tool and part of FMRIB's FSL library (Steven M. Smith, University of Oxford, UK) [8]. It is based on a hidden Markov random field (MRF) model and an associated iterative Expectation-Maximization (EM) algorithm for estimating tissue intensity parameters and spatial intensity bias field. Before this, the images are registered to a standard space brain image, where a mask is used to remove non-brain tissue. SIENAX explicitly estimates PVE by evaluating the tissue intensity model on a particular voxel's neighborhood.

EMS was developed by Koen Van Leemput at the Medical Image Computing Group at KU Leuven, Belgium [9], and builds upon the SPM package (Wellcome Department of Imaging Neuroscience, University College London, UK). Much like SIENAX, EMS relies on unsupervised EM tissue classification, corrects for MR signal inhomogeneities, and incorporates contextual information through MRF modeling. Instead of using a brain mask, a digital brain atlas containing prior expectations about the spatial location of tissue classes is used after mutual information based affine registration to initialize the algorithm.

MBV is simpler than the two other methods in that it does not comprise EM classification, MRF or nonuniformity modeling. Rather, MBV relies on skull stripping and histogram analysis only. More precisely, the following four subsequent steps are performed: (*i*) Interactive definition of a cuboid ROI on three orthogonal and synchronized 2D views. (*ii*) Automatic resampling to an isotropic grid (spacing 0.9 mm³) using a Mitchell filter for x, y, and z directions. (*iii*) Skull stripping using the marker-driven, three-dimensional Interactive Watershed Transform (IWT), which has been described in detail by Hahn and Peitgen [11,12]. (*iv*) Automatic histogram analysis for the 3D region defined by the IWT result [13]. The analysis is based on a model consisting of four Gaussian distributions for pure tissue types (WM, GM, CSF, and bone/air), as well as dedicated partial volume distributions for mixed tissue types. The histogram model

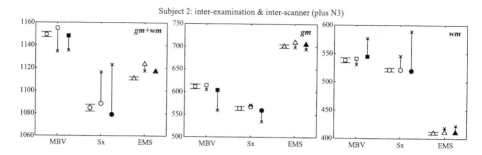

Fig. 2. Inter-examination and inter-scanner characteristics (subject 2). Same categories as Fig. 1, but without inter-examination N3 correction.

corresponds to the assumptions formulated by Santago and Gage [14], i. e. uniform PVE from each pair of two tissues, and is fitted to the histogram by minimizing least square deviations. We use a fourth class to cover air and bone tissue, which is required since the IWT when applied to the original data (interpreted as depth information) includes most of the partial volume regions at the outer brain surface (GM-CSF interface) and extracerebral CSF (CSF-bone interface) [12].

Finally, we investigated the N3 method by John Sled *et al.* [15] in order to improve the volumetric results in presence of a low-frequency image bias field caused by RF inhomogeneity and typical for MR images. N3 employs an iterative approach to estimate both the multiplicative bias field and the true intensity distribution. It requires only two parameters to be selected, one controlling the smoothness of the estimated nonuniformity, the other controlling the tradeoff between accuracy and convergence rate.

3   Results

Several results were acquired on a total of 66 images (phantom: 10, volunteer: 43, N3 corrected: 13). We computed inter-examination mean and standard deviations (SD) of TBV, BPF, GM, and WM volumes for the three subjects (error bars in Figs. 1–3). For subjects 1 and 2, we also assessed inter-scanner variability (candle plots in Figs. 1, 2, and 3 b). For the inter-scanner images and for all images of subject 1, we applied N3 nonuniformity correction using the parameters suggested by J. Sled *et al.* [15] (filled symbols in Figs. 1–3). Figure 4 shows the dependency of inter-examination mean values and variations on the axial image resolution. Figure 5 comprises measured volumes and ground truth for ten phantom images (different noise, nonuniformity, and resolution) in a combined graph. The characteristics for TBV and BPF over all subjects are summarized in Table 1.

Since it is an interactive technique, a second observer (H.K.H.) used MBV to analyze the five original images of subject 3 (diamonds in Fig. 3 a). We found inter-observer differences (mean ± SD) for TBV, GM, and WM volumes to be +4.5 ± 4.9 ml, +3.6 ± 3.4 ml, and +1.0 ± 1.6 ml, respectively. From our experience with MBV, we did not observe significant variations between observers [3], so that we only chose the subject for inter-observer test that required most interaction.

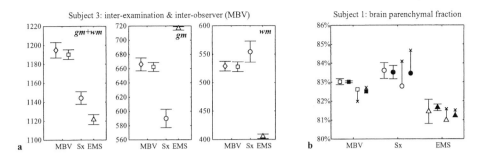

Fig. 3. a: Inter-examination characteristics (subject 3) with results from two observers for MBV (diamonds and squares). **b:** BPF characteristics for subject 1 (cf. Fig. 1).

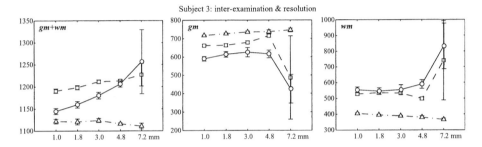

Fig. 4. Inter-examination characteristics for five different axial resolutions (1.0–7.2 mm, subject 3). Each element is computed from five independently acquired and resampled images (mean ± SD, symbols cf. Fig. 1).

We used all methods without modification or – except the N3 correction – image preprocessing (resampling, noise reduction, etc.). SIENAX (FSL 3.1, July 2003) was operated under Linux on a Dual 2.8 GHz Xeon with processing times of approximately eleven minutes per case. For our evaluation, we used the given brain volumes before normalization.   EMS and MBV were operated under Windows 2000 on a 1.7 GHz Pentium III. For EMS, we used SPM99 and Matlab 6.1 with processing times of approximately 26 minutes per case (15 min registration plus 11 min segmentation), including modeling of MRF and fourth-order bias field. EMS volumes were calculated as weighted sum of tissue probability maps. For convergence, we had to manually provide the EMS registration with good initial parameter settings (e. g., 20° frontal rotation was a good starting point in many cases).   For MBV, steps i, ii, plus iv required less than one minute, while the interactive skull stripping (step iii) required approximately 1–4 minutes for marker placement and visual inspection of the actual segmentation, resulting in an overall analysis time of less than five minutes.

For all image processing and evaluation, we paid attention to three important aspects: (a) our own method and its parameters were not altered after the first data set was analyzed; (b) the comparative evaluation of all three methods was conducted exactly once by a person (B.J.), which has not been involved in any method development; and (c) for the phantom, the operator was blinded with respect to the real tissue volumes.

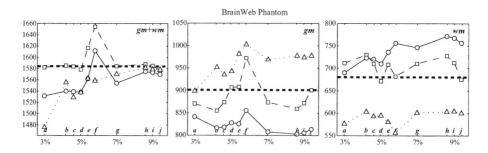

Fig. 5. Volumetric results on ten phantom images. The bold dashed lines indicate the ground truth (symbols cf. Fig. 1). Simulated noise levels are indicated on x-axis. Nonuniformity levels are 0% (b,h), 40% (d,j), and 20% (others). Axial slice thickness is 3 mm (e), 5 mm (f), and 1 mm (others).

4 Discussion

Within our study, each of the three methods revealed advantages and disadvantages. Even though similar in concept, we found considerable differences between SIENAX and EMS. The inter-examination characteristics were slightly better for EMS and MBV than for SIENAX, while EMS performed best for GM and WM (cf. Figs. 1–3) and MBV for TBV and BPF (cf. Table 1 left). In total, including inter-resolution (Fig. 4) and inter-scanner results (cf. Table 1 right), EMS was the most robust method.

One important question, to which a phantom can provide answers to a certain extent, is which method gets closest to the ground truth. Despite its stability, EMS yielded the highest GM volumes and lowest WM volumes on all images, which is consistent with a GM overestimation and WM underestimation compared to the phantom ground truth (Fig. 5). Conversely, SIENAX consistently underestimated GM and overestimated WM volumes compared to the ground truth, and yielded lowest GM volumes on all images. WM volumes were similar for SIENAX and MBV in some cases (Figs. 1 and 2). On the phantom data, MBV was closest to the ground truth on average and yielded values between the other two methods in most cases (cf. Fig. 5). We also analyzed images of AD patients and found similar results (cf. Fig. 6).

The systematic behavior of EMS could be influenced by the atlas based prior tissue probabilities; in Fig. 6 right, a comparably broad GM layer can be discerned. The GM

Table 1. Overall characteristics for TBV and BPF, from left to right: mean inter-examination SD (n=20 images at 1 mm slice thickness: S1, S2, S3, S1+N3); effect of N3 (n=13 images, mean and SD of pair-wise differences); effect of N3 on inter-scanner differences (n=16 images, mean difference $\langle V_A - V_B \rangle$, without → with N3).

	inter-examination SD		N3 effect		inter-scanner N3 effect	
	TBV (ml)	BPF (%)	TBV (ml)	BPF (%)	TBV (ml)	BPF (%)
MBV	3.6	0.17	-0.8 ± 4.2	0.00 ± 0.41	18.0 → 12.2	0.56 → 0.11
Sx	9.7	0.30	-2.0 ± 10.9	0.22 ± 0.52	14.8 → 25.4	1.17 → 1.61
EMS	4.9	0.33	-1.4 ± 9.6	0.09 ± 0.46	8.3 → 4.0	0.34 → 0.16

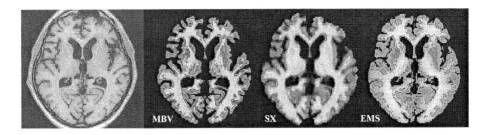

Fig. 6. AD patient (M, 60y). Note that for MBV, partial volume voxels are not shown. The results were (TBV/GM/WM/BPF) 1004.2 / 560.4 / 443.8 / 68.81% for MBV, 972.08 / 475.33 / 496.75 / 77.96% for SX, and 1096.5 / 671.7 / 424.8 / 79.40% for EMS.

underestimation of SIENAX could be caused by a too rigorous brain masking, which removes some of the partial volume voxels at the pial brain surface (cf. Fig. 6 center).

BPF is a normalized measure of brain atrophy, which can be used in cross-group studies. When computing the mean inter-examination SD for BPF, MBV performed slightly better than the other methods (cf. Fig. 3 b and Table 1 left).

Pair-wise comparison of results with and without N3 revealed the least changes of TBV and BPF for the MBV method, showing its high robustness to image nonuniformity (Table 1 middle). Note that this is despite the fact that MBV is the only method that comprises neither nonuniformity correction nor spatial (MRF) regularization, such that we expected it to benefit most from the N3 method. Moreover, N3 did not significantly reduce inter-scanner differences. It yielded some improvements for TBV and BPF, but only for EMS and MBV (Table 1 right); GM and WM differences were mostly worsened by N3 (cf. Figs. 1 and 2).

5 Conclusion and Future Work

In conclusion, EMS was most robust for very large slice thickness and between scanners, and with best inter-examination characteristics for WM and GM. SIENAX has a major advantage in its full and robust automation. MBV showed best inter-examination characteristics for TBV and BPF, and was least influenced by N3. Despite its interactivity, MBV was the fastest of the three methods, but only if a human operator is available. Schubert *et al.*, therefore, investigated a full automation of MBV's remaining interactive steps [16]. Still, we see an advantage in MBV's possibility to interactively control and refine the brain mask and that it does not depend on image registration or anatomical template.

Future work includes a more extensive investigation of these and other methods on a variety of patient images. In particular, the systematic behavior with respect to image resolution (cf. Figs. 4 and 5 e/f) requires further research on a larger set of MR images. Other methods include SIENA (also FSL) that is designed for longitudinal brain volume measurements. One issue that is important for clinical use was not explicitly addressed in this paper, namely sensitivity. While reproducibility is a measure for the robustness of a method, small changes, e. g. associated with GM atrophy, could remain undetected by a highly reproducible method. This needs to be addressed in future studies.

Acknowledgments. We kindly acknowledge the Medical Image Computing Group at KU Leuven (Paul Suetens), for providing their software EMS, the University of Oxford and the Image Analysis Group of FMRIB Oxford (Steven M. Smith) for providing their software FSL, the McCornell Brain Imaging Centre, MNI, McGill University (Alan C. Evans) for providing the BrainWeb phantom as well as their software N3, and Koen Van Leemput for assisting in the use of EMS. We thank our colleagues Florian Link and Tobias Boskamp for their groundbreaking work on MeVisLab.

References

1. Rudick, R.A., Fisher, E., Lee, J.C., et al.: Use of the brain parenchymal fraction to measure whole brain atrophy in relapsing-remitting MS. Neurology **53** (1999) 1698–1704
2. De Stefano, N., Matthews, P.M., Filippi, M., et al.: Evidence of early cortical atrophy in MS: Relevance to white matter changes and disability. Neurology **60** (2003) 1157–1162
3. Lukas, C., Hahn, H.K., Bellenberg, B., et al.: Sensitivity and reproducibility of a new fast 3D segmentation technique for clinical MR based brain volumetry in multiple sclerosis. Neuroradiology (2004) in print
4. Fox, N.C., Freeborough, P.A., Rossor, M.N.: Visualisation and quantification of rates of atrophy in Alzheimer's disease. Lancet **348** (1996) 94–97
5. Brunetti, A., Postiglione, A., Tedeschi, E., et al.: Measurement of global brain atrophy in Alzheimer's disease with unsupervised segmentation of spin-echo MRI studies. J Magn Reson Imaging **11** (2000) 260–266
6. Andreasen, N.C., Rajarethinam, R., Cizadlo, T., et al.: Automatic atlas-based volume estimation of human brain regions from MR images. J Comput Assist Tomogr **20** (1996) 98–106
7. Collins, D.L., Zijdenbos, A.P., Kollokian, V., et al.: Design and construction of a realistic digital brain phantom. IEEE Trans Med Imaging **17** (1998) 463–468, `//www.bic.mni.mcgill.ca/brainweb/`.
8. Smith, S., Zhang, Y., Jenkinson, M., et al.: Accurate, robust and automated longitudinal and cross-sectional brain change analysis. NeuroImage **17** (2002) 479–489, `//www.fmrib.ox.ac.uk/fsl/`.
9. Van Leemput, K., Maes, F., Vandermeulen, D., Suetens, P.: Automated model-based tissue classification of MR images of the brain. IEEE Trans Med Imaging **18** (1999) 897–908, `//bilbo.esat.kuleuven.ac.be/web-pages/downloads/ems/`.
10. MeVisLab development environment available at: `//www.mevislab.de/`.
11. Hahn, H.K., Peitgen, H.O.: IWT – Interactive Watershed Transform: A hierarchical method for efficient interactive and automated segmentation of multidimensional grayscale images. In: Med Imaging: Image Processing. Proc. SPIE 5032, San Diego (2003) 643–653
12. Hahn, H.K., Peitgen, H.O.: The skull stripping problem in MRI solved by a single 3D watershed transform. In: MICCAI – Medical Image Computing and Computer-Assisted Intervention. LNCS 1935, Springer, Berlin (2000) 134–143
13. Hahn, H.K., Millar, W.S., Klinghammer, O., et al.: A reliable and efficient method for cerebral ventricular volumetry in pediatric neuroimaging. Methods Inf Med 43 (2004) in print
14. Santago, P., Gage, H.D.: Quantification of MR brain images by mixture density and partial volume modeling. IEEE Trans Med Imaging **12** (1993) 566–574
15. Sled, J.G., Zijdenbos, A.P., Evans, A.C.: A nonparametric method for automatic correction of intensity nonuniformity in MRI data. IEEE Trans Med Imaging **17** (1998) 87–97
16. Schubert, A., Hahn, H.K., Peitgen, H.O.: Robust fully automated brain segmentation based on a 3D watershed transform. In: Proc. BVM, Springer, Berlin (2002) 193–196, in German.

Anisotropic Interpolation of DT-MRI

Carlos A. Castaño-Moraga[1], Miguel A. Rodriguez-Florido[1], Luis Alvarez[2],
Carl-Fredrik Westin[3], and Juan Ruiz-Alzola[1,3]

[1] Medical Technology Center, Signals & Communications and Telematic Engineering
Departments
[2] Informatics and Systems Department
Universidad de Las Palmas de Gran Canaria
Canary Islands - Spain
{ccasmor,marf,jruiz}@ctm.ulpgc.es;lalvarez@dis.ulpgc.es
http://www.ctm.ulpgc.es
[3] Laboratory of Mathematics in Imaging
Brigham & Women's Hospital and Harvard Medical School
Boston (MA) - USA
westin@bwh.harvard.edu

Abstract. Diffusion tensor MRI (DT-MRI) is an image modality that
is gaining clinical importance. After some preliminaries that describe
the fundamentals of this imaging modality, we present a new technique
to interpolate the diffusion tensor field, preserving boundaries and the
constraint of positive-semidefiniteness. Our approach is based on the use
of the inverse of the local structure tensor as a metric to compute the
distance between the samples and the interpolation point. Interpolation
is an essential step in managing digital image data for many different
applications. Results on resampling (zooming) synthetic and clinical DT-
MRI data are used to illustrate the technique. This new scheme provides
a new framework for anisotropic image processing, including applications
on filtering, registration or segmentation.

1 Introduction

From its advent in the mid-nineties, diffusion tensor MRI (DT-MRI) has become
a powerful imaging modality for many clinical analysis [1]: brain ischemia, multiple sclerosis, leucoencephalopathy, Wallerian degeneration, Alzheimer's disease,
white matter fiber tracking, brain connectivity, etc.

This medical image modality provides a discrete volumetric dataset where
each voxel contains a second-order positive-semidefinite tensor associated with
the effective anisotropic diffusion of water molecules in biological tissues.
This information proves very useful, for example, in fiber tractography where
the trajectories of nerve tracts and other fibrous tissues are followed by the
direction of the eigenvectors associated with the largest eigenvalues of the
diffusion tensors [2].

C. Barillot, D.R. Haynor, and P. Hellier (Eds.): MICCAI 2004, LNCS 3216, pp. 343–350, 2004.
© Springer-Verlag Berlin Heidelberg 2004

A DT-MRI dataset consists of noisy samples drawn from an underlying macroscopic diffusion tensor field, which is assumed continuous and smooth at a coarse anatomical scale. Therefore the measured effective tensor field describes voxel-averaged tensors, and in regions where fibers diverge or converge, bend or twist, branch or merge, there are disparities between the measured macroscopic tensor field and the real heterogeneous microscopic field [3].

In many applications, such as fiber-tract organization or statistical estimation of histological and physiological MRI parameters (e.g. principal diffusivities), it would be desirable to work with higher resolution images. However, a DT-MRI dataset usually have low resolution, and upsampling techniques are needed.

DT-MRI upsampling is a problem that has been discussed before. For example, in [4] a continuous tensor field approximation from a discrete set of noisy DT-MRI measurements is proposed. But the upsampled tensor field is not guaranteed to be positive-semidefinite at all points within the imaging volume and the boundaries, where diffusion properties change abruptly, are not preserved.

In this paper we propose a new anisotropic interpolation technique for DT-MRI and other positive semidefinite (PSD) tensor data. Interpolation is normally performed by weighting local signal samples according to some rule (linear, cubic, etc.). The idea behind the approach presented here is to weigh the samples in the direction of maximum variation (e.g. across and edge) less than in the orthogonal direction (e.g. along the edge) in order to reduce inter-region blurring. In our scheme this is achieved by using a metric defined from a local structure tensor estimated from tensor data. In the experiments below the local structure tensor is obtained following a recent approach proposed in [5].

Furthermore, since weights naturally are constrained to be positive, if the tensors in the input tensor field are PSD, the interpolated tensors will be PSD as well. It is important to note that this idea can be extended to more general anisotropic tensor estimation problems.

This paper is organized as follows: First, we present the tensor data interpolation problem. Then, we briefly review our recently published approach to tensor coding the local structure of tensor fields, which will prove essential in the new interpolator proposed in this paper and presented in the next section. Finally, illustrative results from synthetic and real DT-MRI data are also presented.

2   DT-MRI Interpolation

Interpolating DT-MRI data requires estimating the effective diffusion tensor at unsampled points in order to obtain an upsampled DT-MRI field, with the constraint that the interpolated field is PSD. Of course, it is desirable that boundaries are preserved, something that is not achieved with simple interpolation algorithms.

Our approach to interpolate assumes that the unknown tensor in an upsampled point can be estimated as a linear combination of tensor data sampled from surrounding locations, i.e.,

$$\hat{\mathbf{D}}(\mathbf{x}) = \frac{\sum_{i=1}^{n} \omega_i \mathbf{D}(\mathbf{x_i})}{\sum_{i=1}^{n} \omega_i}, \tag{1}$$

where $\mathbf{x}$ is the interpolation point in our reference system, $\mathbf{x_i}$ the samples position, n the number of samples used to interpolate, and ω_i the weights of those samples. Different interpolators and estimators assign different weights to samples. In some cases it is possible to obtain very efficient separable kernels. Nevertheless, in order to preserve edges, the local structure should be accounted for, and the estimator must be adaptive, with weights changing from one location to another.

Consider for example the weights to be obtained as inversely proportional to the squared distance to the sample,

$$\omega_i = \frac{1}{(\mathbf{x} - \mathbf{x_i})^T (\mathbf{x} - \mathbf{x_i})}. \tag{2}$$

This inverse squared distance interpolator is usual in many applications with conventional scalar images, but it smooths boundaries and other highly structured regions. If only distance to the sample is accounted for, the estimator mixes samples drawn from areas that can be very different even though they are close, eg. samples from two sides of an edge. Therefore an analysis of the local complexity of the signal is necessary prior to assigning weights to samples in order to avoid this behavior. There are several alternatives to local structure analysis in scalar data, including simple gradient computations, and we have selected the one proposed in [6,7] due to its good properties such as phase invariance and its advantages to gradient measures [7]. This scheme encodes local structure from scalar data in a second order PSD tensor field. Our approach to anisotropic interpolation, and presented for the first time here, makes use of the local structure tensor field to adaptively change the interpolation weights.

In order to interpolate tensor data we follow a similar approach, though now we use a generalization of the previous local structure analysis scheme we published recently for tensor data in [5]. Now, again, local structure is encoded in a second order PSD tensor field.

For the sake of simplicity, and in order to keep the computational burden as low as possible, the interpolation is based on the 4 nearest samples in 2D and on the 8 nearest samples in 3D; this could obviously be extended easily to larger neighborhoods. For regular discrete arrays, such as with DT-MRI data, the interpolated point is located in the center of the pixel/voxel or on an edge/side. Interpolation is carried out in successive sweeps for interpolation in centers, edges and sides.

3   Local Structure Estimation in Vector and Tensor Data

Edges in vector and higher order tensor data (multivalued data) can be defined as regions in the dataset where the signal changes abruptly, and similarly to the scalar case, a local structure tensor can be defined and estimated for such data. As will be described in more detail below, the new interpolation scheme presented in this paper uses the local structure to infer a local metric for the calculation of sample distances.

The local structure tensor proposed by Knutsson [6] is coded by a second order symmetric positive-semidefinite tensor $\mathbf{T}$, represented with respect to a tensor basis $\{\mathbf{M}^k\}$: $\mathbf{T} = \sum_k \|q_k\| \, \mathbf{M}^k$. The coordinates $\|q_k\|$ are the magnitudes of the outputs of a set of multidimensional spherically separable quadrature filters applied to the scalar field, which are maximum in the high structure regions.

The set of quadrature filters is defined in the Fourier domain by:

$$Q(\omega)_k = \begin{cases} e^{(\frac{-4}{B^2 ln2})(ln^2(\frac{\|\omega\|}{\|\omega_o\|}))} \cdot (\hat{\omega}^T \hat{\mathbf{n}}_k)^2 & if \; \hat{\omega}^T \hat{\mathbf{n}}_k > 0 \\ 0 & otherwise \,, \end{cases} \tag{3}$$

where $\hat{\mathbf{n}}_k$ is the unitary vector defining the direction of each quadrature filter, and where w denotes the frequency vector. These filters can be seen as an oriented Gaussian function in a logarithmic scale, centered at $\|\omega_o\|$ and with bandwidth B. The tensor basis elements $\mathbf{M}^k$ are defined by the filter directions $\hat{\mathbf{n}}_k$. They are defined as the *dual tensor basis* to the tensor basis defined by the outer products of these filter directions, $\{\hat{\mathbf{n}}_k \hat{\mathbf{n}}_k^T\}$. More details about how to calculate the elements $\mathbf{M}^k$ can be found in [8].

In order to evenly cover the local spectrum of the dataset, Knutsson proposed to use filter directions defined by the vertexes of the hexagon in 2D, and the icosahedron in 3D.

For an n-dimensional scalar dataset, the minimum number of quadrature filters required is $\frac{n(n+1)}{2}$, and the local structure tensor can be written as:

$$\mathbf{T} = \sum_{k=1}^{n(n+1)/2} \|q_k\| \, \mathbf{M}^k \,. \tag{4}$$

Recently we extended the scalar approach to tensor valued data [5] where the local structure tensor is defined by:

$$\mathbf{T} = \sum_{k=1}^{n(n+1)/2} \left(\sum_{xyz..n} \|q_{[k]xyz..n}\|^2 \right)^{\frac{1}{2}} \mathbf{M}^k \,, \tag{5}$$

and subscripts $xyz..n$ are associated to the components of the tensor field.

4   Anisotropic Interpolation Weighted by Local Structure

The local structure tensor field consists of a field of second-order symmetric PSD tensors, which can be associated with ellipsoids. These ellipsoids tend to be big

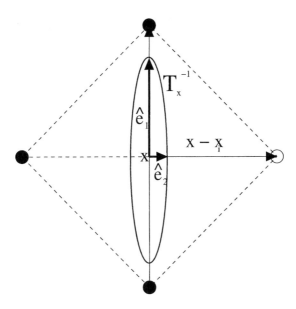

Fig. 1. Regular grid with tensors from different regions represented as white and black dots, respectively.

when there are steep changes in the signal and small otherwise. Moreover, the ellipsoids are elongated in the direction of maximum signal variation. Rounder tensors either mean two or more directions of signal variation (e.g. a corner) or no significant direction of variation (e.g. homogeneous signal). The local structure tensor can therefore be used to control how samples are combined when building signal estimators and, in particular, samples on two different sides of a strong edge should not be combined.

In this work, we propose to use the inverse of the local structure tensor as a metric tensor. The inversion corresponds to a $\pi/2$ radians rotation of the associated ellipsoid, and it is necessary to weigh the samples along the direction of maximum signal variation less than those in the orthogonal one. This is illustrated in Fig. 1, where tensors from different regions are represented as black and white dots in a regular grid. As it can be seen, although the distance between the interpolated point and data samples is the same, their contributions are not.

Hence, the weights for the linear combination in (1) are computed as

$$\omega_i = (\mathbf{x} - \mathbf{x_i})^T \mathbf{T_x}^{-1} (\mathbf{x} - \mathbf{x_i}), \tag{6}$$

where $T_{\mathbf{x}}$ denotes the local structure tensor at the interpolation point.

Since these weights are positive (the metric tensors are positive semidefinite), the interpolated tensors are PSD if input tensors are.

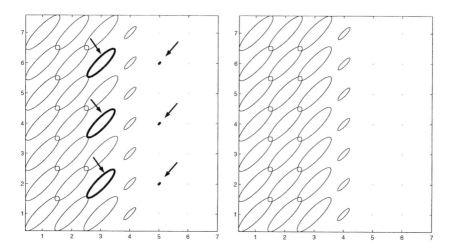

Fig. 2. Results from interpolation of tensor valued data using linear interpolation (left), and anisotropic interpolation (right).

5   Results

In this section, we present some experiments with synthetic and clinical DT-MRI data.

Synthetic Data. To assess our approach in the presence of edges, we perform interpolation of a tensor field consisting of a step edge with constant tensors on one side and zero tensors on the other side. In figure 2 we compare interpolation using linear interpolation (left) with the approach presented in this paper (right). To estimate the local structure tensor field with (5), we use the values $\| \omega_0 \| = \frac{\pi}{8}$, and $B = 2$ in (3). The quadrature filters are oriented in the directions pointing to the vertexes of a hexagon. Notice that the edge is smeared out further using linear interpolation compared to the proposed method using the inverse structure tensor as a local metric.

DT-MRI Data. The DT-MRI data was obtained at Brigham & Women's Hospital (Boston (MA) - USA) from a GE Signa 1.5 Tesla Horizon Echospeed 5.6 system with standard 2.2 Gauss/cm field gradients. The voxel resolution is 0.85 mm×0.85 mm×5 mm.

A central area in an axial slice (see Fig. 3, left) is then zoomed (right). Again edges are correctly preserved by the interpolation algorithm.

6   Conclusions

Interpolation is essential for many important tasks managing digital imagery and, in particular for data of low resolution such as clinical DT-MRI data. In

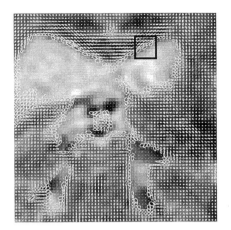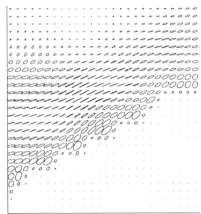

Fig. 3. DT-MRI 64×64 slice of the *corpus callosum* superposed over the corresponding MRI T2 image (left) and a zoomed part of the central area (right).

this paper we present a new method to interpolate a tensor field, preserving boundaries and assuring the positive-semidefinite constraint. Our approach interpolates tensors by using the natural neighbors of the interpolation point, in a regular grid, with weights proportional to the inverse squared distance between the samples and the interpolation point, using the inverse of a generalization of the local structure tensor as a metric to compute the distance.

This scheme has been applied to synthetic and *in vivo* DT-MRI data with very encouraging results.

The ideas presented in this work can be extended to more general problems involving anisotropic estimation from digital image data (scalar, vector, and tensor data). We are currently working on such extensions.

Acknowledgements. This work was supported by a FPU grant at the Spanish Ministry of Education AP2002-2774, the Spanish Ministry of Science and Technology and European Commission, co-funded grant TIC-2001-38008-C02-01, and the US grants NIH P41-RR13218 and CIMIT.

References

1. Le Bihan D., Mangin J.-F., Poupon C., Clark C.A., Pappata S., Molko N. and Chabriat H.: Diffusion tensor imaging: Concepts and applications. Magn. Reson. Imaging J. **13** (2001) 534–546
2. Basser P.J., Pajevic S., Pierpaoli C. and Aldroubi A.: Fiber tract following in the human brain using DT-MRI data. IEICE Trans. Inf. & Sist. **1** (2002) 15–21
3. Pierpaoli C. and Basser P.J.: Toward a quantitative assesment of diffusion anisotropy. Magn. Reson. Med. **36** (1996) 893–906

4. Pajevic S., Aldroubi A., and Basser P.J.: A continuous tensor field approximation of discrete DT-MRI data for extracting microstructural and architectural features of tissue. Journal of Magnetic Resonance **154** (2002) 85–100
5. Rodriguez-Florido M.A., Westin C.-F., and Ruiz-Alzola J.: DT-MRI regularization using anisotropic tensor field filtering. In: 2004 IEEE International Symposium on Biomedical Imaging - April 15-18 - Arlington,VA (USA). (2004) 336–339
6. Knutsson, H.: Representing local structure using tensors. In: 6th Scandinavian Conference on Image Analysis. Oulu, Finland. (1989) 244–251
7. Knutsson H., and Andersson M.: What's so good about quadrature filters? In: 2003 IEEE International Conference on Image Processing. (2003)
8. Westin, C.F., Richolt, J., Moharir, V., Kikinis, R.: Affine adaptive filtering of CT data. Medical Image Analysis **4** (2000) 161–172

3D Bayesian Regularization of Diffusion Tensor MRI Using Multivariate Gaussian Markov Random Fields

Marcos Martín-Fernández[1,2], Carl-Fredrik Westin[2], and
Carlos Alberola-López[1]*

[1] Image Processing Lab. University of Valladolid
47011 Valladolid (SPAIN) {marcma, caralb}@tel.uva.es
[2] Lab. of Mathematics in Imaging, Brighman and Women's Hospital,
Harvard Medical School
02115 Boston, MA. (USA) {marcma,westin}@bwh.harvard.edu

Abstract. 3D Bayesian regularization applied to diffusion tensor MRI is presented here. The approach uses Markov Random Field ideas and is based upon the definition of a 3D neighborhood system in which the spatial interactions of the tensors are modeled. As for the prior, we model the behavior of the tensor fields by means of a 6D multivariate Gaussian local characteristic. As for the likelihood, we model the noise process by means of conditionally independent 6D multivariate Gaussian variables. Those models include inter-tensor correlations, intra-tensor correlations and colored noise. The solution tensor field is obtained by using the simulated annealing algorithm to achieve the maximum *a posteriori* estimation. Several experiments both on synthetic and real data are presented, and performance is assessed with mean square error measure.

1 Introduction

Diffusion Tensor (DT) Magnetic Resonance Imaging (MRI) is a volumetric imaging modality in which the quantity assigned to each voxel of the volume scanned is not a scalar, but a tensor that describes local water diffusion. Tensors have direct geometric interpretations, and this serves as a basis to characterize local structure in different tissues. The procedure by which tensors are obtained can be consulted elsewhere [2]. The result of such a process is, ideally speaking, a 3×3 symmetric positive-semidefinite (psd) matrix.

Tensors support information of the underlying anisotropy within the data. As a matter of fact, several measures of such anisotropy have been proposed using tensors to make things easier to interpret; see, for instance, [2,10]. However, these measures rely on the ideal behavior of the tensors, which may be, in cases, far from reality due to some sources of noise that may be present in the imaging process itself. As was pointed out in [8], periodic beats of the cerebro-spinal fluid and partial volume effects may add a non-negligible amount of noise to the data,

---

* To whom correspondence should be addressed.

C. Barillot, D.R. Haynor, and P. Hellier (Eds.): MICCAI 2004, LNCS 3216, pp. 351–359, 2004.
© Springer-Verlag Berlin Heidelberg 2004

and the result is that the hypothesis of psd may not be valid. The authors are aware of this fact, and that some regularization procedures have been proposed in the past [4,5,6,7,8,10].

In this paper we focus on regularization of DT maps using Markov Random Fields (MRFs) [3]; other regularization philosophies exist (see, for instance, [9] and [11] and references therein) although they will not be discussed in the paper. About MRFs we are aware of the existence of other Markovian approaches to this problem [7,8], in which the method presented is called by the authors the *Spaghetti model*. These papers propose an interesting optimization model for data regularization. We have recently presented two Bayesian MRF approaches to regularization of DT maps [4,5]. The former is a 2D method based on Gaussian assumptions. That method operates independently on each tensor component. The latter approach is also a 2D method in which the psd condition is imposed naturally by the model. In this method two entities are regularized, namely, the linear component of the tensor and the angle of the eigenvector which corresponds to the principal eigenvalue.

In the present work we generalize those models to 3D and, furthermore, we extend them to take into account the intra-tensor relationships. We regularize the 6 elements of each tensor of the volume defining 6D Gaussian statistics for the prior and a 6D Gaussian noise model for the likelihood (transition) under 3D spatial neighborhood Markov system. Then, by means of the maximum *a posteriori* estimation —obtained with the simulated annealing algorithm— the solution tensor field is obtained. A theoretical statistical modeling of tensors is also proposed in [1] by means of a multivariate normal distribution. Nevertheless, this modeling is not presented there as a regularization method but as a statistical model itself, but stressing the idea of using tensor operations to reveal relationships in the tensor components.

2   Prior Model

The non-observable regularized tensor field is represented by a 5D random matrix $\mathbf{X}$ with dimensions $3 \times 3 \times M \times N \times P$ of a volume of dimensions $M \times N \times P$. Each volume element (voxel) is represented by a random tensor given by the 3×3 matrix

$$\mathbf{X}(m,n,p) = \begin{pmatrix} X_{11}(m,n,p) & X_{12}(m,n,p) & X_{13}(m,n,p) \\ X_{21}(m,n,p) & X_{22}(m,n,p) & X_{23}(m,n,p) \\ X_{31}(m,n,p) & X_{32}(m,n,p) & X_{33}(m,n,p) \end{pmatrix} \tag{1}$$

with $1 \leq m \leq M$, $1 \leq n \leq N$ and $1 \leq p \leq P$. Each tensor matrix $\mathbf{X}(m,n,p)$ is symmetric so that $X_{ij}(m,n,p) = X_{ji}(m,n,p)$, with $1 \leq i,j \leq 3$, thus each tensor has 6 distinct random variables. The total number of different random variables of the field $\mathbf{X}$ is $6MNP$. Now, we define a rearrangement matrix operator $\mathbf{LT}$ (lower triangular part) in order to extract the 6 different elements of each tensor and to regroup them as a 6×1 column vector, defining $\mathbf{X}_{LT}(m,n,p)$ as

$$\mathbf{X}_{LT}(m,n,p) = \mathbf{LT}\big[\mathbf{X}(m,n,p)\big] = \begin{pmatrix} X_{11}(m,n,p) \\ X_{21}(m,n,p) \\ X_{31}(m,n,p) \\ X_{22}(m,n,p) \\ X_{32}(m,n,p) \\ X_{33}(m,n,p) \end{pmatrix} \tag{2}$$

By performing the operation just defined to each tensor, a 4D random matrix $\mathbf{X}_{LT}$ with dimensions $6 \times M \times N \times P$ is defined without repeated elements. In order to formulate the probability density function (PDF) of the tensor field we need to rearrange the tensor field $\mathbf{X}_{LT}$ as a column vector, so we define a new rearrangement matrix operator $\mathbf{CV}$ (column vector) to achieve that as

$$\mathbf{X}_{CV} = \mathbf{CV}\big[\mathbf{X}_{LT}\big] \tag{3}$$

so $\mathbf{X}_{CV}$ will be a $K \times 1$ random vector which represents the whole tensor field, with $K = 6MNP$.

Now, we hypothesize that the prior PDF of the non-observable tensor field $\mathbf{X}_{CV}$ will be the K-dimensional multivariate Gauss-MRF with given $K \times 1$ mean vector $\boldsymbol{\mu}_{\mathbf{X}_{CV}}$ and $K \times K$ covariance matrix $\mathbf{C}_{\mathbf{X}_{CV}}$.

As dependencies are local (the field is assumed a spatial MRF) the matrix $\mathbf{C}_{\mathbf{X}_{CV}}$ will be sparse so it is more convenient in practice to work with the local characteristics of the field. To that end, we define a 3D neighborhood system $\boldsymbol{\delta}(m,n,p)$ for each site (voxel), homogeneous and with L neighbors, i.e., each $\boldsymbol{\delta}(m,n,p)$ is a set of L triplet indices. We also define the sets of neighboring random vectors $\boldsymbol{\delta}\mathbf{X}_{LT}(m,n,p)$ as

$$\boldsymbol{\delta}\mathbf{X}_{LT}(m,n,p) = \Big\{ \mathbf{X}_{LT}(m',n',p'), (m',n',p') \in \boldsymbol{\delta}(m,n,p) \Big\} \tag{4}$$

Under these assumptions the local characteristic of the field is given by the following 6-dimensional multivariate conditional Gauss-MRF

$$p\Big(\mathbf{X}_{LT}(m,n,p)\Big|\boldsymbol{\delta}\mathbf{X}_{LT}(m,n,p)\Big) = \frac{1}{8\pi^3\sqrt{\big|\mathbf{C}_{\mathbf{X}_{LT}}(m,n,p)\big|}} \exp\Big\{-\frac{1}{2}\Big(\mathbf{X}_{LT}(m,n,p)$$

$$-\boldsymbol{\mu}_{\mathbf{X}_{LT}}(m,n,p)\Big)^T \mathbf{C}_{\mathbf{X}_{LT}}^{-1}(m,n,p)\Big(\mathbf{X}_{LT}(m,n,p) - \boldsymbol{\mu}_{\mathbf{X}_{LT}}(m,n,p)\Big)\Big\} \tag{5}$$

where the operator T stands for matrix transpose and with

$$\boldsymbol{\mu}_{\mathbf{X}_{LT}}(m,n,p) = \frac{1}{L} \sum_{(m',n',p')\in\boldsymbol{\delta}(m,n,p)} \mathbf{X}_{LT}(m',n',p') \tag{6}$$

the 6×1 local mean vector and

$$\mathbf{C}_{\mathbf{X}_{LT}}(m,n,p) = \frac{1}{L}\sum_{(m',n',p')\in\boldsymbol{\delta}(m,n,p)} \mathbf{X}_{LT}(m',n',p')\mathbf{X}_{LT}^T(m',n',p') - \boldsymbol{\mu}_{\mathbf{X}_{LT}}(m,n,p)\boldsymbol{\mu}_{\mathbf{X}_{LT}}^T(m,n,p) \tag{7}$$

the 6×6 local covariance matrix both estimated with the ML method.

3   Transition Model

The non-regularized observed tensor field $\mathbf{Y}_{CV}$ is given by

$$\mathbf{Y}_{CV} = \mathbf{X}_{CV} + \mathbf{N}_{CV} \tag{8}$$

being $\mathbf{X}_{CV}$ the regularized non-observable tensor field and $\mathbf{N}_{CV}$ the noise tensor field. We suppose that the noise tensor field is independent of the regularized non-observable tensor field. The transition model is given by the conditional PDF of the observed tensor field given the non-observed tensor field which is assumed to be a K-dimensional multivariate Gauss-MRF with given $K \times 1$ mean vector $\mathbf{X}_{CV}$ and $K \times K$ covariance matrix $\mathbf{C}_{\mathbf{N}_{CV}}$.

In the transition model we can also exploit the spatial dependencies of the MRF to determine the transition local characteristic of the tensor field. For that PDF the following conditional independence property will be assumed

$$p\Big(\mathbf{Y}_{LT}(m,n,p)\Big|\mathbf{X}_{LT}(m,n,p), \boldsymbol{\delta}\mathbf{X}_{LT}(m,n,p)\Big) = p\Big(\mathbf{Y}_{LT}(m,n,p)\Big|\mathbf{X}_{LT}(m,n,p)\Big) \tag{9}$$

That PDF is given by a 6-dimensional multivariate conditional Gauss-MRF as

$$p\Big(\mathbf{Y}_{LT}(m,n,p)\Big|\mathbf{X}_{LT}(m,n,p)\Big) = \frac{1}{8\pi^3 \sqrt{|\mathbf{C}_{\mathbf{N}_{LT}}|}} \exp\Big\{ -\frac{1}{2}\Big(\mathbf{Y}_{LT}(m,n,p)$$

$$-\mathbf{X}_{LT}(m,n,p)\Big)^T \mathbf{C}_{\mathbf{N}_{LT}}^{-1} \Big(\mathbf{Y}_{LT}(m,n,p) - \mathbf{X}_{LT}(m,n,p)\Big)\Big\} \tag{10}$$

where the local 6×6 noise covariance matrix $\mathbf{C}_{\mathbf{N}_{LT}} = \mathbf{C}_{\mathbf{Y}_{LT}|\mathbf{X}_{LT}}$ is supposed to be homogeneous, that is, independent of the triplet indices (m,n,p). That covariance matrix has to be estimated from the observed tensor field $\mathbf{Y}_{CV}$. The proposed estimator is

$$\mathbf{C}_{\mathbf{N}_{LT}} = \lambda \mathbf{C}_{\mathbf{N}_{\mathrm{mean}}} + (1-\lambda)\mathbf{C}_{\mathbf{N}_{\mathrm{min}}} \tag{11}$$

with $0 \le \lambda \le 1$ a free parameter setting the degree of regularization (low λ means low regularization). The 6×6 covariance matrix $\mathbf{C}_{\mathbf{N}_{\mathrm{mean}}}$ is given by

$$\mathbf{C}_{\mathbf{N}_{\mathrm{mean}}} = \frac{6}{K} \sum_{m=1}^{M} \sum_{n=1}^{N} \sum_{p=1}^{P} \mathbf{C}_{\mathbf{Y}_{LT}}(m,n,p) \tag{12}$$

where $\mathbf{C}_{\mathbf{Y}_{LT}}(m,n,p)$ is given by the ML method following the equations (6) and (7) replacing all the $\mathbf{X}$ variables with $\mathbf{Y}$. The 6×6 covariance matrix $\mathbf{C}_{\mathbf{N}_{\mathrm{min}}}$ is given by

$$\mathbf{C}_{\mathbf{N}_{\mathrm{min}}} = \mathbf{C}_{\mathbf{Y}_{LT}}(m_1, n_1, p_1) \tag{13}$$

with the triplet indices (m_1, n_1, p_1) given by

$$(m_1, n_1, p_1) = \arg \min_{m,n,p} \mathrm{TR}\big[\mathbf{C}_{\mathbf{Y}_{LT}}(m,n,p)\big] \tag{14}$$

where the TR operator stands for matrix trace.

4   Posterior Model

Bayes' theorem lets us write

$$p\big(\mathbf{X}_{CV}\big|\mathbf{Y}_{CV}\big) = \frac{p\big(\mathbf{Y}_{CV}\big|\mathbf{X}_{CV}\big)p\big(\mathbf{X}_{CV}\big)}{p\big(\mathbf{Y}_{CV}\big)} \tag{15}$$

for the posterior PDF, where $p\big(\mathbf{Y}_{CV}\big)$ depends only on $\mathbf{Y}_{CV}$ known.

The posterior PDF $p\big(\mathbf{X}_{CV}\big|\mathbf{Y}_{CV}\big)$ is a K-dimensional multivariate Gauss-MRF with given $K \times 1$ posterior mean vector $\boldsymbol{\mu}_{\mathbf{X}_{CV}|\mathbf{Y}_{CV}}$ and $K \times K$ posterior covariance matrix $\mathbf{C}_{\mathbf{X}_{CV}|\mathbf{Y}_{CV}}$.

In the Gaussian case the maximum *a posteriori* (MAP) estimation is equal to the minimum mean square error (MMSE) estimation given both by

$$\mathbf{X}_{CV}^{\mathrm{MAP}} = \arg\max_{\mathbf{X}_{CV}} p\big(\mathbf{X}_{CV}\big|\mathbf{Y}_{CV}\big) = \mathbf{X}_{CV}^{\mathrm{MMSE}} = E\big[\mathbf{X}_{CV}\big|\mathbf{Y}_{CV}\big] = \boldsymbol{\mu}_{\mathbf{X}_{CV}|\mathbf{Y}_{CV}} \tag{16}$$

In general $\mathbf{C}_{\mathbf{X}_{CV}}$, $\mathbf{C}_{\mathbf{N}_{CV}}$ and $\boldsymbol{\mu}_{\mathbf{X}_{CV}}$ are unfeasible to determine so we have to resort to the simulated annealing (SA) algorithm to iteratively finding the solution tensor field. These algorithms are based on iteratively visiting all the sites (voxels) by sampling the posterior local characteristic of the field under a logarithmic cooling schedule given by a temperature parameter T. For determining that posterior local characteristic we can resort to the Bayes' theorem again

$$p\Big(\mathbf{X}_{LT}(m,n,p)\Big|\mathbf{Y}_{LT}(m,n,p), \boldsymbol{\delta}\mathbf{X}_{LT}(m,n,p)\Big)$$

$$= \frac{p\Big(\mathbf{Y}_{LT}(m,n,p)\Big|\mathbf{X}_{LT}(m,n,p)\Big)p\Big(\mathbf{X}_{LT}(m,n,p)\Big|\boldsymbol{\delta}\mathbf{X}_{LT}(m,n,p)\Big)}{p\Big(\mathbf{Y}_{LT}(m,n,p)\Big|\boldsymbol{\delta}\mathbf{X}_{LT}(m,n,p)\Big)} \tag{17}$$

where $p\Big(\mathbf{Y}_{LT}(m,n,p)\Big|\boldsymbol{\delta}\mathbf{X}_{LT}(m,n,p)\Big)$ depends only on $\mathbf{Y}_{LT}(m,n,p)$ known.

That posterior local characteristic is a 6-dimensional multivariate Gauss-MRF given by

$$p\Big(\mathbf{X}_{LT}(m,n,p)\Big|\mathbf{Y}_{LT}(m,n,p), \boldsymbol{\delta}\mathbf{X}_{LT}(m,n,p)\Big) = \frac{1}{8\pi^3\sqrt{T\big|\mathbf{C}_{\mathbf{X}_{LT}|\mathbf{Y}_{LT}}(m,n,p)\big|}}$$

$$\cdot \exp\Bigg\{ -\frac{1}{2T}\Big(\mathbf{X}_{LT}(m,n,p) - \boldsymbol{\mu}_{\mathbf{X}_{LT}|\mathbf{Y}_{LT}}(m,n,p)\Big)^T$$

$$\cdot \mathbf{C}_{\mathbf{X}_{LT}|\mathbf{Y}_{LT}}^{-1}(m,n,p)\Big(\mathbf{X}_{LT}(m,n,p) - \boldsymbol{\mu}_{\mathbf{X}_{LT}|\mathbf{Y}_{LT}}(m,n,p)\Big)\Bigg\} \tag{18}$$

with

$$\boldsymbol{\mu}_{\mathbf{X}_{LT}|\mathbf{Y}_{LT}}(m,n,p) = \Big[\mathbf{C}_{\mathbf{X}_{LT}}(m,n,p) + \mathbf{C}_{\mathbf{N}_{LT}}(m,n,p)\Big]^{-1}$$

$$\cdot \Big[\mathbf{C}_{\mathbf{N}_{LT}}(m,n,p)\boldsymbol{\mu}_{\mathbf{X}_{LT}}(m,n,p) + \mathbf{C}_{\mathbf{X}_{LT}}\mathbf{Y}_{LT}(m,n,p)\Big] \tag{19}$$

the 6×1 posterior local mean vector and

$$\mathbf{C}_{\mathbf{X}_{LT}|\mathbf{Y}_{LT}}(m,n,p)=\left[\mathbf{C}_{\mathbf{X}_{LT}}(m,n,p)+\mathbf{C}_{\mathbf{N}_{LT}}(m,n,p)\right]^{-1}\mathbf{C}_{\mathbf{X}_{LT}}(m,n,p)\mathbf{C}_{\mathbf{N}_{LT}}(m,n,p) \tag{20}$$

the 6×6 posterior local covariance matrix. Now, both the local mean vector $\boldsymbol{\mu}_{\mathbf{X}_{LT}|\mathbf{Y}_{LT}}(m,n,p)$ and the local covariance matrix $\mathbf{C}_{\mathbf{X}_{LT}|\mathbf{Y}_{LT}}(m,n,p)$ can be easily determined.

For the SA algorithm we need to sample the posterior local characteristic given by equation (18). First we get a sample of a white normal random vector with zero mean and identity covariance matrix, obtaining the 6×1 vector $\mathbf{U}$. The sample we are looking for is thus given by

$$\mathbf{X}_{LT}(m,n,p) = \sqrt{T}\,\mathbf{D}_{\mathbf{X}_{LT}|\mathbf{Y}_{LT}}(m,n,p)\mathbf{U} + \boldsymbol{\mu}_{\mathbf{X}_{LT}|\mathbf{Y}_{LT}}(m,n,p) \tag{21}$$

with $\mathbf{D}_{\mathbf{X}_{LT}|\mathbf{Y}_{LT}}(m,n,p)$ a 6×6 matrix given by

$$\mathbf{D}_{\mathbf{X}_{LT}|\mathbf{Y}_{LT}}(m,n,p) = \mathbf{Q}_{\mathbf{X}_{LT}|\mathbf{Y}_{LT}}(m,n,p)\boldsymbol{\Lambda}^{1/2}_{\mathbf{X}_{LT}|\mathbf{Y}_{LT}}(m,n,p) \tag{22}$$

where the 6×6 matrix $\mathbf{Q}_{\mathbf{X}_{LT}|\mathbf{Y}_{LT}}(m,n,p)$ has in its columns the eigenvectors of the covariance matrix $\mathbf{C}_{\mathbf{X}_{LT}|\mathbf{Y}_{LT}}(m,n,p)$. The 6×6 matrix $\boldsymbol{\Lambda}_{\mathbf{X}_{LT}|\mathbf{Y}_{LT}}(m,n,p)$ is diagonal having the corresponding eigenvalues in the principal diagonal. The notation $\boldsymbol{\Lambda}^{1/2}_{\mathbf{X}_{LT}|\mathbf{Y}_{LT}}(m,n,p)$ means a 6×6 diagonal matrix having the square root of the eigenvalues in the principal diagonal. The following relationship is satisfied

$$\mathbf{C}_{\mathbf{X}_{LT}|\mathbf{Y}_{LT}}(m,n,p)=\mathbf{Q}_{\mathbf{X}_{LT}|\mathbf{Y}_{LT}}(m,n,p)\boldsymbol{\Lambda}_{\mathbf{X}_{LT}|\mathbf{Y}_{LT}}(m,n,p)\mathbf{Q}^{T}_{\mathbf{X}_{LT}|\mathbf{Y}_{LT}}(m,n,p)$$
$$= \mathbf{D}_{\mathbf{X}_{LT}|\mathbf{Y}_{LT}}(m,n,p)\mathbf{D}^{T}_{\mathbf{X}_{LT}|\mathbf{Y}_{LT}}(m,n,p) \tag{23}$$

In order to assure the psd condition the SA algorithm is modified as follows: after visiting a tensor site, the condition is tested; if the test is not passed then the tensor is discarded and sampled again until the condition is satisfied.

5   Results

Two types of experiments will be presented, namely, a first experiment based on synthetic data to quantitatively measure how the regularization method works and a second experiment, in this case with DT-MRI data, in which we illustrate the extent of regularization this approach can achieve.

In figure 1(a) we can see the surface rendering of the synthetic tensor field used: it is an helix in which the internal voxels are mainly linear (anisotropic) and the external ones are spheric (isotropic). The surface shows the boundary points at which the transition between the linear and the spheric voxels takes place. Then, we have added a non-white noise tensor field, and the surface shown in figure 1(b) has been obtained. This figure clearly shows the presence of noise. The extra spots shown on that figure represent linear voxels which are outside

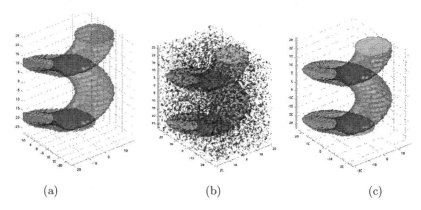

(a)   (b)   (c)

Fig. 1. (a) Linear component for the original synthetic helix tensor field. (b) Linear component for the noisy synthetic helix tensor field. (c) Linear component for the regularized synthetic helix tensor field.

the helix and spheric voxels which are inside. The regularization process allows us to obtain the result shown in figure 1(c). Although by visual inspection it is clear that the original data are fairly recovered, we have quantified the regularization process by measuring the mean square error (MSE) between the original and the noisy data, on one side, and between the original and the regularized field, on the other. The obtained values are 5.6 for the former and 1.9 for the latter. From these figures we can conclude that the noise is cleared out without losing details in the tensor field.

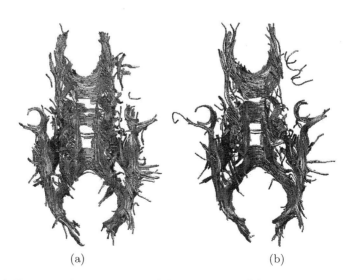

(a)   (b)

Fig. 2. (a) Tractography of the original DT-MRI data. (b) Tractography of the regularized data.

As for the second experiment, a 3D DT-MRI data acquisition is used. This data has an appreciable amount of noise that should be reduced. We have used an application that automatically extracts the tracts from the 3D DT-MRI data. In figure 2(a) we can see the tractography obtained. Due to the presence of noise and non-psd tensors, that application largely fails in the determination of the tracts. After applying the proposed regularization method the achieved result is the one shown in figure 2(b). The performance of the tractography application considerably increases after filtering the data, obtaining tracts which are visually correct. We have used a regularization parameter of $\lambda = 0.1$ and 20 iterations of the SA algorithm.

6   Conclusions

In this paper we have described the application of the multivariate normal distribution to tensor fields for the regularization of noisy tensor data by using a 3D Bayesian model based on MRFs. The prior model, the transition and the posterior are theoretically proven. All the parameters are also estimated from the data during the optimization process. The free parameter λ allows us to select the amount of regularization needed depending on the level of detail. Two experiments have also been presented. The synthetic experiment enables us to measure the MSE improvement to assess the amount of regularization achieved.

Acknowledgments. The authors acknowledge the Comisión Interministerial de Ciencia y Tecnología for the research grant TIC2001-3808-C02-02, the NIH for the research grant P41-RR13218 and CIMIT. The first author also acknowledges the Fulbright Commission for the postdoc grant FU2003-0968.

References

1. P. J. Basser, S. Pajevic, A Normal Distribution for Tensor-Valued Random Variables: Application to Diffusion Tensor MRI, *IEEE Trans. on Medical Imaging*, Vol. 22, July 2003, pp. 785–794.
2. P. J. Basser, C. Pierpaoli, Microstructural and Physiological Features of Tissues Elucidated by Quantitative-Diffusion-Tensor MRI, *J. of Magnetic Resonance*, Ser. B, Vol. 111, June 1996, pp. 209–219.
3. S. Geman, D. Geman, Stochastic Relaxation, Gibbs Distributions and the Bayesian Restoration of Images, *IEEE Trans. on Pattern Analysis and Machine Intelligence*, Vol. 6, Nov. 1984, pp. 721–741.
4. M. Martín-Fernández, R. San José-Estépar, C. F. Westin, C. Alberola-López, A Novel Gauss-Markov Random Field Approach for Regularization of Diffusion Tensor Maps, *Lecture Notes in Computer Science*, Vol. 2809, 2003, pp. 506–517.
5. M. Martín-Fernández, C. Alberola-López, J. Ruiz-Alzola, C. F. Westin, Regularization of Diffusion Tensor Maps using a Non-Gaussian Markov Random Field Approach, *Lecture Notes in Computer Science*, Vol. 2879, 2003, pp. 92–100.
6. G. J. M. Parker, J. A. Schnabel, M. R. Symms, D. J. Werring, G. J. Barker, Nonlinear Smoothing for Reduction of Systematic and Random Errors in Diffusion Tensor Imaging, *J. of Magnetic Resonance Imaging*, Vol. 11, 2000, pp. 702–710.

7. C. Poupon, J. F. Mangin, V. Frouin, J. Regis, F. Poupon, M. Pachot-Clouard, D. Le Bihan, I. Bloch, Regularization of MR Diffusion Tensor Maps for Tracking Brain White Matter Bundles, in *Lecture Notes in Computer Science*, Vol. 1946, 1998, pp. 489–498.
8. C. Poupon, C. A. Clark, V. Frouin, J. Regis, D. Le Bihan, I. Bloch, J. F. Mangin, Regularization Diffusion-Based Direction Maps for the Tracking of Brain White Matter Fascicles, *NeuroImage*, Vol. 12, 2000, pp. 184–195.
9. D. Tschumperlé, R. Deriche, DT-MRI Images: Estimation, Regularization and Application, *Lecture Notes in Computer Science*, Vol. 2809, 2003, pp. 530–541.
10. C. F. Westin, S. E. Maier, H. Mamata, A. Nabavi, F. A. Jolesz, R. Kikinis, Processing and Visualization for Diffusion Tensor MRI, *Medical Image Analysis*, Vol. 6, June 2002. pp. 93–108.
11. C. F. Westin, H. Knuttson, Tensor Field Regularization using Normalized Convolution, *Lecture Notes in Computer Science*, Vol. 2809, 2003, pp. 564–572.

Interface Detection in Diffusion Tensor MRI

Lauren O'Donnell[1,2], W. Eric L. Grimson[1], and Carl-Fredrik Westin[1,3]

[1] MIT CSAIL
[2] Harvard-MIT Division of Health Sciences and Technology,
Cambridge MA, USA
odonnell@ai.mit.edu
[3] Laboratory of Mathematics in Imaging,
Brigham and Women's Hospital, Harvard Medical School, Boston MA, USA
westin@bwh.harvard.edu

Abstract. We present a new method for detecting the interface, or edge, structure present in diffusion MRI. Interface detection is an important first step for applications including segmentation and registration. Additionally, due to the higher dimensionality of tensor data, humans are visually unable to detect edges as easily as in scalar data, so edge detection has potential applications in diffusion tensor visualization. Our method employs the computer vision techniques of local structure filtering and normalized convolution. We detect the edges in the tensor field by calculating a generalized local structure tensor, based on the sum of the outer products of the gradients of the tensor components. The local structure tensor provides a rotationally invariant description of edge orientation, and its shape after local averaging describes the type of edge. We demonstrate the ability to detect not only edges caused by differences in tensor magnitude, but also edges between regions of different tensor shape. We demonstrate the method's performance on synthetic data, on major fiber tract boundaries, and in one gray matter region.

1 Introduction

The problem of interface detection in diffusion tensor imaging (DTI) is more complicated than the problem of interface detection in scalar images. This is because there are two types of interface. In DTI data, one would like to detect both interfaces due to changes in tensor orientation and interfaces due to changes in tensor magnitude. Furthermore, it would be ideal to control the relative effects of tensor magnitude and tensor orientation information on the output interfaces.

Potential applications of interface detection in MRI diffusion data are both the same as those in scalar data, and different. Segmentation and registration are two applications that are already known from scalar data. An application that is different is the detection of interfaces that may not be apparent to the human eye. In scalar data, a radiologist is the gold standard for interface detection. However with tensor data, the higher dimensionality of the data and the limitations of any tensor visualization technique may confound human edge detectors. Consequently it is truly useful to study methods of edge detection in

C. Barillot, D.R. Haynor, and P. Hellier (Eds.): MICCAI 2004, LNCS 3216, pp. 360–367, 2004.
© Springer-Verlag Berlin Heidelberg 2004

tensor fields, not just to automate tasks that could be laboriously performed by a human, but to actually enable localization of the interfaces at all.

There are many anatomical interfaces of interest in DTI. The most obvious are tract boundaries, for example the medial and lateral borders of the optic radiation. Another interface that is obvious is the border between the near-isotropic diffusion tensors in cerebrospinal fluid and neighboring tensors, for example those in white matter which have a more anisotropic shape. A very interesting and less obvious type of interface is that within gray matter. For example, it would be clinically interesting if borders of thalamic nuclei were directly detectable.

Related work on tensor interfaces includes one study which presents a method very similar to ours, but without addressing the difference between magnitude and orientation interfaces [4]. Their application is level set motion in a tensor field, and their results while nice show mainly interfaces due to tensor magnitude and do not address any anatomical features of interest. An earlier investigation of tensor field edge detection defines the tensor field gradient and its generalized correlation matrix, then applies these to point detection in DTI [14]. Another approach to defining edges using local structure in DTI was presented in the context of adaptive filtering [11]. Other interface detection in DTI includes the implied interfaces at the borders of tractographic paths [1,2,16]. Finally, any type of segmentation will output interfaces. Work on DTI segmentation includes two methods that have been presented for automatic segmentation of nuclei in thalamic gray matter. The first technique groups voxels using a combined tensor similarity and distance measure [20]. The second method classifies voxels based on their connection probabilities to segmented cortical regions [2]. Both methods produce beautiful results but to our knowledge there has been no work which looks at the local interface structure within the thalamus.

In this paper we present an extension of the method of local structure estimation to tensor-valued images using normalized convolution for estimating the gradients. We produce a new local structure tensor field which describes the interfaces present in the original data. We use the method of normalized convolution to reduce the overall dependence of our results on the magnitude of the tensors, in order to enable detection of both magnitude and orientation interfaces. We present results of our method on synthetic tensor data and anatomical diffusion tensor data.

2   Materials and Methods

2.1   Data Acquisition

DT-MRI scans of normal subjects were acquired using Line Scan Diffusion Imaging [6] on a 1.5 Tesla GE Echospeed system. The following scan parameters were used: rectangular 22 cm FOV (256x128 image matrix, 0.86 mm by 1.72 mm in-plane pixel size); slice thickness = 3 mm; inter-slice distance = 1 mm; receiver bandwidth = +/-6 kHz; TE = 70 ms; TR = 80 ms (effective TR = 2500 ms); scan time = 60 seconds/section. Between 20 and 40 axial slices were acquired covering the entire brain. This protocol provides diffusion data in 6 gradient directions as well as the corresponding T2-weighted image. All gradients and T2-weighted images are acquired simultaneously, and thus do not need any rigid registration prior to the tensor reconstruction process. Tensors are reconstructed as described in [17].

In addition, a synthetic dataset was created in matlab for the purpose of demonstrating edge detection based on orientation differences. The dataset consisted of a circle of nonzero diffusion tensors in a "sea" of background 0-valued tensors. The left half of the circle contained tensors whose major eigenvectors pointed vertically, while tensors in the right half of the circle had horizontal principal directions. The purpose of this test data is to demonstrate the results of the method on magnitude and orientation differences in the tensor field.

2.2   Local Image Structure

In two dimensions, local structure estimation has been used to detect and describe edges and corners [5]. The local structure in 2D is described in terms of dominant local orientation and isotropy, where isotropy means lack of dominant orientation. In three dimensions, local structure has been used to describe landmarks, rotational symmetries, and motion [7,3,8,12,13]. In addition to isotropy, it describes geometrical properties which have been used to guide the enhancement and segmentation of blood vessels in volumetric angiography datasets [10, 15], bone in CT images [18], and to the analysis of white matter in DTI [17].

Let the operator $\sum_a$ denote averaging in the local neighborhood a about the current spatial location. Then the local structure tensor for a scalar neigborhood can be estimated by

$$\sum_a \nabla I \nabla I^T \tag{1}$$

For multi-valued (vector) data, this formula extends straightforwardly to

$$\sum_k \sum_a \nabla I_k \nabla I_k^T = \sum_a \sum_k \nabla I_k \nabla I_k^T \tag{2}$$

where k indicates the component. For a tensor field with components D_{kl} the generalized local structure is then estimated by

$$T = \sum_a \sum_{kl} \nabla D_{kl} (\nabla D_{kl})^T \tag{3}$$

2.3   Normalized Convolution

Normalized convolution (NC) was introduced as a general method for filtering missing and uncertain data [9,19]. In NC, a signal certainty, c, is defined for the signal. Missing data is handled by setting the signal certainty to zero. This method can be viewed as locally solving a weighted least squares (WLS) problem, where the weights are defined by signal certainties and a spatially localizing mask. Here we estimate image gradients using normalized convolution.

A local description of a signal, f, can be defined using a weighted sum of basis functions b_k. Let B denote a matrix where these basis functions are stacked as column vectors. In NC the basis functions are spatially localized by a positive scalar mask denoted the "applicability function,"or a. Minimizing

$$\left\| W_a W_c (B\theta - f)) \right\| \tag{4}$$

results in the following WLS local neighborhood model:

$$f_0 = B(B^* W_a W_c B)^{-1} B^* W_a W_c f, \tag{5}$$

where W_a and W_c are diagonal matrices containing a and c respectively, and B^* is the conjugate transpose of B.

The coordinates θ describing the local signal $f_0 = B\theta$ are

$$\theta = (B^* W_a W_c B)^{-1} B^* W_a W_c f \tag{6}$$

The estimated coordinates are used in this paper to describe the gradient from planar basis functions, $b_1 = 1$, $b_2 = x$, $b_2 = y$, and $b_2 = z$, where x, y, z are local spatial coordinates. Since normalized convolution calculates the coordinates of data described locally using this basis, the last three coordinates correspond to the derivative in x, y, and z respectively.

2.4   Subvoxel Gradient Estimation

We can effectively calculate the gradient on a higher-resolution grid than the voxel resolution, using the separation of data and certainty to our advantage. The goal of using a higher-resolution grid is to increase the ability to detect edges that may be close together on the original grid. To "expand" the initial grid, we insert zero-valued tensors between data points. The operation of the rest of the algorithm is unchanged, since those points are simply treated as uncertain in the gradient computation. Empirically this gives improved results over a two-step process of first interpolating the tensor data and second calculating the local structure.

2.5   Procedure

First, for each DTI dataset local structure estimation was performed as described above using gradients from normalized convolution. We employed the trace of the diffusion tensors as the certainty measure. This method emphasizes tensor shape edges over diffusion-magnitude edges and aims to suppress border effects. Then regions of interest were expanded as described above for detection of spatially close edges, and the local structure estimation was run on these regions.

The choice of applicability function depends on the width of the edges of interest. Here we use a Gaussian function, and experiments were performed with standard deviations between one and two mm, and neighborhood sizes (in voxels)

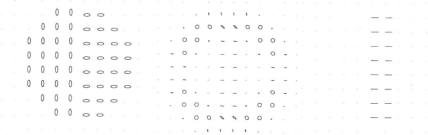

Fig. 1. Simulated data to show unwanted bias in local interface estimation in tensor data close to data borders. The leftmost image shows the input tensor data. The middle image is the local structure tensor estimated without normalized convolution, i.e. with no knowledge of data certainty. Note the unwanted responses on the border of the data, and how this affects the estimation of the interface between the to regions close to the border. The rightmost image shows the shape of the local structure tensors estimated with normalized convolution. Note that the interface is now correctly estimated between regions of tensor data and no border effects are present.

from 9 by 9 by 9 to 21 by 21 by 11. We aimed to match the variance to the size of the features of interest and to the data resolution. The neighborhood sizes were chosen to allow the Gaussian to fall smoothly to near zero at the boundaries. In order to perform subvoxel gradient estimation we found that inserting one or two zero voxels between known data points was useful. In practice, creating a larger grid than that gave little improvement and was computationally expensive.

3   Results

Here we demonstrate the performance of the method on synthetic data and we show selected results from diffusion tensor MRI data.

First we present an experiment showing the performance of the method on the synthetic data described in Section 2.1. The goal is to show that the algorithm will react only to edges that are accompanied by local confidence in the data.

Figure 1 demonstrates the result: the input tensors have both magnitude-type and orientation-type edges, but only the orientation-type edges are detected by the local structure estimation with normalized convolution. The certainty outside of the "circle" is proportional to the tensor trace which is zero there, so the method does not recognize the border of the circle. It detects only the edge caused by differences in tensor shape.

Figure 2 shows slices through the trace of the local structure tensor at many levels in an axial DTI dataset. Anatomical borders, including the following list, are detected. Note the bilateral cingulate bundles running in an anterior-posterior direction in the top middle slice. In the top right and lower left slice the corpus callosum can be seen. The anterior and posterior limbs of the internal capsule are seen in the lower left slice. Additionally the optic radiation and some brainstem structure can be seen in the lower right slice.

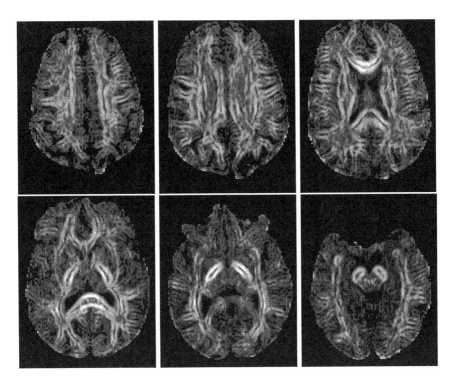

Fig. 2. Trace of the local structure tensor at several levels in an axial DTI dataset. Before filtering, the data was masked with a rough segmentation of the brain. Dark regions inside the brain, however, are not from masking but rather are regions of low edge magnitude.

One motivation for this work was interest in measuring the structure, if any, that is present in gray matter regions of a diffusion tensor dataset. The obvious choice for initial investigation is the thalamus because it is home to many nuclei which have characteristic connections to the rest of the brain, and hence some characteristic tensor orientation. We investigated the local structure in the thalamic region in three diffusion tensor datasets. The results were qualitatively similar and on some slices visually corresponded to the expected nuclear anatomy. One such slice is shown here alongside a 3D diagram of the thalamus and its nuclei.

4   Discussion

We have demonstrated a novel method for tissue interface detection in diffusion tensor MRI. By using a certainty field to define the importance of each tensor data point, it is possible to control the behavior of the edge detection, be insensitive to missing data, and produce subvoxel measurements. Another feature of this approach is that masks defining anatomical regions can be applied to the certainty field, removing the impact of surrounding tissue structures without

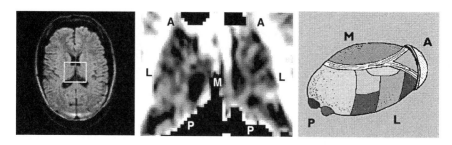

Fig. 3. DTI tissue interface detection in the region of the thalamus. The leftmost image is an axial diffusion-weighted MRI image. The white square outlines the location of the middle image, which displays the magnitude of the trace of the local structure tensor in the thalamic region. The ventricles have been masked and show in black (at the top and bottom of the image), while regions outside of the thalami with higher trace show as white. The image on the right is a diagram of the nuclei of the thalamus, adapted from www.phys.uni.torun.pl/ duch/ref/00-how-brain/. In the images the letters A, P, M, and L signify anterior, posterior, medial, and lateral, respectively.

obtaining erroneous responses from the interface of the segmentation border. This is important since these border effects may be magnitudes stronger than the changes of interest inside the structures. Here we choose to employ the tensor trace as the certainty measure, but it would be informative to compare the behavior of the method using other measures.

The presented method is able to detect boundaries of tracts such as the optic radiation, corpus callosum, cingulate bundles, and internal capsule. In addition preliminary results demonstrate some detectable structure in the gray matter region of the thalamus, but it is not clear at this point that these interfaces represent borders between thalamic nuclei.

Acknowledgments. We would like to thank the HST Neuroimaging Training Grant, NSF ERC CISST 8810-27499, and NAC grant number NIH P41 RR 13218.

References

1. P.J. Basser, S. Pajevic, C. Pierpaoli, J. Duda, and A. Aldroubi. In vivo fiber tractography using DT–MRI data. *Magnetic Resonance in Medicine*, 44:625–632, 2000.
2. TEJ Behrens, H Johansen-Berg, MW Woolrich, SM Smith, CAM Wheeler-Kingshott, PA Boulby, GJ Barker, EL Sillery, K Sheehan, O Ciccarelli, AJ Thompson, JM Brady, and PM Matthews. Non-invasive mapping of connections between human thalamus and cortex using diffusion imaging. *Nature Neuroscience*, 6:750–757, 2003.
3. J. Bigün, G. H. Granlund, and J. Wiklund. Multidimensional orientation: texture analysis and optical flow. *IEEE Transactions on Pattern Analysis and Machine Intelligence*, PAMI–13(8), August 1991.

4. C. Feddern, J. Weickert, and B. Burgeth. Level-set methods for tensor-valued images. In O. Faugeras and N. Paragios, editors, *Proc. Second IEEE Workshop on Variational, Geometric and Level Set Methods in Computer Vision*, pages 65–72, 2003.
5. W. Förstner. A feature based correspondence algorithm for image matching. *Int. Arch. Photogrammetry Remote Sensing*, 26(3):150–166, 1986.
6. H. Gudbjartsson, S. Maier, R. Mulkern, I.A. Morocz, S. Patz, and F. Jolesz. Line scan diffusion imaging. *Magnetic Resonance in Medicine*, 36:509–519, 1996.
7. H. Knutsson. Representing local structure using tensors. In *The 6th Scandinavian Conference on Image Analysis*, pages 244–251, Oulu, Finland, June 1989.
8. H. Knutsson, H. Bårman, and L. Haglund. Robust orientation estimation in 2D, 3D and 4D using tensors. In *Proceedings of Second International Conference on Automation, Robotics and Computer Vision, ICARCV'92*, Singapore, September 1992.
9. H. Knutsson and C-F. Westin. Normalized and differential convolution: Methods for interpolation and filtering of incomplete and uncertain data. In *Computer Vision and Pattern Recognition*, pages 515– 523, 1993.
10. T.M. Koller, G. Gerig, G. Szekely, and D. Dettwiler. Multiscale detection of curvilinear structures in 2D and 3D image data. In *Proc. ICCV'95*, pages 864–869, 1995.
11. Rodriguez-Florido M.A., Westin C.-F., and Ruiz-Alzola J. Dt-mri regularization using anisotropic tensor field filtering. In *IEEE International Symposium on Biomedical Imaging*, number 336339, pages 336–339, 2004.
12. R. Deriche O. Monga, R. Lengagne. Extraction of zero crossings of the curvature derivatives in volumetric 3D medical images: a multi-scale approach. In *Proc. IEEE Conf. Comp. Vision and Pattern Recognition*, pages 852–855, Seattle, Washington, USA, June 1994.
13. K. Rohr. Extraction of 3D anatomical point landmarks based on invariance principles. *Pattern Recognition*, 32:3–15, 1999.
14. J. Ruiz-Alzola, R. Kikinis, and C-F. Westin. Detection of point landmarks in multidimensional tensor data. *Signal Processing*, 81:2243–2247, 2001.
15. Y. Sato, S. Nakajima, N. Shiraga, H. Atsumi, S. Yoshida, T. Koller, G. Gerig, and R. Kikinis. Three-dimensional multiscale line filter for segmentation and visualization of curvilinear structures in medical images. *Medical Image Analysis*, 2(2):143–168, 1998.
16. Dave S. Tuch. *Diffusion MRI of Complex Tissue Structure*. PhD thesis, Division of Health Sciences and Technology, Massachusetts Institute of Technology, 2002.
17. C.-F. Westin, S.E. Maier, H. Mamata, A. Nabavi, F.A. Jolesz, and R. Kikinis. Processing and visualization of diffusion tensor MRI. *Medical Image Analysis*, 6(2):93–108, 2002.
18. C.-F. Westin, J. Richolt, V. Moharir, and R. Kikinis. Affine adaptive filtering of CT data. *Medical Image Analysis*, 4(2):161–172, 2000.
19. Carl-Fredrik Westin. *Multidimensional Signal Processing*. PhD thesis, Linkoping University, 1994.
20. M.R. Wiegell, D.S. Tuch, H.W.B. Larson, and V.J. Wedeen. Automatic segmentation of thalamic nuclei from diffusion tensor magnetic resonance imaging. *Neuroimage*, 19:391–402, 2003.

Clustering Fiber Traces Using Normalized Cuts

Anders Brun[1,4], Hans Knutsson[1], Hae-Jeong Park[2,3,4],
Martha E. Shenton[2], and Carl-Fredrik Westin[4]

[1] Department. of Biomedical Engineering, Linköping University, Sweden
{andbr,knutte}@imt.liu.se
[2] Clinical Neuroscience Division, Laboratory of Neuroscience,
Boston VA Health Care System-Brockton Division, Department of Psychiatry,
Harvard Medical School, Boston, MA
martha_shenton@hms.harvard.edu
[3] Dept. of Diagnostic Radiology, Yonsei University College of Medicine, Seoul, South Korea
parkhj@yumc.yonsei.ac.kr
[4] Laboratory of Mathematics in Imaging, Harvard Medical School, Boston, MA, USA
westin@bwh.harvard.edu

Abstract. In this paper we present a framework for unsupervised segmentation of white matter fiber traces obtained from diffusion weighted MRI data. Fiber traces are compared pairwise to create a weighted undirected graph which is partitioned into coherent sets using the normalized cut (*Ncut*) criterion. A simple and yet effective method for pairwise comparison of fiber traces is presented which in combination with the *Ncut* criterion is shown to produce plausible segmentations of both synthetic and real fiber trace data. Segmentations are visualized as colored stream-tubes or transformed to a segmentation of voxel space, revealing structures in a way that looks promising for future explorative studies of diffusion weighted MRI data.

1 Introduction

Diffusion Weighted MRI (DWI) makes it possible to non-invasively measure water diffusion within tissue. In a volume acquired using DWI, each voxel contains a diffusion tensor or other higher order descriptor for the local water diffusion. In fibrous tissue such as muscles and human brain white matter, water tend to diffuse less in the directions perpendicular to the fiber structure. This makes it possible to study the local fiber orientations indirectly by interpreting the water diffusion within the voxel. From DWI data it is therefore possible to create so called fiber traces from virtual particles, traveling along the direction of maximum diffusion, starting from a set of seed points [1,2,13], a.k.a fiber tracking. Performing fiber tracking in DWI data from the human brain gives valuable insights about fiber tract connectivity, useful in for instance surgical planning and for the study of various diseases such as schizophrenia.

In our experiments we have exclusively used data from so called diffusion tensor MRI (DT-MRI) [9], where the diffusion inside a voxel is described by a second order symmetric positive definite 3×3 tensor, which may be thought of as an ellipsoid. An elongated ellipsoid represent high diffusivity in a particular direction, which may be interpreted as the dominant orientation of the fibers going thru that particular voxel.

C. Barillot, D.R. Haynor, and P. Hellier (Eds.): MICCAI 2004, LNCS 3216, pp. 368–375, 2004.

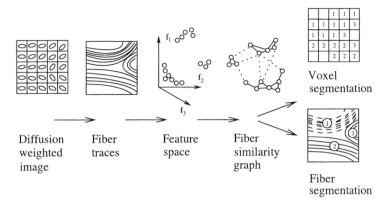

Diffusion   Fiber   Feature   Fiber
weighted   traces   space   similarity
image   graph

Voxel
segmentation

Fiber
segmentation

Fig. 1. An overview of the proposed method. Whether the result should be in voxels or fiber traces depends highly on the application. Fiber traces are flexible, they are for instance able to represent multiple fiber directions going thru a point in space. Voxels are on the other hand more suitable for volume rendering.

From this data, fiber traces were created within the white matter areas using a standard fiber tracking algorithm following the principal direction of diffusion based on a fourth-order Runge-Kutta integration scheme.

The contribution of this paper is a novel post processing method for clustering or segmentation of such fiber traces. Fiber traces are grouped according to a pairwise similarity function which takes into account the shape and connectivity of fiber traces. The clustering method we propose builds on so called normalized cuts, which have previously been introduced in the computer vision community by Shi and Malik [10] for automatic segmentation of digital images. This results in an unsupervised segmentation of human brain white matter, in which fiber traces are grouped into coherent bundles, applicable to any DWI technology able to produce fiber traces. For an overview of the method, see figure 1.

1.1   Previous Work

There are numerous examples where fiber traces from DWI have successfully revealed fiber tracts in the human brain, see for instance [2,3,13]. Stream-tubes have often been used for visualization [14], sometimes in combination with coloring schemes and variation of the stream-tube thickness according to some aspect of the underlying local diffusion descriptor. The idea of using fiber traces to obtain segmentations of white matter fiber tracts, as well as gray matter areas, have been explored in a number of papers recently. In [3] a segmentation of deep gray matter structures is performed using probabilistic fiber tracking, which connects pre-segmented areas of the human cortex with the thalamus. There also exist manual approaches to organize fiber traces into fiber bundles, such as the virtual dissection proposed in [5]. In [4] the idea of pseudo-coloring (soft clustering) fiber traces to enhance the perception of connectivity in visualizations of human brain white matter was presented. Some unsupervised approaches to clustering of fiber traces, similar to the one in this paper, have also been reported. For instance fuzzy c-means clustering [11] and K nearest neighbors [6]. Outside the area of medical image processing, clustering of curves [8] has been reported.

2   Determining Fiber Similarity

Many clustering methods, including the $NCut$ being used in this paper, operate on a graph with undirected weighted edges describing the pairwise similarity of the objects to be clustered. This graph may be described using a weight matrix W, which is symmetric and has values ranging from 0 (dissimilar) to 1 (similar).

A fiber trace, represented as an ordered set of points in space, is a fairly high-dimensional object. Therefore the pairwise comparison of all fiber traces could potentially be a time-demanding task if fiber trace similarity is cumbersome to calculate and the number of fiber traces is high. In this paper we propose to split the computation of similarity into two steps:

1. Mapping high-dimensional fiber traces to a relatively low-dimensional Euclidean feature space, preserving some but not all information about fiber shape and fiber connectivity. This mapping is oblivious, acting on each fiber separately.
2. The use of a Gaussian kernel for comparison of points in the Euclidean feature space. This function acts on pairs of fiber traces.

It is important to point out early that even though the above mapping to a feature space may seem to be crude at a first glance, it works surprisingly well for fiber traces in practice. For a set of N fiber traces the first calculation above cost $O(N)$, while the second calculation cost $O(N^2)$ operations. This is also the reason for pre-processing the fiber data in the first step, making the second calculation more computationally efficient.

2.1   Mapping Fiber Traces to an Euclidean Feature Space

The position, shape and connectivity are important properties of a fiber trace to preserve in the mapping to a feature space. If we regard a fiber trace as just a set of points in space, we capture a sketch of these properties by calculating the mean vector $\mathbf{m}$ and the covariance matrix $\mathbf{C}$ of the points building up the fiber trace. In order to avoid non-linear scaling behavior, we take the square root of the covariance matrix, $\mathbf{G} = \sqrt{\mathbf{C}}$ Now the mapping of a fiber F may be described

$$\Phi(F) = (m_x, m_y, m_z, g_{xx}, g_{xy}, g_{xz}, g_{yy}, g_{yz}, g_{zz})^T, \tag{1}$$

which is a 9-dimensional vector. This mapping has the desirable property that it is rotation and translation invariant in the sense that the Euclidean distance between two fiber traces mapped to the 9-dimensional space is invariant to any rotations or translations in the original space. For applications where mean and covariance is not enough to discriminate between different clusters of fiber traces, higher order central moments [12] could add more feature dimensions to the above mapping. Also, in cases when fiber connectivity is more important than shape, a higher weight could be given to the fiber trace end-points in the calculation of the mean vector and covariance matrix above. Different weights could also be given to the mean vector and the covariance components in the mapping in eq (1).

2.2   Using the Gaussian Kernel for Pairwise Comparison

When fiber traces have been mapped to points in a Euclidean feature space, they may be compared relatively easy for similarity. We choose Gaussian kernels (a.k.a. Radial Basis Functions in Neural Networks literature)

$$K(x, y) = \exp(-\frac{\| x - y \|^2}{2\sigma^2}) \tag{2}$$

which are symmetric and contain a parameter σ which we may use to adjust the sensitivity of the similarity function. This function maps similar points in feature space to unity and dissimilar points to zero.

2.3   Constructing W

By combining the mapping to a Euclidean feature space with the Gaussian kernel, we obtain the weights of an undirected graph describing the similarity between all pairs of fiber traces. The weights are stored in a matrix W defined as

$$w_{ab} = K(\Phi(F_a), \Phi(F_b)). \tag{3}$$

This matrix is expected to be sparse, having most of the values close to zero.

3   Normalized Cut and Clustering

Clustering, segmentation and perceptual grouping using normalized cuts was introduced to the computer vision community by Shi and Malik in [10]. The points to be clustered are represented by a undirected graph $G = (V, E)$, where the nodes correspond to the points to be clustered and each edge has weight $w(i, j)$ which represent the similarity between point i and j. The cut is a graph theoretical concept which for a partition of the nodes into two disjunct sets A and B bipartitioning V is defined as

$$cut(A, B) = \sum_{u \in A, v \in B} w(u, v) \tag{4}$$

Using the cut, an optimal partitioning of the nodes may be defined as one that minimizes the cut. Intuitively this could be used for segmentation, while the minimum cut corresponds to a partitioning which keeps well connected components of the graph together. However, there is no bias in the minimum cut which says it should partition the graph in two parts of equal size. Shi and Malik therefore defined the normalized cut, which is defined as

$$Ncut(A, B) = \frac{cut(A, B)}{asso(A, V)} + \frac{cut(A, B)}{asso(B, V)} \tag{5}$$

where $asso(A, V) = \sum_{u \in A, t \in V} w(u, t)$. This new measure $Ncut$ tries to minimize the cut, while at the same time penalizing partitions in which one set of nodes is only loosely connected to the graph at large. If we define $x_i = 1$ when node $i \in A$, $x_i = -1$ when node $i \in B$, $d(i) = \sum_j w(i,j)$, $k = \frac{\sum_{x_i>0} d_i}{\sum_i d_i}$, D is a matrix with $\mathbf{d} = d(i)$ in it's diagonal and W is the matrix defined by $w(i,j)$ then it is shown in [10] that

$$N cut = \frac{(1+x)^T(D-W)(1+x)}{k\bar{1}^T D\bar{1}} + \frac{(1-x)^T(D-W)(1-x)}{(1-k)\bar{1}^T D\bar{1}}. \tag{6}$$

which can be shown to be equivalent to

$$N cut = \frac{y^T(D-W)y}{y^T Dy} \tag{7}$$

where $y_i \in \{1, -b\}$, $b = k/(1-k)$, for $y = (1+x) - b(1-x)$ while $y^T \mathbf{d} = 0$. Relaxing the problem by allowing y to take any real values results in the minimization of the so called Rayleigh quotient, which can be minimized by solving

$$(D-W)y = \lambda Dy \tag{8}$$

It is shown in [10] that the second smallest eigenvector of eq. (8) minimizes the real valued version of the normalized cut.

In our implementation we used the second smallest eigenvector to obtain a 1-d ordering of the vertices of the graph. A random search was then performed to determine a good threshold for the bipartitioning of the graph. To test the goodness of a specific threshold the true discrete $N cut$ was calculated. When the graph has been split into two, [10] recommends the partitioning continues recursively until the $N cut$ raises above a certain value.

4   Results

The method was tested on both synthetic datasets and fiber traces from real diffusion weighted MRI. Results are visualized using both stream-tubes and color coded voxel data. All algorithms were implemented in Matlab.

- In figure 2 the method is tested on synthetically generated fiber traces in 2-D.
- In figure 3 real fiber traces obtained from DT-MRI was used as input.
- In figure 4 the method was tested with a very large value of σ and direct mapping of the second, third and fourth eigenvector to colors similar to the approach described in [4].

5   Discussion

We have not yet investigated the effects of noise to the clustering. Also, the maximum number of fiber traces we have analyzed so far is only about 5000, due to the current implementation in Matlab which does not fully exploit the sparsity of W. Never the less, the experiments show the potential of the $N Cut$ criterion and the proposed measure of fiber similarity.

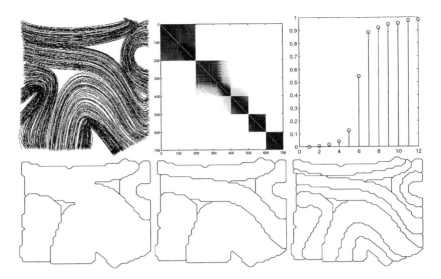

Fig. 2. Top left: A set of synthetic fiber traces in 2-D. **Top middle:** The matrix W. Rows and columns sorted according to the second smallest eigenvector. The Gaussian kernel have been chosen so that five clusters present themselves naturally. **Top right:** The 15 smallest eigenvalues of $(D - W)/D$. **Bottom:** Segmentation obtained from recursive bipartitioning of the fiber traces. Maximum value of the $Ncut$ set to 0.2, 2.5 and 4.5 respectively.

One insight from the experiments is that pseudo-coloring of fiber traces is very effective to reveal errors in fiber tracking algorithms. A collection of fiber traces may look ok at a first glance, but after pseudo-coloring, the anomalies are easily spotted. One example of this is in figure 4 (middle) where the red fiber traces may be identified instantly as outliers because they have a very different color than surrounding fiber traces.

In our experiments we have segmented fiber traces and then sometimes transformed the results back to voxel space. One may ask if it would be possible to segment voxels directly, and what features to use to discriminate voxels. A solution with obvious similarities to the approach presented in this paper would be to perform fiber tracking, possibly stochastic [3], from each voxel inside white matter and regard the fiber traces as a non-local features of the voxels – *macro features*.

The continuous coloring in figure 4 appears to be more visually pleasing than the discrete coloring according to the segmentation in figure 3. One may in fact ask if a structure such as the corpus callosum is meaningful to partition into several clusters or whether it is better described as one fiber bundle parameterized by a coordinate system going from anterior to posterior. One could think of the smoothly varying colors in figure 4 as coordinate systems, parameterizing all fiber traces in the cross bundle directions. It is in fact then also natural to add a parameterization of each bundle in the fiber direction.

In conclusion the proposed clustering method seems to be a promising new way to automatically reveal the global structure of white matter by segmentation of fiber traces obtained from DWI data. We believe this to be useful in for instance explorative studies of the brain and for visualization of DWI data in surgical planning applications.

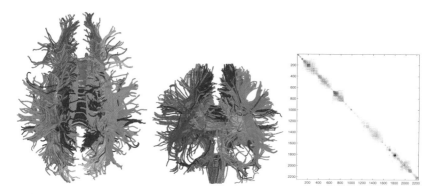

Fig. 3. Left: Axial view of a segmentation obtained from recursive bipartitioning of the white matter fiber traces. Maximum value of the $Ncut$ was set to 1.5 and Gaussian kernel $\sigma = 20.$. The colors of fiber traces indicate cluster membership. **Middle:** Coronal view. **Right:** The matrix W. Rows and columns sorted according to the second smallest eigenvector.

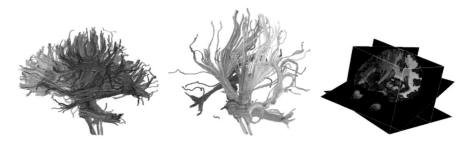

Fig. 4. Pseudo-coloring of fiber traces. RGB colors are derived directly from scaled versions of the 2nd, 3rd and 4th eigenvector of $(D-W)/D$. Using a very large Gaussian kernel, $\sigma = 100$, results in a soft clustering effect. Note the enhanced perception of fiber connectivity and shape, despite the lack of discrete clusters. **Left:** Whole brain white matter visualized using pseudo-colored fiber traces. **Middle:** A subset of the white matter fiber traces visualized using pseudo-colored fiber traces. **Right:** Pseudo-coloring of voxels belonging to white matter enhance perception of connectivity in slices or volumes. To fill in holes in white matter when fiber traces were transformed to voxels, a nearest-neighbor approach combined with a white matter mask was used.

Important to note though is that all post processing methods for fiber traces share the same weakness: they all rely on a good fiber tracking algorithm to perform well.

Acknowledgments. Thanks to Marek Kubicki, Lauren O'Donnell, William Wells, Steven Haker, Stephan Maier, Robert McCarley and Ron Kikinis for interesting discussions and to Raúl San José Estépar for valuable comments on the manuscript.

This work was funded in part by NIH grants P41-RR13218 and R01 MH 50747, and CIMIT. It was also supported in part by the Post-doctoral Fellowship Program of Korea Science & Engineering Foundation (KOSEF).

References

1. P. J. Basser: Inferring microstructural features and the physiological state of tissues from diffusion-weighted images. *NMR in Biomedicine*. 8 (1995) 333-344.
2. P. J. Basser, S. Pajevic, C. Pierpaoli, J. Duda, and A. Aldroubi: In vivo fiber tractography using DT-MRI data. *Magn. Reson. Med.*. 44 (2000) 625-632.
3. T. E. J. Behrens,, H. Johansen-Berg,M. W. Woolrich, S. M. Smith C. A. M. Wheeler-Kingshott, P. A. Boulby, G. J. Barker, E. L. Sillery, K. Sheehan, O. Ciccarelli, A. J. Thompson, J. M. Brady and P. M. Matthews: Non-invasive mapping of connections between human thalamus and cortex using diffusion imaging. *Nature Neuroscience* 6(7):750-757, 2003.
4. A. Brun, H.-J. Park, H. Knutsson and Carl-Fredrik Westin: Coloring of DT-MRI Fiber Traces using Laplacian Eigenmaps. *Computer Aided Systems Theory - EUROCAST 2003*, LNCS, Volume 2809, Las Palmas de Gran Canaria, Spain, February, 2003.
5. M. Catani, R. J. Howard, S. Pajevic, and D. K. Jones: Virtual in vivo interactive dissection of white matter fasciculi in the human brain. *Neuroimage* 17, pp 77-94, 2002.
6. Z. Ding, J. C. Gore, and A. W. Anderson: Classification and quantification of neuronal fiber pathways using diffusion tensor MRI. *Mag. Reson. Med.* 49:716-721, 2003.
7. C. Fowlkes, S. Belongie, and J. Malik: Efficient Spatiotemporal Grouping Using the Nyström Method *CVPR*, Hawaii,December 2001.
8. S. J. Gaffney and P. Smyth: Curve clustering with random effects regression mixtures. in C. M. Bishop and B. J. Frey (eds:) *Proc. Ninth Int. Workshop on AI and Stat.*, Florida, 2003.
9. D. Lebihan, E. Breton, D. Lallemand, P. Grenier, E. Cabanis, and M. LavalJeantet: MR imaging of intravoxel incoherent motions: application to diffusion and perfusion in neurologic disorders. *Radiology* 161, 401–407, 1986.
10. J. Shi and J. Malik: Normalized Cust and Image Segmentation, *PAMI*, vol. 22, no.8, 2000.
11. J. S. Shimony, A. Z. Snyder, N. Lori, and T. E. Conturo: Automated fuzzy clustering of neur-Sonal pathways in diffusion tensor tracking. *Proc. Intl. Soc. Mag. Reson. Med.* 10, Honolulu, Hawaii, May 2002.
12. E. Weisstein: Eric Weisstein's world of mathematics. http://mathworld.wolfram.com/, March 5, 2004.
13. C.-F. Westin, S. E. Maier, H. Mamata, A. Nabavi, F. A. Jolesz, R. Kikinis: Processing and Visualization of Diffusion Tensor MRI, *Medical Image Analysis*, vol. 6, no. 8, 2002.
14. S. Zhang, T. Curry, D. S. Morris, and D. H. Laidlaw: Streamtubes and streamsurfaces for visualizing diffusion tensor MRI volume images. *Visualization '00 Work in Progress* October 2000.

Area Preserving Cortex Unfolding

Jean-Philippe Pons[1], Renaud Keriven[1], and Olivier Faugeras[2]

[1] CERTIS, ENPC,
Marne-La-Vallée, France
Jean-Philippe.Pons@sophia.inria.fr
[2] Odyssée Lab, INRIA,
Sophia-Antipolis, France

Abstract. We propose a new method to generate unfolded area preserving representations of the cerebral cortex. The cortical surface is evolved with an application-specific normal motion, and an adequate tangential motion is constructed in order to ensure an exact area preservation throughout the evolution. We describe the continuous formulation of our method as well as its numerical implementation with triangulated surfaces and level sets. We show its applicability by computing inflated representations of the cortex from real brain data.

1 Introduction

Building unfolded representations of the cerebral cortex has become an important area of research in medical imaging. On a simplified geometry, it becomes easier to visualize and analyze functional or structural properties of the cortex, particularly in previously hidden sulcal regions. Moreover, if some metric properties of the cortical surface can be preserved while eliminating folds, it makes sense to map the data from different subjects in a canonical space for building brain atlases.

Three types of unfolded reprentations have been proposed in the litterature: inflated, that is to say a smoothed version of the cortex retaining its overall shape, spherical and flattened (see [1] and references therein). Three metric properties have been considered: geodesic distances, angles and areas. Unfortunately, preserving distances exactly is impossible because the cortical surface and its simplified version will have different Gaussian curvature [2]. Moreover, it is not possible to preserve angles and areas simultaneously.

As a consequence, early methods for cortex unfolding have settled for variational approaches, leading to a variety of local forces encouraging an approximate preservation of area and angle while smoothing the surface [3,4]. In [1], the authors point out that the result of such methods are not optimal with respect to any metric property, and work out a method which focuses on distances only and minimizes their distortion.

A lot of work has focused on building conformal representations of the cortical surface, i.e. one-to-one, onto, and angle preserving mappings between the cortex and a target surface, often a sphere or a plane (see [5,6] and references

C. Barillot, D.R. Haynor, and P. Hellier (Eds.): MICCAI 2004, LNCS 3216, pp. 376–383, 2004.

therein). These approaches use a well known fact from Riemannian geometry that a surface without any handles, holes or self-intersections can be mapped conformally onto the sphere, and any local portion thereof onto a disk.

In our work we focus on area preservation, motivated by a general result which ensures the existence of an area preserving mapping between two diffeomorphic surfaces of the same total area [7]. A method for building such an area preserving mapping for the purpose of cortex unfolding has been proposed in [8]. In addition, this method allows to pick, among all existing area preserving mappings, a local minimum of metric distortion. This minimum is in some sense the nearest area preserving map to a conformal one. This mathematical formulation is very promising but no numerical experiment is presented in the paper. Moreover, the numerical implementation of their method is feasible only for spherical maps.

We propose a method to evolve the cortical surface while preserving local area, and we use it to build area preserving inflated representations of the cortex. Our method relates both to [8] and [3,4,9]. We evolve a surface in time as in [3, 4,9], whereas the method of [8] is static and generates a single mapping between the cortex and a sphere. We achieve an exact area preservation as in [8], whereas in [3,4,9] area preservation is only encouraged by tangential forces. Furthermore, the latter approaches only have a discrete formulation and are specific to one type of deformable model, whereas ours is continuous and can be applied numerically both to triangulated surfaces and level sets.

To achieve this, we treat the normal and the tangential components of the motion differently. On the one hand, the normal motion controls the geometry of the surface. It is application-specific and is chosen by the user. For example, it can be a mean curvature motion in order to obtain a multiresolution representation of the cortex, or it can be a force pulling the surface towards a target shape, typically a sphere. On the other hand, given the selected normal motion, an adequate tangential motion is constructed in order to ensure an exact area preservation throughout the evolution.

The rest of the paper is organized as follows. In Sect. 2, we present a general method for building an area preserving motion for a codimension one manifold in arbitrary dimensions. Given a desired normal motion, we compute a nontrivial tangential motion such that the evolution is area preserving. In Sect. 3, we demonstrate the applicability of our method by computing area preserving inflated representations of the cortex from real brain data. Finally, we evoke some potential applications of our method in other fields in Sect. 4.

2 Area Preserving Surface Motion

In this section we first explicitly state the mathematical conditions for the preservation of the local area of an evolving codimension one manifold in arbitrary dimensions. This condition ensures that the total area, as well as the area of any patch, is preserved. When the total area needs not to be preserved, we can nonetheless preserve the relative local area, i.e. the ratio between the area of any patch and the total area. We then derive a procedure to build an area preserving or relative area preserving tangential motion. Finally we describe the numerical implementation of our method with two major types of deformable models: triangulated surfaces and level sets. In the following, we make an intensive use of differential geometry. We refer the reader to [2] for the basic theory. Note that, contrary to conformal approaches, our formulation is not limited to a genus zero surface and applies, a priori, to an arbitrary topology.

2.1   The Total, Local, and Relative Area Preserving Conditions

Let us consider an hypersurface Γ in $\mathbb{R}^n$ evolving with speed $\mathbf{v}$. We define the local areal factor J at a point of Γ as the ratio between the initial area and the current area of an infinitesimal patch around this point. So an increasing J indicates local shrinkage and a decreasing one local expansion. The preservation of total area, local area, and relative area respectively write

$$\bar{J} = 1 \ \text{(1a)} \quad ; \quad J = 1 \ \text{(1b)} \quad ; \quad J = \bar{J} \ \text{(1c)} \ , \tag{1}$$

where $^-$ is the average of a quantity along Γ. $\bar{J}$ is related to the variation of the total area through $A_0 = A\,\bar{J}$. The local areal factor J of a material point evolves according to

$$\frac{DJ}{Dt} + J \operatorname{div}_\Gamma \mathbf{v} = 0 \ , \tag{2}$$

where D/Dt denotes the material derivative, and $\operatorname{div}_\Gamma$ denotes the intrinsic divergence operator on Γ. As a consequence, the condition to be verified by the motion for the preservation of total area, local area and relative area are respectively

$$\overline{\operatorname{div}_\Gamma \mathbf{v}} = 0 \ \text{(3a)} \quad ; \quad \operatorname{div}_\Gamma \mathbf{v} = 0 \ \text{(3b)} \quad ; \quad \operatorname{div}_\Gamma \mathbf{v} = \overline{\operatorname{div}_\Gamma \mathbf{v}} \ \text{(3c)} \ . \tag{3}$$

Note that the right-hand side of (3c) is spatially constant but is time-varying. Also, the preservation of local area is the combination of the preservation of total and relative area, so in the sequel we focus on (3a,c) only.

If we decompose $\mathbf{v}$ into its outward normal component v_N and its tangential part $\mathbf{v}_T$, (3a,c) become

$$\overline{H\,v_N} = 0 \ \text{(4a)} \quad ; \quad \operatorname{div}_\Gamma \mathbf{v}_T + (n-1)\,H\,v_N = (n-1)\,\overline{H\,v_N} \ \text{(4b)} \ , \tag{4}$$

where $\mathbf{N}$ is the outward normal and H is the mean curvature. In the left-hand side of (4b), we now better see the two different sources of local expansion/shrinkage: one is tangential motion, the other is the association of normal motion and curvature.

2.2   Designing a Relative Area Preserving Tangential Motion

We now outline our method to build a relative area preserving motion. We are given a normal velocity field v_N. Let us consider the solution η of the following intrinsic Poisson equation on Γ:

$$\Delta_\Gamma \eta = (n-1)\left(H\,v_N - \overline{H\,v_N}\right) \quad, \tag{5}$$

where Δ_Γ denotes the Laplace-Beltrami operator on Γ. Finding a solution of (5) is possible because the right-hand side is of zero average [10]. Moreover, the solution η is unique up to a constant. Then one can check that

$$\mathbf{v} = v_N \mathbf{N} - \nabla_\Gamma \eta \tag{6}$$

verifies (4). Note that the normal motion is not altered since $\nabla_\Gamma \eta$, the intrinsic gradient of η, is purely tangential, and that the resulting velocity is non local: it depends on the whole shape and motion of the interface.

For a given normal velocity, there are in general an infinity of admissible area preserving tangential velocities. The particular solution derived from (5) is a reasonable choice since our method outputs a null tangential motion if the normal motion is already area preserving.

In general, the given normal velocity field v_N does not preserve total area, and our method can only enforce a relative area preservation. If a strict area preservation is required, we can either apply an adequate rescaling at a post processing step, or integrate in the normal motion a rescaling motion $-\overline{H\,v_N}\,(\mathbf{x}\cdot\mathbf{N})\mathbf{N}$ so that the total area is preserved.

2.3   The Area Relaxation Term

Numerical implementations of the above method may yield deceiving results. Indeed, in pratice, (5) can only be solved up to a certain tolerance, and the surface evolution is subject to discretization errors. As a consequence, the area preserving condition cannot be fulfilled exactly and the area of interface patches may drift slowly from its expected values. Thus, area preservation is likely to be broken when the number of iterations increases.

We augment our method with an area relaxation term which encourages a uniform area redistribution whenever area preservation is lost. This feature is crucial to counteract local drifts in area due to numerical errors. We insist on the fact that this additional term is not a numerical heuristic: it is fully consistent with the mathematical formulation given above. Let us now seek the solution of

$$\Delta_\Gamma \eta = (n-1)\left(H\,v_N - \overline{H\,v_N}\right) + \lambda(1 - \frac{J}{\bar{J}}) \quad, \tag{7}$$

where λ is a weighting parameter. We build the velocity from (6) as previously. Using (2) we get that

$$\frac{D(\bar{J}/J)}{Dt} = \lambda(1 - \bar{J}/J) \quad. \tag{8}$$

Hence the ratio $\bar{J}/J$ relaxes exponentially towards unity with time constant $1/\lambda$. In our problem we have $J = \bar{J} = 1$ for $t = 0$ so that the solution of (8) is $J = \bar{J}$ for all t as desired. This was already the case without the relaxation term, so at first sight this term is of no use. But in practice, numerical errors can make $\bar{J}/J$ incidently deviate from unity. Thanks to the area relaxation term, it is now possible to recover from this numerical drift.

2.4   Numerical Methods

For each time step we have to solve the intrinsic Poisson equation (7). Apparently it represents a huge computational cost. Hopefully, only the very first iteration is expensive. Indeed, for subsequent iterations, we use the solution η of time $t - 1$ as the initial guess for time t. If the shape and the normal motion change slowly relatively to the chosen time step, the guess is likely to be very close to the actual solution, and solving (7) is computationally cheap.

Triangulated surfaces: solving a Poisson equation on a triangulated surface can be done with a finite element technique as proposed in [6]. Equation (7) then translates into a linear system with a sparse symmetric positive semi-definite matrix and can be solved efficiently with numerical iterative methods such as the conjugate gradient method [11].

Level sets: at first sight, a level set implementation of cortex unfolding is not feasible. Indeed, a level set representation conveys a purely geometric description of the interface. The tangential part of the velocity vanishes in the level set evolution equation. As a consequence, it is impossible to keep point correspondences or to handle data living on the interface with the straightfoward level set approach. Some hybrid Lagrangian-Eulerian methods have been proposed to circumvent this limitation [12]. However, for sake of stability and topology independence, a completely Eulerian approach should be preferred. Recently, several Eulerian methods based on a system of coupled partial differential equations have been proposed to handle interface data in the level set framework. [13, 14] address the transport and diffusion of general data on a moving interface. In [15], we have described how to maintain explicit backward point correspondences from the current interface to the initial one. Our method consists in advecting the initial point coordinates with the same speed as the level set function. This extension of the level set method makes it applicable to cortex unfolding.

In order to solve the Poisson equation in this framework, we use a finite-difference discretization of the Laplace-Beltrami operator proposed in [16]. Equation (7) then translates into a linear system with a sparse symmetric indefinite matrix suited for a minimum residual method [11]. To compute the average of a quantity along the interface, we use a smoothed version of the Dirac function on the cartesian grid as in [17].

3   Experimental Results

In this section we focus on the level set implementation of our method and we compute inflated representations of the cortex from real brain data. Our method

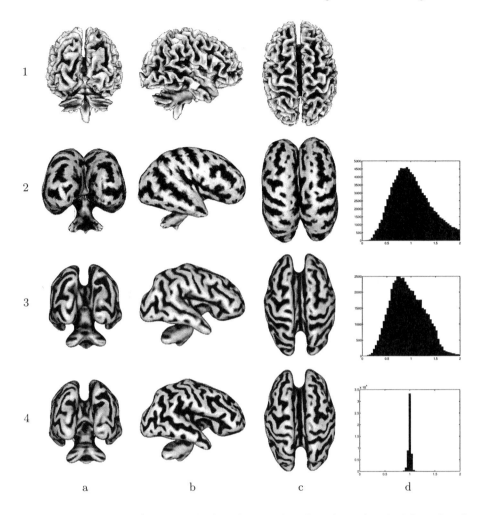

Fig. 1. Several views *(columns a,b,c)* of the initial surface *(row 1)* and of the inflated representations obtained with the popular method of Fischl et al. *(row 2)*, with a standard mean curvature motion *(row 3)* and with our method *(row 4)*. Histograms of the normalized areal factor $J/\bar{J}$ in each case *(column d)*.

is quite flexible through the choice of the normal motion, and we could obtain a sphere or any target shape by designing a force pulling the surface towards the target. In order to obtain smoothed versions of the cortex, we use the well-known and easy-to-implement motion by mean curvature $v_N = -H$ or a variant with an additional rescaling motion $v_N = -H + \overline{H^2}\,(\mathbf{x} \cdot \mathbf{N})$ in order to preserve the total area.

In the following experiments, the input of our algorithm is a $128 \times 128 \times 128$ level set of the pial surface of a human brain extracted from a $256 \times 256 \times 256$ T1 weighted MRI image with a home-made segmentation software combining hidden Markov random fields classification [18] and topology preserving level

Table 1. Standard deviation of $J/\bar{J}$ against λ when using our method.

λ	1	3	5	10
$\sigma(J/\bar{J})$	0.060	0.041	0.035	0.027

set deformable models [19]. To give an idea of the resolution of the surface, the marching cube algorithm produces roughly 100000 triangles from this level set.

In Fig. 1, in order to show the benefits of area preservation, we compare three inflated representations. The first one *(row 2)* was obtained with the nice method of Fischl et al. [1]. This method minimizes metric distortion but does not consider area. The second inflated cortex *(row 3)* was obtained with a standard mean curvature motion with a null tangential motion. The third one *(row 4)* was obtained with a mean curvature motion plus an area preserving tangential motion computed with our method. As expected, the geometries of last two representations are identical since the normal motion is the same in both cases. We display the histograms of the normalized areal factor $J/\bar{J}$ in each case *(column d)*. Not suprisingly, area distortion is far smaller when using our method. In this example, it is less that 5 percent almost everywhere. More interestingly, the overall aspect all the representations is similar, which suggests that our method does not induce a blow-up in metric distortion. Moreover, as shown in Table 1, the amount of area distortion decreases when the area relaxation parameter λ increases. On the other hand, higher values of λ require to use smaller time steps and hence to perform a larger number of iterations.

4   Conclusion and Future Work

We have presented a new method to generate unfolded area preserving representations of the cerebral cortex: depending on the normal motion driving the geometry, an adequate tangential motion is computed to ensure an exact area preservation. A demonstration of the efficiency of the method and a comparison with a popular existing method have been done on real brain data.

Future work includes implementing our method for triangulated surfaces and evaluating its benefits for the evolution of explicit deformable models in other applications. Indeed, our approach involves a good redistribution of control points which is synonymous of numerical stability: we expect it to prevent the merging of grid points or the formation of the so-called swallow tails. Thus, it could be an alternative to the heuristic elastic forces or the delooping procedures typically used to deal with these difficulties.

References

1. Fischl, B., Sereno, M., Dale, A.: Cortical surface-based analysis ii : inflation, flattening, and a surface-based coordinate system. Neuroimage **9** (1999) 195–207
2. DoCarmo, M.P.: Differential Geometry of Curves and Surfaces. Prentice-Hall (1976)

3. Dale, A.M., Sereno, M.I.: Improved localization of cortical activity by combining eeg and meg with mri cortical surface reconstruction: A linear approach. Journal of Cognitive Neuroscience **5** (1993) 162–176

4. Carman, G., Drury, H., Van Essen, D.: Computational methods for reconstructing and unfolding the cerebral cortex. Cerebral Cortex (1995)

5. Gu, X., Wang, Y., Chan, T., Thompson, P., Yau, S.T.: Genus zero surface conformal mapping and its application to brain surface mapping. In Taylor, C., Noble, J.A., eds.: Information Processing in Medical Imaging. Volume 2732 of LNCS., Springer (2003) 172–184

6. Angenent, S., Haker, S., Tannenbaum, A., Kikinis, R.: Laplace-Beltrami operator and brain surface flattening. IEEE Transactions on Medical Imaging **18** (1999) 700–711

7. Moser, J.: On the volume elements on a manifold. AMS Transactions **120** (1965) 286–294

8. Angenent, S., Haker, S., Tannenbaum, A., Kikinis, R.: On area preserving mappings of minimal distorsion. Preprint (2002)

9. Montagnat, J., Delingette, H., Scapel, N., Ayache, N.: Representation, shape, topology and evolution of deformable surfaces. Application to 3D medical image segmentation. Technical Report 3954, INRIA (2000)

10. Rauch, J.: Partial Differential Equations. Springer-Verlag, New York (1991)

11. Barret, R., Berry, M., Chan, T.F., Demmel, J., Donato, J., Dongarra, J., Eijkhout, V., Pozo, R., Romine, C., van der Vonst, H.: Templates for the Solution of Linear Systems: Building Blocks for Iterative Methods. SIAM, Philadelphia (1994) Available from netlib.

12. Hermosillo, G., Faugeras, O., Gomes, J.: Unfolding the cerebral cortex using level set methods. In Nielsen, M., Johansen, P., Olsen, O., Weickert, J., eds.: Scale-Space Theories in Computer Vision. Volume 1682 of Lecture Notes in Computer Science., Springer (1999) 58–69

13. Xu, J., Zhao, H.: An Eulerian formulation for solving partial differential equations along a moving interface. Technical Report 02-27, UCLA Computational and Applied Mathematics Reports (2002)

14. Adalsteinsson, D., Sethian, J.: Transport and diffusion of material quantities on propagating interfaces via level set methods. Journal of Computational Physics **185** (2003)

15. Pons, J.P., Hermosillo, G., Keriven, R., Faugeras, O.: How to deal with point correspondences and tangential velocities in the level set framework. In: Proceedings of the 9th International Conference on Computer Vision, Nice, France, IEEE Computer Society, IEEE Computer Society Press (2003) 894–899

16. Bertalmio, M., Cheng, L., Osher, S., Sapiro, G.: Variational problems and partial differential equations on implicit surfaces. Journal of Computational Physics **174** (2001) 759–780

17. Peng, D., Merriman, B., Osher, S., Zhao, H., Kang, M.: A PDE-based fast local level set method. Journal on Computational Physics **155** (1999) 410–438

18. Zhang, Y., Brady, M., Smith, S.: Segmentation of brain mr images through a hidden markov random field model and the expectation-maximization algorithm. IEEE Transactions on Medical Imaging **20** (2001)

19. Han, X., Xu, C., Prince, J.: A topology preserving level set method for geometric deformable models. IEEE Transactions on Pattern Analysis and Machine Intelligence **25** (2003) 755–768

Cortical Reconstruction Using Implicit Surface Evolution: A Landmark Validation Study

Duygu Tosun[1], Maryam E. Rettmann[2], Daniel Q. Naiman[3],
Susan M. Resnick[2], Michael A. Kraut[4], and Jerry L. Prince[1]

[1] Electrical and Computer Engineering Dept., Johns Hopkins University, MD, USA
[2] National Institute on Aging, National Institutes of Health, MD, USA
[3] Applied Mathematics and Statistics Dept., Johns Hopkins University, MD, USA
[4] Department of Radiology, Johns Hopkins Hospital, MD, USA

Abstract. A validation study was conducted to assess the accuracy of an algorithm developed for automatic reconstruction of the cerebral cortex from T1-weighted magnetic resonance (MR) brain images. Manually selected landmarks on different sulcal regions throughout the cortex were used to analyze the accuracy of three reconstructed nested surfaces – the inner, central, and pial surfaces. We conclude that the algorithm can find these surfaces with subvoxel accuracy, typically with an accuracy of one third of a voxel, although this varies by brain region and cortical geometry. Parameters were adjusted on the basis of this analysis in order to improve the algorithm's overall performance.[1]

1 Introduction

Many brain mapping procedures require automated methods to find and mathematically represent the cerebral cortex in volumetric MR images. Such reconstructions are used for characterization and analysis of the two-dimensional (2-D) geometry of the cortex – e.g., computation of curvatures, geodesic distance, segmenting sulci or gyri, surface flattening, and spherical mapping.

The cerebral cortex is a thin, folded sheet of gray matter (GM), bounded by the cerebrospinal fluid (CSF) on the outside, and by the white matter (WM) on the inside, as illustrated in Fig. 3. The boundary between GM and WM forms the inner surface, and the boundary between GM and CSF forms the pial surface. It is useful to define the central surface as well; it lies at the geometric center between the inner and pial surfaces, representing an overall 2-D approximation to the three-dimensional (3-D) cortical sheet. A 3-D reconstruction method, called Cortical Reconstruction Using Implicit Surface Evolution (CRUISE), has been developed for automatic reconstruction of these three nested cortical surfaces from T1-weighted SPGR volumetric axially acquired MR images.

The goal of the landmark validation study presented in this paper was to evaluate the performance of CRUISE, yielding quantitative measures of accuracy and suggesting optimal parameters. Sect. 2 briefly explains the cascaded

---

[1] This work was supported by the NIH/NINDS under grant R01NS37747.

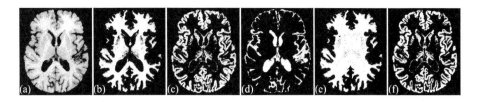

Fig. 1. Sample axial slices from (a) the skull-stripped MR image volume; (b) μ_{WM}; (c) μ_{GM}; (d) μ_{CSF}; (e) $\hat{\mu}_{WM}$; (f) $\hat{\mu}_{GM}$.

algorithms of CRUISE and the relation between its parameters and the location of the surfaces. Next, the paper describes the data and the validation study in Sect. 3. Based on the analysis reported in Sect. 3, a way to select optimal parameters is discussed in Sect. 4 and an analysis to validate the new parameters is presented. In Sect. 5, we summarize with some concluding remarks.

2 CRUISE: Cortical Reconstruction Using Implicit Surface Evolution

CRUISE is a data-driven method combining a robust fuzzy segmentation method, an efficient topology correction algorithm, and a geometric deformable surface model. Overall, the general approach we use in finding cortical surfaces from MR image data is described in [1], and several improvements have been incorporated, as described in [2,3,4]. The algorithm has been targeted toward and evaluated on the MR images acquired by the Baltimore Longitudinal Study of Aging [5] with the following parameters: TE = 5, TR = 35, FOV = 24, flip angle = $45°$, slice thickness = 1.5, gap = 0, matrix = 256×256, NEX = 1.

The first processing step is to re-slice the image volume to axial cross-sections parallel to the line through the manually identified anterior and posterior commissures, followed by removing the cerebellum, extracranial tissue, and brain stem from the image using a semi-automatic algorithm. The remaining image volume is then re-sampled to obtain isotropic voxels each having size 0.9375 mm×0.9375 mm×0.9375 mm using cubic B-spline interpolation in order to make subsequent processing less sensitive to orientation.

The next step in processing this "skull-stripped" MR image volume is to apply a fuzzy segmentation algorithm [6], yielding three membership function image volumes representing the fractions of WM, GM, and CSF within each image voxel – i.e., μ_{WM}, μ_{GM}, and μ_{CSF}, while compensating for intensity inhomogeneity artifacts inherent in MR images, and smoothing noise. A sample axial slice from the skull-stripped MR image volume and its tissue segmentation results are shown in Figs. 1(a)-(d).

Fig. 2 illustrates the one-dimensional profiles of the membership functions. This profile starts in the WM, passes through the GM of the cortex, and ends in the CSF surrounding the cortex. An isosurface of μ_{WM} at an isolevel $\alpha = 0.5$

provides a good approximation to the GM/WM interface. It is apparent from Fig. 1(b), however, that such an isosurface will include non-cortical surfaces such as the subcortical interfaces near the brainstem and within the ventricles. To prevent undesirable parts of the isosurface from being generated, an automatic method [2] called *AutoFill* is used to modify μ_{WM} in order to fill these concavities with WM. The largest $\alpha = 0.5$ isosurface of the edited WM membership, $\hat{\mu}_{WM}$ (Fig. 1(e)), is a close approximation to the GM/WM interface within each hemisphere, connected across the corpus callosum at the top and through the brainstem at the bottom. A graph-based topology correction algorithm [3] followed by a topology-preserving geometric deformable surface model (TGDM) [4] is used to estimate a topologically correct and slightly smoothed "inner surface" on the GM/WM interface, as shown in Fig. 5(a).

The inner surface serves as an initial surface for finding both the central and pial surfaces. These surfaces are difficult to find due to the partial volume averaging effect, which makes adjacent GM banks within narrow sulci barely dis-

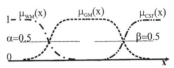

Fig. 2. One-dimensional (1-D) profiles of membership functions.

tinguishable because of the missing evidence of CSF. To compensate for this effect, CRUISE uses *anatomically consistent enhancement* (ACE) [2], which automatically modifies μ_{GM}, creating thin (artificial) CSF separations within tight sulci and yielding $\hat{\mu}_{GM}$ shown in Fig. 1(f). $\hat{\mu}_{GM}$ is used in two ways to find these surfaces. First, a gradient vector flow (GVF) external force [1] is computed directly from $\hat{\mu}_{GM}$, as if it was an edge map itself. A TGDM deformable surface is then initialized at the inner surface and is driven toward the central surface using the GVF forces, yielding a central surface as shown in Fig. 5(c). It is observed that the $\beta = 0.5$ isosurface of $\hat{\mu}_{WM} + \hat{\mu}_{GM}$ is a very good approximation to the pial surface. Accordingly, a region-based TGDM deformable surface model is used to drive the central surface toward the $\beta = 0.5$ isosurface of $\hat{\mu}_{WM} + \hat{\mu}_{GM}$, yielding an estimate of the pial surface as shown in Fig. 5(e).

When surfaces are computed using geometric deformable models such as TGDM, they contain no self-intersections. Also, an extra constraint is used to ensure the proper nesting of these three cortical surfaces with no mutual intersections. Figs. 5(b),(d), and (f) show the contours of these nested cortical surfaces superposed on a skull-stripped MR image (axial) cross-section.

3   Landmark Validation Study on Inner and Pial Surfaces

A validation study on the central surface using a set of 50 manually selected central surface landmarks – 5 on each hemisphere of 5 brains – was reported in our previous work [1]. The distance from each landmark to the central surface estimated by our algorithm served as a measure of accuracy. Overall, the mean landmark error was 0.51 mm with a standard deviation of 0.41 mm illustrating subvoxel accuracy in our reconstruction of the central surface.

The focus of the validation study presented in this paper is to quantify the accuracy of the inner and pial surfaces estimated by CRUISE. In addition, we assess how the accuracy varies both across the cortical surface as well as within different cortical geometries illustrated in Fig. 3 – sulcal "fundi" (the bottom of a cortical fold), "banks" (the sides of the fold), and "gyri"(the top of the fold). Twelve volunteers (three neuroanatomists) participated in this validation study. Each participant identified a series of landmarks at the GM/WM and GM/CSF interfaces on the skull-stripped MR image volumes. The landmarks effectively yielded a "user implied surface" at the corresponding cortical layer. Throughout this study, we refer to these surfaces as the *implied surfaces* and the estimated surfaces by CRUISE as the *reference surfaces*. To quantify the agreement between the reference and implied surfaces, we define a "landmark offset" as the minimum distance between the given landmark and the corresponding reference surface, with the sign negative inside and positive outside (Fig. 4). These measurements will be used to quantify the accuracy of the estimated surfaces and to infer any systematic bias of CRUISE in the inward or outward directions.

The reference surfaces are defined primarily by the 0.5 isolevels of the $\hat{\mu}_{WM}$ and $\hat{\mu}_{GM} + \hat{\mu}_{WM}$ as described in Sect. 2. Thus, the value of $\hat{\mu}_{WM}$ at the GM/WM interface landmarks, and the value of $\hat{\mu}_{GM} + \hat{\mu}_{WM}$ at the GM/CSF interface landmarks could provide insight into a systematic bias of CRUISE. This is made clear by referring back to Fig. 2. Consider the isosurfaces of $\hat{\mu}_{WM}$ and $\hat{\mu}_{GM} + \hat{\mu}_{WM}$ generated at higher

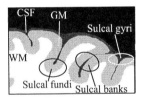

Fig. 3. Illustration of the three cortical geometries.

isolevel values – $\alpha > 0.5$ and $\beta > 0.5$. The isosurfaces estimated at these isolevels would give an inner and pial surface inside the surfaces estimated at $\alpha = 0.5$ and $\beta = 0.5$ indicating an outward bias of CRUISE. We are particularly interested in these measures because α and β are easily changed, to improve the performance of CRUISE.

First, we will conduct an analysis of the landmark offsets and the membership function values at the landmarks to quantify the accuracy of CRUISE as well as any systematic bias. Second, we will select the optimal α and β threshold that best fit the users' data. Finally, we will repeat the landmark validation study with the new thresholds.

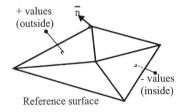

Fig. 4. Illustration of the "landmark offset".

3.1 Interactive Program for Landmark Picking

Our initial landmark validation study on the central surface [1] included only one user who picked a single landmark in each region at integer number coordinates. We have designed a new landmark validation study for the inner and pial surfaces with an extended number of landmarks and users, using two MR image volumes of different individuals. Landmarks are located on the GM/WM and GM/CSF interfaces in eleven cortical regions comprising the Sylvian, superior frontal, superior temporal, cingulate, and parieto-occipital sulci of each hemisphere, and the central sulcus of the left hemisphere. Within each region, landmarks are defined on the three cortical geometries – sulcal "fundi", "banks", and "gyri".

A visualization program was written using Open Data Explorer [7] to provide a standard way of picking the landmarks on the pre-selected axial slices of the skull-stripped MR brain volume so a statistical analysis approach could be used to compare the data of different users. The visualization program has two primary displays. The first display, shown in Fig. 6(a), provides the tissue interface and geometry information required to pick the landmarks on that axial slice. In addition, a counter is incremented after each landmark selection indicating the number of picks remaining. In the second primary display, shown in Fig. 6(b), an enlarged view around a 10×10 voxel region (outlined by the blue box in the first primary display) in which the user is required to pick the landmarks at least 0.50 mm apart from each other is shown. The interface allows the user to adjust several parameters including the center and size of the enlarged view in the second display as well as the colormap scaling – linear or logarithmic (provides more contrast at low intensities) – to improve the contrast between neighboring tissues. Each landmark is selected in this second primary display and the selected point is marked in red in all displays. In order to get a sense of the location of the point in 3-D, the two orthogonal slices through this point are also displayed, as shown in Figs. 6(c) and (d). The landmark is automatically recorded as the physical position of the selected point with floating number coordinates. The user also has the flexibility of removing any of the previously recorded landmarks.

3.2 Data

First six participants picked landmarks on two different MR image volumes and the remaining six participants picked landmarks on only one image volume. Ten landmarks were picked on each of 33 selected axial cross-sections yielding a total of 330 landmarks equally distributed across the cortical regions and geometries for each tissue interface. Two measures were computed in this validation study – the signed distance (SD), or landmark offset, and the surface defining membership function value (SDMFV) defined as the value of $\hat{\mu}_{WM}$ and $\hat{\mu}_{GM} + \hat{\mu}_{WM}$ at the landmark for the inner and pial surface, respectively.

3.3   Statistical Analysis

We first test the effects of variable intensity inhomogeneity and colormap scaling by comparing the algorithm versus user across the two different brains, the three different geometries (sulcal "fundi", "banks", and "gyri"'), and eleven different sulcal regions. Since it is hard to quantify the intensity inhomogeneity and colormap scaling, in the following statistical analysis, differences in SD and SDMFV across "brain", "geometry", and "sulci" provide information on the effects of variation in intensity inhomogeneity and colormap scaling. The GM/WM and GM/CSF interface data are analyzed separately.

Multivariate analysis of variance (MANOVA) [8] is a statistical technique for analyzing correlated measurements (i.e., SD and SDMFV) depending on several kinds of factors (i.e., brain, geometry, sulci) operating simultaneously. The measurements of the first six users were tested separately in a balanced additive MANOVA design with "sulci", "geometry", and "brain" as the factors. Another balanced additive design with "sulci" and "geometry" as the factors was used to test the measurements of the users 7–12 separately because they had completed landmarks for a single brain. MANOVA revealed a significant effect of "geometry" and "sulci" for all twelve users, but "brain" failed to reach significance (5% level) for both GM/WM and GM/CSF interface data of the users 1, 2, 5 and 6. Significant differences in performance of the algorithm relative to user across different aspects of the cortical geometry and across different sulcal regions may reflect variability in noise, intensity inhomogeneity, abnormalities in the original MR brain volume, and colormap scaling function for the different brain features. On the other hand, the absence of an effect for "brain" reflects the intra-rater consistency of picking landmarks in different MR images.

3.4   Landmark Offset on the Inner Surface

The average landmark offsets for the inner surface for different geometries are shown in Table 1. The overall mean landmark offset is -0.35 mm with a standard deviation of 0.65 mm. Only 16% of the landmarks are farther than 1.00 mm from the estimated inner cortical surfaces, indicating that gross errors are not common.

3.5   Landmark Offset on the Pial Surface

The average landmark offsets on the pial surface are also shown in Table 1. The overall mean landmark offset is -0.32 mm with a standard deviation of 0.50 mm, and only 8% of the landmarks are farther than 1.00 mm from the reference surfaces. Smaller standard deviations of the pial surface landmark offsets compared with inner surface landmark offsets indicate a higher stability for the pial surface. The higher stability on the pial surface could be due to the ACE-processing in CRUISE. In separate experiments, we have found that in ACE-processed regions, ACE is more dominant than the membership isolevel criterion in defining the surface location. Smaller landmark offset statistics (-0.16 ± 0.43 mm) are

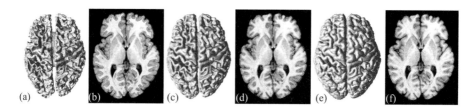

Fig. 5. Estimated surface of a sample brain and the surface superposed on an axial cross-section of the skull-stripped MR image: (a-b) inner, (c-d) central, (e-f) pial.

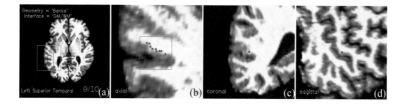

Fig. 6. Interactive program for landmark picking: (a) An example axial cross-section, (b) enlarged view, and (c)-(d) orthogonal cross-sections through the selected point.

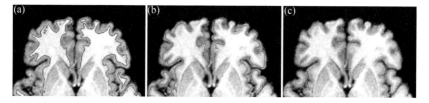

Fig. 7. Estimated surfaces superposed on an axial cross-section of the skull-stripped MR image: (a) inner, (b) central, (c) pial (blue: $\alpha = 0.5$ and $\beta = 0.5$; red: $\alpha = 0.64$ and $\beta = 0.72$).

observed in the ACE-processed regions as compared with the landmark offset statistics $(-0.47 \pm 0.51$ mm) in the regions not processed by ACE.

Consistent negative mean landmark offsets (more pronounced on the sulcal fundi regions) and the mean SDMFVs larger than 0.5 (reported in Table 1) may be interpreted as an outward bias of CRUISE. To address this observation, a simple threshold selection study is described in Sect. 4.

4   Threshold Optimization and Evaluation

In Sect. 3, we reported the landmark offsets on the inner and pial surfaces inferring an outward bias of CRUISE. Based on the observed SDMFV at the landmarks, here we want to estimate the α and β thresholds that best fit the landmark data and repeat the validation analysis with the surfaces estimated with the new thresholds. For these purposes, we divide the landmark data into two groups; the first group (training) is used for thresholds estimation, and the

Table 1. Statistics of Landmark Errors.

Geometry	Inner Surface SD mean	SD stdev	AD >1 mm	AD >2 mm	$\hat{\mu}_{WM}$ mean	$\hat{\mu}_{WM}$ stdev	Pial Surface SD mean	SD stdev	AD >1 mm	AD >2 mm	$\hat{\mu}_{GM}+\hat{\mu}_{WM}$ mean	$\hat{\mu}_{GM}+\hat{\mu}_{WM}$ stdev
Fundus	-0.60	0.60	22%	2.1%	0.73	0.21	-0.48	0.50	14%	0.4%	0.73	0.21
Bank	-0.37	0.55	11%	1.0%	0.68	0.22	-0.30	0.45	6.4 %	0.1 %	0.65	0.22
Gyrus	-0.09	0.70	16%	1.0%	0.61	0.25	-0.16	0.48	5.2 %	0.0 %	0.63	0.23
All	**-0.35**	**0.65**	**16%**	**1.4%**	**0.67**	**0.23**	**-0.32**	**0.50**	**8.4%**	**0.2%**	**0.67**	**0.23**

SD: signed distance in mm, AD: absolute distance in mm

Table 2. Membership function values at the training data landmarks

Geometry	Inner Surface $\hat{\mu}_{WM}$ mean	stdev	Pial Surface $\hat{\mu}_{GM}+\hat{\mu}_{WM}$ mean	stdev
Fundus	0.71	0.21	0.78	0.21
Bank	0.64	0.22	0.69	0.23
Gyrus	0.58	0.25	0.69	0.25
All	**0.64**	**0.23**	**0.72**	**0.23**

second group (test) is used to repeat the analysis. The grouping is based on the intra-user consistency on picking landmarks reported in Sect. 3.3. In particular, the data of the users 1, 2, 5, and 6 form the training data.

SDMFV statistics for the training data are reported in Table 2. Although we observed that the α and β thresholds should be functions of the cortical geometry – i.e., the ideal thresholds are different for different parts of the brain –, in this study, we choose a simpler approach and set α and β to the observed mean SDMFV, and repeated our previous analysis with these thresholds.

The cortical surfaces were estimated using the $\alpha = 0.64$ and $\beta = 0.72$ thresholds, and the landmark validation study was repeated on both inner and pial surfaces. Table 3 gives the landmark offsets of the test data on the surfaces estimated with the original and the new α and β thresholds. Overall, there is a 79% improvement on the inner surface, and a 64% improvement on the pial surface. Different percentile improvements on the different geometries support the idea of defining the thresholds as functions of the cortical geometry. A sample axial cross-section with the surfaces estimated with the original and the new α and β thresholds are shown in Fig. 7. We repeated the central surface landmark validation study reported in [1] with the new central surfaces. Slight differences with no substantial improvement or change were observed on the reported values. These results show the robustness of the central surface reconstruction.

5   Discussion and Future Work

The purpose of this work was to evaluate the accuracy of the CRUISE algorithms developed for the automatic reconstruction of the three nested surfaces of the cerebral cortex from MR brain images. This was accomplished by conducting a validation study using landmarks. The surfaces can be found with subvoxel accuracy, typically with an accuracy of one third of a voxel. Currently, we utilize "user implied surfaces", derived from user selected landmarks, to quantify the

Table 3. Landmark errors for the test data

Geometry	α	Inner Surface SD mean	stdev	AD >1 mm	>2 mm	β	Pial Surface SD mean	stdev	AD >1 mm	>2 mm
Fundus	0.50	-0.64	0.62	24%	2.7%	0.50	-0.52	0.56	18%	1.7%
Bank	0.50	-0.44	0.54	13%	1.0%	0.50	-0.41	0.56	14%	1.3%
Gyrus	0.50	-0.10	0.74	17%	1.1%	0.50	-0.24	0.57	11%	1.3%
All	**0.50**	**-0.39**	**0.68**	**18%**	**1.6%**	**0.50**	**-0.39**	**0.57**	**14%**	**1.4%**
Fundus	0.64	0.38	0.61	12%	1.6%	0.72	-0.39	0.75	18%	4.4%
Bank	0.64	-0.16	0.62	7%	1.9%	0.72	-0.14	0.59	9%	0.1%
Gyrus	0.64	0.29	0.92	20%	6.6%	0.72	0.12	0.59	10%	0.1%
All	**0.64**	**-0.08**	**0.78**	**13%**	**3.4%**	**0.72**	**-0.14**	**0.68**	**12%**	**1.8%**

SD: signed distance in mm, AD: absolute distance in mm

accuracy of CRUISE. In future work, we plan to create a nested surface truth model from the visible human cyrosection and MR image data [9], and validate our methods against this data.

A simple experiment to improve CRUISE by selecting new threshold values which were more in accordance with the user implied surfaces was presented in Sect. 4. Based on the statistics reported in this work, a more extensive study is currently underway to formulate CRUISE thresholds as functions of cortical geometry. We expect a variable threshold scheme – based on local cortical geometry – will provide even higher accuracy in the CRUISE reconstruction algorithms.

References

1. C. Xu, D. L. Pham, M. E. Rettmann, D. N. Yu, and J. L. Prince. Reconstruction of the human cerebral cortex from magnetic resonance images. *IEEE Trans. Med. Imag.*, 18(6):467–480, June 1999.
2. X. Han, C. Xu, M. E. Rettmann, and J. L. Prince. Automatic segmentation editing for cortical surface reconstruction. In *Proc. of SPIE Medical Imaging*, Feb 2001.
3. X. Han, C. Xu, U. Braga-Neto, and J. L. Prince. Topology correction in brain cortex segmentation using a multiscale, graph-based algorithm. *IEEE Trans. Med. Imag.*, 21:109–121, 2002.
4. X. Han, C. Xu, and J. L. Prince. A topology preserving level set method for geometric deformable models. *IEEE Trans. on Pattern Anal. Machine Intell.*, 25:755–768, 2003.
5. S. M. Resnick, A. F. Goldszal, C. Davatzikos, S. Golski, M. A. Kraut, E. J. Metter, R. N. Bryan, and A. B. Zonderman. One-year age changes in MRI brain volumes in older adults. *Cerebral Cortex*, 10(5):464–72, May 2000.
6. D. L. Pham. Robust fuzzy segmentation of magnetic resonance images. In *IEEE Symposium on Computer-Based Medical Systems*, pages 127–131, 2001.
7. OpenDX Developers. http://www.opendx.org/, 1997.
8. H. Scheffe. *The analysis of variance.* Wiley, New York, 1959.
9. V. Spitzer, M. J. Ackerman, A. L. Scherzinger, and D. J. Whitlock. The visible male: A technical report. *J. Am. Med. Informat. Assoc.*, 3:118–130, 1996.

Discriminative MR Image Feature Analysis for Automatic Schizophrenia and Alzheimer's Disease Classification[*]

Yanxi Liu[1][**], Leonid Teverovskiy[1], Owen Carmichael[1], Ron Kikinis[2],
Martha Shenton[2], Cameron S. Carter[3], V. Andrew Stenger[4], Simon Davis[4],
Howard Aizenstein[4], James T. Becker[4], Oscar L. Lopez[4], and
Carolyn C. Meltzer[4]

[1] Carnegie Mellon University
[2] Harvard Medical School
[3] University of California, Davis
[4] University of Pittsburgh

Abstract. We construct a computational framework for automatic central nervous system (CNS) disease discrimination using high resolution Magnetic Resonance Images (MRI) of human brains. More than 3000 MR image features are extracted, forming a high dimensional coarse-to-fine hierarchical image description that quantifies brain asymmetry, texture and statistical properties in corresponding local regions of the brain. Discriminative image feature subspaces are computed, evaluated and selected automatically. Our initial experimental results show 100% and 90% separability between chronicle schizophrenia (SZ) and first episode SZ versus their respective matched controls. Under the same computational framework, we also find higher than 95% separability among Alzheimer's Disease, mild cognitive impairment patients, and their matched controls. An average of 88% classification success rate is achieved using leave-one-out cross validation on five different well-chosen patient-control image sets of sizes from 15 to 27 subjects per disease class.

1 Introduction

Schizophrenia (SZ) is a severe, chronic and persistent mental disorder with onset in late adolescence or early adulthood resulting in lifelong mental, social and occupational disability. Alzheimer's Disease (AD) is a disease of aging, and the financial and social burdens of AD are compounded by recent and continued increases in the average life span. Assisting clinicians in making accurate early diagnostic distinctions for SZ and AD becomes increasingly important with the development of effective treatments for CNS diseases.

Structural Magnetic Resonance (MR) images have an important advantage over other imaging modalities in that they are non-invasive and provide detailed

---

[*] This work is supported in part by NIH grants AG05133 and DA015900-01.
[**] Corresponding Author: yanxi@cs.cmu.edu

C. Barillot, D.R. Haynor, and P. Hellier (Eds.): MICCAI 2004, LNCS 3216, pp. 393–401, 2004.

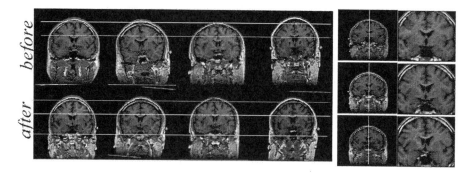

Fig. 1. Left: sample corresponding slices from four subjects (left to right: control, sz, control, sz). Before and after affine registration vertical correspondences are indicated by horizontal lines. Right: input consecutive slices of one subject where the iMSP is aligned with the center of the image and the ROI is cropped uniformly in preparation for brain asymmetry and other image-features computation.

information about gray and white matter parenchyma of the brain, and cerebrospinal fluid (CSF)-filled spaces. Nevertheless, classification of SZ and AD patients using high resolution MR neuroimages remains a challenging task even for the most experienced neuroradiologists. Most work in automatic or semi-automatic MR neuroimage classification [1,5,14,7,16] has been focusing on precise segmentation of various anatomical structures for volumetric and local shape comparisons [14,16]. In both cases of SZ and AD, there are considerable reported group morphological differences in specific anatomical structures of the brain [3, 18]. Due to group overlap, however, few existing methods reliably distinguish whether an *individual* MR image is from a specific disease category (SZ vs. normal or AD vs. normal), particularly in early stages of the disease.

Section 2 gives a general description of our image-feature based classification approach. Section 3 describes our experiments on SZ and AD datasets. In Section 4 we discuss the results and summarize the paper. A more detailed report of this work can be found in [12].

2   General Approach

We propose an image feature based statistical learning approach, in addition to anatomical morphology analysis, to better classify MR image of CNS diseases. We formulate this task as a supervised learning problem, where the MR image labels are given (class decisions are made by doctors based on specific clinical criteria for SZ and AD through behavior and cognitive tests). The key element is to learn those MR image features that best discriminate disease classes. We shall examine both *separability* on the training data to visualize the data distribution, and *generality* in terms of leave-one-out cross validation results to evaluate the predicting power of the selected MR image features. The basic components in our computational framework include:

3D Image Alignment: All MR images for each classification problem in our feasibility study are taken using the same scanner and protocols. We verify image intensity consistency by carrying out an analysis of intensity histograms of all input images. All MR images are deformably registered using an affine registration algorithm [13] to a digital brain atlas (the Harvard brain atlas [9] for schizophrenia study and the Montreal Neurological Institute (MNI) template [4] for Alzheimer's Disease study). Affine deformable registrations normalize all brain images for shape and scale globally. Internal local differences are **not** further corrected intentionally.

An automatic ideal midsagittal plane (iMSP) extraction algorithm [11] is applied to each 3D MR image before and after the affine registration to (1) initialize yaw, roll angles and X-axis translation [11] before the 3D registration for faster convergence and better registration accuracy. (2) validate and reassure the iMSP accuracy after affine registration (Figure 1) in preparation for quantified-brain-asymmetry image feature extraction.

Regions of Interest: Since each brain image is affinely registered with a digital atlas in 3D space, our medical experts can identify a region of interest (ROI) by specifying a stack of 2D slices on the atlas. These are regions which may have potential relevance to disease classification on individual MR scans as indicated in the literature.

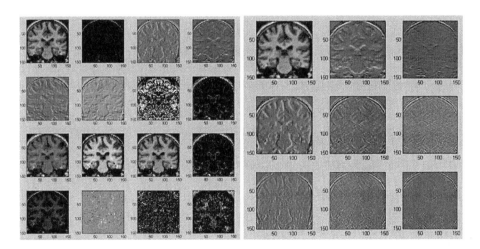

Fig. 2. Left: A sample view of all extracted *statistical features*. From left to right, top to bottom: mean intensity, variance, vertical edge, horizontal edge, diagonal edge, (other) diagonal edge, edge orientation, standard deviation, maximum intensity, minimum intensity, median intensity, range, energy, skewness, kurtosis, entropy. Right: the top-left 3 by 3 2D *texture features* out of the 25 Law's texture features — L5L5, E5L5, S5L5; L5E5, E5E5, S5E5; L5S5, E5S5, S5S5. The five 1D convolution kernels: Level, L5 = [1 4 6 4 1]; Edge, E5 = [-1 -2 0 2 1]; Spot, S5 = [-1 0 2 0 -1]; Wave, W5 = [-1 2 0 -2 1]; and Ripple, R5 = [1 -4 6 -4 1]. Each two-dimensional convolution kernel is generated by convolving a *vertical* 1D kernel with a *horizontal* 1D kernel.

1 mean
2 variance
3 mean Asym
4 variance Asym

5 m	6 m
9 v	10 v
45 mA	46 mA
49 vA	50 vA

8 m	7 m
12 v	11 v
48 mA	47 mA
52 vA	51 vA

13m 17v 53mA 57vA	14m 18v 54mA 58vA	21m 25v 61mA 65vA	22m 26v 62mA 66vA
16m 20v 56mA 60vA	15m 19v 55mA 59vA	24m 28v 64mA 68vA	23m 27v 63mA 67vA
37m 41v 77mA 81vA	38m 42v 78mA 82vA	29m 33v 69mA 73vA	30m 34v 70mA 74vA
40m 44v 80mA 84vA	39m 43v 79mA 83vA	32m 36v 72mA 76vA	31m 35v 71mA 75vA

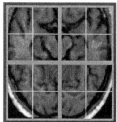

Fig. 3. The three left-panels illustrate the hierarchical decomposition of each slice. For each image feature, we compute the mean(m), variance(v) , asymmetry mean(mA), and asymmetry variance(vA) in each local region (right). We then concatenate all of these local measures into a feature vector. The numbers in each block indicate an index of the feature location (clockwise rotation of the four quarters starting from top-left).

Image Features: Two general categories of 41 image features are used in our feasibility study, including 16 *statistical features* [8] and 25 *Law's texture features* [10] (Figure 2).

For each filtered brain slice $I(x, y)$, we also compute an *asymmetry brain image feature* defined as: $D(x, y) = I(x, y) - I_{vRef}(x, y)$ where I_{vRef} is the vertical reflection of the original feature image $I(x, y)$. Since $I(x, y)$ is already centered by the iMSP, $D(x, y)$ is the intensity difference of the corresponding left and right halves of a brain slice. Left-right asymmetry redundancy is removed during feature screening process.

Image Feature Location: One important aspect of our exploration is to localize where the potential discriminative features lie in the ROI. We subdivide each slice of the registered brain (in coronal or axial direction) hierarchically. Figure 3 shows such a division on three levels (each level has 1, 4 and 16 regions respectively). For each level, we compute the mean and variance of the image feature in each subdivision. Given both original image feature and bilateral asymmetry difference measures, a total of $(1+4+16)*4 = 84$ "location features" are generated for each image feature type on each 2D slice. Therefore we have a total of $41 \times 84 \times \#of slices = 3444 \times \#of slices$ dimensional feature space with regional, asymmetry, statistical and textural information to explore.

Discriminative Feature Evaluation and Screening: A common theme in our research is to use available image features selectively for different image discrimination tasks; this is especially effective when *redundancy* exists among different feature dimensions which is highly characteristic in image feature-based classifications. We define an *augmented variance ratio* (AVR) as

$$AVR(F) = \frac{Var(S_F)}{\frac{1}{C}\sum_{i=1..C} \frac{Var_i(S_F)}{min_{i\neq j}(|mean_i(S_F)-mean_j(S_F)|)}}$$

where $Var(S_F)$ is the cross-class variance of feature F, $Var_i(S_F)$ and $mean_i(S_F)$ are the within-class variance and mean of feature F for class i out of C distinct classes. Similar to Fisher criteria [6], AVR is the ratio of cross-class variance of the feature over within-class variance, with an added penalty to features that have close inter-class means. AVR ranked features provide us with a quantitative basis to screen out non-discriminative features before feature subset selection [2]. Feature subset selection is carried out using Linear Discriminant Analysis (LDA) [6] whose criteria is consistent with AVR.

Separability Analysis: We define *separability* of a given data set D as the classification rate (plus sensitivity and specificity) in a learned discriminative feature subspace on D using a K-nearest neighbor (KNN) classifier [6]. Different feature subspaces are explored using either an exhaustive search for all triplets or a forward sequential selection strategy [2]. The result is a set of image feature subspaces with the highest classification rates indicating best separation among image classes.

Prediction: Given N data points (3D MR images from N different subjects), $N - 1$ are used for training to find discriminative feature subspaces, and the one left out is used as the unseen test sample for evaluating the prediction accuracy of the learned classifier. This process is repeated N times in a round-robin manner.

3   Experiments

3.1   Classification of Schizophrenia Patients

A feasibility study is carried out using (1) an image data set from Dr. Shenton [17] containing MR images of 15 schizophrenia patients (chronicle) and 15 controls; and (2) an image data set from Dr. Carter[1], containing MR images of 24 first episode (FE) schizophrenia patients and 27 normal controls. The controls are matched in age, family background and handedness. From each 3D MR scan a set of 2D coronal slices are sampled around the region of interest. Taking the top 30 most discriminative features from more than 3000 candidates, followed by sequential forward feature subset selection using LDA [2], and LOO using KNN we achieve the results listed in Table 4 and Figure 5.

3.2   Classification of Alzheimer's Disease

A set of 60 subjects are selected by experts from the Alzheimer's Disease Research Center (ADRC - an NIH research center) of University of Pittsburgh, in which 20 are normal controls, 20 are subjects with MCI, and 20 are diagnosed AD patients matched on age, education and sex. The image data are acquired on a 1.5T GE scanner in the coronal plane, with minimized partial voluming effects. This image data set is normalized for intensity mean (0.4 in a 0 to 1 scale) and variance (0.25). See Table 1 and Figure 6 for classification results on this data set.

Combination of Image Features with Shape Features: Using LONI [15] we have hand-segmented hippocampi for each subject in the 20-20-20 (control, MCI and AD) image data set. Several shape features are computed using the hand

---
[1] originally from University of Pittsburgh, now at UC Davis

Disease Class # of Subjects	CTL vs. SZ 15 vs. 15	CTL vs. SZ 27 vs. 24
Separability	100%	90%
Sensitivity	100%	88%
Specificity	100%	92%
LOO Rate	90%	78%
Sensitivity	93%	79%
Specificity	87%	77%

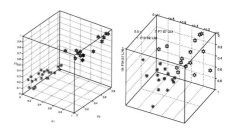

Fig. 4. Experimental Results: Harvard data set contains 15 SZ patients (chronicle) versus 15 normals. UPMC data set contains 24 SZ patients (first episode) versus 27 normals.

Fig. 5. Examples of two automatically selected 3-feature discriminative subspaces for schizophrenia MR image data sets (1) and (2). Stars (lower-left) indicate SZ patients.

Table 1. Alzheimer's Disease Classification Results

Disease Class # of Subjects Features Used	CTL vs. MCI 20 vs. 20 Image	CTL vs. AD 20 vs. 20 Image	MCI vs. AD 20 vs. 20 Image	MCI vs. AD 20 vs. 20 **Image+Shape**
Separability	100%	96%	97%	98%
Sensitivity	100%	95%	100%	100%
Specificity	100%	96%	95%	95%
LOO Rate	93%	93%	78%	88%
Sensitivity	100%	85%	80%	85%
Specificity	85%	100%	75%	90%

traced 3D surface information. They are: hippocampus volume, the coordinate of the centroid of the hippocampus, the x,y, and z dimensions of the bounding box around the hippocampus, the 2nd-order geometric moments of the hippocampus along three axes, and 2nd-order legendre moments of the hippocampus. Adding these shape features to the image feature selection process we have achieved better classification rates (right-most column in Table 1), indicating that the image intensity features and shape features complement each other.

Experiments with Multiple Classifiers: We have also experimented with many standard classifiers including decision trees, decision graphs, decision stumps, instance-based learning, naive Bayes and support vector machines (SVM) with or without bagging or stacking on the top 100 AVR ranked image features. We found the performance depends primarily on the *image features* used. Using the top 30 AVR ranked image features in combination with shape features, for example, decision stumps achieves the best classification rates for control versus AD, 90% (sensitivity and specificity).

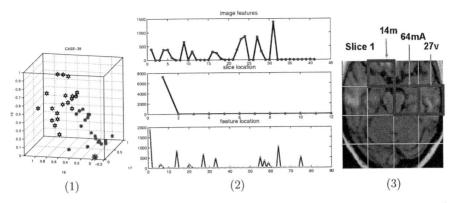

Fig. 6. (1): Sample LOO result showing the predicting power of the learned image feature space for MCIs versus normal controls. The larger star indicates the subject (an MCI patient) *left-out* during the training process. (2): Three plots showing feature type, slice number and geometric location of the most discriminative features selected for MCI vs. normal controls prediction. Top: The most popular image feature is the 15th texture feature (31st on the X axis) composed of ripple and spot. Middle: The most important slice in a 3D image is the most inferior slice in the chosen ROI. Bottom: the top three most discriminative *local features* come from region 64 (mean intensity asymmetry value, hippocampus region), region 14 (mean value of the top left-middle region) and region 27 (the intensity variance). (3): the local regions containing the most discriminative local features are outlined on the most selected brain slice.

4   Discussion and Conclusion

We establish a framework for a computer system to automatically explore very high dimensional image feature spaces in search of a discriminative subspace. The preliminary results suggest that regional image features contain highly discriminative information to separate different CNS diseases, e.g. SZ or AD, from normal brains on several limited (15 to 27 subjects in each disease class) but well-chosen image sets. The LOO cross validation results also suggest the potential to build a disease predictor that uses critically chosen image features to classify an unknown individual image into one of the disease categories with probability much higher than chance. The LOO result of controls versus AD surpasses the result reported in [7], which is based on a one-time division of the input data. Our result, on the other hand, is based upon a statistically justified 40-way division of the input data [6]. Our result on SZ classification (Table 4) also surpasses the performance reported in [16] on the same image set.

One non-intuitive aspect of our approach perhaps lies in the fact that, contrary to most medical image analysis and particularly in SZ and AD MR image studies, no anatomical segmentation of the MR neuroimages is carried out. Instead, we bring all brain images into a common coordinate system where they are affinely registered and their iMSPs coincide, divide each 2D slice into equal sized geometric regions and compute image properties in each region where the true anatomical structures in corresponding patches may or may not correspond. Our method takes advantage of the intensity discrepancy caused by local non-correspondences and examines quantitatively whether such discrepancies are representative of their image semantic class (disease) by statistical learning and cross validation. Another advantage of our method over, e.g. neural network approaches, is that it is not a black-box. We are able to visualize the relative weights in the found discriminative subspace, data points distributions, and trace back the type and the (anatomical) locations of selected image features (Figure 6).

The ultimate goal of our research is to understand the biological implications of the automatically selected discriminative features. Current results, considering local features from temporal lobe asymmetry (for SZ study) and hippocampus asymmetry (for AD/MCI study, Figure 6) highly discriminative, are encouraging. We plan to further validate the consistency of selected image features from LOO, explore the whole 3D brain systematically in future studies using volumetric image features, and test our method on larger MR image data sets.

References

1. R. Bilder, H. Wu, B. Bogerts, M. Ashtari, D. Robinson, M. Woerner, J. Lieberman, and G. Degreef. Cerebral volume asymmetries in schizophrenia and mood disorders: a quantitative magnetic resonance imaging study. *International Journal of Psychophysiology*, 34(3):197–205, December 1999.
2. C. M. Bishop. *Neural Networks for Pattern Recognition*. Clarendon Press, 1995. ISBN:0198538499.
3. R. Buchanan, K. Vladar, P. Barta, and G. Pearlson. Structural evaluation of the prefrontal cortex in schizophrenia. *Am. J. of Psychiatry*, 155:1049–55, 1998.
4. D. L. Collins, A. Zijdenbos, V. Kollokian, J. G. Sled, N. J. Kabani, C. J. Holmes, and A. C. Evans. Design and construction of a realistic digital brain phantom. *IEEE Trans. Med. Imag.*, 17:463–468, 1998.
5. T. Crow. Schizophrenia as an anomaly of cerebral asymmetry. In K. Maurer, editor, *Imaging of the brian in psychiatry and related fields*. Springer-Verlag, 1993.
6. R. Duda, P. Hart, and D. Stork. *Pattern Classification*. John Wiley & Sons, New York, 2001.
7. P. Freeborough and N. C. Fox. MR image texture analysis applied to the diagnosis and tracking of alzheimer's disease. *IEEE Transactions on Medical Imaging*, 17(3):475–479, June 1998.
8. A. Jain, R. Duin, and J. Mao. Statistical pattern recognition: a review. *IEEE Trans. Pattern Analysis and Machine Intelligence*, 22(1):4–37, Jan. 2000.
9. R. Kikinis, M. Shenton, D. Iosifescu, R. McCarley, P. Saiviroonporn, H. Hokama, A. Robatino, D. Metcalf, C. Wible, C. Portas, R. Donnino, and F. Jolesz. A digital brain atlas for surgical planning, model-driven segmentation, and teaching. *IEEE Transactions on visualization and computer graphics*, 2(3):232–240, Sept. 1996.
10. K. Law. *Textured Image Segmentation*. PhD thesis, University of Southern California, January 1980.
11. Y. Liu, R. Collins, and W. Rothfus. Robust Midsagittal Plane Extraction from Normal and Pathological 3D Neuroradiology Images. *IEEE Transactions on Medical Imaging*, 20(3):175–192, March 2001.

12. Y. Liu, L. Teverovskiy, O. Carmichael, R. Kikinis, M. Shenton, C. Carter, V. Stenger, S. Davis, H. Aizenstein, J. Becker, O. Lopez, and M. Meltzer. Discriminative mr image feature analysis for automatic schizophrenia and alzheimer's disease classification. Technical Report CMU-RI-TR-04-15, The Robotics Institute, Carnegie Mellon University, Pittsburgh, PA, 2004.

13. F. Maes, A. Collignon, D. Vandermeulun, G. Marchal, and P. Suetens. Multimodality image registration by maximization of mutual information. *IEEE Transactions on Medical Imaging*, 16(2):187,198, 1997.

14. R. McCarley, C. Wible, Y. Frumin, J. Levitt, I. Fischer, and M. Shenton. MRI anatomy of schizophrenia. *Society of Biological Psychiatry*, 45:1099–1119, 1999.

15. D. Rex, J. Ma, and A. Toga. The LONI pipeline processing environment. *Neuroimage*, 19(3):1033–48, 2003.

16. M. Shenton, G. Gerig, R. McCarley, G. Szekely, and R. Kikinis. Amygdala-hippocampal shape differences in schizophrenia: the application of 3d shape models to volumetric mr data. *Psychiatry Research Neuroimaging*, 115:15–35, 2002.

17. M. Shenton, R. Kikinis, F. Jolesz, S. Pollak, M. Lemay, C. Wible, H. Hokama, J. Martin, B. Metcalf, M. Coleman, M. A. Robert, and T. McCarley. Abnormalities of the left temporal lobe in schizophrenia. response to roth, pfefferbaum and to klimke and knecht. *New England Journal of Medicine*, 327:75–84, 1992.

18. P. Thompson, D. MacDonald, M. Mega, C. Holmes, A. Evans, and A. Toga. Detection and mapping of abnormal brain structure with a probabilistic atlas of cortical surfaces. *Journal of Computer Assisted Tomography*, 21(4):567–81, 1997.

Left Ventricular Segmentation in MR Using Hierarchical Multi-class Multi-feature Fuzzy Connectedness

Amol Pednekar[1], Uday Kurkure[1], Raja Muthupillai[2], Scott Flamm[3], and Ioannis A. Kakadiaris[1]*

[1] Visual Computing Lab, Dept. of Computer Science,
University of Houston, Houston, TX, USA
[2] Philips Medical Systems North America, Bothell, WA, USA
[3] Dept. of Radiology, St. Luke's Episcopal Hospital, Houston, TX, USA

Abstract. In this paper, we present a new method for data-driven automatic extraction of endocardial and epicardial contours of the left ventricle in cine bFFE MR images. Our method employs a hierarchical, multi-class, multi-feature fuzzy connectedness framework for image segmentation. This framework combines image intensity and texture information with anatomical shape, while preserving the topological relationship within and between the interrelated anatomical structures. We have applied this method on cine bFFE MR data from eight asymptomatic and twelve symptomatic volunteers with very encouraging qualitative and quantitative results.

1 Introduction

Magnetic resonance imaging (MRI) is the preferred cardiac imaging technique as it acquires images in oblique planes; obviating geometric assumptions regarding the shapes of the ventricles providing high blood-to-myocardium contrast. However, the cine cardiac MR (CMR) images are not incisive; they are fuzzy due to patient motion, background variation, and partial voluming. Left ventricle (LV) myocardial delineation allows the computation of critical LV functional descriptors (e.g., ejection fraction and wall thickening). The manual contour tracing used in current clinical practice is labor-intensive, time-consuming, and involves considerable inter- and intra-observer variations [1]. The development of computer-assisted myocardial contour extraction will reduce the analysis time and, more importantly, will produce unbiased and consistent results. The segmentation of CMR data typically faces two challenges: the determination of the inter-tissue boundaries (blurred due to partial voluming), and the delineation of

---

* This material is based upon work supported in part by the National Science Foundation under Grants IIS-9985482 and IIS-0335578. Any opinions, findings, and conclusions or recommendations expressed in this material are those of the authors and do not necessarily reflect the views of the National Science Foundation.

C. Barillot, D.R. Haynor, and P. Hellier (Eds.): MICCAI 2004, LNCS 3216, pp. 402–410, 2004.

the boundaries of anatomical structures composed of the same tissue type (e.g., trabeculae carnae and papillary muscles projecting out of the myocardium).

Most of the research towards automated segmentation of CMR data follows one of three major approaches: 1) active contour-based methods - positioning of a two-dimensional (2D) contour near the strongest local image features using the principle of energy minimization [2,3] (these methods rely on user interaction for initialization of the shape and location of the ventricle's boundaries); 2) deformable model-based methods - three-dimensional (3D) shape fitting for functional analysis of cardiac images using physics-based deformable models [4,5, 6] ; and 3) active appearance-based methods - fitting with models that provide a statistical description of local shape (geometry) and appearance (brightness) [7, 8] (these methods could be biased towards a "too normal" pattern of the LV shape and its dynamics). Research is ongoing in developing hybrid segmentation methods for the extraction of LV endocardial boundary surfaces by combining edge, region, and shape information [9,10,11,12]. Our hybrid segmentation approach is data-driven and hence works across a wide range of patient data. It is an extension of the fuzzy connectedness-based image segmentation framework developed by Udupa and Samarasekera [13], which effectively captures the fuzzy "hanging togetherness" of image elements specified by their strength of connectedness. That framework has been further extended with the introduction of object scale, relative strength of connectedness, multiple objects, and multi-dimensional images. The idea of using dynamic adaptive weights for affinity components was introduced in our previous work [14].

In this paper, we present a new method for segmenting the LV myocardium automatically. The main steps are the following: 1) automatic localization of the LV and myocardium using multi-view, intensity, and shape information; 2) employing a hierarchical, multi-class, multi-feature fuzzy connectedness framework to overcome the low contrast between interfacing tissues; 3) integrating shape-oriented coordinate transforms, myocardial fuzzy affinity, and optimal path computation using dynamic programming to overcome anatomy-specific challenges (such as those posed by papillary muscles projecting out of the myocardium). Our data-driven method does not require any user interaction at either the LV identification or the myocardial segmentation phases. Our contributions include the development of a hierarchical, multi-class, multi-feature fuzzy connectedness framework for image segmentation, which combines the image intensity and texture information with the shape of the anatomy, while preserving the topological relationship within and between the interrelated anatomic structures. The main attributes of this framework are the following: 1) computing multi-class affinity that takes into consideration the affinity component distributions of all the neighboring objects (which allows competition between different objects); 2) computing multi-feature affinity; and 3) integrating multi-class affinity and multi-feature affinity components to compute fuzzy affinity, where the weights for individual affinity components are determined automatically.

2　Method

In this section, we present our hierarchical, multi-class, multi-feature fuzzy connectedness framework and its application to the segmentation of the LV myocardium.

2.1　Hierarchical Multi-class Multi-feature Fuzzy Connectedness

We describe our formulation of hierarchical, multi-class multi-feature fuzzy connectedness using the terminology introduced by Udupa and Samarasekera [13]. The aim of image segmentation is to capture the local and global "hanging-togetherness" that is, the perception of a coherent object region in spite of heterogeneity of scene intensity) of pixels. For any relationship ρ, the strength of ρ between any two pixels c and d in digital space Z^2 is represented by a membership function $\mu_\rho(c, d)$.

Local Fuzzy Spel Affinity: Any fuzzy relation κ in a scene domain C is a *fuzzy pixel affinity* in a scene $\mathcal{C}$ if it is reflexive and symmetric. We define the *local fuzzy spel affinity* (μ_κ) to consist of three components: 1) the object feature intensity component (μ_ϕ); 2) the intensity homogeneity component (μ_ψ); and 3) the texture feature component (μ_φ). This can be expressed in the following form:

$$\mu_\kappa(c, d) = \mu_\alpha(c, d)g(\mu_\phi(c, d), \mu_\psi(c, d), \mu_\varphi(c, d)) \tag{1}$$

where $\mu_\alpha(c, d)$ is a hard adjacency relation. Thus, the fuzzy relation κ in a digital space Z^2 indicates the degree of local hanging togetherness of pixels c and d in the space of the feature vector:

$$\mathbf{x} = [\frac{1}{2}(f(c) + f(d)), f(c) - f(d), \frac{1}{2}(t(c) + t(d))]^\top \tag{2}$$

where $f(c)$ and $f(d)$ are the image intensities, and $t(c)$ and $t(d)$ are the texture features at pixels c and d. The similarity of the pixels' feature vectors is computed using the Mahalanobis metric:

$$md^2_{(\mathbf{c} \to \mathbf{d})} = (\mathbf{x}_{(\mathbf{c} \to \mathbf{d})} - \bar{\mathbf{x}}_{(\mathbf{c} \to \mathbf{d})})^\top S^{-1}_{(\mathbf{c} \to \mathbf{d})}(\mathbf{x}_{(\mathbf{c} \to \mathbf{d})} - \bar{\mathbf{x}}_{(\mathbf{c} \to \mathbf{d})}), \tag{3}$$

where $\mathbf{x}_{(\mathbf{c} \to \mathbf{d})}$, $\bar{\mathbf{x}}_{(\mathbf{c} \to \mathbf{d})}$, $S_{(\mathbf{c} \to \mathbf{d})}$ are the feature vector, the mean feature vector, and the covariance matrix in the direction from c to d, respectively. The bias in intensity in a specific direction is accounted for by allowing different levels and signs of intensity homogeneities in different directions of adjacency [14]. The advantage of using the Mahalanobis metric is that it weighs the differences in various feature dimensions by the range of variability in the direction of the feature dimension. These distances are computed in units of standard deviation from the mean. This allows us to assign a statistical probability to the measurement. The local fuzzy spel affinity is computed as: $\mu_\kappa(c, d) = \frac{1}{1 + md_{(\mathbf{c} \to \mathbf{d})}}$ to ensure $\mu_\kappa(c, d) \in Z^2 \to [0, 1]$ and it is reflexive and symmetric.

Global Object Affinity: *Fuzzy connectedness* captures the global hanging-togetherness of pixels by using the local affinity relation and by considering all possible paths between two, not necessarily nearby, pixels in the image. *Fuzzy κ-connectedness* in $\mathcal{C}$, denoted K, is a fuzzy relationship in $\mathcal{C}$ that assigns to every pair $(c, d) \in C$ a value $\mu_K(c, d) = \max_{p_{cd} \in P_{cd}} \{ \min_{1 \leq i \leq m} [\mu_\kappa(c_{(i)}, c_{(i+1)})] \}$, which is the largest of the weakest affinities between the successive pairs of pixels along the path p_{cd} of all possible paths P_{cd} in $\mathcal{C}$ from c to d. For any seed pixel $o \in C$, the $\kappa - connectivity$ $scene$ of o in $\mathcal{C}$ is the scene $\mathcal{C}_{K_o} = (C, f_{K_o})$ such that, for any $c \in C$, $f_{K_o}(c) = \mu_K(o, c)$. For any strength $\theta \in [0, 1]$, the binary relationship defined by $\mu_K(c, d) \geq \theta$, denoted K_θ, and defined in C is an equivalence relation in C [13]. For any seed pixel $o \in C$, let $O_{K_\theta}(o)$ be an equivalence class of K_θ in C that contains o. A *fuzzy $\kappa\theta$-object* of o in $\mathcal{C}$ is a fuzzy subset $O_{K_\theta}(o)$ of C such that, for any $c \in C$

$$\mu_{O_{K_\theta}(o)}(c) = \begin{cases} \eta(f(c)) & \text{if } \mu_K(o, c) \geq \theta \\ 0 & \text{otherwise} \end{cases}, \tag{4}$$

where η is an objectness function with range $[0, 1]$. Since $\mu_\kappa(c, d) = \frac{1}{1 + m_{d(c \rightarrow d)}}$, $\theta \leq 0.25$ denotes a probability of 0.01 or less and can be used to define the binary object. Thus, $\mu_\kappa(c, d)$ defines the probability of pixel pair belonging to the target object class. The threshold for the object definition can be set based on the probability distribution in a specific feature space for a particular application.

Global Class Affinity: In our framework the global object affinity and local pixel affinity are assigned only if the probability of c and d belonging to the neighboring objects' classes is much less than 0.01. The neighboring objects are defined as the objects with common boundaries in Euclidean space. For a given pixel pair (c, d), we compute the discrepancy measure with respect to the pre-determined or existing distributions (covariance matrices) of neighboring classes in terms of its Mahalanobis distance. Then, the minimum discrepancy measure $J(c, d) = \min_{1 \leq i \leq b} m_d(c, d)$, where b is the number of neighboring classes of the target object, gives the maximum probability of a pixel pair belonging to a certain class. If the $J(c, d) < 3$, and the class to which the pixel pair belongs is not the target object class, then local pixel affinity $\mu_{\kappa(c,d)} = 0$, else the pixel pair is a candidate to be considered to belong to the target object, hence its local pixel and global object affinity is computed as described earlier.

2.2   Left Ventricular Segmentation in MR

To apply our hierarchical, multi-class, multi-feature fuzzy connectedness algorithm for LV segmentation, first we determine the relevant classes and features. The training is performed only once for this application. Next, we compute the target object seed pixel and sample regions, and extract the LV myocardial contours. We further refine the myocardial contours to overcome the papillary muscles by using dynamic programming on the polar representation of the data.

A. Determination of Relevant Classes and Features

Step 1 - Compute the intensity and texture features: In the case of bFFE CMR data, the contrast between blood and myocardium is high. However, the tissue contrast between myocardium and air, and myocardium and liver is not adequate for intensity-based discrimination. Thus, we compute the Laws [15] and Gabor [16] texture features of these neighboring tissue types to increase the discrimination. Laws texture features are generated by using the 2D convolution kernels obtained by convolving five one-dimensional (1D) kernels with one another. Gabor features are obtained by filtering the original images with filter banks of four scales and six orientations of quazi-orthogonal Gabor filters. Currently, we employ the data from 10 subjects using three mid-ventricular end-diastolic (ED) slices per subject. In these 30 images, we manually delineated the myocardium, blood, liver, and air.

Step 2 - Compute the most discriminant texture features: From the feature images, we extract pixel features for the following classes: myocardium, blood, liver, and air. The texture features are ranked according to their individual ability to discriminate myocardium from all the neighboring tissues using the Fisher's criterion and the Mahalanobis distance measure. We found that spot-spot (ss) and spot-average intensity level (sl) Laws features are individually the most discriminating. Laws spot and level 1D kernels represent a second derivative filter and an averaging filter, respectively. The convolution of spot with spot, and spot with level kernels provide the ss and sl filters. Further, we found that combining intensity and intensity gradient with the ss feature provided higher discrimination between myocardium and other neighboring tissues. However, the discrimination between the myocardial muscle and the liver tissue remains low because the $T2$ values of these tissues are very similar. Thus, our feature vector (Eq. (2)) consists of pixel pair intensity, directional gradients, and the ss feature in a 5x5 neighborhood.

B. Extraction of the LV Myocardial Contours

Step 1 - Determine the LV medial axis: First, we determine the LV centroids in the blood region. In CMR imaging, the short-axis view is planned from vertical long-axis, two chamber (2CH), and approximate four chamber (4CH) scouts.

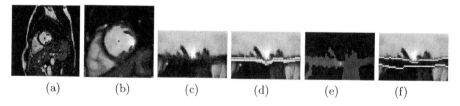

(a)   (b)   (c)   (d)   (e)   (f)

Fig. 1. (a) Original MRI (with LV center localization), (b) cropped (with LV center localization), and (c) polar image of mid-ventricular slice of Subject-1. Corresponding (d) sample region, (e) affinity image, and (f) endo- and epicardial contours for myocardium.

This multi-view information along with intensity, shape, and temporal information is used to localize the 3D medial axis of the LV. Specifically, we map the end-diastolic (ED) lines corresponding to the 2CH and the 4CH scouts onto the ED short-axis as a cross-hair. Due to patient motion between acquisitions and the curved nature of the LV, the cross-hair does not necessarily fall into LV in all the slices. We then crop the ED short-axis images around the cross-hair intersection point (Fig. 1(b)). Thresholding the cropped images using the threshold provided by Otsu's algorithm [17] provides the blood regions. This threshold is obtained by maximizing a function of the ratio of the between-class variance and the total variance of the intensity levels. The LV region is extracted from the binary image using the cost function based on the larger blood area and the minimum distance of the center of blood regions from the cross-hair. The LV centroids detected in each slice are then updated using a cost function which maintains 3D continuity of the LV medial axis along the entire volume from base to apex. These ED LV medial axis points are then propagated along time as the initial LV centroids in all the phases, and they are then updated using the above cost function to maintain the temporal continuity of the LV medial axis. Figures 2(a,b) depict the estimated centroids in the ED and the ES phases for Subject-1.

Step 2 - Compute myocardium seed pixel and sample regions: In the second step, we determine the seed point for the LV myocardium and the sample regions for all the classes. In cine CMR data, tissue types (due to their feature responses) and LV myocardium (due to its spatial adjacency in polar coordinates) form clusters in a feature space, thus providing clues for LV blood and myocardium classification. We convert images into polar coordinates (Fig. 1(c)) and form the feature space of (p, i) (Fig. 2(c)). The p coordinate is formed by appending rows of pixels in the polar image according to their radius value. We use subtractive clustering [18] in the (p, i) space to identify the different clusters. Starting from zero radius, the first centroid with the highest intensity value and the last centroid with the lowest intensity value are identified as the centroids for the LV blood and the air clusters, respectively. Next, we take the derivative of the line connecting the centroids of the detected clusters with respect to the intensity and the first negative peak from zero radius is identified as the centroid for the myocardial cluster. The intensity values in these clusters along with their position provide the myocardial seed pixel with the sample region (Fig. 1(d)) and the feature distribution for all the classes.

Step 3 - Segmentation: Having determined the feature vector distributions and seed regions for LV blood, myocardium and air, we segment the LV myocardium using our framework. The segmented region includes the papillary muscles and occasionally the liver. Thus, we employ dynamic programming-based border detection in polar coordinates on the segmented region to exclude the papillary muscles and obtain the endocardial and epicardial contours (Figs. 1(e,f)) [12].

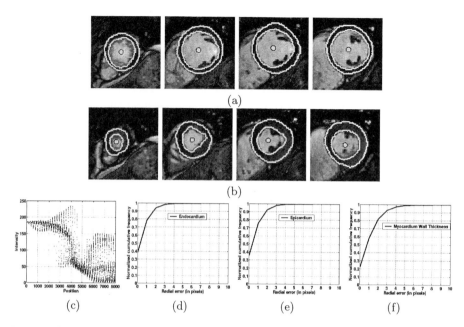

Fig. 2. The automatically estimated centroids and myocardial contours in (a) ED and (b) ES slices for Subject-1. (c) Cluster centers in (p, i). Cumulative distribution of radial distance error for (d) endocardium, (e) epicardium, and (f) wall thickness.

3   Results

We applied our framework for extracting the LV myocardial contours in three mid-ventricular ED slices of 20 subjects. Volunteers were imaged on a 1.5T commercial scanner (Philips Gyroscan NT-Intera) using vector-cardiographic gating. The bFFE short-axis sequence was acquired to cover the entire LV. The acquisition parameters for a cine bFFE sequence were TE/TR/flip: 3.2/1.6/55 deg; 38-40 msec temporal resolution. The endocardial and epicardial contours determined by our algorithm for Subject-1 are depicted in Figs. 2(a,b). We validated our results against the endocardial and epicardial contours drawn manually by experts from St. Luke's Episcopal Hospital. The automatically detected contours are quantitatively assessed for the border positioning error in terms of radial distance of each point from the corresponding point on the manually traced contour. The radial error magnitude effectively captures the effect of the error on the LV volume, EF, and WT computations. Figures 2(d-f) depict the cumulative radial distance errors between automatic and manual contours. Note that maximum error of three or more pixels for endo- and epicardial contours and five pixels for wall thickness are observed less than 1% of the time.

4   Conclusion

Our data-driven method does not require any user interaction at either the LV identification or the myocardial segmentation phases. This method allows accurate extraction of endocardial and epicardial contours of the LV in cine bFFE MR images. The results of our algorithm are consistent with the manual tracings of clinical experts. This method allows unbiased and consistent computation of the following LV functional parameters: cardiac output, ejection fraction, end-diastolic and end-systolic volumes, stroke volume, wall thickness, and wall thickening.

References

1. Matheijssen, N., Baur, L., Reiber, J., der Velde, E.V., Dijkman, P.V., der Geest, R.V., de Ross, A., der Wall, E.V.: Assessment of left ventricular volume and mass by cine magnetic resonance imaging in patients with anterior myocardial infarction: Intra-observer and inter-observer variability on contour detection. International Journal of Cardiac Imaging **12** (1996) 11–19
2. Paragios, N.: Shape-based segmentation and tracking in cardiac image analysis. IEEE Transactions on Medical Imaging **22** (2003) 773–776
3. Lelieveldt, B., van der Geest, R., Rezaee, M.R., Bosch, J., Reiber, J.: Anatomical model matching with fuzzy implicit surfaces for segmentation of thoracic volume scans. IEEE Trans. on Medical Imaging **18** (1999) 218–230
4. Frangi, A., Niessen, W., Viergever, M.: Three-dimensional modeling for functional analysis of cardiac images: A review. IEEE Trans. Med. Imaging **20** (2001) 2–25
5. Singh, A., Goldgof, D., Terzopoulos, D.: Deformable Models in Medical Image Analysis. IEEE Computer Society, Los Alamitos, CA (1998)
6. Park, J., Metaxas, D., Young, A., Axel, L.: Deformable models with parameter functions for cardiac motion analysis from tagged MRI data. IEEE Trans. Medical Imaging **15** (1996) 278–289
7. Mitchell, S., Bosch, J., Lelieveldt, B., van der Geest, R., Reiber, J., Sonka, M.: 3-D active appearance models: segmentation of cardiac MR and ultrasound images. IEEE Trans. on Medical Imaging **21** (2002) 1167 –1178
8. Sonka, M., Lelieveldt, B., Mitchell, S., Bosch, J., der Geest, R.V., Reiber, J.: Active appearance motion model segmentation. In: Second International Workshop on Digital and Computational Video, Tampa, Florida, (2001) 64–68
9. Paragios, N.: A variational approach for the segmentation of the left ventricle in cardiac image analysis. Int. Journal of Computer Vision **50** (2002) 345–362
10. Jolly, M.: Combining edge, region, and shape information to segment the left ventricle in cardiac MR images. In: Proc. of the 4th Int. Conference on Medical Image Computing & Computer-Assisted Intervention, Utrecht, The Netherlands, (2001) 482–490
11. Imielinska, C., Metaxas, D., Udupa, J., Jin, Y., Chen, T.: Hybrid segmentation of anatomical data. In: Proc. of the 4th Int. Conference on Medical Image Computing & Computer-Assisted Intervention, Utrecht, The Netherlands, (2001) 1048–1057
12. Pednekar, A., Kakadiaris, I., Kurkure, U., Muthupillai, R., Flamm, S.: Intensity and morphology-based energy minimization for the automatic segmentation of the myocardium. In: Proc. of IEEE Workshop on Variational and Level Set Methods, Nice, France, (2003) 185-192
13. Udupa, J., Samarasekera, S.: Fuzzy connectedness and object definition: theory, algorithms, and applications in image segmentation. Graphical Models and Image Processing **58** (1996) 246–261

14. Pednekar, A.S., Kakadiaris, I., Kurkure, U.: Adaptive fuzzy connectedness-based medical image segmentation. In: Proceedings of the Indian Conference on Computer Vision, Graphics, and Image Processing, Ahmedabad, India (2002) 457–462
15. Laws, K.: Textured Image Segmentation. PhD thesis, USC (1980)
16. Manjunath, B.S., Ma, W.Y.: Texture features for browsing and retrieval of image data. IEEE Trans. Pattern Anal. Mach. Intell. **18** (1996) 837–842
17. Otsu, N.: A threshold selection method from gray-level histograms. IEEE Transactions on Systems, Man, and Cybernetics **SMC-9** (1979) 62–66
18. Chiu, S.: Fuzzy model identification based on cluster estimation. Journal of Intelligent Fuzzy Systems **2** (1994) 267–278

3D Cardiac Anatomy Reconstruction Using High Resolution CT Data

Ting Chen[1], Dimitris Metaxas[1], and Leon Axel[2]

[1] Rutgers, the State University of New Jersey, Piscataway, NJ 08854, USA,
chenting@gradphics.cis.upenn.edu,
dnm@cs.rutgers.edu
[2] New York University, School of Medicine, 550 first Avenue, New York, NY, 10016, USA,
leon.axel@med.nyu.edu

Abstract. Recent advances in CT technology have allowed the development of systems with multiple rows of detectors and rapid rotation. These new imaging systems have permitted the acquisition of high resolution, spatially registered, and cardiac gated 3D heart data. In this paper, we present a framework that makes use of these data to reconstruct the 3D cardiac anatomy with resolutions that were not previously possible. We use an improved 3D hybrid segmentation framework which integrates Gibbs prior models, deformable models, and the marching cubes method to achieve a sub-pixel accuracy of the reconstruction of cardiac objects. To improve the convergence at concavities on the object surface, we introduce a new type of external force, which we call the scalar gradient. The scalar gradient is derived from a gray level edge map using local configuration information and can help the deformable models converge into deep concavities on object's surface. The 3D segmentation and reconstruction have been conducted on 8 high quality CT data sets. Important features, such as the structure of papillary muscles, have been well captured, which may lead to a new understanding of the cardiac anatomy and function. All experimental results have been evaluated by clinical experts and the validation shows the method has a very strong performance.

1 Introduction

Cardiovascular disease is the most common cause of death in America and there is a strong need to detect and diagnose such disease in its early stages. The automated analysis of cardiac images has been improved dramatically in the past few year and provides a way to get detailed anatomic and functional information of the heart. One of the pre-requisites of quantitative analysis of cardiac images is the accurate location of the surfaces of the ventricles and the myocardium. The segmentation and the subsequent reconstruction of the ventricular-myocardium surface is not trivial because of the noise, blurring effects at edges, and motion artifacts. In addition, the segmentation should be automated and time-efficient in order to be clinically applicable.

C. Barillot, D.R. Haynor, and P. Hellier (Eds.): MICCAI 2004, LNCS 3216, pp. 411–418, 2004.
© Springer-Verlag Berlin Heidelberg 2004

Recently, several methodologies have been proposed by different research groups to solve the cardiac segmentation problem. In [8], [9] deformable models are integrated with statistical models or atlases to enable the use of both intensity and spatial information. Several techniques derived from the Active Shape Model (ASM)[4] and the Active Appearance Model (AAM)[7] have been used in [10] to improve the reliability and consistency of the segmentation process. However, all of these approaches aim to solve 2D problems, so that the segmentation and reconstruction may miss important features distributed along the cardiac long axis.

In [5], a 3D ventricular surface is constructed using a deformable model from tagged MRI data. This approach has succeeded in capturing the data related to the strain and stress distribution on the surface of the myocardium. However, the reconstructions, especially of the endocardial surface, are limited by the sparsity of the data and the low quality of the shape model. Important anatomic structures, such as the papillary muscles and valves, can be missed in this model. In [11] a 3D statistical model for atria and ventricles has been built using a 3D AAM. However, the deformable model does not converge well to the data at concavities and convexities on the ventricular surface because of: 1) the smoothing effect of the deformable surface at concavities, and 2) the lack of corresponding details in the initialization of the deformable model.

In [6], the Gradient Vector Flow approach has been proposed to address the problem of deformable model convergence at concavities. The use of the Gradient Vector Flow can extend the attraction range of the gradient information by diffusing a gray level or binary edge map. The extended gradient flow enables the deformable model to fit into concavities on the object surface. However, the computation process of the Gradient Vector Flow is tedious. Moreover, the Gradient Vector Flow's performance degrades as the concavity becomes deeper.

In previous work [2], we have proposed a 3D hybrid framework that is capable of achieving sub-pixel accuracy segmentation of medical images. In this paper, we improve the framework by using a new type of external force during model deformation, which derives from the idea of "scale" in [3]. The new external force has a superior performance in concavity convergence.

The remaining parts of this paper are organized as follows. In section 2, we present the acquisition of the high quality CT data. In section 3, the hybrid framework will be explained. Related improvements, such as the definition of the new external force, will also be given. Section 4 shows some representative high quality 3D reconstructions of cardiac objects produced by our framework. We will also discuss an interesting anatomical structure based on the 3D reconstruction result. Section 5 presents the validation results and the final conclusion.

2   Data Acquisition

Image acquisition with multi-detector CT (MDCT) with continuous table motion is accomplished using cardiac gating. Current MDCT systems permit coverage of the chest in a breath hold, with effective temporal resolution on the order of

120 ms of the cardiac cycle and isotropic spatial resolution in three dimensions on the order of 0.75 mm; a 16 detector-row CT system (Siemens Sensation 16, SMS, Malvern, PA) with these specifications was used to acquire the images used in this study. The images were acquired during the intravenous infusion of radiographic contrast agent (Visipaque 320) at 4 ml/s; image acquisition was timed to coincide with the maximum opacification of the cardiac chambers. The heart rate was slowed using beta blockers, preferably to 60 BPM or less, in order to minimize motion blurring; image acquisition was gated from mid to late diastole to minimize motion blurring and to capture the ventricles in a relatively relaxed state. The data created have 512 by 512 by 281 pixels.

3   Methodology

The hybrid framework proposed in [2] consists of 4 internal modules: the region segmentation module driven by high order Gibbs prior models, the deformable model, marching cubes, and the parameter updating module.

The acquired high quality CT data (in DICOM format, refer to section 2) are translated into raw data sets using the image reader provided by Insight Toolkit (ITK) for further processing.

During the segmentation process, we first apply the Gibbs prior models onto the image. The joint distribution of the medical image is expressed in the following Gibbsian form:

$$\Pi(X) = Z^{-1} \exp(-H(X)) \tag{1}$$

where we use $\mathbf{X}$ to denote the set of all possible configurations of the image X, z is an image in the set of $\mathbf{X}$, $Z = \sum_{z \in \mathbf{X}} \exp(-H(z))$ is a normalizing factor, and $H(X)$ is the energy function of image X. The image is segmented by constructing a suitable energy function for the image and minimizing it. A Gibbs prior energy is defined as follows:

$$H_{prior}(X) = H_1(X) + H_2(X) \tag{2}$$

where $H_1(X)$ models the piecewise pixel homogeneity statistics and $H_2(X)$ models the object boundary continuity. In studying the CT data, we find that the ventricular-myocardium surfaces are not smooth; instead, the surface features many small concavities and convexities. In addition, the existence of the papillary muscle and cardiac valves makes the surface even more irregular. In our implementation, such surface features have been modelled by assigning low potential to local configurations that ensemble a continuous surface with angles so that during the energy minimization the Gibbs model is capable of capturing the saw-like cardiac chamber surface structure.

According to Bayesian framework, the final energy function we minimized is a posterior energy which is in the form of:

$$H_{posterior}(X,Y) = H_{prior}(X) + H_{observation}(X,Y) \tag{3}$$

where $H_{observation}(X,Y) = \vartheta_3 \sum_{s \in X}(y_s - x_s)^2$ if we assume the image has been distorted by Gaussian noise, y_s is the observation of pixel s, x_s is the estimated value, $\vartheta_3 = 2\sigma^2$ is the weight for the constraint of observation, and σ is the standard deviation.

The 3D binary mask output by the region segmentation module is used as the input to the marching cubes module. A 3D mesh consisting of triangular elements is created along the surface of the binary mask. The 3D mesh is used as the initial geometry of the deformable model.

We use Langrange dynamics to deform our model as follows:

$$\dot{\mathbf{d}} + \mathbf{K}\mathbf{d} = \mathbf{f}_{ext} \tag{4}$$

where $\mathbf{d}$ is the displacement, $\mathbf{K}$ is the stiffness matrix, and f_{ext} are the external forces.

The deformable model deforms under the effect of the internal force $\mathbf{K}\mathbf{d}$ and external forces $\mathbf{f}_{ext}$. The internal forces keep the deformable model surface smooth and continuous during its deformation. The external force will lead the model to the object surface using image information such as the gradient. In [2], the external force is derived from the second order derivative of a diffused gradient map. In this paper, we describe a new type of external force that will improve the convergence at concavities (refer to section 3.1).

To solve equation (4) we use the Euler integration as follows:

$$\mathbf{d}_{new} = \dot{\mathbf{d}} \cdot \Delta t + \mathbf{d}_{old} \tag{5}$$

where Δt is the time step. The deformation stops when the force equilibrate or vanish.

The deformable model segmentation will then be used to update the parameters of the Gibbs prior model, which includes mean intensity, standard deviation, and the local potentials (refer to [2]). Then we will start a new loop of the segmentation framework. In most cases, we can achieve a good segmentation result within 2 iterations.

We show the process of our segmentation-reconstruction method in figure 1.

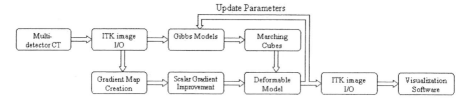

Fig. 1. Hybrid Segmentation Framework

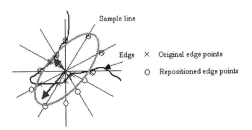

Fig. 2. 2D scalar gradient vector construction

3.1   Scalar Gradient

During the process of fitting the deformable model to the cardiac surface, we use a new type of external force, which we call the 'scalar gradient', to achieve better convergence at concavities. The scalar gradient is derived from the definition of 'tensor scale' in [3]. The tensor scale at an image pixel is the parametric representation of the largest ellipse (for 2D) centered at the pixel and containing only the homogeneous region under prior criterion. It contains information of the orientation, anisotropy, and thickness of local structures.

In a 2D implementation, to calculate the scale at a pixel, we first find the closest edge points to the pixel along a group of sample lines that are normally distributed over the entire angular space around the pixel. Different from the computation of the tensor scale, for each conjugate pair of sample lines, we reposition the sampled edge points by selecting the point that is further from the pixel and reflect it on its complementary sample line. Let the coordinates of the edge points on sample lines be $(x_1, y_1), (x_2, y_2), \ldots, (x_{2m}, y_{2m})$, and that of the pixel be (x_0, y_0); we can compute the local covariance matrix $\mathbf{M}$, where

$$\mathbf{M}_{1,1} = \tfrac{1}{2m} \sum_{i=1,2,\ldots,2m} (x_i - x_0)^2, \mathbf{M}_{2,2} = \tfrac{1}{2m} \sum_{i=1,2,\ldots,2m} (y_i - y_0)^2,$$
$$\mathbf{M}_{1,2} = \mathbf{M}_{2,1} = \tfrac{1}{2m} \sum_{i=1,2,\ldots,2m} (x_i - x_0)(y_i - y_0) \tag{6}$$

$\mathbf{M}$ is a symmetric matrix with positive diagonal elements so it has two orthogonal eigenvectors and two positive eigenvalues λ_1, λ_2 associated with the eigenvectors. We use the direction of the principal radius as the direction of the scalar gradient vector, and the magnitude of the scalar gradient is proportional to $\frac{\lambda_1}{\lambda_2}$, where $\lambda_1 > \lambda_2$. The computation of the 2D scalar gradient is shown in figure 2, and it is simple to extend it into 3D.

For simplicity, we derive the scalar gradient field using the edge map of the original image. The threshold of the edge can be calculated using the result of the Gibbs segmentation. This map will be used to locate those edge points around pixels during the computation of local ellipses. We then combine the scalar gradient with the original gradient flow to form the external force field.

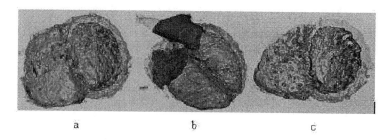

Fig. 3. We show the LV and RV atria in blue, the ventricles in green, and the epicardial surface in transparent red. a) shows a view of the heart from the bottom. b) shows a view of the heart from the front. In c) we intersect the 3D reconstruction using a plane that is vertical to the long axis of the heart and show the resulting endocardial and epicardial surface from the top.

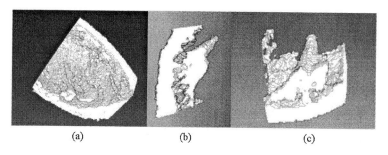

Fig. 4. Anatomic structure of the papillary muscle. 3 views of the papillary muscle being cut by user-defined planes. The white plane is the intersection of cutting plane to the 3D reconstruction of myocardium. Notice that there are tunnels for blood between the papillary muscle and the myocardium.

4   Experimental Results and Discussion

We applied our method to eight different cardiac datasets. In figure 3, we show the 3D reconstructions of cardiac surfaces based on the segmentation result of one dataset. The data size is 256 by 256 by 140. Our segmentation method has succeeded in capturing the surface features and the global shape of the cardiac chambers. The whole segmentation process takes about 10 minutes on a P4 2.2G Hz desktop.

Figure 4 illustrates the anatomic structure of the papillary muscle. The rendered 3D images of the segmented heart wall show the structures of the trabeculae carnae and papillary muscles very clearly on the endocardial surface of the ventricular cavity. The three-dimensional nature of these structures and their anatomical relationships are much more readily appreciated with such a rendering than from the original image data, even with interactive reformatting of the displayed image plane. In particular, it can be appreciated how the rope-like trabeculae carnae course over the inner surface of the heart wall, and how the papillary muscles are attached to the trabeculae carnae by branching structures at their bases, rather than directly to the solid portion of the heart wall, as has been conventionally believed.

5   Validation and Conclusion

The experimental results of our segmentation and reconstruction framework has been qualitatively evaluated by clinical experts. According to them, in most cases our segmentation framework achieves an excellent agreement with the manual segmentation, while the segmentation time is dramatically decreased compared to manual segmentation. More validation results will be available soon to prove the possible clinical usage of this method. We also plan to use the framework on other image modules with different noise levels. Currently, we tried the framework on a 192 by 192 by 18 MRI cardiac data to reconstruct the endocardial surface of the LV. The result has also been approved by clinical experts.

Although the inner surface of the cardiac chambers is well known to be rough, the three-dimensional structure of the endocardial surface has not been previously well demonstrated non-invasively in vivo. In particular, the relationship of the papillary muscles to the heart wall can be seen with our high resolution CT images to be not a simple joining of the base of the papillary muscles with the solid portion of the wall, as has been conventionally believed, but rather a branching connection of the base with the trabeculae carnae lining the ventricular cavity. This has not been appreciated with previous tomographic imaging methods, which have had insufficient resolution to demonstrate these structures and limited 3-D registration between different image planes. Study of ex vivo specimens has also not demonstrated this relationship, due to the typically highly contracted state of these specimens. The ability to efficiently and accurately segment these high resolution 3D CT images for full 3D demonstration of the structural relationships of the interior of the heart should provide us with a valuable new tool for the study of normal and abnormal cardiac anatomy. It should also lead us to new insights as to the functional significance of these anatomical relationships.

Our 3D hybrid segmentation framework has provided high resolution segmentation results of the complex cardiac structure. This is the first time that the roughness on the endocardial surface has been so fully reconstructed in 3D. Its time efficiency should enable us to apply it to more clinical use. The high convergence at concavities shows the advantage of the hybrid framework and the strength of the scalar gradient. Our aim is to make further improvements to the methodology so that it can be used as a standard method for 3D cardiac data segmentation and reconstruction.

References

1. D.N. Metaxas.: Physics-Based Deformable Models: Application to Computer Vision, Graphics and Medical Imaging. (1996)

2. Chen, T., Metaxas, D.: Gibbs prior models, marching cubes, and deformable Models: A hybrid framework for 3D medical image segmentation. Proceedings of MICCAI Montreal **6** (2003) 703–710
3. P. K. Saha, J. K. Udupa: Tensor-scale-based fuzzy connectedness image segmentation. SPIE**4.23** (2003) 1580–1590
4. T. Cootes, C. Taylor, D. Cooper, J. Graham, Active shape model - their training and application. Computer Vision, Graphics, and Image Process: Image Understanding, 1(61): 38-59, 1994.
5. Jinah Park, Dimitris Metaxas, and Leon Axel, Volumetric deformable models with parameter functions: A new approach to the 3D motion analysis of the LV from MRI-SPAMM, in Proceedings of International Conference on Computer Vision pp 700-705, 1995.
6. C. Xu and J. L. Prince, Snakes, shapes and gradient vector flow, IEEE Trans. Image Processing, vol7, no. , pp. 359-369, 1998.
7. T. Cootes, G J. Edwards, and C. J. Taylor. Active appearance models. In Proc. of ECCV'98, volume 2, pp 484-498. 1998
8. M. R. Kaus, V. Pekar, C. Lorenz, R. Truyen, S. Lobregt, and J. Weese. Automated 3D PDM construction from segmented images using deformable models. IEEE Trans. Med. Imag., 22(8): 1005-1013, 2003.
9. M. Lorenzo-Valdes, G. I. Sanchez-Ortiz, R. Mohiaddin, and D. Rueckert. Segmentation of 4D cardiac MR images using a probabilistic atlas and the EM algorithm. In Proc. MICCAI 2003. 440-447
10. S. C. Mitchell, B. P. F. Lelieveldt, R. J. van der Geest, H. G. Bosch, J. H. C. Reiber, and M. Sonka. Multistage hybrid active appearance model matching: Segmentation of left and right ventricles in cardiac MR images. IEEE Trans. Med. Imag., 20(5): 415-423, 2001
11. J. Lotjonen, J. Koikkalainen, D. Smutek, S. Kivisto, and K. Lauerma. Four-chamber 3-D statistical shape model from cardiac short-axis and long axis MR data. MICCAI 2003. pp 459-466.
12. K. Park, D. Metaxas, L. Axel. A finite element model for functional analysis of 4D cardiac-tagged MR images. MICCAI 2003. pp 491-498

3D/4D Cardiac Segmentation Using Active Appearance Models, Non-rigid Registration, and the Insight Toolkit

Robert M. Lapp[1], Maria Lorenzo-Valdés[2], and Daniel Rueckert[2]

[1] Institute of Medical Physics, University of Erlangen-Nürnberg,
Henkestrasse 91, 91052 Erlangen, Germany
[2] Visual Information Processing Group, Department of Computing, Imperial College
London, 180 Queen's Gate, London SW7 2BZ, United Kingdom

Abstract. We describe the design of a statistical atlas-based 3D/4D cardiac segmentation system using a combination of active appearance models (AAM) and statistical deformation models with the Insight Toolkit as an underlying implementation framework. Since the original AAM approach was developed for 2D applications and makes use of manually set landmarks its extension to higher dimensional data sets cannot be easily achieved. We therefore apply the idea of statistical deformation models to AAMs and use a deformable registration step for establishing point-to-point correspondences. An evaluation of the implemented system was performed by segmenting the left ventricle cavity, myocardium and right ventricle of ten cardiac MRI and ten CT datasets. The comparison of automatic and manual segmentations showed encouraging results with a mean segmentation error of 2.2±1.1 mm. We conclude that the combination of a non-rigid registration step with the statistical analysis concepts of the AAM is both feasible and useful and allows for its application to 3D and 4D data.

1 Introduction

A number of different segmentation approaches have been proposed that make use of statistical evaluations of the variations observed in one subject over time or across subjects. This allows to derive a probabilistic atlas of the possible variations which provides the means to produce *plausible* approximations of the objects stored. Recent applications of such statistical techniques to the domain of cardiac segmentation have been published [1,2,3,4] and also other new cardiac segmentation algorithms have been proposed [5].

1.1 Active Appearance Models

One promising statistical modeling approach are active appearance models (AAM), which were first proposed by Cootes *et al.* [6] in 1999 and have since received a lot of attention. In contrast to other techniques they utilize both shape and texture information of the object and lead to a unified description of possible *appearances* of the object.

C. Barillot, D.R. Haynor, and P. Hellier (Eds.): MICCAI 2004, LNCS 3216, pp. 419–426, 2004.

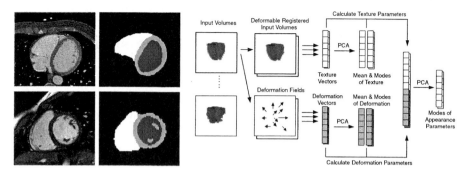

Fig. 1. CT and MRI input data and segmentations.

Fig. 2. Statistical atlas-building procedure.

Numerous applications have been published recently which apply the original concept with its manually identified landmarks to 2D segmentation problems and extensions to incorporate time have been proposed, as for example [7,8]. Also, a hybrid AAM and active shape model approach [9] was published recently for 2D, which demonstrates a fully automated segmentation of the left and right ventricle. However, these approaches are mainly applied to 2D data since they require a manual or semi-automatic localization of landmarks. Due to the lack of a sufficient number of uniquely identifiable points, establishing a dense map of point to point correspondences becomes significantly more difficult in higher dimensions.

Very few approaches for such higher dimensional data have been published and often depend on special geometrical models, which were customized for the specific application domain. For example, Mitchell *et al.* [1] show the application of AAM to 3D cardiac data. Their algorithm adapts a cylindrical model of the heart to the actual patient data thereby facilitating the identification of corresponding landmarks.

1.2   Statistical Deformation Models

Statistical deformation models (SDM) [10] aim to overcome this limitation and generalize the method of identifying corresponding points over various patients. They extend the concept of statistical shape models to allow their application in 3D and higher dimensions without manual landmarking. Instead, a deformable registration algorithm is used to register the reference object onto the training datasets. The resulting description of the dense mapping is then either used directly for the statistical analysis or is applied to transfer landmarks from one dataset onto the other. However, SDMs only consider the shape information of the object while the texture information is not utilized.

1.3   Contribution

We combined the concepts of active appearance motion models and statistical deformation models. To validate our ideas, we implemented a segmentation

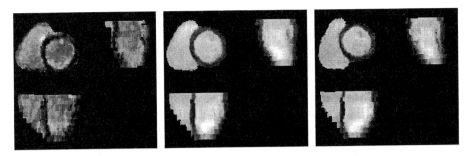

Fig. 3. Variation of the first mode of appearance parameters between $\pm 1.5\sigma$

system based on the Insight Segmentation and Registration Toolkit (ITK) [11] and applied it in 3D and 4D for the segmentation of the left ventricular (LV) myocardium, LV cavity and right ventricle (RV) of ten cardiac computed tomography (CT) and ten magnetic resonance imaging (MRI) datasets (cp. Fig. 1). For evaluation purposes we compared the volume overlap of the segmented voxels and calculated the mean distances between the automatic segmentation results and the manual segmentations which served as the gold standard.

2   Methods

2.1   Global Registration

Prior to the alignment of the data, the four dimensional training datasets and the corresponding manual segmentations are resampled to achieve the same 4D voxel and image size over all datasets. The training datasets are globally registered onto one arbitrary reference dataset using affine registration with an initial starting estimate generated by aligning the centers of mass. The registration is implemented within ITK's multi-resolution registration framework using a mutual information similarity measure and a linear interpolation scheme. In case of 4D datasets, these are split into their 3D time frames and registered separately. The mean transform over all time frames is subsequently calculated and applied to the 4D training datasets.

2.2   Local Registration

First, an average reference dataset for the local registration is created using an iterative procedure of deformable registering the datasets onto one (first arbitrary) dataset and subsequently calculating the mean appearance parameters. This new mean dataset is used as the new reference for the next iteration.

All training datasets are warped onto the reference subject using deformable registration. In particular, ITK's implementation of Thirion's *demons* algorithm [12] is applied which uses deformation fields as underlying representation, i.e. n-dimensional images with n-dimensional vectors as voxels which describe the correspondence mapping of voxels between the training and reference images. These serve as the basis for the statistical analysis.

Two different approaches are available for deformable registration. In the first method, the datasets are split into their 3D time frames which are then registered separately. The resulting 3D deformation fields are assembled to a pseudo 4D deformation field with an additional zero element in the fourth dimension. This 4D field then actually describes a deformation where no influence between time frames exists. Alternatively, the non-rigid registration is directly performed on the 4D training datasets resulting in a genuine 4D deformation field.

The memory footprint of the resulting deformation fields is four times larger than the original image since the offset in every dimension has to be stored for every voxel. Therefore, a size reduction of the deformation field becomes necessary which is achieved by reducing the sample density by an arbitrary factor. Further memory saving measures include the introduction of automatic bounding boxes for deformation and texture regions.

2.3   Atlas Building Stage

As a first step, all training datasets and their segmentations are warped onto the standard shape using the result of the local registration, i.e. the deformation field. The texture information of every voxel from within the manually segmented standard shape is then concatenated to one texture vector t. As shape information, the voxels of the deformation field within a bounding box around the LV and RV of the heart are concatenated to a deformation vector d.

The subsequent statistical analysis follows the procedure as presented in the original AAM publication [6]. The principal component analysis (PCA) performs a dimensionality-reducing decomposition of the vectors into $t = \bar{t} + P_t b_t$ and $d = \bar{d} + P_d b_d$ with $\bar{t}$ and $\bar{d}$ being the mean texture and deformation vectors, P being the orthogonal modes of variation and b being the texture and deformation parameter vectors respectively. As a result, a mean model of shape and texture is created together with modes of variation, which capture the entire information about texture and shape of the training data. To incorporate both shape and greylevel information into one model both parameters b_d and b_t are concatenated and a further PCA is applied, i.e.

$$\begin{pmatrix} W_d\, b_d \\ b_t \end{pmatrix} = \begin{pmatrix} Q_d \\ Q_t \end{pmatrix} c = Q\, c \qquad (1)$$

where W_d is a diagonal matrix with weights allowing for different units in deformation and texture parameters, c is the appearance parameters vector which controls both shape and greyscale of the model and Q represents the resulting eigenvectors of the PCA. Because of the linear nature of the problem, Q can be split into Q_d and Q_t as indicated above. This statistical atlas of the heart allows the creation of arbitrary plausible images of the heart within the variations of the training datasets. Fig. 2 gives an overview of the performed steps and Fig. 3 shows the variation of the first mode of variation of the appearance parameters between $\pm 1.5\sigma$ of one example cardiac MRI atlas.

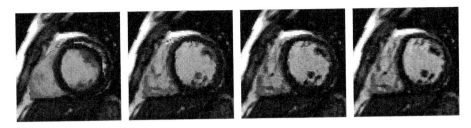

Fig. 4. Current hypothesis image within the enclosing target image while optimizing the appearance parameters: initial approximation, after few iterations, final approximation, target image (from left to right).

2.4 Image Segmentation

The statistical atlas is subsequently used for the actual image segmentation procedure. Given the results from before, any plausible image can be described by one appearance vector c using the following equations

$$d = \bar{d} + P_d W_d^{-1} Q_d c \tag{2}$$

$$t = \bar{t} + P_t Q_t c . \tag{3}$$

To synthesize new images a shape-free texture image is created from the resulting vector t and warped by the deformation field d. An iterative optimization process is now applied to adapt the appearance parameters to the actual image. A root-mean-square measure is calculated to determine the correspondence between the target image and the approximated image. The gradient information, required by the gradient descent optimization method, is calculated by forward differencing. Fig. 4 shows exemplary an iterative approximation of the shape and texture during the appearance optimization process. Finally, to obtain the segmentation result, the deformation field which is defined by the optimized appearance parameter set is used to deform the standard segmentation. The result is the approximated segmentation for the given target dataset.

3   Results

The performance of the system was evaluated using 10 MRI and 10 CT datasets. The cardiac MRI short-axis datasets had an original pixel size of between $1.37 \times 1.37 \times 10\,\text{mm}^3$ and $1.48 \times 1.48 \times 10\,\text{mm}^3$ and between 10 and 19 time frames each. The MRI cardiac short-axis datasets were acquired at the Royal Brompton Hospital, London, UK in a study with 10 healthy volunteers. A 1.5T Magnetom Sonata scanner (Siemens Medical Solutions, Erlangen, Germany) with a TrueFisp sequence was used with a total acquisition time of 15 minutes. For eight datasets manual segmentations and for two datasets semi-automatic segmentations were available.

The CT datasets were acquired during normal clinical practice using a Sensation 16 scanner (Siemens Medical Solutions, Forchheim, Germany) with a rotation time of 0.42 seconds and 12 slices acquired simultaneously. They were kindly provided by the Institute of Diagnostic Radiology and the Department of Internal Medicine II, University of Erlangen-Nürnberg, Germany. The rawdata was reconstructed using a dedicated cardiac CT image reconstruction software (VAMP GmbH, Möhrendorf, Germany) using retrospective gating with 5 reconstructed cardiac phases and an initial isotropic voxel size of $(2\,\mathrm{mm})^3$. One CT dataset was segmented manually in 3D to provide an initial reference segmentation. To be able to calculate quantitative measures, also single slices of all other CT datasets were segmented manually.

3.1 Quantitative and Qualitative Performance

The performance of the system was evaluated qualitatively by visual inspection and quantitatively using two different measures. The distance between the manual reference segmentation and the automatic segmentation was measured in 3D and used to calculate maximum, mean and standard deviation of the absolute distance of surface points of the segmented volume to the closest point of the reference segmentation.

Also voxel volume percentages of correctly assigned voxels were calculated and used for evaluation. The measure *volume overlap* Δ was defined as

$$\Delta = \min \left(\frac{V_{M \cap A}}{V_M}, \ \frac{V_{M \cap A}}{V_A} \right) \tag{4}$$

with V_M being the volumes of the true (manual) segmentation, V_A the volume of the automatic segmentation and $V_{M \cap A}$ the volume of the correctly labeled regions, i.e. where the automatically computed segmentation values match the manual reference segmentation. While this volume measure is easily calculated and gives an indication of the quality of volumetric accuracy, the distance measure gives a more intuitively understandable result of the quality of the segmentation.

Figs. 5 and 6 show the results of the quantitative evaluation after global registration and segmentation using leave *one* out and leave *none* out schemes using all eigenmodes. The correlation for the segmented volumes for LV cavity, myocardium and RV in the MRI datasets is $r = 0.95$, $r = 0.83$ and $r = 0.94$, respectively. The mean absolute distance measure shows a segmentation error of 2.2 ± 1.1 mm for the leave-none-out scheme, which increases to 4.0 ± 1.6 mm for the leave-one-out test. For the CT segmentation, the volume overlap was calculated for one slice per volume only since no 3D segmentations were available. The evaluations show only a slight increase in segmentation accuracy when compared to the initial segmentation estimate which in our case originated mainly from poor deformable registration results.

The automatic segmentation of a typical $256\times256\times128$ volume with 8 time frames took approximately 20 minutes on a standard PC with 3 GHz and 2 GB main memory.

MAD MRI [mm]	Mean	Std Dev	Max
Initialization	4.6	2.3	56.1
AAM (one out)	4.0	1.6	29.4
AAM (none out)	2.2	1.1	25.4

Overlap MRI	LV cav	LV myo	RV
Initialization	0.66	0.42	0.71
AAM (one out)	0.72	0.49	0.73
AAM (none out)	0.86	0.68	0.86

Overlap CT	LV cav	LV myo	RV
Initialization	0.82	0.57	0.72
AAM (one out)	0.77	0.59	0.72
AAM (none out)	0.85	0.65	0.73

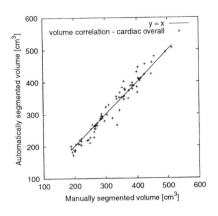

Fig. 5. Achieved segmentation accuracy in terms of mean absolute distance (MAD) and volume overlap.

Fig. 6. Correlation of segmented volumes of MRI datasets using AAM segmentation and manual segmentation.

4   Discussion and Conclusion

We developed and implemented a statistical atlas-based 3D/4D cardiac segmentation system based on the ITK and incorporating both texture and shape information. The problem of landmarking was solved by using the idea of statistical deformation models, i.e. using deformable registration to obtain point-correspondence information and taking the deformation information as shape description.

The implemented system proved to achieve satisfactory segmentation results with mean errors of about 2.2±1.1 mm for the cardiac MRI images. The accuracy is comparable to [2] and slightly worse than the results presented by Kaus *et al.* [3]. Nevertheless, the full utilization of the time dimension did not show the expected improvement of the segmentation results, which was probably due to the limited temporal resolution of the datasets. Also, when working with high-resolution data, memory problems originated from the large texture vectors. This matter leaves room for improvement and will be investigated further.

The extensive use of the ITK leaves a positive impression and can especially be recommended for new researchers working in the field of image analysis. A migration to ITK may also be worthwhile because of its good architecture, multi-platform capabilities and the prospect of a broad developer basis. However, at many points a good command of C++ is required, especially for optimizing the relatively large memory footprint and the execution speed of the algorithms. One aspect that could be criticized is the software documentation. Nevertheless, there has been much improvement over the last months and a lot of effort has been put into the excellent software guide [11].

Interesting aspects of future work include the evaluation of other machine learning algorithms as e.g. the recent *locally linear embedding* approach [13] or *support vector machines* [14]. Desired properties include a better preservation of neighborhood information and improved results for small numbers of training datasets. Also, CT and MRI datasets could be combined to a multi-modality atlas offering an increased number of available training datasets and cross-training, i.e. the refinement of the atlas for one modality by another imaging modality. Thereby, specific advantages of each modality, e.g. the high isotropic resolution of CT images, could be incorporated into a common atlas.

Acknowledgements. This work benefited from the use of the ITK, an open source software developed as an initiative of the U.S. National Library of Medicine. R.M. Lapp is funded by a grant from the DFG, Germany. M. Lorenzo-Valdés is funded by a grant from CONACyT, México.

References

1. Mitchell, S., Bosch, J., Lelieveldt, B., Geest, R., Reiber, J., Sonka, M.: 3-D active appearance models: Segmentation of cardiac MR and ultrasound images. IEEE Trans. Med. Imag. **21** (2002) 1167–1178
2. Lorenzo-Valdés, M., Sanchez-Ortiz, G., Mohiaddin, R., Rueckert, D.: Segmentation of 4D cardiac MR images using a probabilistic atlas and the EM algorithm. In: MICCAI 2003, Springer (2003) 440–450
3. Kaus, M., Berg, J., Niessen, W., Pekar, V.: Automated segmentation of the left ventricle in cardiac MRI. In: MICCAI 2003, Springer (2003) 432–439
4. Stegmann, M.B., Ersbøll, B., Larsen, R.: FAME - a flexible appearance modeling environment. IEEE Trans. Med. Imag. **22** (2003) 1319–1331
5. Noble, N., Hill, D., Breeuwer, M., Schnabel, J., Hawkes, D., Gerritsen, F., Razavi, R.: Myocardial delineation via registration in a polar coordinate system. In: MICCAI 2002, Springer (2002) 651–658
6. Cootes, T., Beeston, C., Edwards, G., Taylor, C.: A unified framework for atlas matching using active appearance models. In: International Conference on Information Processing in Medical Imaging. LNCS, Springer (1999) 322–333
7. Sonka, M., Lelieveldt, B., Mitchell, S., Bosch, J., Geest, R., Reiber, J.: Active appearance motion model segmentation. In: Second International Workshop on Digital and Computational Video, IEEE (2001)
8. Bosch, J., Mitchell, S., Lelieveldt, B., Nijland, F., Kamp, O., Sonka, M., Reiber, J.: Automatic segmentation of echocardiographic sequences by active appearance motion models. IEEE Trans. Med. Imag. **21** (2002)
9. Mitchell, S., Lelieveldt, B., Geest, R., Bosch, H., Reiber, J., Sonka, M.: Multistage hybrid active appearance model matching: Segmentation of left and right ventricles in cardiac MR images. IEEE Trans. Med. Imag. **20** (2001)
10. Rueckert, D., Frangi, A., Schnabel, J.: Automatic construction of 3D statistical deformation models of the brain using non-rigid registration. IEEE Trans. Med. Imag. **22** (2003) 1014–1025
11. Ibanez, Schroeder, Ng, Cates: The ITK Software Guide. Insight Consortium. (2003) http://www.itk.org.
12. Thirion, J.P.: Non-rigid matching using demons. In: Computer Vision and Pattern Recognition. (1996)
13. Roweis, S., Saul, L.: Nonlinear dimensionality reduction by locally linear embedding. Science **290** (2000)
14. Golland, P., Grimson, W., Shenton, M., Kikinis, R.: Small sample size learning for shape analysis of anatomical structures. In: MICCAI 2000, Springer (2000) 72–82

Segmentation of Cardiac Structures Simultaneously from Short- and Long-Axis MR Images

Juha Koikkalainen[1], Mika Pollari[1], Jyrki Lötjönen[2], Sari Kivistö[3], and Kirsi Lauerma[3]

[1] Laboratory of Biomedical Engineering, Helsinki University of Technology, P.O.B. 2200, FIN-02015 HUT, Finland
{Juha.Koikkalainen,Mika.Pollari}@hut.fi
[2] VTT Information Technology, P.O.B. 1206, FIN-33101 Tampere, Finland
Jyrki.Lotjonen@vtt.fi
[3] Helsinki Medical Imaging Center, University of Helsinki, P.O.B. 281, FIN-00029 HUS, Finland

Abstract. We introduce a framework for the automatic segmentation of the ventricles, atria, and epicardium simultaneously from cardiac magnetic resonance (MR) volumes. The basic idea is to utilize both short-axis (SA) and long-axis (LA) MR volumes. Consequently, anatomical information is available from the whole heart volume. In this paper, the framework is used with deformable model based registration and segmentation methods to segment the cardiac structures. A database consisting of the cardiac MR volumes of 25 healthy subjects is used to validate the methods.

The results presented in this paper prove that by using both the SA and LA MR volumes the ventricles and atria can be simultaneously segmented from cardiac MR volumes with a good accuracy. The results show that notably better segmentation results are obtained when the LA volumes are used in addition to the SA volumes. For example, this enables accurate segmentation of the ventricles also in the basal and apical levels.

1 Introduction

Cardiac MR imaging provides accurate information on the anatomy of the heart. This information can be used to study and analyze the cardiac function [1]. Segmentation of cardiac structures is a pre-requisite for the determination of quantitative measurements, such as the volume of the ventricles, wall thickness, or ejection fraction. Automated segmentation algorithms are needed to produce objective, reproducible segmentations, and to avoid the need for the time-consuming manual segmentation of large amount of data.

Cardiac MR volumes have often low quality: the signal is lost due to the blood flow and partial volume effect, and the volumes are noisy and corrupted with artifacts. Therefore, *a priori* knowledge is usually utilized in segmentation. In model-based segmentation, for example, atlases or statistical models can be

C. Barillot, D.R. Haynor, and P. Hellier (Eds.): MICCAI 2004, LNCS 3216, pp. 427–434, 2004.
© Springer-Verlag Berlin Heidelberg 2004

used. In [2], an anatomical atlas was constructed from a set of healthy subjects, and the atlas was used to give an *a priori* estimate in the non-rigid registration-based segmentation of the ventricles. In [3], a probabilistic anatomical atlas was used to initialize the parameters of expectation maximization algorithm. Statistical shape (Active Shape Model, ASM) [4] and appearance (Active Appearance Model, AAM) [5] models are popular methods in cardiac segmentation. Kaus *et al.* [6] used a statistical shape model to regularize the deformable model-based segmentation of the left ventricle. In [7], Mitchell *et al.* combined ASM and AAM approaches in the cardiac segmentation, and in [8], they presented fully 3D AAM algorithm for the same problem.

Most of the recent cardiac segmentation studies using MR images deal with the segmentation of the left ventricle and epicardium [6,8,9,10]. In some studies, also the right ventricle is segmented [2,3,7,11]. These studies have been done using short-axis MR images. In this study, we utilize simultaneously both short-axis and long-axis MR volumes. The SA and LA volumes are first transformed into same coordinate system using image header information. Then, the segmentation takes place in this coordinate system. The use of two volumes provides supplementary information that enables more accurate segmentation of the ventricles in the basal and apical levels.

In this paper, we apply a deformable model-based segmentation method in this context. A mean shape and grey-level model, which is constructed from a database, is deformed using deformation spheres [12]. Previously, we have used similar framework in the tracking of cardiac MR images [13], and in the construction of statistical shape model [14]. Lelieveldt *et al.* constructed an AAM from three MR views, and used the model to segment the left ventricle simultaneously from all three views in [15]. However, to our knowledge, the simultaneous segmentation of the ventricles and atria from SA and LA MR volumes has not been reported earlier.

2   Material

The cardiac MR volumes of 25 healthy control persons of two separate clinical studies formed the database of this study. The volumes were obtained with 1.5 T Siemens Vision and Siemens Sonata MR devises with a phased array coil (Siemens, Erlangen, Germany) at the Helsinki Medical Imaging Center in the University of Helsinki. A standard turboflash cine imaging series was obtained with ECG-gating during a breath hold. SA volumes contained ventricles from the valve level until the last level where the apex is still visible, and LA volumes contained atria and ventricles. The pixel size of both SA and LA image slices was either 1.0×1.0 mm or 1.4×1.4 mm, and the slice thickness was $6 - 7$ mm. The number of slices in the SA volumes was $4 - 5$, and in the LA volumes $4 - 7$. Examples of the SA and LA image slices are given in Fig. 1 for one database subject. The ventricles, atria, and epicardium were manually segmented from the volumes by an expert. Thereafter, triangle surface models were constructed from the manual segmentations (Fig. 1c).

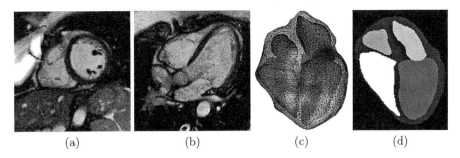

Fig. 1. a) A short-axis, b) long-axis slice, and c) a triangle surface model of one database subject. d) A slice from a labeled volume constructed from the manual segmentation

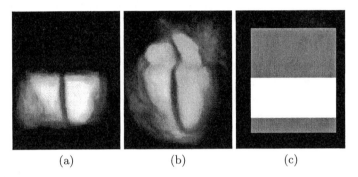

Fig. 2. a) A short-axis, b) long-axis mean model. c) A mask used in the calculation of the similarity measure

2.1 Mean Shape and Grey-Level Model

A mean shape and grey-level model (Fig. 2) was constructed from the database using the procedure presented in [16]. One subject was randomly selected as a reference. The remaining database volumes were registered with the reference volume using translation, rotation, and isotropic scaling. The registration method used for this purpose is presented in Section 3.3. Next, the reference volume was non-rigidly registered to the database volumes. The non-rigid registration method based on deformation spheres was used in this step [12]. Labeled volumes constructed from the manual segmentations (Fig. 1d) were used instead of the real grey-level volumes to ensure accurate registrations of the object surfaces [17]. From the resulting deformation fields, a mean deformation field was computed, and it was applied to the reference volume. This produced a mean shape model. To end up with a mean grey-level volume, the deformation fields of the non-rigid registrations were used to register the database volumes to the mean shape model, and the grey-level values were averaged voxel-wise. This procedure was repeated twice by using the obtained mean model as the reference to reduce the bias of the mean shape towards the selected reference subject.

3   Methods

The basic idea of the segmentation and registration methods studied in this paper is to deform an *a priori* model to match with the target volume. The deformations are determined based on a voxel similarity measure that is computed from both the SA and LA volumes. The mean model that was constructed in Section 2.1 is used as an *a priori* model.

3.1   Preprocessing

Because both the SA and LA volumes are used simultaneously in segmentation, the correspondence between the SA and LA volumes has to be determined. The necessary information is available in the image headers. Based on this information, the translation, rotation, and scaling parameters that transform the LA volumes to the coordinate system of the SA volumes, or vice versa, can be computed [13]. In this study, this procedure is used to transform the LA volumes into the coordinate system of the SA volumes.

There are several sources of motion artifacts (e.g., breathing) in the cine cardiac MR imaging. Consequently, the slices may be misaligned, and the correspondence between the SA and LA volumes may be inaccurate. The motion artifacts are corrected from the data using a registration-based method that moves the slices, and optimizes the normalized mutual information (NMI) between the SA and LA volumes [18]. After this, the voxel-by-voxel correspondence between the SA and LA volumes is guaranteed.

3.2   Similarity Measure

The initial alignment and image segmentation are implemented using normalized mutual information (NMI) as a similarity measure [19]. The NMI is defined as

$$I(S, T_i) = \frac{H(S) + H(T_i)}{H(S, T_i)}, \tag{1}$$

where $H(S)$ and $H(T_i)$ are the marginal entropies and $H(S, T_i)$ is the joint entropy of the source data S and the target data T_i.

In this study, the source data consist of both SA and LA source data, $S = \{S_{SA}, S_{LA}\}$, and the target data consist of the SA and LA data of the target subject, $T_i = \{T_{i,SA}, T_{i,LA}\}$. For example, the histogram that is used to calculate the joint entropy $H(S, T_i)$ is built from both the SA and LA volumes. The volume in which the SA source volume has meaningful information constitutes the SA source data, S_{SA}. Similarly, a part of the LA source volume constitutes the LA source data, S_{LA}. A mask is made to determine these regions (Fig. 2c). The SA volume information is used in the white regions, and the LA volume information in both the white and grey regions of Fig. 2c.

3.3   Affine Registration

The transformation parameters for the initial alignment of the database volumes with the mean model are optimized using the similarity measure presented in Section 3.2, and the Simplex optimization algorithm. Both seven- (rigid plus isotropic scaling) and nine-parameter (rigid plus anisotropic scaling) affine transformations were studied. The seven-parameter affine transformation was selected because it proved to be more robust and accurate than the nine-parameter affine transformation.

3.4   Non-rigid Registration-Based Segmentation

The mean model and the affinely registered database volumes are used as source and target volumes, respectively, in a deformable model-based segmentation method. The method registers non-rigidly the mean model to the database volumes using deformation spheres [12]. In this method, smooth deformations are applied to the voxels inside a sphere in such a way that the NMI (Section 3.2) is maximized. The location of the sphere is randomly chosen from the surfaces of the ventricles, atria, and epicardium, and it is varied during the iteration. The radius of the sphere is iteratively decreased from 30 voxels to 10 voxels. The deformation can be regularized in several ways in the segmentation tool. In this study, the directions of the normal vectors of the surfaces are regularized.

3.5   Evaluation Methods

The registration and segmentation methods presented in this section are evaluated using the database presented in Section 2. Leave-one-out cross-validation is used: each database subject is once regarded as a target, and the mean model used as an *a priori* model is constructed from the remaining 24 database subjects. For comparison, identical segmentations were performed using only the SA volumes.

The segmentation/registration error is defined as the mean distance from the manually segmented target surface to the deformed mean model's surface:

$$E \equiv \frac{1}{N_t} \sum_{i=1}^{N_t} d\left(\mathbf{t}_i, S\right), \tag{2}$$

where N_t is the number of the nodes in the target triangle surface model, $\mathbf{t}_i$ is the ith target node, and $d\left(\mathbf{t}_i, S\right)$ is the Euclidean distance from the point $\mathbf{t}_i$ to the triangle surface of the deformed mean model, S. The error of the epicardium is computed only from the surface below the valve level.

4   Results

The results for the segmentation using only the SA volumes and for the segmentation using both the SA and LA volumes are given in Table 1. For one

Table 1. The segmentation/registration errors (mean $\pm$ standard deviation) after the affine registration and after the non-rigid registration-based segmentation

	E (mm) after affine registration		E (mm) after segmentation	
organ	only SA	SA+LA	only SA	SA+LA
LV	4.20 ± 1.64	2.97 ± 0.77	3.12 ± 1.40	2.62 ± 0.75
RV	4.84 ± 2.06	3.75 ± 1.01	4.13 ± 2.68	3.66 ± 1.04
LA	5.71 ± 2.50	3.26 ± 1.34		2.62 ± 1.11
RA	7.14 ± 4.15	3.76 ± 1.08		2.85 ± 0.89
epicardium	4.38 ± 1.88	3.30 ± 0.72	3.62 ± 1.46	3.21 ± 0.65
all	5.25 ± 2.22	3.41 ± 0.66		2.99 ± 0.58

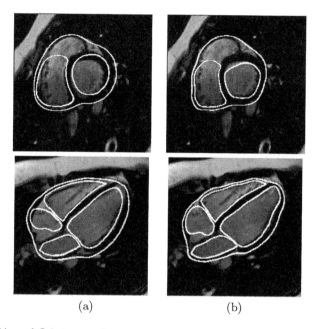

(a)   (b)

Fig. 3. An SA and LA image slice of the results for one database subject a) after the affine registration ($E = 3.83$ mm), and b) after the non-rigid registration-based segmentation ($E = 2.96$ mm)

database subject, the method using only the SA volumes produced totally incorrect segmentation. To enable reasonable comparison, this database subject was excluded from the results presented in Table 1. Therefore, the error values in Table 1 are the mean errors of 24 target subjects. The removed database subject gave the worst accuracy also for the segmentation using both the SA and LA volumes. When all 25 database subjects were used as a target, the mean segmentation error of all organs was $E = 3.09 \pm 0.75$ mm. The results for one database subject after the affine registration and the non-rigid registration-based segmentation are shown in Fig. 3.

The segmentation using both the SA and LA volumes was performed also by using a randomly selected database subject as an *a priori* model instead of the mean model. The mean errors of all organs, which are comparable to the results in Table 1, were $E = 5.72 \pm 2.32$ after the affine registration and $E = 4.22 \pm 1.83$ after the non-rigid registration-based segmentation.

5   Discussion

The results in Table 1 showed that by utilizing both the short-axis and long-axis MR volumes the ventricles and atria can be simultaneously segmented. Especially, the segmentation accuracy of the atria was improved from the affine registration. The superiority of using both the SA and LA volumes instead of just the SA volumes was demonstrated. The reason for the improved segmentation accuracy is that the comprehensive information on the SA and LA volumes is utilized to produce more accurate spatial transformations. In addition, the LA volumes include areas which are not visible in the SA volumes. It is worth of noting that the SA volumes used in this study did not contain atria. Therefore, when only the SA volumes were used in the affine registration, the transformation parameters had to be estimated from the ventricle data only. Furthermore, this is why the segmentation errors in Table 1 are reported only for the ventricles and epicardium when only the SA volumes were used.

We also proved that better accuracy is obtained by using a mean model as an *a priori* model instead of a randomly selected database subject. Naturally, if another database subject had been selected, the results could have been different.

In this study, the LA volumes were transformed into the coordinate system of the SA volumes (Section 3.1), in which the segmentation was performed. When the LA volumes were transformed into the coordinate system of the SA volumes, interpolation errors were produced. The registration and segmentation could have been performed with the LA volumes in their own coordinate system, but this would have increased the computational complexity.

Acknowledgements. Research was supported by Tekes, the National Technology Agency, Finland, the Finnish Cultural Foundation, and the Foundation for Advancement of Technical Sciences, Finland.

References

1. A.F. Frangi, W.J. Niessen, M.A. Viergever. Three-Dimensional Modeling for Functional Analysis of Cardiac Images: A Review. *IEEE Trans. Med. Imag.*, vol. 20(1), pp. 2–25, 2001.
2. M. Lorenzo-Valdés, G.I. Sanchez-Ortiz, R. Mohiaddin, D. Rueckert. Atlas-Based Segmentation and Tracking of 3D Cardiac MR Images Using Non-rigid Registration. *Proc. MICCAI'02*, 642–650, 2002.
3. M. Lorenzo-Valdés, G.I. Sanchez-Ortiz, R. Mohiaddin, D. Rueckert. Segmentation of 4D Cardiac MR Images Using a Probabilistic Atlas and the EM Algorithm. *Proc. MICCAI'03*, 440–450, 2003.

4. T.F. Cootes, C.J. Taylor, D.H. Cooper, J. Graham. Active Shape Models - their training and application. *Comput. Vis. Image Underst.*, vol. 61(1), 38–59, 1995.

5. T.F. Cootes, G.J. Edwards, C.J. Taylor. Active Appearance Models. *Proc. European Conference on Computer Vision*, 484–498, 1998.

6. M.R. Kaus, J. von Berg, W. Niessen, V. Pekar. Automated Segmentation of the Left Ventricle in Cardiac MRI. *Proc. MICCAI'03*, 432–439, 2003.

7. S.C. Mitchell, B.P.F. Lelieveldt, R.J. van der Geest, H.G. Bosch, J.H.C. Reiber, M. Sonka. Multistage Hybrid Active Appearance Model Matching: Segmentation of Left and Right Ventricles in Cardiac MR Images. *IEEE Trans. Med. Imag.*, vol. 20(5), pp. 415–423, 2001.

8. S.C. Mitchell, J.G. Bosch, B.P.F. Lelieveldt, R.J. van der Geest, J.H.C. Reiber, M. Sonka. 3-D Active Appearance Models: Segmentation of Cardiac MR and Ultrasound Images. *IEEE Trans. Med. Imag.*, vol. 21(9), pp. 1167–1178, 2002.

9. J.S. Suri. Computer Vision, Pattern Recognition and Image Processing in Left Ventricle Segmentation: The Last 50 Years. *Pattern Analysis & Applications*, vol. 3, 209–242, 2000.

10. N. Paragios. A Level Set Approach for Shape-Driven Segmentation and Tracking of the Left Ventricle. *IEEE Trans. Med. Imag.*, vol. 22(6), pp. 773–776, 2003.

11. D.T. Gering. Automatic Segmentation of Cardiac MRI. *Proc. MICCAI'03*, 524–532, 2003.

12. J. Lötjönen, T. Mäkelä. Elastic matching using a deformation sphere. *Proc. MICCAI'01*, 541–548, 2001.

13. J. Lötjönen, D. Smutek, S. Kivistö, K. Lauerma. Tracking Atria and Ventricles Simultaneously from Cardiac Short- and Long-Axis MR Images. *Proc. MICCAI'03*, 467–474, 2003.

14. J. Lötjönen, J. Koikkalainen, D. Smutek, S. Kivistö, K. Lauerma. Four-Chamber 3-D Statistical Shape Model from Cardiac Short-Axis and Long-Axis MR Images. *Proc. MICCAI'03*, 459–466, 2003.

15. B.P.F. Lelieveldt, M. Üzümcü, R.J. van der Geest, J.H.C. Reiber, M. Sonka. Multiview Active Appearance Models for Consistent Segmentation of Multiple Standard Views: Application to Long and Short-axis Cardiac MR Images. *Computer Assisted Radiology and Surgery*, vol. 1256, 1141–1146, 2003.

16. A. Guimond, J-P. Thirion. Average Brain Models. A Convergence Study. *Computer Vision and Image Understanding*, vol. 2, 192–210, 2000.

17. A.J. Frangi, D. Rueckert, J.A. Schnabel, W.J. Niessen. Automatic Construction of Multiple-Object Three-Dimensional Statistical Shape Models: Application to Cardiac Modeling. *IEEE Trans. Med. Imag.*, vol. 21(9), pp. 1151–1166, 2002.

18. J. Lötjönen, M. Pollari, S. Kivistö, K. Lauerma. Correction of movement artifacts from 4-D cardiac short- and long-axis MR data. *Proc. MICCAI'04*, 2004. In press.

19. C. Studholme, D.L.G. Hill, D.J. Hawkes. Automated three-dimensional registration of magnetic resonance and positron emission tomography brain images by multiresolution optimization of voxel similarity measures. *Medical Physics*, vol 24(1), 71–86, 1997.

Segmentation of Left Ventricle via Level Set Method Based on Enriched Speed Term

Yingge Qu, Qiang Chen, Pheng Ann Heng, and Tien-Tsin Wong

Department of Computer Science and Engineering
The Chinese University of Hong Kong, Shatin, Hong Kong
ygqu@cse.cuhk.edu.hk

Abstract. Level set methods have been widely employed in medical image segmentation, and the construction of speed function is vital to segmentation results. In this paper, two ideas for enriching the speed function in level set methods are introduced, based on the problem of segmenting left ventricle from tagged MR image. Firstly, a relaxation factor is introduced, aimed at relaxing the boundary condition when the boundary is unclear or blurred. Secondly, in order to combine visual contents of an image, which reflects human visual response directly, a simple and general model is introduced to endow speed function with more variability and better performance. Promising experimental results in MR images are shown to demonstrate the potentials of our approach.

1 Introduction

Computer-aided diagnosis is an important application domain of medical image analysis. Segmentation and tracking of cardiac structures are advanced techniques used to assist physicians in various states of treatment of cardiovascular diseases.

There have been many methods for segmentation purpose. Snake-driven approaches [1] are popular in medical image segmentation; however it cannot perform well around a cusp or in topology changing cases. B-splines, deformable templates, and Fourier descriptors are common ways to describe the structure of interest. Level set representation is an emerging technique to represent shapes and track moving interfaces [5]. Such techniques are applicable to segmentation and tracking [4]. Dealing with local deformations, multicomponent structures and changes of topology are the main strengths of these representations.

In the level set method, the construction of speed function is vital to the final result. The speed function is designed to control the movement of curve; and in different application problems, the key is to determine the appropriate stopping criteria for the evolution [6]. In case of segmentation, the segmentation precision depends on when and where the evolving curved surface stops, and the termination of the evolving curved surface also depends on the speed term. So the construction of speed term is critical to the segmentation results.

In this paper, two ideas for enriching the speed function are introduced, based on the problem of segmenting left ventricle from tagged MR image. Relaxation

C. Barillot, D.R. Haynor, and P. Hellier (Eds.): MICCAI 2004, LNCS 3216, pp. 435–442, 2004.
© Springer-Verlag Berlin Heidelberg 2004

factor is first introduced. It provides a force to stop evolving curve at ventricle boundary even when the boundary is blurred. As visual contents of image, including color, shape and texture reflect human visual response directly, various image content based speed terms have been introduced to tackle different application problems. Here, we derive a simple and general model, through introducing the image content items, to endow speed function with more variability and better performance.

The rest of this paper is organized as follows. In Section 2, level set method and segmentation procedure are introduced. Section 3 focuses on the speed term improvement and presents experimental results. Conclusion is given in Section 4.

2   Level Set Method and Left Ventricle Segmentation

2.1   Level Set

Level set method, developed by Osher and Sethian, is a zero equivalent surface method [5]. Its basic idea is to change movement track of planar curve into movement track of three-dimensional curved surface. Though this conversion complicates the solution, it has many other merits; and the main merit is that it can deal with the change of topological structure easily.

The classical level set boundary is defined as the zero level set of an implicit function Φ defined on the entire image domain. The dimensionality of the level set function Φ is one higher than the evolving boundary, which in this case for a 2-D image domain is a 3-D surface. The level set method tracks the evolution of a front that is moving normal to the boundary with a speed $F(x, y)$. The speed function can be dependent on the local or global properties of the evolving boundary or from forces external to the boundary. The level set function Φ is defined such that the location of the boundary Γ and the region enclosed by the boundary Ω are functions of the zero-level set of Φ, namely,

$$\Phi_t + F|\nabla\Phi| = 0 . \tag{1}$$

It is the basic equation of level set, and the zero level set denotes object contour curve

$$\Gamma(t) = \{x|\Phi(x, t) = 0\} . \tag{2}$$

Generally, Φ represents the signed distance function to the front. That is,

$$\Phi(x, y) = \pm d(x, y) , \tag{3}$$

where $d(x, y)$ is the smallest distance from the point to the boundary, and the sign is chosen such that points inside the boundary have a negative sign and those outside have a positive sign.

The function Φ is initialized based on a signed distance measure to the initial front. In the case of a single point this is simply the euclidian distance to that point. The evolution of the boundary is defined via a partial differential equation on the zero level set of Φ

$$\frac{\partial\Phi}{\partial t} = -F|\nabla\Phi| . \tag{4}$$

Finally, level set methods may be easily adapted to a discrete grid implementation for efficient processing. Refer to [6] for a more detailed description on level set methods and their applications.

2.2 Left Ventricle Segmentation

The level set framework has been adapted to a number of applications beyond front propagation of physical phenomena, including the denoising of images, object recognition, and shortest path identification. Key to the success of these approaches is to determine the appropriate stopping criteria for the evolution [6]. The level set will continue to propagate as long as the speed function $F(x, y) > 0$. Therefore, the speed function must be properly designed such that $F(x, y) \rightarrow 0$ as the boundary approaches the desired location. For the segmentation problem, it is desirable for $F(x, y) \rightarrow 0$ at the edges of the left ventricle boundary. The algorithm flow is:

```
1. Initialize the narrow band;
2. Resolve the level set equation (4);
3. Track the zero level set curve, and reinitialize the narrow band;
4. Repeat step 3 and 4, and enter the calculations of the next time step.
```

The Hamilton-Jacobi equation (4) can be resolved according to the *hyperbolic conservation law*. When the curve evolves to the boundary of the narrow band, the narrow band should be reinitialized. If the point difference between sequential times is smaller than the designed threshold in narrow band, the propagating speed will be set to zero. When the narrow band is not reinitialized within some time, it means that the curve evolvement has stopped. So the iteration ends, and the final zero level curve is the boundary of the left ventricle.

3 Improvement on Speed Term

Much of the challenge in interface problems comes from producing an adequate model for speed term [6]. As mentioned above, the construction of speed function is vital to final results. The speed function is designed to control the movement of curve; and in different problems, the key is to determine the appropriate stopping criteria for the evolution. In a segmentation case, the segmentation precision depends on when and where the evolving curved surface stops, and the stop of the evolving curved surface also depends on the speed term F. So the construction of F is critical to the segmentation results.

In this section, based on the problem of segmenting left ventricle from tagged MR image, two ideas to enrich the speed function are introduced. Relaxation factor is first introduced, followed by an introduction to image content items.

3.1 Relaxation Factor

In [4], the construction of speed term is described as: $F = F_A + F_G$, where F_A is a constant. It does not depend on the geometry of the front, but its sign determines the movement direction of the front. F_G depends on the geometry of the front. It is ignored in this case, so supposing $F_G=0$. In [4] a negative speed term is constructed as equation (5), and then constructs the speed term as: $F = F_A + F_I$, where F_I is defined as

$$F_I(x,y) = \frac{-F_A}{M_1 - M_2}\{|\nabla G_\sigma \cdot I(x,y)| - M_2\} . \tag{5}$$

The expression $G_\sigma \cdot I(x,y)$ denotes the image convolved with a Gaussian smoothing filter whose characteristic width is σ. M_1 and M_2 are the maximum and minimum values of the magnitude of image gradient $|\nabla G_\sigma \cdot I(x,y)|$. So the speed term F tends to be zero when image gradient is large.

However, in practical, gradient on object boundary are impossible of the same maximum value (M_1). In other word, the evolvement cannot stop at the object boundary. Especially for MR images whose boundaries are blurry, the results are more unsatisfactory. To solve this problem, here, a *relaxation factor* δ is introduced to relax the bounding of $M_1 - M_2$:

$$r = \frac{|\nabla G_\sigma \cdot I(x,y)| - M_2}{M_1 - M_2 - \delta} , \tag{6}$$

where $\delta \in [0, M_1 - M_2]$. Let $r = \begin{cases} r \text{ if } r < 1 \\ 1 \text{ if } r \geq 1 \end{cases}$, and the reconstructed negative speed term will be $F'_I(x,y) = -r \cdot F_A$.

By introducing this relaxation factor, when the front propagates to places where the gradient of object boundary are close to M_1, but not exactly M_1, the speed F drops to zero and the evolving curve will be stopped soundly. Fig. 1 shows the result of solving this problem by introducing the relaxation factor δ. Here, $\delta=0.23$.

3.2   Image Content Items

Visual content of an image includes color, shape, texture, and spatial layout, reflecting human visual response directly. Based on them, image/object feature extraction techniques have been fully developed. In typical level set methods, the construction of speed function mainly uses the gradient information. However, as medical imaging technique advances, more clear and detailed images have brought more difficulties to level set based segmentation methods. As a response, various image content based speed items have been introduced to solve different application problems. In this paper, we derive a simple yet general model, through combining the image content items, to endow the speed function with more variability and better performance.

The form of speed function can be written as [4]: $F = F_A + F_G$. By adding control items or other image force, it can be expressed as a general but simple model:

$$F = A(F_A + F_G) + B \tag{7}$$
$$A = C_{img}/C_{front} \; or \; A = 1 - dist(C_{img}, C_{front}) \tag{8}$$
$$B = dist(C_{img}, C_{front}) \tag{9}$$

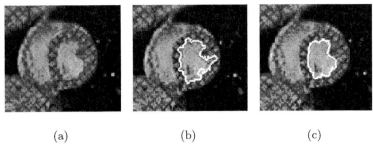

(a)   (b)   (c)

Fig. 1. (a) is the original MR image. In (b), the white line is the propagated front get by original level set speed term. It easily gets across the true boundary due to the blurred boundary. (c) is the result by introducing the relaxation factor into the speed term.

The $dist()$ could be an arbitrary distance function. It is engaged to measure the difference of image features between the propagating front and the target image. B stands for the additional forces come from image content. C stands for the image content model, including any of color, shape, and texture features. A is used to balance the force from front and the force from additional items, and $A \rightarrow 1$.

3.3   The Enriched Speed Terms

For example, when curve movement is relative to curvature, namely $F_G \neq 0$, literatures [4] and [8] introduce the stop term based on image gradient:

$$K_I(x,y) = \frac{1}{1 + |\nabla G_\sigma \cdot I(x,y)|} \tag{10}$$

Here, gradient can be treated as the difference measure of gray/brightness value. To adjust the image gradient's influence on the speed term, we can overwrite it:

$$K_I'(x,y) = \frac{1}{1 + |\nabla G_\sigma \cdot I(x,y)|^p} = 1 - \frac{|\nabla G_\sigma \cdot I(x,y)|^p}{1 + |\nabla G_\sigma \cdot I(x,y)|^p}, \tag{11}$$

where the constant $p \geq 1$. When p is larger, K_I' will be smaller, so it will control the speed to decrease faster. Then the speed term can be written as

$$F = K_I'(K + F_A), \tag{12}$$

where $K = \frac{\phi_{yy}\phi_x^2 - 2\phi_x\phi_y\phi_{xy} + \phi_{xx}\phi_y^2}{(\phi_x^2 + \phi_y^2)^{3/2}}$ is the curvature of the front at point (x,y).

Other examples: To resolve boundary leak problem, Kichenassamy et al. [2] and Yezzi et al. [9] introduced a pull-back term $(\nabla c \cdot \nabla \phi)$ due to edge strength, here $c(x,y) = \frac{1}{1 + |\nabla G_\sigma \cdot I(x,y)|}$. It is an additional force term based on the color feature. To provide an additional attraction force when the front was in the vicinity of an edge, Siddiqui et al. [7] introduced an extra term $\frac{1}{2} div \left[\begin{pmatrix} x \\ y \end{pmatrix} \phi \right]$

according to the area minimization. It is an additional force term based on the shape feature.

In tagged MR image case, new feature also can be introduced based on this idea. High clarity of tag lines makes segmentation more complex than untagged image. According to human response, texture is the most distinguish feature, see Fig. 2(a). In this example, the tag lines are on vertical direction, hence we design an additional term B based on texture feature BPV [3].

$$BPV(x,y) = \frac{1}{N} \sum_{y-\lceil\frac{N-1}{2}\rceil}^{y+\lceil\frac{N-1}{2}\rceil} (I(x,i) - M)^2 \,, M = \frac{1}{N} \sum_{y-\lceil\frac{N-1}{2}\rceil}^{y+\lceil\frac{N-1}{2}\rceil} |I(x,i) - I(x,y)| \tag{13}$$

Here, the distance is measured by the standard deviation. $BPV(x,y)$ is the BPV value of point (x,y), $1 \leq x \leq m$, $\frac{N-1}{2} \leq y \leq n - \frac{N-1}{2}$, m and n are height and width of image, and N is the width of window, which is appropriate to be 7 or 9 according to the width of tag lines. $I(x,y)$ is the intensity value of the block center. Meaning of the above equation is: When the intensity value of some point is quite different from that of points which are on the same line and whose center is the point, this BPV value of the point is smaller, and vice verse. Now, the speed function has been enriched to:

$$F = K_I'(\varepsilon K + F_A + F_I') + \beta \frac{\nabla c \cdot \nabla \phi}{|\nabla \phi|} + \mu \, div \left[\begin{pmatrix} x \\ y \end{pmatrix} \phi \right] + \gamma(BPV) \,, \tag{14}$$

where K_I' is the A item, used to control the balance between the original speed term and the additional speed term. Larger K_I' will speedup the decrease of the speed term. The coefficients β, μ, and γ are constant, which should be defined according to the contribution of their following part. In equation (14), image features, such as curvature, shape and texture information, have been combined into the speed term. Experiment with this enriched speed item is carried in the following section.

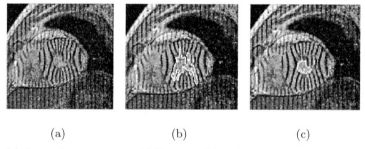

(a)   (b)   (c)

Fig. 2. (a) shows the strong tagged MR image (b) is the result obtained by the standard level set method. This result has a serious leak phenomenon due to the affection from strong tag lines. (c) is the improved result by using the BPV feature to control the propagation of the front.

3.4   Experiments and Results

The first experiment focused on the left ventricle MR image with tag lines. Because of the blood flow, tag lines within the left ventricle decrease fast in the last stage of the cardiac shrink, until they disappear; But tag lines in the myocardium decrease slowly, which can be seen from Fig. 2(a). In other words, within the left ventricle the intensity changes are smaller and the relative BPV value is larger; in the myocardium the intensity changes are larger and the relative BPV value is smaller. As for images like Fig. 2(a) whose tag lines are very strong, the weight of BPV should be larger in the construction of speed term.

In the above experiment, the spatial step length is 1, the temporal step length is 0.001, $F_A=-20$, $\beta=5$, $\mu = 0.0025$, $\gamma = 280$, $\delta = 0.23$. The number of iterations is 150. As the tag lines in Fig. 2 are strong, constant γ should be set large. While in other cases, it could be set small. For MR images without tag lines, we do not have to impose the BPV term (namely $\gamma=0$). These parameters are fine tuned empirically and adjusted manually. An automatic process to estimate the parameters could be further studied in future work [10].

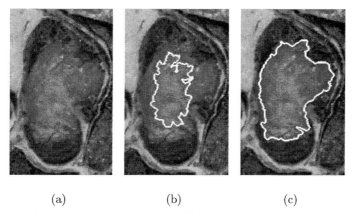

(a)   (b)   (c)

Fig. 3. (a) is the original color slide image. (b) shows that propagate front stop at the non-boundary area. (c) is the result after incorporating color and texture features into the speed function.

This model can be applied to various cases. For example, in color slide image case, another experiment result can be seen in Fig. 3. The original segmentation result is far from ideal (Fig. 3(b)) because that the stronger image details could stop the propagation easily. In this case, the introduction of color and texture into the speed term makes the result closer to user's expectation. So we introduce block color histogram and BPV texture feature. The distance measures are: the histogram intersection, as a measure of the block wised histogram; and the Euclidean distance, as a measure in BPV item. Balancing items are: $F_A=-15$, $\beta = 5$, $\mu = 0.002$, $\gamma = 20$, $\delta = 0.2$.

4   Conclusion

In medical image segmentation problems, image features vary much. Gradient and gray level information are far from enough to describe proper stopping condition of the speed term. Introducing new speed item to control the propagating is necessary and important. In this paper, two ideas for enriching the speed function are introduced. Relaxation factor is first introduced. It provides a relaxing boundary condition, so as to stop the evolving curve at a blurred or unclear boundary. Secondly, the speed term is enriched by introducing visual content items. A simple and general model is proposed to incorporate the image features into the speed item in order to improve the flexibility and performance of the speed function. Promising experiment shows that the incorporation of powerful distance measure and proper image features in speed function can improve the segmentation result significantly.

Acknowledgement. This work was supported by the Research Grants Council of the Hong Kong Special Administrative Region, under RGC Earmarked Grants (Project CUHK 4180/01E, CUHK 1/00C).

References

1. M. Kass, A. Witkin, and D. Terzopoulos. Snakes: Active contour models. *IJCV*, pages 321–332, 1988.
2. S. Kichenassamy, A. Kumar, P. Olver, A. Tannenbaum, and A. Yezzi. Conformal curvature flows: from phase transitions to active vision. *Archive of Rational Mechanics and Analysis*, 134(3):275–301, 1996.
3. C. G. Looney. *Pattern Recognition Using Neural Networks*, chapter 10. Oxford University Press, 1997.
4. R. Malladi, J. Sethian, and B. Vemuri. Shape modeling with front propagation: A level set approach. *IEEE Pattern Anal. Machine Intell.*, 17:158–175, 1995.
5. Stanley Osher and James A. Sethian. Fronts propagating with curvature-dependent speed: algorithms based on hamilton-jacobi formulations. *J. Comput. Phys.*, 79(1):12–49, 1988.
6. J.A. Sethian. *Level Set Methods and Fast Marching Methods: Evolving Interfaces in Computational Geometry, Fluid Mechanics, Computer Vision, and Materials Science.* Cambridge University Press, 1999.
7. K. Siddiqui, Y.B. Lauriere, A. Tannenbaum, and S. W. Zucker. Area and length minimizing flows for shape segmentation. *IEEE Trans. on Image Processing*, 7(3):433–443, 1998.
8. J. Suri, K. Liu, S. Singh, S. Laxminarayana, and L. Reden. Shape recovery algorithms using level sets in 2-d/3-d medical imagery: A state-of-the-art review. *IEEE Trans. in Information Technology in Biomedicine (ITB)*, 6(1):9–12, 2001.
9. A. Yezzi, S. Kichenassamy, A. Kumar, P. Olver, and A. Tannenbaum. A geometric snake model for segmentation of medical imagery. *IEEE Trans. on Medical Imaging*, 16(2):199–209, 1997.
10. A. J. Yezzi, A. Tsai, and A. S. Willsky. Binary and ternary flows for image segmentation. In *Proc. Int. Conf. on Image Processing*, volume 2, pages 1–5, 1999.

Border Detection on Short Axis Echocardiographic Views Using a Region Based Ellipse-Driven Framework

Maxime Taron[1], Nikos Paragios[1], and Marie-Pierre Jolly[2]

[1] Ecole Nationale des Ponts et Chaussees,
Champs-sur-Marne, France
{taron,nikos}@cermics.enpc.fr
[2] Imaging & Visualization Department,
Siemens Corporate Research, Princeton, NJ, USA
marie-pierre.jolly@scr.siemens.com

Abstract. In this paper, we propose a robust technique that integrates spatial and temporal information for consistent recovery of the endocardium. To account for the low image quality we introduce a local variant of the Mumford-Shah that is coupled with a model of limited parameters to describe the ventricle, namely an ellipse. The objective function is defined on the implicit space of ellipses, separates locally the blood pool from the heart wall and explores geometric constraints on the deformations of the endocardium to impose temporal consistency. Promising experimental results demonstrate the potentials of our method.

1 Introduction

Ultrasonic imaging provides time-varying two-dimensional imagery of the heart and is an important modality in medical image analysis [11] because of the low acquisition cost and the portability of the device. However, such images present low signal-to-noise (SNR) ratio resulting in poor signal quality and therefore model-based approaches are suitable to deal with such a modality.

Cardiovascular diseases are an important cause of death in the United States. Segmenting the left ventricle is a challenging component of computer aided diagnosis. Recovering the systolic and diastolic form of the endocardium is often the target of echocardiographic segmentation. Learning appropriate organ models [4] is an important pre-segmentation step for model-based techniques. The objective is to recover a compact structure that consists of limited parameters and can describe most of the examples within the training set.

Segmentation techniques for ultrasonic images consist of model-free [7,1] and model-based approaches [3,9]. Model-free techniques can better capture the variations of the endocardium while suffering from not being able to deal with the corrupted data. Model-based approaches are more efficient when dealing with echocardiographic images due to the high signal-to-noise ratio. One can also separate the techniques that perform filtering/segmentation in the polar [7] or in the raw space [1]. Markov random fields formulations [7], active shape and appearance models [4,9], snakes [3], deformable models and templates [8] and level set techniques [1] are well established techniques considered to address the segmentation of the left ventricle in echocardiographic images.

C. Barillot, D.R. Haynor, and P. Hellier (Eds.): MICCAI 2004, LNCS 3216, pp. 443–450, 2004.
© Springer-Verlag Berlin Heidelberg 2004

In this paper we propose a local variant of an ellipse driven Mumford-Shah framework where data terms are considered locally. Such an approach is well suited to echocardiography when data is heavily corrupted. Furthermore, the use of prior knowledge is introduced in a simple and efficient manner according to a continuous (in the temporal domain) elliptic model. Segmentation is then equivalent to the recovery of a limited set of parameters (5) that are continuous in time.

The remainder of this paper is organized as follows. In the next section, we introduce the local variant of the Mumford-Shah framework. Segmentation that involves the recovery of the ellipse parameters is presented in section 3 while temporal segmentation is considered in section 4. Results are discussed in section 5.

2   Object Extraction Through Curve Propagation

Curve evolution is a popular technique in image analysis for object extraction and segmentation. The Mumford-Shah framework [10] and the snake model [8] are the basis of a wide range of segmentation techniques. To this end, the evolution of a closed contour C is associated with the minimization of a cost function (energy) that accounts for certain image properties while respecting the internal geometric properties of the contour. In the most general case, the objective is to segment the image while restoring the signal [10]. That is equivalent to optimizing an objective function of the following form:

$$E(u, C) = E_{image}(u, C) + E_{smooth}(C) + E_{shape}(C)$$

E_{image} depends on the image features along a planar curve C that creates a partition of the domain into two regions (Ω_1 and Ω_2). This term also depends on a function u that has to be smooth on the domains Ω_1 and Ω_2 while approximating the image f. The smoothness term E_{smooth} depends on the internal curve properties. In our case we use $E_{smooth}(C) = \nu L(C)$ according to the L^2 norm as in [6].
Last, E_{shape} put constraints on the contour according to some prior knowledge.

We consider the image part of the Mumford-Shah functional to be the basis of our approach [10] :

$$E_{image}(u, C) = \frac{1}{2} \int_{\Omega} (f - u)^2 d\omega + \lambda^2 \frac{1}{2} \int_{\Omega - C} |\nabla u|^2 d\omega \qquad (1)$$

The first component is a matching term between the image f and the approximation function u, while the second term enforces the regularity (smoothness) of the u function. Most of existing segmentation techniques are based on the assumption of homogeneity of visual features. Therefore, under certain conditions, u could be considered as piecewise constant. This is equivalent to considering $\lambda \to \infty$ and simplifies the objective function as follows :

$$E_{image}(u, C) = \frac{1}{2} \int_{\Omega} (f - u)^2 d\omega$$

The function u that minimizes the energy for a fixed contour corresponds to the average intensity within the regions Ω_1 and Ω_2 :

$$u(x) = \begin{cases} \frac{1}{\Omega_1} \int_{\Omega_1} f(\omega) d\omega & \text{if } \omega \in \Omega_1 \\ \frac{1}{\Omega_2} \int_{\Omega_2} f(\omega) d\omega & \text{if } \omega \in \Omega_2 \end{cases}$$

The assumption of homogeneity is not valid when dealing with ultrasonic images. Speckle, presence of papillary muscles, and other structures violate such assumptions. Consequently, the scenario where the two image classes are well separated using their means is unrealistic. On the other hand, such condition is valid within local image patches. The Mumford-Shah framework can now be considered in local patches. The calculation of the approximation function u only takes into account the pixel intensities in a local neighborhood.

Let ω be the radius of the local neighborhood and $\mathcal{K}_{x,y}$ be a local image patch centered at location (x,y) :

$$\mathcal{K}_{x,y} = [x-\omega, x+\omega] \times [y-\omega, y+\omega]$$

Then, using prior definitions on Ω_1 and Ω_2, we can introduce a local partition as shown on the side figure according to:

$$\mathcal{K}_{x,y} = \Omega_{1,L}(x,y) \bigcup \Omega_{2,L}(x,y)$$
$$\Omega_{1,L}(x,y) = \mathcal{K}_{x,y} \bigcap \Omega_1$$
$$\Omega_{2,L}(x,y) = \mathcal{K}_{x,y} \bigcap \Omega_2$$

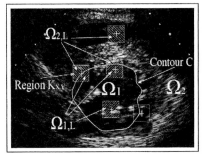

Using this local partition, we introduce the following functional :

$$
\begin{aligned}
E_{image}(u,C) = &\tfrac{1}{2} \int \int_{\Omega} (f(x,y) - u(x,y))^2 dx\,dy \\
&+ \tfrac{1}{2}\lambda \left[\int \int_{\Omega_1} \left(\int \int_{\Omega_{1,L}(X,Y)} (f(x,y) - u(X,Y))^2 \, dx\,dy \right) dX\,dY \right. \\
&\left. + \int \int_{\Omega_2} \left(\int \int_{\Omega_{2,L}(X,Y)} (f(x,y) - u(X,Y))^2 \, dx\,dy \right) dX\,dY \right]
\end{aligned}
\tag{2}
$$

Where the last two terms are optimized when u corresponds to the average image intensity over the $\Omega_{1,L}$ and $\Omega_{2,L}$. Considering the limit case when $\lambda \to \infty$, the energy can be rewritten and simplified :

$$E_{image}(u,C) = \tfrac{1}{2} \int \int_{\Omega} (f(x,y) - u(x,y))^2 dx\,dy \tag{3}$$

$$\text{with : } \quad u(x,y) = \begin{cases} \frac{1}{|\Omega_{1,L}(x,y)|} \int \int_{\Omega_{1,L}(x,y)} f(X,Y) dX\,dY & \text{if } (x,y) \in \Omega_1 \\ \frac{1}{|\Omega_{2,L}(x,y)|} \int \int_{\Omega_{2,L}(x,y)} f(X,Y) dX\,dY & \text{if } (x,y) \in \Omega_2 \end{cases} \tag{4}$$

Such a definition makes u a piecewise smooth function on Ω_1 and Ω_2 and discontinuous across the contour C.

Minimizing the energy (3) using gradient descent results in the following evolution equation :

$$\frac{\partial C}{\partial t} = [e^+(s,t) - e^-(s,t)].n(s,t) = 0 \quad \forall s \in [0,1].$$

Where $n(s)$ is the outer normal to the contour and $e^{-/+}$ denotes the energy density outside and inside the contour :

$$e^{-/+} = (f(C(s)) - u(C(s)))^2$$

Quite often, image derived terms are not sufficient to perform segmentation since noisy and corrupted data could lead to non optimal results. Prior knowledge on the geometric form of the structure to be recovered could address such a limitation.

Statistical analysis of a set of training examples is the most common technique to derive compact representations used to encode prior knowledge. Given a training set, we compute the statistics on the deformations of the endocardium using Principal Component Analysis (PCA) [5]. These statistics are then used to compute the likelihood of the contour C in the energy term $E_{shape}(C)$ [6]. Since the orientation and scale of the endocardium are also unknown, the energy seeks for a similarity transformation between the contour and the average model. Such an analysis could provide an adequate framework to introduce prior knowledge on the segmentation.

However, the complexity of the model and the large number of training examples are difficult issues. Instead, one can model the endocardium in short axis views as an ellipse. Such a statement is supported by the PCA where the mean model is an ellipse with a small eccentricity and the modes of variation do not significantly alter this. Therefore, it is adequate to consider short axis segmentation in the space of ellipses. Such an approach is a good compromise between complexity and fair approximation of the ventricle shape.

3   Ventricle Recovery Through an Elliptic Structure

The segmentation according to an ellipse is equivalent to the recovery of five parameters parameters. Therefore, we consider the following space to be optimized :

$$\Theta = [a, \lambda, \phi, x_0, y_0]$$

where :

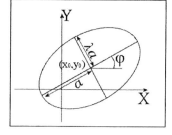

- a is the length of the main axis.
- λ is the aspect ratio between the two axes.
- ϕ is the aspect rotation between the main axis and the abscissa.
- x_0, y_0 the coordinates of the center.

Given this parameter space, the parametric and implicit form of the ellipse are defined as follows :

$$R_\Theta(\theta) = R_{a,\lambda,\phi,x_0,y_0}(\theta) = \begin{cases} x(\theta) = a(cos(\theta)cos(\phi) - \lambda sin(\theta)sin(\phi)) + x_0 \\ y(\theta) = a(cos(\theta)sin(\phi) + \lambda sin(\theta)cos(\phi)) + y_0 \end{cases}$$

$$F_\Theta(x,y) = 0 = \left(\frac{(x-x_0)*cos(\phi)+(y-y_0)*sin(\phi)}{a} \right)^2 + \left(\frac{-(x-x_0)*sin(\phi)+(y-y_0)*cos(\phi)}{\lambda a} \right)^2 - 1$$

Knowledge based segmentation is now equivalent to deforming an ellipse according to Θ, so it is attracted to the desired image features. Within such a concept, the smoothness is ensured by the parametrisation; therefore the energy term $E_{smooth}(C)$ can be omitted. An ellipse (Θ) creates an image partition (Ω_1, Ω_2). We use a similar energy term as in section 2, also considering the limit case in equation (2) when $\lambda \to \infty$ leading to the following simplified energy :

$$E_1(u, \Theta) = \frac{1}{2} \int \int_\Omega (f(x,y) - u(x,y))^2 dx\, dy \qquad (5)$$

where for the approximation function u an interpretation as the one presented in equation (4) is considered.

In order to explicitly introduce the ellipse parameters, we define a C^1 function H_σ (that converges toward a Heaviside distribution when $\sigma \to 0$):

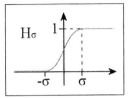

$$H_\sigma(x) = \begin{cases} 0 & \text{if } x \in]-\infty, -\sigma] \\ 0.5(1 + sin(\frac{\pi x}{2\sigma})) & \text{if } x \in]-\sigma, \sigma[\\ 1 & \text{if } x \in [\sigma, \infty[\end{cases}$$

Then the cost function could be rewritten :

$$E_1(u, \Theta) = \lim_{\sigma \to 0} \int_\Omega [H_\sigma(F_\Theta - \sigma) + H_\sigma(-F_\Theta - \sigma)] (f - u)^2 dx$$

and be differentiated leading to the following expression :

$$\frac{\partial E_1(\Theta, u)}{\partial \Theta} = \int_0^{2\pi} \frac{\partial (F_\Theta(R_\Theta(\theta)))}{\partial \Theta} \frac{1}{|\nabla F_\Theta(R_\Theta(\theta))|} k(\theta) h(\theta) d\theta$$

with $k(\theta) = ((f_{ext}(R_\Theta(\theta)) - u_{ext}(R_\Theta(\theta)))^2 - (f_{int}(R_\Theta(\theta)) - u_{int}(R_\Theta(\theta)))^2)$
and $h(\theta) = a\sqrt{(sin(\theta))^2 + (\lambda cos(\theta))^2}$
The calculation of the gradient of the implicit representation ($|\nabla F_{1,\Theta}(R(\theta))|$) and the derivative of $\nabla F_{1,\Theta}$ with respect to the parameters of the ellipse is straightforward.

Up to this point, regional information was considered to perform segmentation. While in general boundary information is not reliable, there are areas where the boundaries on the endocardium are visible. Towards exploring such a visual cue, a term based on gradient information can be considered. This information was considered in various papers dealing with boundary detection on short axis views after a preprocessing of the ultrasound image [12].

Let g be a monotonically decreasing function that depends on the image gradient defined at the pixel level. A common form of boundary term refers to the sum over the whole contour of the edge function g :

$$E_2(\Theta) = \int_{\theta=0}^{\theta=2\pi} g(R_\Theta(\theta)) \, d\theta \tag{6}$$

The speckle that transforms the myocardium wall into a collection of small bright dots generates strong values of the gradient magnitude almost everywhere on the heart muscle. Therefore, using the gradient magnitude to compute g could lead to inconsistent results. So, rather than seeking important gradient magnitude along the contour, we also expect the gradient to be directed toward the outside of the ventricle as proposed in [2]. Such a condition will eliminate most of the gradients due to speckle and the ones oriented in other directions will be eliminated. We use the center of the initial contour to determine an outward unit vector $\overrightarrow{n}$ at each point of the image. Then, we compute g as follows :

$$g(z) = \frac{1}{1 + (\nabla(G * I(z)).\overrightarrow{n})^2}$$

where G is a large Gaussian kernel that aims at removing partly the speckle noise.

The global energy for the contour is therefore composed of region based and gradient based terms :

$$E(\Theta, u) = \alpha_1 E_1(\Theta, u) + \alpha_2 E_2(\Theta)$$

A gradient descent method, starting from a manually drawn initial contour, can be used to recover the optimal ellipse parameters associated to the lowest potential of this function.

4   Temporal Segmentation

Temporal information can be valuable in echocardiography. Quite often, parts of the endocardium border are visible in only some of the frames of the cardiac cycle. Therefore, knowledge accumulation within local time intervals can be very beneficial when dealing with corrupted data. To this end, we propose an energy to be minimized on a set of frames so that it leads to the segmentation of the endocardium on a complete sequence.

The heart sits in a sac (the pericardium) filled with serous liquid; therefore the movement relatively to the other organs is restricted. Moreover, the effort made by the myocardium occurs simultaneously in every directions, so the global movement of the heart relative to the transducer (fixed during the recording process) will remain negligible compared with the inner movements of the heart muscles. Consequently, the coordinate of the center as well as the orientation of the ellipse can be considered constant over short sequences of frames. Moreover, the eccentricity of the ellipses approximating the endocardium varies very little so that the scale factor will be considered as the only temporal variable.

We consider the vectors of parameters Θ_t, defining an elliptic contour on the frame at time t. The motion constraints mean that the parameters $[\lambda, \phi, x_0, y_0]$ are constant over a set of frames and the only parameter depending on time is the length of the main axis a_t :

$$\Theta_t = [a_t, \lambda, \phi, x_0, y_0] = [a_t, \Theta^*]$$

Then one can define the following energy computed on a sequence of frames :

$$E(\Theta) = \sum_{\tau=t-\Delta t}^{\tau=t+\Delta t} \{\alpha_1 E_{1,\tau}(a_\tau, \Theta^*) + \alpha_2 E_{2,\tau}(a_\tau, \Theta^*)\} \tag{7}$$

That consists of $5 + 2\Delta t$ parameters. The minimization of such a functional using a gradient descent leads to the segmentation of the endocardium for $2\Delta t + 1$ frames.

$E_{1,\tau}$ is an energy term similar to the one presented in (5) for the frame at time τ. Therefore, it depends on the ellipse with parameters Θ_τ and the approximation function u. Assuming that the contour is tracking some features, one can also consider that these features have about the same intensity on consecutive frames. Therefore, the approximation function u combined information from neighboring frames:

$$\frac{\partial E_1(\Theta, u)}{\partial \Theta_t^*} = \sum_{\tau=t-\Delta t}^{\tau=t+\Delta t} \int_0^{2\pi} \frac{\partial (F_{\Theta_\tau}(R_{\Theta_\tau}(\theta)))}{\partial \Theta_t^*} \frac{1}{|\nabla F_{\Theta_\tau^*}(R_{\Theta_\tau}(\theta))|} g_\tau(\theta) h_\tau(\theta) d\theta$$

with $h_\tau(\theta) = a_\tau \sqrt{(\sin(\theta))^2 + (\lambda \cos(\theta))^2}$

and $g_\tau(\theta) = [f_{ext,\tau}(R_{\Theta_\tau}(\theta)) - v_{ext,\tau}(\theta)]^2 - [f_{int,\tau}(R_{\Theta_\tau}(\theta)) - v_{int,\tau}(\theta)]^2$

$v_{side,\tau}(\theta) = 0.2 u_{side,\tau-1}(R_{\Theta_{\tau-1}}(\theta)) + 0.6 u_{side,\tau}(R_{\Theta_\tau}(\theta)) + 0.2 u_{side,\tau+1}(R_{\Theta_{\tau+1}}(\theta))$

$v_{side,\tau}$ is calculated on frame τ with $side$ either equal to ext or int.

In practice, an initial ellipse is positioned in the vicinity of the endocardium in one of the frames (t) of the cardiac cycle. Then, segmentation is performed within a temporal window of five frames. Upon convergence of the process, the temporal window is shifted and centered at the next frame. The segmentation parameters on the previous step are used to initialize the process, and a new solution is recovered for frame $t+1$. The process is repeated until the entire clip is segmented.

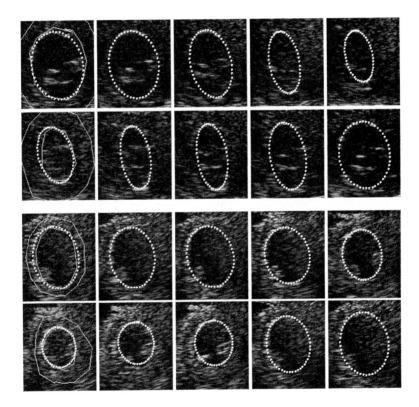

Fig. 1. Segmentation using the ellipse model on a complete cardiac cycles for two different patients. The dotted ellipse shows the recovered endocardium. The thin line shows the ground truth for both endocardium and epicardium on two frames as drawn by an expert.

5 Discussion and Perspectives

The proposed technique was considered to segment several short axis echocardiographic clips. Preliminary results - as shown in figure 1 - demonstrate the potentials of the method. From a set of 15 patients, the method recovered successfully the endocardium in 5 cases. While a more in depth validation is required, we conclude that the use an ellipse is a good compromise between complexity and performance. In addition, local image-driven terms improve significantly the segmentation results. However, more complicated statistical methods are required to capture the complex structure of the visual features, a promising direction to be explored. Moreover, introducing visual motion and tracking in a coherent manner along with existing geometric consistency will further improve the results and provide the clinical user with tools for better diagnosis.

References

1. E. Angelini, A. Laine, S. Takuma, J. Holmes, and S. Homma. LV volume quantification via spatio-temporal analysis of real-time 3D echocardiography. *IEEE Transactions on Medical Imaging*, 20:457–469, 2001.
2. S. Birchfield. Elliptical head tracking using intensity gradient and color histograms. *IEEE Computer Vision, Pattern Recognition*, 1998.
3. V. Chalana, D.T. Linker, D.R. Haynor, and Y. Kim. A multiple active contour model for cardiac boundary detection on echocardiographic sequences. *MedImg*, 15(3):290–298, June 1996.
4. T. Cootes, A. Hill, C. Taylor, and J. Haslam. Use of Active Shape Models for Locating Structures in Medical Imaging. *Image Vision and Computing*, 12:355–366, 1994.
5. T.F. Cootes, C.J. Taylor, D.H. Cooper, and J. Graham. Active shape models, their training and applications. *Computer vision and image understanding*, 61(1):38–59, 1995.
6. D. Cremers, F. Tischhäuser, J. Weickert, and C. Schnörr. Diffusion snake : Introducing statistical shape knowledge into the mumford-shah functional. *IJCV*, 3:295–313, 2002.
7. I. Herlin and N. Ayache. Feature extraction and analysis methods for sequences of ultrasound images. In *European Conference in Computer Vision*, pages 43–55, 1992.
8. M. Kass, A. Witkin, and D. Terzopoulos. Snakes: Active Contour Models. *International Journal of Computer Vision*, 1:321–332, 1988.
9. S.C. Mitchell, J.G. Bosch, B.P.F. Lelieveldt, R.J. van der Geest, J.H.C Reiber, and M. Sonka. 3-d active appearance models: Segmentation of cardiac mr and ultrasound images. *IEEE Trans. Med. Img.*, 21:1167–1178, 2003.
10. D. Mumford and J. Shah. Optimal approximations by piecewise smooth functions and associated variational problems. *Comm. Pure Appl. Math.*, 42:577–685, 1989.
11. C. Rumack, S. Wilson, and W. Charboneau. *Diagnostic Ultrasound*. Mosby, 1998.
12. Y. Kim V. Chalana, D. R Haynor. Left ventricular detection from short axis echocardiograms : the use of active contour models. *SPIE*, 2167:787–798, 1994.

A Data Clustering and Streamline Reduction Method for 3D MR Flow Vector Field Simplification

Bernardo S. Carmo[1], Y.H. Pauline Ng[2], Adam Prügel-Bennett[1], and Guang-Zhong Yang[2]

[1] Department of Electronics and Computer Science,
University of Southampton, SO17 1BJ, UK
{b.carmo, apb}@soton.ac.uk
[2] Department of Computing, Imperial College London,
180 Queen's Gate, London SW7 2BZ, UK
{yhpn, gzy}@doc.ic.ac.uk

Abstract. With the increasing capability of MR imaging and Computational Fluid Dynamics (CFD) techniques, a significant amount of data related to the haemodynamics of the cardiovascular systems are being generated. Direct visualization of the data introduces unnecessary visual clutter and hides away the underlying trend associated with the progression of the disease. To elucidate the main topological structure of the flow fields, we present in this paper a 3D visualisation method based on the abstraction of complex flow fields. It uses hierarchical clustering and local linear expansion to extract salient topological flow features. This is then combined with 3D streamline tracking, allowing most important flow details to be visualized. Example results of the technique applied to both CFD and *in vivo* MR data sets are provided.

1 Introduction

Blood flow patterns in vivo are highly complex. They vary considerably from subject to subject and even more so in patients with cardiovascular diseases. Despite the importance of studying such flow patterns, the field is relatively immature primarily because of previous limitations in the methodologies involved in acquiring and calculating expected flow details. The parallel advancement of MRI and CFD has now come to a stage that their combined application allows for a more accurate and detailed measurement of complex flow patterns. Velocity Magnetic resonance imaging was originally developed in the mid 1980's [1,2] and is now available on most commercial scanners. The accuracy of the method has been validated for the quantification of volume flow and delineation of flow patterns. There are now a wide range of clinical applications in acquired and congenital heart disease as well as general vascular disease.

Computational fluid dynamics, on the other hand, involves the numerical solution of a set of partial differential equations (PDEs), known as the Navier

C. Barillot, D.R. Haynor, and P. Hellier (Eds.): MICCAI 2004, LNCS 3216, pp. 451–458, 2004.
© Springer-Verlag Berlin Heidelberg 2004

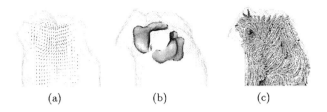

(a)   (b)   (c)

Fig. 1. Different flow field visualisation methods. (**a**) Arrow plot. (**b**) Interactive iso-vorticity plot. (**c**) Streamline plot.

Stokes (N-S) equations. The application of CFD has become important in cardio-vascular fluid mechanics as the technique has matured in its original engineering applications. Moreover, with the parallel advancement of MR velocity imaging, their combination has become an important area of research [3]. The strength of this combination is that it enables subject-specific flow simulation based on in vivo anatomical and flow data [4]. This strategy has been used to examine flows in the left ventricle [5], the descending aorta, the carotid and aortic arterial bifurcation [6], aortic aneurysms and bypass grafts.

With the availability of a detailed 3D model capturing the dynamics of the LV and its associated inflow and outflow tracts, it is now possible to perform patient specific LV blood flow simulation. For many years, techniques based on CFD have been used to investigate LV flow within idealised models. The combination of CFD with non-invasive imaging techniques has proven to be an effective means of studying the complex dynamics of the cardiovascular system as it is able to provide detailed haemodynamic information that is unobtainable by using direct measurement techniques.

With the increasing use of combined MRI/CFD approach, the amount of data needs to be interpreted is becoming significant and becomes challenging to anal-yse and visualise (Figure 1). This is true especially when flow in major cardiac chambers through the entire cardiac cycle needs to be simulated. To examine detailed changes in flow topology, data reduction based on feature extraction needs to be applied. Streamlines give a good indication of the transient pattern of flow [7]. However, for 3D datasets these plots can be highly cluttered and for complex flow they tend to intertwine with each other, limiting their practical value [8]. The purpose of this paper is to present a new method for velocity MR flow field visualisation based on flow clustering and automatic streamline selec-tion. Flow clustering enables data simplification and compression. The method assumes linearity around critical points to ensure that these are preserved by the simplification process. Each cluster therefore contains points sharing a common flow feature. Automatic streamline selection is then applied to determine the salient flow features that are important to the vessel morphology.

2   Materials and Methods

2.1   Clustering

Several methods based on hierarchical clustering have been proposed in recent years. Current methods can be divided into two categories: top-down [9] and bottom-up strategies [10,11] strategy. More recently, Garcke et al. [12] have proposed a continuous clustering method for simplifying vector fields based on the Cahn-Hilliard model that describes phase separation and coarsening in binary alloys. In general, all these methods use a single vector to represent a cluster and are well suited for visualisation purposes, however, given a set of such clusters, it is difficult to recover the original vector field.

To generate an abstract flow field from a dense flow field, the dense flow field is partitioned into a set of flow regions each containing a cluster of vectors. Local linear expansion is employed to represent the clustered flow vectors. Using gradients to represent a flow field is particularly suitable for regions near critical points, and thus this representation technique intrinsically preserves critical points.

A hierarchical clustering algorithm merges flow vectors in an iterative process. The fitting error, $E(C)$, for each cluster C is defined as the total square distance between the original data points and the those fitted by the gradients. The cost M_C of merging two clusters, C_1 and C_2, to form a new cluster C_{new} is:

$$M_C(C_1, C_2) = E(C_{new}) - [E(C_1) + E(C_2)] \ . \tag{1}$$

Initially, each vector forms its own cluster and the neighbouring vectors are used to approximate the local linear expansion of this cluster. Subsequently, the associated cost of merging a pair of clusters is calculated and stored in a pool for each pair of neighbouring clusters. The following steps are then repeated until all clusters are merged to form one single cluster enclosing the entire flow field. First, the pair of clusters with the smallest merging cost in the pool is removed and merged to form a new cluster. Then, the cost of merging the latter with its neighbours is calculated and inserted into the pool. By repeatedly merging clusters, a hierarchical binary tree is constructed in the process, with each node representing a cluster and its children representing its sub-clusters. Once the hierarchical tree is constructed, abstract flow fields at various clustering levels can then be obtained from this tree efficiently.

2.2   Local Linear Expansion

The flow field near critical points is assumed here to be linear. In order to enclose regions around critical points, each cluster joins points with approximately the same velocity gradients. Local linear expansion is carried out to determine these gradients inside each cluster.

We assume that the velocity in a region, $\mathcal{R}$, is given by

$$v = \mathbf{A}(x - x_0)$$
$$= \mathbf{A}\,x - v_0 \tag{2}$$

where $v_0 = \mathbf{A}\,x_0$.

We know the velocity v at a set of cluster points. We therefore perform a least squares fitting over the lattice points in each cluster's region $\mathcal{R} = \{x(i)\}_{i=1}^{N}$, where $x(i)$ designates the coordinates of each cluster point, and N is the size of the cluster. Least squares is equivalent to minimising the energy

$$E = \frac{1}{N}\sum_{i=1}^{N}\left\|v(i) - \mathbf{A}x(i) + v_0\right\|^2. \tag{3}$$

where $v(i) = v(x(i))$ (i.e. the value of the velocity at the cluster point $x(i)$). Optimising with respect to v_0 we obtain

$$v_0 = \mathbf{A}\left\langle x\right\rangle - \left\langle v\right\rangle, \tag{4}$$

where $\left\langle \cdots \right\rangle$ denotes averaging over the points in the cluster.

Substituting the optimal value of v_0 into the energy and differentiating with respect to $\mathbf{A}$, we can compute $\mathbf{A}$ using

$$\mathbf{A} = \mathbf{W}^{\mathsf{T}}\mathbf{V}^{-1} \tag{5}$$

where

$$\mathbf{W} = \frac{1}{N}\sum_{i=1}^{N}\left(x(i) - \left\langle x\right\rangle\right)\left(v(i) - \left\langle v\right\rangle\right)^{\mathsf{T}}$$

$$\mathbf{V} = \frac{1}{N}\sum_{i=1}^{N}\left(x(i) - \left\langle x\right\rangle\right)\left(x(i) - \left\langle x\right\rangle\right)^{\mathsf{T}}.$$

To be able to reconstruct the flow field, we store v_0 and the contents of $\mathbf{A}$ for each cluster. Retrieving the field's velocities then simply involves applying equation (2).

2.3   Topology Display

Streamlines are generated in the same way as steady flow streamlines, but they must be interpreted as transient in time as they do not result from steady flow. Used in conjunction with clustering, however, they can be used to convey the overall topology of the field.

After clusters have been formed from the flow field, streamlines are grown from equally spaced points throughout the image and stored in a streamline array. Each streamline passes through one or several clusters, and this is recorded in a list. A streamline "correlation" matrix $\mathbf{C}_{cluster}$ is then built by computing the ratio between common clusters occupied by streamlines and the total number of clusters spanned by each streamline:

$$\mathbf{C}_{cluster}(e, v) = \frac{\tau_{cluster}(e, v)}{\gamma_{cluster}(e)} \tag{6}$$

where e, v are streamline array indices, $\tau_{cluster}(e, v)$ is the number of clusters occupied by both e and v and $\gamma_{cluster}(e)$ is the total number of clusters occupied by streamline e.

The most representative streamlines can then be selected by setting a maximum streamline correlation $T_{cluster}(e)$, the value of which is interactively chosen by the user. This is defined as:

$$T_{cluster}(e) = \sum_{\substack{v=1 \\ v \neq e}}^{N} \mathbf{C}_{cluster}(e, v) \tag{7}$$

where N is the total number of streamlines in the streamline array.

3   Results and Discussions

The proposed method was applied to 3D flow through the human heart simulated from a CFD model [13]. The model after mesh processing contained 54,230 nodes and 41,000 cells. A total of 16 meshes representing the LV across the complete cardiac cycle were generated from the original image data. In order to permit CFD simulation, it was necessary to increase the temporal resolution of the model. This ensured that none of the constituent cells underwent excessive deformation or displacement between adjacent time steps. To this end, cubic spline interpolations were performed to generate a total of 49 meshes across the cardiac cycle. The Navier-Stokes equations for 3D time-dependent laminar flow with prescribed wall motion was solved using a finite-volume based CFD solver - CFX4 (CFX international, AEA technology, Harwell). The blood was treated as an incompressible Newtonian fluid with a constant viscosity of 0.004 Kg/(ms). The simulation was started from the beginning of systole with the pressure of the aortic valve plane set to zero and with the mitral valve plane treated as a non-slip wall. At the onset of diastole, the aortic valve was closed by treating it as a solid wall, whilst the mitral valve was opened by using a combination of pressure and flow boundaries.

As can be seen in Figure 2, the choice of the maximum total correlation is important for the rendering result. If that value is too low, this results in too few streamlines being selected and flow features being missed (Figure 2(c)); if the value is too high, the display is cluttered by excessive streamlines (Figure 2(a)). This visualisation method was also applied along the time series data of the same dataset. The previous results depict the flow during diastole showing flow through the mitral valve, as shown in Figure 3. The proposed method was also applied to 2D *in vivo* MR velocity data acquired with sequential examination following myocardial infarction using a Marconi whole body MR scanner operating at 1.5T. Cine phase contrast velocity mapping was performed using a FEER sequence with a TE of 14ms. The slice thickness was 10mm and the field of view was 30-40cm. The dataset has a temporal resolution of 45ms and the diastolic phase is covered in about 5-10 frames, five of which are shown here.

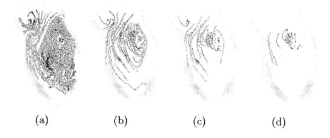

(a)   (b)   (c)   (d)

Fig. 2. Effect of interactively changing the maximum total correlation threshold. **(a)** No threshold - all streamlines selected. **(b)** $T_{cluster}(e)_{MAX}$ = 20; **(c)** $T_{cluster}(e)_{MAX}$ = 10; **(d)** $T_{cluster}(e)_{MAX}$ = 5, the smaller vortex is now invisible.

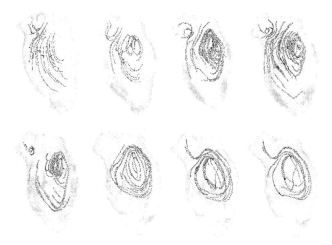

Fig. 3. Simplified streamline rendering of 3D simulated flow inside the human cardiac left ventricle. Time samples 9 to 16 of a set of 33.

The dataset was denoised using the restoration scheme described in [14]. Figure 4 shows a comparison between our automatically selected streamlines and arrow plots overlayed on the corresponding conventional MR images. In order to quantify the error introduced by the clustering process we measured the root-mean-square difference between the original velocity field and that reconstructed by the cluster gradients using equation (2). The results are plotted in Figure 5 for clustering of the 12th frame (540ms) of the 2D *in vivo* dataset and time sample 12 of the 3D simulated dataset. The number of clusters used to produce all streamline plots in this paper was 10 for both datasets. The size of the region of interest was 3536 pixels and 47250 voxels for the 2D and 3D datasets, respectively.

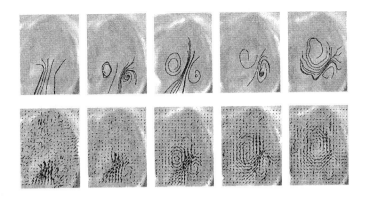

Fig. 4. Flow pattern within the left ventricle of a patient following myocardial infarction, from 450ms to 630ms after onset of ECG R wave, depicting vortical flow rendered by streamlines selected by clustering (top row) and 2D arrows where arrow size is proportional to velocity magnitude (bottom row). A 3-spaced grid was used to select the arrow data.

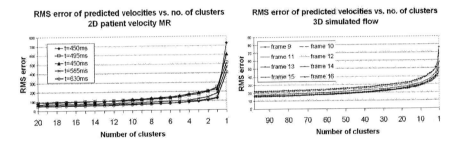

Fig. 5. Root mean square error between original and cluster velocity predicted from gradients (see text) for the 2D frames of Figure 4 (left) and 3D simulated time samples of Figure 3 (right).

4   Conclusion

We have presented a novel method for velocity MR flow simplification and display. Flow simplification is achieved by clustering, where each cluster contains points with similar local linear approximation gradients. This ensures that each cluster encloses points sharing relevant flow features. Streamlines are then generated over the flow field and selected using a measure of inter-streamline cluster overlap, interactively thresholded. The rendered streamlines depict the important features of the flow and present the observer with an overview of the general flow topology of the field.

Acknowledgements. BSC is supported by a Portuguese FCT grant and a British EPSRC grant. YHPN is funded by the Croucher Foundation in Hong Kong.

References

1. van Dijk, P.: Direct cardiac NMR imaging of heart wall and blood flow velocity. J Comput Assist Tomogr 1984; 8: 429-36.
2. Bryant, D.J., Payne, J.A., Firmin, D.N., Longmore, D.B.: Measurement of flow with NMR imaging using a gradient pulse and phase difference technique. J Comput Assist Tomogr 1984; 8: 588-93.
3. Papaharilaou, Y., Doorly, D.J., Sherwin, S.J., Peiro, J., Anderson, J., Sanghera, B., Watkins, N., Caro C.G.: Combined MRI and computational fluid dynamics detailed investigation of flow in a realistic coronary artery bypass graft model, pp 379 Proc. Int. Soc. Mag. Res. Med. 2001.
4. Gill, J.D., Ladak, H.M., Steinman, D.A., Fenster, A.: Accuracy and variability assessment of a semi-automatic technique for segmentation of the carotid arteries from 3D ultrasound images. Med Phys 2000;27:1333-1342.
5. Saber, N.R., Gosman, A.D., Wood, N.B., Kilner, P.J., Charrier, C. L., Firmin, D. N.: Computational flow modelling of the left ventricle based on in vivo MRI data - Initial experience. Annals Biomed Engineering 2001; 29:275-283.
6. Long, Q., Xu, X.Y., Ariff, B., Thom, S.A., Hughes, A.D., Stanton, A.V.: Reconstruction of blood flow patterns in a human carotid bifurcation: A combined CFD and MRI study. JMRI 2000; 11:299-311.
7. Yang, G. Z., Kilner, P. J., Mohiaddin, R. H., Firmin, D. N.: Transient streamlines: texture synthesis for in vivo flow visualisation. Int. J. Card. Imag. **16**: 175-184, 2000.
8. Interrante, V., Grosch C.: Strategies for effectively visualizing 3D flow with volume LIC. Proc. Visualization '97 421-424, 1997.
9. Heckel, B., Weber, G., Hamann, B., Joy, K.I: Construction of vector field hierarchies. Proc. IEEE Visualization'99, 19-25, October 1999.
10. Telea, A., van Wijk, J.: Simplified representation of vector fields. IEEE Visualization 1999: 35-42.
11. Lodha, S.K., Renteria, J.C., Roskin, K.M.: Topology preserving compression of 2D vector fields. Proc. IEEE Visualization'00, 343-350, October 2000.
12. Garcke, H., Preußer, T., Rumpf, M., Telea, A., Weikard, U., van Wijk, J.J.: A phase field model for continuous clustering on vector fields. IEEE Trans. Visualization and Computer Graphics, 7(3): 230-241, 2001.
13. Long, Q., Merrifield, R., Yang, G.Z., Kilner, P.J., Firmin, D.N., Xu, X.Y.: The influence of inflow boundary conditions on intra left ventricle flow predictions. J Biomech Eng. 2003 Dec;125(6):922-7.
14. Ng, Y.H.P., Yang, G.Z.: Vector-valued image restoration with application to magnetic resonance velocity imaging. Journal of WSCG **11**(2): 338-345, 2003.

Velocity Based Segmentation in Phase Contrast MRI Images*

Jan Erik Solem, Markus Persson, and Anders Heyden

School of Technology and Society
Malmö University, Sweden
{jes,markus.persson,heyden}@ts.mah.se

Abstract. Phase contrast MRI is a relatively new technique that extends standard MRI by obtaining flow information for tissue in the human body. The output data is a velocity vector field in a three-dimensional (3D) volume. This paper presents a method for 3D segmentation of blood vessels and determining the surface of the inner wall using this vector field. The proposed method uses a variational formulation and the segmentation is performed using the level set method. The purpose of this paper is to show that it is possible to perform segmentation using only velocity data which would indicate that velocity is a strong cue in these types of segmentation problems. This is shown in experiments. A novel vector field discontinuity detector is introduced and used in the variational formulation. The performance of this measure is tested with satisfactory results.

1   Introduction

Magnetic Resonance Imaging (MRI) provides three-dimensional (3D) images that are useful for diagnostic purposes. Phase contrast MRI also provides velocity measurements that can be used for analysis of the blood flow and tissue motion. Segmentation is a well studied problem within medical image analysis and have great impact on diagnostic performance. This paper presents a method for 3D segmentation of blood vessels. After segmentation, when the shape of the vessels has been determined, volumetric flow data can be obtained from the velocities. Blood volume, pressure and velocity of the blood flow and the motion and shape of the vessel walls are examples of useful measurements that can aid in the diagnosis and are also important for research within the medical field.

This paper deals with the problem of segmentation using velocity data without the assumption that the walls are stationary. This is the case for many medical images taken for diagnostic purposes, such as dynamic cardiac images. Many different approaches have been proposed to analyze and extract shape information from cardiac images and 3D model-based methods have shown to improve the diagnostic value [1].

The most basic approach to segmentation is to threshold the images. However, this method only works on very simple images. Later approaches makes

---

* This work has been supported by the SRC project 621-2002-4822.

C. Barillot, D.R. Haynor, and P. Hellier (Eds.): MICCAI 2004, LNCS 3216, pp. 459–466, 2004.
© Springer-Verlag Berlin Heidelberg 2004

use of moving interfaces, e.g. snakes and other active contours, cf. [2]. During the latest years level set approaches have become popular, since they can handle global properties and are based on a solid mathematical framework, cf. [3,4].

The level set method [5] is a popular technique for representing and tracking dynamic interfaces. The surface is represented implicitly as a level set of a function. The sign of the level set function gives a natural partitioning and is frequently used in segmentation. Our segmentation problem is solved using a variational level set framework. The optimal solution, i.e. the optimal position of the surface separating the blood from the vessel walls, corresponds to the minimum of a functional driven by the velocity data.

1.1   Relation to Previous Work

In [6] blood is segmented in cardiac phase contrast MR images using the fact that the heart wall has a periodic motion and resumes its position after a completed heart cycle. The method is based on a particle trace technique for time-resolved 3D velocity vector fields, combined with magnitude image data. In [7] the myocardium is segmented from MRI intensity and phase contrast images. The segmentation is performed in 2D images using level set curve evolution. Three different constraints determine the curve motion, the intensity gradient, the velocity magnitude and the coherence of the velocity direction. In [8] segmentation of curvilinear structures in MR angiography images is performed using evolution techniques for implicit curves. In [9] blood vessels are segmented from MR angiography images using the criterion that the normal of the blood vessel boundary should be orthogonal to the vector flow field and thus minimizes the flux through the surface. The underlying assumption is that the velocity of the vessel wall is zero. Our proposed method solves the segmentation problem with moving vessel walls. An approach like the one in [9] would not work since the velocity field of the walls are approximately orthogonal to the blood flow.

1.2   Contribution of the Paper

This paper presents a method for three-dimensional segmentation of blood vessels and determining the surface of the vessel wall using the vector field obtained from phase contrast MRI measurements. It improves upon the performance of previous methods in that it can handle wall motion, a feature that is lacking in e.g. [9]. A measure for finding discontinuities in this vector field is introduced. The segmentation problem is then formulated as a variational problem with a new functional using this measure. The proposed method uses only the information contained in the velocity vector field and this gives support to the claims that velocity is an important cue for these types of segmentation problems.

2   Background

2.1   Phase Contrast MRI

Phase contrast MRI is based on the property that a uniform motion of tissue in a magnetic field gradient produces a change in the MR signal phase, Φ. This change is proportional to the velocity of the tissue, $\mathbf{v}$. The MR signal from a volume element accumulates the phase [10]

$$\Phi(r,t) = \gamma B_0 T + \gamma \mathbf{v} \cdot \int_0^T \mathbf{G}(r,t)t\,dt \ ,$$

$$\Phi(r,t) = \gamma B_0 T + \gamma \mathbf{v} \cdot \overline{\mathbf{G}} \ , \tag{1}$$

during time T, where B_0 is a static magnetic field, γ the gyro-magnetic ratio and $\mathbf{G}(r,t)$ is the magnetic field gradient. Notice that $\overline{\mathbf{G}}$ is exactly the first moment of $\mathbf{G}(r,t)$ with respect to time. If the field gradient is altered between two consecutive recordings, then by subtracting the resulting phases

$$\Phi_1 - \Phi_2 = \gamma \mathbf{v} \cdot (\overline{\mathbf{G}}_1 - \overline{\mathbf{G}}_2) \ , \tag{2}$$

the velocity in the $(\overline{\mathbf{G}}_1 - \overline{\mathbf{G}}_2)$-direction is implicitly given. In this way a desired velocity component can be calculated for every volume element simultaneously. To construct the velocity vector in 3D, the natural way is to apply appropriate gradients to produce the x-, y- and z-components respectively.

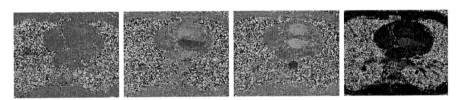

Fig. 1. Examples of the velocity vector field for a transversal slice with the heart in the center of the image. (left to right) v_x, v_y, and v_z-velocity component and velocity magnitude $|\mathbf{v}|$.

2.2   Level Set Formulation

The level set method was introduced in [5] as a tool for capturing moving interfaces. The time dependent surface $\Gamma(t)$ is implicitly represented as the zero level set of a function $\phi(\mathbf{x}, t) : R^3 \times R_+ \to R$ as

$$\Gamma(t) = \{\mathbf{x} \ ; \ \phi(\mathbf{x}, t) = 0\} \ , \tag{3}$$

where ϕ is defined such that

$$\phi(\mathbf{x}, t) \begin{cases} < 0 \text{ inside } \Gamma \\ = 0 \text{ on } \Gamma \\ > 0 \text{ outside } \Gamma . \end{cases} \tag{4}$$

Using the definition above, the outward unit normal $\mathbf{n}$ and the mean curvature κ of Γ are[1]

$$\mathbf{n} = \frac{\nabla \phi}{|\nabla \phi|} \quad \text{and} \quad \kappa = \nabla \cdot \frac{\nabla \phi}{|\nabla \phi|} . \tag{5}$$

The zero set of $\phi(\mathbf{x}, t)$ represents $\Gamma(t)$ at all times t. This means that $\phi(\mathbf{x}(t), t) \equiv 0$ for a curve $\mathbf{x}(t) \in \Gamma(t)$. Differentiating with respect to t gives

$$\phi_t + \mathbf{u} \cdot \nabla \phi = 0 \iff \phi_t + u_n |\nabla \phi| = 0 , \tag{6}$$

where $\mathbf{u} = d\mathbf{x}(t)/dt$ and u_n is the normal component of the surface velocity. To move the surface according to some derived velocity, a PDE of the form (6) is solved. One of the advantages of this representation is that the topology of the surface is allowed to change as the surface evolves, thus making it easy to represent complex surfaces that can merge or split and also surfaces that contain holes. For a more thorough treatment of level set surfaces, see [3,4].

3 Problem Formulation

Given velocity data and basic dynamic characteristics of the flow, the problem consists of finding the boundary between the blood and the vessel walls. This boundary should be a closed surface within the domain of interest i.e. within the measured volume. The segmentation is then determined by the interior of the surface representing the vessels. The interior of Γ will be denoted Ω and the exterior Ω^c. The solution is found by maximizing the discontinuity of the flow at the surface and maximizing the flow inside the surface (or equivalently, minimizing the flow outside).

3.1 Using Velocity as a Cue

As mentioned above, phase contrast MRI provides velocity measurements in three directions (x,y,z) in an arbitrary coordinate system. The velocity can be expressed in vector form $\mathbf{v} = (v_x, v_y, v_z)^T$, and the velocity magnitude is

$$|\mathbf{v}| = \sqrt{\mathbf{v} \cdot \mathbf{v}} = \sqrt{v_x^2 + v_y^2 + v_z^2} .$$

There are two important reasons why the velocity field $\mathbf{v}$ should be used for segmentation. First, $\mathbf{v}$ is discontinuous across the vessel boundary since the fluid inside moves parallel to the boundary surface and the walls move roughly normal to the boundary. Second, it has been noted, e.g. by [7], that the velocity magnitude, $|\mathbf{v}|$, of the fluid is large compared to the magnitude of the wall motion. These observations constitute the foundation for the variational formulation introduced in this paper.

---

[1] Here $\nabla \phi$ denotes the gradient of ϕ and $\nabla \cdot$ denotes the divergence.

3.2   Measure for Discontinuities

To encode the information in the vector field $\mathbf{v}$ we define a field of matrices $\mathbf{M_v} = \mathbf{M_v}(\mathbf{x})$, $\mathbf{x} \in R^3$ where $\mathbf{M_v}$ is the positive semi-definite, symmetric matrix defined by

$$\mathbf{M_v} = \mathbf{v}\mathbf{v}^T = \begin{bmatrix} v_x \\ v_y \\ v_z \end{bmatrix} \begin{bmatrix} v_x & v_y & v_z \end{bmatrix} = \begin{bmatrix} v_x^2 & v_x v_y & v_x v_z \\ v_x v_y & v_y^2 & v_y v_z \\ v_x v_z & v_y v_z & v_z^2 \end{bmatrix} . \tag{7}$$

$\mathbf{M_v}$ has rank one with eigenvalues $\lambda_1 = |\mathbf{v}|^2$ and $\lambda_2 = \lambda_3 = 0$. Let $W \geq 0$ be a weight function (typically a Gaussian filter G_σ) and define the average matrix field to be the convolution

$$\overline{\mathbf{M}}_{\mathbf{v}} = W * \mathbf{M_v} ,$$

taken componentwise. We denote this matrix field the *density matrix field*. Depending on the values of $\mathbf{v}$ in the region of interest there are three cases.

i) 1 dominant direction. If $\mathbf{v} \approx$ constant in a region we will have a case of $\overline{\mathbf{M}}_{\mathbf{v}}$ similar to (7) with eigenvalues $\lambda_1 \approx |\mathbf{v}|^2$ and $\lambda_2 \approx \lambda_3 \approx 0$.

ii) 2 dominant directions. This is the interesting case since we want to detect discontinuities in the vector field originating from the motion of the blood and the motion of the walls. Basically, the motion of the blood is orthogonal to the normal of the wall surface and the motion of the wall is approximately in the normal direction. With two dominant directions, $\overline{\mathbf{M}}_{\mathbf{v}}$ will have approximately rank two and only one small eigenvalue, $\lambda_3 \approx 0$.

iii) 3 dominant directions. $\overline{\mathbf{M}}_{\mathbf{v}}$ will have full rank and this is the case where there are three prominent directions of $\mathbf{v}$ or when there is no prominent direction at all, e.g. where there is high noise.

To discriminate i) from ii), the following real valued function is introduced, inspired by [11] and [12],

$$R = \frac{4\lambda_1 \lambda_2}{(\lambda_1 + \lambda_2)^2} , \tag{8}$$

where $\lambda_1 \geq \lambda_2 \geq 0$ are the two largest eigenvalues of $\overline{\mathbf{M}}_{\mathbf{v}}$ and $0 \leq R \leq 1$. For case i) $R \approx 0$ and for ii) R will be large, i.e. $R \approx 1$. It turns out that this measure is an excellent detector for discontinuities in $\mathbf{v}$. This will be used in the next section.

4   Variational Formulation

In this section the segmentation problem is formulated as a variational problem. A functional is introduced and minimized using the level set framework. The desired surface should enclose as much of the flow in $\mathbf{v}$ as possible and the flow should be discontinuous over the surface. This leads to the minimization of the following energy functional

$$E(\Gamma) = \underbrace{\int_{\Omega^c} \chi(\mathbf{v}) d\mathbf{x}}_{\text{flow outside the surface}} - \underbrace{\int_{\Gamma} R(\mathbf{x}) dS}_{\text{discontinuities at the surface}} \quad , \tag{9}$$

where Γ is the surface, Ω^c the exterior of the surface, $R(\mathbf{x})$ is the measure for discontinuities from Section 3.2 and $\chi(\mathbf{v})$ is a C^2 approximation to the translated Heaviside function defined by

$$\chi(\mathbf{v}) = \chi(|\mathbf{v}|) = H(|\mathbf{v}| - \delta) = H_\delta(|\mathbf{v}|) \ , \tag{10}$$

where $\delta \in R_+$. Here H is defined as in [13]

$$H(x) = \begin{cases} 1 & x > \epsilon \\ 0 & x < -\epsilon \\ \frac{1}{2}[1 + \frac{x}{\epsilon} + \frac{1}{\pi} \sin(\frac{\pi x}{\epsilon})] & |x| \le \epsilon \ . \end{cases} \tag{11}$$

This is commonly used in level set based segmentation, cf. [14]. The definition above will make $\chi(\mathbf{v})$ equal to zero for very low velocities and one otherwise. This makes it an approximate characteristic function for $\mathbf{v}$ and the measure of the first integral in (9) is then in volume units.

Representing the surface using the zero level set of a function ϕ, the energy (9) becomes

$$E(\phi) = \int \chi(\mathbf{v}) H(\phi) d\mathbf{x} - \int R(\mathbf{x})|\nabla \phi| \delta(\phi) d\mathbf{x} \ , \tag{12}$$

where $H(\phi)$ is again the approximation to the Heaviside function and therefore a characteristic function for Ω^c. The term $|\nabla \phi| \delta(\phi) d\mathbf{x}$ in the second integral is the surface area element and $\delta(\cdot)$ is the one dimensional delta function. From the Euler-Lagrange equation for (12), the motion PDE for the surface, as a gradient descent, is then

$$\phi_t = (-\chi + \kappa R + \nabla R \cdot \mathbf{n})|\nabla \phi| \ , \tag{13}$$

where ϕ_t denotes derivative with respect to the evolution time and κ is the mean curvature of the surface. This acts as a natural regularizer of the boundary.

5   Experiments

The performance of the response function for vector field discontinuities R was tested on both real and synthetic phase contrast MRI data. The value of R is shown for a transversal slice of a human heart, see Fig 2. The results are very satisfactory. The heart walls are clearly shown in white (R=1), and the heart cavities in black, indicating only one prominent flow direction.

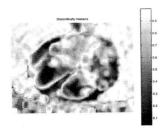

Fig. 2. The value for R, shown for a transversal cross section of the heart.

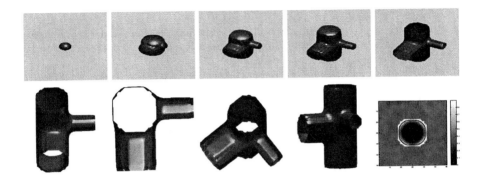

Fig. 3. (top row) The surface evolution at initial value, 300 iterations, 500 iterations, 700 iterations and final surface. (bottom row) Different views of the resulting surface and value of R for a cross section with the resulting boundary marked in black.

Experiments to determine the viability of the proposed variational method were also performed. Unfortunately we are not allowed to use the data for publication. We therefore present results on synthetic data here. We intend to show results on clinical data in the near future.

The synthetic data consists of a double T-junction in a volume of resolution $60 \times 60 \times 60$. The velocity of the walls was 30% of the maximum blood velocity and noise with amplitude $\pm 20\%$ of the maximum blood velocity was added to the whole volume.

6   Conclusions

The experiments in the previous section confirm that velocity data is a valuable cue for this segmentation problem. We also find the performance of the flow discontinuity measure introduced in Section 3.2 to be quite satisfactory.

Future work will include: incorporating other cues such as the gradient of intensity MRI images as boundary information, integrating prior information using statistical shape models [15,16] and analysis of methods for initialization.

Acknowledgements. The authors would like to thank the Department of Clinical Physiology, Lund University, especially Erik Bergvall and Karin Markenroth at Philips Medical Systems, for interesting discussions regarding MRI.

References

1. Frangi, A., Niessen, W., Viergever, M.: Three-dimensional modeling for functional analysis of cardiac images: A review. IEEE Trans. on Med. Imag. **20** (2001) 2–25
2. Kass, M., Witkin, A., Terzopoulos, D.: Snakes: Active contour models. Int. J. Computer Vision **1** (1987) 321–331
3. Osher, S.J., Fedkiw, R.P.: Level Set Methods and Dynamic Implicit Surfaces. Springer Verlag (2002)
4. Sethian, J.: Level Set Methods and Fast Marching Methods Evolving Interfaces in Computational Geometry, Fluid Mechanics, Computer Vision, and Materials Science. Cambridge University Press (1999)
5. Osher, S., Sethian, J.A.: Fronts propagating with curvature-dependent speed: Algorithms based on Hamilton-Jacobi formulations. Journal of Computational Physics **79** (1988) 12–49
6. Ebbers, T.: Cardiovascular Fluid Dynamics. PhD thesis, Departments of Biomedical Engineering & Medicine and Care, Linkoping University, Sweden (2001)
7. Wong, A., Liu, H., Shi, P.: Segmentation of myocardium using velocity field constrained front propagation. In: IEEE Applications in Computer Vision, Orlando, Fl (2002)
8. Lorigo, L., Faugeras, O., Grimson, W., Keriven, R., Kikinis, R., Nabavi, A., Westin, C.F.: Curves: Curve evolution for vessel segmentation. IEEE Transactions on Medical Image Analysis **5** (2001) 195–206
9. Vasilevskiy, A., Siddiqi, K.: Flux maximizing geometric flows. In: Proc. Int. Conf. on Computer Vision, Vancouver, Canada (2001)
10. Pelc, N.J., Herfkens, R.J., Shimakawa, A., Enzmann, D.: Phase contrast cine magnetic resonance imaging. Magnetic Resonance Quarterly **4** (1991) 229–254
11. Harris, C., Stephens, M.: A combined corner and edge detector. In: Proc. Alvey Conf. (1988) 189–192
12. Knutsson, H.: Representing local structure using tensors. In: The 6th Scandinavian Conference on Image Analysis, Oulu, Finland (1989) 244–251 Report LiTH–ISY–I–1019, Computer Vision Laboratory, Linköping University, Sweden, 1989.
13. Zhao, H., Chan, T., Merriman, B., Osher, S.: A variational level set approach to multiphase motion. J. Computational Physics 127 (1996) 179–195
14. Paragios, N.: A level set approach for shape-driven segmentation and tracking of the left ventricle. IEEE Transactions on Medical Imaging **22** (2003) 773–776
15. Rousson, M., Paragios, N.: Shape priors for level set representations. In: Proc. European Conf. on Computer Vision. Volume 2351 of LNCS., Springer (2002)
16. Cremers, D.: Statistical Shape Knowledge in Variational Image Segmentation. PhD thesis, Dept. of Mathematics and Computer Science, University of Mannheim, Germany (2002)

Multi-scale Statistical Grey Value Modelling for Thrombus Segmentation from CTA

Silvia D. Olabarriaga[1], Marcel Breeuwer[2], and Wiro J. Niessen[1]

[1] University Medical Center Utrecht, Image Sciences Institute,
Heidelberglaan 100, 3584 CX Utrecht, NL {silvia,wiro}@isi.uu.nl
[2] Philips Medical Systems, Medical IT - Advanced Development, Best, NL

Abstract. In this paper we present, evaluate, and discuss two multi-scale schemes for modelling grey-level appearance in a deformable model for the segmentation of abdominal aortic aneurysm thrombus from CT angiography scans. The methods are initialised with the lumen boundary, and the image-based deformation force is based on a non-parametric statistical grey level model built from training data obtained at multiple scales. The image force direction and magnitude are based on a fit between the trained model and the data. Two multi-scale schemes are used for deformation. In one scheme, the boundary is progressively refined based on training data obtained at each scale, in a coarse-to-fine approach, and in the other, the training data obtained at all scales are used simultaneously to drive the deformation. The two schemes are evaluated and compared to the single scale scheme based on a leave-one-out study of nine patients.

1 Introduction

Abdominal aortic aneurysm (AAA) is a relatively common disease among the elderly population. Because the rupture of an AAA can be fatal, there is clinical interest in risk analysis, simulation, surgery planning, and treatment follow-up based on minimally invasive imaging, such as CT angiography (CTA). Segmentation of lumen, thrombus and calcifications is necessary for the reconstruction of a patient-specific model based on CTA scans. While lumen and calcifications can be rather easily isolated with thresholding techniques, this is not true for the thrombus. Due to the low contrast between thrombus and surrounding tissue, automated segmentation methods have difficulty to delineate the correct boundary. Only a few thrombus segmentation methods have been reported in the literature [1,2,3,4]. The methods proposed by De Bruijne et al. [1,3] are based on an active shape model (ASM), while those proposed by Subasic et al. [2] and Giachetti & Zanetti [4] are based on deformable models. These methods, however, suffer from shortcomings: either they require significant amount of user intervention [1,3,4], or the reported results are not sufficiently accurate [2].

In [5] we introduced a new AAA segmentation method in which the lumen and thrombus are segmented automatically based on two positions clicked by the user. The lumen surface is used to initialize the thrombus segmentation

C. Barillot, D.R. Haynor, and P. Hellier (Eds.): MICCAI 2004, LNCS 3216, pp. 467–474, 2004.
© Springer-Verlag Berlin Heidelberg 2004

method, which is based on a discrete deformable model approach. A statistical grey level model built from training data is adopted to generate the image-based deformation force. This force expands (or shrinks) the boundary to include (or exclude) image locations with intensity patterns that correspond to the inside (or outside) of the object, respectively. A non-parametric technique is used for intensity pattern classification, and the most likely class determines the force direction (inwards or outwards the boundary). That method is now extended by determining the force magnitude also from the class with largest likelihood, creating a natural link between training and deformation in a multi-scale framework. In this paper, we propose two multi-scale schemes and investigate their added value with respect to the single-scale case. The first scheme consists of progressively refining the boundary based on models built from training data, using a coarse-to-fine approach. The second is a new scheme in which a single model, built at multiple scales simultaneously, is used to guide deformation. In both schemes, the image force direction and magnitude are determined based on training data. The schemes are evaluated on nine CTA scans, and the results are compared with manual segmentations.

2 Thrombus Segmentation Method

The proposed method is based on a deformable model approach, in particular the discrete formulation proposed in [6] and extended in [7]. The deformation of an initial boundary, represented with a polygonal mesh, is performed at discrete time steps t by changing the position of its vertices $\mathbf{x}_j$ according to the evolution equation:

$$\mathbf{x}_j^{t+1} = \mathbf{x}_j^t + (1 - \lambda)(\mathbf{x}_j^t - \mathbf{x}_j^{t-1}) + \lambda \left(\alpha_j F_{int}(\mathbf{x}_j^t) + \beta_j F_{ext}(\mathbf{x}_j^t) \right), \qquad (1)$$

where λ is a damping factor, F_{int} and F_{ext} are respectively the internal (shape-based) and external (image-based) forces acting on the vertex, and α_j and β_j indicate the forces relative importance in the deformation process. The initial boundary is the lumen surface obtained automatically with another deformable model initialised with minimal user interaction (see details in [5]). The adopted internal force (continuity of mean curvature) enforces mesh smoothness and regularization. The external force moves the mesh into image positions with "boundary-like" properties. Typically, this force would be determined from the thrombus edge (e.g. image gradient) because object boundaries are expected at locations of sharp intensity variation. In the case of the AAA thrombus, however, this assumption does not hold. Firstly, several other neighbouring structures (e.g., spine and calcifications) appear with strong contrast in an abdominal CTA image and may attract the boundary to the wrong position. Secondly, the contrast between thrombus and background can be extremely weak in some regions (e.g. bowels), and image derivatives at such locations are not easily distinguishable from noise. Therefore, a more complex image force is required for AAA thrombus segmentation.

2.1   Multi-scale Image Force

The image force adopted in this work corresponds to an inflating (or shrinking) vector along the vertex normal $\mathbf{n}_j$:

$$F_{ext}(\mathbf{x}_j) = \begin{cases} S\mathbf{n}_j & : & \mathbf{x}_j \text{ is inside the object} \\ -S\mathbf{n}_j & : & \mathbf{x}_j \text{ is outside the object} \\ 0 & : & \mathbf{x}_j \text{ is at the object boundary} \end{cases} \qquad (2)$$

where S is the magnitude of the force (deformation step size). A non-parametric pattern classification approach, namely k-nearest neighbours (kNN [8]), is used to determine the most likely class (inside/outside/boundary) corresponding to the intensity pattern at the vertex. The posterior probability of an intensity pattern $\mathbf{y}$ belonging to class ω is determined as follows:

$$P(\omega|\mathbf{y}) = \frac{k_\omega}{k} \qquad (3)$$

where k_ω is the number of points with class label ω among the k nearest neighbours (closest training points) of $\mathbf{y}$. The classification features are image intensity values (intensity profiles of length l and sampling spacing δ) collected along the vertex normal $\mathbf{n}$ – see fig. 1.

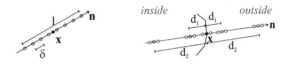

Fig. 1. Profile sampling. Left: normal vector $\mathbf{n}$, profile length l and sampling spacing δ. Right: Multi-scale training scheme with 5 classes ($n = 2$).

During training, profile samples are collected at the correct boundary (delineated manually) and at shifted positions inside and outside the thrombus. In our previous work [5], a three-class model is adopted, in which two shifted samples are collected respectively at $\mathbf{x} - d\mathbf{n}$ and $\mathbf{x} + d\mathbf{n}$. Here we extend this notion to a $2n + 1$-class model in which shifted samples are collected at increasing distances $d_q, q \in [1, n]$ from the boundary position $\mathbf{x}$ – see fig. 1. The class labels are assigned as follows: ω_0 for boundary samples, ω_{-q} for inside samples and ω_{+q} for outside ones.

During deformation, the image force at a vertex $\mathbf{x}_j$ is calculated in the following way: the intensity profile $\mathbf{y}_j$ at the vertex is sampled, and the most likely class ω_i is determined by $\max_{i \in [-n, +n]} P(\omega_i|\mathbf{y}_j)$ – see eq. 3. The class label ω_i indicates directly whether the vertex is most likely to be inside ($i < 0$), outside ($i > 0$) or at the boundary ($i = 0$) – see eq. 2. The image force strength is also scaled according to the most likely class ω_i:

$$S = d_q c f \qquad (4)$$

where d_q is the shift distance for class ω_i, with $q = |i|$; $c = P(\omega_i|\mathbf{y}_j)$ is the confidence in the classification step; and f is a factor that regulates the maximum force magnitude. Note that larger (or smaller) deformation steps are taken when the intensity pattern best fits a class sampled far from (or near to) the correct boundary. Moreover, the force magnitude is reduced when the intensity pattern does not clearly indicate the situation at hand. Note that the multiple training samples obtained at varying d_q could be used in several ways during deformation. Here we consider two possibilities:

- A refinement scheme in which the surface is progressively deformed by running the method n times using the non-boundary training profiles obtained at $d_p, p \in [n, 1]$ (similarly to [9,3]), and
- A new multi-scale modelling scheme in which the training profiles obtained at all scales d_q are used simultaneously, in a single deformation run.

3   Evaluation Study

The method is tested on nine contrast-enhanced CTA scans of different patients in which the AAA is located between the renal and the iliac arteries and no implants. The scans consist of a random sample of patients from the University Medical Centre Utrecht (UMCU) endovascular aneurysm repair programme [10]. All images are acquired with Philips Medical Systems (PMS) spiral CT scanners with resolution of $0.5 \times 0.5 \times 2$ mm and contain circa 125 slices of 512×512 voxels.

The training samples are collected based on manual segmentations performed by experts of the Dept. of Vascular Surgery and the Image Sciences Institute, UMCU, using the PMS EasyVision workstation contouring facilities. The original manual meshes are smoothed and resampled before profile extraction and comparison with the obtained results. The leave-one-out strategy is used, i.e., the segmented scan is never part of the training set. Each training set contains 80 000 to 200 000 profiles.

The profile configuration is constant in all experiments, with $l = 5$ mm and $\delta = 1.0$ mm (6 features per sample). The number of neighbours is fixed to $k = 21$, since the behaviour with respect to k in the multi-scale schemes is rather robust [5]. The thrombus deformable model parameters are set as follows: $\lambda = 0.8$, $\beta = 0.1$, and $\alpha = 1 - \beta$ (see eq. 1); and $f = 0.5$ mm (see eq. 4). The deformation stops automatically if the volume difference between two iterations is smaller than 0.1%.

In the experiments we investigate the behaviour of each multi-scale scheme with respect to the shift distance d_n and to the number of scales ($n = 1, 2, 3$). The closest sample is obtained at $d_1 = 0.5$ mm (in-slice image resolution) and the farthest at varying distances ($d_n \in \{1, 2, 3, 4, 5\}$ mm). Distances increase exponentially for $n = 3$, with $d_2 \in \{0.7, 1.0, 1.2, 1.4, 1.6\}$ mm. Results are analysed separately for the single scale, refinement and the multi-modelling schemes, and finally the schemes are compared. The error measure adopted in the evaluation corresponds to the distance (in mm) between vertices in a given result and

Table 1. Segmentation error (mm) for the single and multi-scale schemes for varying n and d_n: mean $\pm$ standard deviation of rmse for nine scans. The star marks the configuration with smallest average error.

d_n	Single Scale	Refinement		Multi-model	
		$n = 2$	$n = 3$	$n = 2$	$n = 3$
1	4.3±2.2	4.3±2.2	4.3±2.2	5.2±2.2	5.0±2.2
2	2.0±1.4	2.0±1.4	2.0±1.4	2.9±2.1	2.9±2.1
3 (*)	1.4±0.4	1.2±0.3	1.2±0.4	1.2±0.3	1.2±0.4
4	3.0±3.2	3.0±3.3	2.7±3.4	2.6±2.8	2.3±2.5
5	3.1±3.1	2.8±3.3	2.5±3.4	3.2±3.1	2.8±3.2

the surface obtained with manual segmentation. The root mean squared error (rmse) of all vertices characterizes the overall segmentation quality. The statistical significance of differences between results obtained with different settings is evaluated with a paired T-test and expressed by the null hypothesis probability (p value). The relative volume of overlap between a segmentation A and the manual segmentation B is calculated with $2\frac{V(A \cap B)}{V(A)+V(B)}$.

4   Results

Table 1 summarizes the segmentation errors obtained for all scans with varying number of scales n, shift distance d_n, and deformation schemes.

In average, smaller errors are obtained for $d_n = 3$ mm in all configurations. The difference is more significant with respect to $d_n = 1, 2$ ($p < 0.05$) than to $d_n = 4, 5$ ($p > 0.15$). Figure 2 illustrates a typical case: for larger d_n, the boundary erroneously deforms into neighbouring structures, while for smaller d_n, it stays near the lumen boundary. In the remainder of the paper we only compare results obtained with $d_n = 3$ mm.

Figure 3 presents the segmentation error (rmse) obtained for each scan in all deformation schemes. Although a small reduction in error is obtained with the multi-scale schemes in comparison to single scale, the difference is not significant. The same observation holds for the improvement obtained by adopting 3 scales instead of 2 in both multi-scale schemes ($n = 2, 3$). Note, however, that the segmentation error is rather small in all schemes, with rmse$\leq$ 2.2 mm, and that this is significantly smaller than the initial error (rmse$\geq$ 2.8 mm). Table 2 presents the average volume of overlap between these segmentation results and the manual segmentations and the errors in the volume calculated based on these segmentations. Note that the average segmentation error (rmse), volume accuracy and volume errors are comparable to those reported in [3] (respectively 1.9 mm, 95% and 4.1%).

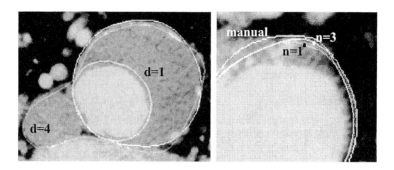

Fig. 2. Illustration of segmentation results and manual segmentation at selected slices of different scans. Left: varying d_n (monoscale). Right: varying n (refinement scheme, $d_n = 3$).

Table 2. Volume of overlap (%) and difference in volume calculation (%) between segmentation results and manual segmentation ($d_n = 3$ mm).

	Single Scale	Refinement $n = 2$	Refinement $n = 3$	Multi-model $n = 2$	Multi-model $n = 3$
Overlap	95.5±1.3	96.2±1.0	96.7±1.2	96.2±1.3	96.3±1.6
Error	3.9±2.9	2.6±2.9	2.7±3.1	2.9±3.1	3.1±3.6

5   Discussion and Conclusions

The image force adopted here for segmentation is inspired by approaches in which an appearance model built from training data is fit to the image. In ASMs, as introduced by Cootes et al. [11], a parametric statistical model is adopted for modelling grey values along the boundary profile; the model is built based on training samples of correct boundary profiles only. Such a simple model is not applicable for AAA thrombus segmentation, as shown in [3]. Extensions to grey level modelling for ASMs are proposed by Ginneken et al. [9] and De Bruijne et al. [3], in which the training is based on profile samples obtained at boundary positions and at multiple positions inside and outside the object. In both cases, a non-parametric classification technique (kNN) is used to determine the fit between model and data, and the landmark is moved into a position with best fit among a number of considered options. While in [9] the classification features are automatically selected from a large bank of Gaussian filters to discriminate between patterns inside and outside the object, in [3] image intensity is adopted. Finally, in the deformable model method proposed by Pardo et al. [12], the model is trained in one slice based on a 2-D contour, with samples at boundary and non-boundary positions. The most discriminating classification features are selected automatically from a Gaussian bank, and the model fit is measured with a parametric model for deformation in the adjacent slice. The methods above [11,9,3,12] are similar with respect to the following aspects: (1)

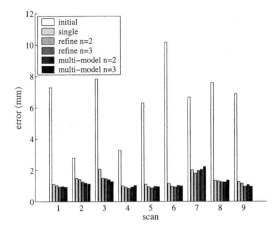

Fig. 3. Root mean squared error for the initial boundary (lumen) and the segmentation results obtained with all schemes ($d_n = 3$ mm).

the deformation is driven by a quality of fit that only takes into account the boundary/non-boundary distinction, and (2) a coarse-to-fine scheme is adopted, in which the boundary is progressively refined with grey level models built at increasing resolution. Compared to these works, two novelties are introduced here. First, the method uses a three-type class model that also distinguishes inside and outside non-boundary profiles, and in this way steers both the direction and magnitude of deformation. Our approach imposes fewer requirements on the initial surface than when an on-off boundary model is adopted. In particular, no successful AAA thrombus segmentation could be obtained when using such an on-off boundary model for deformation starting from the lumen boundary. Secondly, a novel multi-scale modelling approach is introduced that simultaneously considers profiles trained at multiple distances.

The method was evaluated on nine scans using a leave-one-out strategy, and the results were compared to manual segmentations. A limited number of parameters for the coarse-to-fine and multi-scale modelling schemes were considered. With respect to the largest shift distance d_n, better results were obtained in average with $d_n = 3$ mm in both schemes. Accurate results were obtained with all schemes; segmentation errors ($[1.2, 1.4]$mm) and volume accuracy ($[95.5, 96.5]\%$) are in the same range as reported in [3] (1.9 mm and 95%), and the volume error ($[2.6, 3.9]\%$) is comparable to the intra-observer variability reported in [13] (3.2%).

In conclusion, the results indicate that the three-type class model, that distinguishes inside and outside profiles, is very well suited for thrombus segmentation in CTA. With the lumen as initialization, the thrombus was found as accurate as the previously reported variability in manual outlining. We have shown previously [5] that the lumen can automatically be obtained using only two mouse clicks as initialization. The three-type class model was essential for obtaining these results: we found that these results could not be obtained with an on-off boundary profile training. Interestingly, the multi-scale approaches only slightly improved on the single scale approach, as long as an appropriate scale is selected. It remains to be investigated what the additional value of multi-scale schemes is in other applications.

Acknowledgments. We thank Prof. Dr. J. Blankensteijn and M. Prinssen, formerly with the Dept. of Vascular Surgery at the UMCU, for kindly providing datasets and manual segmentations. We also thank Dr. de Bruijne for the valuable discussions and suggestions. Finally, we are grateful to the developers of several libraries: 3D Active Objects, by Philips Research Paris; Approximate Nearest Neighbors (ANN), by Univ. of Maryland; and isiImage library, by Image Sciences Institute, UMCU.

References

1. M. de Bruijne et al. Active shape model based segmentation of abdominal aortic aneurysms in CTA images. In *SPIE Medical Imaging*, volume 4684, pages 463–474. SPIE, 2002.
2. M. Subasic, S. Loncaric, and E. Sorantin. 3-D image analysis of abdominal aortic aneurysm. In *SPIE Medical Imaging - Image Processing*, pages 1681–1689, 2002.
3. M. de Bruijne et al. Adapting active shape models for 3D segmentation of tubular structures in medical images. In *Information Processing in Medical Imaging (IPMI)*, volume 2732 of *LNCS*, pages 136–147. Springer, 2003.
4. A. Giachetti and G. Zanetti. AQUATICS reconstruction software: the design of a diagnostic tool based on computer vision algorithms. In *CVAMIA and MMBIA Workshop*, 2004.
5. S.D. Olabarriaga, M. Breeuwer, and W.J. Niessen. Segmentation of abdominal aortic aneurysms with a non-parametric appearance model. In *CVAMIA and MMBIA Workshop*, 2004.
6. H. Delingette. General object reconstruction based on simplex meshes. *International Journal of Computer Vision*, 32(2):111–146, 1999.
7. O. Gérard et al. Efficient model-based quantifications of left ventricular function in 3-d echocardiography. *IEEE Trans. Medical Imaging*, 21(9):1059–1068, 2002.
8. R. Duda, P. Hart, and D. Stork. *Pattern Classification*. John Wiley & Sons, 2001.
9. B.v.Ginneken et al. Active shape model segmentation with optimal features. *IEEE TMI*, 21(8):924–933, 2002.
10. M. Prinssen et al. Concerns for the durability of the proximal abdominal aortic aneurysm endograft fixation from a 2-year and 3-year longitudinal computed tomography angiography study. *J Vasc Surg*, 33:64–69, 2001.
11. T.F. Cootes et al. The use of active shape models for locating structures in medical images. *Imaging and Vision Computing*, 12(6):355–366, 1994.
12. X.M. Pardo, P. Radeva, and D. Cabello. Discriminant snakes for 3d reconstruction of anatomical organs. *Medical Image Analysis*, 7(3):293–310, 2003.
13. J.J. Wever et al. Inter- and intraobserver variability of CT measurements obtained after endovascular repair of abdominal aortic aneurysms. *American Journal of Roentgenology*, 175:1279–1282, 2000.

Local Speed Functions in Level Set Based Vessel Segmentation

Rashindra Manniesing and Wiro Niessen

Image Sciences Institute
University Medical Center Utrecht
The Netherlands {rashindra,wiro}@isi.uu.nl

Abstract. A new segmentation scheme is proposed for 3D vascular tree delineation in CTA data sets, which has two essential features. First, the segmentation is carried out locally in a small volume of interest (VOI), second, a global topology estimation is made to initialize a new VOI. The use of local VOI allows that parameter settings for the level set speed function can be optimally set depending on the local image content, which is advantageous especially in vascular tree segmentation where contrast may change significantly, especially in the distal part of the vascular. Moreover, a local approach is significantly faster. A comparison study on five CTA data sets showed that our method has the potential to segment larger part of the vessel tree compared to a similar global level set based segmentation, and in substantially less computation time.

1 Introduction

Vessel segmentation in computed tomography angiography (CTA) data sets remains an important image processing task. Usually, segmentation is the first step in quantification, visualization, pre-operative planning, 3D vessel modeling or in the design of computer aided diagnostic systems. Given its importancy, numerous methods have been developed; an attempt in [6] is made to categorize the different methods that have appeared in literature. In this work we consider level set based approaches [9,13] for vessel segmentation. Level set evolution is a way of describing the movement of surfaces by embedding them as the zero level set of a higher dimensional function, thereby obtaining an intrinsic, *i.e.* parameter free representation, gaining topological flexibility, and allowing for a simple calculation of geometrical properties, such as curvature, of the moving surfaces. These properties make the level set framework a suitable choice for describing the complex structures of vessel trees.

The crucial factor that determines the success of level set segmentation is the speed function that evolves the surface to the desired boundaries. Typically, most of these speed functions are of a *global* nature, *i.e.* , the same speed function is used at all voxel locations in the image and is often completely pre-computed. There are two important reasons for changing from a global to a local perspective, especially in the case of angiography data sets. First, image contrast is often varying owing to different concentrations of contrast agent, vessel resolution, or

C. Barillot, D.R. Haynor, and P. Hellier (Eds.): MICCAI 2004, LNCS 3216, pp. 475–482, 2004.
© Springer-Verlag Berlin Heidelberg 2004

in case of magnetic resonance imaging, coil inhomogeneities. Second, the vessel voxels only count for a few percentage of all voxels in the data sets and therefore a local approach would be computationally more efficient. In this paper we propose such a local scheme which is based on level set evolution for carrying out the local segmentation.

The idea of a local adaptive segmentation scheme is certainly not new. However, to the best of our knowledge, only very few adaptive local approaches are proposed in literature. This is perhaps due to the fact that local segmentation is often considered as merely a technical, or implementation issue of a (global) segmentation method. Still, the most closely related work we have found, is given by [5, 11, 1]. Generally speaking, these methods do have a variant of a locally adapting function for segmentation (for instance, the adaptive thresholding technique described in Jiang et al. [5] or the speed function based on statistics that is periodically updated during evolution, in Pichon et al. [11]), but differ essentially in the *dependency* that exist of each local segmentation function on the previous functions at every global iteration step, while we assume a complete independent segmentation function (*i.e.* speed function) for each local volume of interest (VOI).

Our contribution is twofold; first, selection of the next local VOI is done in a novel way by simply estimating the topology of the global segmentation result by skeletonization, and marking those skeleton points which have largest distance from the root point as the new seed points for a subsequent local segmentation. Second, we have applied our proposed method to five realistic, CTA data sets of the brain vasculature, and evaluated these local results with the result obtained by evolving a similar, global level set evolution with constant speed function.

2   Method

The proposed method is as follows (see also Figure 1).

0. Initialization. The user is required to place the first seed point at the root of the vessel tree of interest.
1. VOI selection and local speed function determination. A boxed VOI symmetrical around the seed point is determined for carrying out the local segmentation. An intensity histogram from voxels around a rough segmentation of the vasculature is used to construct the local speed function.
2. Local segmentation by level set evolution. The speed function is used to steer a level set which is iterated until convergence.
3. Topology extraction and labeling. Topology extraction is performed by skeletonization of the global segmentation results, followed by a labeling of the skeleton points. The selection of the next seed points is based on the resulting labeling and distances. Of interest are these end points having the largest distances from the seed point.

Steps 1-3 are repeated. The *global* stopping criteria for a locally adaptive scheme becomes crucial now, since we want to prevent the method to adapt to

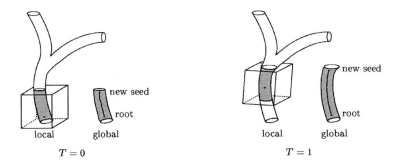

Fig. 1. The local segmentation result adds up to the global segmentation result of which the topology is estimated by skeletonization; the end points from this skeleton are then selected as the next seed points. This way, the orientation of the next volume of interest is implicitly taken into account. Disadvantage is that subsequent local volumes may overlap, for at most half their sizes.

background. Since this a research topic on its own, the discussion is postponed, and we simply set an upper limit on the overall number of local segmentations, as stopping criteria.

2.1   VOI Selection and Local Speed Function Determination

Given a seed point, the VOI is simply chosen symmetrical around this point, and its size should be such, that in this volume the intensity values of vessel and background are approximately homogeneously distributed. This is determined once for a data set by visual inspection. The size can not be too small since then the resulting histogram would not be properly defined. This is important, because the speed function depends on this histogram. The size remains fixed throughout execution of the algorithm. After the VOI has automatically been selected, an initial threshold value is applied to get a rough segmentation of vessel voxels. This initial threshold value is obtained by taking the mean voxel value in a small neighborhood of a few millimeters around the seed point. This neighborhood is set approximately equal to the distance of the seed point to the vessel border. After thresholding, the morphological operations erosion of one voxel width (to remove any noise voxel that may have occurred) and subsequentially dilation of three voxels width (to ensure we include the background, *i.e.* voxels surrounding the vessel voxels, as well), are applied. The resulting histogram is then used to construct the speed function - from now on denoted as the external, image based speed function F_{ext}, as follows[1], see also Figure 2 (the derivation follows the line of a previous paper on this subject [8]).

Two Gaussian distributions g_v and g_b are fitted, using an expectation maximization algorithm [2], and the histogram is then described as (approximately)

---

[1] Including spatial and higher order information could in principle, improve the results, but for showing the the main ideas of our method, intensity information suffices.

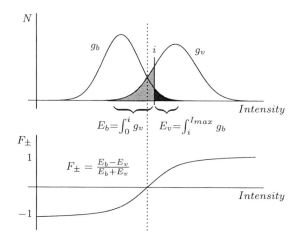

Fig. 2. From histogram to speed functions by classification error functions.

the sum of these functions. The Gaussian distributions overlap and therefore thresholding the image results in misclassifications of voxels; denote E_b and E_v as the fraction of voxels erroneously denoted as background and vessel voxels, i.e. $E_b(i) := \int_0^i g_v(x)\,dx$ and $E_v(i) := \int_i^{Imax} g_b(x)\,dx$. We propose the following function for F_{ext}

$$F_{ext} := \frac{E_b - E_v}{E_b + E_v} \qquad (1)$$

with range $[-1, 1]$ and with $E_b + E_v$ as a normalization factor. F_{ext} is zero at the optimal threshold value (optimal with respect to the total error given by the sum of E_b and E_v), has positive value if the number of misclassified background voxels is larger than the number of misclassified vessel voxels, and vice versa, thus giving rise to positive speed function values inside the vessel, zero at the boundary, and negative values outside the vessel. The negative range of the speed function combined with a smoothness constraint on the evolving level set, is particular effective in preventing possible leaking of the level set evolution through the vessel boundaries when started within the vessel.

2.2   Local Segmentation

Segmentation in the local volume is performed by applying level set evolution [9,13]. The basic partial differential equation is given by $u_t + F|\nabla u| = 0$, with u the signed distance function, u_t the partial derivative to time, and F some general speed function. In image segmentation, F is often defined as $F := F_{ext}(c - \epsilon\kappa)$ (first proposed in [3,7]), with F_{ext} the image based term (previously defined in Equation 1), $c := 1$ a constant advection term (similar to a balloon force [4]), and $\epsilon\kappa$ a weighted curvature term assuring smoothness of the surface. See [4,12] for more detailed derivations and motivations of the same and related PDEs and related image based speed functions. The curvature on a point on a 3D surface can be decomposed in two directions perpendicular to each other, in which the curvature takes minimal and maximal value; these extremal curvatures are called the principal curvatures. For vessel structures we prefer a smoothness along the longitudinal direction in which the curvature term is minimal, and therefore we define κ as $\kappa := \kappa_{min}$. Together, they yield our final differential equation

$$u_t + F_{ext}(1 - \epsilon\kappa_{min})|\nabla u| = 0 \qquad (2)$$

Evolution is started at the seed point and continued until convergence, *i.e.* stopped if there was no change in segmented volume.

2.3   Topology and Labeling

After convergence of the level set evolution, the zero level set is extracted and combined with the previous segmentation results by the boolean operator OR to get the global segmentation result. OR-ing the results is fast and accurate enough for topology estimation, however, a much cleaner and consistent approach, especially for obtaining the final global segmentation result, would be to merge the borders by applying level set evolutions again, but now initialized by the local results. For now, we choose the first solution. The topology of the global segmentation is then estimated by a 3D skeletonization algorithm [10] based on thinning. Thinning deletes border points of the object satisfying certain criteria until the resulting object does not change any more. The final result of the thinning procedure is a connected, topological preserving skeleton of the original object that is a representation of the central vessel axis part of the vascular tree. In [10] they are called the medial lines, *i.e.* 1D structures in 3D space, making this 3D skeleton algorithm particular suitable for representing the vessel structures.

The resulting medial lines are of only one voxel thick which simplifies labeling. The purpose of labeling is to provide sufficient information to select the next seed points for continuation of the global segmentation. A straight forward algorithm is depicted. First, labeling is started at the root point, which is the seed point or the nearest skeleton point if the seed point is not in the set of skeleton points. The root point is then initialized with distance zero. From the root we traverse the skeleton and for every skeleton point the Euclidean distance is updated and a label is given, either {(E)nd, (S)egment, (B)ranch}, depending on the number of neighbors. That is, if the number of neighbors of a given point minus one equals zero, the point is labeled 'E', equals one, the point is labeled 'S', equals two or more, the point is labeled 'B'. Giving the labeling and distances for each skeleton point, the next seed points are simply those end points having the largest distance from the root point.

3   Experiments and Results

The method is applied to cerebral CTA data sets acquired at the radiology department of the University Medical Center (UMC), Utrecht. A large num-

ber of scans of patients are made on a 16-slice CT scanner (Philips), resulting in data sets of 512×512 by approximately 300 slices, with voxel sizes of
0.3125×0.3125×0.5 mm. Five scans of patients are selected who are examined
for screening and showing no signs of hemorrhage (bleeding). Of each patients
two scans are made; a low dose scan without contrast, showing bone only, and a
high dose scan with contrast, showing bone and vasculature. First bone masking
is applied [14]; which consists of rigid registration (based on mutual information
and trilinear interpolation), erosion/dilation for noise removal and compensating
for inaccuracy of registration, and finally thresholding with T_{bone} and masking.
T_{bone} is not critical because the gap between the upper bound of vessel intensity
(∼500 Hounsfield Units HU) and the lower bound of bone intensity (∼800 HU)
is around 300 HU. Bone masking is not mentioned as part of our method since
it is not essential for communicating the main idea of our method. Then, each
data set was split into two region of interests - denoted left and right, because
the method expects only one seed point for initialization (conveniently chosen
at the internal carotid arteries) and which indeed is, of only a technical limitation, and will be removed in a future implementation of our method. The
user required input consist of (i) setting T_{bone} (we choose $T_{bone} := 600$ HU),
(ii) selection of the initial seed point at the root of the vessel tree, (iii) setting
of the global parameters (by lack of an appropriate stopping criteria, the maximum number of local segmentations is set at 25, the size of the local VOI is set
at 100×100×100) and finally, (iv) setting of the local, $i.e.$ level set parameters.
Their values are empirically determined; the number of iterations $n := 1500$
(all local level set evolutions converged before n either by reaching the vessel
boundaries, or reaching the bounding box of the VOI in case of adapting to
background that sometimes happened during the last VOIs), time step $t := 0.1$,
bandwidth $b := 6$, and $\epsilon := 0.35$. Initializiation of the level sets occur in a small
sphere of radius two voxels around the seed points. The level set evolution has
been implemented using the narrow band method [13].

The evaluation of segmentation methods is important and difficult, and this
work forms no exception. A comparison study is conducted and we evaluated the
results of our method with the results of a similar global level set evolution, by
visual inspection. This global level set evolution starts at the same seed points
and has the same parameters as the local level set, except for the number of
iterations that now was set at $n := 10000$. To get an impression of the data sets
and results, maximum intensity projections of three typical results out of five
data sets are shown in Figure 3; the first column gives the original data set (bone
masked), the second column the result of the global level set evolution and the
third column the results of the locally adaptive segmentations. On average and
based on all five results, the local segmentation method captures more vessel
structures than the global level set evolution does. In the figure some typical
regions of interests are denoted with arrows. For example, the arrow of the first
row points at a region the method is erroneously adapting to background. The
arrow of the second row points a vessel at which the method discontinues the
selection of next VOIs. This is due to seed point selection which only consider

those end points with maximal distance from the root point, thereby running the risk of missing some important end points. The improvement in computation time was significant, about 500 minutes on average for the global segmentation compared to 130 minutes on average for both local segmentations (left and right summed up) of each data set, on the same machine. Clearly, these results are very pleminary, but still gives an indication of the potential of the method.

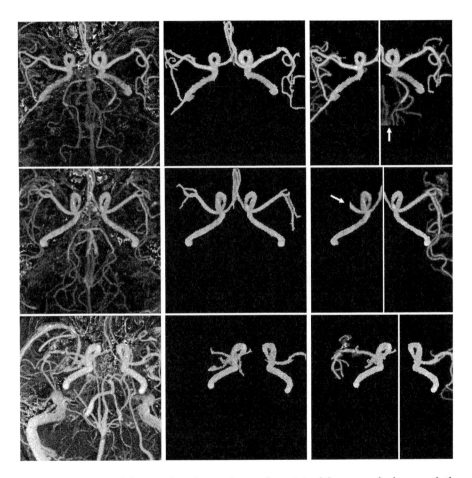

Fig. 3. Three out of five results; first column the original bone masked, second the global result, third the local results. The local results are splitted for technical reasons. Some regions of interest are denoted by arrows, see the main text for an explanation.

4   Conclusions

A new local adaptive segmentation scheme is proposed based on level set evolution for carrying out the local segmentation, and topology estimation by skeletonization of the global segmentation for selection of the next volume of interest. A comparison study of our method to a similar global level set evolution on five real, CTA data sets, showed that on average larger parts of the vessel tree are segmented initialized by a single seed point only, and showed a significant decrease in computation time. Future work is to devise a more intelligent, global stopping criteria, to refine the next seed point selection, to include bone masking in the local segmentation, and to conduct a better evaluation study based on a larger patient groups.

References

1. S.R. Aylward and E. Bullit. Initialization, noise, singularities, and scale in height ridge traversal for tubular object centerline extraction. *IEEE Transactions on Medical Imaging*, 21(2):61–75, February 2002.
2. C.M. Bishop. *Neural Networks for Pattern Recognition.* Oxford University Press Inc, New York, 1995.
3. V. Caselles, F. Catte, T.Coll, and F.Dibos. A geometric model for active contours. *Num. Math*, 66:1–31, 1993.
4. V. Caselles, R. Kimmel, and G. Sapiro. Geodesic active contours. *International Journal of Computer Vision*, 22(1):61–79, 1997.
5. X. Jiang and D. Mojon. Adaptive local thresholding by verification-based multithreshold probing with application to vessel detection in retinal images. *IEEE Transactions on Pattern Analysis and Machine Intelligence*, 25(1):131–137, January 2003.
6. C. Kirbas and F.K.H. Quek. Vessel extraction techniques and algorithms: A survey. In *Proceedings of the Third IEEE Symposium on BioInformatics and BioEngineering (BIBE)*, 2003.
7. R. Malladi, J.A. Sethian, and B.C. Vemuri. Evolutionary fronts for topology independent shape modeling and recovery. In *Proceedings of the Third European Conference on Computer Vision*, pages 3–13, 1994.
8. R. Manniesing, B. Velthuis, M. van Leeuwen, and W. Niessen. Skeletonization for re-initialization in level set based vascular tree segmentation. In *SPIE Medical Imaging*. SPIE, SPIE, 2004.
9. S.J. Osher and J.A. Sethian. Fronts propagation with curvature dependent speed: Algorithms based on Hamilton-Jacobi formulations. *Journal of Computational Physics*, 7:12–49, 1988.
10. K. Palágyi and A. Kuba. A 3d 6-subiteration thinning algorithm for extracting medial lines. *Pattern Recognition Letters*, 19:613–627, 1998.
11. E. Pichon, A. Tannenbaum, and R. Kikinis. A statistically based surface evolution method for medical image segmentation: Presentation and validation. In *Medical Image Computing and Computer-Assisted Intervention*, volume 2, pages 711–720, 2003.
12. Guillermo Sapiro. *Geometric Partial Differential Equations and Image Analysis.* Cambridge University Press, 2001.
13. J.A. Sethian. *Level Set Methods and Fast Marching Methods.* Cambridge University Press, second edition, 1999.
14. H.W. Venema, F.J.H. Hulsmans, and G.J. den Heeten. CT angiography of the Circle of Willis and intracranial internal carotid arteries: Maximum intensity projection with matched mask bone elimination - feasibility study. *Radiology*, 218:893–898, 2001.

Automatic Heart Peripheral Vessels Segmentation Based on a Normal MIP Ray Casting Technique

Charles Florin[1], Romain Moreau-Gobard[2], and Jim Williams[2]

[1] Ecole Nationale des Ponts et Chaussees,
Champs-sur-Marne, France
`florin@cermics.enpc.fr`
[2] Imaging & Visualization Department,
Siemens Corporate Research, Princeton, NJ, USA
{`romain.moreau-gobard,jim.williams`}`@scr.siemens.com`

Abstract. This paper introduces a new technique to detect the coronary arteries as well as other heart's peripheral vessels. After finding the location of the myocardium through a graph theoretic segmentation method, the algorithm models the heart with a biaxial ellipsoid. For each point of this ellipsoid, we compute the collection of intensities that are normal to the surface. This collection is then filtered to detect the cardiovascular structures. Ultimately, the vessels centerline points are detected using a vessel tracking algorithm, and linked together to form a complete coronary artery tree.

1 Introduction

In the USA, someone suffers a vascular failure every 29 seconds according to the American Federation of Aging Research. The cost of treating congestive heart failure (CHF) resulting from blocked coronary arteries is between \$20 and \$50 billion a year for 4.7 million Americans. Computer Tomography (CT) is more precise than echocardiography, but one can claim that no tool is presently available for the detection of heart peripheral vessels in CT. That is the reason why this new technique for heart vessels segmentation is of relevance for a quicker and more accurate diagnosis of CHF. Vessels segmentation allows the early detection of plaques, aneurysms and abnormal configuration of coronary arteries.

In this paper, we propose a heart peripheral vessels reconstruction solution that assumes the existence of a segmented volume representing the heart myocardium. The method is based upon the fact that the vessels are parallel to the heart surface. Therefore, segmenting the heart wall gives an important piece of information about the blood vessels. We consider a multi-stage approach to achieve this task. The first step consists of segmenting the heart, and acquiring the heart wall shell. Then the surface is modeled by a simple geometrical volume, such as a spheroid. In the next step, a ray is cast from each point on the spheroid surface, and the intersected intensities are recorded. During the next step, the ray collection in 3D is used as a pre-segmentation tool. Each vessel crossed by a ray generates a peak of intensity on the ray's profile curve. This is a simple technique to detect voxels belonging to vessels. High-intensity tubular structures in this voxel space can then be used to detect the vessels. During the last step, a full vessel tree is built, using vessel tracking techniques and minimum spanning tree.

C. Barillot, D.R. Haynor, and P. Hellier (Eds.): MICCAI 2004, LNCS 3216, pp. 483–490, 2004.
© Springer-Verlag Berlin Heidelberg 2004

2   Ray Collection

2.1   Heart Segmentation and Distance Map Computation

We consider a segmentation algorithm driven from the graph optimization technique [2] with a shape constraint. The idea lying behind this "graphcut" segmentation is to minimize an energy function that is defined on a graph, according to the cut of minimum weight. The energy is written as the sum of two terms : $E_{smooth}(f)$ that imposes smoothness constraints on the segmentation map, and $E_{data}(f)$ measuring how the label f is adapted to the data:

$$E(f) = E_{smooth}(f) + E_{data}(f) , \tag{1}$$

$$E_{smooth}(f) = \sum_{p,q \in neighbors} V_{p,q}(f(p), f(q)), \tag{2}$$

$$E_{data}(f) = \sum_{p \in P} D_p(f(p)). \tag{3}$$

$V_{p,q}$ in (2) is the interaction function between the pair of neighboring pixels $\{p, q\}$, and D_p in (3) measures how close the label f is to the pixel p intensity. It is known [2] that such a method provides a global optimal solution for the case of binary valued $f(p)$. There are also a couple of other methods that can be used to isolate the heart, e.g. a model-based segmentation [3] or segmentation algorithms based on level set methods [8] [10].

The segmentation produces a 3D mask (pixels labeled "object" and "background"). The distance map [6] from this surface can provide valuable constraints during the recovery of the peripheral vessels. For instance, as they stay parallel to the surface of the heart, their distance in the distance map varies smoothly. The distance map is computed by parsing the mask twice, in one direction and in the other one, and then filtering each voxel on an edge (object-background) by a 3D chamfer mask M and is then used to model the heart by a simpler geometrical object, such as an ellipsoid, in order to flatten its surface easily using cartography algorithms.

2.2   Modelization of the Shell by a Spheroid

In the next step, the distance map is used to model the heart wall by an ellipsoid or a biaxial spheroid. Although one may consider a more accurate model like a triaxial ellipsoid, a major drawback is that there is no simple mathematical solution to the 3D-2D projection. The biaxial ellipsoid projection is a well known technique in cartography. Nevertheless, the biaxial spheroid reduces the deformations we could have using a sphere. For a biaxial ellipsoid, of semi-axes length a and b, the surface equation is

$$\frac{x^2}{a^2} + \frac{y^2}{a^2} + \frac{z^2}{b^2} = 1 \tag{4}$$

or, in a parametric form: $x = a \, cos(\lambda) sin(\phi), y = a \, sin(\lambda) sin(\phi), z = b \, cos(\phi)$ where $\lambda \in [0, 2\pi]$ and $\phi \in [0, \pi]$. In reference to cartography, λ and ϕ are called longitude and

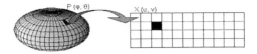

Fig. 1. 3D onto 2D projection, from an ellipsoid onto a plane

latitude respectively. The ellipsoid center is computed as the center of gravity G of all the points located on the distance map isosurface 0 (the heart shell). The large axis $\mathbf{Z}$ is the vector $\overrightarrow{GM}$, where M is the point on the isosurface maximizing the length $\| \overrightarrow{GM} \|$. Similarly, the small axis $\mathbf{X}$ is the vector $\overrightarrow{GN}$, where $\mathbf{N}$ is the point on the isosurface minimizing the length $\| \overrightarrow{GN} \|$. The axis $\mathbf{Y}$ is deduced to have a direct orthogonal base, $B = (G, \mathbf{X}, \mathbf{Y}, \mathbf{Z})$.

Note that the quality of the modeling does not rely on the quality of the segmentation, which makes the method described in this paper independent from the selection of the segmentation algorithm, and robust to noise. Moreover, unlike other organs, one can claim that the heart naturally has the shape of an ellipsoid. From the ellipsoid surface, rays are cast to compute a 2D view of the heart surface.

2.3   Ray Casting and n-MIP Projection

Once the distance map is computed, we cast rays from the ellipsoid, and collect the voxel intensities in a predefined direction and range inside and outside the heart wall. A very similar method is used for visualization purposes solely and applied to the cerebral cortex [7]. The distribution of the nodes on the ellipsoid used to cast rays is recovered through a simple transformation: for each point $P(\lambda, \phi)$ in 3D-space (Figure 1), the 2D-point X(u, v) is computed according to

$$[-\pi, \pi] \times [-\pi/2, \pi/2] \longmapsto [0, W] \times [0, H],$$

$$(\lambda, \phi) \longmapsto (u = \frac{W}{2\pi}\lambda, v = \frac{H}{\pi}\phi).$$

One could think about casting rays directly from the distance map itself, but in this case, the rays would not be homogeneous enough to be exploitable. Indeed, because of the heart surface irregularities, the rays would miss many vessels. For comparison purposes, we also implemented another solution, based on transverse Mercator projection for a biaxial ellipsoid. The drawback of such a method is that the volume has to be an ellipsoid of revolution, meaning the semi-minor axis is on the polar plane, and the semimajor axes are on the equatorial plane. Examples of unfolded n-MIP view are shown for different patients (Figure 2) with inverted colors. As the intensities have been inverted for the views to look like angiograms, the coronary arteries appear darker, compared to the other heart components. Each pixel I(x, y) on the 2D view is the normalized sum of each intensity, I_n, of the ray

$$I(x, y) = \frac{1}{N} \sum_{0 < n < N+1} In \tag{5}$$

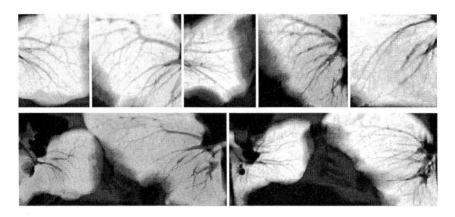

Fig. 2. Unfolded n-MIP (normal MIP) views of heart peripheral vessels for various patients, with inverted colors

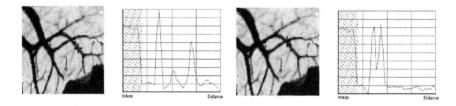

Fig. 3. Profile curves at two different locations on the heart's surface - Myocardium area indicated in crosshatched area

A profile matching technique is used to detect whether or not a ray crosses a vessel structure. As shown in Figure 3, the ray profile curve starts in the heart wall, which is represented as a large, flat, high intensity area. The vascular structures appear as peaks of high intensity, of limited diameter, and at a certain distance from the pericardium.

Next, peaks are processed to determine if they are suitable candidates for a vessel point, according to the following criteria:

1. It respects certain intensity properties (intensity value and peak shape)
2. It is within a certain distance from the heart wall

The intensity peaks, added to the local maximum (a ridge detection [11]), allow a fair detection of the vessels on the rays' profile curve (Figure 3). In order to detect peaks, we used a zero-crossing of the Laplacian, with the following kernel: [-1 2 -1].

Upon completion of such a procedure, a set of 3D points that are on a vessel, but not necessarily represent the vessel centerline is available (Figure 4). Such a condition has its origin in the ray-casting effect, as the rays are homogeneously distributed through space. Therefore, the next step will center these candidate points, filter the noise out, and track the detected vessels.

3   Heart Peripheral Vessel Detection

3.1   Refining the Vessel Candidate Points to Find the Centerlines

Vessel candidate voxels can be assumed to be next to or within a vessel's lumen. Nevertheless, they are not yet on the vessel's centerline (Figure 4). Furthermore, one can claim that the peak detection could be sensitive to noise (as one can see in Figure 4). Therefore, additional processing is required to center these points and to eliminate the noise as well. The refinement operation consists of an eigenvalues analysis [9] for each 3D-point within its corresponding local intensity space neighbors. With

$$A_{ij} = \frac{\partial^2 I}{\partial i \partial j}, \tag{6}$$

where i and j are equal to x, y or z, and the image intensity function I. At point P in space, the Hessian matrix M is defined as

$$M(P) = [A_{ij}]_{[i=x..z, j=x..z]}.$$

As the matrix M is defined, symmetric and positive, the computation of the eigenvalues is straightforward. At the center of the vessels, the three eigenvalues λ_1, λ_2 and λ_3 verify the following equations [1]

$$\lambda_1 \approx 0 \tag{7}$$

$$\lambda_2 \approx \lambda_3 << 0. \tag{8}$$

There are two principal directions given by the eigenvectors. The vector $\vec{v_1}$ associated with λ_1 corresponds to the local vessel orientation, whereas $\vec{v_2}$ and $\vec{v_3}$ define the vessel tangential plane.

For each candidate point P, the intensity function on the tangential cut plane defined by $\vec{v_2}$ and $\vec{v_3}$ is filtered by Gaussian functions, G_σ, with increasing variance σ. The G_σ minimizing the L^2 norm of $(I - G_\sigma)$ is kept as model. Then, a potential function V_σ is built and minimized [5]. V_σ represents how well a Gaussian vessel model fits for a variance σ at point P

$$A = \frac{|\lambda_2|}{|\lambda_3|}$$

$$B = \frac{|\lambda_1|}{\sqrt{|\lambda_3 \lambda_2|}}$$

$$S = \sqrt{\lambda_1 + \lambda_2 + \lambda_3}$$

$$V_\sigma(p) = \left(1 - e^{-\frac{A^2}{2\alpha^2}}\right) e^{-\frac{B^2}{2\beta^2}} \left(1 - e^{-\frac{S^2}{2\gamma^2}}\right) + \int |G_\sigma - I|^2$$

where α, β and γ are used to control the sensitivity of V_σ to the diverse ratio A, B and S. This approach is based on an intensity analysis. Other approaches would consist, for instance, in averaging the candidate points over a neighborhood. However, noise and high spacing between the points depending on the density of rays make these methods unsuitable for our application. To account for the high spacing between vessel points, we consider a vessel tracking technique to increase the number of points, and link them together to get the complete coronary arteries tree.

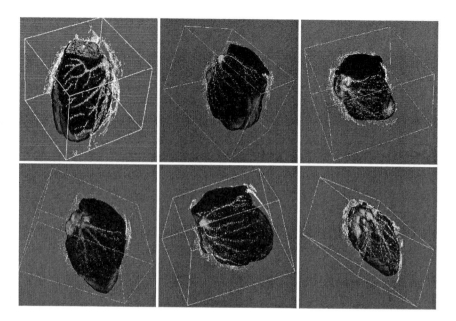

Fig. 4. Vessel Candidates displayed in 3D are not aligned on the vessels centerline

3.2 Points Densification

After the eigenanalysis, we assume we have the points, correctly placed, even though their number is not sufficient to track a vessel's centerline. Thus, in order to place more points, a simple vessel tracking operation is performed for each 3D candidate point, under the conditions of linear intensity variation, consistent distance from the segmented heart wall, and consistent orientation. In other words, from a point resulting from the eigenanalysis, we build another point and link it to the previous one, thus tracking the vessel. The speed vector $\vec{v_t}$ is the weighted sum of two vectors, the speed vector $\vec{v_{t-1}}$ and the local orientation vector $\vec{v_1}$ from 7

$$\vec{v_t} = \lambda \times \vec{v_{t-1}} + (1-\lambda) \times \vec{v_1}$$

where $\lambda \in [0,1]$. This speed vector, as well as intensity and distance to the heart, has to be homogeneous. We detected edges through a Laplacian analysis:

$$\int \left| \vec{\nabla} I \, \vec{dl} \right| < I_{coronary} - I_{exterior}.$$

If such an inequality is not satisfied for the distance function D and the image intensity I, an edge has been detected, and the tracking operation stops. Otherwise this tracking operation is performed until we reach the end of the vessel, or we can link all the chains to another point. At this stage, the candidate points are centered and homogeneously distributed on the centerline of the vessel. They are linked by a minimum spanning tree

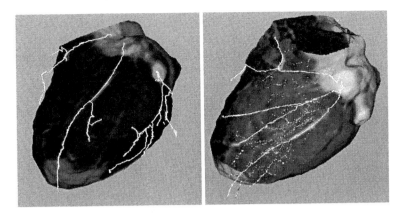

Fig. 5. The points on the vessels centerline are linked together

[13] algorithm, minimizing the following cost function E between two points P_1 and P_2

$$E_{P_1 P_2} = |D(P_1) - D(P_2)|^2 + |I(P_1) - I(P_2)|^2 + \left\| \overrightarrow{P_1 P_2} \right\|^2 + |\overrightarrow{v_1}(P_1).\overrightarrow{v_1}(P_2)|,$$

and result in the peripheral vessel's centerline (Figure 5).

Other algorithms are available to group together connect components [4] [14] [15]. These algorithms will be implemented in further studies. An interesting approach is based on a supervised region expansion [12].

4 Results and Conclusion

A heart peripheral vessel segmentation algorithm was presented in this paper, based on a ray filtering algorithm. In a step-by-step approach, the heart is first segmented using an algorithm based on graph cuts and geodesic surfaces, and a 3D distance map is computed out of the segmentation's output. Then, from this distance map, the biaxial ellipsoid modeling the heart is computed, and rays are cast from its surface toward the heart. Then, candidate points likely belonging to vessels are detected along the n-MIP rays' profiles. Finally, the vessel's centerline is tracked from the candidate points. This method can be used, for example, to visualize the full peripheral vessel tree, and detect plaques and aneurysms. Once segmented, the vascular structures can be unfolded, and the quantification of the stenosis and the aneurysms is straightforward. The segmentation results support efficient reporting by enabling automatic generation of overview visualizations, guidance for virtual endoscopy, generation of curved MPRs along the vessels, or cross-sectional area graphs. Moreover, applied to CT data sets, this algorithm detected vascular structures (Figure 5) quickly enough for industrial applications (60 seconds for a bi-processor 900MHz, 1GB RAM). Beside time constraints, the main advantage of this method compared to techniques relying on front propagation is its robustness to noise.

We are currently working on a hybrid front propagation algorithm that combines the above-mentioned technique with a multiscale vesselness measure. Moreover, another surface to model the heart is under investigation, to minimize the distortions introduced by the ellipsoid.

Acknowledgments. The authors would like to thank Christophe Chefdhotel for his help with the minimum spanning tree algorithm, Yuri Boykov for his precious help with his Graphcut segmentation algorithm, and the reviewers for their advice.

References

1. Stephen Aylward, Elizabeth Bullitt, Stephen Pizer, and Charles Chung. Tubular objects in 3d medical images: Automated extraction and sample application. In *1999 Radiology Research Review*, 1999.
2. Yuri Boykov, Olga Veksler, and Ramin Zabih. Fast approximate energy minimization via graph cuts. In *ICCV*, pages 377–-384, 1999.
3. T.F. Cootes, C.J. Taylor, D.H. Cooper, and J. Graham. Active shape models: Their training and application. *CVIU*, 61(1):38–59, January 1995.
4. T. Deschamps and L.D. Cohen. *Geometric Methods in Bio-Medical Image Processing*, chapter Grouping connected components using minimal path techniques. Mathematics and Visualization. Springer, 2002.
5. Alejandro F. Frangi, Wiro J. Niessen, Koen L. Vincken, and Max A. Viergever. Multiscale vessel enhancement filtering. *Lecture Notes in Computer Science*, 1496:130–??, 1998.
6. S. F. Frisken Gibson. Calculating the distance map for binary sampled data. Technical Report TR99-26, Mitsubishi, 1999.
7. Junfeng Guo, Alexandru Salomie, Rudi Deklerck, and Jan Cornelis. Rendering the unfolded cerebral cortex. In *MICCAI*, pages 287–296, 1999.
8. M. Kass, A. Witkin, and D. Terzopoulos. Snakes: Active contour models. In *Proc. of IEEE Conference on Computer Vision*, page 259–268, London, England, 1987.
9. K. Krissian, G. Malandain, N. Ayache, R. Vaillant, and Y. Trousset. Model based detection of tubular structures in 3d images. *Computer Vision and Image Understanding*, 80(2):130–171, November 2000.
10. M. Leventon, O. Faugeras, and W. Grimson. Level set based segmentation with intensity and curvature priors. In *Workshop on Mathematical Methods in Biomedical Image Analysis Proceedings (MMBIA)*, pages 4–11, June 2000.
11. T. Lindeberg. Edge detection and ridge detection with automatic scale selection. *Int. J. of Computer Vision*, 1996.
12. Cristian Lorenz, Steffen Renisch, Thorsten Schlathlter, and Thomas Bulow. Simultaneous segmentation and tree reconstruction of the coronary arteries in msct images. In *SPIE International Symposium on Medical Imaging*, volume 5031, 2003.
13. Seth Pettie and Vijaya Ramachandran. An optimal minimum spanning tree algorithm. *J. ACM*, 49(1):16–34, 2002.
14. G. Shechter, F. Devernay, A. Quyyumi, E. Coste-Mani'ere, and E.R. McVeigh. Three–dimensional motion tracking of coronary arteries in biplane cineangiograms. *IEEE Trans. Med. Imaging*, 22(4):493–603, April 2003.
15. Alexander Vasilevskiy and Kaleem Siddiqi. Flux maximizing geometric flows. *IEEE Trans. Pattern Anal. Mach. Intell.*, 24(12):1565–1578, 2002.

A New 3D Parametric Intensity Model for Accurate Segmentation and Quantification of Human Vessels

Stefan Wörz and Karl Rohr

School of Information Technology, Computer Vision & Graphics Group
International University in Germany, 76646 Bruchsal
{woerz,rohr}@i-u.de

Abstract. We introduce an approach for 3D segmentation and quantification of vessels. The approach is based on a new 3D cylindrical parametric intensity model, which is directly fit to the image intensities through an incremental process based on a Kalman filter. The model has been successfully applied to segment vessels from 3D MRA images. Our experiments show that the model yields superior results in estimating the vessel radius compared to approaches based on a Gaussian model. Also, we point out general limitations in estimating the radius of thin vessels.

1 Introduction

Heart and vascular diseases are one of the main causes for the death of women and men in modern society. An abnormal narrowing of arteries (stenosis) caused by atherosclerosis is one of the main reasons for these diseases as the essential blood flow is hindered. Especially, the blocking of a coronary artery can lead to a heart attack. In clinical practice, images of the human vascular system are acquired using different imaging modalities, for example, ultrasound, magnetic resonance angiography (MRA), X-ray angiography, or ultra-fast CT. Segmentation and quantification of vessels (e.g., estimation of the radius) from these images is crucial for diagnosis, treatment, and surgical planning.

The segmentation of vessels from 3D medical images, however, is difficult and challenging. The main reasons are: 1) the thickness (radius) of vessels depends on the type of vessel (e.g., relatively small for coronary arteries and large for the aorta), 2) the thickness typically varies along the vessel, 3) the images are noisy and partially the boundaries between the vessels and surrounding tissues are difficult to recognize, and 4) in comparison to planar structures depicted in 2D images, the segmentation of curved 3D structures from 3D images is much more difficult. Previous work on vessel segmentation from 3D image data can be divided into two main classes of approaches, one based on differential measures (e.g., Koller *et al.* [6], Krissian *et al.* [7], Bullitt *et al.* [2]) and the other based on deformable models (e.g., Rueckert *et al.* [10], Noordmans and Smeulders [8], Frangi *et al.* [3], Gong *et al.* [5]). For a model-based 2D approach for measuring

C. Barillot, D.R. Haynor, and P. Hellier (Eds.): MICCAI 2004, LNCS 3216, pp. 491–499, 2004.
© Springer-Verlag Berlin Heidelberg 2004

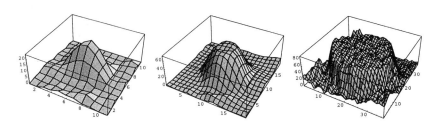

Fig. 1. Intensity plots of 2D slices of a thin vessel in the pelvis (left), the artery iliaca communis of the pelvis (middle), and the aorta (right) in 3D MR images.

intrathoracic airways see Reinhardt *et al.* [9]. The main disadvantage of differential measures is that only local image information is taken into account, and therefore these approaches are relatively sensitive to noise. On the other hand, approaches based on deformable models generally exploit contour information of the anatomical structures, often sections through vessel structures, i.e. circles or ellipses. While these approaches include more global information in comparison to differential approaches, only 2D or 3D contours are taken into account.

We have developed a new 3D parametric intensity model for the segmentation of vessels from 3D image data. This analytic model represents a cylindrical structure of variable radius and directly describes the image intensities of vessels and the surrounding tissue. In comparison to previous contour-based deformable models much more image information is taken into account which improves the robustness and accuracy of the segmentation result. In comparison to previously proposed Gaussian shaped models (e.g., [8],[5]), the new model represents a Gaussian smoothed cylinder and yields superior results for vessels of small, medium, and large sizes. Moreover, the new model has a well defined radius. In contrast, for Gaussian shaped models the radius is often heuristically defined, e.g., using the inflection point of the Gaussian function. We report experiments of successfully applying the new model to segment vessels from 3D MRA images.

2   3D Parametric Intensity Model for Tubular Structures

2.1   Analytic Description of the Intensity Structure

The intensities of vessels are often modeled by a 2D Gaussian function for a 2D cross-section or by a 3D Gaussian line (i.e. a 2D Gaussian swept along the third dimension) for a 3D volume (e.g., [8],[7],[5]). However, the intensity profile of 2D cross-sections of medium and large vessels is plateau-like (see Fig. 1), which cannot be well modeled with a 2D Gaussian function. Therefore, to more accurately model vessels of small, medium, and large sizes, we propose to use a Gaussian smoothed 3D cylinder, specified by the radius R (thickness) of the vessel segment and Gaussian smoothing σ. A 2D cross-section of this Gaussian smoothed 3D cylinder is defined as

$$g_{Disk}(x, y, R, \sigma) = \text{Disk}(x, y, R) \ * \ G_\sigma^{2D}(x, y) \tag{1}$$

where $*$ denotes the 2D convolution, $\text{Disk}(x, y, R)$ is a two-valued function with value 1 if $r \leq R$ and 0 otherwise (for $r = \sqrt{x^2 + y^2}$), as well as the 2D Gaussian function $G_\sigma^{2D}(x, y) = G_\sigma(x)\, G_\sigma(y)$, where $G_\sigma(x) = \left(\sqrt{2\pi}\sigma\right)^{-1} e^{-\frac{x^2}{2\sigma^2}}$. By exploiting the symmetries of the disk and the 2D Gaussian function as well as the separability of the 2D convolution, we can rewrite (1) as

$$g_{Disk}(x, y, R, \sigma) = 2 \int_{-R}^{R} G_\sigma(r - \eta)\, \Phi_\sigma\left(\sqrt{R^2 - \eta^2}\right)\, d\eta$$
$$- \left(\Phi_\sigma(r + R) - \Phi_\sigma(r - R)\right) \tag{2}$$

using the Gaussian error function $\Phi(x) = \int_{-\infty}^{x} (2\pi)^{-1/2}\, e^{-\xi^2/2}\, d\xi$ and $\Phi_\sigma(x) = \Phi(x/\sigma)$. Unfortunately, a closed form of the integral in (2) is not known. Therefore, the exact solution of a Gaussian smoothed cylinder cannot be expressed analytically and thus is computationally expensive. Fortunately, in [1] two approximations $g_{Disk<}$ and $g_{Disk>}$ of g_{Disk} are given for the cases $R/\sigma < T_\Phi$ and $R/\sigma > T_\Phi$, respectively (using a threshold of $T_\Phi = 1$ to switch between the cases). Note that the two approximations are generally not continuous at the threshold value T_Φ. However, for our model fitting approach a continuous and smooth model function is required (see Sect. 3 for details). Therefore, based on these two approximations, we have developed a combined model using a Gaussian error function as a blending function such that for all ratios R/σ always the approximation with the lower approximation error is used. The blending function has two fixed parameters for controlling the blending effect, i.e. a threshold T_Φ which determines the ratio R/σ where the approximations are switched and a standard deviation σ_Φ which controls the smoothness of switching. We determined optimal values for both blending parameters (see Sect. 2.2 for details). The 3D cylindrical model can then be written as (using $\mathbf{x} = (x, y, z)^T$)

$$g_{Cylinder}(\mathbf{x}, R, \sigma) = g_{Disk<}(r, R, \sigma)\left(1 - \Phi_{\sigma_\Phi}\left(\frac{R}{\sigma} - T_\Phi\right)\right) +$$
$$g_{Disk>}(r, R, \sigma)\, \Phi_{\sigma_\Phi}\left(\frac{R}{\sigma} - T_\Phi\right) \tag{3}$$

where

$$g_{Disk<}(r, R, \sigma) = \frac{2R^2}{4\sigma^2 + R^2}\, e^{-\frac{2r^2}{4\sigma^2 + R^2}}, \tag{4}$$

$$g_{Disk>}(r, R, \sigma) = \Phi\left(\frac{c_2 - 1}{c_1} + c_1\right), \tag{5}$$

$$c_1 = \frac{2}{3}\sigma\frac{\sqrt{\sigma^2 + x^2 + y^2}}{2\sigma^2 + x^2 + y^2}, \quad \text{and} \quad c_2 = \left(\frac{R^2}{2\sigma^2 + x^2 + y^2}\right)^{1/3}. \tag{6}$$

Fig. 2 shows 1D cross-sections (for different ratios R/σ) of the exact Gaussian smoothed cylinder g_{Disk} (numerically integrated), the two approximations $g_{Disk<}$ and $g_{Disk>}$, and our new model $g_{Cylinder}$. It can be seen that our model approximates the exact curve very well (see the *positive* axis). In addition, we include in our model the intensity levels a_0 (surrounding tissue) and a_1 (vessel)

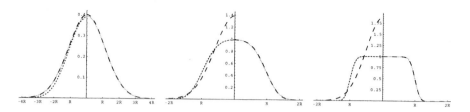

Fig. 2. For different ratios of $R/\sigma = 1.0; 3.0; 8.0$ (from left to right), the exact curve g_{Disk} of a 1D cross-section of a Gaussian smoothed disk is given (grey curve) as well as the approximations $g_{Disk<}$ and $g_{Disk>}$ (dashed resp. dotted curve for the *negative* axis) and the new model $g_{Cylinder}$ (dashed curve for the *positive* axis).

as well as a 3D rigid transform $\mathcal{R}$ with rotation parameters $\boldsymbol{\alpha} = (\alpha, \beta, \gamma)^T$ and translation parameters $\mathbf{t} = (x_0, y_0, z_0)^T$. This results in the parametric intensity model with a total of 10 parameters $\mathbf{p} = (R, a_0, a_1, \sigma, \alpha, \beta, \gamma, x_0, y_0, z_0)$:

$$g_{M,Cylinder}\left(\mathbf{x}, \mathbf{p}\right) = a_0 + (a_1 - a_0)\, g_{Cylinder}\left(\mathcal{R}\left(\mathbf{x}, \boldsymbol{\alpha}, \mathbf{t}\right), R, \sigma\right) \tag{7}$$

2.2   Optimal Values T_Φ and σ_Φ for the Blending Function

In order to determine optimal values T_Φ and σ_Φ for the blending function used in (3), we computed the approximation errors of the approximations $g_{Disk<}$ and $g_{Disk>}$ for different values of $\sigma = 0.38, 0.385, \ldots, 0.8$ and fixed radius $R = 1$ (note, we can fix R as only the ratio R/σ is important). The approximation errors were numerically integrated in 2D over one quadrant of the smoothed disk (using Mathematica). From the results (see Fig. 3 left and middle) we found that the approximation errors intersect at $\sigma/R = 0.555 \pm 0.005$ in the L1-norm and at $\sigma/R = 0.605 \pm 0.005$ in the L2-norm. We here chose the mean of both intersection points as threshold, i.e. $T_\Phi = 1/0.58 \approx 1.72$. It is worth mentioning that this value for T_Φ is much better than $T_\Phi = 1$ originally proposed in [1]. For σ_Φ we chose a value of 0.1. From further experiments (not shown here) it turns out that these settings give relatively small approximation errors in both norms. It nicely turns out (see Fig. 3 left and middle) that our model not only combines the more accurate parts of both approximations but also has a lower error in the critical region close to T_Φ, where both approximations have their largest errors.

2.3   Analysis for Thin Structures

For thin cylinders, i.e. $R/\sigma < T_\Phi$, our model $g_{Cylinder}$ is basically the same as the approximation $g_{Disk<}$, which has the following remarkable property for some factor f with $0 < f \leq f_{max} = \sqrt{1 + 4\sigma^2/R^2}$:

$$a\, g_{Disk<}\left(r, R, \sigma\right) = \frac{a}{f^2}\, g_{Disk<}\left(r,\ R' = fR,\ \sigma' = \frac{1}{2}\sqrt{4\sigma^2 + R^2\left(1 - f^2\right)}\right) \tag{8}$$

where a represents the contrast $a_1 - a_0$ of our model $g_{M,Cylinder}$ and $a' = a/f^2$. This means that this function is identical for different values of f, i.e. different

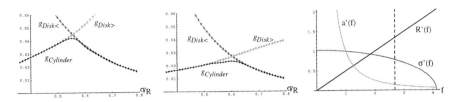

Fig. 3. For different values of $\sigma = 0.38, 0.385, \ldots, 0.8$ and radius $R = 1$, the errors of the approximations $g_{Disk<}$ and $g_{Disk>}$ (dark resp. light gray) as well as the error of the new model $g_{Cylinder}$ (black) are shown for the L1-norm (left) and L2-norm (middle). The right diagram shows $R'(f)$, $\sigma'(f)$, and $a'(f)$ for a varying factor f between 0 and f_{max} (for fixed $R = 0.5$, $\sigma = 1$, $a = 1$). The vertical dashed line indicates the ratio $f = R/\sigma = T_\Phi$, i.e. only the left part of the diagram is relevant for $g_{Disk<}$.

settings of $R'(f)$, $\sigma'(f)$, and $a'(f)$ generate the same intensity structure. This relation is illustrated for one example in Fig. 3 (right). As a consequence, based on this approximation it is *not* possible to unambiguously estimate R, σ, and a from intensities representing a thin smoothed cylinder. In order to uniquely estimate the parameters we need additional information, i.e. a priori knowledge of one of the three parameters. With this information and the ambiguous estimates we are able to compute f and subsequently the remaining two parameters.

Obviously, it is unlikely that we have a priori knowledge about the radius of the vessel as the estimation of the radius is our primary task. On the other hand, even relatively accurate information about the smoothing parameter σ will not help us much as can be seen from (8) and also Fig. 3 (right): $\sigma'(f)$ is not changing much in the relevant range of f. Therefore, a small deviation in σ can result in a large deviation of f and thus gives an unreliable estimate for R. Fortunately, the opposite is the case for the contrast $a'(f)$. For given estimates $\hat{R}$ and $\hat{a}$ as well as a priori knowledge about a, we can compute $f = \sqrt{a/\hat{a}}$ and $R = \hat{R}/f = \hat{R}\sqrt{\hat{a}/a}$. For example, for an uncertainty of $\pm 10\%$ in the true contrast a the computed radius is only affected by ca. $\pm 5\%$, and for an uncertainty of -30% to $+56\%$ the computed radius is affected by less than 20%. Note, this consideration only affects thin vessels with a ratio $R/\sigma < T_\Phi = 1.72$, i.e. for typical values of $\sigma \approx 1$ voxel and thus a radius below 2 voxels, the error in estimating the radius is below 0.2 voxels even for a large uncertainty of -30% to $+56\%$.

We propose two strategies for determining a. In case we are segmenting a vessel with varying radius along the vessel, we can use the estimate of the contrast in parts of the vessel where $R/\sigma > T_\Phi$ (here the estimates of the parameters are unique) for the other parts as well. In case of a thin vessel without thicker parts we could additionally segment a larger close-by vessel for estimating the contrast, assuming that the contrast is similar in this region of the image.

Standard approaches for vessel segmentation based on a Gaussian function (e.g., [8],[7],[5]) only estimate two parameters: the image contrast a_g and a standard deviation σ_g. Assuming that the image intensities are generated by a Gaussian smoothed cylinder based on $g_{Disk<}$, we can write $a_g = 2aR^2/(4\sigma^2 + R^2)$ and $\sigma_g = \sqrt{4\sigma^2 + R^2}/2$, see (4). Often, the radius of the vessel is defined by the

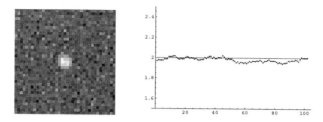

Fig. 4. Estimated radius R for 102 segments of a smoothed straight 3D cylinder with settings $R = 2$, $\sigma = 1$, $a_0 = 50$, and $a_1 = 150$ as well as added Gaussian noise ($\sigma_n = 10$). In addition, one 2D cross-section of the 3D synthetic data is shown.

estimated standard deviation σ_g, which implies that $\sigma = R\sqrt{3}/2$ holds. However, this is generally not the case and therefore leads to inaccurate estimates of R.

3   Incremental Vessel Segmentation and Quantification

To segment a vessel we utilize an incremental process which starts from a given point of the vessel and proceeds along the vessel. In each increment, the parameters of the cylinder segment are determined by fitting the cylindrical model in (7) to the image intensities $g(\mathbf{x})$ within a region-of-interest (ROI), thus minimizing

$$\sum_{\mathbf{x} \in \text{ROI}} (g_{M,Cylinder}(\mathbf{x}, \mathbf{p}) - g(\mathbf{x}))^2 \tag{9}$$

For the minimization we apply the method of Levenberg-Marquardt, incorporating 1st order partial derivatives of the cylindrical model w.r.t. the model parameters. The partial derivatives can be derived analytically. The length of the cylinder segment is defined by the ROI size (in our case typically 9-21 voxels). Initial parameters for the fitting process are determined from the estimated parameters of the previous segment using a linear Kalman filter, thus the incremental scheme adjusts for varying thickness and changing direction.

4   Experimental Results

4.1   3D Synthetic Data

In total we have generated 388 synthetic 3D images of straight and curved tubular structures using Gaussian smoothed discrete cylinders and spirals (with different parameter settings, e.g., for the cylinders we used radii of $R = 1, \ldots, 9$ voxels, smoothing values of $\sigma = 0.5, 0.75, \ldots, 2$ voxels, and a contrast of 100 grey levels). We also added Gaussian noise ($\sigma_n = 0, 1, 3, 5, 10, 20$ grey levels). From the experiments we found that the approach is quite robust against noise and produces accurate results in estimating the radius as well as the other model parameters (i.e. contrast and image smoothing as well as 3D position and orientation). As an example, Fig. 4 shows the estimated radius for 102 segments of a

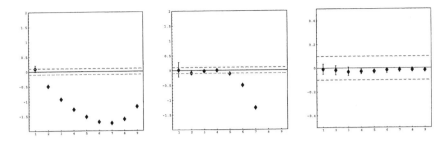

Fig. 5. Differences of the estimated radius (mean over ca. 99 segments) and the true radius for a synthetic straight cylinder with different radii $R = 1, \ldots, 9$ for the uncalibrated (left) and calibrated Gaussian line model (middle), as well as for the new cylindrical model (right). The dashed lines highlight the interval from -0.1 to 0.1 voxels.

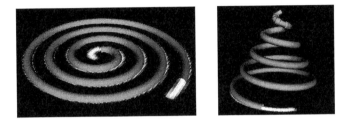

Fig. 6. Segmentation results of applying the cylindrical model to 3D synthetic data of a spiral (left) and a screw-like spiral (right). For visualization we used 3D Slicer [4].

relatively thin smoothed cylinder. The correct radius could be estimated quite accurately within ±0.06 voxels along the whole cylinder. Fig. 5 (right) shows the differences of the estimated radius to the true radius of smoothed cylinders for a range of different radii (for $\sigma = 1$ and $\sigma_n = 10$). It can be seen that the error in the estimated radius is in all cases well below 0.1 voxels. As a comparison we also applied a standard approach based on a 3D Gaussian line. To cope with the general limitations of the Gaussian line approach (see Sect. 2.3), we additionally calibrated the estimated radius (assuming an image smoothing of $\sigma = 1$, see [5] for details). It can be seen that the new approach yields a significantly more accurate result in comparison to both the uncalibrated and calibrated Gaussian line approach (Fig. 5 left and middle). Fig. 6 shows segmentation results of our new approach for a spiral and a screw-like spiral (for a radius of $R = 2$ voxels). It turns out that our new approach accurately segments curved structures of varying curvature, i.e. the estimated radius is within ±0.1 voxels to the true radius for nearly all parts of the spirals. Larger errors only occur for the last part of the innermost winding, where the curvature is relatively large.

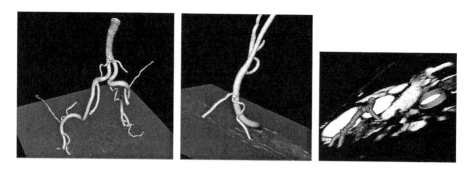

Fig. 7. Segmentation results of applying the new cylindrical model to arteries of the pelvis (left and middle) as well as to coronary arteries and the aorta (right).

4.2   3D Medical Images

With our approach both position and shape information (radius) are estimated from 3D images. Fig. 7 shows segmentation results of applying the new cylindrical model to 3D MRA images of the human pelvis and heart. Note that for the segmentation of the vessel trees we used starting points at each bifurcation. It can be seen that arteries of quite different sizes and high curvatures are successfully segmented. As a typical example, the computation time for segmenting an artery of the pelvis (see Fig. 7 left, main artery in left branch including the upper part) using a radius of the ROI of 10 voxels is just under 4min for a total of 760 segments (on a AMD Athlon PC with 1.7GHz, running Linux).

5   Discussion

The new 3D cylindrical intensity model yields accurate and robust segmentation results comprising both position and thickness information. The model allows to accurately segment 3D vessels of a large spectrum of sizes, i.e. from very thin vessels (e.g., a radius of only 1 voxel) up to relatively large arteries (e.g., a radius of 14 voxels for the aorta). Also, we pointed out general limitations in the case of thin structures and disadvantages of approaches based on a Gaussian function.

Acknowledgement. The MRA images are courtesy of Dr. med. T. Maier and Dr. C. Lienerth, Gemeinschaftspraxis Radiologie, Frankfurt/Main, Germany, as well as Prof. Dr. T. Berlage and R. Schwarz from the Fraunhofer Institute of Applied Information Technology (FIT), Sankt Augustin, Germany.

References

1. M. Abramowitz and I. Stegun, *Pocketbook of Mathematical Functions*, Verlag Harri Deutsch, 1984

2. E. Bullitt, S. Aylward, K. Smith, S. Mukherji, M.Jiroutek, K. Muller, "Symbolic Description of Intracerebral Vessels Segmented from MRA and Evaluation by Comparison with X-Ray Angiograms", *Medical Image Analysis*, 5, 2001, 157-169.
3. A. F. Frangi, W. J. Niessen, R. M. Hoogeveen, *et al.*, "Model-Based Quantitation of 3D Magnetic Resonance Angiographic Images", *T-MI*, 18:10, 1999, 946-956
4. D.T. Gering, A. Nabavi, R. Kikinis, *et al.*, "An integrated Visualization System for Surgical Planning and Guidance using Image Fusion and Interventional Imaging", *Proc. MICCAI'99*, 1999, 808-819
5. R.H. Gong, S. Wörz, and K. Rohr, "Segmentation of Coronary Arteries of the Human Heart from 3D Medical Images", *Proc. BVM'03*, 2003, 66-70
6. Th.M. Koller, G. Gerig, G. Székely, and D. Dettwiler, "Multiscale Detection of Curvilinear Structures in 2D and 3D Image Data", *Proc. ICCV'95*, 1995, 864-869
7. K. Krissian, G. Malandain, N. Ayache, R. Vaillant, and Y. Trousset, "Model Based Detection of Tubular Structures in 3D Images", *CVIU*, 80:2, 2000, 130-171
8. H.J. Noordmans, A.W.M. Smeulders, "High accuracy tracking of 2D/3D curved line structures by consecutive cross-section matching", *Pattern Recogn. Letters*, 19:1, 1998, 97-111
9. J.M. Reinhardt, N.D. D'Souza, and E.A. Hoffman, "Accurate Measurement of Intrathoracic Airways", *IEEE Trans. on Medical Imaging*, 16:6, 1997, 820-827
10. D. Rueckert, P. Burger, S.M. Forbat, R.D. Mohiaddin, G.Z. Yang, "Automatic Tracking of the Aorta in Cardiovascular MR Images Using Deformable Models", *IEEE Trans. on Medical Imaging*, 16:5, 1997, 581-590

Geometric Flows for Segmenting Vasculature in MRI: Theory and Validation

Maxime Descoteaux[1], Louis Collins[2], and Kaleem Siddiqi[1]

McGill University, Montréal, QC, Canada
[1] School of Computer Science & Centre For Intelligent Machines
{mdesco,siddiqi}@cim.mcgill.ca
[2] McConnell Brain Imaging Centre, Montréal Neurological institute
{louis}@bic.mni.mcgill.ca

Abstract. Often in neurosurgical planning a dual spin echo acquisition is performed that yields proton density (PD) and T2-weighted images to evaluate edema near a tumor or lesion. The development of vessel segmentation algorithms for PD images is of general interest since this type of acquisition is widespread and is entirely noninvasive. Whereas vessels are signaled by black blood contrast in such images, extracting them is a challenge because other anatomical structures also yield similar contrasts at their boundaries. In this paper, we present a novel multi-scale geometric flow for segmenting vasculature from standard MRI which can also be applied to the easier cases of angiography data. We first apply Frangi's vesselness measure [3] to find putative centerlines of tubular structures along with their estimated radii. This measure is then distributed to create a vector field which is orthogonal to vessel boundaries so that the flux maximizing geometric flow algorithm of [14] can be used to recover them. We perform a quantitative cross validation on PD, phase contrast (PC) angiography and time of flight (TOF) angiography volumes, all obtained for the same subject. A significant finding is that whereas more than 80% of the vasculature recovered from the angiographic data is also recovered from the PD volume, over 25% of the vasculature recovered from the PD volume is *not* detected in the TOF data. Thus, the technique can be used not only to improve upon the results obtained from angiographic data but also as an alternative when such data is not available.

1 Introduction

A three-dimensional (3D) representation of vasculature can be extremely important in image-guided neurosurgery, pre-surgical planning and clinical analysis. It is unfortunately often the case that in order to obtain such representations from an MRI volume an expert has to interact with it manually, coloring regions of interest and connecting them using image processing operations. This process is extremely laborious, is prone to human error and makes large scale clinical studies of vasculature infeasible. In computer vision there has been a significant amount of work towards automating the extraction of vessels or vessel centerlines, typical examples of which include [10,6,5,1]. However, most of these methods have been developed for 2D projection angiography or 3D CT and MR angiography, several of which require the injection of contrast agents. To our knowledge no method currently exists for the automatic extraction of vessel boundaries

C. Barillot, D.R. Haynor, and P. Hellier (Eds.): MICCAI 2004, LNCS 3216, pp. 500–507, 2004.

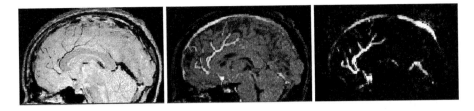

Fig. 1. A mid-sagittal slice of a proton density (PD) weighted MRI volume, a time of flight (TOF) MR angiogram and a phase contrast (PC) MR angiogram of the same subject. The spaghetti-like structures in the PD correspond to vasculature, which is more easily detected in the angiograms where there are sharp bright to dark contrast changes *only* at vessel boundaries.

in standard MRI volumes, such as the proton density (PD) image in Figure 1. Here it is clear that a signal decrease is present in the vascular regions (the spaghetti-like structures), but the contrast between blood vessels and surrounding tissue is not limited to vessel boundaries as it is in the corresponding angiographic sequences. The problem of recovering vessels from image intensity contrast alone on PD images is a challenge and requires shape information to constrain the segmentation. If successful, such a procedure could result in a vascular model that could be used in surgical planning while eliminating the need for an additional scan thus saving time during image acquisition and easing the burden on the patient.

   In this paper we introduce a novel algorithm for vessel segmentation which is designed for the case of PD images, but can be applied as well to angiographic data or Gadolinium enhanced volumes. The algorithm is motivated in part by the approach in [12] where Frangi's vesselness measure [3] is thresholded to find centerlines. However, rather than threshold this measure we extend it to yield a vector field which is locally normal to putative vessel boundaries. This in turn allows the flux maximizing geometric flow of [14] to be applied to recover vessel boundaries. This approach allows for a type of local integration, while affording the ability to connect branching structures. The flow has a formal motivation, is topologically adaptive due to its implementation using level set methods, and finally is computationally efficient. We perform a quantitative comparison of segmentations from PD, PC and TOF volumes, all obtained for the same subject (Figure 1).

2   A Multi-scale Geometric Flow for Segmenting Vasculature

2.1   Modeling Vasculature Using the Hessian

Several multi-scale approaches to modeling tubular structures in intensity images have been based on properties of the Eigen values $\lambda_1, \lambda_2, \lambda_3$ of the Hessian matrix $\mathbf{H}$ [8,13, 3]. These methods exploit the fact that at locations centered within tubular structures the smallest Eigen value of $\mathbf{H}$ is close to zero, reflecting the low curvature along the direction of the vessel, and the two other Eigen values are high and are close to being equal because the cross-section of the vessel is approximately circular. The corresponding Eigen vectors span the vessel direction and the cross-sectional plane.

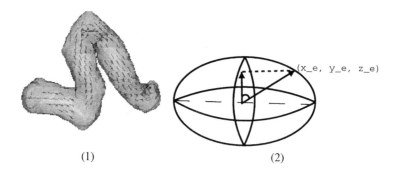

Fig. 2. (1) The superimposed vectors on the synthetic helix indicate the estimated vessel orientation at locations where the multi-scale vesselness measure (Eq. 1) is high. (2) The vector from the center of the ellipsoid to the surface voxel (x_e, y_e, z_e), as well as its projection onto the cross-sectional plane, taken to be the xy plane. We distribute the vesselness measure to all (x_e, y_e, z_e) on the ellipsoid by scaling it by the magnitude of this projection.

We choose to focus here on Frangi's vesselness measure [3] because it incorporates information from all three Eigen values. With the Eigen values sorted such that $|\lambda_1| \leq |\lambda_2| \leq |\lambda_3|$, three quantities are defined to differentiate blood vessels from other structures: $R_B = \frac{|\lambda_1|}{\sqrt{|\lambda_2\lambda_3|}}$, $R_A = \frac{|\lambda_2|}{|\lambda_3|}$, and $S = \sqrt{\lambda_1^2 + \lambda_2^2 + \lambda_3^2}$. R_B is non zero only for blob-like structures, the R_A ratio differentiates sheet-like objects from other structures and S, the Frobenius norm, is used to ensure that random noise effects are suppressed from the response. For a particular scale σ the intensity image is first convolved by a Gaussian $G(\sigma)$ at that scale[1]. The vesselness measure is then defined by

$$V(\sigma) = \begin{cases} 0 & \text{if } \lambda_2 < 0 \text{ or } \lambda_3 < 0 \\ (1 - \exp\left(-\frac{R_A^2}{2\alpha^2}\right))\exp\left(-\frac{R_B^2}{2\beta^2}\right)\left(1 - \exp\left(-\frac{S^2}{2c^2}\right)\right) \end{cases}.$$

(1)

This measure is designed to be maximum along the centerlines of tubular structures and close to zero outside vessel-like regions.

In our implementation we set the parameters α, β and c to 0.5, 0.5 and half the maximum Frobenuis norm, respectively, as suggested in [3]. At each voxel we compute vesselness responses using ten log scale increments between $\sigma = 0.2$ and $\sigma = 2.5$ (in our data the maximum radius of a vessel is 2.5 voxels) and select the maximum vesselness response along with its scale. The chosen scale gives the estimated radius of the vessel and the Eigen vector associated with the smallest Eigen value its local orientation. This process is illustrated in Figure 2 (left) for a synthetic helix. The grey surface coincides with a particular level set of the vesselness measure. Within this surface locations of high vesselness are indicated by overlaying the Eigen vectors which correspond to the estimated vessel orientation.

---

[1] In practice we directly compute the entries which comprise the Hessian matrix by using derivatives of Lindeberg's γ-parametrized normalized Gaussian kernels [7]. This allows us to compare responses at different scales.

2.2   Extending the Vesselness Measure to Vessel Boundaries

We now construct a vector field which is both large in magnitude at vessel boundaries as well as orthogonal to them, so that the flux maximizing flow of [14] can be applied. Since the vesselness measure is concentrated at centerlines, we need to first distribute it to the vessel boundaries which are implied by the local orientation and scale. At each voxel (x, y, z) where this measure is a local maximum in a 3x3x3 neighborhood we consider an ellipsoid with its major axis oriented along the estimated orientation and its two other axes equal to the estimated radius. The vesselness measure is then distributed over every voxel (x_e, y_e, z_e) on the boundary of the ellipsoid by scaling it by the projection of the vector from (x, y, z) to (x_e, y_e, z_e) onto the cross-sectional plane, as illustrated in Figure 2 (right). This process of distributing the vesselness measure to the implied boundaries clearly favors voxels in the cross-sectional plane. We define the addition of the extensions carried out independently at all voxels to be a scalar function ϕ. The extended vector field is given by the product of the normalized gradient of the original intensity image with ϕ:

$$\vec{V} = \phi \frac{\nabla \mathcal{I}}{|\nabla \mathcal{I}|}. \tag{2}$$

2.3   The Multi-scale Geometric Flow

We now apply the flux maximizing geometric flow of [14], which is the gradient flow that evolves a curve (2D) or a surface (3D) so as to increase the inward flux of a fixed (static) vector field through its boundary as fast as possible. With S an evolving surface and $\vec{V}$ the vector field, this flow is given by

$$S_t = div(\vec{V})\vec{N} \tag{3}$$

where $\vec{N}$ is the unit outward normal to each point on S. The motivation behind this flow is that it evolves a surface to a configuration where its normals are aligned with the vector field.

In their original formulations, the above flow and the related co-dimension 2 flow developed [9] are both quite restrictive since they are designed specifically for angiographic data. They are both initialized essentially by thresholding such data, and thus would fail when vasculature cannot be identified from contrast alone. Furthermore, neither has an explicit term to model tubular structures. Rather, each flow relies on the assumption that the gradient of the intensity image yields a quantity that is significant *only* at vessel boundaries. Finally, neither of these methods takes into account explicitly the multi-scale nature of vessels boundaries as they appear in all modalities.

With regard to the flux maximizing flow, these limitations can be overcome by choosing as the static vector field in Eq. 3 the construction defined in Eq. 2. This vector field embodies two important constraints. First, the magnitude of ϕ is maximum on vessel boundaries and the ellipsoidal extension performs a type of local integration. Second, $\frac{\nabla \mathcal{I}}{|\nabla \mathcal{I}|}$ captures the direction information of the gradient, which is expected to be high at boundaries of vessels as well as orthogonal to them[2]. The surface evolution equation works out to be

$$S_t = div(\overrightarrow{V})\overrightarrow{N} = \left[\left\langle \nabla\phi, \frac{\nabla\mathcal{I}}{|\nabla\mathcal{I}|} \right\rangle + \phi div\left(\frac{\nabla\mathcal{I}}{|\nabla\mathcal{I}|}\right)\right]\overrightarrow{N} = \left[\left\langle \nabla\phi, \frac{\nabla\mathcal{I}}{|\nabla\mathcal{I}|} \right\rangle + \phi\kappa_{\mathcal{I}}\right]\overrightarrow{N},$$

(4)

where $\kappa_{\mathcal{I}}$ is the Euclidean mean curvature of the iso-intensity level set of the image. This is a hyperbolic partial differential equation since all terms depend solely on the vector field and not on the evolving surface. The first term $\left\langle \nabla\phi, \frac{\nabla\mathcal{I}}{|\nabla\mathcal{I}|} \right\rangle$ acts like a doublet because at vessel boundaries $\nabla\phi$ has a zero-crossing while $\nabla\mathcal{I}$ does not change sign. Hence, when the evolving surface overshoots the boundary slightly, this term acts to push it back towards the boundary. The second term behaves like a geometric heat equation [4] since $\kappa_{\mathcal{I}}$ is the mean curvature of the iso-intensity level set of the original intensity image. The flow cannot leak in regions outside vessels since by construction both ϕ and $\nabla\phi$ are zero there.

In our implementation we compute the Hessian operator over 10 log scales and select the maximum vesselness response, using Jacobi's method for symmetric matrices to find the Hessian's Eigen values. The geometric flow in Eq. 4 is then simulated using a first-order in time discretized level-set version of the flow [11]:

$$\Psi_n = \Psi_{n-1} - \Delta t * \mathcal{F} * ||\nabla\Psi_{n-1}||.$$

(5)

Here $\mathcal{F} = \left\langle \nabla\phi, \frac{\nabla\mathcal{I}}{|\nabla\mathcal{I}|} \right\rangle + \phi div\left(\frac{\nabla\mathcal{I}}{|\nabla\mathcal{I}|}\right)$, Ψ is the embedding hypersurface typically initialized as a signed Euclidean distance function to the initial seed boundaries, Δt is the step size and the evolving surface S is obtained as the zero level set of the Ψ function.

3   Experiments

3.1   Image Acquisition

In order to validate our algorithm we acquired four different volumes from the same subject on a Siemens 1.5 Tesla system at the Montréal Neurological Institute. We first used a PD/T2-weighted dual turbo spin-echo acquisition with sagittal excitation (2mm thick slices, 50% overlap 1mm^3 isotropic voxels, TE = 0.015s TR = 3.3s). Following this, a 3D axial phase-contrast (PC) volume (0.47mm x 0.47mm x 1.5mm resolution, TE = 0.0082s TR = 0.071s) and a 3D axial time-of-flight (TOF) volume (0.43mm x 0.43mm x 1.2 mm resolution, TE = 0.0069s TR = 0.042s) were acquired. Each data set was registered to a standardized coordinate system and re-sampled onto a 0.5mm^3 isotropic voxel grid to facilitate processing and comparisons (Figure 1).

In the PC data, contrast is determined by tissue motion. Static tissue yields no signal, and is therefore black. In the TOF data, vessel brightness is proportional to blood flow velocity. However complex flow or turbulence can cause some signal loss in the vessels

---

[2] It is important to normalize the gradient of the image so that its magnitude does not dominate the measure in regions of very low vesselness. Without this normalization structures such as white and gray matter boundaries could get significant unwanted contributions.

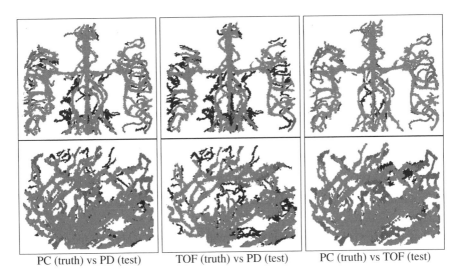

| PC (truth) vs PD (test) | TOF (truth) vs PD (test) | PC (truth) vs TOF (test) |

Fig. 3. Each column shows a pair-wise comparison of reconstructions obtained on different modalities, with transverse views in the top row and saggital views in the bottom row. White labels correspond to the background, red labels to locations common to the ground truth and test data, green labels to locations in the ground truth only and blue labels to locations in the test data only.

in such images. In the data presented here, vessel/background contrast is greatest for the PC data (white on black tissue), intermediate for the PD data (black on grey) and slightly less for the TOF data (white on grey).

3.2 Vessel Extraction

Owing to the high resolution of the scans, the volumes lead to significant memory costs when processed in their entirety. Hence we chose to work with a common 259 x 217 x 170 voxel region cropped from each volume, which had vessels of different widths and contrasts in the three modalities. The segmentation process was carried out by computing the vesselness measure, constructing the extended vector field $\overrightarrow{\mathcal{V}}$ for a selected vesselness threshold and finally applying the geometric flow (Eq. 4), initializing it by placing seeds at locations where the vesselness measure was above a high threshold so that the evolution began from within vessels.

Figure 3 compares the reconstructions obtained on the three different modalities, with transverse views shown in the top row and saggital views in the bottom row. To allow for slight alignment errors due to the process by which the initial volumes were scaled we consider two locations to be in common if the Euclidean distance between them is no greater than 3 voxels (1.5 mm). In each column red labels indicate locations common to the two data sets, green labels indicate locations present in the ground truth data set but not in the test set and blue labels locations in the test data set which are not in the ground truth data set. It is clear from the first column that most of reconstructed vessels in the PD and PC data agree. The PC reconstruction has some finer vessels apparent in the transverse view where small collaterals branch off the posterior aspects of the middle cerebral artery in the lateral fissure. On the other hand, the PD reconstruction has

Table 1. A pair-wise comparison between the different modalities, treating one as the ground truth and the other as the test data. See the text for an explanation of the measures computed.

Data Sets		Validation Measures			
Ground Truth	Test Data	kappa	ratio	alignment (voxels)	(mm)
PC	PD	0.84	0.80	0.95	0.48
TOF	PD	0.81	0.89	0.66	0.33
PD	PC	0.84	0.89	0.56	0.28
PD	TOF	0.81	0.74	0.60	0.30
PC	TOF	0.81	0.72	0.82	0.41
TOF	PC	0.81	0.94	0.88	0.44

more vasculature visible in the sagittal view with vessels branching off the callosal and supra-callosal arteries. The second and third column of Figure 3 indicate that the TOF reconstruction is missing a large number of vessel labels when compared to the PC and PD reconstructions.

3.3 Cross Validation

We now carry out a quantitative analysis of these segmentation results by computing a number of statistics between each pair of modalities, treating one as the ground truth data set and the other as the test data set. These comparisons are shown in Table 1 and include the following measures:

1. The kappa coefficient defined by $\frac{2a}{2a+b+c}$ where a is the number of red voxels, b is the number of green voxels and c the number of blue voxels. This measure tests the degree to which the agreement exceeds chance levels[2].
2. The ratio $\frac{a}{a+b}$, where a and b are as before. This measure indicates the degree to which the ground truth data is accounted for by the test data.
3. The alignment error, defined by taking the average of the Euclidean distance between each voxel in the ground truth data set and its closest voxel in the test data set (for the red voxels). This measure also indicates the degree to which the test data explains the ground truth data, but in terms of an average distance error.

It is clear from Table 1 that the vasculature obtained from the PD volume accounts for more than 80% of that obtained from either of the angiographic sequences. Furthermore a signficant proportion (over 25%) of vessel voxels recovered from the PD and PC volume are not seen in the TOF angiographic sequence. The results also indicate that the segmentations are closely aligned, with an average alignment error less than 0.5mm.

4 Conclusions

We have presented what to our knowledge is the first multi-scale geometric flow that can be applied for segmenting vasculature in proton density weighted MRI volumes. The key idea is to incorporate a multi-scale vesselness measure in the construction of an appropriate vector field for a geometric flow. We have performed a quantitative cross validation of the flow by applying the algorithm on PD, PC and TOF volumes obtained for the same subject and computing several measures. The results indicate that the vessels segmented from the PD data alone account for 80% and 89% of the vasculature segmented from PC and TOF angiographic data sets respectively, but also that over 25% of the vasculature obtained from the PD data are not recovered from either of the angiographic volumes. This suggests that our algorithm can be used to both improve upon the results obtained from angiographic data but also as a promising alternative when such data is not available, since the PD-weighted MRI data are often acquired when planning brain tumour surgery.

References

1. E. Bullitt, S. Aylward, A. Liu, J. Stone, S. K. Mukherjee, C. Coffey, G. Gerig, and S. M. Pizer. 3d graph description of the intracerebral vasculature from segmented mra and tests of accuracy by comparison with x-ray angiograms. In *Information Processing in Medical Imaging*, pages 308–321, 1999.
2. L. R. Dice. Measures of the amount of ecologic association between species. *Ecology*, 26(3):297–302, 1945.
3. A. Frangi, W. Niessen, K. L. Vincken, and M. A. Viergever. Multiscale vessel enhancement filtering. In *MICCAI'98*, pages 130–137, 1998.
4. M. Grayson. The heat equation shrinks embedded plane curves to round points. *Journal of Differential Geometry*, 26:285–314, 1987.
5. T. M. Koller, G. Gerig, G. Székely, and D. Dettwiler. Multiscale detection of curvilinear structures in 2-d and 3-d image data. In *International Conference On Computer Vision*, pages 864–869, 1995.
6. K. Krissian, G. Malandain, and N. Ayache. Model-based detection of tubular structures in 3d images. *Computer Vision and Image Understanding*, 80(2):130–171, November 2000.
7. T. Lindeberg. Edge detection and ridge detection with automatic scale selection. *International Journal of Computer Vision*, 30(2):77–116, 1998.
8. C. Lorenz, I. Carlsen, T. Buzug, C. Fassnacht, and J. Weese. Multi-scale line segmentation with automatic estimation of width, contrast and tangential direction in 2d and 3d medical images. In *CVRMED-MRCAS'97, Lecture Notes in Computer Science*, volume 1205, pages 233–242, 1997.
9. L. M. Lorigo, O. D. Faugeras, E. L. Grimson, R. Keriven, R. Kikinis, A. Nabavi, and C.-F. Westin. Curves: Curve evolution for vessel segmentation. *Medical Image Analysis*, 5:195–206, 2001.
10. T. McInerney and D. Terzopoulos. T-snakes: Topology adaptive snakes. *Medical Image Analysis*, 4:73–91, 2000.
11. S. J. Osher and J. A. Sethian. Fronts propagating with curvature dependent speed: Algorithms based on hamilton-jacobi formulations. *Journal of Computational Physics*, 79:12–49, 1988.
12. L. Ostergaard, O. Larsen, G. Goualher, A. Evans, and D. Collins. Extraction of cerebral vasculature from mri. In *9th Danish Conference on Pattern Recognition and Image Analysis*, 2000.
13. Y. Sato, S. Nakajima, N. Shiraga, H. Atsumi, S. Yoshida, T. Koller, G. Gerig, and R. Kikinis. 3d multi-scale line filter for segmentation and visualization of curvilinear structures in medical images. *Medical Image Analysis*, 2(2):143–168, 1998.
14. A. Vasilevskyi and K. Siddiqi. Flux maximizing geometric flows. *IEEE Transactions on Pattern Analysis and Machine Intelligence*, 24(12):1–14, 2002.

Accurate Quantification of Small-Diameter Tubular Structures in Isotropic CT Volume Data Based on Multiscale Line Filter Responses

Yoshinobu Sato[1], Shuji Yamamoto[2], and Shinichi Tamura[1]

[1] Division of Interdisciplinary Image Analysis
Osaka University Graduate School of Medicine, Japan
yoshi@image.med.osaka-u.ac.jp, http://www.image.med.osaka-u.ac.jp/yoshi
[2] Department of Radiology, Osaka University Hospital, Japan

Abstract. A method fully utilizing multiscale line filter responses is presented to estimate the point spread function (PSF) of a CT scanner and diameters of small tubular structures based on the PSF. The estimation problem is formulated as a least square fitting of a sequence of multiscale responses obtained at each medial axis point to the precomputed multiscale response curve for the ideal line model. The method was validated through phantom experiments and demonstrated to accurately measure small-diameter structures which are significantly overestimated by conventional methods based on the full width half maximum (FWHM) and zero-crossing edge detection.

1 Introduction

Diameter measurement of tubular structures in 3D medical data is an essential tool for quantitative evaluations of blood vessels, bronchial airways, and other similar anatomical structures. A typical method is to extract medial axes of the structures and then quantitate the width of the contour of cross-section orthogonal to the axis [1],[2],[3]. The diameters of small-diameter structures are known to be overestimated when they are measured based on the cross-sectional contours [3]. There are inherent limits on the accuracy of diameter measurement due to finite resolution of imaging scanners [4] and blurring involved in edge detectors. The influences of these limits are also discussed on thickness measurement of thin sheet structures [5],[6],[7]. In order to overcome these limits, Reinhardt *et al.* [8] incorporated the effects of the point spread function (PSF) of an imaging scanner into a measurement procedure for two diameters of the cross-sectional pattern specific to bronchial airways based on model fitting of one-dimensional original intensity profiles. Its main drawbacks, however, are as follows.

- The PSF width is assumed to be known.
- The direct use of the original intensity profiles is sensitive to noise.

In this paper, we propose a method for measurement of small-diameter tubular structures based on model fitting of multiscale Gaussian blurred second derivatives along intensity ridges. The proposed method has the following advantages.

C. Barillot, D.R. Haynor, and P. Hellier (Eds.): MICCAI 2004, LNCS 3216, pp. 508–515, 2004.
© Springer-Verlag Berlin Heidelberg 2004

- The PSF width is estimated in the method, and thus any pre-calibration process is unnecessary.
- The use of Gaussian blurred responses along intensity ridges is expected to be relatively insensitive to noise.
- Scale-dependent constraints can be incorporated into a measurement procedure so as to improve the measurement accuracy and stability.

In our current formulation, it is assumed that 3D data sets are acquired from a CT scanner whose PSF is approximated by an isotropic Gaussian function and the cross section of tubular structure is approximated by a pill-box function (although either of these assumptions can be potentially removed). We compare the proposed method with the full width half maximum (FWHM) measure and diameter measurement based on zero-crossing contours of cross-sections.

2   Method

2.1   Modeling Multiscale Line Filter Response of Ideal 3D Line

A 3D tubular structure (line) orthogonal to the xy-plane is modeled as

$$\text{Line}(\boldsymbol{x}; D) = \text{Pill-Box}(x, y; D), \tag{1}$$

where $\boldsymbol{x} = (x, y, z)^\top$, D is the line diameter, and

$$\text{Pill-Box}(x, y; D) = \begin{cases} 1 & \sqrt{x^2 + y^2} < \frac{D}{2} \\ 0 & \sqrt{x^2 + y^2} > \frac{D}{2} \end{cases}. \tag{2}$$

Here, line structures are assumed to be brighter than surrounding regions.

The point spread function (PSF) of a CT scanner is assumed to be described by $\text{Gauss}(\boldsymbol{x}; \sigma_{psf})$, where $\text{Gauss}(\boldsymbol{x}; \sigma)$ is the isotropic 3D Gaussian function, and σ_{psf} denotes the PSF width. The intensity function of 3D data, $f_{line}(\boldsymbol{x}; D, \sigma_{psf})$, of line diameter D imaged by a CT scanner of PSF width σ_{psf} is given by

$$f_{line}(\boldsymbol{x}; D, \sigma_{psf}) = \text{Line}(\boldsymbol{x}; D) * \text{Gauss}(\boldsymbol{x}; \sigma_{psf}), \tag{3}$$

where $*$ denotes the convolution operation.

When the Gaussian filters are applied to the acquired 3D data by post-processing, the Gaussian filtered 3D data of a line are described by

$$f_{line}(\boldsymbol{x}; D, \sigma_{psf}, \sigma_f) = \text{Line}(\boldsymbol{x}; D) * \text{Gauss}(\boldsymbol{x}; \sigma_{psf}) * \text{Gauss}(\boldsymbol{x}; \sigma_f), \tag{4}$$

where σ_f is the filter width. The Gaussian filtered line with intensity height H is described by $H \cdot f_{line}(\boldsymbol{x}; D, \sigma_{psf}, \sigma_f)$. In our problem, D, H, and σ_{psf} are unknown and need to be estimated from 3D data while σ_f is known.

In the proposed approach, we fully utilize the scale-dependency of the line filter responses in order to estimate line diameter D as well as PSF width σ_{psf}

and line height H. We consider the line filter responses, $R(\sigma; D)$, of the ideal 3D line at the line axis, that is, $\boldsymbol{x} = (0, 0, z)$, which is given by

$$R(\sigma; D) = \sigma^2 \cdot \frac{\partial^2}{\partial x^2} f_{line}(0, 0, z; D, \sigma_{psf}, \sigma_f), \qquad (5)$$

where $\sigma = \sqrt{\sigma_{psf}^2 + \sigma_f^2}$. As shown in the previous work [9], σ^2 is multiplied for scale-normalization of the responses. Given D, σ_{psf}, and σ_f, $R(\sigma; D)$ can be calculated using Eq. (5). Fig. 1 shows an example of $R(\sigma; D)$ calculated numerical simulation.

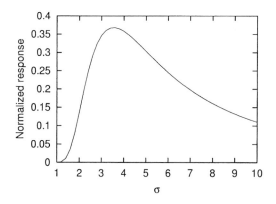

Fig. 1. Normalized line filter responses, $R(\sigma; D)$, of ideal 3D line at line axis. This plot shows $R(\sigma; D)$ for $D = 10$. Normalized line filter responses have the maximum when $\sigma = 0.36D$ for line structures with a pill-box cross-section.

2.2   Extracting a Sequence of Multiscale Line Filter Responses on Medial Axis from 3D Data

A method for localizing the medial axis element [3] is summarized, and then a procedure for extracting a sequence of multiscale filter responses on each medial axis element is described. Hereafter, we call the axis element "*axel*". It should be noted that the *axels* are not grouped and only fragmentally detected at each voxel.

Let the intensity function of Gaussian filtered 3D data be $f(\boldsymbol{x}; \sigma_{psf}, \sigma_f)$ or $f(\boldsymbol{x}; \sigma)$, where $\sigma = \sqrt{\sigma_{psf}^2 + \sigma_f^2}$. The gradient vector of $f(\boldsymbol{x}; \sigma)$ is defined as $\nabla f(\boldsymbol{x}; \sigma) = (f_x(\boldsymbol{x}; \sigma), f_y(\boldsymbol{x}; \sigma), f_z(\boldsymbol{x}; \sigma))^\top$, where partial derivatives of $f(\boldsymbol{x}; \sigma)$ are represented as $f_x(\boldsymbol{x}; \sigma) = \frac{\partial}{\partial x} f(\boldsymbol{x}; \sigma)$, and so on. The Hessian matrix of $f(\boldsymbol{x}; \sigma)$ is given by

$$\nabla^2 f(\boldsymbol{x}; \sigma) = \begin{bmatrix} f_{xx}(\boldsymbol{x}; \sigma) & f_{xy}(\boldsymbol{x}; \sigma) & f_{xz}(\boldsymbol{x}; \sigma) \\ f_{yx}(\boldsymbol{x}; \sigma) & f_{yy}(\boldsymbol{x}; \sigma) & f_{yz}(\boldsymbol{x}; \sigma) \\ f_{zx}(\boldsymbol{x}; \sigma) & f_{zy}(\boldsymbol{x}; \sigma) & f_{zz}(\boldsymbol{x}; \sigma) \end{bmatrix}, \qquad (6)$$

where partial second derivatives of $f(x; \sigma)$ are represented as $f_{xx}(x; \sigma) = \frac{\partial^2}{\partial x^2} f(x; \sigma)$, $f_{yz}(x; \sigma) = \frac{\partial^2}{\partial y \partial z} f(x; \sigma)$, and so on.

Let the eigenvalues of $\nabla^2 f(x; \sigma)$ be $\lambda_1, \lambda_2, \lambda_3$ ($\lambda_1 \geq \lambda_2 \geq \lambda_3$) and their corresponding eigenvectors be e_1, e_2, e_3 ($|e_1| = |e_2| = |e_3| = 1$), respectively. e_1 is expected to give the tangential direction of the line and the line filter response is obtained as the combination of λ_2 and λ_3 [9], directional second derivatives orthogonal to e_1.

We assume that the tangential direction of line is given by e_1 at the voxel around the medial axis. The 2-D intensity function, $c(u)$ ($u = (u, v)^\top$), on the cross-sectional plane of $f(x; \sigma)$ orthogonal to e_1, should have its peak on the medial axis. The second-order local approximation of $c(u)$ is given by

$$c(u) = f(x_0; \sigma) + u^\top \nabla c_0 + \frac{1}{2} u^\top \nabla^2 c_0 u, \tag{7}$$

where $u e_2 + v e_3 = x - x_0$, $\nabla c_0 = (\nabla f \cdot e_2, \nabla f \cdot e_3)^\top$ (∇f is the gradient vector, that is, $\nabla f(x_0; \sigma)$), and

$$\nabla^2 c_0 = \begin{bmatrix} \lambda_2 & 0 \\ 0 & \lambda_3 \end{bmatrix}. \tag{8}$$

$c(u)$ should have its peak on the medial axis of the line. The peak is located at the position satisfying

$$\frac{\partial}{\partial u} c(u) = 0 \quad \text{and} \quad \frac{\partial}{\partial v} c(u) = 0. \tag{9}$$

By solving Eq. (9), we have the offset vector, $p = (p_x, p_y, p_z)^\top$, of the peak position from x_0 given by $p = s e_2 + t e_3$, where $s = -\frac{\nabla f \cdot e_2}{\lambda_2}$ and $t = -\frac{\nabla f \cdot e_3}{\lambda_3}$. For the medial axis to exist at the voxel x_0, the peak of $c(u)$ needs to be located in the territory of voxel x_0. Thus, the medial axis element, that is, medial axel, is detected only if $|p_x| \leq 0.5$ & $|p_y| \leq 0.5$ & $|p_z| \leq 0.5$ (voxels). By combining the voxel position x_0 and offset vector p, the medial axel is localized at subvoxel resolution.

We define the line filter response as $\sigma_f^2 \sqrt{\lambda_2 \lambda_3}$ in this paper, where σ_f^2 is multiplied to normalize the responses (although additional normalization will be incorporated in the later section when the PSF is considered). A sequence of multiscale line filter responses, R_i, of different filter widths σ_{f_i} ($i = 1, 2, 3, ...$) is extracted at each detected medial axel as follows.

1. The medial axel detection and line filtering are performed at different scales σ_{f_i} ($i = 1, 2, 3, ..., n$).
2. The medial axel having the strongest line filter response is selected among all the detected axels irrespective to scales. Let the strongest axel be found at x_0 of $\sigma_{f_{i_0}}$.
3. The axels nearest and within one-voxel distance to position x_0 are extracted at adjacent scales $\sigma_{f_{i_0}+1}$ and $\sigma_{f_{i_0}-1}$. Similarly, the axels are extracted in larger and smaller scales until no axels are found.
4. The above three steps are repeated for the axels to be extracted until all the axels are completed.

2.3   Estimation Processes

The basic strategy is to find D, H, and σ_{psf} minimizing the square sum of differences between the model $H \cdot R(\sigma; D)$ (more precisely, $H \cdot R(\sqrt{\sigma_{psf}^2 + \sigma_f^2}; D)$) and the data set at each axel, that is, a sequence of multiscale line filter responses, R_i, of different filter widths σ_{f_i} $(i = i_s, ...i_e)$ where i_s and i_ℓ are the smallest and largest scales, respectively, in the sequence at the axel of interest.

   The estimation processes consist of two stages. During the first stage, σ_{psf} and H are estimated using the axels which have relatively large diameters and whose positions are close to the voxel center. During the second stage, D is estimated for every sequence of multiscale filter responses using σ_{psf} and H estimated in the first stage.

Estimating PSF of CT imaging and intensity height of line. To accurately estimate PSF width σ_{psf} and intensity height H, R_i needs to be fit to the model $R(\sigma; D)$ in a wide range of scale σ including the range around maximum values of $R(\sigma; D)$. Furthermore, the axel position localized in subvoxel accuracy should be close to the voxel center to guarantee the response is the peak response or close to it. We selected the sequences satisfying the following conditions.

1. $i_t < \arg\max_i R_i$, where $\sigma_{f_{i_t}}$ should be sufficiently large (at least twice as large as the minimum filter scale σ_{f_1}).
2. $\sqrt{|p_x|^2 + |p_y|^2 + |p_z|^2} < d_t$, where d_t is a constant representing the maximum distance to the voxel center to be allowed. In the experiment, we used $d_t = 0.3$ (voxels).

   For the sequences of multiscale filter responses satisfying the above conditions, σ_{psf}, D, and H are searched which minimize

$$E_1(\sigma_{psf}, H, D) = \sum_{i=i_s}^{i_\ell} \{H \cdot R(\sqrt{\sigma_{psf}^2 + \sigma_{f_i}^2}; D) - \frac{\sigma_{psf}^2 + \sigma_{f_i}^2}{\sigma_{f_i}^2} R_i\}^2, \qquad (10)$$

where i_s and i_ℓ are the smallest and largest scales in the extracted sequence of multiscale filter responses at the axel of interest.

   In the experiments, exhaustive search was applied to D and σ_{psf}. D was discretized from 0.02 to 24.0 voxels with 0.02 voxel interval, and σ_{psf} was discretized from 0.02 to 4.0 voxel with 0.02 voxel interval. For all the combinations of discretized D and σ_{psf}, H was estimated by minimizing Eq. (10). With known D and σ_{psf}, the estimation of H minimizing Eq. (10) is formulated as a linear square problem. Thus, D, σ_{psf}, and H are obtained for each sequence of multiscale responses. We assume that σ_{psf} and H are not locally variable. σ_{psf} and H are obtained as averages of all the results from the sequences of multiscale responses considered at this stage.

Diameter estimation. For all the extracted sequences of multiscale filter responses, using known H and σ_{psf}, D is searched minimizing

$$E_2(D) = \sum_{i=i_s}^{i_\ell} \{H \cdot R(\sigma; D) - \frac{\sigma^2}{\sigma_{f_i}^2} R_i\}^2, \tag{11}$$

where $\sigma = \sqrt{\sigma_{psf}^2 + \sigma_{f_i}^2}$. In the experiments, exhaustive search was applied to D. D was discretized from 0.02 to 24.0 voxels with 0.02 voxel interval,

3   Results

CT volume data of several diameters of acrylic rods were acquired using a Toshiba Aquilion CT scanner. Isotropic voxel imaging was performed with voxel size of 0.5 mm^3. The diameters of acrylic rods were 3.0, 1.6, 1.0, 0.75, and 0.5 mm. A cross-sectional image in the yz-plane of the acquired CT data and its volume rendered image are shown in Fig. 2(a). The rods were straight and the angle of their axes was approximately 20 degrees to the xy-plane of the CT coordinate system. The volume data were trimmed and sinc-interpolated so that the voxel interval was 0.25 mm. The multiscale filter widths were $\sigma_{f_i} = 2^{\frac{i-1}{4}}$ (voxels), where $i = 1, 2, ..., 11$ (the voxel size is 0.25 mm^3).

The estimation results in the first stage were $\sigma_{psf} = 1.61$ (voxels) $= 0.40$ (mm) and $H = 1054$, where the voxel size was that of the interpolated volume data, that is, 0.25 mm^3. Fig. 2(b) shows the results of diameter estimation at the second stage. The averages and standard deviations of the experimentally estimated diameters of five rods are indicated in Fig. 2(b). Since the results of the proposed method were experimentally measured, the averages and standard deviations for diameters 3.0, 1.6, 1.0, 0.75, and 0.5 mm are indicated as error-bars. (The standard deviations were very small for diameters 3.0 and 1.6, and thus their error-bars collapsed.) The ideal relation was plotted as a dotted line. Fig. 2(b) also shows simulation results of the diameters estimated using full width half maximum (FWHM) and using zero-crossings of radial directional second derivatives orthogonal to medal axis. These results are plotted as dashed lines since they are numerically computed. In the simulations, $\sigma_{psf} = 0.40$ (mm) was used. In the simulations of zero-crossings, computation of second derivatives was assumed to be combined with Gaussian blurring of standard deviation of 1.2 (voxels) $= 0.3$ (mm). In diameter estimations using FWHM and zero-crossings, significant overestimation was observed when the actual diameter was 1.0 mm or less. In the proposed diameter estimation, accurate measurement was realized even for diameters 1.0 mm, 0.75 mm, and 0.5 mm.

4   Discussion and Conclusions

We have described a method for accurate measurement of small-diameter tubular structures. This work provides a unified approach based on multiscale filter

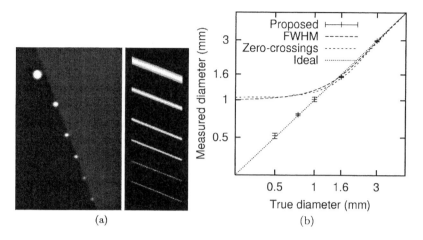

Fig. 2. Phantom experiments. (a) CT volume data of several diameters of acrylic rods. Cross-sectional image in the yz-plane (left) and volume rendered image (right). (b) Results of diameter measurement. Averages and standard deviations of experimentally estimated diameters of five rods using the proposed method are indicated as error-bars. The ideal relation is plotted as a dotted line. Estimated diameters based on full width half maximum (FWHM) and zero-crossing edge detection were numerically computed and are plotted as dashed lines.

responses to the estimation of the point spread function (PSF) of a CT scanner as well as the estimation of diameters. The method is validated through phantom experiments and demonstrated to accurately measure small-diameter structures which are significantly overestimated by conventional methods based on full width half maximum (FWHM) and zero-crossing edge detection.

Because the method is based on second derivatives, it is insensitive to the DC component, that is, the background level, of image intensity. However, inaccuracy in the estimated intensity height H may affect the estimated diameter accuracy (although previous methods based on FWHM and zero-crossings are insensitive to H). We are planning to quantitatively evaluate this effect. Future work will also include the effects of inaccuracy in the PSF width σ_{psf}. In this paper, we have assumed isotropic imaging and circular cross-section of the straight tubular structures on a uniform background. The validation needs to be completed on the robustness with respect to anisotropic resolution, non-circular cross-section, the curvature of the structure, and a non-uniform background. (The effects of curvatures on line filter responses were partly evaluated in [9].)

The proposed method is related to the heuristics that the scale at which the maximum normalized response is obtained is selected as the optimal scale of the tubular structures [9],[10],[11]. The optimal scale σ_{opt} is regarded as the true radius, that is, $\sigma_{opt} = 0.5D$, when cross-sectional intensity distributions are Gaussian [9], while the relation $\sigma_{opt} = 0.36D$ is observed when they have pill-box shapes (as shown in Fig. 1). In this heuristics, the effect of the imaging scanner PSF is not considered. When the effect of PSF is considered, the maximum response is inherently not obtainable for small-diameter structures which do not satisfy the condition $\frac{1}{0.36}\sigma_{psf} < D$. Further, the output of this heuristics is discrete. In the proposed method, by least square fitting of multiscale responses to the theoretical multiscale response curve, accurate, continuous estimates are obtained even for small-diameter structures not satisfying $\frac{1}{0.36}\sigma_{psf} < D$.

For clinical application, a multiscale tracking method for tubular structures in 3D data as described in [11] can be effectively combined with the proposed method. We are now developing a method for scale-space tracking of extracted axels to combine with the proposed method.

Acknowledgment. The authors would like to thank Dr. H. Shikata for the permission of using CT volume data of the acrylic rod phantom.

References

1. Frangi AF, Niessen WJ, Hoogeveen RM, *et al.*: Model-based quantitation of 3-D magnetic resonance angiographic images, *IEEE Trans Med Imaging*, 18(10):946-956, 1999.
2. Wink O, Niessen WJ, Viergever MA: Fast delineation and visualization of vessels in 3-D angiographic images, *IEEE Trans Med Imaging*, 19(4):337-346, 2000.
3. Sato Y, Tamuras S: Detection and quantification of line and sheet structures in 3-D images, *Lecture Notes in Computer Science (Proc. Third International Conference on Medical Image Computing and Computer Assisted Intervention (MICCAI2000)*, Pittsburgh, Pennsylvania), 1935: 154-165, 2000.
4. Hoogeveen RM, Bakker CJG, Viergever MA: Limits to the accuracy of vessel diameter measurement in MR angiography, *JMRI – J Magn Reson Imaging*, 8(6):1228–1235, 1998.
5. Prevrhal S, Engelke K, Kalender WA: Accuracy limits for the determination of cortical width and density: the influence of object size and CT imaging parameters, *Phys Med Biol*, 44(3):751–764, 1999.
6. Dougherty G and Newman DL: Measurement of thickness and density of thin structures by computed tomography: A simulation study, *Med Phys*, 25(7):1341-1348, 1999.
7. Sato Y, Tanaka H, Nishii T, *et al.*: Limits on the accuracy of 3D thickness measurement in magnetic resonance images — Effects of voxel anisotropy —, *IEEE Trans Med Imaging*, 22(9):1076-1088, 2003.
8. Reinhardt JM, D'Souza ND, Hoffman EA: Accurate measurement of intrathoracic airways *IEEE Trans Med Imaging*, 16(6):820-827, 1997.
9. Sato Y, Nakajima S, Shiraga N, *et al.*: Three dimensional multi-scale line filter for segmentation and visualization of curvilinear structures in medical images, *Med Image Anal*, 2(2):143-168, 1998.
10. Krissian K, Malandain G, Ayache, N, *et al.*: Model-based detection of tubular structures in 3D images, *Comput Vis Image Und*, 80(2):130-171, 2000.
11. Aylward SR, Bullitt E: Initialization, noise, singularities, and scale in height ridge traversal for tubular object centerline extraction, *IEEE Trans Med Imaging*, 21(2):61-75, 2002.

A Methodology for Validating a New Imaging Modality with Respect to a Gold Standard Imagery: Example of the Use of 3DRA and MRI for AVM Delineation

Marie-Odile Berger[1], René Anxionnat[1,2], and Erwan Kerrien[1]

[1] LORIA/INRIA Lorraine, France
[2] CHU Nancy, France
{berger,anxionna,kerrien}@loria.fr

Abstract. Various medical treatments require an accurate determination of the shape of a considered anatomic structure. The shape is often recovered from several delineations performed on a two-dimensional gold standard imagery. Using true 3D imagery is attractive to supplement this gold standard. However, before using 3D modalities in clinical routine, it must be proved that these modalities are well suited to the delineation task. We propose in this paper a methodology for validating a new imaging modality with respect to a reference imagery.

1 Introduction

Numerous clinical treatments, such as radiotherapy, require an accurate definition of the true three-dimensional size and shape of a given anatomic structure. Depending on the pathology, a reference imagery, so-called Gold Standard imagery, is classically used by physicians for the definition of the target. Other imaging modalities, especially emerging modalities, may complement this reference imagery to better understand the architecture of the targeted organ. However, prior to using these modalities for the delineation task, it must be proved that they bring more than or at least equal information to the reference imagery.

This paper focuses on the case where the reference imagery is two-dimensional. This is especially true for vascular imaging (cardiology, neurology,...) where 2D angiographic (DSA) images are still the gold standard. The difficulty of obtaining a good approximation of the shape from its delineation in a small number of views is well known. For this reason, several groups have reverted to using true three dimensional data from either computed tomography (CT) or magnetic resonance imaging (MRI). Unfortunately, these 3D modalities present with a lower spatial and temporal resolution than conventional DSA. A better identification of vascular structures in these images is therefore not guaranteed. This important problem of validating the use of a new imaging modality using standardized protocols has been little addressed in the literature.

In this paper, we propose a methodology for validating a new 3D image modality with respect to a Gold Standard imagery in the clinical context of the

C. Barillot, D.R. Haynor, and P. Hellier (Eds.): MICCAI 2004, LNCS 3216, pp. 516–524, 2004.

delineation task of a target. This methodology is applied to validate the use of 3D image modalities to delineate cerebral arteriovenous malformation (AVM). The clinical context of this application is depicted in section 2. The overall methodology is described in section 3. Application of our framework to the use of 3D rotational angiography (3DRA) and magnetic resonance imaging (MRI) for AVM delineation is shown in section 4.

2   Clinical Context

The efficiency of our methodology is illustrated by the clinical problem of cerebral arteriovenous malformation delineation. A cerebral arteriovenous malformation (AVM) is defined as a localized arteriovenous shunt consisting of a tangle of capillaries and veins, also called nidus. The treatment of complex AVMs is classically a two stage process. Embolization or endovascular treatment is first performed. It reduces the size of the AVM but is usually not sufficient to cure it completely. This step is then followed by a stereotactic irradiation of the remnant through the intact skull. Therefore, accurate definition of the target is of crucial importance for the efficacy of the treatment.

For many years, 2D angiography has been the gold standard for the diagnosis and the delineation of the AVMs: the AVM is delineated in at least two calibrated views and the volume of interest is limited by the intersection of X-ray cones defined by each delineation [7]. This method only provides an approximation of the shape since only a small number of views is allowable (from 2 to 5 views), due to clinical and technical limitations. This procedure overestimates the volume, by an amount depending on the shape of the AVM and on the considered viewpoints (Fig. 1).

For these reasons, several groups have attempted to supplement conventional angiography with true 3D data for defining the vascular lesion: MRI helps to exclude vulnerable tissues, MR angiography is a fast, non invasive 3D imaging that provides information on vascular and parenchymal brain anatomy important for optimal dose planning [6,5]. 3DRA has been also used for AVM delineation with promising results [3]. In all these studies, the evaluation often rests on a visual inspection of the delineations and is thus partly subjective. The volume of the target derived from different modalites also often grounds the comparison: because the AVM size is somewhat overestimated in angiography and to avoid irradiation of safe tissues, methods leading to the smallest volumes are preferred. Unfortunately, though unnecessary irradiation of adjacent safe tissue is important to avoid, the reduction of the volume does not necessarily prove that the complete detection of the nidus has been achieved.

All these modalities have a lower temporal resolution than conventional angiography. Though the use of a 3D modality theoretically allows us to increase the accuracy on the target, it must be proved that the information available in the volume effectively allows for a complete detection of the nidus. Indeed, nidus are identified from the arterial phase, just as the draining vein begins to fill. As all the considered 3D modality are acquired during the whole progression of the opaque mixture (around 5 seconds for 3DRA, much more for MRA), it is not

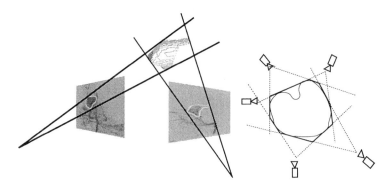

Fig. 1. AVM reconstruction using conventional angiography.

clear whether all the parts of the nidus will be appearant in the 3D images, in particular those presenting with a fast blood flow.

If the development of MR and 3DRA will no doubt improve the evaluation of the AVM in the near future, a meticulous assessment of both the target delineation and the treatment outcome has to be performed. This problem has not yet been studied in the medical community and we propose in the next section a general methodology to this aim.

3   Methodology

3.1   Evaluating the Relevance

This section addresses the general problem of validating a 3D modality with respect to a 2D reference imagery. The shape inferred from the 3D modality (which is called *new 3D shape* in the following) must be proven better than or at least as good as the shape inferred from the reference imagery. Phantoms are commonly used to compare imaging modalities. However, no phantom currently enables a realistic simulation of the complexity of the vascular phenomena occuring in the nidus.

In the absence of ground truth, the only standards available to assess the quality of a new 3D shape are the delineations produced by expert observers in the 2D reference imagery. Comparison can be achieved either directly in 2D - by comparing the projection of the new shape to the expert curves in each reference image - or in 3D. In this latter case, the shape delineated in the 3D modality must be compared to the 3D shape recovered from expert delineations, which is only a rough approximation of the actual shape due to the small number of considered views. In addition, delineating a vascular structure is a difficult task especially when some parts of the boundary are hidden by vessels superposition. Such difficulties prevent from delineating the true boundary and lead to inaccurate reconstruction. Hence, direct comparison in 3D is not well founded.

We therefore propose to validate the use of a 3D imaging modality by a direct comparison of the projected shape with experts delineations. The problem of evaluating a curve with respect to expert delineations was previously addressed in [2]. Their methodology strongly relied on the existence of a metric between curves which is supposed to reflect their similarity. In our clinical application, preliminary investigations indicated that manual delineations suffer from observer bias and large inter and intra-observer variability [1] (Fig. 2): large consensus areas alternate with high variability areas, preventing us from defining a reliable metric between curves and to use [2]. Fortunately, a statistical model of the variability derived from the set of expert curves can be computed [4]: it is then possible to learn what are plausible variations in the shapes and what are not, allowing us to check if a projected shape is compatible with expert delineations.

3.2   Building a Statistical Shape Model

Statistical shape models were introduced by Cootes [4] in order to capture variability in shape. Such a models is built by analyzing shape variations over a training set of 2D curves $C_{i\{1 \leq i \leq N\}}$ drawn by experts. Dense correspondences were established using a semi-interactive interface. A curve C_i is represented with a set of n 2D points $C_i = (x_i^1, ..., x_i^n)$. Let $\bar{C} = \frac{1}{N} \sum_{i=1}^{i=N} C_i$ be the mean of the curves, computed from point-to-point correspondences, and $S = \frac{1}{N-1} \sum (C_i - \bar{C})(C_i - \bar{C})^t$ be the covariance of the data. Following Cootes [4], a linear eigen-model can be built through a principal component analysis (PCA) that provides the t principal modes of variation. These modes are represented by the $N \times t$ matrix P of eigenvectors of S corresponding to the t largest eigenvalues. A particular curve C is then approximated by:

$$C \approx C' = \bar{C} + Pb \qquad \text{where } b = P^t(C - \bar{C}) \tag{1}$$

The squared error on this approximation is therefore:

$$r^2(C) = ||C - C'||^2 = (C - \bar{C})^t(C - \bar{C}) - b^t b \tag{2}$$

The value of t is classically chosen so that the model represents a suitable proportion of the variation in the training set (95%).

3.3   A Framework for Validation

The relevance of a 3D imaging modality is estimated by comparing the shape recovered with this modality to the statistical 2D shape model built from a set of experts in the same viewing conditions. A two stage process is proposed:

1. **Building the database and the statistical models.** A set of patients is considered. The standard clinical technique is used and 2D calibrated images are acquired using the reference modality. N_e experts delineate the shape in each view and a statistical model of the 2D shape is built from these expert delineations for each view.

2. **Validating the 3D modality.** The projection of the new 3D shape is computed with the same viewing parameters as used for the acquisition of the reference images. Each obtained 2D shape is then tested to check if it can be considered as an instance of the statistical model built from the experts.

The second stage requires to decide how a new delineation matches the model. A first measure of the quality of fit is classically deduced from the PCA:

$$fit_1(\mathcal{C}) = \sum_{i=1}^{i=t} \frac{b_i^2}{\lambda_i} \tag{3}$$

where λ_i is the i-th largest eigenvalue in the PCA and $b = (b_i)$. This criterion only measures the distance of the shape from the mean along the modes of the model but it does not consider the distance of the delineation from the linear model given by the residual in eq. 2.

To cope with this problem, a complementary measure must be defined to decide if this residual is compatible with the delineations of the experts $\{\mathcal{C}_e\}_{e \in Experts}$ for a given reference view. Any measure which involves $\{r(\mathcal{C}_e)\}_{e \in Experts}$ is not a convenient measure of the performance of the model because it comes down to estimate the model from data which were used to build the model. A better measure is given by cross-validation and especially miss-one-out experiments: for each expert e, a reduced PCA model is built from all the data except $\mathcal{C}_e$. The residual of this reduced PCA is denoted r_e. $r_e^2(\mathcal{C}_e)$ is thus a good measure of the compatibility of a given expert with the others. Estimating the compatibility of a new curve $\mathcal{C}$ is then better achieved by comparing $r_e^2(\mathcal{C})$ with $r_e^2(\mathcal{C}_e)$ on the set of experts. Therefore, we propose to statistically assess a delineation $\mathcal{C}$ using:

$$fit_2(\mathcal{C}) = \frac{\sum_{e \in Expert} r_e^2(\mathcal{C})}{\sum_{e \in Expert} r_e^2(\mathcal{C}_e)} \tag{4}$$

The complete measure of fit is then defined as the sum $fit(\mathcal{C}) = fit_1(\mathcal{C}) + fit_2(\mathcal{C})$. In order to design a statistical test for acceptance/rejection of new delineations, the distribution of the measure of fit must be studied on the particular clinical application. Using bootstrap techniques [4], we found experimentally that the distribution of fit for AVM detection could be modeled with a χ square distribution with t degrees of freedom.

4   Validating 3D Modalities for AVM Delineation

4.1   Clinical Material

Twelve patients with AVM were treated using embolization and radiotherapy at Nancy University Hospital (France). According to the complexity of the AVM shape, between 2 to 5 2DSA views were considered for delineation (antero-posterior, lateral and oblique views). Overall, 45 2DSA images were available

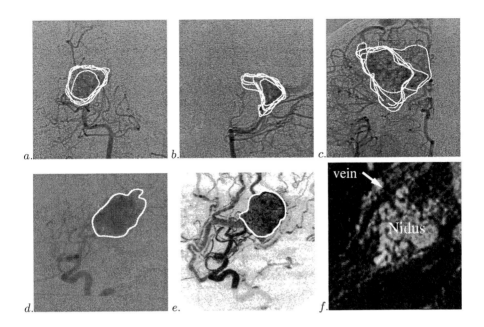

Fig. 2. Angiographic views of AVMs
First raw: Examples of AVM delineation realized by the experts for 2D angiographic views for type A (a and b) and type B (c) AVMs. **Second raw**: Example of (d) an original 2DSA view and (e) the MIP view computed from 3DRA along with the expert delineations. (f) is a slice of the 3DRA volume through the AVM.

for this study. In addition, the 3DRA and the MRI volumes were available for each patient. These images were acquired in stereotactic conditions, allowing for 2DSA/3DRA/MRI image registration.

The AVMs considered in this study were complex pathological cases. In order to assess a possible bias due to inner medical difficulties, each AVM was labelled with A or B according to the complexity of the delineation task: type A is for fairly difficult AVMs (5 patients) whereas type B is for very difficult AVMs (7 patients).

Three experts in interventional neuroradiology from Nancy University Hospital (France) and Karolinska Institute (Stockholm, Sweden) were involved in this study. They manually delineated the AVMs twice on the 45 2DSA images.

3D Rotational angiography. 3DRA is a new emerging imaging modality [8] and physicians are used to analyzing this volume using 3D rendering techniques, such as MIP (Maximum Intensity Projection). However, they are unable to delineate the shape directly in 3D because the appearance of one slice does not allow them to identify the nidus properly (Fig.2.f). Hence, for each patient, MIP images of the 3DRA were generated with the same viewing parameters as the original 2DSA images. An example of a MIP view, together with the original

2DSA image are shown in Fig. 2.d,e. The same three experts were asked to delineate the AVMs in these MIP views. These contours were then tested using the statistical model built from the six experts delineations.

MRI modality. Though used by several groups for AVM delineations [6,5], the clinical superiority of MRI over DSA has never been proved. These previous experimental studies concerned small patient series. They suggest that MR can be of great value in widening radiosurgical indications to large AVM but seems inadequate for previously embolized AVMs. Our results will partly confirm these impressions. Our three experts delineated the AVMs slice by slice to get the 3D shapes. These shapes were then projected onto the reference views.

4.2   Results

Validating the Use of 3DRA

Results are summarized in table 1 which indicates the acceptance rate of the MIP contours on the whole database (type A and B) and on type A AVMs. As in section 3.3, these results are compared to the acceptance rate of each expert curve when compared to the statistical model built from the other experts.

For type A AVMs, the results are equivalent for DSA and for 3DRA, proving that 3DRA can be used for nidus delineation. On the other hand, delineations are not equivalent for type B AVMs. Differences mainly originate in the large size of type B AVMs and in multiple vessels superposition in 2D, making the true boundary very difficult to assess in a single 2D view. Fortunately, the use of several views often allows us to get a fair target reconstruction despite these errors: an erroneous part delineated in one view is often removed by a contour drawn in another view due to cone intersections (Fig. 3.a). Hence, a more coherent database is given by the reprojection of the 3D shape recovered from expert delineations onto the reference images (see Fig. 3).

Results of the evaluation of 3DRA against this new database are given in Table 2. The global acceptance rates are nearly similar for both modalities. Though the imaging set up for large AVMs must certainly be improved to get a better image quality, these results still prove that 3DRA can be used for AVM delineation.

Validating the Use of MRI Modality

The validation framework was also applied to assess MRI images. The contours were considered in our statistical framework with the same confidence as for 3DRA (95 %). Table 2 shows that globally, only 44% of the contours were accepted. This rate improved to 60% for type A AVMs. It must be noted that the difficulty of the delineation task depends on the considered image modality. Only 3 AVMs were considered as fairly difficult (type A) for MRI delineation. They were also classified type A in DSA. For type A AVMs, the volume recovered from DSA and MRI are quite similar. On the contrary, the volume computed for type B AVMs are significantly larger than those computed from DSA. A careful examination of the target proves that previously embolized areas are included in the MRI delineations. The large number of previously embolized patients in our dataset (10/11) thus explains these poor results. This study proves that

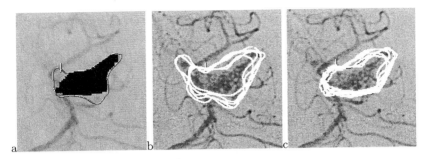

Fig. 3. (a)Reprojection of the recovered 3D shape on a reference image in black along with the expert delineation.(b) The set of expert curve delineations. (c) The new database using the reprojection of the 3D shape recovered from expert delineations for the same view.

MRI cannot be used alone for AVM delineation for previously embolized AVMs. Though this study should be extended to incorporate more non embolized AVMs, these results also tend to prove that the delineation of the nidus in MRI and DSA presents a similar level of difficulty for simple non embolized AVMs.

Table 1. Acceptance rate of 3DSA contours compared to the acceptance rate of 2DSA contours computed by cross validation.

Contours	global acceptance rate (type A & B)	acceptance for type A AVMs
2DSA	77.5%	77%
3DRA	64%	76%

Table 2. Acceptance rate of 3DSA and MRI contours with the corrected database.

Contours	global acceptance rate (type A & B)	acceptance for type A AVMs
2DSA	83%	85%
3DRA	77%	83%
MRI	44 %	60 %

5   Conclusion

In this paper, we have proposed a methodology for validating a new imaging modality with respect to a reference imagery. We have applied this protocol to prove that 3DRA can be used for AVM delineation. We believe that the objective and quantitative evaluation of new image modalites is an important step toward their acceptance in clinical use. We are currently investigating the use of 3DRA to improve AVM delineation through the definition of virtual 2D views which can be generated from the 3DRA volume for any position. Hence, the physician could potentially use an arbitrary number of views to delineate the AVM without further dose exposure for the patient.

References

1. R. Anxionnat, M-O. Berger, E. Kerrien, S. Bracard, and L. Picard. Intra- and inter-observer variability in the angiographic delineation of brain arterio-venous malformations (AVM). In *CARS, London (UK)*,1297–1298, 2003.
2. V. Chalana and Y. Kim. A methodology for evaluation of boundary detection algorithms on medical images. *IEEE Trans. Med. Imag.*, 16(5):642–652, 1997.
3. F. Colombo, C. Cavedon, P. Francescon, L. Casentini, U. Fornezza, L. castellan, F. Causin, and S. Perini. Three-dimensional angiography for radiosurgical treatment planning for AVMs. *Journal of Neurosurgery*, 98:536–543, 2003.
4. T. Cootes, C. Page, C. Jackson, and C. Taylor. Statistical grey-level models for object location and identification. *Image and Vision Computing*, 14:533–540, 1996.
5. W. Guo. Application of MR in Stereotactic Radiosurgery. *JMRI*, 8:415–420, 1998.
6. Douglas Kondziolka, Dade Lunsford, Emanuel Kanal, and lalith Talagala. Stereotactic magnetic resonance angiography for targeting in arteriovenous malformations radiosurgery. *Neurosurgery*, 35:585–591, 1994.
7. M. Soderman, B. Karlsson, L. Launay, B. Thuresson, and K. Ericson. Volume measurement of cerebral arteriovenous malformations from angiography. *Neuroradiology*, 42:697–702, 2000.
8. K. Wiesent, K. Barth, N. Navab, P. Durlak, T. Brunner, O. Schuetz, and W. Seissler. Enhanced 3-d- Reconstruction Algorithm for C-Arm Systems Suitable for Interventional Procedures. *IEEE Transations on Medical Imaging*, 19(5):391–403, 2000.

VAMPIRE: Improved Method for Automated Center Lumen Line Definition in Atherosclerotic Carotid Arteries in CTA Data

H.A.F. Gratama van Andel, E. Meijering, A. van der Lugt,
H.A. Vrooman, and R. Stokking*

Biomedical Imaging Group Rotterdam
Erasmus MC – University Medical Center Rotterdam
Departments of Medical Informatics and Radiology
P.O. Box 1738, 3000 DR Rotterdam, The Netherlands
* Corresponding Author, Tel.: +31-10-4088187
r.stokking@erasmusmc.nl

Abstract. We evaluate a new method, called VAMPIRE, for automated definition of a center lumen line in vessels in cardiovascular image data. VAMPIRE is based on detection of vessel-like structures by analyzing first-order and second-order image derivatives combined with a minimal cost path algorithm. The image derivatives are obtained using Canny edge detection and an improved ridge filter for detecting elongated structures. We compared VAMPIRE with an established technique in a multi-observer evaluation study involving 40 tracings in slabbed MIP images of multislice CTA datasets of atherosclerotic carotid arteries. The results show that VAMPIRE, in comparison with the established technique, presents considerably more successful tracings and improved handling of stenosis, calcifications, multiple vessels and nearby bone structures. We conclude that VAMPIRE is highly suitable for automated path definition in vessels in (clinical) cardiovascular image data and we expect to improve VAMPIRE to yield paths that are adequate enough to directly serve as center lumen lines in accordance with standards provided by clinicians.

1 Introduction

Cardiovascular disease causes millions of deaths every year. Visualization and quantification of the vasculature in patients suspected of atherosclerosis is of great importance and determining the degree of stenosis in arteries is crucial when considering therapeutical options. Increasingly, magnetic resonance angiography (MRA) and computed tomography angiography (CTA), both three-dimensional (3D) imaging techniques, are being used for diagnostic purposes on vessels [1]. In general, measurements on the MRA and CTA data are performed manually, which is time consuming and highly user dependent [2]. This has motivated the development of automated methods for fast, robust and reproducible segmentation, quantification and visualization of vessels in CTA and MRA data of patients suspected of athero-sclerosis. Automated quantification of a stenosis generally involves definition of a

C. Barillot, D.R. Haynor, and P. Hellier (Eds.): MICCAI 2004, LNCS 3216, pp. 525–532, 2004.
© Springer-Verlag Berlin Heidelberg 2004

center lumen line (CLL), either directly, by path tracing or, indirectly, by first segmenting the lumen (or vessel). Here we focus on direct path tracing.

Several methods have been proposed and evaluated for automated tracing of blood vessels. Direct vessel tracking [3] applies a local search algorithm based on detection of the edges of the lumen. This method has difficulties in dealing with vessels of high curvature and vessels where the lumen area does not change gradually, such as in the transition to a stenosis or an aneurysm. Another class is based on filtering of vessel-like structures [4-8] by convolving the image with Gaussian-derivative filters on different scales and subsequent analysis of the Hessian (second-order derivative matrix) at every pixel. The resulting information can be applied for definition of a CLL and/or segmentation of the vasculature. Definition of a CLL generally involves a minimal cost path algorithm [7] or a B-spline curve fitting procedure [6]. The high computational cost of the Hessian analysis on multiple scales in 3D data is a problem, which can be surpassed by performing the Hessian analysis locally instead of globally [8]. Unfortunately, this requires presegmentation of the vasculature based on thresholding, which can be a cause of errors. Alternatively, segmentation of blood vessels can be performed by statistical inference using a priori information of the vasculature as a tree-like structure and a Gaussian intensity profile of the vessels [9].

Typical problems reported in automated path tracing are areas with stenoses, aneurysms, calcifications, other vessels and bone. Given these problems, we have developed a new method for automated definition of a CLL in cardiovascular image data which is based on first-order (edges) as well as second-order (ridges) image features combined with a minimal cost path algorithm. The edges are obtained using Canny edge detection and the ridges by means of an improved steerable filter for detecting elongated image structures [10, 11]. In this paper we present the results of an evaluation of our method for (clinical) cardiovascular image data.

2 Materials and Methods

Our method for automated definition of a CLL in vessels in cardiovascular image data is called 'VAMPIRE' (Vascular Analysis using Multiscale Paths Inferred from Ridges and Edges). It is based on an improved ridge filter enhancing elongated structures [10, 11]. This filter was initially applied for neurite tracing and uses a modified Hessian which, in theory, is more sensitive to elongated structures compared to techniques based on normal Hessian analysis such as described by Frangi [6,12] (a visual comparison of the two ridge-filters is shown in Figure 1).

VAMPIRE uses a multiscale implementation of the ridge filter in combination with a Canny edge filter [13] to make the technique suitable for cardiovascular data. A cost image is calculated from the resulting edge and ridge information (as illustrated in Figure 2). With this cost image and the vector information obtained from the Hessian analysis (see Figure 3), a minimal cost path is calculated with an implementation of Dijkstra's shortest path algorithm [14] (see also [7]).

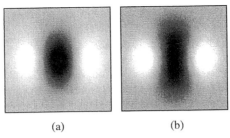

(a)   (b)

Fig. 1. Impression of the shapes of the used ridge filters: (a) filter based on normal Hessian analysis [12], (b) filter used in VAMPIRE. Clearly, the latter is more elongated and should, in theory, be more sensitive to vessel-like structures

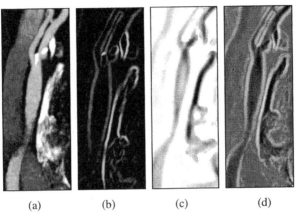

(a)   (b)   (c)   (d)

Fig. 2. Calculation of the cost image (d) from the original image (a) is based on the results of edge filtering (b) as well as ridge filtering (c)

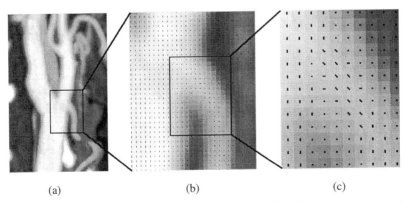

(a)   (b)   (c)

Fig. 3. The vector information computed with the Hessian analysis from (a) is shown in (b) and (c) as black lines for each pixel

We compare VAMPIRE to a method based on the filter using normal Hessian analysis as described by Frangi et al. [12] for the enhancement of vessels, combined with a minimal cost path algorithm (same algorithm as VAMPIRE) as described by Wink et al. [7]. In the sequel, we refer to this latter method as the Frangi-Wink method. Both methods were implemented in Java™ [15] in the form of a plugin for use with ImageJ [16], a public domain image processing program.

The data used for the evaluation are 21 "slabbed" (volume of interest) maximum intensity projections (MIPs) of multislice CTA datasets from 14 patients with internal carotid artery (ICA) stenosis. These MIPs showed the bifurcation of the common carotid artery (CCA), the ICA with the stenosis and (part of) the external carotid artery (ECA) yielding a total of 40 CLLs (24 ICA paths and 16 ECA paths).

As reference, four qualified observers performed manual path tracings by placing points in the image, which were automatically connected by straight lines. The path tracings had to start as early as possible in the CCA and follow the ICA or ECA as long as possible. The paths were stored for further analysis and the mean tracing of the four observers for each vessel was calculated. In addition, the required time and number of points were registered so as to further evaluate the benefits of automating the definition of a CLL. The datasets were blinded and offered to the observers in different order to minimize distortion by learning effects.

As an intuitive measure of deviation of the automated tracings (VAMPIRE and the Frangi-Wink method) from the reference tracings (mean of the four observers) we used the area spanned between the automated tracing and corresponding reference tracing, divided by the length of the latter tracing (area/length).

3 Results

In Table 1 the results for the 40 path tracings are presented. The mean deviation of the paths manually defined by the four observers was 1.00mm. The deviation for each observer was assessed using the tracings of the other observers as reference. The mean deviation of VAMPIRE and the Frangi-Wink method was, respectively, 2.66mm and 16.33mm. This difference is primarily caused by the fact that the path tracings obtained using the Frangi-Wink method left the target vessel in 29 out of 40 cases, compared to only 7 out of 40 cases with VAMPIRE.

Table 1. Deviations (in mm) of all 40 path tracings based on 2 initialization points

	Obs. 1	Obs. 2	Obs. 3	Obs. 4	Manual mean	VAMPIRE	Frangi-Wink
Mean deviation	1.08	1.02	0.90	0.99	1.00	2.66	16.33
Standard deviation	0.33	0.29	0.29	0.33	0.31	2.32	19.91

In Table 2, the results of VAMPIRE and the Frangi-Wink method are presented in three categories: (i) 'direct' tracings, initialized by one start and one end point that do not leave the vessel, (ii) 'direct & extra click' tracings, requiring one additional point to stay in the vessel, and (iii) 'not in vessel' tracings, leaving the vessel even after an additional point is placed. In our opinion, the 'direct & extra click' category can be considered to contain successful path definitions of the target vessel.

Table 2. Deviations (in mm) in three categories

Category	VAMPIRE	Frangi-Wink
direct	1.71 sd. 0.51 (n=33)	1.58 sd. 0.64 (n=11)
direct & extra click	1.70 sd. 0.52 (n=40)	1.61 sd. 0.75 (n=20)
not in vessel	- -	7.06 sd. 4.28 (n=20)

VAMPIRE successfully defined a path in the target vessel in all 40 cases including only 7 cases requiring an additional point. In 20 out of 40 cases the Frangi-Wink method successfully defined a path in the desired vessel including 9 cases requiring an additional point. Figure 4 presents cases where the Frangi-Wink method resulted in paths leaving the target vessel because of bone, calcifications, or another vessel. The paths defined using VAMPIRE did not leave the target vessel. Both methods were initialized with the same start and end point. Figure 5 presents cases indicating three problems of the current implementation of VAMPIRE in defining a CLL.

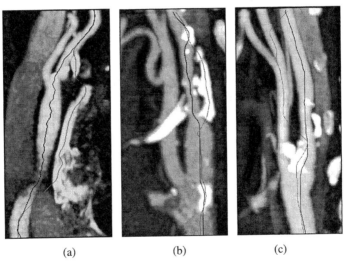

(a)   (b)   (c)

Fig. 4. Three examples of tracings in which the Frangi-Wink method (gray tracings) resulted in gross errors in path definition because it was attracted to (a) bone, (b) calcifications, or (c) another vessel. Paths defined using VAMPIRE (black tracings) did not leave the target vessels

The average time required for manual vessel tracing in these MIP images was 42 seconds and the average number of points used was 16. The time needed for calculation of the cost-image (essentially preprocessing) was 12 seconds on a Pentium IV 2 GHz, after which a minimal cost path was calculated almost instantly. In the 40 cases it took an average of 2-4 seconds for path-definition using VAMPIRE.

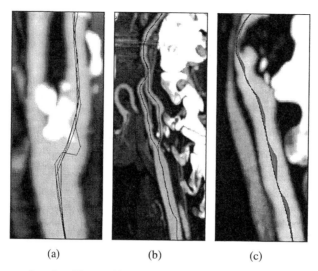

(a)   (b)   (c)

Fig. 5. Three examples of problems with definition of a CLL: (a) tracings of a CLL by multiple observers, (b) a VAMPIRE tracing through the wrong vessel caused by the proximity of vessels in the image, and (c) occasional swaying behavior in the tracings defined by VAMPIRE

4 Discussion

As a proof of concept we decided to first evaluate a 2D implementation of VAMPIRE on clinical data. This allowed us to save considerably on time and effort, not only in implementing and testing the method, but also in the manual definition of paths by the clinicians. Our results show that VAMPIRE, in comparison with the Frangi-Wink method, presents considerably more successful tracings and improved handling of stenosis, calcifications, multiple vessels and nearby bone structures. However, the design of the present study prevents a conclusion whether these improvements are primarily caused by the use of an improved ridge filter or by the addition of edge information. The Frangi-Wink method yielded a slightly lower mean deviation and a higher standard deviation in the successful tracings (1.61mm sd. 0.75) compared to VAMPIRE (1.70mm sd. 0.52). The difference in mean deviation is probably due to the swaying behavior (see Figure 5(c)) of the tracings by VAMPIRE, which appears to result from multiple factors (edges in the lumen caused by inhomogeneous contrast filling, edges of the vessel itself, calcifications and nearby bone structures). The current version of VAMPIRE makes use of thresholding as a way to suppress edge responses in the lumen, but we expect to dispense with this step in the future. The differences in standard deviation indicate that VAMPIRE results in more consistent tracings than the Frangi-Wink method.

Additional experiments were carried out to test the applicability of our method on images in other clinical cardiovascular applications. Results of VAMPIRE for these cases are depicted in Figure 6. VAMPIRE was successful in finding a path through the vessels upon initialization of a startpoint and endpoint.

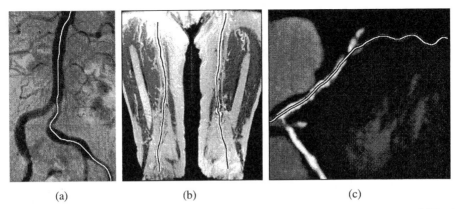

(a)   (b)   (c)

Fig. 6. Examples of tracings with VAMPIRE in (a) a DSA of aorta-iliac arteries, (b) a MIP of an MRA of the peripheral arteries, and (c) a MIP of a CTA of the coronary arteries

While it may be possible to uniquely (mathematically) define a CLL in simulated and phantom data of vessels, there is no unique way of defining *the* CLL of a vessel in clinical cases. The latter was exemplified by the variation in the paths manually defined by the observers (all trained in the same department), especially in areas involving e.g. a bifurcation, stenosis, or calcification (see the manually defined paths in Figure 5(a)). In addition, the definition of an 'optimal' CLL (or path) may be dependent on the clinical question at hand: for example, the optimal path defined for stent placement may be different from the path defined for quantification of stenoses. In order to further improve VAMPIRE, one of the key issues will be to develop standards for CLL definition in clinical cases.

We emphasize our finding that the dependency on the observer in tracing a path with VAMPIRE is virtually absent. In the MIP images of the carotids only two or three points were required and it is easy to use those points as a first guess, whereupon VAMPIRE is able to define the optimal points based on the available edge and ridge information (snapping). This means that no observer-critical decision is required to define a path in these images. In the future, the remaining observer input can be replaced by using an atlas or (CLL) model (e.g. based on statistical analysis) in combination with nonlinear registration so as to provide the relevant initialization data. This would result in completely user-independent vessel tracing and the observer will only be required to verify the results of the path tracing.

We conclude that the VAMPIRE approach has a high potential for automated path definition in vessels in (clinical) cardiovascular image data and we expect to further develop the technique to yield paths (also in 3D) that may directly serve as CLLs in accordance with standards provided by clinicians.

References

[1]   P. J. Nederkoorn, W. P. Th. M. Mali, B. C. Eikelboom, O. E. Elgersma, E. Buskens, M. G. Hunink, L. J. Kappelle, P. C. Buijs, A. F. Wust, A. van der Lugt, Y. van der Graaf. Preoperative Diagnosis of Carotid Artery Stenosis: Accuracy of Noninvasive Testing. *Stroke* 33(8):2003-8, 2002.

[2]   G. D. Rubin. Data Explosion: The Challenge of Multidetector-Row CT. *European Journal of Radiology* 36(2):74-80, 2000.

[3]   O. Wink, W. J. Niessen, M. A. Viergever. Fast Delineation and Visualization of Vessels in 3-D Angiographic Images. *IEEE Transactions on Medical Imaging* 19(4):337-46, 2000.

[4]   Y. Sato, S. Nakajima, N. Shiraga, H. Atsumi, S. Yoshida, T. Koller, G. Gerig, R. Kikinis. Three-Dimensional Multi-Scale Line Filter for Segmentation and Visualization of Curvilinear Structures in Medical Images. *Medical Image Analysis* 2(2):143-68, 1998.

[5]   C. M. van Bemmel, L. Spreeuwers, M. A. Viergever, W. J. Niessen. Central Axis Based Segmentation of the Carotids. In: *Proceedings of the International Society of Magnetic Resonance in Medicine*, ISMRM-2002, p. 1797.

[6]   A. F. Frangi, W. J. Niessen, R. M. Hoogeveen, T. van Walsum, M. A. Viergever. Model-Based Quantitation of 3-D Magnetic Resonance Angiographic Images. *IEEE Transactions on Medical Imaging* 18(10):946-56, 1999.

[7]   O. Wink, A. F. Frangi, B. Verdonck, M. A. Viergever, W. J. Niessen. 3D MRA Coronary Axis Determination using a Minimum Cost Path Approach. *Magnetic Resonance Imaging* 47(6):1169-75, 2002.

[8]   S. R. Aylward, E. Bullitt. Initialization, Noise, Singularities, and Scale in Height Ridge Traversal for Tubular Object Centerline Extraction. *IEEE Transactions on Medical Imaging* 21(2):61-75, 2002.

[9]   A. Bhalerao, E. Thönnes, W. Kendall, R. Wilson. Inferring Vascular Structure from 2D and 3D Imagery. In: *Proceedings of Medical Image Computing and Computer-Assisted Intervention*, MICCAI-2001, pp 820-828.

[10] M. Jacob, M. Unser. Design of Steerable Filters for Feature Detection using Canny-Like Criteria. *IEEE Transactions on Pattern Analysis and Machine Intelligence*, 2004. In press.

[11] E. Meijering, M. Jacob, J.-C. F. Sarria, P. Steiner, H. Hirling, M. Unser. Design and Validation of a Tool for Neurite Tracing and Analysis in Fluorescence Microscopy Images. *Cytometry*, 2004. In press.

[12] A. F. Frangi, W. J. Niessen, K. L. Vincken, M. A. Viergever. Mutiscale Vessel Enhancement Filtering. In: *Proceedings of Medical Image Computing and Computer-Assisted Intervention*, MICCAI-1998, pp. 130-137.

[13] J. Canny. A Computational Approach to Edge Detection. *IEEE Transactions on Pattern Analysis and Machine Intelligence* 8(6):679-698, 1986.

[14] T. H. Cormen, C. E. Leiserson, R. L. Rivest, C. Stein. Introduction to Algorithms. 2nd edition. Cambridge, MA, MIT Press, 2001.

[15] Sun Microsystems, Inc. Java^{TM} Platform Standard edition, http://java.sun.com/

[16] W. Rasband. ImageJ: Image Processing and Analysis in Java. U.S. National Institutes of Health, http://rsb.info.nih.gov/ij/

A General Framework for Tree Segmentation and Reconstruction from Medical Volume Data

Thomas Bülow, Cristian Lorenz, and Steffen Renisch

Philips Research Laboratories
Roentgenstrasse 24-26, D-22335 Hamburg, Germany

Abstract. Many anatomical entities like different parts of the arterial system and the airway system are of tree-like structure. State of the art medical imaging systems can acquire 3D volume data of the human body at a resolution that is sufficient for the visualization of these tree structures. We present a general framework for the simultaneous segmentation and reconstruction of the abovementioned entities and apply it to the extraction of coronary arteries from multi detector-row CT data. The coronary artery extraction is evaluated on 9 data-sets with known ground truth for the centerlines of the coronary arteries.

1 Introduction

Modern medical imaging devices like multi detector-row computed tomography (MDCT) scanners and magnetic resonance imaging (MRI) devices provide us with high resolution volume data of the human body. Among the anatomic entities with diagnostic relevance that become visible by these means are the vessel trees and the bronchial tree. Depending on the quality of the data wrt. noise, artifacts, spatial resolution etc. tree extraction can be a very challanging task.

In this paper we propose a general framework for the extraction of tree structures from 3D data. Due to the modularity of our approach it can be tailored to specific applications with minor changes. Two implementations of the method – for airways extraction [1], and a preliminary approach to coronary artery segmentation [2] both from MDCT data – have been presented in earlier work. The main contributions of this paper are (i) the presentation of the general framework underlying the abovementioned works (ii) an automated evaluation environment for vessel tree segmentations based on manually extracted ground-truth, and (iii) an extended and improved version of the coronary artery segmentator for MDCT data based on a comparison of several configurations of the general segmentation algorithm. It is crucial that this comparison is not based on visual inspection datasets but rather on the use of an automated evaluation environment.

For the detection of vessels measures of *vesselness* have been designed most of which are based on the eigen-values of the Hesse matrix (second derivative matrix) of the local gray-value structure [4,5]. However, the latter methods are likely to fail at rapid gray-value changes along the vessel which can, e.g., occur in our example application of cardiac MDCT, due to the presence of calcified plaques.

C. Barillot, D.R. Haynor, and P. Hellier (Eds.): MICCAI 2004, LNCS 3216, pp. 533–540, 2004.

Another class of approaches is based on front propagation. Starting from a seed-point a front is expanded according to a given speed function. This expansion can efficiently be implemented using fast marching and level set methods [3]. Speed functions have been designed according to the abovementioned vesselness measures [7,8]. Besides *segmentation* we are interested in the *reconstruction* of the tree-structure, including proper labeling of connectedness of different segments and parent-child relationships. In the past this has sometimes been dealt with as a separated problem building upon the segmentation results [6].

The framework proposed here allows for the simultaneous segmentation and reconstruction of tree-like structures. Our hierarchical approach consists of three levels ranging from a voxel level to an abstract tree-reasoning level with an intermediate segment level. On each level we have exchangable modules that allow the adaptation of the methodology to specific applications.

2   The General Framework

There are two major advantages of starting with this general approach rather than dealing with the specific application directly. First, this allows us to adapt the method to different applications easily. Second, it allows to test various configurations for one specific application. This is especially useful since the interplay of different components – each intuitive on its own – can be hard to predict.

2.1   Assumptions

We assume that the tree structure to be segmented stands out against the background according to some image feature $f : (v, I) \mapsto \mathbb{R}$ where $v \in D \subset \mathbb{Z}^3$ is a voxel in the image domain and $I : D \to \mathbb{R}^N$ is the volumetric data ($N = 1$ for gray scale data). Thus, segments of the tree can in general be segmented locally from the background by a thresholding operation with respect to the local feature value $f(v, I)$. The appropriate threshold can vary within the data volume. Furthermore we assume that segments of the tree roughly comply with certain geometric restrictions, e.g., being elongated cylindrical objects

2.2   The Segmentation Process

We distinguish between *branches* and *segments*, where one branch consists of one or more segments (see Fig. 1). Here, *segments* have merely algorithmic significance. The tree is extracted segment by segment with the main components of the algorithm being *segment initialization*, *segment growing*, and *segment evaluation*. The set of voxels belonging to the tree structure will be denoted by V_{tree}. A segment S is defined as the tuple $S = (V, w, c, p)$ where $V \subset D$ is the set of voxels belonging to S, $w \subset V$ constitutes the *wave front*, $c = (c_1, \ldots, c_m)$ with $c_i \in \mathbb{R}^3$ is the centerline of S, and p is a set of parameters used in the expansion and evaluation process.

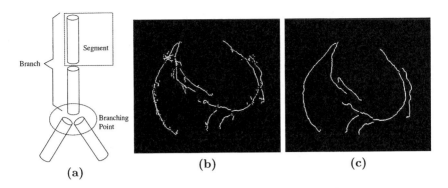

Fig. 1. (a) A *branch* is one component of the tree to be segmented. A branch starts either at the *root* of the tree or at a *branching point* and ends at a *branching point* or at a *termination point*. It can be broken into several *segments*. (b) A raw coronary centerline tree result. (c) The centerline tree after pruning.

Initialization. The segmentation process is started from one or more *seed-voxels* $s_i \in D, i \in \{1, \ldots, N\}$. For each seed, a segment $S_i^0 = (s_i, s_i, s_i, p_i)$ is initialized and put into the *segment queue*. The parameter set p_i contains an initial feature threshold t_f based on which acceptable voxels ($f(v, I) > t_f$) are recognized.

The Segment Queue is a sorted list $(S_i^0, S_{i+1}^0, \ldots, S_m^0)$ of initialized but yet unprocessed segments. The first segment S_i^0 is removed from the queue, expanded, and its child segments $S_{m+1}^0, \ldots$, if any, are added to the queue. This process is repeated as long as there are segments in the queue or until terminated interactively by the user.

The Wave Front and its Propagation. The prototypical wave front of a segment S can be visualized as a mainly disk-shaped flat subset of V. A propagation function $P^{I,p}$ transforms a wave front w_i into a new wave front w_{i+1} such that for each voxel $v \in w_{i+1}$ the voxel itself or one of its 6-neighbors is contained in w_i. None of the new voxels may be in the set of already segmented voxels V_{tree}, i.e., $\{w_{i+1} \backslash w_i\} \cap V_{tree} = \emptyset$.

Segment Expansion. *Front propagation* is used to expand a segment $S^t = (V, w^t, c, p)$ to $S^{t+1} = (V \cup w^{t+1}, w^{t+1}, (c, center(w^{t+1})), p)$, with $w^{t+1} = P^{I,p}(w^t)$. At this stage the centerline information is built up. We use the notation $P^{I,p}(S^t) = S^{t+1}$. A segment S^t can be reset to its initial state $S^0 = reset(S^t)$.

Segment Evaluation. We evaluate segments in order to determine whether they are part of the desired structure. An application dependent *segment evaluation function* $E(S)$ decides whether a segment should be accepted, rejected or growing should be continued. Depending on the results – especially if S is rejected – the segment can be reset to its initial state and regrown using a different parameter set $p_m = U(p_{m-1}, E(S))$, where U is a parameter update function. Since U can depend on the reason why a segment was rejected we allow for different *reject* and *accept* return values in addition to the *continue* results of E. As soon as the front does no longer consist of a single connected component the segment is not expanded further, i.e., $E(S) \neq continue$. This allows us to keep track of the tree-structure.

Child Segment Initialization. After growing an acceptable segment S one new segment $S_{new} = (w_i, w_i, center(w_i), \Pi(S))$ per connected front component w_i is initialized. Here Π determines the parameter set of the new segment.

Tree Processing. During the segmentation process the centerline tree is built. Domain knowledge can be used in order to accept/reject segments or whole sub-trees based on the centerline tree. This can be done either during the segmentation or as a postprocessing step pruning the raw centerline tree.

The pseudo-code for the whole process is shown below. Note, that U needs a termination criterion, e.g., a counter that guarantees that $p = U(p, E(S))$ eventually occurs.

```
initialize segments from seed-voxels
put new segments into segment queue
while ( queue not empty )
        retrieve segment S from queue
        do {  S = reset(S)
              while ( E(S) == continue ) {  S = P^{I,p}(S) }
              p_i = U(p_{i-1}, E(S))
              p = p_i
        } while ( p ≠ p_{i-1} )
        V_{tree} = V_{tree} ∪ V^S
        initialize child segments and include in segment queue
```

3   Coronary Artery Extraction

In coronary CTA the coronary arteries are imaged by MDCT using an intraveneous contrast injection and a special acquistion and reconstruction protocol. Thus, we use the HU-value, i.e., the gray-value as feature $f(v, I) = I(v)$. The extraction of coronary arteries is of use, e.g., in visualization, lumen measurement, computer aided detection (CAD), navigation, and intervention planning. There exists little literature on segmentation of the coronary tree from MDCT data. A previous version of the algorithm presented here has been published [2]. Recently an algorithm for the segmentation of a single vessel with user defined seed-points at the both ends of the vessel has been presented [9].

Difficulties in this domain are that along with the coronary arteries the heart chambers are filled with contrast agent. Due to motion artifacts the delineation between a vessel and a heart chamber may in some cases become almost completely blurred. Furthermore the vessels may be of inhomogeneous gray-value appearance due to calcifications.

The wave-front propagation follows a fast marching approach [3] that simulates the propagation of a wave-front according to the Eikonal equation from geometric optics. We use a binary velocity function with $v = 1$ for voxels above the feature threshold and $v = 0$ else. For the numerical details we refer to [2].

The segment evaluation function for coronary artery segments consists of several modules.

$$E(S) = \begin{cases} reject_{frontsize} & \text{if} \quad \frac{N_{front}}{N_{initial}} > t_{fs} \\ reject_{radius} & \text{else if} \quad \mathcal{R}(S) > t_r \\ reject_{collisions} & \text{else if number of collisions} > t_c \\ E'(S) & \text{else if front split} \\ E'(S) & \text{else if} \quad \frac{\mathcal{L}(S)}{\mathcal{R}(S)} > t_{lr} \\ E'(S) & \text{else if segment is unchanged.} \\ continue & \text{else.} \end{cases}$$

Here $E'(S)$ is a secondary evaluation function that is only computed when the segment is fully grown. It has no *continue* return value. The objective of including E' is that it is only computed once, when the segment is complete, rather than after each expansion step. Here E' is given by

$$E'(S) = \begin{cases} reject_{vesselness} & \text{if} \quad \max_{v \in V}\left(\mathcal{V}(v, I)\right) < t_v \\ reject_{splintering} & \text{if} \quad N(frontparts) > t_s \\ reject_{frontexplosion} & \text{if} \quad \frac{N_{front}}{\mathcal{L}(S)N_{initial}} > t_{fe} \\ accept & \text{else.} \end{cases}$$

The different components in the evaluation functions have the following meaning. Whenever the number of front voxels N_{front} exceeds the number of voxels in the initial front by more then a factor of t_{fs} the segment is rejected. This prevents leakage in many cases. The limitation of the radius $\mathcal{R}(S)$ by t_r has a similar reason. The "number of collisions" is the number of segments in direct vicinity to S. Since, e.g., leakage into the myocardium leads to many collisions of small segments, we limit the number of allowed collisions by t_c. Whenever the front disintegrates or the segment length exceeds its radius by more then t_{lr} the segment expansion is stopped and a final evaluation is done by E'. The same is done in case the segment has not changed in the last expansion step. This happens if there are no voxels above the current gray-value threshold available and consequently the front propagation yields an empty voxel set as new front.

The reason for stopping as soon as the front decomposes is simply that we wish to keep track of the branching structure of the tree. The length/radius ratio is limited in order to save "good" parts of the vessel and not to reject too much whenever the process leaks out of the vessel.

The final evaluation by E' involves a measure of vesselness $\mathcal{V}(v, I)$ that investigates the local gray-value structure and is based on the eigenvalues of the Hessian at different scales [4,5]. Note that we use the maximal vesselness value within the segment rather than the mean vesselness. This helps to account for inhomogeneous appearance of the vessel which leads to low vesselness values for many actual vessel voxels. Also since we use vesselness just as one of several components the threshold t_{vs} is usually chosen to be rather low.

Splintering of the front, i.e., front decomposition into many parts, usually occurs in the presence of noise and can be avoided by raising the gray value

Table 1. 30 vessels compared to ground truth. The table shows the numbers of vessels for which a certain percentage was found for various parameter settings. **(a)** The default parameter setting (see text). **(b)** $N_{nec} = 3$ and $N_{prob} = 1$. **(c)** Number of front components is unlimited. **(d)** Front growth is not restricted. **(e)** Without *front explosion* restriction. **(f)** Maximally 20 segment generations allowed.

		Percentage of vessel found				
		$0-20\%$	$20-40\%$	$40-60\%$	$60-80\%$	$80-100\%$
	(a)	3	4	3	3	17
	(b)	10	5	3	3	9
Parameter	(c)	4	4	5	0	17
setting	(d)	3	5	9	5	8
	(e)	4	5	3	3	15
	(f)	0	5	8	10	7

threshold. Finally, the segment is rejected if "front explosion" occurs, i.e., if the front grows too fast. This is measured by normalizing the front size ratio $N_{front}/N_{initial}$ by the length of the segment.

The threshold values used in E and E' are all in the parameter set of the segment S. We also include N_{prob}, a counter of *probationary parameter adaptations*, and N_{nec}, a counter of *necessary parameter adaptations*. The parameter update function U for this application acts merely on the three parameters (t_g, N_{prob}, N_{nec}).

$$
U((t_g, N_{prob}, N_{nec}), E(S))
$$
$$
= \begin{cases}
(t_g + \Delta g, N_{prob}, N_{nec} + 1) & \text{if } E(S) = reject \text{ and } N_{nec} < max_{nec} \\
(t_g - \Delta g, max_{prob}, max_{nec}) & \text{if } E(S) = reject \text{ and } N_{nec} = max_{nec} \\
(t_g - \Delta g, N_{prob} + 1, N_{nec}) & \text{if } E(S) = accept \text{ and } N_{prob} < max_{prob} \\
(t_g, N_{prob}, N_{nec}) & \text{if } E(S) = accept \text{ and } N_{prob} = max_{prob}
\end{cases}
$$

For a rejected segment the gray value threshold is increades by Δ_g and N_{nec} is incremented. If the maximum number max_{nec} is reached t_g is reduced in order to return to an acceptable state of the segment that might have existed in the previous round. If the segment has been accepted the threshold is reduced probationarily in order to reach distal vessel parts with lower contrast.

4   Results

For evaluation purposes nine cardiac MDCT datasets with manually extracted centerlines of the three main vessels (LAD, LCX, and RCA) were available. For two of the datasets additional marginal and diagonal branches were extracted. This gave us a whole of 30 vessels with known ground truth. For each of the nine datasets two seed-points were placed one in left and right ostium, respectively. The results for each vessel was evaluated   by comparison to a ground-truth centerline $c^{true} = (c_0^{true}, \ldots, c_N^{true})$. For each point c_i^{true} we checked whether the automatically extracted centerline contains a corresponding point. We allow for a distance of up to 2 mm in order to account for small inaccuracies of the manually and automatically extracted centerlines. Let c^{found} be the found part

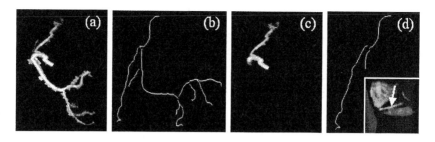

Fig. 2. **(a)** and **(b)**: MIP and vessel centerlines of a right coronary artery tree segmented using the default parameter setting (see text). **(c)** and **(d)**: Results for the same dataset at a reduced number of threshold adaptation steps $max_{nec} = 3$, $max_{prop} = 1$. The lower right corner of (d) shows where the segmentation process gets blocked if insufficient threshold adaptation steps are used. In the vicinity of the ventricle the vessel can only be segmented at a higher threshold in this case.

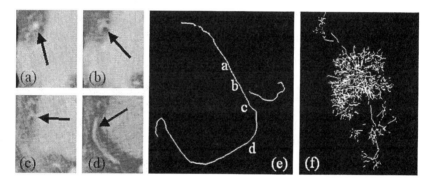

Fig. 3. **(a)-(d)** Four axial sections from top to bottom. The arrows indicate the RCA. (Clearly visible in (a) and (d), blurred and distorted due to motion artifacts in (c) and (d)). **(e)** Vessel centerlines after segmentation with default parameter setting. **(f)** Segmentation without using the vesselness criterion. In this case, severe leakage occurs at blurred portions.

of the centerline corresponding to c^{true}. We judge the result of the segmentation by the ratio $length(c^{found})/length(c^{true})$. We thus identify *true positives*. On the contrary we do not have an automated way to tell for a centerline found by the algorithm but not contained in the ground truth whether it is a *false* or a *true positive*. For this kind of evaluation the results need to be inspected visually. However, the automated results yield some means to rate the quality of an algorithm. For the results of our algorithm please refer to Tab. 1. The default settings used in Tab. 1 **(a)** were, $t_{fs} = 4$, $t_c = 10$, $t_{lr} = 5$, $t_v = 0.2$, $t_s = 4$, $t_{fe} = 1/mm$, $max_{nec} = 12$, $max_{prob} = 3$, and $\Delta g = 10HU$. From Tab. 1 it can be seen that the default parameter settings as described above yield the best overall results. Reducing the number of threshold adaptation cycles (Tab. 1 **(b)**) reduces the number of completely found vessels ($> 80\%$) almost by half.

Not restricting front growth (Tab. 1 (d)) leads to more severe leakage and to self blockage, once a segment gets rejected by another criterion. Figures 2 and 3 visualize the effects of different parameter settings (see captions for details).

5   Conclusion and Outlook

It has been shown how the introduced general segmentation scheme can be applied to coronary tree extraction from MDCT data. Due to its modularity we were able to modify the algorithm in order to perform optimally for the given application. This was possible due to the automatic evaluation environment proposed in Sect. 4 in combination with given ground truth for the vessel centerlines. The methodology presented here has also been sucessfully applied to the extraction of the bronchial tree [1]. In future work we are going to apply the presented approach to other domains, different vessel-trees and other modalities.

Acknowledgement. We thank the clinical science group from Philips Medical Systems CT for helpful discussions and for providing the MSCT data.

References

1. T. Schlathölter, C. Lorenz, I. Carlsen, S. Renisch, T. Deschamps. "Simultaneous Segmentation and Tree Reconstruction of the Airways for Virtual Bronchoscopy" SPIE Conf. on Medical Imaging, Proc. of SPIE Vol. 4684, pp. 103-113 (2002)
2. C. Lorenz, S. Renisch, Th. Schlathölter, Th. Bülow. "Simultaneous Segmentation and Tree Reconstruction of the Coronary Arteries in MSCT Images" SPIE Conference on Medical Imaging, Proceedings of SPIE Vol. 5031, pp. 167-177, (2003)
3. D. Adalsteinsson, J.A. Sethian. "A Fast Level Set Method for Propagating Interfaces", J. Comp. Phys., 118 (2), pp. 269-277, (1995)
4. C. Lorenz, I.-C. Carlsen, T.M. Buzug, C. Fassnacht and J. Weese. "A Multi-scale Line Filter with Automatic Scale Selection Based on the Hessian Matrix for Medical Image Segmentation", Scale-Space '97, LNCS 1252, pp. 152-163 (1997)
5. A.F. Frangi, W.J. Niessen, K.L. Vincken, M.A. Viergever. "Muliscale Vessel Enhancement Filtering", MICCAI 1998, pp. 130-137 (1998)
6. E. Bullitt, S. Aylward, A. Liu, J. Stone, S.K. Mukherji, Ch. Coffey, G. Gerig, S.M. Pizer. "3D Graph Description of the Intracerebral Vasculature from Segmented MRA and Tests of Accuracy by Comparison with X-ray Angiograms", IPMI 99, Springer, LNCS 1613, pp. 308-321 (1999)
7. O. Wink, W.J. Niessen, B. Verdonck, M.A. Viergever. "Vessel Axis Determination Using Wave Front Propagation Analysis". MICCAI 2001, Springer, LNCS 2208, pp. 845-853 (2001)
8. S. Young, V. Pekar, J. Weese. "Vessel Segmentation for Visualization of MRA with Blood Pool Contrast Agent." MICCAI, Springer, LNCS 2208, pp. 491-498 (2001)
9. S. Wesarg, E. Firle. "Segmentation of Vessels: The Corkscrew Algorithm", SPIE Conference onf Medical Imageing, Proc. of the SPIE (2004) to appear.

Shape-Based Curve Growing Model and Adaptive Regularization for Pulmonary Fissure Segmentation in CT

Jingbin Wang[1], Margrit Betke[1], and Jane P. Ko[2]

[1] Computer Science Department, Boston University, Boston MA 02215, USA
[2] Department of Radiology, New York University, New York NY 10016, USA
{jingbinw,betke}@cs.bu.edu, www.cs.bu.edu/groups/ivc

Abstract. This paper presents a shape-based curve-growing algorithm for object recognition in the field of medical imaging. The proposed curve growing process, modeled by a Bayesian network, is influenced by both image data and prior knowledge of the shape of the curve. A maximum a posteriori (MAP) solution is derived using an energy-minimizing mechanism. It is implemented in an adaptive regularization framework that balances the influence of image data and shape prior in estimating the curve, and reflects the causal dependencies in the Bayesian network. The method effectively alleviates over-smoothing, an effect that can occur with other regularization methods. Moreover, the proposed framework also addresses initialization and local minima problems. Robustness and performance of the proposed method are demonstrated by segmentation of pulmonary fissures in computed tomography (CT) images.

1 Introduction

Enormous demands for automatically recognizing complicated anatomical structures in medical images have been raised in recent years. The medical community has seen many benefits from computer aided diagnosis (CAD) systems [5] and computer visualizations [7]. A large body of literature on segmentation of anatomical structures has been published [14]. Low-level image processing methods, for example, thresholding or edge detection, by themselves, were often not sufficient to segment such structures. Many methods have attempted to introduce prior knowledge of the shape of a structure into the object recognition process. A widely known technique, the "snake" or active contour method [8], used a deformable spline contour to capture the boundary of an object in an iterative energy minimizing process. The assumption of a smooth object boundary was guaranteed implicitly by the geometry of the spline contour. The level set method [12] was later proposed as a more powerful solution for handling instability and allowing changes in object topology. However, for objects with high curvatures or large boundary discontinuities, the smoothness assumption by itself is not sufficient for modeling object shape. Thus, some high-level prior knowledge is needed to guide the object segmentation process. Statistics based methods (e.g., [4]) used training data for recognizing objects with complicated

C. Barillot, D.R. Haynor, and P. Hellier (Eds.): MICCAI 2004, LNCS 3216, pp. 541–548, 2004.

shapes. Recently several methods (e.g., [11]) have incorporated shape priors into existing segmentation methods, e.g., [8,12], and presented promising results for applications in which closed contours can be used to model objects. For an object modeled by an open contour, Berger and Mohr's curve-growing method [2] can be applied. A shape model can also be used in the deformation of open contours, for example, as proposed by Akgual et al. [1].

A pulmonary fissure is a boundary between the lobes in the lungs. Its segmentation is of clinical interest because pulmonary nodules are frequently located adjacent to the fissure, whose identification would benefit computer aided diagnosis systems. Moreover, the ability to segment the lobes has additional clinical implications that include automated quantitative assessment of regional lung pathology and image registration. Few systems [9,15,17] have addressed the problem of fissure segmentation. The main contributions of our paper are (1) an approach to include a shape prior in a curve-growing method for object segmentation (2) an adaptive regularization framework, (3) a process to address curve initialization and alleviate the local minima problem, (4) a successful application of the proposed method to the problem of segmenting fissures in CT. With the introduced shape prior, meaningful segmentation results are produced in the presence of uncertainties, such as ambiguous image features or high curvature variation on the object boundary. The adaptive regularization alleviates over-smoothing, an effect encountered by classical regularization methods. Our method also provides a solution for the initialization problem by taking advantage of the shape prior. It also alleviates the local minima problem effectively by a revised definition of the "image force."

2   Method

2.1   Bayesian Formulation of Curve Growing

Bayesian networks [13] have been applied to many applications that involve reasoning processes, as they succinctly describe causal dependencies using probabilities. Suppose that an object is modeled by a piecewise spline curve $\mathcal{C}$. A random variable I, representing the observed image data, and a random variable $\mathcal{C}^*$, representing prior information about the object shape, are considered as two causal predecessors of the random variable $\mathcal{C}$, the curve to be estimated. This relation can be modeled by the Bayesian network shown in Fig. 1A. The curve is represented as a collection of curve segments $\mathcal{C} = \{S_1, \ldots, S_K, \ldots, S_N\}$, where S_K represents the K-th curve segment and is also considered a random variable. The curve $\mathcal{C}$ is created by adding curve segments S_K one at a time. Random variable S_K is assumed to be only dependent on the most recently added curve segment S_{K-1} and not on earlier segments. We call this the "Markovianity assumption" [10] on subsequent curve segments. The corresponding Bayesian network is shown in Fig. 1B. Estimating the curve $\mathcal{C}$ is equivalent to finding the maximum of the joint probability $P(S_1, S_2, ..., S_N, \mathcal{C}^*, I)$ defined by the Bayesian network. By applying the Markovianity assumption, this is

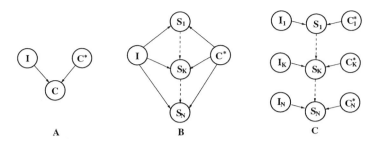

Fig. 1. A Hierarchy of Bayesian Networks for Curve Growing

$$P(S_1, ..., S_N, \mathcal{C}^*, I) = P(\mathcal{C}^*, I)P(S_1|\mathcal{C}^*, I)P(S_2|S_1, \mathcal{C}^*, I) \ldots P(S_N|S_{N-1}, \mathcal{C}^*, I). \quad (1)$$

This product includes the prior distribution $P(\mathcal{C}^*, I)$, which is generally assumed to be uniform, the posterior probability $P(S_1|\mathcal{C}^*, I)$, which models the probability of the initial curve placement and relates to the curve initialization problem, and the remaining posterior probabilities $P(S_K|S_{K-1}, \mathcal{C}^*, I)$, for $K = 1, \ldots N$. The maximum of the joint probability given in Eq. 1 is approximated by the product of the maximum of $P(S_1|\mathcal{C}^*, I)$ and each $P(S_K|S_{K-1}, \mathcal{C}^*, I)$, where

$$
\begin{aligned}
P(S_K|S_{K-1}, \mathcal{C}^*, I) &= P(S_K|S_{K-1}, \mathcal{C}_K^*, I_K) \\
&= P(I_K|S_K, S_{K-1})P(\mathcal{C}_K^*|S_K, S_{K-1}, I_K)P(S_K, S_{K-1}) \, / \, P(S_{K-1}, \mathcal{C}_K^*, I_K).
\end{aligned}
\quad (2)
$$

Here I_K is the local image region containing S_K and is considered to be the only relevant part of the image I for estimating S_K (Fig. 2). Similarly, $\mathcal{C}_K^*$ is the part of the shape prior $\mathcal{C}^*$ relevant to estimating S_K. The normalizing factor $P(S_{K-1}, \mathcal{C}_K^*, I_K)$ is considered irrelevant to S_K and thus omitted. The corresponding Bayesian network is shown in Fig. 1C.

2.2 Energy Function of Curve Growing Model

The conditional probability $P(I_K|S_K, S_{K-1})$ in Eq. 2 is defined as

$$\mathbf{P}(I_K|S_K, S_{K-1}) \propto \exp(-|E_{img}(S_K) - E_{img}^{min}|), \quad (3)$$

where $E_{img}(S_K) = -\sum_i |\nabla I(V_K^i)|$ is the associated image energy of curve segment S_K, ∇I defines the image force, in many applications, the intensity gradient, V_K^i represents the i-th spline point in the segment S_K, and E_{img}^{min} is a lower bound on the values of E_{img} that can occur in an image. In contrast to previous methods [8,16], the image energy is evaluated on the curve segment instead of a singular spline point, which reduces the possibility that the curve-growing process is trapped in off-curve local image energy minima.

In Eq. 2, the probability $P(\mathcal{C}_K^*|S_K, S_{K-1}, I_K)$ is used to model the similarity of the Kth segment of curve C and prior curve $\mathcal{C}^*$. It is a function of S_K, S_{K-1} and I_K, and can be defined by a Gaussian distribution:

$$P(\mathcal{C}_K^*|S_K, S_{K-1}, I_K) \propto \exp(-\alpha(I_K)f_{sim}(S_K, S_{K-1}, C_K^*))$$
$$= \exp(-|\mu(S_K, S_K^*) - \mu(S_{K-1}, S_{K-1}^*)|/(2\sigma^2)) \text{ with} \tag{4}$$
$$\mu(S_K, S_K^*) = \tfrac{1}{n}\sum_i |V_K^i - V_K^{i*}|, \; S_K^* = \{V_K^{i*}|V_K^i \in S_K\}, \text{ and } C_K^* = S_K^* \cup S_{K-1}^*,$$

where $f_{sim}(S_K, S_{K-1}, C_K^*)$ is a function measuring the similarity between (S_K, S_{K-1}) and the shape prior C_K^*, (V_K^i, V_K^{i*}) is a pair of corresponding points on $\mathcal{C}$ and $\mathcal{C}^*$ (correspondence is established by a closest-point search), $\mu(S_K, S_K^*)$ is the mean difference vector between two corresponding curve segments, n is the number of points included in S_K, and $\alpha(I_K)$ is a function of I_K used to control the magnitude of the Gaussian deviation $(\alpha(I_K) \propto 2\sigma^2)$.

The smoothness constraint on the curve is modeled by:

$$P(S_K, S_{K-1}) \propto \exp(-|f_{curv}(S_K, S_{K-1})|), \tag{5}$$

where $f_{curv}(S_K, S_{K-1})$ is a function measuring the curvature between S_{K-1} and S_K, e.g. as in Ref. [16]. By incorporating the Eqs. 3-5 into Eq. 2 and taking the logarithm, the curve energy function

$$\mathbf{E}(\mathcal{C}) = \mathbf{E}_{shape}(\mathcal{C}) + \mathbf{E}_{curv}(\mathcal{C}) + \mathbf{E}_{img}(\mathcal{C}) \propto$$
$$\sum_{K=1}^{N}(\alpha(I_K)f_{sim}(S_K, S_{K-1}, C_K^*) + \beta_K f_{curv}(S_K, S_{K-1}) + \gamma_K E_{img}(S_K)) \tag{6}$$

is obtained, where α, β and γ regularization factors, whose ratios are constrained by the variances of the underlying Gaussian distributions. Each of E_{shape}, E_{curv} and E_{img} is normalized as suggested by Ref. [16]. The energy minimum of $\mathbf{E}(\mathcal{C})$ is considered an approximate MAP solution of the curve segmentation problem.

2.3   Causal Confidence Approximation and Adaptive Regularization

Ill-suited values for α, β and γ in Eq. 6 can cause the curve C to become overly smoothed. Regularization factors can be estimated by various approaches, for instance, a cross-validation method [10], which requires a large amount of off-line computation and is then static during the segmentation phase. To obtain

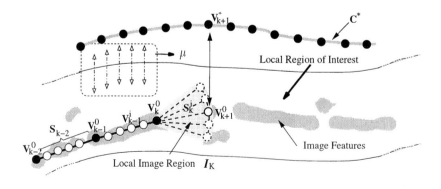

Fig. 2. Curve Growing with Adaptive Regularization

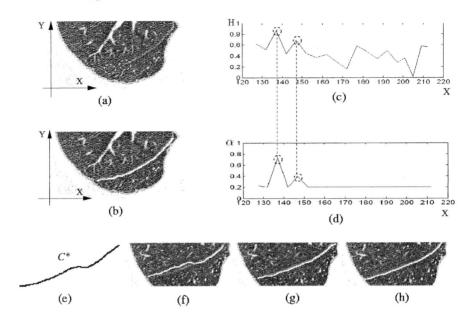

Fig. 3. Image features, entropy and adaptive regularization: Example 1: (a) Region of interest in a CT image. (b) Ground truth curve. (c) Entropy H along the curve. (d) Corresponding value of α. The two highest values of H and α and the corresponding locations in the image are circled. Example 2: (e) Shape prior. (f) Curve obtained with static regularization, $\alpha = 1.2$ and $\gamma = 1.4$. (g) Curve obtained with adaptive regularization. (h) Ground truth curve.

a well-behaved regularizer, we propose an adaptive regularization framework. A revised factor $\alpha(I_K)$ is introduced to weigh adaptively the influence of image region I_K versus the influence of prior shape C_K^*. This also reflects the causal dependencies in the Bayesian network (Fig. 1c). The adaptive regularization parameter $\alpha(I_K)$ can be related to the entropy

$$H(I_K) = -F \sum_{i=1}^{n} P(I_K|S_K^i, S_{K-1}) \log_2 P(I_K|S_K^i, S_{K-1}) \qquad (7)$$

of image region I_K, where S_K^i is the i-th sample of S_K in I_K (Fig. 2) and F is a normalizing factor. The entropy $H(I_K)$ can be interpreted as the amount of uncertainty contained in image region I_K. For regions with large entropy values, the prior shape term should be weighted higher than for regions with small entropy values. The adaptive regularization parameter $\alpha(I_K)$ is thus defined as

$$\alpha(I_K) = \max\{\epsilon, (H(I_K) - \lambda)/(1 - \lambda)\}, \qquad (8)$$

where λ is the threshold that corresponds to a desirable feature in I_K and can be learned offline from a set of training examples, and where ϵ defines the minimum value of $\alpha(I_K)$. The values $\lambda = 0.5$ and $\epsilon = 0.1$ were chosen in the current implementation. Fig. 3(a)– 3(e) gives an example where adaptive regularization satisfactorily strengthened the influence of the prior shape (circled areas).

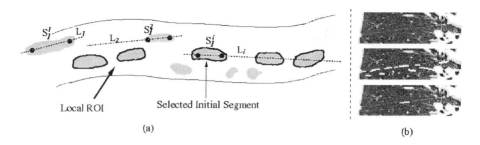

(a)   (b)

Fig. 4. Curve Initialization: (a) Alignments of relevant portions $\{L_i\}$ of prior curve C^* with candidate segments $\{S_1^i\}$. (b) Local region of interest in CT (top), candidate segments $\{S_1^i\}$ (middle), and the selected initial curve segment S_1 (bottom).

Fig. 3(f)– 3(i) shows a second example, where adaptive regularization is clearly superior to static regularization.

2.4   Curve Initialization

The curve-growing process starts after a segment belonging to the curve is selected. The Bayesian formulation $P(S_1|C^*, I)$ suggests that both the prior curve C^* and the current image data I should be considered in selection of S_1. In our work, the positions of salient image features, for example, local minima of the brightness gradient, are collected to form a set of candidate segments $\{S_1^i\}$. To choose S_1 among them, the prior curve C^* is translated onto each $\{S_1^i\}$. A confidence weight is assigned to each candidate segment by accumulating image feature values along the relevant portion of translated C^* (Fig. 4(a)). The segment with the highest confidence weight among all segments is chosen as the initial curve segment S_1. An example of the selection of an initial curve segment on CT is shown in Fig. 4(b). Our method provided more effective start conditions for the curve-growing process than Berger and Mohr's method [2] for most of our data.

3   Results for Pulmonary Fissure Segmentation

On CT, a fissure often looks like a ribbon structure with variable width due to respiratory motion and the partial volume effect. Fissures have been demonstrated as frequently incomplete on imaging [6] – they may appear as collections of discontinuous curve segments. Tissue surrounding the fissure, e.g., adjacent vessels or nodules, and clutter due to noise in the imaging process can result in off-curve local minima of the image energy. Traditional active contour methods [8,2] typically cannot overcome these difficulties.

The proposed method has been tested to segment pulmonary fissures on 11 thin-section CT scans of 4 patients. On each slice, a morphological operation was applied to generate a feature map of the local region of interest containing the fissure. The prior shape C^* was estimated from fissures previously segmented in

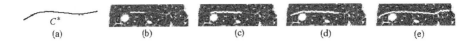

Fig. 5. Curve growing process: (a) Prior curve C^*. (b) Image region with initial curve segment S_1. (c)–(e) Intermediate results after 4, 8, and 18 iterations.

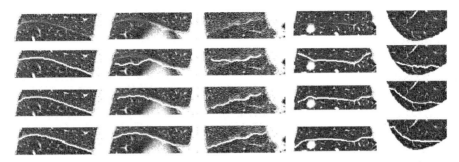

Fig. 6. Comparison of curve-growing results: Row 1: Original images. Row 2: Curve by method in Ref. [2]. Row 3: Curve by proposed method. Row 4: Ground-truth curve.

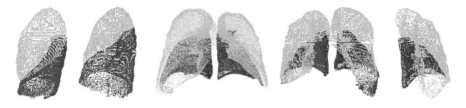

Fig. 7. Visualization of the segmented lung lobes of four patients.

other images of the same scan. For each CT scan, the fissure on a single slice was segmented semi-automatically; the fissures on the remaining slices were then segmented fully automatically (Figs. 5 and 6). The average time for segmenting fissures in one CT scan was less than 5 min on a PIII 1.2 GHz PC. Among 509 slices sampled from a total 1432 slices, the proposed method successfully segmented the fissures on 460 slices. The overall success rate was $460/509 = 90.4\%$. The method then interpolated the segmentation of fissures on the remaining slices. Berger and Mohr's method [2] produced comparable results in the few cases where image features were sufficiently salient (Fig. 6). In many other cases, where image features were ambiguous, our method produced more meaningful results. Finally, the lung lobes were fully segmented by combining the segmented fissures with lung contours [3], as visualized in Fig. 7.

4   Conclusion and Future Work

We described a shape-based curve-growing method and its application to pulmonary fissure segmentation. Effectively selecting the location of the next curve segment in each iteration of the curve-growing process is a critical part of our solution. It overcomes some of the difficulties encountered by other methods [8, 2]. Moreover, the idea of adaptive regularization may be generalized and applied to other model-based energy-minimizing mechanisms. This will be investigated in future work involving different applications, possibly in higher dimensional spaces.

References

1. Y.S. Akgul, C. Kambhamettu, and M. Stone. Automatic extraction and tracking of the tongue contours. *IEEE Trans Med Imag*, 18:1035–1045, 1999.
2. M.O. Berger and R. Mohr. Towards autonomy in active contour models. In *Tenth International Conference on Pattern Recognition*, 847–851, Atlantic City, U.S., 1990.
3. M. Betke, J.B. Wang, and J.P. Ko. An integrated chest CT image analysis system – "BU-MIA." *Tech. Report, Boston University, Computer Science Department*, 2003.
4. T.F. Cootes, C.J. Taylor, D.H. Cooper and J. Graham. Active shape models - their training and application. *Comput Vis Image Underst*, 61:38–59, 1995.
5. M.L. Giger and C.J. Vyborny. Computers aid diagnosis of breast abnormalities. *Diagn Imaging*, 15:98–102, 1993.
6. H.S. Glazer, D.J. Anderson, J.J. DiCroce, et al. Anatomy of the major fissure: evaluation with standard and thin-section CT. *Radiology*. 180:839–44, 1991
7. P. Golland, R. Kikinis, M. Halle, et al. AnatomyBrowser: A Novel Approach to Visualization and Integration of Medical Information. *J Computer Assisted Surg*, 4:129–143, 1999.
8. M. Kass, A. Witkin, and D. Terzopoulos. Snakes: Active contour models. *Int J Comput Vis*, 1:321–331, 1987.
9. M. Kubo, Y. Kawata, N. Niki et al. Automatic extraction of pulmonary fissures from multidetector-row CT images. In *Proceedings of the IEEE International Conference on Image Processing*. 1091–1094, Thessaloniki, Greece, 2001.
10. S.Z. Li. Markov Random Field Modeling in Computer Vision. Springer, 1995.
11. M.E. Leventon, W.E.L. Grimson, and O. Faugeras. Statistical shape influence in geodesic active contours. In *Proceedings of the IEEE Conference on Computer Vision and Pattern Recognition*, I:316–323, Hilton Head, U.S., 2000.
12. R.Malladi, J.A. Sethian and B.C. Vemuri. Shape modeling with front propagation: A level set approach. In *IEEE Trans Pattern Anal Mach Intell*, 17:158–175, 1995.
13. J. Pearl. Probabilistic reasoning in intelligent systems: Networks of plausible inference. San Mateo, California. Morgan Kaufmann, 1988.
14. D.L. Pham, C. Xu, and J.L. Prince. Current Methods in Medical Image Segmentation. *Annual Review of Biomedical Engineering*, 2:315+, 2000.
15. J. Wang, M. Betke, and J.P. Ko. Segmentation of pulmonary fissures on diagnostic CT – preliminary experience. In *Proceedings of the International Conference on Diagnostic Imaging and Analysis*, 107–112, Shanghai, China, 2002.
16. D.J. Williams and M. Shah. A fast algorithm for active contours and curvature estimation. *CVGIP: Image Understanding*, 55:14–26, 1992.
17. L. Zhang. Atlas-driven lung lobe segmentation in volumetric X-ray CT images. Ph.D. Thesis, University of Iowa. 2002.

A Fully Automated Method for the Delineation of Osseous Interface in Ultrasound Images

Vincent Daanen[1], Jerome Tonetti[2], and Jocelyne Troccaz[1]

[1] Joseph Fourier University,
TIMC Laboratory, GMCAO Department
Institut d'Ingénierie de l'Information de Santé (IN3S)
Faculty of Medecine - 38706 La Tronche cedex - France
[2] University Hospital
Orthopaedic Surgery Department
CHU A Michallon, BP217
38043 Grenoble

Abstract. We present a new method for delineating the osseous interface in ultrasound images. Automatic segmentation of the bone-soft tissues interface is achieved by mimicking the reasoning of the expert in charge of the manual segmentation. Information are modeled and fused by the use of fuzzy logic and the accurate delineation is then performed by using general a priori knowledge about osseous interface and ultrasound imaging physics. Results of the automatic segmentation are compared with the manual segmentation of an expert.

1 Introduction

In computer-aided orthopaedic surgery (CAOS), the knowledge of the bone volume position and geometry in the operative room is essential. The usual way to acquire it is to register pre-operative data with intra-operative data. For the last years, the use of ultrasound imaging as intra-operative imaging has significantly increased ([1,2,3,4]) because such imaging investigations are inexpensive and riskless ; and using 6D localized ultrasound probe makes it possible to reconstruct the 3D shape of a structure after its delineation. The extraction of structures from ultrasound data appears to be a delicate key point in CAOS. Several automatic or semi-automatic methods have been proposed to achieve the delineation of features in ultrasound images but these methods apply to specific parts of the human body ([2,3]) because of the poor quality of the ultrasound images (low contrast, low signal-to-noise ratio and speckle noise). We propose a fully automated method in order to achieve the delineation of the bone-soft tissues interface in ultrasound images based on data fusion : data available in images are modeled and fused by the use of fuzzy logic. We then mimic the expert's reasoning to accurately delineate the osseous interface.

C. Barillot, D.R. Haynor, and P. Hellier (Eds.): MICCAI 2004, LNCS 3216, pp. 549–557, 2004.

2   Material and Method

2.1   Material

Ultrasound imaging is achieved using a linear US probe, 25 mm large, working at a frequency of 7.5 MHz. The probe is localized in 3D space by an optical localizer. The US probe is calibrated according to the technique described in [5] (the pixel size is about 0.1mm/pixel). The position of an image pixel is known in 3D space with a precision in the range of the optical localizer (i.e. 1mm).

2.2   Method

In this section, we introduce the expert's reasoning and the way we mimic it in order to achieve an accurate segmentation of the osseous interface.

Expert's reasoning. The expert's reasoning is based on one hand on the physics of the ultrasound imaging and on the other hand on his knowledge of anatomy. Five properties can be pointed out :

1 - bones appear to be hyper-echoic
> the great difference of acoustical impedance between bones and surrounding soft-tissues generates an important echo.

2 - bones are said to 'stop' ultrasound waves
> this is due to the high absorption rate of bones.

3 - the reflection is almost completely specular
> only interfaces almost perpendicular to the direction of the ultrasound beam will reflect so features of interest appear to be composed of horizontal (or near horizontal) parts.

4 - non-broken bone surface do not present major discontinuities
> the found osseous interface should be as smooth as possible.

5 - among an osseous interface, the contrast appears to be homogeneous

We propose a method that models these information and mimics the reasoning of the expert. The method is divided into 3 steps :

- **the image processing step**
  > which aims at modeling the information available in the images and then concentrate them into one image representing the membership of the pixel to a given property. This stage models and fuses points 1,2 and 3 cited above.
- **the 'continuity-ness' cost function computation step**
  > which aims at finding continuous osseous interfaces from the fuzzy image. We model here the point 4.
- **the contrast computation and decision making**
  > which purpose is to select the optimal osseous interface from the candidates at the previous step from the fifth property.

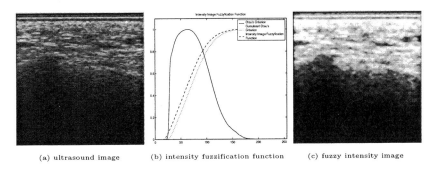

(a) ultrasound image   (b) intensity fuzzification function   (c) fuzzy intensity image

Fig. 1. Computation of FII from the original ultrasound image (pelvic bone)

Image Processing Step

Fuzzy Intensity Image: this image attempts to model the first property, i.e. in ultrasound imaging, bones appear as hyper-echoic and therefore *bright* pixels constitute an indication of the location of the osseous interface. In a previous development [6], we pointed out that binarizing the initial ultrasound image using the Otsu's threshold (T_{Otsu}) gives a good approximation of the echogenic area and so, of the position of the osseous interface.

We make use of this information to build the fuzzification function μ_{Int} : the criterion (we call V_{Otsu} : Fig.1-b, *solid curve*), needed to compute T_{Otsu}, is used as follows ; first, V_{Otsu} is normalized and cumulated (Fig.1-b, *dotted curve*) and it is then shifted in order to force the membership function value :

$$\mu_{Int}(T_{Otsu}) = 0.5 \qquad (1)$$

The fuzzification function (Fig.1-b, *dashed curve*) is finally applied over the gray-level image in order to achieve the construction of the fuzzy intensity image $FII(p)$ which gives for a pixel p of the intensity image its membership degree to the echogenic area.

Fig.1-a shows an ultrasound image[1] of the sacrum part, the intensity fuzzification function and the Intensity Fuzzy Image (Fig.1-c).

Fuzzy Gradient Image: the gradient information constitutes another important part in the determination of the osseous interface and so the fuzzy gradient image $FGI(p)$ is of great interest. Indeed, the transition from the bone to the acoustic shadow area suggests to search for highly contrasted pixels (properties 1 and 2) and because ultrasound imaging should only 'detect' structure changes which are perpendicular to the ultrasound beam (point 3: Fig. 2-a), we make use a 5x5 'horizontal-direction' MDIF edge detector, which is a first-order derivative filter obtained by the convolution of the 4-connexity 3×3 mean lowpass filter with the Prewitt's derivative kernels.

---

[1] All the images have been cropped to half their length because the inferior part does not present any interest

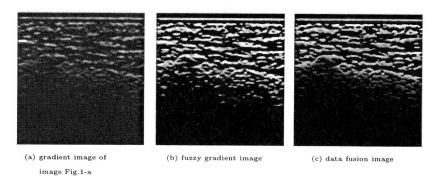

(a) gradient image of   (b) fuzzy gradient image   (c) data fusion image
image Fig.1-a

Fig. 2. Gradient image, *FGI* and Fusion Image of the original ultrasound image

The resulting image is then thresholded in order to remove the transition from *dark-to-bright*. Finally, we use the S-shape function to perform the *fuzzification* of the gradient image and obtain the *Fuzzy Image Gradient FGI(p)* (Fig. 2-b). The parameters of the S-shape function are computed such that $S(x)$ is the closest s-shape function to the normalized cumulative histogram.

Data Fusion: a pixel of the US image may belong to the osseous interface if both its gray-level and gradient are 'high'. This combination is achieved by the use of the 'conjunctive-type' combination operator *min* . The membership of a pixel to the osseous interface is then given by :

$$FI(p) = min(FII(p), FGI(p))\qquad(2)$$

$FI(p)$ denotes the global degree of membership of the pixel p to the echogenic area and to an highly contrasted image area (Fig.2-c).

Determination of the osseous interface. According to the expert's reasoning, the optimal threshold described a continuous interface where the local contrast is maximum and homogeneous. For each membership degree $0 < \mu < 1$ (μ space is discretized with a step $\delta_\mu = 0.005$), the defuzzification of $FI(p)$ is performed and the 'continuity-ness' of the profile is evaluated. We then choose the membership degree which maximizes the local contrast and its homogeneity, and also ensures a local maximum continuity of the profile.

Defuzzification at a given membership degree μ: the defuzzification process aims at extracting from the fuzzy image $FI(p)$ the osseous interface related to a membership degree μ_{ref}. To achieve this task, we make use of a priori knowledge about the physics of ultrasound imaging. As mentioned earlier, bones 'stop' the US-waves and so, for a column of the image, the pixel of the osseous interface related to a membership value μ_{ref} is the last (from the top) pixel which has a membership equal to μ_{ref}. At the end of this *defuzzification* process, at the most one pixel per column is highlighted. The 'curve' described by these pixels is called *profile* in the rest of the paper.

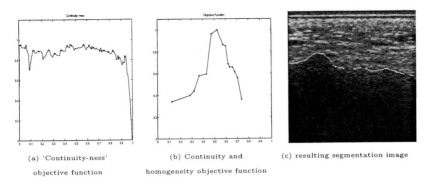

(a) 'Continuity-ness'
objective function

(b) Continuity and
homogeneity objective function

(c) resulting segmentation image

Fig. 3. Computation of FII from the original ultrasound image

Evaluation of the 'continuity-ness' of the profile: because, actual osseous interfaces do not present discontinuities, the osseous interface we detect should be as smooth as possible. We use this property to determine the optimal defuzzification threshold by computing a function that reflects the 'continuity-ness' of a computed osseous interface.

The measure of the 'continuity-ness' of a profile is achieved by applying the wavelet transform to it : the wavelet transform decomposes the profile with a multiresolution scale factor of two providing one low-resolution approximation (A_1) and one wavelet detail (D_1). We then apply the wavelet transform to A_1 and get a second order low-resolution approximation (A_2) and wavelet detail (D_2). The *Detail* signals are then used to quantify the discontinuities of the original profile. The 'amount' of discontinuities in the profile is computed as follows :

$$\varepsilon(\mu) = E(D_1) + E(D_2) + Pen \qquad (3)$$

where $E(s)$ is the energy of a signal $s(t)$.

Experimentally, we choose the Daubechies-4 wavelet basis (several other bases have been tested and no dependence was pointed out at the exception of the Haar Basis). *Pen* is a penalization term related to the length of the profile which is used to reject small osseous interfaces detected when μ_{ref} is unsuitable (i.e. too high).

Finally, $\varepsilon(\mu)$ is normalized (giving $\varepsilon'(\mu)$) and we compute the 'continuity-ness' of the profile as :

$$C(\mu) = 1 - \varepsilon'(\mu) \qquad (4)$$

As one can see (Fig.3-a), the 'continuity-ness' function $C(\mu)$ presents several local maxima. Each of them locates a membership degree μ where the associated profile is more continuous than the profiles of its neighbors and so each of them may be the optimal defuzzification threshold. We detect them by computing the watershed transform of $C(\mu)$. For each local maxima, the image is defuzzed to the corresponding membership degree μ and the local contrast is computed.

Local contrast computation: for each pixel p belonging to a profile, the local contrast $LC(p)$ associated to the pixel p is computed by :

$$LC(p) = \frac{\overline{Up} - \overline{Down}}{\overline{Up} + \overline{Down}} \tag{5}$$

where $\overline{Up}$ (resp. $\overline{Down}$) is the mean value of the above (resp. underneath) region-of-interest[2]. The global contrast along the profile $Contrast(\mu)$ is then computed by :

$$Contrast(\mu) = \sum_p LC(p) \tag{6}$$

We also evaluate the homogeneity of the local contrasts along a profile by computing the standard deviation of the values along it. This gives us a function $StdDev(\mu)$.

Optimal defuzzification threshold determination: Finally, the optimal membership degree is the one that maximized $Cost(\mu)$:

$$\mu_{Optimal} = \arg\max Cost(\mu)) \tag{7}$$

where

$$Cost(\mu) = Contrast(\mu) + \frac{1}{StdDev(\mu)} \tag{8}$$

Fig.3-b shows the objective function computed by (8) and the resulting segmentation is shown in Fig.3-c.

3   Results

The proposed method has been tested on ultrasound images of sacrum coming from cadaver datasets or patient datasets : about 300 images have been processed. For each image, the manual segmentation of the expert is available and constitutes our bronze-standard.

For each image within a dataset, we compute the error between the manual segmentation and the segmentation computed by our method. We then compute the mean error for each image (Table 1-column 1) and the Hausdorff distance and mean absolute distance (average of all the maximum errors within a subset) (Table 1-column 2). In order to evaluate the ability of the proposed method to delineate the osseous interface in strongly corrupted images, we also compute the *Signal-to-Mean Squared Error* ratio (Table 1-column 3)(see [7] for more information about the S/MSE).

---

[2] A *roi* is an area of 10 pixels long-by-1 pixel large

Table 1. Segmentation differences

Dataset	Segmentation Error mean/SD (pixel)	Max Errors mean/max (pixel)	S/mse mean/SD (dB)
Patient 1 (51 images)	7.808 / 1.995	12.137 / 22	5.052 / 0.185
Patient 2 (49 images)	8.807 / 3.177	16.905 / 25	5.206 / 0.428
Patient 3 (69 images)	4.545 / 3.874	17.0789 / 35	8.905 / 0.283
Cadaver 1 (37 images)	3.495 / 1.931	9.830 / 36	8.786 / 0.340
Cadaver 2 (41 images)	2.679 / 1.456	7.294 / 19	9.019 / 0.259
Cadaver 3 (39 images)	4.056 / 3.213	12.14 / 38	7.984 / 0.177

pixel size is 0.112mm x 0.109mm

As one can see (table 1), as compared to the manual delineation of the expert:

- the mean error of segmentation is always less than 10 pixels (i.e. 1mm) even on highly corrupted images. However, it is clear that the accuracy of the delineation is correlated within the amount of noise and therefore, we think that taking into account the noise (measured by the S/sme ratio by example) during the fusion and/or delineation process may be a way to improve the delineation.

- the maximum errors still remain important but, according to us, it is not the error we should focus on : we point out that these errors occur at more or less one pixel on complex shapes (such as medial sacral crest or sacral hiatus) giving thus an important maximum error comparatively the manual delineation but the overall error on the global shape still remains negligible and has very limited impact on the registration step which follows.

- the proposed method is also sufficiently fast to be used during the intra-operative stage of a CAOS : the time needed to delineate one image is less than 4 s on a *Pentium III*-800 MHz PC. The processing of large datasets such as *Patient 3* takes about 4 minutes whereas it would take more than 30 minutes in the case of a manual delineation (according to [1]).

This method have also been used to delineate the osseous interface in femur and vertebrae ultrasound images and the osseous interface was well delineated in particular the spinous process in vertebrae images.

4   Discussion

Recently, lots of methods dedicated to the *indirect* delineation of the bone surface in ultrasound images have been proposed in the literature ([2,3]) but these methods have not been tested on real patients' datasets yet. Moveover, the ultrasound imaging is constrained by the use of a mechanical system ([2]) ; and a good initial estimation of the rigid registration matrix between the CT and US datasets is often required to achieve the bone surface segmentation in the ultrasound images ([3,4]).

The method described in this paper does not require neither a dedicated ultrasound images acquisition system nor an estimation of the rigid registration matrix between the CT and US datasets to perform the delineation of the osseous interface in ultrasound images. Moreover, it has been extensively tested on images acquired on cadavers (about 120 images) and on real patients (about 170 images). We point out that although the method is sensible to noise, the mean errors are still acceptable : we measure a maximum mean error of 8.8 pixels (i.e. 0.8 mm) with a S/mse ratio of 5.206 dB which corresponds to a highly corrupted image (according to [7]).

We do not notice any dependence of the results to the visualization parameters tuning at the exception that the osseous interface should not get bogged down in noise. We think that this condition is acceptable since the physician has to validate the images during the acquisition stage (and so, this validation can only be done if he is able to localize the osseous interface).

We think that an important point has also to be made clear : the validation, based on the comparison to a single expert segmentation, may appear limited. However, segmenting bones on ultrasound images is very unusual for physicians and it is difficult to find several expert users. Moreover, gold-standard does not exist and tests on phantoms or isolated bones would not allow to draw conclusions applicable to real data. Thus, we consider that this evaluation is a first step.

5 Conclusion

In this paper, we presented a method for automatic delineation of the osseous interface in ultrasound image. The method is based on the fusion of the pixels intensity and gradient properties in a first step and then on the fusion of information extracted from the physics of ultrasound imaging and a priori knowledge. The method has been used to delineate osseous interface in ultrasound images of the sacrum which may present several shapes ; we also use it to delineate the osseous interface in vertebrae images and good results were obtained in all cases. As it is independent of the shape to be recovered we think that the described method is a first step toward robust delineation of the osseous interface in ultrasound images.

References

1. L. Carrat, J.Tonetti, S. Lavallée, Ph. Merloz, L. Pittet, and JP. Chirosset. Treatment of Pelvic Ring Fractures : Percutaneous Computer Assisted Iliosacral Screwing. In *CS Serie, Springer Verlag, MICCAI*, volume 1496, pages 84–91, 1998.
2. B. Brendel, S. Winter, A. Rick, M. Stockheim, and H. Ermert. Registration of 3D CT and Ultrasound Datasets of the Spine using Bone Structures. *Computer Aided Surgery*, 7(3):146–155, 2002.
3. D.V. Amin, T Kanade, A.M. DiGioia III, and B. Jaramaz. Ultrasound Registration of the Bone Surface for Surgical Navigation. *Computer Aided Surgery*, (8):1–16, 2003.

4. G. Ionescu, S.Lavallée, and J. Demongeot. Automated Registration of Ultrasound with CT Images : Application to Computer Assisted Prostate Radiotherapy and Orthopedics. In *CS Serie, Springer Verlag, MICCAI*, volume 1679, pages 768–777, 1999.
5. T. Lang . *Ultrasound Guided Surgery : Image Processing and Navigation*. PhD thesis, Norwegian University of Science and Technology, Trondheim, Norway, 2000.
6. V. Daanen, J. Tonetti, J. Troccaz, and Ph. Merloz. Automatic Determination of the Bone-Soft Tissues Interface in Ultrasound Images. First Results in Iliosacral Screwing Surgery. In *Proceedings of Surgetica-CAMI 2002*, pages 144–151, 2002.
7. A. Achim, A. Bezerianos, and P. Tsakalides. Novel Bayesian Multiscale Method for Speckle Removal in Medical Ultrasound Images. *IEEE Transactions on Medical Imaging*, 20(8):772–783, 2001.

Registration-Based Interpolation Using a High-Resolution Image for Guidance

Graeme P. Penney[1], Julia A. Schnabel[1], Daniel Rueckert[2], David J. Hawkes[1], and Wiro J. Niessen[3]

[1] Imaging Sciences Division, Guy's, King's and St. Thomas' Schools of Medicine, King's College London, UK. graeme.penney@kcl.ac.uk

[2] Visual Information Processing Group, Department of Computing, Imperial College London, UK.

[3] Image Sciences Institute, University Medical Center Utrecht (UMCU), The Netherlands.

Abstract. A method is presented for interpolation between neighbouring slices in a grey-scale tomographic data set, when a high-resolution image of the same patient is also available. Spatial correspondence between adjacent slices in the high-resolution image are established using a voxel-based non-rigid registration algorithm. These spatial correspondences are used to calculate a set of vectors, which are transferred from the high-resolution image to the lower resolution image by rigidly registering the image volumes together. Linear interpolation is then carried out along these vector directions between neighbouring slices in the low-resolution image. This method has been compared to standard linear interpolation, shape-based interpolation and registration-based interpolation in MR head volumes. Results using a mean square difference error measure show that the proposed method outperforms the other three interpolation techniques.

1 Introduction

Three-dimensional medical imaging devices typically produce images as a set of slices. The distance between neighbouring pixels in a slice is often smaller than the centre-to-centre slice separation, and therefore the voxel dimensions are generally not isotropic. In a number of image processing, analysis and visualization tasks it is advantageous to have voxel dimensions which are close to isotropic.

This paper describes a method which can use information from a high-resolution image to aid in the interpolation of a low-resolution image. Example clinical scenarios include: functional MR, where a high-resolution anatomical scan is typically acquired before a number of lower resolution functional images; and studies which involve both CT and MR imaging, where a large CT slice thickness has been used to keep the radiation exposure to the patient at an acceptable level. The terms high- and low-resolution used in this paper refer specifically to the resolution in the image 'Z' direction, i.e. the direction perpendicular to the image slices.

Interpolation techniques can be divided into two groups: scene-based and object-based methods [4]. In scene-based methods the interpolated intensity is determined only from the image intensities: examples include nearest neighbour, linear and spline-based

C. Barillot, D.R. Haynor, and P. Hellier (Eds.): MICCAI 2004, LNCS 3216, pp. 558–565, 2004.

interpolation. These methods can produce large artifacts when the in-plane position of anatomical features shift considerably between slices.

In object-based interpolation some additional information is extracted from the images, and used to help guide the interpolation process. These techniques can be further subdivided into methods which operate on extracted features, and into methods which operate on image intensities. An example of object-based interpolation which uses features is shape-based interpolation [6,12] which has been extended by allowing registration between slices [7] and using feature guidance [9]. These techniques provide a practical way to interpolate between segmented slices. However, they are unable to interpolate grey-scale images. An example of an object-based method which directly uses the image intensities is the extension to shape-based interpolation proposed by Grevera and Udupa [3]. There are also published methods where non-rigid registration is used to register adjacent slices, and then interpolation is carried out between corresponding positions in each slice [2]. We have recently shown how a registration-based method can outperform both linear and shape-based interpolation [11]. This paper describes an extension to our registration-based method which makes use of information from a high-resolution image to guide the interpolation process.

2   Description of Algorithm

For registration-based interpolation two assumptions are made: that adjacent slices contain similar anatomical features, and that the registration algorithm is capable of finding the transformation which maps these similar features together. If the first assumption is violated, and an anatomical feature disappears from one slice to the next, then the advantages of a registration-based approach will be lost. The second assumption is concerned with the types of transformation that the registration algorithm is capable of. If the transformation between features in adjacent slices is outside of the capabilities of the registration algorithm, then the results will be sub-optimum. Examples for this would be: if the underlying model assumes a smooth deformation field, whereas the "true" transformation requires a discontinuity; or if the transformation required by the algorithm is outside of its capture range.

The inputs into the algorithm are shown at the top of Figure 1: a high-resolution (HR) image (a) and a low-resolution (LR) image (b). Figure 1 (c) shows a schematic of a zoomed region defined as lying inside the white rectangle in (a). Some major image features, such as the brain and skull boundary, are represented by the thick lines and the HR slice planes are represented by the dotted lines. The algorithm proceeds as follows:

1. Each slice in the HR image is registered to the adjacent slice using a 2D voxel-based non-rigid registration algorithm (described in section 2.1). This produces a non-rigid transformation T_{NR_i} for each pair of slices $i, i+1$ (where $i = 1, \ldots, N_{HR} - 1$ and N_{HR} is the number of slices in the HR image). The T_{NR_i} are used to calculate a set of interpolation lines L. These lines connect the centre of each pixel $\mathbf{u}$ in slice i with its corresponding position, $T_{NR_i}(\mathbf{u})$ in slice $i+1$, see Figure 1 (c).
2. The HR and LR images are rigidly registered together to calculate T. This transformation is used to transform two adjacent LR slices and an interpolation plane into the HR coordinate system, as shown in Figure 1 (d).

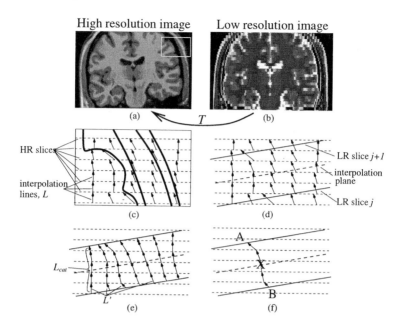

Fig. 1. Interpolation method: low-resolution (LR) image (b) is interpolated using prior information from high-resolution (HR) image (a). Adjacent HR slices are registered together to give interpolation lines (c). Adjacent LR slices are transformed, using T, into the HR image (d). The interpolation lines are concatenated from LR slice j to LR slice $j + 1$ (e). The intensity value at **X** is calculated using linear interpolation between the intensity values at **A** and **B** (f).

3. For each pixel in LR slice j the closest interpolation line is calculated. This line is then translated (parallel to the HR slice planes) so that it intercepts this pixel. These lines form set L'.

4. The non-rigid transformations T_{NR_i} are then successively applied to each interpolation line in L' to extend it from LR slice j to LR slice $j + 1$. This produces a set of concatenated lines L_{cat} as shown in Figure 1 (e).

5. To interpolate a value at position **X** on the interpolation plane, the closest concatenated line in L_{cat} is found, and translated parallel to the LR slices until it intercepts **X**. This line is used to calculate positions **A** and **B** in Figure 1 (f).

6. The pixel intensity value at **X** is calculated using linear interpolation between the intensity values at **A** and **B**.

This new approach has two main advantages over standard registration-based interpolation: Firstly, the standard approach assumed that features in adjacent slices were connected by straight lines, whereas this method follows the path of connected features in the HR image. Secondly, because the HR slices are closer together there is less chance of the non-rigid registration algorithm finding a local minimum.

Potential disadvantages of the new approach are: Firstly, that errors may be introduced by the rigid registration T. Secondly, the interpolation method requires a number of non-rigid transformations to be concatenated, and so the overall error will be an aggregate of the individual non-rigid registration errors.

2.1 Matching Process

The registration algorithm is a two-dimensional version of the non-rigid registration algorithm of Rueckert *et al.* [13]. The algorithm models deformations based on a set of B-splines controlled by a regular lattice of control points. The similarity measure was normalized mutual information, and no regularization was used (λ in [13] set to zero).

Three parameters define the optimization process: step size (s) to calculate the finite difference values; grid spacing (g) between the control points; and the maximum number of iterations. The following pairs of g and s values were used for all the experiments described in this paper: $g = 20$ and $s = 5$, $s = 2.5$, $s = 1.25$, $s = 0.625$; then $g = 10$ and $s = 5$, $s = 2.5$, $s = 1.25$, $s = 0.625$; then $g = 5$ and $s = 5$, $s = 2.5$, $s = 1.25$, $s = 0.625$ (all values are in mm). For each pair of g and s values, when either a minimum of the similarity measure is found, or more than 20 iterations occur, the algorithm then moves along to the next pair of g and s values.

3 Experimental Evaluation

The evaluation of our new interpolation method has been carried out in conformity with the paradigm proposed by Grevera and Udupa [4]. We have compared our new approach with three other interpolation methods: linear interpolation, shape-based interpolation (or more specifically, shape-based averaging [3]) and a registration-based method [11]. Linear intensity interpolation was implemented in a standard fashion. The shape-based algorithm was implemented using information from [3], the weighting between pixel dimensions and intensity values (called the intensity scale factor μ in [3]) was set equal to 0.25. Euclidean distance transforms were generated by using the method described in [10]. The registration-based algorithm is described in [11]. It uses the registration algorithm and optimization described in Section 2.1 to obtain corresponding positions in each slice, and then carries out linear interpolation between these positions.

3.1 Data

Experiments have been carried out using the BrainWeb simulated Brain Database [8, 1][1]. MR T1, T2 and proton density (PD) images were generated with zero noise and image sizes $181 \times 217 \times 181$ with voxel dimensions $1 \times 1 \times 1$ mm^3. The T1 image was used as the high-resolution image. To simulate the effect of registration errors, this image was translated and rotated by 5mm and 5° in all six degrees of freedom, and then reformatted in this new coordinate system using trilinear interpolation. Each of the slices from this image were then registered to the neighbouring slice. The T2 and PD images were transformed into low-resolution images by removing three from every four slices, resulting in images with a slice thickness of 1mm and a centre-to-centre slice separation

---

[1] http://www.bic.mni.mcgill.ca/brainweb/

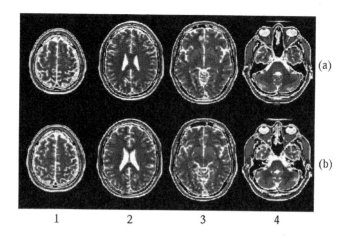

Fig. 2. The four pairs of superior (a) and inferior (b) adjacent slices chosen from the low-resolution T2 data set.

of 4mm. Each LR image was then registered to the high-resolution T1 volume, using a rigid registration algorithm based on normalised mutual information [14], to calculate transformation T.

3.2 Method

Four pairs of adjacent slices were chosen from the low-resolution T2 and PD data sets, as shown in Figure 2. A position was chosen near the top of the head to produce the pair of slices labelled as 1 in Figure 2. Three other pairs of slices were then extracted at 32mm intervals below this top pair of slices. Each interpolation algorithm was used to produce a slice midway between the chosen slices. This interpolated slice was then compared to the corresponding slice from the original high-resolution T2 and PD data sets. Initially visual inspection was used to compare the slices, and then the mean square difference (MSD) between the intensity values of the two slices was calculated, as given by Equation (1), where N_R is the number of interpolated pixels in the slice, and $I_i(\mathbf{u})_{int}$ and $I_i(\mathbf{u})_{orig}$ are the interpolated and original intensity values at pixel position $\mathbf{u}$.

$$\text{MSD} = \frac{1}{N_R} \sum_{\mathbf{u} \in R} (I_i(\mathbf{u})_{int} - I_i(\mathbf{u})_{orig})^2 \qquad (1)$$

Following Grevera and Udupa [4] we have used a measure called statistical relevance, which essentially shows the percentage difference between two interpolation techniques, e.g. the statistical relevance r between linear MSD_{lin} and shape-based averaging MSD_{sba} is given by Equation 2.

$$r_{sba/lin} = \begin{cases} +100 \times [1 - \text{MSD}_{sba}/\text{MSD}_{lin}] & , \quad \text{if} \ \ \text{MSD}_{lin} > \text{MSD}_{sba} \\ -100 \times [1 - \text{MSD}_{lin}/\text{MSD}_{sba}] & , \quad \text{otherwise} \end{cases} \qquad (2)$$

Table 1. Statistical relevance values, comparing four interpolation techniques using a mean square difference (MSD) error measure.

interpolation methods	MSD statistical relevance r								mean value
	T2 slice number				PD slice number				
	1	2	3	4	1	2	3	4	
hrg/reg	12.9	32.2	33.1	23.1	1.0	15.9	8.9	19.1	18.3
hrg/sba	80.4	46.1	49.8	41.9	81.9	34.4	20.9	34.5	48.7
hrg/lin	85.2	53.2	49.9	46.5	88.8	53.2	32.4	48.2	57.2
reg/sba	77.5	20.5	25.0	24.4	81.7	22.0	13.2	18.9	35.4
reg/lin	83.0	31.0	25.1	30.4	88.7	44.4	25.9	35.9	45.6
sba/lin	24.7	13.2	0.1	7.9	38.1	28.7	14.6	21.0	18.5

4   Results

Table 1 shows the MSD statistical relevance (r) values which compare the four interpolation algorithms: high-resolution guided (hrg), registration-based (reg), shape-based (sba) and linear (lin). Results are given for both the T2 and PD data sets for each of the four slices individually. All the values in Table 1 are positive, which means that (using MSD as an error measure, and for the data used in this paper) we can rank the interpolation methods from best to worse as: high-resolution guided, registration-based, shape-based and linear.

Figure 3 shows difference or subtraction images for each of the 4 slices in the T2 data set and for each interpolation technique. At the top of the head (slice 1), where the skull diameter changes significantly between slices, large errors were observed when using linear interpolation. Shape-based interpolation accurately interpolated the outer boundary of the skull in this region, but did not perform so well in interpolating structures immediately inside the skull boundary, whereas both the registration-based and high-resolution guided methods performed more accurately in this region.

Slice 2 cuts through the ventricles, which can be seen to change greatly in size and shape between the two slices (see Figure 2). Predictably, the linear interpolation algorithm is unable to interpolate these features accurately. The registration-based algorithm also had difficulties, and failed to completely recover the large changes in size and shape of the ventricles. The shape-based algorithm performed well in the region of the ventricles, however, larger differences elsewhere in the images still resulted in a larger MSD value compared to the registration-based method (see Table 1). The best result visually, both near the ventricles and in the surrounding image, was achieved using the high-resolution guided method.

In slices 3 and 4 a general improvement in the interpolation methods can be seen with the images becoming a more uniform grey colour with fewer residual features remaining as you look from the bottom to the top of Figure 3.

5   Discussion and Future Work

We have presented a novel interpolation algorithm which can use a high-resolution image to guide the interpolation. Although experiments have only been carried out to interpolate

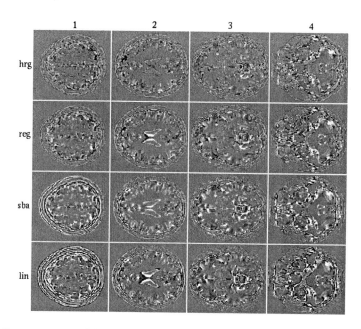

Fig. 3. Difference images $I(u)_{orig} - I(u)_{int}$ for each interpolated slice from the T2 image, and for each interpolation technique.

eight slices, these preliminary results are encouraging, showing an average improvement in statistical relevance of 18.3 compared to registration-based interpolation, 48.7 compared to shape-based averaging and 57.2 compared to linear interpolation.

The algorithm assumes that corresponding structures in adjacent slices from one modality will line up in the same way as corresponding structures from a second modality. This is a reasonable assumption if both of the images are anatomical i.e. MR T1 or T2 weighted, or CT. However, the validity of using a high-resolution T1 image to help interpolate a functional MR image requires further investigation. In addition, problems may arise if the high-resolution image does not depict structures present in the low-resolution image. This could occur if a high-resolution CT image was used to guide the interpolation of soft-tissue structures in a low-resolution MR image.

We have used a very general error measure to compare the interpolation techniques. In future it may be advantageous to tailor the error measure to a particular clinical problem. This type of approach has been proposed by Grevera *et al.* [5] where, as an example, they examine how interpolation methods influence the accuracy of multiple sclerosis lesion volume measurement.

The algorithm described in this paper requires a rigid-body relationship between the high- and low-resolution images. We are currently working on an algorithm which can allow a non-rigid relationship between the images. This should greatly increase the flexibility of this method. Particularly in areas such as cardiac imaging where it is possible to acquire end-diastolic high-resolution images, where the heart is moving relatively slowly, whereas at other points in the cardiac cycle, as the heart is moving more quickly, lower resolution images are usually acquired. We currently believe the greatest benefit of moving to a system which allows a non-rigid relationship between the high- and low-resolution images, would be the possibility of replacing the high-resolution image with an atlas image and, therefore, removing the requirement of a high-resolution image altogether.

Acknowledgements. Thanks go to Calvin Maurer Jr. for providing fast distance transfer software; Medical IT – Advanced Development, Philips Medical Systems BV, Best, The Netherlands for funding J.A. Schnabel; and to the Netherlands Organization for Scientific Research (NWO) VENI grant programme for sponsoring W.J.Niessen.

References

1. D.L. Collins, A.P. Zijdenbos, V. Kollokian, J.G. Sled, N.J. Kabani, C.J. Holmes, and A.C. Evans. Design and construction of a realistic digital brain phantom. *IEEE Trans. Med. Imaging*, 17(3):463–468, 1998.
2. A. Goshtasby, D.A. Turner, and V. Ackerman. Matching of tomographic slices for interpolation. *IEEE Trans. Med. Imaging*, 11(4):507–516, 1992.
3. G.J. Grevera and J.K. Udupa. Shape-based interpolation of multidimensional grey-level images. *IEEE Trans. Med. Imaging*, 15(6):881–892, 1996.
4. G.J. Grevera and J.K. Udupa. An objective comparison of 3-D image interpolation methods. *IEEE Trans. Med. Imaging*, 17(4):642–652, 1998.
5. G.J. Grevera, J.K. Udupa, and Y. Miki. A task-specific evaluation of three-dimensional image interpolation techinques. *IEEE Trans. Med. Imaging*, 18(2):137–143, 1999.
6. G.T. Herman, J. Zheng, and C.A. Bucholtz. Shape-based interpolation. *IEEE Comput. Graph. Appl.*, 12(3):69–79, 1992.
7. W.E. Higgins, C. Morice, and E.L. Ritman. Shape-based interpolation of tree-like structures in three-dimensional images. *IEEE Trans. Med. Imaging*, 12(3):439–450, 1993.
8. R.K.-S. Kwan, A.C. Evans, and Pike G.B. MRI simulation-based evaluation of image-processing and classification methods. *IEEE Trans. Med. Imaging*, 18(11):1085–1097, 1999.
9. T.-Y. Lee and C.-H. Lin. Feature-guided shape-based image interpolation. *IEEE Trans. Med. Imaging*, 21(12):1479–1489, 2002.
10. C.R. Maurer, Jr., R. Qi, and V. Raghavan. A linear time algorithm for computing exact Euclidean distance transforms of binary images in arbitrary dimensions. *IEEE Trans. Pattern Anal. Mach. Intell.*, 25(2):265–269, 2003.
11. G.P. Penney, J.A. Schnabel, D. Rueckert, M.A. Viergever, and W.J. Niessen. Registration-based interpolation. *IEEE Trans. Med. Imaging*. Accepted for publication.
12. S.P. Raya and J.K. Udupa. Shape-based interpolation of multidimensional objects. *IEEE Trans. Med. Imaging*, 9(1):32–42, 1990.
13. D. Rueckert, L.I. Sonoda, C. Hayes, D.L.G. Hill, M.O. Leach, and D.J. Hawkes. Nonrigid registration using free-form deformations: application to breast MR images. *IEEE Trans. Med. Imaging*, 18(8):712–721, 1999.
14. C. Studholme, D.L.G. Hill, and D.J. Hawkes. An overlap invariant entropy measure of 3D medical image alignment. *Pattern Recognition*, 32:71–86, 1999.

Surface-Based Registration with a Particle Filter

Burton Ma and Randy E. Ellis

School of Computing, Queen's University at Kingston, Canada K7L 3N6

Abstract. We propose the use of a particle filter as a solution to the rigid shape-based registration problem commonly found in computer-assisted surgery. This approach is especially useful where there are only a few registration points corresponding to only a fraction of the surface model. Tests performed on patient models, with registration points collected during surgery, suggest that particle filters perform well and also provide novel quality measures to the surgeon.

1 Introduction

Preoperative 3D medical images, such as CT and MRI scans, can be registered intraoperatively to a patient's anatomy by estimating a transformation from surfaces in image coordinates to anatomical points in patient coordinates for use in image-guided surgery. Two notable limitations of current algorithms are: (a) most algorithms are non-incremental and process an additional anatomical point by reconsidering the entire set of anatomical points gathered during surgery; and (b) most algorithms report errors such as root-mean-square (RMS) or target registration (TRE) but do not report the probable distribution of errors. Particle filters offer an incremental method for computing probability distributions of the rotational and translational components of a rigid registration.

Most registration algorithms attempt to find the registration parameters that maximize the likelihood of the registration given the anatomical points, surface model, and measurement noise. This results in an *a posteriori* problem that admits a solution by expectation maximization, which has been solved by Chui and Rangarajan [2], Granger and Pennec [6], Dellaert [4], and even by Besl and McKay [1] (the ICP algorithm).

We propose to solve the registration problem by estimating a *filter distribution*. For a state vector $\mathbf{x}_t$ at time t that represents the state of rotation and translation of the registration transformation, and given the observations $\mathbf{y}_1, ..., \mathbf{y}_t \equiv \mathbf{y}_{1:t}$, the filter distribution $p(\mathbf{x}_t|\mathbf{y}_{1:t})$ is the conditional probability distribution over the state vector given the observations. We use a particle filter (PF), specifically the unscented particle filter (UPF) described by van der Merwe et al. [13], to estimate the filter distribution. A PF represents the posterior distribution of the states as a set of weighted *particles* (or samples), making it easy to calculate statistical estimates of the state. This means that we can estimate the registration parameters using the mean, or any other statistical measure of location, and the precision of the parameters in terms of their standard deviations, confidence intervals, or any other statistical measure of spread. All of these estimates are updated *incrementally* as new registration points become available, which gives the surgeon an indication of whether or not more anatomical points are needed to achieve the desired level of precision. Multiple peaks in the distribution indicate

C. Barillot, D.R. Haynor, and P. Hellier (Eds.): MICCAI 2004, LNCS 3216, pp. 566–573, 2004.

that there are multiple plausible registrations and that some action should be taken to resolve the ambiguity; broad peaks indicate that the anatomical points do not provide good localization and that the surgeon should take this into account while operating. Our framework can incorporate any prior knowledge, such as the location and localization uncertainty of landmarks, into the estimation process.

2 Previous Work

Particle filtering is a Monte Carlo method for estimating the posterior distribution of a state space model. The technique has been independently described by many different authors; a survey of sequential sampling methods for Bayesian filtering has been written by Doucet et al. [5]. An example of more recent work is the mixture particle filter of Vermaak et al. [15] and its application to multi-target tracking by Okuma et al. [11].

The state space model at time t, is described by a state transition model, $p(\mathbf{x}_t|\mathbf{x}_{t-1})$, and an observation model, $p(\mathbf{y}_t|\mathbf{x}_t)$. The state is modeled as a first-order Markov process, and the observations are conditionally independent given the states. We can express the state transition model (often called the process model), $\mathbf{F}$, and the observation model, $\mathbf{H}$, as

$$\mathbf{x}_t = [x_{1_t}\ x_{2_t}\ x_{3_t}\ x_{4_t}\ x_{5_t}\ x_{6_t}]^T$$
$$\mathbf{x}_{t+1} = \mathbf{F}(\mathbf{x}_t, \mathbf{u}_t, \mathbf{v}_t)$$
$$\mathbf{y}_t = \mathbf{H}(\mathbf{x}_t, \mathbf{u}_t, \mathbf{n}_t) \tag{1}$$

where the registration state has three rotation parameters $x_{1_t}, x_{2_t}, x_{3_t}$ and three translation parameters $x_{4_t}, x_{5_t}, x_{6_t}$; $\mathbf{u}_t$ is a known control input; and $\mathbf{n}_t$ is the observation noise. The process noise, $\mathbf{v}_t$, influences the system dynamics. The distribution of the initial state, $p(\mathbf{x}_0)$, is the prior distribution and must also be specified. The equations $\mathbf{F}$ and $\mathbf{H}$ need not be linear functions of their parameters.

The basic idea underlying the PF is that the posterior distribution $p(\mathbf{x}_{0:t}|\mathbf{y}_{0:t})$ can be approximated by a weighted sum of particles from the posterior distribution. We cannot in general sample directly from the posterior, so instead we sample from a *proposal* distribution $q(\mathbf{x}_{0:t}|\mathbf{y}_{0:t})$. The weights are called the importance weights; particles with high weights correspond to regions of high density in the posterior. Under certain assumptions, the weights at time t can be computed sequentially using the weights at time $t - 1$ to yield an incremental registration algorithm. It is inefficient to keep particles with low importance weights, so a resampling step is performed to remove particles with low weights and multiply particles with high weights. An optional Markov-chain Monte-Carlo step can be introduced after the resampling step to smooth the distribution of particles. The output of the PF is a set of equally weighted samples that approximate the posterior $p(\mathbf{x}_{0:t}|\mathbf{y}_{0:t})$. The filter distribution is simply the marginal distribution $p(\mathbf{x}_t|\mathbf{y}_{0:t})$.

The UPF uses the unscented Kalman filter (UKF) of Julier and Uhlmann [10] (see also [16] and the Gaussian filters of Ito and Xiong [8]) to compute a Gaussian approximation of the posterior for each particle; the proposal is drawn from the resulting Gaussian distribution. The UKF is a filter that assumes a state space model given by Equation 1.

- Initialize the filter by drawing $i = 1, ..., N$ particles $\mathbf{x}_0^i$ from the prior distribution of the states $p(\mathbf{x}_0)$. Assign to each particle a covariance matrix $\mathbf{P}_0^i$ (which will be propagated through the UKF).
- For time $t = 1, 2, 3, ...$
  - For $i = 1, ..., N$
    * Filter particle $\mathbf{x}_{t-1}^i$ with covariance $\mathbf{P}_{t-1}^i$ using the UKF to get an updated estimate $\bar{\mathbf{x}}_t^i$ and $\hat{\mathbf{P}}_t^i$
    * Sample $\hat{\mathbf{x}}_t^i$ from the Gaussian proposal $q(\mathbf{x}_t^i | \mathbf{x}_{0:t-1}^i, \mathbf{y}_{0:t}) = \mathcal{N}(\bar{\mathbf{x}}_t^i, \hat{\mathbf{P}}_{t-1}^i)$
    * Compute the observation likelihood $p(\mathbf{y}_t | \hat{\mathbf{x}}_t^i)$
    * Compute the state transition prior $p(\hat{\mathbf{x}}_t^i | \mathbf{x}_{t-1}^i)$
    * Compute the importance weight $w_t^i \propto \frac{p(\mathbf{y}_t | \hat{\mathbf{x}}_t^i) p(\hat{\mathbf{x}}_t^i | \mathbf{x}_{t-1}^i)}{q(\hat{\mathbf{x}}_t^i | \mathbf{x}_{0:t-1}^i, \mathbf{y}_{0:t})}$
  - Normalize the importance weights $w_t^i = w_t^i / \sum_{i=1}^N w_t^i$
  - Apply a resampling scheme to remove particles with low weights and multiply particles with high weights if necessary.
  - Output the N particles $\mathbf{x}_t^i$, or more generally the particle trajectories $\mathbf{x}_{0:t}^i$

Fig. 1. The unscented particle filter algorithm.

It propagates the state mean and covariance through the (possibly non-linear) process and observation models by using a set of deterministically sampled points called sigma points. The previously cited references provide evidence of the superior performance of the UKF compared to the well known extended Kalman filter.

Figure 1 is an abbreviated version of the UPF algorithm; the algorithm is discussed in much greater detail by van der Merwe et al. [13] and the application of the filter to object tracking is given by Rui and Chen [12].

3   UPF Registration

We use the state space model

$$\mathbf{x}_{t+1} = \mathbf{F}(\mathbf{x}_t, \mathbf{v}_t) = \mathbf{x}_t + \mathcal{N}(\mathbf{0}, \mathbf{Q}_t) \tag{2}$$

$$\mathbf{y}_t = \mathbf{H}(\mathbf{x}_t, \mathbf{u}_t, \mathbf{n}_t) = \begin{bmatrix} \mathbf{r}(x_{1_t}, x_{2_t}, x_{3_t})(\mathbf{u}_1 + [x_{4_t} \ x_{5_t} \ x_{6_t}]^T) \\ \vdots \\ \mathbf{r}(x_{1_t}, x_{2_t}, x_{3_t})(\mathbf{u}_t + [x_{4_t} \ x_{5_t} \ x_{6_t}]^T) \end{bmatrix} + \mathcal{N}(\mathbf{0}, \mathbf{R}_t) \tag{3}$$

Equation 2 is the process model for estimating the registration state of the three rotation parameters and the three translation parameters; the model has time-invariant state, except for the additive process noise, because we are estimating a constant. The zero-mean Gaussian process noise with covariance $\mathbf{Q}_t$ allows us to move from possibly poor initial estimates of the state to successively better estimates. We anneal $\mathbf{Q}_t$ towards $\mathbf{0}$ over time as our estimates become better. For this article, we took $\mathbf{Q}_t$ to be uncorrelated with initial variances of $1.22 \times 10^{-3} \text{rad}^2$ and 4mm^2 for the rotational and translational components; we annealed by a factor of 0.7 after each time step. We prefer to use rotation parameters that surgeons are most familiar with, measured as order-independent angles of rotation in the coronal, sagittal, and horizontal planes. Iyun et al. [9][1] presented a simplified version of this rotation matrix.

Our observation model is given by Equation 3 where $\mathbf{r}(x_{1_t}, x_{2_t}, x_{3_t})$ is a rotation matrix, $[x_{4_t}\ x_{5_t}\ x_{6_t}]^T$ is a translation vector, $\mathbf{u}_i$ is the ith registration point in patient coordinates. The model is simply the estimated registration transformation applied to the registration points (which we supply as the control input) concatenated into a single vector; the length of the vector at time t is $3t$. We assume additive, zero-mean Gaussian noise with covariance $\mathbf{R}_t$; the noise is the displacement of each transformed registration point to the surface of the model. For this article, we took $\mathbf{R}_t$ to be uncorrelated with initial variances of 4mm^2 and annealed by a factor of 0.8 after each time step.

The actual observation, $\mathbf{y}_t$, should be the vector formed by the concatenation of the model points corresponding to the registration points; of course, these correspondences are unknown. We used the nearest-neighbor approximation made popular by Besl and McKay [1]; computationally more expensive alternatives such as the Mahalanobis distance (Granger and Pennec [6]) or Gaussian weighted distance (Chui and Rangarajan [2], Grimson et al. [7]) could also be used.

The prior distribution $\mathbf{x}_0$ depends on how the initial estimate of the registration transformation was obtained, e.g., by performing a Monte Carlo simulation of the initial estimation process. If anatomic landmarks or fiducial markers are present then the prior should reflect this information.

4 Experiments

We performed experiments to test for accuracy and precision using synthetic and intraoperatively digitized registration points for the proximal tibia, distal radius, and proximal femur. All surface models were derived from CT scans of patients who consented to surgery and research use of data in a study approved by the Research Ethics Board of Queen's University and Kingston General Hospital.

4.1 Synthetic Points and the Proximal Tibia

We tested for registration accuracy and precision by massively subsampling points from a realistic surgical exposure of the proximal tibia. Fifteen points were selected from the surface model generated from a CT scan of a patient that underwent high tibial osteotomy (HTO). We generated 500 random transformations by drawing from the uniform distribution $\mathcal{U}(\pm 20°, \pm 20°, \pm 20°, \pm 10\text{mm}, \pm 10\text{mm}, \pm 10\text{mm})$; each transformation was applied to the points to which we added random noise drawn from the uniform distribution $\mathcal{U}(\pm 0.5\text{mm}, \pm 0.5\text{mm}, \pm 0.5\text{mm})$. The range of angles and displacements are large compared to the error of the initial estimate that we typically obtain in surgery; the mean total angular displacement was $19°$ and mean total translation was 10mm. We used 5000 particles and a prior of $\mathcal{U}(\pm 25°, \pm 25°, \pm 25°, \pm 12\text{mm}, \pm 12\text{mm}, \pm 12\text{mm})$. We used the UPF to register the transformed point sets, taking the mean of the posterior distribution for the registration parameters. The distribution of rotation and translation errors are shown in Figure 2.

---

[1] There is a typographical error in this reference; in Equation 1, page 235, the term $dc - af$ should be $af - dc$

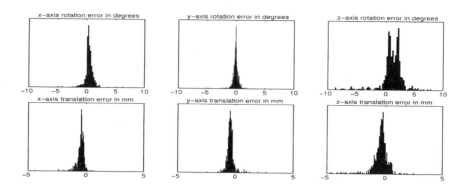

Fig. 2. Proximal tibia and synthetic data results. Error distributions for 500 UPF registrations; standard deviations are $0.98°$, $0.49°$, $2.02°$ for the x, y, z axis rotation errors, and 0.39mm, 0.36mm, 0.77mm for the x, y, z axis translation errors.

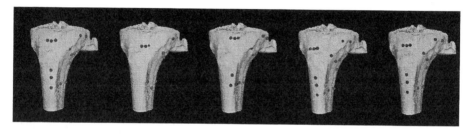

Fig. 3. Proximal tibia and synthetic data results. Left: the registration data points. The other four images are of registrations with large rotation and/or translation errors. The spheres indicating the registration points are 4mm in diameter.

The consistency of the registrations was good, particularly in the rotations about and the translations along the x and y axes. Rotation errors about and translation errors along the z axis (the long axis of the bone) were worse, but this was expected given the shape of the proximal tibia and the location of the surgically accessible region. The registrations that were far from the correct registrations still produced small RMS errors between the registered points and the surface model; the filter simply found a different fit of the very small number of registration points to the model. Figure 3 illustrates the potential difficulty in finding the correct registration.

The evolution of the posterior distribution of the rotation about the z axis for one trial is shown in Figure 4. When there are only a few registration points, the UPF finds a few different possible values for the angle of rotation. As more points are added, the ambiguity is resolved and the posterior converges to narrow range of values.

4.2   Intraoperative Points and the Distal Radius

We performed a retrospective analysis of registration data from seven patients who underwent computer-assisted distal radius osteotomy (Croitoru et al. [3]). We used the registration data collected intraoperatively using a calibrated pointer and an Optotrak

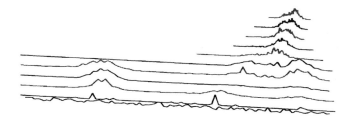

Fig. 4. Proximal tibia and synthetic data results. The evolution of the posterior distribution of the z-axis rotation. The prior distribution, sampled from $\mathcal{U}(\pm 25°)$ is at the bottom. Moving towards the top of the page are the posteriors after $6, 7, ..., 15$ registration points have been processed.

Table 1. Distal radius and intraoperative registration points experimental results. Standard deviations, over 100 trials, of the registration state using the UPF to register to the distal radius. The z axis is the long axis of the bone.

Num. Reg. Pts.	θ_x	θ_y	θ_z	t_x	t_y	t_z
11	0.74°	0.54°	2.48°	0.36mm	0.20mm	0.50mm
10	0.51°	0.83°	1.26°	0.10mm	0.06mm	0.31mm
11	0.54°	0.37°	0.69°	0.08mm	0.10mm	0.30mm
11	0.36°	0.48°	0.42°	0.14mm	0.12mm	0.80mm
10	0.38°	0.27°	0.66°	0.16mm	0.07mm	0.65mm
11	0.26°	0.52°	1.47°	0.05mm	0.06mm	0.13mm
12	0.14°	0.33°	0.69°	0.07mm	0.03mm	0.11mm

3020 localizer (NDI, Waterloo, Canada) and examined the consistency of the UPF registrations. Lister's tubercle is a prominent anatomic landmark on the distal radius. We can use the tubercle to directly estimate the translation component of the registration, thus reducing the range of the translation component of the prior.

We generated 100 random transformations, starting from the surgical registration, for each bone by drawing from the uniform distribution $\mathcal{U}(\pm 10°, \pm 10°, \pm 10°, \pm 1\text{mm}, \pm 1\text{mm}, \pm 3\text{mm})$. We applied these transformations to the registration points and computed the UPF registrations using 2000 particles and a prior of $\mathcal{U}(\pm 12°, \pm 12°, \pm 12°, \pm 3\text{mm}, \pm 3\text{mm}, \pm 5\text{mm})$; standard deviations over the 100 trials are shown in Table 1.

4.3   Intraoperative Points and the Proximal Femur

We examined the utility of obtaining the filter distribution by retrospectively calculating the distribution of probable drill paths for a computer-assisted minimally invasive removal of a deep bone tumor. The registration points for this procedure were collected through a small incision on the lateral side of the hip and percutaneously using a needle-tipped probe. The cylindrical shape of the proximal femur makes it difficult to precisely estimate the axial rotation component of the registration transformation; the standard deviation for this component was $3.34°$. Figure 5 illustrates the osteoma, planned drill

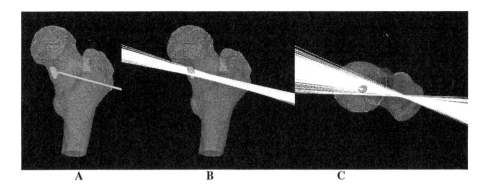

Fig. 5. Proximal femur and intraoperative registration points experimental results. **A** an osteoid osteoma located in the neck of the femur and the planned drill path. **B** predicted drill paths after registration viewed in the frontal plane. **C** predicted drill paths in the axial plane; the axial rotation component has the highest uncertainty due to the almost cylindrical shape of the proximal femur.

path, and the drill path predicted by each of the 2000 particles. It is easy to appreciate the consequences of uncertainty in the axial rotation by direct visualization of the drill paths; target registration error (TRE) is a single number that is less informative.

5   Discussion

UPF registration offers notable advantages to most alternative approaches. Because it is iterative, a surgeon can collect only as many points as needed, which can reduce operative time. More importantly, the surgeon can directly visualize the *quality* of the registration, by examining either the posterior distribution (which gives an overall view of the error space) or of the transformation of a planned trajectory (which gives a task-specific view of error effects). For example, had UPF registration been available when the osteoid osteoma case was performed, the surgeons would have been vividly aware that they were well on target but that the drill bit was more likely to track posteriorly.[2]

Limitations of our study include running times, an unoptimized implementation, and unknown robustness to statistical outliers. The UPF runs in an acceptable period of time when using a small number of registration points. For example, using an Intel Pentium 4 PC (2.8 GHz) we updated the state estimate with 2000 particles and 15 registration points in 1.5 seconds; much of the time was spent performing nearest-neighbor searches. We have not thoroughly investigated the relationship between the number of particles and the estimation process; it may be possible to safely reduce the number of particles. It may even be possible to avoid particle filtering altogether by estimating the posterior density using a Gaussian mixture filter (van der Merwe and Wan [14] or Ito and Xiong [8]). We also have not addressed the issue of robustness to outliers, but we believe that the PF framework will allow us to improve our algorithm in this respect.

---

[2] The tumor was successfully excised using robust registration for guidance.

We have illustrated an application of estimating the filter distribution for surgical removal of an osteoid osteoma. Any quantities that depend on having a registration transformation, such as instrument trajectories, can also be estimated and the uncertainty of the registration can be propagated into the estimations. We believe that UPF registration will allow us to estimate the stability of surface-based registration, which is an important but poorly understood part of computer-assisted surgical systems.

Acknowledgments. This research was supported in part by the Institute for Robotics and Intelligent Systems, the Ontario Research and Development Challenge Fund, and the Natural Sciences and Engineering Research Council of Canada.

References

[1] P. Besl and N. McKay. A method for registration of 3-D shapes. *IEEE Trans Pattern Anal*, 14(2):239–256, 1992.

[2] H. Chui and A. Rangarajan. A feature registration framework using mixture models. In *IEEE Workshop on Math Methods in Biomed Im Anal*, pages 190–197, 2000.

[3] H. Croitoru, R. E. Ellis, C. F. Small, R. Prihar, and D. R. Pichora. Fixation-based surgery: A new technique for distal radius osteotomy. *J Comp Aided Surg*, 6:160–169, 2001.

[4] F. Dellaert. *Monte Carlo EM for Data-Association and its Applications in Computer Vision*. PhD thesis, Carnegie Mellon University, 2001.

[5] A. Doucet, S. Godsill, and C. Andrieu. On sequential Monte Carlo sampling methods for Bayesian filtering. *Stat Comp*, 10:197–208, 2000.

[6] S. Granger and X. Pennec. Multi-scale EM-ICP: A fast and robust approach for surface registration. In *ECCV 2002*, pages 418–432, 2002.

[7] W. E. L. Grimson, G. J. Ettinger, S. J. White, T. Lozano-Pérez, W. M. Wells III, and R. Kikinis. An automatic registration method for frameless stereotaxy, image guided surgery, and enhanced reality visualization. *IEEE Trans Med Imaging*, 15(2):129–140, 1996.

[8] K. Ito and K. Xiong. Gaussian filters for nonlinear filtering problems. *IEEE Trans Automat Con*, 45(5):910–927, 2000.

[9] O. Iyun, D. P. Borschneck, and R. E. Ellis. Computer-assisted correction of bone deformities. In T. Dohi and R. Kikinis, editors, *MICCAI 2002*, pages 232–240, Tokyo, 2002.

[10] S. Julier and J. Uhlmann. A new extension of the Kalman filter to nonlinear systems. In *Proc. of AeroSense*, Orlando, Florida, 1997.

[11] K. Okuma, A. Taleghani, N. de Freitas, J. Little, and D. Lowe. A boosted particle filter: Multitarget detection and tracking. In *ECCV 2004*, 2004.

[12] Y. Rui and Y. Chen. Better proposal distributions: Object tracking using unscented particle filter. In *Proc. of IEEE Conf on Comp Vis and Patt Recog*, pages 786–793, 2001.

[13] R. van der Merwe, A. Doucet, N. de Freitas, and E. Wan. The unscented particle filter. Technical Report CUED/F-INFENG/TR 380, Cambridge Univ. Dept. of Eng., 2000.

[14] R. van der Merwe and E. Wan. Gaussian mixture sigma-point particle filters for sequential probabilistic inference in dynamic state-space models. In *Proc of the Int Conf on Acous, Speech, and Sig Proc*, 2003.

[15] J. Vermaak, A. Doucet, and P. Pérez. Maintaining multi-modality through mixture tracking. In *Int. Conf. on Computer Vision*, Nice, France, 2003.

[16] E. Wan and R. van der Merwe. The unscented kalman filter for nonlinear estimation. In *Proc of Sym on Adapt Sys for Sig Proc, Comm and Control*, Lake Louise, Canada, 2000.

Standardized Evaluation of 2D-3D Registration

Everine B. van de Kraats[1], Graeme P. Penney[1], Dejan Tomaževič[2],
Theo van Walsum[1], and Wiro J. Niessen[1]

[1] Image Sciences Institute, University Medical Center Utrecht, The Netherlands,
{everine,theo,wiro}@isi.uu.nl, http://www.isi.uu.nl
[2] Faculty of Electrical Engineering, University of Ljubljana, Slovenia

Abstract. In the past few years a number of 2D-3D registration algorithms have been introduced. However, these methods have not been directly compared or only work for specific applications. Understanding and evaluating their performance is therefore an open and important issue. To address this challenge we introduce a standard evaluation method, which can be used for all types of methods and different applications. Our method uses the geometry of the 3D Rotational X-ray (3DRX) imaging system in combination with 3D-3D registration for attaining a highly accurate ground truth for 2D multiple X-ray to 3D MR/CT/3DRX registration. The data and ground truth transformations will be made available on the Internet. Furthermore, we propose starting positions and failure criteria to allow future researchers to directly compare their methods. As an illustration, the proposed method has been used to evaluate the performance of two 2D-3D registration techniques, viz. a gradient-based and an intensity-based method, in spinal applications.

1 Introduction and Background

2D-3D registration has been proposed to help in a number of clinical areas, such as radiotherapy planning and treatment verification, spinal surgery, hip replacement, neurointerventions and aortic stenting.

Several researchers have described and evaluated such methods, but the results are not directly comparable. The use of different datasets, different starting positions, different failure criteria and different error calculation methods hampers direct comparison. To address the challenge of comparing 2D-3D registration algorithms, we introduce a standard validation method, which can be used for different algorithms and different applications. In the field of rigid 3D-3D registration, the availability of the Vanderbilt dataset has already shown the importance of a common database, validation statistics, and error measure for comparison of multiple algorithms [1].

As an illustration of the method we focus on registering images of vertebral bodies using two registration algorithms: an intensity-based method [2] and a gradient-based method [3].

C. Barillot, D.R. Haynor, and P. Hellier (Eds.): MICCAI 2004, LNCS 3216, pp. 574–581, 2004.

2   Validation Method

In the following paragraphs prerequisites for 2D-3D registration methods, the ground truth, accuracy determination, capture range and starting positions, and data preparation of the validation method will be described in detail.

Prerequisites for 2D-3D Registration Methods. The presented evaluation method assumes that the intrinsic parameters of the X-ray device are known and that the X-ray images are corrected for distortion. Therefore six degrees of freedom are left in the 2D-3D registration problem, which are the parameters that describe the position of the 3D volume in space: translations in x, y and z directions (T_x, T_y, T_z) and the orientation of the 3D volume in space: rotations around x-, y- and z-axis (R_x, R_y, R_z).

Ground Truth. Data is acquired with a clinical floor-mounted 3D Rotational X-ray (3DRX) C-arm system (Integris BV5000, Philips Medical Systems, Best, The Netherlands). During an 8 second run of 180 degrees around the patient the 3DRX system acquires 100 projection images, which are used to reconstruct a high resolution 3D volume using a filtered-back projection reconstruction technique [4].

The C-arm system needs to be calibrated for 3DRX imaging [5]. Two calibration runs are required: one run to determine the image intensifier distortion and the position of the focal spot of each projection and a second run to establish the projection parameters of the different projections. The accuracy of the derived geometrical parameters for this calibration method was demonstrated in [6], where the three-dimensional image quality was evaluated in terms of spatial resolution and geometrical accuracy. It was shown that the system can obtain an almost isotropic three-dimensional resolution of up to 22 lp/cm (line pairs per cm). Furthermore, it was shown that the three-dimensional geometrical accuracy is in the order of the spatial resolution of the resulting images.

Since the position of the X-ray images with respect to the reconstructed volume is known from the calibration procedure and since the system is calibrated for distortion [7] of the X-ray images, we can use the 3D volume and the 100 corresponding distortion corrected X-ray images as a ground truth dataset. The use of the standard system calibration enables the acquisition of ground truth datasets for all kinds of anatomical structures without extra or online calibration.

Ground truth registrations for other modalities can be obtained by registering corresponding CT or MR data to the 3DRX data; thereby indirectly obtaining the transformation to the X-ray images. Voxel based 3D-3D registration methods have been described thoroughly in literature and can be performed to subvoxel accuracy. In a previous study we showed that, for spinal images, registration of MR data to 3DRX data based on maximization of mutual information is at least as accurate as marker-based registration [8].

Accuracy of Registration. The accuracy of the registration defines how well the objects of interest coincide after registration. It is measured using the target registration error (TRE) [9]. The 'targets' to be used in the TRE calculation can be predefined locations (either fiducials or landmarks), surface points, or arbitrary chosen points inside a region of interest.

We propose to use a set of evenly distributed points in a region centered around the object of interest to determine a mean TRE (mTRE) over a region. For all points p_i on a regular grid P inside the region, the distance between the point p_i transformed with T_{ground}, the ground truth registration, and the same point transformed with T_{reg}, the transformation determined by the registration algorithm, is computed. The average distance between the points defines the mTRE:

$$\text{mTRE}(P, T_{\text{reg}}, T_{\text{ground}}) = \frac{1}{n} \sum_{i=0}^{n} \| T_{\text{reg}}\, p_i - T_{\text{ground}}\, p_i \| \quad . \tag{1}$$

Capture Range and Starting Positions. The capture range defines the range of starting positions from which the algorithm finds a sufficiently accurate transformation. Two factors are involved here: the definition of a misregistration, and the fraction of allowed misregistrations.

Several approaches are possible for the determination of the initial distance to the ground truth of a starting position. We choose to use the mTRE at the starting position as a measure for the initial distance. By using the same quantity for initial distance and final result, a direct comparison of the effect of the algorithm is possible.

The starting positions are offsets from the ground truth position centered around a specified 'center of rotation' per object of interest. Given our definition of capture range, and the use of the initial mTRE as the distance measure for the registration starting positions, the starting parameter values must be generated such that several transformations are within several ranges of mTRE. This is achieved by:

1. First choosing intervals for the starting position distance, e.g. 0-1, 1-2 mm.
2. Then, for each interval, for each of the six transformation parameters, the range is determined that will yield a mTRE less than or equal to the interval upper bound. E.g. for a starting mTRE between 1 and 2 mm, the range for each translation is 0-2 mm. Since the region used to determine the starting mTREs is not always cubic, rotations around different axes do not have the same effect on the mTRE. This is taken into account by determining the angle of rotation that results in an mTRE of 1 mm for each individual rotation. For the next intervals small angle approximation is used which implies that rotations are assumed to linearly relate to the resulting mTRE.
3. Next, for each interval, transformations are generated, where the transformation parameters are chosen randomly (uniformly distributed) from their predetermined range. Subsequently, the mTRE of the composite transformation is determined, and if that mTRE is within the interval it is kept, otherwise the transformation is discarded.

The last step is continued until each interval contains a sufficient number of starting positions.

Table 1. Parameter values for the registration methods.

Gradient-based			Intensity-based		
Parameter	3DRX	CT	Parameter	3DRX	CT
(σ=Blur volume)	0.5	0.3	MinStep	0.125	0.125
(σ=Blur X-ray)	0.5/1.0	0.5/1.0	Threshold	13000/11000	7000 ($\approx 400\,\mathrm{HU}$)
SampleStep	1.0 mm	1.0 mm			
Threshold	25	18			

Data Preparation. Most registration algorithms only use a part of the available image data because only the object of interest is relevant and less data results in lower computational costs. Since some algorithms use regions of interest (ROIs) in the 2D projection images and others VOIs in the 3D volume, it is difficult to have exactly the same data input available for both types of algorithms. For the presented evaluation method the VOIs are manually determined in the 3DRX volume. When performing intermodality comparison the VOIs are transformed to the corresponding CT or MR dataset using the ground truth image-based 3D-3D registration. Furthermore, ROIs are determined in the X-ray images, which are not directly related to the VOIs in the 3D volumes.

3   Comparison of Two Methods

The validation method described above has been applied to compare two previously published methods, viz. gradient-based and intensity-based registration. For both algorithms the original implementations were available, though the intensity-based algorithm had to be adapted so it could use multiple X-ray images simultaneously.

The gradient-based 2D-3D registration method [3] registers 3D volumes to 2D images by searching for the best match between surface normals in the 3D volume and back projected gradients of the 2D X-ray images. The surface normals and positions are extracted from the 3D image in a preprocessing step. In this preprocessing step the volume is blurred with a Gaussian filter, isotropically resampled and the locations with a gradient magnitude larger than some predefined threshold are extracted. The gradient-based registration method needs the following parameters: volume blur, X-ray image blur, sample step and a gradient threshold. See Table 1 for the parameter values used in this evaluation.

The intensity-based 2D-3D registration method [2] compares digitally reconstructed radiographs (DRRs) to X-ray images using a similarity measure based on gradient difference. The algorithm has two parameters: bone threshold and minimal stepsize. The bone threshold is determined such that the gray values above the threshold correspond to bone tissue projected in the X-ray image. The minimal stepsize is the smallest step that the algorithm takes in the optimization procedure. It is a factor by which the parameter values can change in the optimization procedure. The rotations, which are in radians, need an extra

Table 2. Image data.

Modality	Segment	Resolution	Size
CT	1	$0.31 \times 0.49 \times 0.31 \, \text{mm}^3$	$320 \times 260 \times 320$
	2	$0.31 \times 0.49 \times 0.31 \, \text{mm}^3$	$280 \times 300 \times 300$
3DRX	1	$0.87 \times 0.87 \times 0.87 \, \text{mm}^3$	256^3
	2	$0.52 \times 0.52 \times 0.52 \, \text{mm}^3$	256^3
X-ray	1	$0.63 \times 0.63 \, \text{mm}^2$	512^2
	2	$0.53 \times 0.53 \, \text{mm}^2$	512^2

factor of 0.02 to make the steps comparable to the translation steps, which are in millimeters. The optimization uses a multi resolution approach, where initially coarse resolution 256×256 pixel X-ray images are used, and then finer 512×512 pixel images are used. See Table 1 for the parameter values.

Image Data. Two defrosted segments of a vertebral column, both fixed in foam, were imaged with two modalities: 3DRX and CT. The 3DRX images were obtained with a clinical 3DRX system (Integris BV5000, Philips Medical Systems, Best, The Netherlands). The CT images were made with a clinical 16-detector-row multislice CT scanner (MSCT, Philips Medical Systems, Best, The Netherlands). Spinal segment 1 consists of 3 thoracolumbal vertebral bodies and segment 2 consists of 5 thoracic vertebral bodies. Some soft tissue around the spinal segments was still present. See Table 2 for details on image sizes and resolutions. The CT images were registered to the corresponding 3DRX images, using an algorithm which maximizes mutual information, to establish the ground truth for the CT-to-X-ray registration.

In the 3DRX volumes VOIs were determined (for vertebral bodies in spinal segment 1 approx. $100 \times 50 \times 100$ voxels, and vertebral bodies in spinal segment 2 approx. $120 \times 50 \times 150$ voxels) that were used by the gradient-based method. These VOIs were transformed to the CT data using the ground truth image-based 3D-3D registration. In the X-ray images ROIs around the vertebral bodies were determined (approx. 170×70 pixels) that were used by the intensity-based method. See Fig. 1 for examples of the data with corresponding VOIs and ROIs.

Experiments and Evaluation. For each of the eight vertebral bodies, centers of rotation were determined in the world coordinate system (directly linked to the 3DRX data). In this experiment the starting positions were generated as described in Sect. 2, with 10 starting positions per 1 mm interval up to 20 mm, resulting in 200 starting positions.

From the 100 acquired X-ray images per spinal segment two images were selected, one anterior-posterior and one lateral, which were used for the registration experiment for both CT and 3DRX to X-ray registration. The mTRE was determined in a VOI of $82 \times 39 \times 82 \, \text{mm}^3$ centered around a vertebral body (as

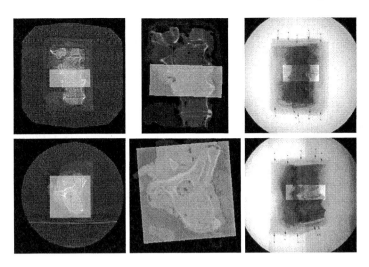

Fig. 1. Left: 3DRX AP and transversal planes with VOIs. Middle: CT AP and transversal planes with corresponding VOIs. Right: two X-ray images with ROIs.

in Sect. 2). Registrations were classified as successful when the end mTRE was smaller than 2 mm. The capture range was defined as the 95 % success range.

4   Results and Discussion

We performed 200 registrations per vertebral body (8), per modality (2) and per registration algorithm (2) resulting in a total of 6400 registrations. The average registration time was approx. 25 seconds for the gradient-based method and approx. 9 minutes for the intensity-based method. The algorithms ran on different machines and they were not optimized for speed. The individual registration results, the percentages of successful registrations, the average end mTRE of all the registrations, and the average end mTRE for the successful registrations, all per method and modality, are displayed in Fig. 2.

From the results several conclusions can be drawn. The average error for successful registrations is stable for the gradient-based method, while the intensity-based method has increasing difficulty in finding the optimal position when the initial offset from the ground truth position increases (Fig. 2D,H). This makes failure determination easier for the gradient-based method (Fig. 2A,E) than for the intensity-based method (Fig. 2B,F) because the difference between correct and incorrect registrations is quite large. E.g. when displaying the DRR belonging to the registration position together with the X-ray image, misregistrations can be visually assessed. In both cases the average error is larger for CT to X-ray registration than for 3DRX to X-ray registration.

The capture ranges for 3DRX and CT respectively are 0–6 mm and 0–3 mm for the gradient-based method and 0–4 mm and 0–3 mm for the intensity-based

580   E.B. van de Kraats et al.

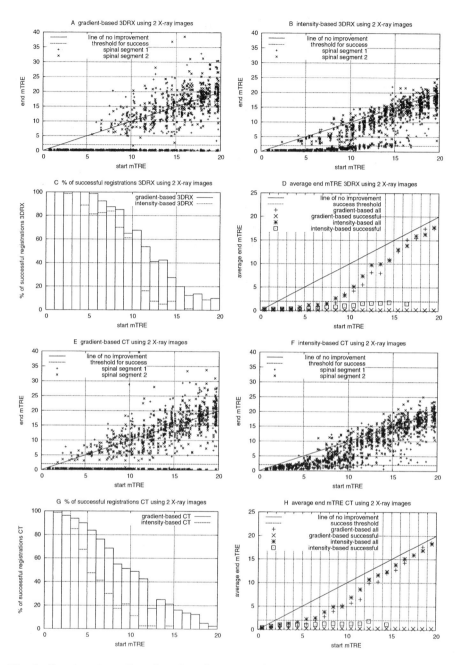

Fig. 2. Results of gradient-based and intensity-based 2D-3D registration, both for 3DRX to X-ray and CT to X-ray registration.

method. See Fig. 2C,G. Within the capture range the average end mTREs for 3DRX and CT respectively are 0.19 mm and 0.38 mm for the gradient-based method and 0.39 mm and 0.75 mm for the intensity-based method.

Better results for 3DRX to X-ray registration could be explained by greater similarity between the 2D and 3D modalities: both X-ray images and 3D volume are produced using X-rays at the same energy (around 60 keV), whereas CT uses 80 keV. Another reason could be an error introduced by the ground truth registration between CT and 3DRX data.

5   Conclusion

The accurate ground truth for 3DRX data and X-ray data in combination with 3D-3D CT/MR-to-3DRX registration, results in a ground truth for objective intermethod and intermodality 2D-3D registration comparison, as is shown in this paper for 2D-3D spine registration.

The ground truth datasets for MR, CT and 3DRX data and corresponding X-ray images, along with starting positions and centers of rotations will be made available on the web. In the future, other applications and anatomical regions can be included in this database.

References

1. West, J., et al.: Comparison and evaluation of retrospective intermodality brain image registration techniques. J Comput Assist Tomogr **21** (1997) 554–566
2. Penney, G., et al.: A Comparison of Similarity Measures for Use in 2-D-3-D Medical Image Registration. IEEE Trans Med Imaging **17** (1998) 586–595
3. Tomaževič, D., et al.: 3-D/2-D Registration of CT and MR to X-Ray Images. IEEE Trans Med Imaging **22** (2003) 1407–1416
4. Grass, M., et al.: Three-dimensional reconstruction of high contrast objects using C-arm image intensifier projection data. Comput Med Imaging Graph **23** (1999) 311–321
5. Koppe, R., et al.: 3D Vessel Reconstruction Based on Rotational Angiography. In: CAR. (1995) 101–107
6. Rasche, V., et al.: Performance of image intensifier-equipped X-ray systems for three-dimensional imaging. In: CARS. (2003) 187–192
7. Haaker, P., et al.: Real-time distortion correction of digital X-ray II/TV-systems: an application example for Digital Flashing Tomosynthesis (DFTS). Int J Card Imaging **6** (1990) 39–45
8. van de Kraats, E.B., et al.: Noninvasive Magnetic Resonance to Three-Dimensional Rotational X-ray Registration of Vertebral Bodies for Image-Guided Spine Surgery. Spine **29** (2004) 293–297
9. Fitzpatrick, J.M., et al.: The Distribution of Target Registration Error in Rigid-Body Point-Based Registration. IEEE Trans Med Imaging **20** (2001) 917–927

Image Registration by Hierarchical Matching of Local Spatial Intensity Histograms

Dinggang Shen

Section of Biomedical Image Analysis, Department of Radiology,
University of Pennsylvania, Philadelphia, PA 19104
dgshen@rad.upenn.edu

Abstract. We previously presented a HAMMER image registration algorithm that demonstrated high accuracy in superposition of images from different individual brains. However, the HAMMER registration algorithm requires pre-segmentation of brain tissues, since the attribute vectors used to hierarchically match the corresponding pairs of points are defined from the segmented images. In many applications, the segmentation of tissues might be difficult, unreliable or even impossible to complete, which potentially limits the use of the HAMMER algorithm in more generalized applications. To overcome this limitation, we use local spatial intensity histograms to design a new type of attribute vector for each point in an intensity image. The histogram-based attribute vector is rotationally invariant, and more importantly it captures spatial information by integrating a number of local histograms that are calculated from multi-resolution images. The new attribute vectors are able to determine corresponding points across individual images. Therefore, by hierarchically matching new attribute vectors, the proposed registration method performs as successfully as the previous HAMMER algorithm did in registering MR brain images, while providing more general applications in registering images of other organs. Experimental results show good performance of the proposed method in registering MR brain images and CT pelvis images.

1 Introduction

Deformable registration of images has been an active topic of research for over a decade [1,10-15]. We previously presented a HAMMER image registration method that demonstrated high accuracy in superposition of images from different individual brains [2,3]. However, the HAMMER algorithm requires that the images be segmented, before image registration can be performed, since the attribute vectors that are used to hierarchically match the corresponding pairs of points are defined from the segmented image. For images in certain modalities and from certain organs, the segmentation of tissues may be difficult, unreliable or even impossible to complete, which unavoidably limits the applications of the HAMMER algorithm.

It would be very attractive to use the deformation techniques developed in the HAMMER algorithm to directly register two intensity images, without pre-segmentation of images. One immediately available method uses wavelet-based feature extraction to characterize the geometric features around each point [4]. However, wavelet features are computationally expensive, and actually not invariant to rotations of the image. Importantly, in image matching and classification, more features will not always produce better results. It is particularly true in brain

C. Barillot, D.R. Haynor, and P. Hellier (Eds.): MICCAI 2004, LNCS 3216, pp. 582–590, 2004.

matching, where the relatively high variability of brain structures makes some features, such as detailed features, vary dramatically across individual brains, thus confusing the image matching. Accordingly, features used for image matching are not necessarily very detailed, but they must be robust to structural variations across individuals.

In this paper, we design a new type of attribute vector for each point in an intensity image, based on local spatial intensity histograms. The histogram-based attribute vectors are very fast to compute, and also invariant to image rotation. Importantly, since local histograms are calculated from the intensity image at multiple resolutions, the new attribute vector captures sufficient spatial image information [5], thereby enabling the discrimination of the corresponding points across the individual images. By hierarchically matching new attribute vectors, the proposed registration method performs as successfully as the previous HAMMER algorithm did in registering MR brain images, while providing more generalized applications in the images of other organs or other modalities. Experimental results show good performance of the proposed method in registering MR brain images and CT pelvis images.

2 Method

2.1 Histogram-Based Attribute Vector

Definition: An attribute vector is defined for each point in the image, and used to best characterize the geometric features around that point, in order to reduce the ambiguities in determining the matching pairs of points during the image registration procedure. In this study, local intensity histograms of multi-resolution images around each point are computed and further used as attributes of that point. Moreover, boundary information, i.e., edgeness, is also extracted from each resolution image and used as additional spatial attribute, for discriminating boundary points from others. Therefore, the attribute vector $\mathbf{a}(v)$ of a point v in an image $f(v)$ includes both histogram-based attributes and boundary information, all of which are calculated from multi-resolution images respectively, as detailed next.

Histogram-based attributes are established by the following three steps. *Firstly*, the original image $f(v)$ is down-sampled by a factor of s, resulting in several down-sampled images, $f_s(v_s)$, where $v_s = [v/s]$ and thus $f_s(v_s) = f(v)$ when $s = 1$. For a point v in the original image $f(v)$, its correspondence in the down-sampled image $f_s(v_s)$ is v_s. Gaussian filter is used here to down-sample an image, and a total of three resolution levels, i.e., $s = 1,2,4$, are used. *Secondly*, for each resolution image $f_s(v_s)$, a local histogram $\mathbf{h}_s(v_s)$ of intensities in a spherical region of point v_s is computed. The radius of the spherical region is set to be identical across different resolutions. Therefore, for each point v in the original image $f(v)$, we can obtain several local histograms, i.e., $\{ \mathbf{h}_s(v_s) | s = 1,2,4 \}$, which capture different levels of spatial image information. *Thirdly*, the shape features, such as regular geometric moments [6], are respectively extracted from each histogram $\mathbf{h}_s(v_s)$, and then used as geometric attributes for the point v. Importantly, by extracting shape features from histograms, we can obtain a relatively shorter vector of attributes (including both mean and variance of intensities in the spherical region) for each point in the image, thereby facilitating the fast and efficient matching of the corresponding points during the image registration procedure. For convenience, let $\mathbf{a}_s^{\text{Hist}}(v)$ represent a vector of low-frequency moments, obtained from a histogram $h_s(v_s)$. Notably, vector $\mathbf{a}_1^{\text{Hist}}(v)$ captures relatively local features, while vector $\mathbf{a}_4^{\text{Hist}}(v)$ captures relatively global features.

Boundary attributes $b_s(v_s)$, used to measure the edge strongness, are computed from each resolution image $f_s(v_s)$ by the Canny edge detector [7], and encoded as boundary attributes in the attribute vector. For each point v in the original image $f(v)$, its corresponding boundary features in the three resolution images are $b_s(v_s)$, where $s = 1,2,4$, since $v_s = [v/s]$ is a corresponding point of v in the down-sampled image $f_s(v_s)$. For consistent representation of attributes, we use $b_s^{\text{Bound}}(v) = b_s(v_s)$ to represent the boundary attribute obtained at resolution s.

Therefore, the attribute vector of a point v can be finally represented as

$$\mathbf{a}(v) = \left[[\mathbf{a}_1^{\text{Hist}}(v) \quad b_1^{\text{Bound}}(v)], \quad [\mathbf{a}_2^{\text{Hist}}(v) \quad b_2^{\text{Bound}}(v)], \quad [\mathbf{a}_4^{\text{Hist}}(v) \quad b_4^{\text{Bound}}(v)] \right],$$

which includes three different levels of geometric features, with $[\mathbf{a}_1^{\text{Hist}}(v) \quad b_1^{\text{Bound}}(v)]$ as local features, $[\mathbf{a}_2^{\text{Hist}}(v) \quad b_2^{\text{Bound}}(v)]$ as middle-level features, and $[\mathbf{a}_4^{\text{Hist}}(v) \quad b_4^{\text{Bound}}(v)]$ as global features. Each attribute has been normalized between 0 and 1. By comparing the similarity of attribute vectors, we can determine the correspondences for points in the images. The similarity of two attribute vectors, $\mathbf{a}(u)$ and $\mathbf{a}(v)$, of two points, u and v, are defined as follows:

$$m(\mathbf{a}(u),\mathbf{a}(v)) = \prod_s \left(\left(1 - \left| b_s^{\text{Bound}}(u) - b_s^{\text{Bound}}(v) \right| \right) \cdot \prod_i \left(1 - \left| \mathbf{a}_{s,i}^{\text{Hist}}(u) - \mathbf{a}_{s,i}^{\text{Hist}}(v) \right| \right) \right),$$

where $\mathbf{a}_{s,i}^{\text{Hist}}$ is the i-th element of $\mathbf{a}_s^{\text{Hist}}$.

It is worth noting that the histogram-based attributes are invariant to rotational transformations of the image. Furthermore, by normalizing histograms both globally and locally, we can make the histogram-based attributes also robust to intensity inhomogeneities in the image. For example, by normalizing the global histogram, we can make any individual image have intensity distribution similar to that of a model image. Currently, histogram normalization is completed by first linearly transforming an individual's histogram to best match the model's histogram, and then using the optimally-estimated linear transformation parameters to map the intensities of the individual image. In the future, we plan to use a nonlinear histogram normalization method, by firstly using an elastic method to non-linearly establish the correspondences between the histograms of the model and the individual, and then using the established correspondences of intensities to map the intensities in the individual image.

Discrimination ability: In the problem of image matching and registration, it is important to make sure that the corresponding points in the different individuals have the similar attribute vectors. To demonstrate this, in Fig 1, the attribute vector of a circled point in the left image is compared with the attribute vectors of all points in the middle image. According to the similarity map in the right, where white represents the high similarity, the circled point in the left image is similar only to its corresponding point, as indicated by a circle, in the middle image. Therefore, this example visually demonstrates that our histogram-based attribute vectors are able to determine the correspondences across different individuals.

It is worth noting the importance of including different levels of spatial geometric features into a single attribute vector for image matching and registration. Otherwise, it is impossible to discriminate different points by using only local/global attributes.

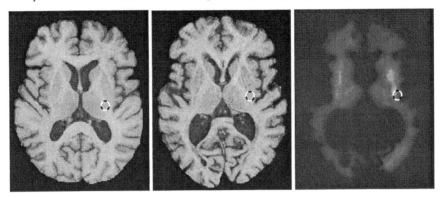

Fig. 1. Similarity of the corresponding points in the two individuals. The attribute vector of a circled point in the left image is compared with the attribute vectors of all points in the middle image. The resulting similarity map is shown in the right. The white represents high similarity, while the black denotes low similarity. The circled point in the middle image is a detected point with the highest degree of similarity.

2.2 Energy Function

Our energy function is formulated very similar to that of the HAMMER algorithm, i.e., it is designed to match the corresponding attribute vectors in the two images. Therefore, the optimization of our energy function can be completed by employing the exactly same deformation strategies developed in the HAMMER algorithm. Let $\mathbf{a}_T(u)$ denote the attribute vector of a point u in the template image $T(u)$, and let $\mathbf{a}_S(v)$ represent the attribute vector of a point v in the subject image $S(v)$. The template image $T(u)$ is deformed to match with the subject $S(v)$ by a displacement field $d(u)$, or equally a forward transformation $h(u) = u + d(u)$. The backward transformation from the subject to the model is $h^{-1}(u)$, which is the inverse of the forward transformation $h(u)$. The following is the energy function that our image registration algorithm will minimize:

$$E = \sum_u \omega_T(u) \left(\frac{\sum\limits_{z \in n(u)} \varepsilon(z)\left(1 - m\left(\mathbf{a}_T(z), \mathbf{a}_S(h(z))\right)\right)}{\sum\limits_{z \in n(u)} \varepsilon(z)} \right)$$

$$+\sum_{v}\omega_{s}(v)\left(\frac{\sum_{z\in n(v)}\varepsilon(z)\left(1-m\left(\mathbf{a}_{T}(h^{-1}(z)),\mathbf{a}_{s}(z)\right)\right)}{\sum_{z\in n(v)}\varepsilon(z)}\right)+\beta\sum_{u}\left\|\nabla^{2}d(u)\right\|.$$

There are three energy terms in this energy function. The first energy term evaluates the match of template with subject, by using forward transformation $h(\cdot)$; while the second energy term evaluates the match of subject with template, by using backward transformation $h^{-1}(\cdot)$. Apparently, our energy function requires the consistent transformations that give identical mapping between two images, regardless of which of the two images is treated as the template [8,2,3].

The first energy term is defined as the weighted summation of neighborhood matching degrees of all points u in the template image. $\omega_{T}(u)$ is used as a weight for the point u, which can be adaptively adjusted by boundary attributes during the image registration procedure. Notably, this design allows the hierarchical selection of active points to focus on, thus enabling the approximation of a very-high-dimensional (equal to the number of points in the two images) cost function by a significantly lower-dimensional function of only the active points. This latter function has fewer local minima, because it is a function of the coordinates of active points, for which relatively unambiguous matches can be found. Accordingly, we can speed up the performance of image registration and also reduce the chances of local minima. For a point u, the degree of its neighborhood match is defined as the similarity of all attribute vectors in the neighborhood, $n(u)$. This design thereby allows the neighborhood matching during the image registration, which effectively increases the robustness to potentially false matches of active points. Here, z is a neighboring point of u, and its attribute vector $\mathbf{a}_{T}(z)$ is compared with the attribute vector $\mathbf{a}_{s}(h(z))$ of its corresponding point $h(z)$ in the subject; the similarity is defined as $m(\cdot,\cdot)$, thereby the difference is $1-m(\cdot,\cdot)$. The term $\sum_{z\in n(u)}\varepsilon(z)$ is used for normalization. Notably, the design of the second energy term is the same as the first.

The third energy term is used to make sure that the resulting displacement fields $d(\cdot)$ be smooth, by requiring the total Laplacian value of displacement fields to be as small as possible. The parameter β controls the smoothness of the deformation fields.

3 Experimental Results

The performance of the proposed registration method is evaluated by using MR brain images and CT pelvis images. All experiments are performed on the volumetric images.

3.1 MR Brain Images

The brains images used in this study are obtained from our project, the Baltimore Longitudinal Study of Aging (BLSA) [9]. These images of elderly subjects pose several difficulties in image matching, including reduced tissue contrast, significant atrophy, and motion artifacts.

Averaging 18 individual brains: The sharpness of the average image of the normalized individuals is often used as a visual display of the accuracy of the normalization algorithm. We selected the 18 individual brains used in our previous HAMMER paper [2]. Notably, the ventricles and also other structures in these 18 brains are of various shapes and sizes [2]. By normalizing these 18 brains to the space of a selected model, we can obtain an average image of these normalized 18 brains, as shown in Fig 2. By comparing this average image with the model as in Fig 2, we can observe the close similarity of these two images. Moreover, we can see that the average image is very clear, for example, in the regions of ventricles, caudate nucleus and lenticular nucleus. Therefore, the accuracy of our image registration method in registering MR brain images can be confirmed in part through this simple visual verification.

We also compare the average image of the proposed registration method, with that obtained by our previous HAMMER warping algorithm. As shown in Fig 2, the two average images possess almost the same level of sharpness, indicating the comparable accuracy of the proposed method to that of HAMMER method. Importantly, the registration method proposed in this paper does not require tissue segmentation, thereby making our registration method independent of the tissue-segmentation methods that may produce segmentation errors. Notably, for certain images in certain modalities, the segmentation of tissues may be difficult, unreliable or even impossible

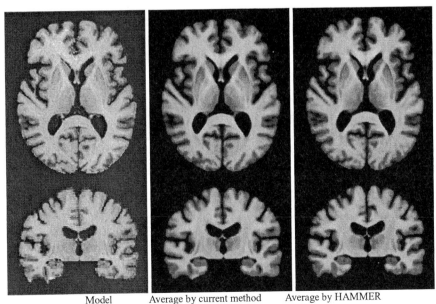

Model   Average by current method   Average by HAMMER

Fig. 2. Demonstration of the accuracy of the proposed method in averaging 18 individual brains. The average brain obtained by the proposed method is compared with that obtained by the HAMMER algorithm, indicating almost the same level of registration accuracy for the two methods.

to complete. Therefore, methods that directly register the intensity images, such as our proposed method, have the potential for success in more generalized applications, as is a major goal of this study.

3.2   CT Pelvis Images

Our registration method is also applicable in registering CT images of human pelvises, as shown in Fig 3. Before registration, the shapes of two individual pelvises and as well as their internal structures are very different, according to the cross-sectional images and 3D renderings in Figs 3a and 3c. After image registration, the two individual images become very similar, not only in their global shapes but in their representation of internal tissues, as shown in Fig 3b.

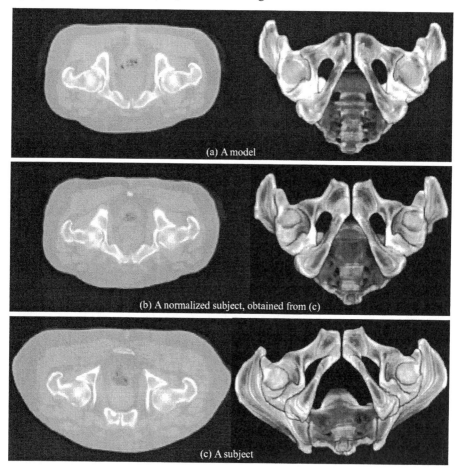

Fig. 3. Demonstration of the proposed method in registering CT images of pelvises. A subject in (c) is normalized to the space of a model in (a), resulting in a spatially normalized image in (b), which is very similar to the model. Both cross-sectional images and 3D renderings are provided.

4   Conclusion

We have presented a method for the direct registration of intensity images that generalizes our previous HAMMER algorithm and eliminates the need to segment images before registration, thereby making the algorithm applicable to a variety of image sources and image modalities. Attribute vectors are used to characterize the local anatomy of each image point in a hierarchical fashion, in order to robustly match the corresponding points during the image registration procedure. The attribute vector in the HAMMER algorithm was defined from tissue-segmented images. In this paper, it is directly computed from the intensity images, by using the local spatial intensity histograms of multi-resolution images as geometric attributes. The histogram-based attribute vector is fast to compute and invariant to rotations of the image. Most importantly, our new type of attribute vector can distinguish between different points in the image, as long as a sufficient number of spatial features are captured from the local spatial histograms of a sufficient number of multi-resolution images.

Acknowledgement. The author would like to thank Dr. Susan Resnick and the BLSA for providing the brain datasets, Dr. Russell Taylor for providing pelvis datasets, and Dr. Christos Davatzikos for very helpful discussion.

References

1. T. McInerney, D. Terzopoulos. "Deformable models in medical image analysis: a survey", *Medical Image Analysis*, 1(2):91-108, 1996.
2. D. Shen, C. Davatzikos. "HAMMER: Hierarchical Attribute Matching Mechanism for Elastic Registration". *IEEE Trans. on Medical Imaging*, Nov 2002.
3. D. Shen, C. Davatzikos. "Very High Resolution Morphometry Using Mass-Preserving Deformations and HAMMER Elastic Registration". *NeuroImage*, 18(1): 28-41, Jan 2003.
4. Z. Xue, D. Shen, C. Davatzikos. "Correspondence Detection Using Wavelet-Based Attribute Vectors", *MICCAI'03*, Canada, Nov 2003.
5. E. Hadjidemetriou, M. Grossberg, and S.K. Nayar. "Spatial information in multiresolution histograms", *IEEE Conference on Computer Vision and Pattern Recognition*, 2001.
6. D. Shen and H.H.S. Ip. "Generalized affine invariant image normalization". *IEEE Trans. on Pattern Analysis and Machine Intelligence*, 19(5):431-440, May 1997.
7. J. Canny. "A computational approach to edge detection", *IEEE Trans. on PAMI*, Vol 8, No. 6, Nov 1986.
8. G.E. Christensen and H.J. Johnson. "Consistent Image Registration", *IEEE Trans. on TMI*, 20(7), 2001, pp. 568-582.
9. S.M. Resnick, A.F. Goldszal, C. Davatzikos, S. Golski, M.A. Kraut, E.J. Metter, R.N. Bryan, and A.B. Zonderman. "One-year age changes in MRI brain volumes in older adults", *Cerebral Cortex*, 10:464-472, 2000.
10. H. Chui, L. Win, R. Schultz, J. Duncan, and A. Rangarajan. "A Unified Feature Registration Method for Brain Mapping". *IPMI*, p.300-314, Davis, CA, USA, June 18-22, 2001.
11. J.P. Thirion, O. Monga, S. Benayoun, A. Gueziec and N. Ayache. "Automatic registration of 3-D images using surface curvature". *SPIE Proc., Mathematical Methods in Medical Imaging*, volume 1768, p.206-216, 1992.

12. P. Thompson and A.W. Toga. "A surface-based technique for warping three-dimensional images of the brain". *IEEE Trans. on Med. Imaging*, volume 15, p.402-417, 1996.
13. J.C. Gee, C. Barillot, L.L. Briquer, D.R. Haynor and R. Bajcsy. "Matching structural images of the human brain using statistical and geometrical image features". *Proc. SPIE Visualization in Biomedical Computing*, vol. 2359, pp.191-204, 1994.
14. S.C. Joshi, M.I. Miller, G.E. Christensen, *et al.* "Hierarchical brain mapping via a generalized Dirichlet solution for mapping brain manifolds". *SPIE Conf. on Geom. Methods in Applied Imaging*, vol 2573, p.278-289, July 1995.
15. A.C. Evans, W. Dai, L. Collins, P. Neeling and S. Marett. "Warping of a computerized 3-D atlas to match brain image volumes for quantitative neuroanatomical and functional analysis". *SPIE Proc., Image Processing*, volume 1445, p.236-246, 1991.

Volume Preserving Image Registration

Eldad Haber[1] and Jan Modersitzki[2*]

[1] Dept. of Mathematics and Computer Science, Emory University, Atlanta GA
30322, haber@mathcs.emory.edu
[2] Inst. of Mathematics, University of Lübeck, Germany
modersitzki@math.uni-luebeck.de

Abstract. In this paper we discuss image registration techniques with a focus on volume preserving constraints. These constraints can reduce the non-uniqueness of the registration problem significantly. Our implementation is based on a constrained optimization formulation. To solve the problem we use a variant of the Sequential Quadratic Programming method. Moreover, we present results on synthetic as well as on real-life data.

1 Introduction

Image registration is one of the fundamental tasks in today's image processing and in particular in medical imaging; see, e.g., [1,2] and references therein. The objective of image registration is to make images which are taken at different times, from different perspectives, and/or from different devices to be more alike. Loosely, the goal of image registration is to find a *"reasonable"* deformation such that the *"distance"* between a reference image R and a deformed version of a template image T becomes small.

An application of particular clinical interest is the registration of pairs of images acquired before and after contrast administration; see, e.g., [3] and references therein. A typical example is depicted in Fig. 1. In this application, magnetic resonance images of a female breast are taken at different times (images from Bruce Daniel, Lucas Center for Magnetic Resonance Spectroscopy and Imaging, Stanford University). The first image shows an MRI section taken during the so-called wash-in phase of a radiopaque marker and the second image shows the analogous section during the so-called wash-out phase. A comparison of these two images indicates a suspicious region in the upper part of the images. This region can be detected easily if the images have been registered: tissue located at a certain position in the wash-in image is related to the tissue at the same position in the wash-out phase. Generally, however, a quantitative analysis is a delicate matter since observable differences are not only related to contrast uptake but also due to motion of the patient, like, for example, breathing or heart beat.

---

* Jan Modersitzki was supported by the US National Institutes of Health under Grant NIHR01 HL 068904.

C. Barillot, D.R. Haynor, and P. Hellier (Eds.): MICCAI 2004, LNCS 3216, pp. 591–598, 2004.

As pointed out by Rohlfing et al. [3], there is a substantial difficulty with the registration of pre and post-contrast images. Bright regions seem to enlarge during the so-called wash-in phase. This enhancement is due to contrast uptake but not to movement of the patient. Fig. 3 illustrates an ideal situation. Without external information, it is impossible to answer whether the white area has been enlarged or the grey area turned to white.

In this paper, we present a flexible constrained image registration approach. It has three main ingredients: a distance measure, a regularizer, and the constraints. Our framework is general enough to handle a variety of distance measures, including the most popular ones, like those based on the sum of squared differences (SSD) (cf., e.g., [4]), mutual information (MI) (cf., e.g., [5,6]), or correlation, as long as a Gâteaux derivative exists; see, e.g., [7,8]. For presentation purposes, we explicitly discuss the approach only for the SSD measure.

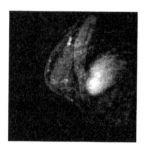 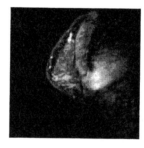 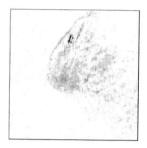

Fig. 1. MRI's of a female breast, LEFT: during the wash-in phase, MIDDLE: during the wash-out phase, and RIGHT: difference image.

2   Mathematical Setup and Discretization

With $d \in \mathbb{N}$ we denote the spatial dimension of the given images $R, T : \mathbb{R}^d \to \mathbb{R}$. Thus, $T(\boldsymbol{x})$ gives a gray value at a spatial position $\boldsymbol{x}$. We assume that the supports of the images are contained in a bounded domain $\Omega :=]0, L[^d$, i.e. $R(\boldsymbol{x}) = T(\boldsymbol{x}) = 0$ for $\boldsymbol{x} \notin \Omega$.

Our goal is to find a *"reasonable"* deformation $\boldsymbol{u}$ such that the *"distance"* between the reference image R and the deformed template image $T(\boldsymbol{x} + \boldsymbol{u}(\boldsymbol{x}))$ becomes small. It is well-known that this problem is ill-posed and therefore needs to be regularized, see, e.g., [9,10]. A formulation of the (VP) constrained problem thus reads

$$\text{minimize } \mathcal{D}[R, T; \boldsymbol{u}] + \alpha \mathcal{S}[\boldsymbol{u}] \tag{1a}$$

$$\text{subject to } \mathcal{C}[\boldsymbol{u}](\boldsymbol{x}) := \det(I_d \nabla \boldsymbol{u}(\boldsymbol{x})) - 1 = 0 \quad \text{for all} \quad \boldsymbol{x} \in \Omega, \tag{1b}$$

where $\mathcal{D}$ is some distance measure (e.g. the sum of squared difference) and $\mathcal{S}$ is some regularization term (e.g. the elastic regularizer). Here, $\alpha > 0$ is a regularization parameter and compromises between similarity and regularity. For ease of presentation, we assume that S is defined via a bilinear form, at it is the case for popular regularizer, like, e.g., the elastic [11,12,13], fluid [12,14], diffusion [15], or curvature regularizers [16].

Choosing a stable discretization method for an optimization problem with a differential constraint is a delicate matter. Similar to [17,18], we use staggered grids. Though staggered grids seem to be natural for the discretization of the registration problem on a regular grid, we are not aware of any registration scheme where this discretization is used.

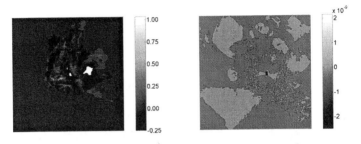

Fig. 2. Volume preservation of the unconstrained (LEFT) and constrained (RIGHT) registration results for the MRI example.

3   Solving the Discrete Optimization Problem

Let U, D, S, and C denote the discrete analogs of $u, \mathcal{D}, \mathcal{S}$, and $\mathcal{C}$. The discrete analog of the image registration problem (1) is phrased as follows,

$$\text{minimize}\quad D(U) + \alpha S(U) \tag{2a}$$
$$\text{subject to}\quad C(U) = 0. \tag{2b}$$

In order to solve problem (2) numerically we use the framework of Sequential Quadratic Programming (SQP); see [19] for a detailed discussion. With the Lagrange multiplier P, the Lagrangian of the problem is

$$L(U, P) = D(U) + \alpha S(U) + C(U)^{\top} P.$$

Differentiating with respect to U and P, we obtain the Euler-Lagrange equations

$$0 = L_U(U, P) = D_U(U) + \alpha S_U(U) + C_U(U)^{\top} P, \tag{3a}$$
$$0 = L_P(U, P) = C(U). \tag{3b}$$

We can now solve the nonlinear system (3) numerically by using a Newton-type method; see [18] for details.

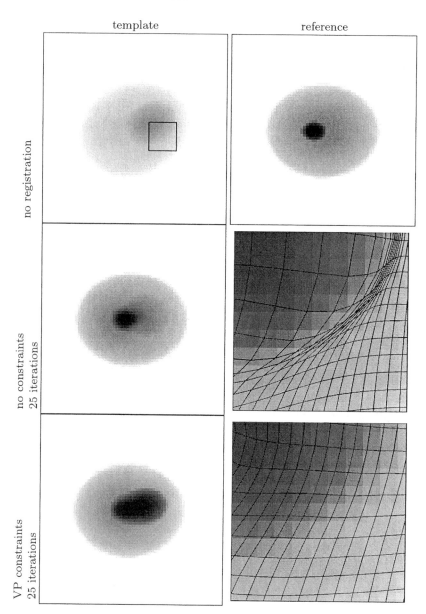

Fig. 3. Synthetic example, LEFT COLUMN: deformed template, RIGHT COLUMN: reference and detail of the deformed grid; TOP ROW: template and reference, no registration, MIDDLE ROW: deformed template and details with grid after unconstrained registration, BOTTOM ROW: deformed template and details with grid after VP constrained registration. For both schemes, we choose $\alpha = 10^3$ and stopped after 25 iterations.

deformed T difference difference with
nodal grid

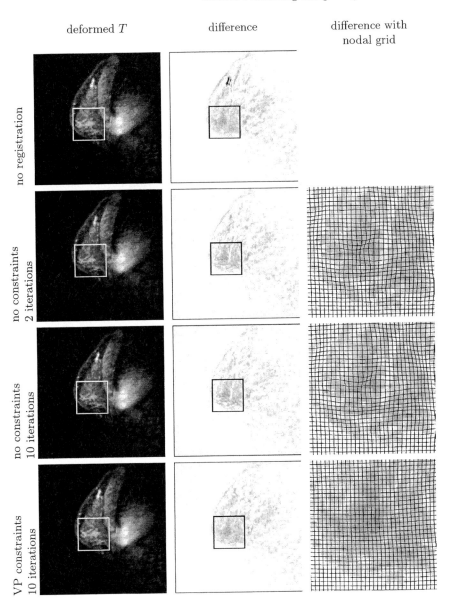

Fig. 4. Registration results for the images of Fig. 1. LEFT COLUMN deformed template images T_u, MIDDLE COLUMN difference image $|R - T_u|$ with region of interest (ROI), RIGHT COLUMN ROI with nodal grid, vertices connected by straight lines ; ROW 1: no registration, ROW 2: no constraints two iterations, ROW 3: no constraints ten iterations, and ROW 4: volume preserving constraints ten iterations.

4   Numerical Examples

The Blob: To illustrate the potential of the volume preserving registration we present a synthetic example; see Fig. 3. The reference image (top right) shows an elliptic global structure which contains a small almost circular object. The template (top left) shows a rotated version of the global ellipse, where the inner structure is translated and considerably enlarged. Note that this example mimics the situation for contrast enhanced images: slightly deformed global structures, where inner structures may change drastically due to contrast uptake.

As it is apparent from Fig. 3, the unconstrained registration gives very good results if we are looking at the difference between the reference and deformed template images alone. However, as expected, the inner structure has been re-

Table 1. Computation time (using MATLAB 6.5 on a DELL Inspiron 8600 Notebook) and iterations for the unconstraint and VP constraint registrations. The stopping criteria is $\|\boldsymbol{u}^{\text{old}} - \boldsymbol{u}\| \leq \text{tol}_U := 10^{-1}$.

image size	unconstraint	VP constrained
64×64	28s, #38	69, #21
128×128	296s, #68	846, #23

Table 2. Numerical results for the un- and VP-contrained registrations; k is the number of iteration performed.

		k	$D(\boldsymbol{U}^{(k)})/D(0)$	$\|C(\boldsymbol{U}^{(k)})\|_\infty$
blob	unconstrained	25	0.21	0.87
	VP constrained	25	0.73	$\leq 10^{-6}$
MRI	unconstrained	2	0.81	1.36
	unconstrained	10	0.78	1.36
	VP constrained	10	0.87	$\leq 10^{-6}$

duced so as to fit the one in the reference image. This results in a drastic change of volume, which can be observe from the visualization of a part of the grid in Fig. 3 (middle right) corresponding to a region of interest emphasized in the template image (top left). Thus, for contrast enhanced images, the registration gives meaningless results, though the difference is small.

Fig. 3 also shows the results of the volume preserving registration (bottom left). As is apparent from this figure, the global deformation has been resolved, the inner ellipse has been moved to match the inner ellipse in the reference image. However, the volume of the inner ellipse has not been altered, which leads to a larger difference as in the unconstrainted case but also to a more realistic registration; see also the deformed grid (bottom right). Computation time and numerical values for the difference D and the constraints C for the un- and VP-constrained registration are summarized in Table 1 and 2.

MRI scans: In our second example, we discuss results obtained for the images shown in Fig. 1. Fig. 4 shows the results after two (2nd row) and ten iterations (3rd row) of the unconstrained registration as well as after ten iterations of the VP constrained registration (4th row). After at most ten iteration both schemes have converged.

Although the numbers (cf. Table 2) indicate a larger reduction of the difference by the unconstrained registrations, the ranking is not so clear if one looks at the difference images, cf. Fig. 4. Here, the difference after ten steps un- and VP constrained registration looks pretty much the same. After two steps of the unconstrained registration the bright spot in the top part of the image has not been resolved satisfiably. The explanation is that small spots which are related to noise in the MRI images and hardly visible in the images are registered in the unconstrained registration. This leads to a large reduction though it is hardly visible. To remove this small spots, the volume has to be changed locally. However, the registration of these small spots does not contribute to a meaningful solution for this problem.

In Fig. 2, we display the pointwise map of the change of volume. Using the unconstrained approach, we observe a considerable change of volume for the breast with a peak value of 1.36. Thus, part of the breast has been enlarged by a factor of 2.36. For the constrained approach, we observe that the volume change is below a user supplied threshold (here, $tol_C = 1o^{-6}$) everywhere. In fact, since we used a quasi-Newton scheme for projection, the numbers are around 10^{-9}.

References

1. Maurer, C.R., Fitzpatrick, J.M.: A Review of Medical Image Registration. In: Interactive Image-Guided Neurosurgery. Park Ridge, IL, American Association of Neurological Surgeons (1993) 17–44
2. Fitzpatrick, J.M., Hill, D.L.G., Jr., C.R.M.: Image registration. In Sonka, M., Fitzpatrick, J.M., eds.: Handbook of Medical Imaging, Volume 2: Medical Image Processing and Analysis, SPIE (2000) 447–513
3. Rohlfing, T., Maurer, Jr., C.R., Bluemke, D.A., Jacobs, M.A.: Volume-preserving nonrigid registration of MR breast images using free-form deformation with an incompressibility constraint. IEEE Transactions on Medical Imaging **22** (2003) 730–741
4. Brown, L.G.: A survey of image registration techniques. ACM Computing Surveys **24** (1992) 325–376
5. Collignon, A., Vandermeulen, A., Suetens, P., Marchal, G.: 3d multi-modality medical image registration based on information theory. Kluwer Academic Publishers: Computational Imaging and Vision **3** (1995) 263–274
6. Viola, P., Wells III, W.M.: Alignment by maximization of mutual information. (1995) 16–23 IEEE 1995.
7. Roche, A.: Recalage d'images médicales par inférence statistique. PhD thesis, Université de Nice, Sophia-Antipolis, France (2001)
8. Hermosillo, G.: Variational methods for multimodal image matching. PhD thesis, Université de Nice, France (2002)
9. Clarenz, U., Droske, M., Rumpf, M.: Towards fast non–rigid registration. In: Inverse Problems, Image Analysis and Medical Imaging, AMS Special Session Interaction of Inverse Problems and Image Analysis. Volume 313., AMS (2002) 67–84
10. Modersitzki, J.: Numerical Methods for Image Registration. Oxford University Press (2004)
11. Broit, C.: Optimal Registration of Deformed Images. PhD thesis, Computer and Information Science, University of Pensylvania (1981)

12. Christensen, G.E.: Deformable Shape Models for Anatomy. PhD thesis, Sever Institute of Technology, Washington University (1994)
13. Fischer, B., Modersitzki, J.: Fast inversion of matrices arising in image processing. Num. Algo. **22** (1999) 1–11
14. Bro-Nielsen, M.: Medical Image Registration and Surgery Simulation. PhD thesis, IMM, Technical University of Denmark (1996)
15. Fischer, B., Modersitzki, J.: Fast diffusion registration. AMS Contemporary Mathematics, Inverse Problems, Image Analysis, and Medical Imaging **313** (2002) 117–129
16. Fischer, B., Modersitzki, J.: Curvature based image registration. J. of Mathematical Imaging and Vision **18** (2003) 81–85
17. Yee, K.: Numerical solution of initial boundary value problems involving Maxwell's equations in isotropic media. IEEE Trans. on Antennas and Propagation **14** (1966) 302–307
18. Haber, E., Modersitzki, J.: Numerical methods for volume preserving image registration. Technical Report TR-2004-012-A, Department of Mathematics and Computer Science, Emory University, Atlanta GA 30322 (2004) Submitted to Inverse Problems.
19. Nocedal, J., Wright, S.: Numerical optimization. Springer, New York (1999)

Multiresolution Image Registration Based on Kullback-Leibler Distance

Rui Gan[1], Jue Wu[2], Albert C.S. Chung[1],
Simon C.H. Yu[3], and William M. Wells III[4,5]

[1] Department of Computer Science, and
[2] Bioengineering Program, School of Engineering,
Hong Kong University of Science and Technology, Hong Kong.
{raygan, johnwoo, achung}@cs.ust.hk
[3] Dept. of Diagnostic Radiology and Organ Imaging, Prince of Wales Hospital, HK.
[4] Brigham & Women's Hospital, Harvard Medical School, Boston, MA, U.S.A.
[5] MIT CSAI Laboratory, Cambridge, MA, U.S.A.

Abstract. This paper extends our prior work on multi-modal image registration based on the *a priori* knowledge of the joint intensity distribution that we expect to obtain, and Kullback-Leibler distance. This expected joint distribution can be estimated from pre-aligned training images. Experimental results show that, as compared with the Mutual Information and Approximate Maximum Likelihood based registration methods, the new method has longer capture range at different image resolutions, which can lead to a more robust image registration method. Moreover, with a simple interpolation algorithm based on non-grid point random sampling, the proposed method can avoid interpolation artifacts at the low resolution registration. Finally, it is experimentally demonstrated that our method is applicable to a variety of imaging modalities.

1 Introduction

In this paper, we extend our prior work on multi-modal image registration method based on the *a priori* knowledge of the joint intensity distribution that we expect to obtain. This expected joint distribution can be estimated from aligned training images [3,10]. Unlike Mutual Information (MI) based image registration method [7,11], our method makes use of the expected joint intensity distribution between two pre-aligned training images as a reference distribution. Two novel images of the same or different acquisitions are aligned when the expected and observed joint intensity distributions are well matched. The difference between distributions is measured using the Kullback-Leibler distance (KLD). The registration procedure is a multiresolution iterative process. The procedure at the current image resolution is terminated when the KLD value becomes sufficiently small. Then, based on the current estimated transformation, the next higher resolution registration continues until the original image resolution is reached.

C. Barillot, D.R. Haynor, and P. Hellier (Eds.): MICCAI 2004, LNCS 3216, pp. 599–606, 2004.
© Springer-Verlag Berlin Heidelberg 2004

Based on the results on T1, T2, PD, CT, and 3DRA image volumes, it is experimentally shown that our method has significantly longer capture range[1] than that of MI based and Approximate Maximum Likelihood (MLa) [6,12] based methods, which can make the multiresolution image registration more robust. Moreover, our method can avoid the problem of interpolation artifact in the low resolution registration. Finally, the experiments demonstrate that our method can be applicable to a variety of imaging modalities.

2   Method

2.1   Estimation of the Joint Intensity Distributions

Let I_f and I_r be the intensity values of two images of the same or different acquisitions (f and r represent respectively the floating and reference images), and X_f and X_r be their image domains respectively. Assume that the intensity values of image voxels are independent of each other.

The expected joint distribution can be estimated from a pre-aligned training image pair, which can be obtained from experienced clinicians or other image registration methods (e.g., an MI based method). Given two precisely aligned training image volumes, samples of intensity pairs $\hat{\mathcal{I}} = \{i_f(x), i_r(x^r)|i_f \in I_f, i_r \in I_r\}$ can be drawn from I_f and I_r, where x are the grid point coordinates in X_f (i.e. the sampling domain is equal to X_f) and x^r are the corresponding coordinates of x in X_r. Histogram partial volume (PV) interpolation [7] is used to achieve subvoxel accuracy in registration results. The expected joint intensity distribution $\hat{P}(I_f, I_r)$ can be approximated by either Parzen windowing or histogramming [1]. Histogramming is employed in this paper because the approach is computationally efficient.

For the observed joint intensity distribution, given a novel testing image pair with a hypothesized transformation T, samples of intensity pairs $\mathcal{I}_o = \{i_f(x), i_r(T(x))|i_f \in I_f, i_r \in I_r\}$ can be drawn from I_f and I_r, where x are the coordinates in X_f. Note that the observed joint intensity distribution $P_o^T(I_f, I_r)$ is dependent on the transformation T and changes during the registration. The histogramming approach is used to estimate the distribution P_o^T.

According to our experiments, interpolation artifacts may occur if we only draw samples at grid positions from X_f and apply PV interpolation in X_r, especially for the same voxel-size image pair of low resolution (see Section 3.1 for more details). Similar observations for the problem have been reported in [8]. In this paper, we propose a simple improvement of PV interpolation based on random sampling to avoid interpolation artifacts and increase the robustness of our method. It can be outlined as follows. Instead of drawing samples at grid positions, we randomly draw samples from X_f. If the sample is a grid position, we update the joint distribution by using the same method as before; otherwise, i.e. a non-grid position, we perform PV interpolation both in X_f and X_r. In

---

[1] Capture range represents the range of positions from which a registration algorithm can converge to the correct minimum or maximum.

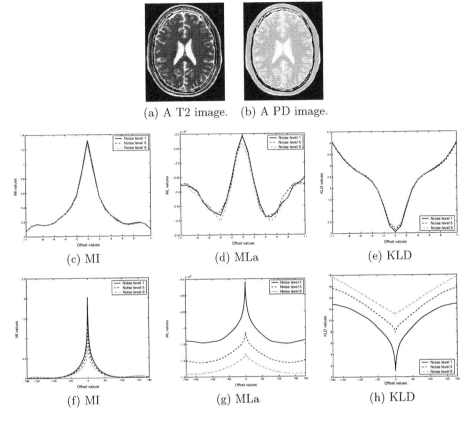

(a) A T2 image.   (b) A PD image.

(c) MI   (d) MLa   (e) KLD

(f) MI   (g) MLa   (h) KLD

Fig. 1. (a) A slice of BrainWeb T2 image volume. (b) A slice of BrainWeb PD image volume. Translational probes for registering low resolution (Level 4) image pairs with different noise levels (1%, 5% and 9%): (c) MI, (d) MLa, and (e) KLD. Translational probes for registering the original resolution (Level 0) image pairs: (f) MI, (g) MLa, and (h) KLD. Training dataset was 0% noise level for all probes.

practice, the sampling rate can be set to $10\% - 50\%$ of the total number of voxels in the floating image.

For a further illustration, suppose that s is a non-grid position in X_f. Let $\mathcal{N}_s$ be a set of neighboring grid positions of s in X_f and $\tilde{\mathcal{N}}_{T(s)}$ be that of $T(s)$ in X_r. Then, the update of P_o^T is given by

$$\forall n \in \mathcal{N}_s \text{ and } \forall \tilde{n} \in \tilde{\mathcal{N}}_{T(s)} \; : \; P_o^T\Big(i_f(n), i_r(\tilde{n})\Big)+ = \frac{w_n \cdot \tilde{w}_{\tilde{n}} \cdot D(T(n), \tilde{n})}{Z}, \quad (1)$$

where w_n and $\tilde{w}_{\tilde{n}}$ are respectively the corresponding fractions of position n and position $\tilde{n}$ in PV interpolation and can be determined via the trilinear interpolation [7], $D(T(n), \tilde{n})$ is a decreasing function with respect to the Euclidean distance between positions $T(n)$ and $\tilde{n}$, and Z is a normalizing factor which keeps $\sum_{\tilde{n} \in \tilde{\mathcal{N}}_{T(s)}} \sum_{n \in \mathcal{N}_s} P_o^T\Big(i_f(n), i_r(\tilde{n})\Big) = 1$. In this paper, we set $D(s_1, s_2)$

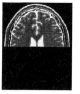 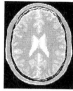 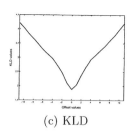 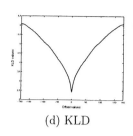

(a) A T2 image   (b) A PD image.

with occlusion.   (c) KLD   (d) KLD

Fig. 2. (a) An occluded slice of BrainWeb T2 image volume. (b) A slice of Brain-Web PD image volume. Translational probes for registering image pairs with different resolutions: (c) KLD level 4 (low resolution), (d) KLD level 0 (original resolution).

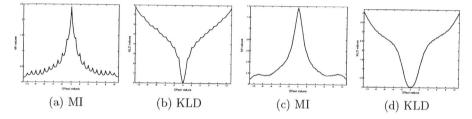

(a) MI   (b) KLD   (c) MI   (d) KLD

Fig. 3. Interpolation artifacts in the low resolution (level 4) image registration. Results of translational probing experiments based on sampling on grid points: (a) MI and (b) KLD. Results based on non-grid point random sampling: (c) MI and (d) KLD.

to $(2 \cdot L_d^r - d_{s_1,s_2})$, where L_d^r is the diagonal length of voxels in X_r and d_{s_1,s_2} represents the Euclidean distance between positions s_1 and s_2.

2.2 Kullback-Leibler Distance (KLD) and Multiresolution Optimization

Given the expected $\hat{P}$ and observed P_o^T joint intensity distributions, the Kullback-Leibler distance between the two distributions is given by

$$D(P_o^T || \hat{P}) = \sum_{i_f, i_r} P_o^T(i_f, i_r) \log \frac{P_o^T(i_f, i_r)}{\hat{P}(i_f, i_r)}. \qquad (2)$$

KLD may be used to measure the similarity between two distributions. According to [5], the KLD value is non-negative and becomes zero if and only if two distributions are equivalent. The more similar the two distributions are, the smaller the KLD value is. Therefore, when the two testing images I_f and I_r are not perfectly registered, the value of KLD, D, will be positive and relatively large because P_o^T and $\hat{P}$ are not similar. On the other hand, if the testing images are well registered, then the value of KLD becomes small or is equal to zero (i.e. P_o^T is very similar or equal to $\hat{P}$).

The goal of registration is to find the optimal transformation $\hat{T}$ by minimizing the difference between the observed P_o and expected $\hat{P}$, which is formulated as

$$\hat{T} = \arg \min_{T} D(P_o^T || \hat{P}). \tag{3}$$

The proposed method is conceptually different from the MI based registration method, which encourages functional dependence between the two image random variables, I_f and I_r. The KLD based registration method guides the transformation T based on the difference between the expected $\hat{P}$ and observed P_o^T joint intensity distributions, or, in other words, based on the expected outcomes learned from the training data.

In order to accelerate the registration process and ensure the accuracy and robustness of the proposed method, we exploit a multiresolution approach based on the Gaussian Pyramid representation [2,11]. Rough estimates of $\hat{T}$ can be found using downsampled images and treated as starting values for optimization at higher resolutions. Then, the fine-tuning of the solution can be derived at the original image resolution.

In this paper, the value of KLD for each resolution is minimized by Powell's method with a multiresolution strategy [9] because it does not require calculations of gradient and, hence, is simpler in terms of implementation. Powell's method iteratively searches for the minimum value of KLD along each parameter axis T (1D line minimization) while other parameters are kept constant.

3   Experimental Results

3.1   T2 – PD (3D – 3D) Registration

Four pairs of T2 and PD image volumes were used for the registration experiments. The images were obtained from the BrainWeb Simulated Brain Database [4] ($181 \times 217 \times 181$ voxels, $1 \times 1 \times 1$ mm^3 and noise levels were 0%, 1%, 5% and 9%). Figures 1a and 1b show T2 and PD image slices respectively. An image pair with 0% noise level was used as the training image pair and the others were the testing image pairs. Figures 1c, 1d and 1e plot the translational probes for registering the low resolution [2] (Level 4) testing image pairs with different noise levels for the Mutual Information (MI) [7,11], Approximate Maximum Likelihood (MLa) [6,12] and Kullback-Leibler Distance (KLD) respectively. Similarly, Figures 1f, 1g and 1h plot the translational probes for registering the original resolution (Level 0) image pairs. Figures 1e and 1h show that the capture ranges of KLD are significantly longer than those of MI and MLa.

To study the effect of occlusion, as shown in Figure 2a, only half of the T2 image volume was used for registration experiments. Another PD image volume (Figure 2b) and the training image pair were unchanged. Results (Figures 2c and 2d) show that our method works when the testing image is occluded.

---

[2] The definition of resolution levels in the Gaussian Pyramid representation follows the same line as in [2]. The smoothing filter was $\{1, 4, 6, 4, 1\}$ in our experiments.

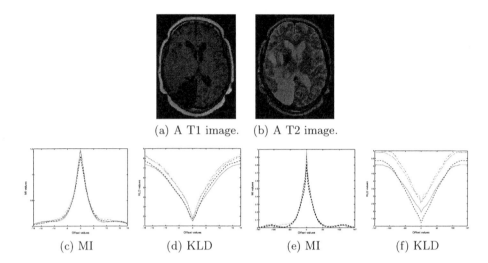

Fig. 4. (a) A slice of Vanderbilt T1 image volume. (b) A slice of Vanderbilt T2 image volume. Translational probes for registering the low resolution (Level 3) image pairs from different testing datasets: (c) MI and (d) KLD. Translational probes for registering the original resolution (Level 0) image pairs: (e) MI and (f) KLD. Training datasets were from patient #001.

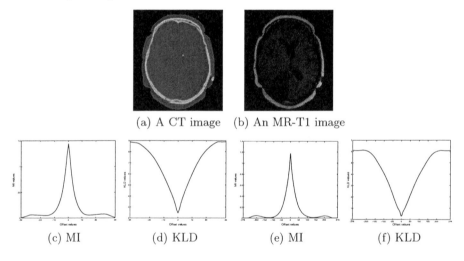

Fig. 5. (a) A slice of Vanderbilt CT image volume. (b) A slice of Vanderbilt MR-T1 image volume. Translational probes for registering the low resolution (Level 3) image pair: (c) MI and (d) KLD. Translational probes for registering the original resolution (Level 0) image pair: (e) MI and (f) KLD.

Figures 3a and 3b illustrate that, when we only draw samples at grid positions for the estimation of joint distributions, interpolation artifacts occur for both MI and KLD based methods at the low resolution (level 4). With the random sam-

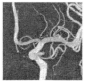
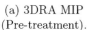

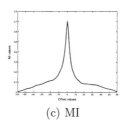
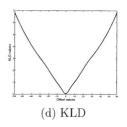

(a) 3DRA MIP   (b) 3DRA MIP
(Pre-treatment).   (Post-treatment).   (c) MI   (d) KLD

Fig. 6. (a) Maximum intensity projection (MIP) of a pre-treatment 3D rotational angiography (3DRA). (b) MIP of a post-treatment 3DRA. Translational probes for registering the image volume pair: (c) MI and (d) KLD.

pling on non-grid positions, Figures 3c and 3d show that interpolation artifact can be avoided. This can make the low resolution registration more robust.

3.2   T1, T2, and CT (3D – 3D) Registration

Five pairs of T1 and T2 image volumes were obtained from the Retrospective Registration Evaluation Project [3] (160×160×26 voxels and 1.25×1.25×4 mm^3). Image volumes from patient #001 were used as the training image pair.

Figures 4a and 4b show T1 and T2 slices respectively. Figures 4c (MI) and 4d (KLD) plot the translational probes for registering four low resolution (Level 3) image pairs. At the original image resolution (Level 0), Figures 4e and 4f plot the translational probes based on MI and KLD respectively. Figures 4d and 4f illustrate that the KLD based method consistently gives longer capture range than that of the MI based method (Figures 4c and 4e).

Two pairs of T1 and CT image volumes from the same project were used for the registration experiments. Figures 5a and 5b show CT and T1 image slices respectively. Probes along the horizontal direction are shown in Figures 5c and 5d for the low resolution (Level 3) registration and in Figures 5e and 5f for the original resolution (Level 0) registration. Similar results for the capture range were obtained as compared with the T1 and T2 registration as shown above.

3.3   Pre-treatment 3DRA – Post-treatment 3DRA Registration

Two pairs of 3D rotational angiographic (RA) image volumes of the same patient were obtained from the Prince of Wales Hospital, Hong Kong for the registration experiments (256×256×256 voxels and 0.19×0.19×0.19 mm^3). Figures 6a and 6b show two maximum intensity projections (MIP) of the pre-treatment and post-treatment image volumes respectively. (Note that the MIPs are for visualization purposes only, not part of the registration process.) The figures show that our method can be applied to 3DRA image registration and useful for interventional treatment assessments because 3DRA volumes can be compared quantitatively.

---

[3] Images were provided as part of the project, "Evaluation of Retrospective Image Registration", National Institutes of Health, Project Number 1 R01 NS33926-01, Principle Investigator, J. Michael Fitzpatrick, Vanderbilt University, Nashville, TN.

4   Summary and Conclusions

This paper has proposed a multiresolution multi-modal image registration method based on minimizing the Kullback-Leibler distance (KLD) between the observed and expected joint intensity distributions until the two testing datasets are aligned. The results consistently show that our method has a longer capture range than that of MI and MLa based methods. The proposed simple non-grid point random sampling method has been experimentally shown that it can avoid the problem of interpolation artifact in the low resolution registration based on histogram partial volume (PV) interpolation. Future work will include a further validation of the proposed algorithm by applying it to a large number of datasets.

Acknowledgements. W. Wells would like to acknowledge support from the NSF ERC grant (JHU Agreement #8810-274) and the NIH (grant #1P41RR13218). A. Chung would like to acknowledge support from the HK RGC grants (HKUST6155/03E and HKUST6209/02E).

References

1. C.M. Bishop. *Neural Networks for Pattern Recognition*. Oxford U. Press, 1995.
2. P.J. Burt and E.H. Adelson. The Laplacian Pyramid as a Compact Image Code. *IEEE Trans. Comms.*, 31(4):532–540, 1983.
3. A.C.S. Chung, W.M. Wells II, and et. al. Multi-Modal Image Registration by Minimising Kullback-Leibler Distance. In *MICCAI*, pages 525–532, 2002.
4. D.L. Collins, A.P. Zijdenbos, and et al. Design and Construction of a Realistic Digital Brain Phantom. *IEEE Trans. Med. Img.*, 17(3):463–468, 1998.
5. T.M. Cover and J.A. Thomas. *Elements of Information Theory*. John Wiley & Sons, Inc., 1991.
6. M.E. Leventon and W.E.L. Grimson. Multi-Modal Volume Registration Using Joint Intensity Distributions. In *MICCAI*, pages 1057–1066, 1998.
7. F. Maes, A. Collignon, and et al. Multimodality Image Registration by Maximization of Mutual Information. *IEEE Trans. Med. Img.*, 16(2):187–198, 1997.
8. J.P.W. Pluim, J.B.A. Maintz, and M.A. Viergever. Interpolation Artefacts in Mutual Information-Based Image Registration. *CVIU*, 77:211–232, 2000.
9. W.H. Press, S.A. Teukolsky, and et al. *Numerical Recipes in C, 2nd Edition*. Cambridge University Press, 1992.
10. S. Soman, A.C.S. Chung, and et. al. Rigid Registration of Echoplanar and Conventional MR Images by Minimizing Kullback-Leibler Distance. In *WBIR*, pages 181–190, 2003.
11. W.M. Wells, P. Viola, and et al. Multi-Modal Volume Registration by Maximization of Mutual Information. *Medical Image Analysis*, 1(1):35–51, 1996.
12. L. Zöllei, J.W. Fisher III, and W.M. Wells III. A Unified Satistical and Information Theoretic Framework for Multi-modal Image Registration. In *IPMI*, pages 366–377, 2003.

Empirical Evaluation of Covariance Estimates for Mutual Information Coregistration

Paul A. Bromiley, Maja Pokric, and Neil A. Thacker

Imaging Science and Biomedical Engineering, Stopford Building, University of Manchester, Oxford Road, Manchester, M13 9PT.

Abstract. Mutual information has become a popular similarity measure in multi-modality medical image registration since it was first applied to the problem in 1995. This paper describes a method for calculating the covariance matrix for mutual information coregistration. We derive an expression for the matrix through identification of mutual information with a log-likelihood measure. The validity of this result is then demonstrated through comparison with the results of Monte-Carlo simulations of the coregistration of T1-weighted to T2-weighted synthetic and genuine MRI scans of the brain. We conclude with some observations on the theoretical basis of the mutual information measure as a log-likelihood.

1 Introduction

The use of mutual information (MI) as a similarity measure for multi-modality coregistration was first proposed in 1995 [1], and since then has become the most popular information-theoretic approach to this problem. Research into coregistration has generally focused on the definition of similarity metrics or on the representation of the transformation model. There is however a growing recognition that characterisation of the accuracy of coregistration is essential if further quantitative processing of the images is to be performed using the resultant transformation model. For example, Crum et. al. [2] state that "...the veracity of studies that rely on non-rigid registration should be keenly questioned when the error distribution is unknown and the results are unsupported by other contextual information". We present an analytical expression for the covariance matrix of the parameters of MI coregistration, based on the identification of the measure as a log-likelihood. This is only the first step towards a full characterisation of the error for the general coregistration problem: for example, it takes no account of the difference between image similarity and biological correspondence. However, it provides a lower bound on the error, which may be attainable for certain coregistration problems and definitions of correspondence.

Mutual information $\mathcal{I}(I;J)$ measures the Kullback-Leibler divergence between the joint probability distribution $p(i,j)$ of two images I and J and the product of their marginal distributions $p(i).p(j)$ [3],

$$\mathcal{I}(I;J) = \sum_{i,j} p(i,j) \log \frac{p(i,j)}{p(i).p(j)}.$$

C. Barillot, D.R. Haynor, and P. Hellier (Eds.): MICCAI 2004, LNCS 3216, pp. 607–614, 2004.
© Springer-Verlag Berlin Heidelberg 2004

i.e. the divergence of the joint distribution from the case of complete independence of the images, where the sum is performed over a joint histogram. Therefore, maximisation of this measure with respect to a set of coregistration parameters will optimise the image alignment. Following [4], we can write

$$\mathcal{I}(I; J) = \sum_i p(i) \log \frac{1}{p(i)} + \sum_{i,j} p(i, j) \log \frac{p(i, j)}{p(j)}.$$

Recognising that the first term on the R.H.S. is the entropy $H(I)$ of image I [3] and that $p(i, j) = N_{ij}/N$, where N_{ij} is the number of entries in histogram bin (i, j) and N is the total number of entries in the histogram, we obtain

$$\log P(I|J) = N[\mathcal{I}(I; J) - H(I)] = \sum_v \log \frac{p(i, j)}{p(j)} \qquad (1)$$

where v represents a sum over voxels rather than histogram bins. At this point we can make the arbitrary definition that I is the target (fixed) image and J the source image i.e. the image altered by the transformation model. If we ensure that the overlapping regions of the images always include the whole of the target image, for example by excluding an appropriately sized border around the reference image, $H(I)$ will be a constant, giving

$$logP(I|J) = N(\mathcal{I}(I; J)) + const.$$

Therefore the MI is a monotonic function of the log-probability of image I given image J.

The covariances for a maximum likelihood technique are given by the minimum variance bound [5]

$$C_\theta^{-1} = -\left.\frac{\partial^2 \log L}{\partial \theta_m \partial \theta_n}\right|_{\theta_0}$$

where θ represent parameters of some model, θ_O represents the parameters for optimal alignment, and L represents the likelihood function. This bound becomes exact if the log-likelihood is quadratic i.e. the likelihood function in Gaussian. Assuming a Gaussian likelihood function

$$L = \prod_d A_d e^{-\frac{(I_d - I_M)^2}{2\sigma_d^2}} \quad \Rightarrow \quad \log L = \sum_d -\frac{(I_d - I_M)^2}{2\sigma_d^2} + logA_d$$

$$\Rightarrow \quad \left.\frac{\partial^2 \log L}{\partial \theta_r \partial \theta_s}\right|_{\theta_0} = \sum_d -\frac{1}{\sigma_d^2}\frac{\partial I_M}{\partial \theta_r}\frac{\partial I_M}{\partial \theta_s}\bigg|_{\theta_0}$$

where A_d is the normalisation of the Gaussian, I_d are the data and I_M the corresponding model predictions, and σ_d are the standard deviations of the data. Note that any constant normalisation of the Gaussian (A_d) disappears upon differentiation. In simple maximum likelihood techniques e.g. linear least-squares fitting, the normalisation of L will indeed be constant. However, MI is constructed from a so-called "bootstrapped" likelihood, constructed from the joint histogram rather than an explicit model. In that case, the usual normalisation (to the area under the distribution) may no longer be constant: for example, simply altering the histogram bin size will alter the normalisation. Fortunately, a solution is available in the form of the χ^2 metric. If we normalise to the peak of the distribution, then A_d becomes 1 and disappears upon taking logs. The maximisation of the log-likelihood is then directly equivalent to minimisation of the χ^2

$$\log L = \sum_d -\frac{(I_d - I_M)^2}{2\sigma_d^2} = -\frac{\chi^2}{2}$$

Whilst this is explicitly true for a Gaussian L, we would suggest that this statistic has higher utility regardless of the form of the underlying distribution as it provides appropriate normalisation.

The χ^2 can be written in terms of a sum over individual data terms, the so-called χ of the χ^2

$$\chi^2 = \sum_d \chi_d^2 = \sum_d -2\log(L_d) \Rightarrow \chi_d = \sqrt{-2\log L_d} \tag{2}$$

The expression for the minimum variance bound can also be rewritten in this form, through comparison with the previous result for a Gaussian likelihood

$$\chi_d = \frac{(I_i - I_M)}{\sigma_d} \quad \Rightarrow \quad \sum_d \frac{\partial \chi_d}{\partial \theta_r} \frac{\partial \chi_d}{\partial \theta_s} = \sum_d \frac{1}{2\sigma_d} \frac{\partial I_M}{\partial \theta_r} \frac{\partial I_M}{\partial \theta_s}$$

Comparing this to the previous expression for the covariances of a Gaussian likelihood, we can write,

$$\Rightarrow \quad C_\theta^{-1} = \sum_d 2(\nabla_\theta \chi_d)^T \otimes (\nabla_\theta \chi_d)\bigg|_{\theta=\theta_{max}} \tag{3}$$

The Gaussian assumption need only be true over a sufficient range around the minimum that the derivatives can be calculated, and since in rigid coregistration we are dealing with a likelihood composed from ≈ 100000 voxels we would expect, via. the Central Limit Theorem, that this would be a good approximation.

In order to identify the equivalent χ^2 term in the MI measure, we can split Eq. 1 into two terms

$$-\log P(I|J) = -\sum_v \log \frac{p(i,j)}{p(i_{max},j)} - \sum_v \log \frac{p(i_{max},j)}{p(j)} \tag{4}$$

The first term on the RHS is the χ^2 metric, normalised to the distribution peak as required. The second is a bias term dependent on the non-uniform normalisation of the likelihood distribution. This expression elucidates the behaviour of the MI measure: it is a maximum likelihood measure biased with a term that maximises the "peakiness" of the distributions in the joint histogram, in order to maximise the correlation between equivalent structures in the images. If we assume that the bias term varies slowly compared to the χ^2 term, which is reasonable since it depends on the marginal distribution, then Eq. 3 can be used: expanding using the chain rule, substituting for the differential of χ_v from Eq. 2, using Eq. 2 and Eq. 4 to substitute for L_v, and remembering that the model terms I_M in this case are represented by the source image voxels J_v gives

$$C_\theta^{-1} = 2\sum_v (\frac{\partial \chi_v}{\partial L_v})^2 (\frac{\partial L_v}{\partial J_v})^2 (\nabla_\theta J_v)^T \otimes (\nabla_\theta J_v)\Big|_{\theta=\theta_{max}}$$

$$C_\theta^{-1} = -\sum_v \frac{(\frac{\partial p(i,j)}{\partial J_v} - \frac{p(i,j)}{p(i_{max},j)}\frac{\partial p(i_{max},j)}{\partial J_v})^2}{2p(i,j)^2 \log \frac{p(i,j)}{p(i_{max}|j)}} (\nabla_\theta J_v)^T \otimes (\nabla_\theta J_v)\Big|_{\theta=\theta_{max}} \quad (5)$$

2   Method

The covariance estimation technique was first tested on the rigid coregistration of T2 to T1 weighted simulated MR of a normal brain, obtained from Brainweb [6]. Each volume consisted of 55 slices of 217 by 195 voxels, with Gaussian random noise added at 1% of the dynamic range of the images. The technique was repeated on the coregistration of genuine T2 to T1 weighted MR from a normal volunteer. These image volumes consisted of 29 3mm thick slices of 256 by 256 (0.89mm by 0.89mm) voxels. The noise on the images, measured using the width of zero crossings in horizontal and vertical gradient histograms, was again approximately 1% of the dynamic range of the images. MI coregistration was implemented within the TINA machine vision software package (www.tina-vision.net), using simplex minimisation, and allowing the coregistration to optimise the rotation (as Euler angles), translation and scaling of the images. A rotation offset of 5° was added to the floating images before coregistration, but the coregistration was started from the correct alignment. This followed the suggestion by Pluim et. al. [7] regarding the suppression of interpolation artefacts. These artefacts arise at points where large portions of the voxel grid for both images coincide, and so large numbers of voxels from the source image are used without interpolation. Since interpolation inevitably smooths the data, such points lead to sudden jumps in the value of the similarity measure.

Monte-Carlo simulations were run by adding random Gaussian noise to the reference image at levels of 0.25 to 2.5 times the original image noise, in ten steps of 0.25σ. One thousand coregistrations were performed at each noise level, and the results used to estimate the covariance matrix of the coregistration parameters. Then, the above estimate was applied at each noise level, taking the median of 1000 estimate of the covariances over a range around the minimum that represented a change of around 0.5% in the χ^2 in order to stabilise the calculation against the effects of interpolation artefacts, local minima etc. Finally,

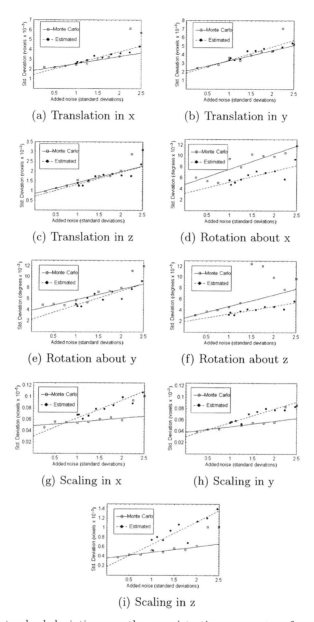

Fig. 1. The standard deviations on the coregistration parameters for the Brainweb data. The lines show least-squares linear fits to the data, omitting the top two points from the Monte-Carlo experiments due to evidence of bimodality around the minimum (see main text).

the two covariance estimates at each noise level were compared. Since each covariance matrix is prepared from a set of $1 \times n$ vectors of parameters, it has only n degrees of freedom despite containing n^2 parameters. Therefore, it is sufficient

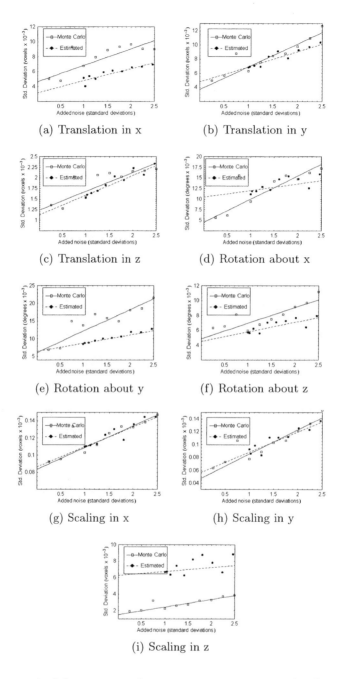

Fig. 2. The standard deviations on the coregistration parameters for the genuine MR data. The lines show least-squares linear fits to the data.

to examine only n parameters, and so we will limit the discussion of the results to the n diagonal elements (the variances) alone.

3   Results

Fig. 1. shows the standard deviations on the parameters for the Brainweb data. In each case, the Monte-Carlo estimates scale linearly with the addition of noise as expected. Linear least-squares fits to the data are shown. The two points for the highest levels of added noise show a departure from the trend. This was due to bimodality in the Monte-Carlo results i.e. the added noise destabilised the coregistration enough that a local minimum close to the global minimum began to contribute. Therefore, these points were omitted from the fitting process. The estimates from the analytical expression are also shown together with linear fits. The covariance estimates on the translation parameters are identical between the Monte-Carlo results and the analytical estimate to within the noise on the data. The results for the rotational parameters show some divergence, and are also notably noisier, due to the non-linear nature of rotational transformations. The results for the scaling parameters show the greatest divergence at the higher noise levels. This is due to an effective underestimate of the covariance through the Monte-Carlo experiments. The scaling parameters are more susceptible to interpolation artefacts than the other parameters, leading to oscillations in the similarity metric around the global minimum. The Monte-Carlo results tend to fall into the local minima generated by these oscillations, leading to underestimates of covariances, whereas the estimated covariance was stabilised against this effect by taking the median value over 1000 points around the global minimum. Overall, all of the estimated covariances either match the Monte-Carlo results closely, or converge at low noise levels, and are always within a factor of two of the Monte-Carlo results.

Fig. 2 shows the standard deviations on the coregistration parameters for the genuine MR data. Again, all results scale linearly with noise as expected. The image content and noise were roughly equivalent to the Brainweb data, but the genuine MR volumes contained only half as many voxels, implying that the variances should be roughly twice as large, and this can indeed be seen in the results. The other features of the results are all broadly similar: the estimated covariances either match the Monte-Carlo results or converge with them at low noise levels. An exception is seen in the scaling parameter in the z direction: here the estimated covariances are significantly higher. This was due to artefacts in the similarity metric around the minimum, which made it impossible to produce a stable covariance estimate.

4   Conclusion

This paper has provided a derivation of an analytical expression for the covariances in the parameters of mutual information (MI) coregistration. The validity of the result has been demonstrated through comparison with the results of

Monte-Carlo simulations on both simulated and genuine MR images of the brain. The estimated variances are consistent between the two techniques, confirming that the equation for variance estimation is valid and that our assumption that the bias term is negligible is justified.

The derivation also illustrates some features of MI in general. Most important is the relationship between MI and log-likelihood. The consistency between the estimated covariances and the practical coregistration performance confirms that this interpretation is valid. We maintain that this is the true theoretical basis of the method, rather than its relationship to concepts of entropy. It is the link to maximum likelihood that allows the theory to support calculation of a covariance matrix. The likelihood interpretation may also provide new perspectives on MI and associated similarity measures, suggesting alternatives based on quantitative statistics. For instance, normalised MI measures [7] are currently used for coregistration problems with varying sample sizes. The approach adopted here suggests using a χ^2 metric i.e. an appropriately normalised log-likelihood, in which the variation in sample size can be accommodated as a variation in the number of degrees of freedom. Ultimately, this could lead to a coregistration algorithm implemented in expectation-maximisation form.

Acknowledgements. The authors would like to acknowledge the support of the EPSRC and the MRC (IRC: From Medical Images and Signals to Clinical Information), and of the European Commission(An Integrated Environment for Rehearsal and Planning of Surgical Interventions). All software is freely available from our web site www.tina-vision.net.

References

1. Viola, P., Wells, W.M.: Alignment by maximisation of mutual information. International Journal of Computer Vision **24** (1997) 137–154
2. Crum, W.R., Griffin, L.D., Hill, D.V.G., Hawkes, D.J.: Zen and the art of medical image registration: correspondence, homology, and quality. Neuroimage **20** (2003) 1425–1437
3. Cover, T.M., Thomas, J.A.: Elements of Information Theory. John Wiley and Sons, New York (1991)
4. Roche, A., Malandain, G., Ayache, N., Prima, S.: Towards a better comprehension of similarity measures used in medical image registration. In: Proceedings MICCAI'99. (1999) 555–566
5. Barlow, R.J.: Statistics: A Guide to the use of Statistical Methods in the Physical Sciences. John Wiley and Sons Ltd., UK (1989)
6. Cocosco, C.A., Kollokian, V., Kwan, R.K.S., Evans, A.C.: Brainweb: Online interface to a 3D MRI simulated brain database. Neuroimage **5** (1997) S425
7. Pluim, J.P.W., Antoine Maintz, J.B., Viergever, M.A.: Interpolation artefacts in mutual information-based image registration. Computer Vision and Image Understanding **77** (2000) 211–232

Deformation Based Representation of Groupwise Average and Variability

Natasa Kovacevic[1], Josette Chen[1,2], John G. Sled[1,2], Jeff Henderson[2], and Mark Henkelman[1,2]

[1] Mouse Imaging Centre, Hospital For Sick Children
555 University Ave., Toronto ON M5G 1X8, Canada
[2] University Of Toronto, Canada

Abstract. This paper presents a novel method for creating an unbiased and geometrically centered average from a group of images. The morphological variability of the group is modeled as a set of deformation fields which encode differences between the group average and individual members. We demonstrate the algorithm on a group of 27 MR images of mouse brains. The average image is highly resolved as a result of excellent groupwise registration. Local and global groupwise variability estimates are discussed.

1 Introduction

Brain atlases together with warping algorithms represent an important tool for the analysis of medical images. For example, an annotated atlas is typically used as a deformable template. Image registration enables warping of the atlas image onto other brain images. Subsequently, the anatomical knowledge about the atlas image is transfered and customized for arbitrary subjects [3,9,11]. Experience shows, however, that the choice of an individual brain as a template leads to biasing. This is because the registration errors are large for brains with morphology that is significantly different from the template. For such brains, the accuracy of the anatomical knowledge obtained through the registration with the template is less accurate. To somewhat alleviate this problem, the authors in [5] have proposed a method for optimizing an individual template brain with respect to a group of subjects. Other methods reduce the dependence on a particular subject by creating a template as an average across a group of subjects (MNI305 - an average of 305 affinely registered brains, [4]). Existing averaging methods can be considered according to two criteria: (i) the number of degrees of freedom in inter-subject registrations and (ii) the dependence on a particular group member. On one end of the spectrum, methods based on affine registrations only, with up to 12 degrees of freedom, give rise to an unbiased common average space [13]. In this case, the average image is blurry because its constituents are matched in terms of the global size and shape only, while residual morphological differences remain. On the opposite end, methods based on a maximum number of degrees of freedom, with an unique deformation vector per image voxel,

C. Barillot, D.R. Haynor, and P. Hellier (Eds.): MICCAI 2004, LNCS 3216, pp. 615–622, 2004.

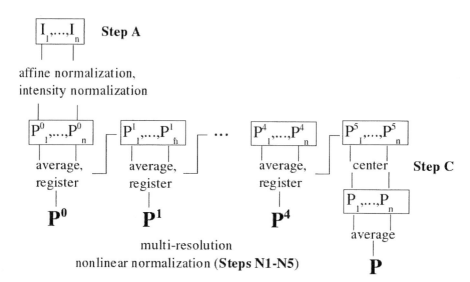

Fig. 1. Atlas creation algorithm

depend on the choice of a single group member as a target for registrations of the remaining images [4]. In this case the average image is crisp as a result of highly resolved morphological matching, but the common space is biased toward the target brain. To this end, an excellent advancement in reducing the impact of such biasing is proposed in [4]. The work of [7] is an interesting compromise between these two extremes, because they derive an optimal common representation using knotpoint based registration ("medium" number of degrees of freedom). A template-free image alignment using the joint image intensity histogram across a group of images was proposed in [8]. This method is best suited for group-wise registration of low-noise, multi-modality images.

In this paper we describe a method for groupwise registration which creates both a high-dimensional and unbiased common representation. The output of the algorithm consists of: (i) the *average image*, as a group average in terms of both image intensities and geometry, and (ii) the *variational component*, as a set of individual deformation fields that encode the morphological differences between the group average and the individual brains. The variational component captures the distribution of anatomical locations across the group. By making an analogy with one-dimensional measurements, we can say that the average image represents an estimate of the sample mean, while magnitudes of the deformation vectors in the variational component can be used to estimate "error bars" (spheres) for anatomical locations. We demonstrate the algorithm on a set of 27 high resolution mouse brain MR images.

2 Atlas Creation Algorithm

The input to the algorithm is a set of n images denoted $I_1, \ldots, I_n$. The algorithm consists of seven steps which are outlined in Fig. 1. In Step A we define a common affine space. Subsequently, individual images are resampled into this common space and intensity normalized. At the end of Step A, only extrinsic and anatomically insignificant differences are removed. The following five steps (N1-N5) assume nonlinear registration models with increasing levels of resolution. Each nonlinear registration step uses the average image of the previous step as the source. The common average nonlinear space evolves iteratively until a fully resolved groupwise alignment is reached. Finally, in Step C, the common space is geometrically centered with respect to the affinely normalized images. The details are given next.

Step A (Affine spatial normalization). We start by performing all pairwise affine registrations among the input images. We use a full affine (12 parameter) model with Levenberg-Marquardt minimization of the ratio image uniformity cost function [12]. The unbiased common affine space is defined by matrix averaging and reconciliation [13]. Each individual image I_k is transformed into this common space and is denoted J_k.

In order to ensure unbiased intensity averaging, we first perform intensity normalization of images $J_1, \ldots, J_n$. We begin by correcting image intensity non-uniformity using the method of [10]. We then apply the method of [6] to estimate the mean gray matter intensity in all images. The images are subsequently normalized to the average mean gray matter intensity using linear intensity rescaling. Images thus produced represent spatially (via an affine transformation model) and intensity normalized versions of the initial raw images and are denoted $P_1^0, \ldots, P_n^0$. The initial average image $\mathbf{P^0}$ is created as their voxel-by-voxel intensity average.

Steps N1-N5 (Nonlinear spatial normalization). The structure of all nonlinear steps is the same: in Step Ni, the output individual images from the previous step, $P_1^{i-1}, \ldots, P_n^{i-1}$, are registered with the most recent average image $\mathbf{P^{i-1}}$ (the intensity average of $P_1^{i-1}, \ldots, P_n^{i-1}$). The nonlinear registration optimizes a similarity function based on a cross-correlation statistic within local neighborhoods which are centered on a regular grid [2]. The nonlinear steps of the algorithm are scheduled in a multi-resolution/multi-scale fashion. The resolution refers to the grid resolution measured by nodal distances. In conjunction with grid resolution, the similarity function is evaluated for extracted image features at appropriate scales (gaussian blur and/or gradient magnitude). Step N1, for example, uses two levels of resolution, first based on 12-voxel grid (nodal distance = 12 voxels in each direction) and second on a 10-voxel grid. The final resolution in Step N5 is maximal, i.e., the grid density equals the image resolution (nodal distance = 1 voxel). The parameters of the multi-resolution schedule have been initially selected similarly as in [2], and then experimentally optimized for maximum registration accuracy and robustness. Full details are given in Table 1.

Step C (Centering). A desirable property of any common space is to be minimally distanced from all group members [5]. If $\mathbf{g}_k$ denotes the cumulative transform of Steps N1-N5 so that $P_k^5 = \mathbf{g}_k(P_k^0)$ then the corresponding inverse transforms $\mathbf{g}_k^{-1}$ are vector fields originating in the same space, that of $\mathbf{P}^5$. The average inverse transform $\mathbf{G}$ is defined as

$$\mathbf{G}(x) = \frac{1}{n} \sum_k \mathbf{g}_k^{-1}(x), \quad x \in \mathbf{P}^5. \tag{1}$$

By composing transforms we define $\mathbf{F}_k = G \circ g_k$ and corresponding images $P_k = \mathbf{F}_k(P_k^0)$, $k = 1, \ldots, n$. Their voxel-by-voxel intensity average image $\mathbf{P}$ is our final average image. By construction, the space of $\mathbf{P}$ is at the centroid position with respect to $P_1^0, \ldots, P_n^0$. The set of inverse transforms $\mathbf{F}_k^{-1}$ represents the variational component; as vector fields, they originate in the $\mathbf{P}$-space and transform into affinely normalized individual images. For any anatomical location $x \in \mathbf{P}$, the distribution of the homologous locations across individual images is given by $\{\mathbf{F}_k^{-1}(x)\}_{k=1,\ldots,n}$.

Table 1. Schedule of nonlinear registrations in Steps N1-N5. The middle column represents grid resolutions in terms of the nodal distance. The right column lists feature extracted images used in each step; the feature scales are measured by the size of the convolving Gaussian kernels, measured in voxels

	Grid resolution	Gaussian fwhm/feature
Step N1.1	12	4/blur
Step N1.2	10	4/gradient magnitude
Step N2.1	8	3/blur
Step N2.2	6	3/gradient magnitude
Step N3.1	4	3/blur
Step N3.2	3	3/gradient magnitude
Step N4.1	3	2/blur
Step N4.2	2	2/gradient magnitude
Step N5.1	2	2/blur
Step N5.2	1	2/gradient magnitude

3 Experimental Validation

We demonstrate the algorithm on the set of $n = 27$ MR images of excised mouse brains with different genetic backgrounds. The animals were selected from three well established mouse strains, 129SV, C57BL6 and CD1, with 9 animals per strain. *In vitro* imaging was performed using a 7.0-T, 40-cm bore magnet with modified electronics for parallel imaging [1]. The parameters used were as follows: T2-weighted, 3D spin-echo sequence, with TR/TE $= 1,600/35$ ms, single average, $FOV = 24 \times 12 \times 12$ mm and matrix size $= 400 \times 200 \times 200$ giving an image with $(60 \ \mu m)^3$ isotropic voxels. The total imaging time was 18.5 hrs. The atlas creation algorithm has been applied to the entire data set.

The progression of the algorithm can be observed in gradual sharpening of the average image updates (Fig. 2). This shows how groupwise consensus has been achieved with an increasing level of detail. In fact, the final average image is so well delineated in all major structures (e.g., corpus callosum, fimbria of the hippocampus, anterior commissure) that it surpasses any of the individual images. This effect is similar to the improvement in signal-to-noise ratio in the case when several images of the same subject are averaged together. In this experiment, however, the input images have significantly different morphologies, which means that a high level of delineation in the average image is due to excellent groupwise registration. Two exceptions to this rule are: small and highly variable internal structures (diameter $< 120 \ \mu m = 2$ voxels, e.g., blood vessels, striatal white matter tracks) and the outer brain surface where unresolved differences remain due to inconsistencies in sample preparation and imaging.

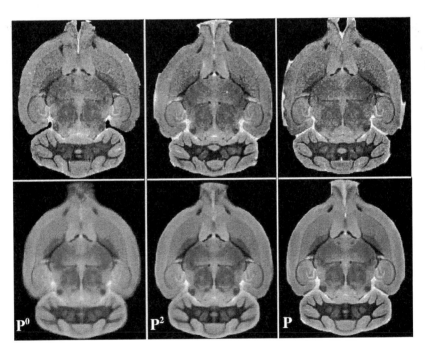

Fig. 2. Examples of individual and average images. Top row: images of 3 different individual mouse brains after global affine normalization. Bottom row: average image updates at different stages of the algorithm.)

The variability of the group in terms of the local morphological differences is captured by the variational component: for each P-voxel, there are $n = 27$ deformation vectors, each consisting of 3 spatial components. In order to summarize and visualize this vast amount of data (~ 5 GB, assuming floating point representation) we estimate the standard deviation of deformation magnitudes ($SDDM$) within the average space:

$$SDDM(x) = \sqrt{\frac{1}{n-1} \sum_k ||x - F_k^{-1}(x)||^2}, \quad x \in P. \tag{2}$$

In other words, $SDDM$ can be treated as an "image" in the same spatial domain as P, such that the voxel intensities represent distances. By displaying the $SDDM$ image in conjunction with the average image, we are able to classify anatomical regions according to the spatial variability (Fig. 3). The highest variability ($SDDM$ values up to $\sim 900 \ \mu m$) is found in the olfactory bulbs and at the posterior end of the brain stem. This is expected because these regions are most affected by the inconsistencies in sample preparation. For the rest of the brain, the average $SDDM$ value is 183 μm. Among interior regions, the most variability is found in the ventricles, corpus callosum, fimbria of the hippocampus and far branches of arbor vita.

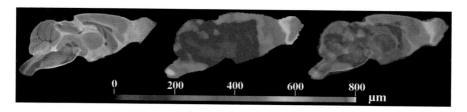

Fig. 3. Morphological variability of the group. Average image (left), $SDDM$ image (middle) and overlay (right)

While the full validation of the methodology is outside the scope of this paper, we present two experiments in this direction. The first one is a cross-validation for the average $SDDM$, based on the *a priori* known genetic background of the samples. For this purpose we created six sub-atlases, each based on 9 images. A sub-atlas is obtained by running the algorithm on the selected image subset only. Each sub-atlas has its own geometrically centered average image and variability component. The first 3 sub-atlases were created to represent a single mouse strain. The other 3 sub-atlases were created by randomly selecting 3 subjects from each of the three strains, totaling to 9 subjects. The variability of the sub-atlases is evaluated using the average $SDDM$ measure. The results are given in Table 2. They confirm the expectation that pure strain atlases have significantly smaller variability than any of the mixed ones. Also, the variability of the mixed sub-atlases is approximately the same as the variability of the full mixed atlas, as it should, since the weights of the three strains within each mixed sub-atlas are the same as in the full atlas. These result indicate that the variabilty estimate is sensitive to group hetreogenity and inter-group differences.

In the second validation experiment we examined atlas bias, rather than registration accuracy. We started with a single brain image, resampled to $(120 \ \mu m)^3$

Table 2. Average $SDDM$ value of the full atlas and 6 sub-atlases (in μm)

Full mixed	129SV	C57BL6	CD1	mixed1	mixed2	mixed3
183	158	145	127	173	180	184

resolution, and 70 regularly spaced landmarks. We used a Gaussian random noise model to displace the landmarks and deform the image in 40 different ways, using thin-plate splines. In addition, we applied random Gaussian noise (8% of the mean brain signal) to image intensities of the 40 deformed images. The resulting images represent a sample with a known mean shape and a known shape variation (with ~ 5 voxels mean displacement over all landmarks and brains). We applied our algorithm to these 40 images in order to measure how accurately it calculates the average shape. For each landmark and each synthetic image we calculated the distance between the known deformation into the space of the sample mean to the calculated deformation into the average space produced by the algorithm. The average distance between the two target positions, across all landmarks and all brains, was found to be 110 μm. This means that the true mean shape and the one recovered by the algorithm are identical, up to a subvoxel distortion on average.

4   Conclusions

We have developed a methodology for creating an unbiased nonlinear average model from a group of images. There is no dependence on a particular member of the group, and at the same time, the groupwise registration is highly resolved, as demonstrated in the Experimental Validation. The novelty of our approach lies in using an evolving intensity average image as the source for nonlinear registrations with the individual images. In this way we avoid problems associated with attempts to fully localize anatomical differences of the group members with respect to a single individual. Instead, we use a multi-resolution strategy to gradually refine the group-wide consensus.

The space of the average image is constructed so that every anatomical location lies at the centroid of the homologous locations across the individual group members. Therefore, the $SDDM$ of deformation magnitudes can be used as a measure of local spatial variability. We have shown that the average $SDDM$ value across the brain can be used as a robust global variability estimate.

The methodology presented here has several implications within the general context of deformation based morphometry. For example, atlases based on normal populations can be used for the detection and characterization of abnormal/pathological deviations. Such questions are particularly interesting in the context of mouse phenotyping, where the power of detection becomes greatly amplified through the use of strictly controlled, genetically uniform populations. Furthermore, there is a clear potential for inter-group comparisons. To this end, population or disease specific atlases can be constructed and compared using registration. The deformation field that warps one atlas onto another can then be parsed for significant deformations, i.e., those that surpass the variational components of the two atlases.

Acknowledgments. This work was supported by the Canada Foundation for Innovation, the Ontario Innovation Trust and the Burroughs Wellcome Fund. The authors would like to thank Nir Lifshitz for technical assistance.

References

1. N.A. Bock, N.B. Konyer and R.M. Henkelman: Multiple-mouse MRI. Magn. Res. Med. **49** (2003) 158-167
2. D.L. Collins and A.C. Evans: Animal: Validation and applications of non-Linear registration-based segmentation. Int. J. Pattern Recogn. **11** (1997) 1271-1294
3. A.C. Evans, W. Dai, D.L. Collins, P. Neelin and S. Marrett: Warping of a computerized 3D atlas to match brain image volumes for quantitative neuroanatomical and functional analysis. SPIE Medical Imaging **1445** (1991) 236-247
4. A. Guimond, J. Meunier and J.P. Thirion: Average brain models: a convergence study. Comput. Vis. Image. Und. **77** (2000) 192-210
5. P. Kochunov, J.L. Lancaster, P. Thompson, R. Woods, J. Mazziotta, J. Hardies and P. Fox: Regional spatial normalization: Towards an optimal target. J. Comput. Assist. Tomogr. **25** (2001) 805-816
6. N. Kovacevic, N.J. Lobaugh, M.J. Bronskill, B. Levine, A. Feinstein and S.E. Black: A robust method for extraction and automatic segmentation of brain images. Neuroimage **17** (2002) 1087-1100
7. S. Marsland, C.J. Twining and C.J. Taylor: Groupwise non-rigid registration using polyharmonic clamped-plate splines. MICCAI (2003) LNCS **2879** 771-779
8. C. Studholme: Simultaneous Population Based Image Alignment for Template Free Spatial Normalisation of Brain Anatomy. WBIR (2003) LNCS **2717** 81-90
9. J.C. Mazziotta, A.W. Toga, A.C. Evans, P. Fox and J. Lankaster: A probabilistic atlas of the human brain: theory and rationale for its development. Neuromiage **2** (1995) 89-101
10. J.G. Sled, A.P. Zijdenbos and A.C. Evans: A nonparametric method for automatic correction of intensity nonuniformity in MRI data. IEEE Trans. Med. Imaging **17** (1998) 87-97
11. P.M. Thompson, A.W. Toga: A Framework For Computational Anatomy. Comput. Visual. Sci. **5** (2002) 13-34
12. R.P. Woods, S.T. Grafton, C.J. Holmes, S.R. Cherry and J.C. Mazziotta: Automated Image Registration: I. General methods and intrasubject, intramodality validation. J. Comput. Assist. Tomogr. **22** (1998) 139-152
13. R.P. Woods, S.T. Grafton, J.D.G. Watson, N.L. Sicotte and J.C. Mazziotta: Automated Image Registration: II. Intersubject validation of linear and nonlinear models. J. Comput. Assist. Tomogr. **22** (1998) 153-165

Spatial-Stiffness Analysis of Surface-Based Registration

Burton Ma and Randy E. Ellis

School of Computing, Queen's University at Kingston, Canada K7L 3N6

Abstract. We have developed a new approach for preoperative selection of points from a surface model for rigid shape-based registration. This approach is based on an extension of our earlier spatial-stiffness model of fiducial registration. We compared our approach with the maximization of the noise-amplification index (NAI), using target registration accuracy (TRE) as our comparison measure, on models derived from computed tomography scans of volunteers. In this study, our approach was substantially less expensive to compute than maximizing the NAI and produced similar TREs with smaller variances. Optimal incremental selection shows promise for improving the preoperative selection of registration points for image-guided surgical procedures.

1 Introduction

A patient's anatomy can be registered to preoperative 3D medical images for use in image-guided surgery by digitizing anatomical registration points on the patient and matching them to surface models derived from the images. We propose a method for choosing model registration points from the preoperative medical image, based on an extension of the method we described in Ma and Ellis [5] for fiducial registration. We view the registration points as the points where an elastic suspension system is attached to a rigid mechanism. By analyzing the stiffness matrix of the mechanism using the techniques developed by Lin et al. [3], we are able to compute a stiffness-quality measure that characterizes the least constrained displacement of the mechanism with respect to a target. The analysis yields the direction of translation or the axis of rotation of the least constrained displacement. The form of the stiffness matrix suggests a way to add a new point to stiffen this displacement thereby improving the quality measure. An unresolved problem is how to relate these preoperative registration points to anatomical registration points derived from the patient.

2 Stiffness of a Passive Mechanical System

The background material, from the robotics literature, is mainly from Lin et al. [3] and is a condensed version of one from our previous work [5]. This material is also related to the compliant axes given by Patterson and Lipkin [9].

A general model of the elastic behavior of a passive unloaded mechanism is a rigid body that is suspended by linear and torsional springs, which leads to analysis of the spatial stiffness or compliance of the mechanism. For a passive mechanism in local equilibrium, a twist displacement $\mathbf{t}$ of a rigid body is related to a counteracting wrench force $\mathbf{w}$ by a 6×6 spatial stiffness matrix $\mathbf{K}$:

$$\mathbf{w} = \mathbf{Kt} = \begin{bmatrix} \mathbf{A} & \mathbf{B} \\ \mathbf{B}^T & \mathbf{D} \end{bmatrix} \mathbf{t} \tag{1}$$

C. Barillot, D.R. Haynor, and P. Hellier (Eds.): MICCAI 2004, LNCS 3216, pp. 623–630, 2004.

where $\mathbf{A}, \mathbf{B}$, and $\mathbf{D}$ are 3×3 matrices. The twist is a vector $\mathbf{t} = [v^T \ \omega^T]^T$ where $v^T = [v_x \ v_y \ v_z]$ is linear displacement and $\omega^T = [\omega_x \ \omega_y \ \omega_z]$ is rotational displacement. The wrench is a vector $\mathbf{w} = [\mathbf{f}^T \ \tau^T]^T$ where $\mathbf{f}^T = [f_x \ f_y \ f_z]$ is force and $\tau^T = [\tau_x \ \tau_y \ \tau_z]$ is torque. Equation 1 is simply a general, vectorial expression of Hooke's Law. We can obtain $\mathbf{K}$ by evaluating the Hessian of the potential energy U of the system at equilibrium (Mishra and Silver [6]).

$\mathbf{K}$ is a symmetric positive-definite matrix for stable springs and small displacements from equilibrium. The eigenvalues of $\mathbf{K}$ are not immediately useful because their magnitudes change with the coordinate frame used to define $\mathbf{K}$; however, it can be shown that the eigenvalues of

$$\mathbf{K}_V = \mathbf{D} - \mathbf{B}^T \mathbf{A}^{-1} \mathbf{B} \tag{2}$$
$$\mathbf{C}_W = \mathbf{A}^{-1} \tag{3}$$

are frame invariant. The eigenvalues μ_1, μ_2, μ_3 of $\mathbf{K}_V$ are the principal rotational stiffnesses, and the eigenvalues $\sigma_1, \sigma_2, \sigma_3$ of $\mathbf{C}_W^{-1}$ are the principal translational stiffnesses.

The screw representation of a twist is a rotation about an axis followed by a translation parallel to the axis. The screw is usually described by the rotation axis, the net rotation magnitude M, with the independent translation specified as a pitch, h, that is the ratio of translational motion to rotational motion. For a twist (Murray et al. [7]) $h = \omega \cdot v / \|\omega\|^2$, $M = \|\omega\|$, and the axis of the screw is parallel to ω passing through the point $\mathbf{q} = \omega \times v / \|\omega\|^2$. A pure translation (where $\omega = 0$) has $h = \infty$ and $M = \|v\|$, with the screw axis parallel to v passing through the origin. A unit twist has magnitude $M = 1$, in which case, for $\omega \neq 0$, $h = \omega \cdot v$ and $\mathbf{q} = \omega \times v$. For a small screw motion with $M = \alpha$ and $\omega \neq 0$, a point located at a distance ρ from the screw axis will be displaced by length

$$l \approx |\alpha| \sqrt{\rho^2 + (\omega \cdot v)^2} \tag{4}$$

Equation 4 is the basis of the frame-invariant quality measure for compliant grasps described by Lin et al. [3]. Because the principal rotational and translational stiffnesses have different units, they cannot be directly compared to one another. One solution is to scale the principal rotational stiffnesses by an appropriate factor (see Lin et al. [3] for details) to yield the so-called equivalent stiffnesses, $\mu_{\text{eq},i}$:

$$\mu_{\text{eq},i} = \mu_i / (\rho_i^2 + (\omega_i \cdot v_i)^2) \qquad i = 1, 2, 3 \tag{5}$$

where, μ_i is an eigenvalue of $\mathbf{K}_V$ with an associated eigenvector ω_i, and ρ_i is the distance between the point of interest and the screw axis of the twist $[v_i^T \ \omega_i^T]^T$. The equivalent stiffnesses can be compared to the principal translational stiffnesses which leads to the stiffness quality measure $Q = \min(\mu_{\text{eq},1}, \mu_{\text{eq},2}, \mu_{\text{eq},3}, \sigma_1, \sigma_2, \sigma_3)$. Q characterizes the least constrained displacement of the mechanism. Therefore, maximizing the smallest rotational and translational stiffnesses will minimize the worst-case displacement of the mechanism.

3   Spatial Stiffness and Surface Registration

Our spatial-stiffness model of surface-based registration is parameterized by N surface points with locations $\{\mathbf{p}_i\}$ and unit normal vectors $\{\mathbf{n}_i\}$ for $i = 1, \ldots N$. Suppose

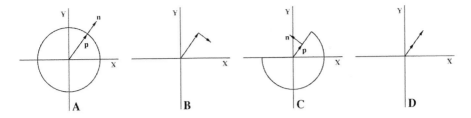

Fig. 1. Two examples of the dot product $\mathbf{d}_{xy}$. (A) A point $\mathbf{p}$ on a circle in the xy plane and its associated surface normal $\mathbf{n}$. (B) The projection of $\mathbf{p}$ onto the xy plane; $\mathbf{n}$ is also projected but then rotated $90°$ in the plane. The dot product of the two vectors shown is $\mathbf{d}_{xy} = 0$; $\mathbf{p}$ provides no rotational constraint about the z axis. (C)A point $\mathbf{p}$ on an edge in the xy plane and its associated surface normal $\mathbf{n}$. (D) The projection of $\mathbf{p}$ onto the xy plane; $\mathbf{n}$ is also projected but then rotated $90°$ in the plane. The dot product of the two vectors shown is $\mathbf{d}_{xy} = \|\mathbf{p}\|$; $\mathbf{p}$ provides good constraint about the z axis.

each point is displaced by a small translation $\boldsymbol{\delta} = [t_x\ t_y\ t_z]^T$ and a small rotation $\mathbf{R} = \mathbf{R_z}(\omega_z)\mathbf{R_y}(\omega_y)\mathbf{R_x}(\omega_x)$. The locations $\mathbf{q}_i$ of the displaced points are given by $\mathbf{q}_i = \mathbf{R}\mathbf{p}_i + \boldsymbol{\delta}$. Because the displacement is small, we can take the region around each $\mathbf{p}_i$ to be locally planar. The squared distance to the point on the surface nearest to $\mathbf{q}_i$ is given by $((\mathbf{q}_i - \mathbf{p}_i) \cdot \mathbf{n}_i)^2$. Assuming a spring constant of unity, the potential energy U_i stored in each linear spring is $U_i = \frac{1}{2}((\mathbf{q}_i - \mathbf{p}_i) \cdot \mathbf{n}_i)^2$. It can be shown that the upper triangular part of the symmetric Hessian matrix $\mathbf{H}_i$ of U_i evaluated at equilibrium is:

$$\mathbf{H}_i = \mathbf{H}(U_i; \boldsymbol{v} = \boldsymbol{\omega} = \mathbf{0})$$

$$= \begin{bmatrix} n_{x_i}^2 & n_{x_i}n_{y_i} & n_{x_i}n_{z_i} & n_{x_i}\mathbf{d}_{yz_i} & -n_{x_i}\mathbf{d}_{xz_i} & n_{x_i}\mathbf{d}_{xy_i} \\ & n_{y_i}^2 & n_{y_i}n_{z_i} & n_{y_i}\mathbf{d}_{yz_i} & -n_{y_i}\mathbf{d}_{xz_i} & n_{y_i}\mathbf{d}_{xy_i} \\ & & n_{z_i}^2 & n_{z_i}\mathbf{d}_{yz_i} & -n_{z_i}\mathbf{d}_{xz_i} & n_{z_i}\mathbf{d}_{xy_i} \\ & & & \mathbf{d}_{yz_i}^2 & -\mathbf{d}_{xz_i}\mathbf{d}_{yz_i} & \mathbf{d}_{xy_i}\mathbf{d}_{yz_i} \\ & & & & \mathbf{d}_{xz_i}^2 & -\mathbf{d}_{xy_i}\mathbf{d}_{xz_i} \\ & & & & & \mathbf{d}_{xy_i}^2 \end{bmatrix} \quad (6)$$

where $\mathbf{p}_i = [x_i\ y_i\ z_i\ ]^T$, $\mathbf{n}_i = [n_{x_i}\ n_{y_i}\ n_{z_i}\ ]^T$, $\mathbf{d}_{xy_i} = [x_i\ y_i] \cdot [n_{y_i}\ -n_{x_i}]$, $\mathbf{d}_{xz_i} = [x_i\ z_i] \cdot [n_{z_i}\ -n_{x_i}]$, and $\mathbf{d}_{yz_i} = [y_i\ z_i] \cdot [n_{z_i}\ -n_{y_i}]$.

The dot products, $\mathbf{d}_{xy_i}$, $\mathbf{d}_{xz_i}$, $\mathbf{d}_{yz_i}$, have important geometric interpretations. For example, $\mathbf{d}_{xy_i}$ can be computed by projecting the vectors $\mathbf{p}_i$ and $\mathbf{n}_i$ onto the xy-plane; $\mathbf{d}_{xy_i}$ is the dot product of the projected $\mathbf{p}_i$ and a vector in the xy-plane that is perpendicular to the projected $\mathbf{n}_i$. An example of the dot products is illustrated in Figure 1. The dot products can also be interpreted as the $x, y,$ and, z components of the cross product $\mathbf{p}_i \times \mathbf{n}_i$.

The spatial-stiffness matrix for surface registration is:

$$\mathbf{K} = \sum_{i=1}^{N} \mathbf{H}_i = \sum_{i=1}^{N} \begin{bmatrix} \mathbf{A}_i & \mathbf{B}_i \\ \mathbf{B}_i^T & \mathbf{D}_i \end{bmatrix} = \begin{bmatrix} \mathbf{A} & \mathbf{B} \\ \mathbf{B}^T & \mathbf{D} \end{bmatrix} \quad \text{where } \mathbf{A}_i = \begin{bmatrix} n_{x_i}^2 & n_{x_i}n_{y_i} & n_{x_i}n_{z_i} \\ n_{x_i}n_{y_i} & n_{y_i}^2 & n_{y_i}n_{z_i} \\ n_{x_i}n_{z_i} & n_{y_i}n_{z_i} & n_{z_i}^2 \end{bmatrix}$$

$$\mathbf{B}_i = \begin{bmatrix} n_{x_i} \mathbf{d}_{yz_i} & -n_{x_i} \mathbf{d}_{xz_i} & n_{x_i} \mathbf{d}_{xy_i} \\ n_{y_i} \mathbf{d}_{yz_i} & -n_{y_i} \mathbf{d}_{xz_i} & n_{y_i} \mathbf{d}_{xy_i} \\ n_{z_i} \mathbf{d}_{yz_i} & -n_{z_i} \mathbf{d}_{xz_i} & n_{z_i} \mathbf{d}_{xy_i} \end{bmatrix} \quad \mathbf{D}_i = \begin{bmatrix} \mathbf{d}_{yz_i}^2 & -\mathbf{d}_{xz_i} \mathbf{d}_{yz_i} & \mathbf{d}_{xy_i} \mathbf{d}_{yz_i} \\ -\mathbf{d}_{xz_i} \mathbf{d}_{yz_i} & \mathbf{d}_{xz_i}^2 & -\mathbf{d}_{xy_i} \mathbf{d}_{xz_i} \\ \mathbf{d}_{xy_i} \mathbf{d}_{yz_i} & -\mathbf{d}_{xy_i} \mathbf{d}_{xz_i} & \mathbf{d}_{xy_i}^2 \end{bmatrix} \quad (7)$$

In [5] we showed that aligning the centroid of the fiducial markers with the origin results in $\mathbf{B} = \mathbf{B}^T = [\mathbf{0}]$ which means that the rotational stiffnesses are decoupled from the translational stiffnesses. Although in general this cannot be done for surface registration or for stiffness matrices, Lončarić [4] showed that one can almost always choose a coordinate frame that maximally decouples rotational and translational aspects of stiffness, and that $\mathbf{B}$ is diagonal in this frame.

In [5] we also showed that a single fiducial marker provided equal translational stiffness in all directions. Inspection of $\mathbf{A}_i$ in Equation 7 shows that a single surface point only contributes to the translational stiffness in the $\pm \mathbf{n}_i$ direction. Thus, at least three surface points with linearly independent normal vectors are required to ensure that the principal translational stiffnesses (the eigenvalues of $\mathbf{A}$) are positive; the translation component of the registration transformation is well-constrained only if all of the translational stiffnesses are positive. Also note that the translational stiffnesses are independent of the locations of the surface points; only the orientations of the surface at the points are relevant. Given this observation it is easy to see how to stiffen a displacement with direction $\mathbf{d}$: simply choose a point where the surface has normal direction most closely aligned to $\pm \mathbf{d}$. Alternatively, apply a coordinate frame rotation so that $\mathbf{d}$ is parallel to the z axis and find the point with normal vector that has the largest value of n_z^2.

The analysis of the rotational stiffnesses is complicated by their being coupled to the translational stiffnesses. Let us focus on the matrix $\mathbf{D}$ which relates torque to rotational displacement. There exists a coordinate frame rotation that diagonalizes $\mathbf{D}$ because it is a symmetric matrix. The eigenvalues of this diagonal matrix are equal to the diagonal elements which are the squared dot products $\mathbf{d}_{xy}^2$, $\mathbf{d}_{xz}^2$, and $\mathbf{d}_{yz}^2$. Suppose we want to stiffen the rotation about the z axis; this can be done by choosing a new point $\mathbf{p}_i$ with normal vector $\mathbf{n}_i$ so that $\mathbf{d}_{xy_i}^2$ is maximized. This leads to a heuristic for stiffening the rotation about the least-constrained rotational axis: apply a coordinate frame transformation so that the axis passes through the origin and is aligned with the z axis, then find the point with normal vector that maximizes $\mathbf{d}_{xy_i}^2$. This heuristic is not optimal because it ignores the coupling with the translational stiffnesses, but it may work in practice.

Simon [12] derived an expression for what he called a scatter matrix, Ψ; this 6×6 matrix characterizes the sum of squared distance errors between a surface and a set of points from the surface displaced by a small rigid transformation. The expression for the scatter matrix is:

$$\Psi = \sum_{i=1}^{N} \begin{bmatrix} \mathbf{n}_i \\ \mathbf{p}_i \times \mathbf{n}_i \end{bmatrix} \begin{bmatrix} \mathbf{n}_i & \mathbf{p}_i \times \mathbf{n}_i \end{bmatrix} \quad (8)$$

Expanding Equation 8 and simplifying terms yields exactly the same expression as the stiffness matrix in Equation 7. An alternative and simpler derivation in the context of mechanism stiffness is already known (Huang and Schimmels [2]).

4   Strategies for Registration Point Selection

Simon [12] addressed the problem of choosing N points for registration by maximizing the noise amplification index (NAI)

$$\text{NAI} = \frac{\lambda_{min}^2}{\lambda_{max}} \tag{9}$$

where λ_{min} and λ_{max} are the smallest and largest eigenvalues of $\mathbf{K}$. The NAI was described by Nahvi and Hollerbach [8], and Simon [12] found that are there were four important problems that must be addressed when using the NAI as a criterion for point selection.

The first problem is that the units of rotational and translational displacement are different. This means that the eigenvalues cannot be used unless they are scaled to compensate for the differing units. Simon [12] addressed this problem by translating the surface model so that its centroid was coincident with the origin, and isotropically scaling the model so that the average distance between the origin and the surface points was one. This solution is correct only for those scaled points that actually have unit distance from the origin. For long thin bones, this results in the NAI being less sensitive to rotations about the long axis of the bone.

The second problem is that $\mathbf{K}$ and its eigenvalues are dependent on the coordinate frame; Simon [12] argued that the origin should be chosen to minimize λ_{min}, although he also noted that this did not result in large differences from simply centering the bone at the origin. The third problem is that the eigenvalues of $\mathbf{K}$, and thus the NAI, are sensitive to variations in the normal directions of the surface points; Simon [12] was forced to eliminate regions of high curvature from consideration for registration point selection. The fourth problem is that maximizing the NAI is a problem with combinatorial complexity; Simon [12] used hillclimbing and evolutionary techniques to solve this optimization problem. These algorithms are too time consuming to use online, and are not guaranteed to find the global maximum of the NAI.

Rusinkiewicz and Levoy [10] suggested choosing points so that the normal vector direction was uniformly sampled. This heuristic is generally inapplicable for typical surgical exposures. Recently, Gelfand et al. [1] suggested a technique called covariance sampling that uses an eigenanalysis of $\mathbf{K}$ that is not frame invariant. Their stability measure is the condition number $\lambda_{max}/\lambda_{min}$.

Our approach to point sampling is to build a point set with a greedy algorithm that iteratively stiffens the least-constrained component found by the stiffness analysis of $\mathbf{K}$. Our algorithm can be described as follows:

- Manually choose an initial set of 6 registration points. We have found that the 3:2:1 fixturing concept (Shirinzadeh [11]) is a useful rule for choosing these 6 points.
- For $i = 7, 8, ...N$
  - Compute the stiffness matrix $\mathbf{K}$.
  - Compute the quality measure Q.
  - If Q corresponds to a translational stiffness
    * Rotate the surface model so that least-constrained translational axis is parallel to the z axis.

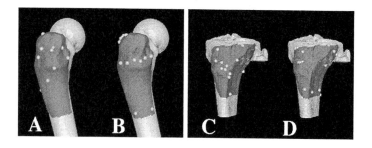

Fig. 2. Models, regions, and example point sets of size 15 used in our experiments. The proximal femur with (A) points chosen using the NAI and (B) our algorithm. The proximal tibia with (C) points chosen using the NAI and (D) our algorithm.

* Choose $\mathbf{p}_i$ with $\mathbf{n}_i$ from the rotated model such that n_z^2 is maximized.
* Undo the rotation applied to $\mathbf{p}_i$ and $\mathbf{n}_i$.
- If Q corresponds to a rotational stiffness
  * Translate and rotate the surface model so that least-constrained rotational axis passes through the origin and is parallel to the z axis.
  * Choose $\mathbf{p}_i$ with $\mathbf{n}_i$ from the translated and rotated model such that $\mathbf{d}_{xy_i}^2 = ([x_i \; y_i] \cdot [n_{y_i} \; -n_{x_i}])^2$ is maximized.
  * Undo the transformation applied to $\mathbf{p}_i$ and $\mathbf{n}_i$.

5   Experiments

We conducted experiments using our algorithm and by maximizing the NAI for point selection. We implemented the hillclimbing method described by Simon [12] for maximizing the NAI; we used the point set with the highest NAI after 10 restarts of the hillclimbing algorithm and allowed the algorithm to converge before each restart.

We used both methods to generate point sets of size $N = 6, 9, ..., 30$. The running time of our algorithm is between two and three orders of magnitude smaller than the next ascent hillclimbing algorithm when run in Matlab on a SunBlade2000 workstation; all of the point sets for our experiments could be generated in approximately forty seconds when using the stiffness-based algorithm.

We used surface models of the proximal femur and the proximal tibia derived from CT scans of volunteers. For the femur, we chose points from the region surrounding the greater trochanter; this region was similar to the one we have used for several clinical cases of computer-assisted bone-tumor excisions. We used the location of a tumor from one of our clinical cases as the target; this point was located inside the neck of the femur. For the tibia, we chose points on the anterior and lateral surfaces consistent with the surgical exposure of a closing-wedge high tibial osteotomy. We used a point on the proximal medial side of the tibia as a target; this is a point on the hinge of osteotomy. The models, regions, and examples of point sets are shown in Figure 2.

To each point set we added noise drawn from the normal distribution with mean zero and standard deviation 0.5mm, and then applied a rotation of $1°$ about a random axis and

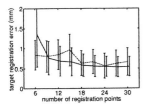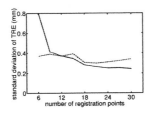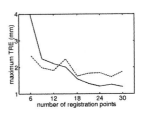

Fig. 3. Results for the proximal femur. Dashed lines are results using the NAI and solid lines are results for our algorithm. (Left) Mean TRE versus number of points; error bars are at ± 1 standard deviation. (Middle) Standard deviation versus number of points. (Right) Maximum TRE versus number of points.

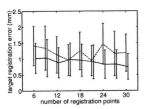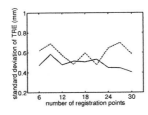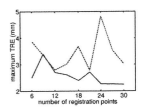

Fig. 4. Results for the proximal tibia. Dashed lines are results using the NAI and solid lines are results for our algorithm. (Left) Mean TRE versus number of points; error bars are at ± 1 standard deviation. (Middle) Standard deviation versus number of points. (Right) Maximum TRE versus number of points.

a translation of magnitude 0.5mm along a random direction; the point set was registered to the model using ICP and the TRE was computed. This process was repeated 500 times for each point set. The displacements we used were small because both our analysis and the NAI are based on the assumption of small displacements. The results are shown in Figures 3 and 4.

6 Discussion

Our heuristic algorithm, based on the stiffness quality measure, appears to perform as well as maximizing the NAI in terms of the mean TRE, and slightly better in terms of the maximum and variance of the TRE, for small displacements from the true registration; more tests, on a wider variety of surfaces, must be conducted before one can be confident in this conclusion. The behaviour of the TRE as a function of the number of registration points is much smoother for our algorithm than for the NAI-based algorithm, in part because the point set with N points is a superset of the one for $N - 1$ points when using our algorithm whereas the NAI-based algorithm always computes an entirely new point set. The most important advantage that our algorithm has over the NAI-based algorithm is that our algorithm is fast enough for online construction of point sets.

A limitation of our study is that the next-ascent hillclimbing algorithm is not guaranteed to converge to the global maximum of the NAI: the optimization of the NAI is a serious challenge for any algorithm that attempts to use it as a point selection criterion. Also, we have not shown that our point-selection scheme improves registration accuracy in practice, because our analysis of the matrix $\mathbf{K}$ is limited to small displacements around the true registration. Simon [12] has provided empirical evidence that increasing the NAI by careful point selection tends to decrease the worst-case correspondence error. Perhaps the major limitation of our study is that we examine *model* registration points, whereas in practice a surgeon selects *anatomical* registration points; the critical, and unresolved, difference between the two is that the correspondence between model registration points and the model is known perfectly, while the correspondence between anatomical registration points and the model must be inferred. We postulate that resolving this difference will result in an algorithm for optimally analyzing the quality of a registration intraoperatively, and incidentally can suggest to a surgeon anatomical regions that might incrementally improve a registration for image-guided surgery.

Acknowledgments. This research was supported in part by the Institute for Robotics and Intelligent Systems, the Ontario Research and Development Challenge Fund, and the Natural Sciences and Engineering Research Council of Canada.

References

[1] N. Gelfand, L. Ikemoto, S. Rusinkiewicz, and M. Levoy. Geometrically stable sampling for the icp algorithm. In *Proc 3DIM 2003*, 2003.

[2] S. Huang and J. Schimmels. The bounds and realization of spatial stiffnesses achieved with simple springs connected in parallel. *IEEE Trans Robot Automat*, 14(3):466–475, 1998.

[3] Q. Lin, J. Burdick, and E. Rimon. A stiffness-based quality measure for compliant grasps and fixtures. *IEEE Trans Robot Automat*, 16(6):675–688, Dec 2000.

[4] J. Lončarić. Normal forms of stiffness and compliance matrices. *IEEE J Robot Automat*, RA-3(6):567–572, Dec 1987.

[5] B. Ma and R. E. Ellis. A spatial-stiffness analysis of fiducial registration accuracy. In R. E. Ellis and T. M. Peters, editors, *MICCAI2003*, volume 1 of LNCS 2879, pages 359–366. Springer, November 2003.

[6] B. Mishra and N. Silver. Some discussion of static gripping and its stability. *IEEE Trans Sys Man Cyber*, 19(4):783–796, Jul/Aug 1989.

[7] R. M. Murray, Z. Li, and S. S. Sastry. A Mathematical Introduction to Robotic Manipulation. *CRC Press*, 1994.

[8] A. Nahvi and J. M. Hollerbach. The noise amplification index for optimal pose selection in robot calibration. In *Proc Int Conf Robot and Automat*, 1996.

[9] T. Patterson and H. Lipkin. Structure of robot compliance. *ASME J Mech Des*, 115(3): 576–580, Sep 1993.

[10] S. Rusinkiewicz and M. Levoy. Efficient variants of the ICP algorithm. In *Proc 3DIM 2001*, pages 145–152, 2001.

[11] B. Shirinzadeh. Issues in the design of the reconfigurable fixture modules for robotic assembly. J Man Sys, 12(1):1–14, 1993.

[12] D. A. Simon. *Fast and Accurate Shape-Based Registration*. PhD thesis, Carnegie Mellon University, Pittsburgh, Pennsylvania, Dec 1996.

Progressive Attenuation Fields: Fast 2D-3D Image Registration Without Precomputation

Torsten Rohlfing[1], Daniel B. Russakoff[1,2], Joachim Denzler[3], and
Calvin R. Maurer, Jr.[1]

[1] Image Guidance Laboratories, Stanford University, Stanford CA, USA,
rohlfing@stanford.edu, calvin.maurer@igl.stanford.edu
[2] Computer Science Department, Stanford University, Stanford CA, USA
dbrussak@stanford.edu
[3] Fakultät für Mathematik und Informatik, Universität Passau, Passau, Germany
denzler@fmi.uni-passau.de

Abstract. This paper introduces the progressive attenuation field (PAF), a method
to speed up computation of digitally reconstructed radiograph (DRR) images during intensity-based 2D-3D registration. Unlike traditional attenuation fields, a PAF
is built on the fly as the registration proceeds. It does not require any precomputation time, nor does it make any prior assumptions of the patient pose that would
limit the permissible range of patient motion. We use a cylindrical attenuation field
parameterization, which is better suited for medical 2D-3D registration than the
usual two-plane parameterization. The computed attenuation values are stored in
a hash table for time-efficient storage and access. Using a clinical gold-standard
spine image dataset, we demonstrate a speedup of 2D-3D image registration by a
factor of four over ray-casting DRR with no decrease of registration accuracy or
robustness.

1 Introduction

The rate-limiting step in intensity-based 2D-3D image registration is the computation
of digitally reconstructed radiograph (DRR) images, which are synthetic x-ray images
generated from CT images. A common method to speed up the process is to precompute
projection values, which can then be looked up from a table during the registration phase.
For storing the projection values, LaRose [1] used a data structure called "Transgraph"
based on the "Lumigraph" introduced by Gortler *et al.* [2] for rendering. Similarly,
Russakoff *et al.* [3,4] used an "attenuation field" (AF), which is based on the principle of
"light field" rendering introduced by Levoy & Hanrahan [5] simultaneously with Gortler
et al. [2].

Two major issues arise in the use of precomputation methods: they require time for
precomputation, and, for memory efficiency, assumptions have to be made regarding
expected viewing angles. Substantially more projections are precomputed than are actually used. It is our experience that only about 10 percent of all rays in an AF are typically
used, and the rays which are used are, on average, accessed about 1,000 times (unpub-
lished results). In the present paper we introduce the concept of a progressive AF (PAF),
which is not precomputed but instead constructed on the fly as the registration proceeds.

C. Barillot, D.R. Haynor, and P. Hellier (Eds.): MICCAI 2004, LNCS 3216, pp. 631–638, 2004.
© Springer-Verlag Berlin Heidelberg 2004

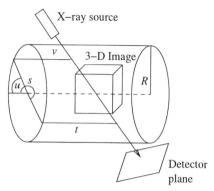

Fig. 1. Cylindrical attenuation field parameterization. Any valid ray through the image volume is parameterized by four parameters. Parameters u and s are rotation angles around the axis of the coordinate system (*dashed line*). Parameters v and t are distances along the axis with respect to an arbitrary reference level.

A PAF effectively acts as a cache for projection values once they are computed, rather than as a lookup table for precomputed projections like standard AFs.

Our novel method eliminates the drawbacks of traditional precomputation methods mentioned above. These benefits come at the cost of higher computational cost during the actual registration compared to precomputed attenuation fields. However, we demonstrate in this paper that there is still a substantial performance increase over unaccelerated computation of DRRs. Also, the speedup provided by our method increases in subsequent serial registrations, which is important for patient tracking applications.

2   Methods

In an AF, each ray through the 3D image is parameterized by a tuple of four real numbers, (u, v, s, t). In traditional light fields in computer graphics, these numbers are most commonly defined as coordinates in two parallel planes where the ray intersects the respective plane [5]. The PAF, like a light field, samples the space of parameter 4-tuples at discrete intervals. Let δ_u, δ_v, δ_s, and δ_t be the step sizes of the discretization of parameters u through t. Then a ray with continuous parameters (u, v, s, t) is stored in the PAF at the discrete index

$$(U, V, S, T) = (\lfloor u/\delta_u \rfloor, \lfloor v/\delta_v \rfloor, \lfloor s/\delta_s \rfloor, \lfloor t/\delta_t \rfloor). \tag{1}$$

Projection values are only computed and stored for rays with parameters that are multiples of the discretization factors and that coincide with grid points in the discretized parameter space. Projection values for all rays in between are obtained by quadrilinear interpolation.

2.1   Cylindrical Parameterization of Attenuation Field

For 2D-3D registration, we define the AF parameterization using a cylinder of radius R around the image volume, the cylinder axis aligned with the body axis. Each ray of the projection geometry is parameterized by four coordinates, which correspond to the two intersection points where the ray enters and exits this cylinder (Fig. 1). Two parameters, u and s, are rotation angles around the cylinder axis, the other two, v and t, are distances along the cylinder axis. Let L be a ray from $\mathbf{a}$ to $\mathbf{b}$, parameterized as $L(c) = \mathbf{a} + \lambda\mathbf{d}$ with $\mathbf{a} = (a_x, a_y, a_z)$, $\mathbf{b} = (b_x, b_y, b_z)$, and $\mathbf{d} = \mathbf{b} - \mathbf{a}$. The AF parameters of R are computed as follows. First the parameters λ_{uv} and λ_{st} of the intersecting points of R with the coordinate cylinder are computed by solving the system

$$R^2 = (a_x + \lambda d_x)^2 + (a_y + \lambda d_y)^2 \qquad (2)$$

for λ. The resulting two solutions λ_{uv} and λ_{st} describe the two intersecting points as

$$\mathbf{p}_{uv} = \mathbf{a} + \lambda_{uv}\mathbf{d},$$
$$\mathbf{p}_{st} = \mathbf{a} + \lambda_{st}\mathbf{d}.$$

From these, the actual AF parameters of the ray can be computed by inverting the following expressions for computing points on the cylinder from a parameter 4-tuple:

$$\mathbf{p}_{uv} = (R\cos u, R\sin u, v),$$
$$\mathbf{p}_{st} = (R\cos s, R\sin s, t).$$

The coordinate system is fixed with respect to the 3D image. The cylinder axis is parallel to the z coordinate and runs through the image center. Note that since the cylinder is infinite, the reference level along the axis can be defined arbitrarily, and therefore the absolute values of v and t are irrelevant. The radius R is chosen as the difference between the center of the 3D image and its projection onto the initial location of the x-ray projection plane. Note that we assume here a stationary 3D image and moving 2D projection devices. In reality, one typically encounters the opposite situation, that is, a moving 3D image that is tracking the patient movement in space, while the x-ray projections are stationary (or at least in a known position). For rigid motion, both situations are easily translated into each other by applying the inverse 3D image transformation to the projection geometry, and vice versa.

Compared to the common two-plane parameterization, the cylindrical coordinate space is capable of describing full 360 degree rotations around the cylinder axis. A spherical parameterization would also be possible and provide full rotational freedom. However, two faces of a medical image volume are virtually always truncation surfaces. Rays entering or exiting through these surfaces are not physically possible and therefore irrelevant to the computation (see Fig. 2). The cylindrical parameterization is naturally suited for rotating imaging systems such as gantry-based systems and C-arm fluoroscopes.

2.2 Storage Data Structure

An efficient data structure is the key to a successful implementation of a PAF. Unlike the case of a precomputed AF, it is important that not only lookup but also storage operations are time-efficient. Memory efficiency is also important, in particular since we cannot

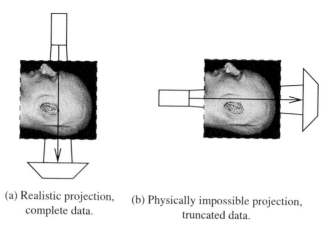

(a) Realistic projection,   (b) Physically impossible projection,
complete data.   truncated data.

Fig. 2. Illustration of physical limitations to projection geometry and data truncation.

use data compression, which prevents a preallocated 4D array. A hash table allows both lookup and insertion operations in constant time and can grow incrementally as necessary. To store the ray attenuation for a given ray, we use the binary-OR composition of the respective lowest 8 bits of the integer values of U, V, S, and T as the hash function. In order to minimize collisions, the binary representation of V is shifted by 8 bits, that of S by 16 bits, and that of T by 24 bits.

For applications with two or more projection geometries, one can either use a single combined PAF for all of them, or one PAF per projection. Both options have their merits, depending on the actual setup. As an example, when two projections are (nearly) orthogonal, it is virtually impossible that the AFs for both will ever intersect. One should therefore use two separate AFs, one for each projection, and thereby reduce the likelihood of hash collisions. On the other hand, when the projection geometries are arranged closer to each other, or when excessive patient motion is possible, it may be advantageous to use only a single AF to share computed attenuation values among all available projections.

2.3 Multi-resolution Progressive Attenuation Fields

Generating a DRR from a PAF takes more time as the sampling of the AF parameters becomes finer. At the same time, the coarser these parameters, the more blurred are the resulting DRR images. It is conceivable to exploit this in an additional layer of multi-resolution computation by starting the registration process with a relatively coarse AF sampling and successively refining it. On the other hand, however, it is desirable to continue using the information stored in the coarse AF when switching to a finer one. Finally, converting the AF to finer coordinate samplings takes time and should be avoided.

Let (U,V,S,T) be the discrete hash table indices for the continuous parameter tuple (u,v,s,t), discretized with samplings δ_u, δ_v, δ_s, and δ_t as before. Also, let $c \in \mathbb{N}^+$ be any positive integer. Then

$$(U', V', S', T') = (c \lfloor u/c\delta_u \rfloor, c \lfloor v/c\delta_v \rfloor, c \lfloor s/c\delta_s \rfloor, c \lfloor t/c\delta_t \rfloor) \qquad (5)$$

is a super-discretization of the previous AF with upsampling factor c. This means that we can initially start building a PAF with an upsampling factor $c > 1$ and later refine the discretization to $c = 1$ without having to convert any entries in the hash table. Note also that c can be different for each of the four parameters.

3   Evaluation Study

3.1   Methods

We evaluate the usefulness of the PAF algorithm by using it to compute DRRs in the intensity-based 2D-3D registration of spine images. We compare the execution speed and the registration accuracy and robustness to that obtained by computing DRRs with traditional ray casting. The registration algorithm has been described previously [3]. In summary, the algorithm searches for the six parameters of the rigid transformation that produces the DRR that is most similar to the real x-ray projection image. We crop the projection images to a region of interest that includes the vertebra of interest plus the two adjacent vertebrae. We optimize the mutual information (MI) image similarity measure, which we have previously found to be both accurate and robust [6]. There are two x-ray projection images and two corresponding DRRs; the similarity measure is the sum of the MI for each of the real-synthetic image pairs. The transformation parameters are optimized using a simple best neighbor search strategy [8]. The registration process is performed in two passes, the first with smoothed versions of the projection images, and the second with the original images.

We use spine image data from two patients who underwent treatment of spinal cord lesions with the CyberKnife Stereotactic Radiosurgery System (Accuray, Sunnyvale, CA). These patients had four to five metal fiducial markers implanted percutaneously before pre-treatment CT scanning in the posterior bony elements of the vertebral levels adjacent to the lesions. For each patient, we obtained: 1) a pre-treatment CT image, 2) a pair of orthogonal projection x-ray images obtained with flat-panel silicon x-ray cameras (Flashscan 20, dpiX, Palo Alto, CA), 3) the camera calibration model and parameters for the two x-ray cameras, 4) positions (3D) of four metal fiducial markers in the CT image, and 5) positions (2D) of the four markers in the projection x-ray images. Additional details can be found in [3,6].

The metal fiducial markers were used to compute a gold-standard transformation. The target registration error (TRE) of an intensity-based registration transformation being evaluated is computed as the difference between the positions of a target mapped by the evaluated transformations and the gold-standard transformation. The TRE values are computed for each voxel inside a rectangular box bounding the vertebra and then averaged. Initial transformations were generated by perturbing the gold-standard reference transformation by adding randomly generated rotations and translations. The initial transformations were characterized by computing the TRE for the transformation and grouped into eight 2 mm intervals: 0–2, 2–4, ..., 14–16 mm. We run the registration algorithm twice for each of twenty random initial transformations from each interval group, once using DRRs computed using PAF and once using DRRs computed using traditional ray casting.

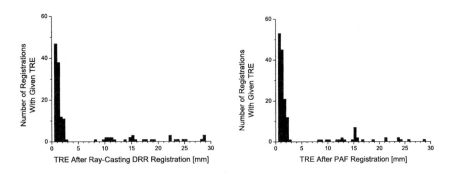

Fig. 3. Histograms of TRE after registration using ray-casting DRR (*left*) and PAF (*right*). Bin width is 0.5 mm in both histograms.

Table 1. Target registration errors (mean ± standard deviation) for patient #1 in millimeters after registration with ray-casting DRR and PAF. Statistics include 20 registrations with random initial transformation per class (failed registrations excluded).

Initial TRE	0–2 mm	2–4 mm	4–6 mm	6–8 mm
DRR	0.95±0.16 mm	1.33±0.55 mm	1.37±0.55 mm	1.36±0.45,mm
PAF	0.99±0.21 mm	1.19±0.50 mm	1.28±0.44 mm	1.43±0.34 mm

Initial TRE	8–10 mm	10–12 mm	12–14 mm	14–16 mm
DRR	1.17±0.38 mm	1.51±0.70 mm	1.20±0.77 mm	1.29±0.39 mm
PAF	1.31±0.46 mm	1.66±0.73 mm	1.70±0.61 mm	1.12±0.29 mm

3.2   Results

Computational Efficiency. A comparison of computation times between ray-casting DRRs and PAF on a per-case basis is not very meaningful, because the number of steps in the search for the optimum transformation varies between the two methods, and so does the number of DRR computations. Over all registrations, the average registration time using ray-casting DRR was 2,357 seconds (standard deviation 1,168 seconds). The average time to complete a PAF registration was 604 seconds (std. dev. 312 seconds). The maximum time using ray-casting DRR was 13,772 seconds, and 2,584 seconds using PAF.

Accuracy and Robustness. Registration can sometimes fail, and the further away from the correct transformation the algorithm is started, the more likely failure becomes. Since the "accuracy" of failed registrations is basically random, these registrations need to be excluded from the accuracy analysis and instead treated in a separate robustness analysis. As Fig. 3 shows, final TRE values using both PAF and ray-casting DRR are either below 3 mm or above 8 mm. We therefore select a final TRE of 3 mm as the threshold for successful vs. failed registrations.

Fig. 4 shows the relative number of failed registrations vs. the initial TRE. All registrations were successful, based on the above threshold of 3 mm, for both PAF and

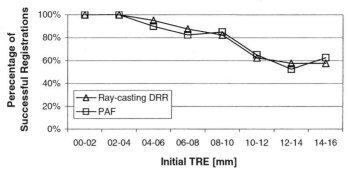

Fig. 4. Robustness vs. initial TRE for registration using ray-casting DRR computation and PAF. The graph shows the relative number of successful registrations (TRE less than 3.0 mm) for initial TREs from 0 through 16 mm (20 registrations with random initial transformation per class and per patient).

Table 2. Target registration errors (mean ± standard deviation) for patient #2 in millimeters after registration with ray-casting DRR and PAF. Statistics include 20 registrations with random initial transformation per class.

Initial TRE	0–2 mm	2–4 mm	4–6 mm	6–8 mm
DRR	1.61±0.07 mm	1.61±0.06 mm	1.60±0.06 mm	1.61±0.08 mm
PAF	1.62±0.06 mm	1.63±0.05 mm	1.60±0.05 mm	1.63±0.06 mm

Initial TRE	8–10 mm	10–12 mm	12–14 mm	14–16 mm
DRR	1.61±0.05 mm	1.61±0.05 mm	1.61±0.05 mm	1.65±0.21 mm
PAF	1.61±0.05 mm	1.64±0.06 mm	1.62±0.09 mm	1.62±0.06 mm

ray-casting DRR as long as initial TRE was less then 4 mm. For initial TREs between 4 mm and 8 mm PAF produced slightly more failed registrations than ray-casting DRR, while between 8 mm and 12 mm it produced slightly less. Overall, the robustness of registration using ray-casting DRR and PAF are approximately the same. The accuracy statistics of all successful registrations are shown in Table 1 for patient #1 and in Table 2 for patient #2. Again, the resulting values are virtually identical for both methods.

Note that for patient #2, the vast majority of TRE values are very close to 1.6 mm. Since the registration results appear visually convincing, this is probably due to inaccuracy of the gold standard transformation rather than errors of the intensity-based registration method. For medical reasons, fiducial markers in actual patients cannot be implanted in mathematically optimal locations that would maximize the accuracy of the computed transformation. Unfortunately, there is currently no more accurate method to compute "correct" coordinate transformations from clinical data than fiducial markers either. The spine as a whole moves nonrigidly, which can only be approximately detected using a small number of markers that are placed on different vertebrae.

4   Discussion

We have described a novel approach to increase the computational efficiency of intensity-based 2D-3D registration with no precomputation and virtually no restriction of the permissible patient movement. Both accuracy and robustness of the registration using PAF are essentially the same as those of registration using ray-casting DRR.

Our method is easily implemented and performs on average about four times faster than registration using ray-casting DRR. Our absolute computation times are still fairly large, which is due to a sub-optimal ray-casting DRR implementation. However, since in our method all attenuation values are computed as they are needed, rather than in a precomputation step, it benefits directly from faster ray casting methods during the registration phase. For example, Mori *et al.* [9] recently presented a fast CPU-based volume rendering method that computes DRRs several times faster than our relatively sub-optimal ray-casting DRR implementation.

Acknowledgment. This research was performed as part of a collaboration established with support from the Bavaria California Technology Center (BaCaTec).

References

1. D. LaRose, *Iterative X-ray/CT Registration Using Accelerated Volume Rendering*, Ph.D. thesis, Robotics Institute, Carnegie Mellon University, 2001.
2. S. J. Gortler, R. Grzeszczuk, R. Szeliski, M. F. Cohen, "The lumigraph," in *Proc. 23rd Annu. Conf. Computer Graphics and Interactive Techniques*, New York, NY, 1996, ACM SIGGRAPH, pp. 43–54, ACM Press.
3. D. B. Russakoff, T. Rohlfing, C. R. Maurer, Jr., "Fast intensity-based 2D-3D fluoroscopy-to-CT registration of clinical data using light fields," in *Ninth IEEE Int. Conf. Computer Vision*, 2003, pp. 416–422.
4. D. B. Russakoff, T. Rohlfing, D. Rueckert, C. R. Maurer, Jr., "Fast calculation of digitally reconstructed radiographs using light fields," in *Medical Imaging: Image Processing*, 2003, vol. 5032 of *Proc. SPIE*, pp. 684–695.
5. M. Levoy and P. Hanrahan, "Light field rendering," in *Proc. 23rd Annu. Conf. Computer Graphics and Interactive Techniques*, New York, NY, 1996, ACM SIGGRAPH, pp. 31–42, ACM Press.
6. D. B. Russakoff, T. Rohlfing, A. Ho, *et al.* "Evaluation of intensity-based 2D-3D spine image registration using clinical gold-standard data," in *Biomedical Image Registration – WBIR 2003*, 2003, vol. 2717 of *LNCS*, pp. 151–160, Springer-Verlag.
7. G. P. Penney, J. Weese, J. A. Little, *et al.* "A comparison of similarity measures for use in 2D-3D medical image registration," *IEEE Trans. Med. Imag.*, vol. 17, no. 4, pp. 586–595, 1998.
8. C. Studholme, D. L. G. Hill, D. J. Hawkes, "Automated three-dimensional registration of magnetic resonance and positron emission tomography brain images by multiresolution optimization of voxel similarity measures," *Med. Phys.*, vol. 24, no. 1, pp. 25–35, 1997.
9. K. Mori, Y. Suenaga, J. Toriwaki, "Fast volume rendering based on software optimization using multimedia instructions on PC platforms," in *Computer Assisted Radiology and Surgery*, Berlin, 2002, pp. 467–472, Springer-Verlag.

Nonrigid Image Registration Using Free-Form Deformations with a Local Rigidity Constraint

Dirk Loeckx, Frederik Maes*, Dirk Vandermeulen, and Paul Suetens

Medical Image Computing (Radiology–ESAT/PSI), Faculties of Medicine and
Engineering, University Hospital Gasthuisberg, Herestraat 49, B-3000 Leuven,
Belgium. Dirk.Loeckx@uz.kuleuven.ac.be

Abstract. Voxel-based nonrigid image registration can be formulated
as an optimisation problem whose goal is to minimise a cost function,
consisting of a first term that characterises the similarity between both
images and a second term that regularises the transformation and/or
penalties improbable or impossible deformations. Within this paper, we
extend previous works on nonrigid image registration by the introduction
of a new penalty term that expresses the local rigidity of the deformation.
A necessary and sufficient condition for the transformation to be locally
rigid at a particular location is that its Jacobian matrix $J_\mathbf{T}$ at this location is orthogonal, satisfying the orthogonality condition $J_\mathbf{T} J_\mathbf{T}^T = 1$.
So we define the penalty term as the weighted integral of the Froben-
ius norm of $J_\mathbf{T} J_\mathbf{T}^T - 1$ integrated over the overlap of the images to be
registered. We fit the implementation of the penalty term in a multidimensional, continuous and differentiable B-spline deformation framework
and analytically determine the derivative of the similarity criterion and
the penalty term with respect to the deformation parameters. We show
results of the impact of the proposed rigidity constraint on artificial and
clinical images demonstrating local shape preservation with the proposed
constraint.

1 Introduction

Image registration is a common task in medical image processing. The problem
of registration arises whenever medical images, e.g. acquired from different scanners, at different time points or pre- and post contrast, need to be combined for
analysis or visualisation. For applications were a rigid or affine transformation
is appropriate, several fast, robust and accurate algorithms have been reported
and validated [1]. However, in many cases the images to be registered show local
differences, e.g. due to intra-subject tissue changes over time or inter-subject
morphological differences, such that overall affine registration is insufficient and
non-rigid image matching is required for accurate local image alignment. Voxel-
based nonrigid image registration can be formulated as an optimisation problem

---

* Frederik Maes is Postdoctoral Fellow of the Fund for Scientific Research - Flanders
(FWO-Vlaanderen, Belgium).

C. Barillot, D.R. Haynor, and P. Hellier (Eds.): MICCAI 2004, LNCS 3216, pp. 639–646, 2004.
© Springer-Verlag Berlin Heidelberg 2004

whose goal is to minimise a cost function, consisting of a first term that characterises the similarity between both images and a second term that regularises the transformation and/or penalties improbable or impossible deformations. The first term is the driving force behind the registration process and aims to maximise the similarity between the two images. The second term, which is often referred to as the regularisation or penalty term, constrains the transformation between the source and target images to avoid impossible or improbable transformations.

In current literature, the penalty term is often expressed as a global energy term that imposes deformation smoothness by modelling the deforming image as a thin plate [2] or membrane [3]. However, in some applications there is a need to explicitly impose the constraint that some structures in the images to be registered should be treated as rigid objects that do not deform and can only be displaced between both images without changing shape. This is the case for instance with bony structures or contrast-enhancing lesions in intra-subject registration of pre- and post contrast images, e.g. for CT subtraction angiography. Several authors have presented different approaches for incorporating local rigidity constraints in non-rigid image registration. Tanner et al. [4] proposed a solution that locally couples the control points of a B-spline free-form deformation field such as to make the transformation rigid within the specified image region of interest. Little et al. [5] incorporate independent rigid objects in a modified thin-plate spline nonrigid registration. Both approaches require explicit identification of the rigid structures prior to or during registration. Also, they enforce the considered structures to be totally rigid, even in cases where they actually might have deformed slightly. Rohlfing et al. [6] proposed a penalty term that imposes local tissue incompressibility and volume preservation overall in the image without need for segmentation, by constraining the local Jacobian determinant to be close to unity everywhere in the image.

In this paper, we extend the approach of Rohlfing et al. [6] and propose a new penalty term that punishes transformations that are not locally equivalent to a rigid transformation by imposing the local Jacobian matrix to be orthogonal. Local rigidity is controlled by a spatially varying weight factor that depends on tissue type, such that the proposed rigidity constraint can be tuned locally and tailored to the problem at hand.

2   Methods

2.1   Transformation Model

To register a floating image F to a reference image R we need to determine the optimal set of parameters ϕ_ι for the transformation $\mathbf{T}(\Phi) = [T_x, T_y, T_z]$ such that $F'(\mathbf{x}_r) = F(\mathbf{T}(\mathbf{x}_r; \Phi))$ is in correspondence with R. For the nonrigid transformation $\mathbf{T}$, we use an independent implementation of the B-spline model introduced by Rueckert *et al.* [2]. The transformation model is a multilevel formulation of a free-form deformation based on tensor product B-splines of degree d (order $d + 1$). Usually, d is chosen to be 3 for cubic B-splines. The transformation $\mathbf{T}$ is defined by a control point grid Φ, i.e. a lattice of uniformly spaced control points $\phi_{i,j,k}$, where $-1 \leq i \leq n_x - 1$, $-1 \leq j \leq n_y - 1$, $-1 \leq i \leq n_z - 1$. The constant spacing between the control points in the x, y and z direction is denoted by δ_x, δ_y, δ_z. At any position $\mathbf{x} = (x, y, z)$ the deformation is computed from the positions of the surrounding $(d+1) \times (d+1) \times (d+1)$ neighbourhood of control points

$$\mathbf{T}(\mathbf{x}) = \mathbf{x} + \sum_{l=0}^{d} \sum_{m=0}^{d} \sum_{n=0}^{d} B_l^d(u) B_m^d(v) B_n^d(w) \phi_{i+l,j+m,k+n}. \tag{1}$$

Here, i, j and k denote the index of the control point cell containing $\mathbf{x} = (x, y, z)$, and u, v and w are the relative positions of x, y and z inside that cell in three dimensions, e.g. $i = \lfloor x/\delta_x \rfloor - 1$ and $u = x/\delta_x - (i+1)$. The functions B_n^d are the B-splines of degree d. The parameters ϕ_ι of the transformation $\mathbf{T}$ are the coordinates of the control points $\phi_{i,j,k} = \phi_\iota = [\phi_{\iota,x}, \phi_{\iota,y}, \phi_{\iota,z}]$.

2.2   Cost Function

The proposed cost function E consists of a similarity measure E_s and a penalty energy E_p, each weighted with a weight factor

$$E_c = \omega_s E_s + \omega_p E_p. \tag{2}$$

The similarity measure E_s is the driving force behind the registration process and aims to maximise the similarity between the two images, whereas the penalty term E_p tries to discourage certain improbable or impossible transformations. The main contribution of this article is the introduction of a new penalty term (and it's derivative) that constrains the transformation between the source and target image to locally rigid transformations.

Similarity Measure. We use mutual information of corresponding voxel intensities [7,8] as the similarity measure. To improve the smoothness of the similarity measure and to make the criterion derivable, we construct the joint histogram using Parzen windowing as proposed by Thévenaz et al. [9]

$$\forall r \in B_R, f \in B_F :$$

$$p(r, f; \Phi) = \sum_{\mathbf{x}_i \in (R \cap F')} w\left(\frac{f - I_F(\mathbf{T}(\mathbf{x}_i; \Phi))}{\epsilon_f}\right) \cdot w\left(\frac{r - I_R(\mathbf{x}_i)}{\epsilon_r}\right) \tag{3}$$

$$p(f; \Phi) = \sum_{r \in B_R} p(r, f; \Phi), \quad p(r) = \sum_{f \in B_F} p(r, f; \Phi) \tag{4}$$

with B_f and B_r the number of bins and using the dth degree B-spline as window function w. From the joint histogram, we can calculate the mutual information, which we will use as similarity measure

$$E_s = I(R, F; \Phi) = \sum_{r \in B_R} \sum_{f \in B_F} p(r, f; \Phi) \log\left(\frac{p(r, f; \Phi)}{p(r) \cdot p(f; \Phi)}\right). \tag{5}$$

Penalty Term. The main contribution of this paper is the introduction of a local rigidity constraint penalty term, based on the Jacobian matrix. In a small neighbourhood of the point $\mathbf{x}$, the non-rigid transformation $\mathbf{T}$ can be approximated by means of the Jacobian matrix $J_{\mathbf{T}}(\mathbf{x})$, which is the local first order or affine approximation to $\mathbf{T}(\mathbf{x})$.

$$J_{\mathbf{T}}(\mathbf{x}; \Phi) = \begin{bmatrix} \frac{\partial T_x(\mathbf{x};\Phi)}{\partial x} & \frac{\partial T_x(\mathbf{x};\Phi)}{\partial y} & \frac{\partial T_x(\mathbf{x};\Phi)}{\partial z} \\ \frac{\partial T_y(\mathbf{x};\Phi)}{\partial x} & \frac{\partial T_y(\mathbf{x};\Phi)}{\partial y} & \frac{\partial T_y(\mathbf{x};\Phi)}{\partial z} \\ \frac{\partial T_z(\mathbf{x};\Phi)}{\partial x} & \frac{\partial T_z(\mathbf{x};\Phi)}{\partial y} & \frac{\partial T_z(\mathbf{x};\Phi)}{\partial z} \end{bmatrix} \tag{6}$$

where

$$J_{\mathbf{T}}^{T} = \begin{bmatrix} \frac{\partial \mathbf{T}}{\partial x} \\ \frac{\partial \mathbf{T}}{\partial y} \\ \frac{\partial \mathbf{T}}{\partial z} \end{bmatrix} = \mathbf{1} + \sum_{l,m,n=0}^{d} \begin{bmatrix} \frac{1}{\delta_x} \frac{dB_l^d(u)}{du} B_m^d(v) B_n^d(w) \\ \frac{1}{\delta_y} B_l^d(u) \frac{dB_m^d(v)}{dv} B_n^d(w) \\ \frac{1}{\delta_z} B_l^d(u) B_m^d(v) \frac{dB_n^d(w)}{dw} \end{bmatrix} \phi_{i+l,j+m,k+n}. \tag{7}$$

Using the B-spline derivative properties, $dB^d(u)/du$ can be computed analytically [10] as

$$\frac{dB^d(u)}{du} = B^{d-1}(u + 1/2) - B^{d-1}(u - 1/2). \tag{8}$$

To obtain a locally rigid transformation, a necessary and sufficient condition is that $J_{\mathbf{T}}$ is an orthogonal matrix, satisfying the orthogonality condition $J_{\mathbf{T}} J_{\mathbf{T}}^{T} = \mathbf{1}$. This condition constrains the deformation to be either a rigid rotation $(\det(J_{\mathbf{T}}) = 1)$ or a rotoinversion $(\det(J_{\mathbf{T}}) = -1)$. Since both kinds of transformations form separated subsets and as we initiate $\mathbf{T}$ with the identity matrix, we assume we will not reach any rotoinversion. Therefore, we define the rigidity penalty term as the integral of the Frobenius norm of $J_{\mathbf{T}} J_{\mathbf{T}}^{T} - \mathbf{1}$ integrated over the overlap of the reference and the transformed floating image. Alternatively, one could multiply the orthogonality condition with $\det(J_{\mathbf{T}})$.

As different structures in the images may have different deformation properties and thus do not need to deform similarly, a local weight term $w(\mathbf{x})$ is added. This weight can be intensity based, e.g. $w(\mathbf{x})$ is a function of $F(\mathbf{T}(\mathbf{x}; \Phi))$, or based upon a prior segmentation of the floating or reference image. Finally, the total penalty term is given by

$$E_p = \int_{R \cap F'} w(\mathbf{x}) \left\| J_{\mathbf{T}} J_{\mathbf{T}}^{T} - \mathbf{1} \right\|_F d\mathbf{x}. \tag{9}$$

Similar to Rohlfing et al. [6], we compute the penalty term as a discrete approximation to the continuous integral calculated over the set of sampled voxels contained in $R \cap F'$.

2.3 Optimization

We use an optimization method similar to Rueckert et al. [2] and Rohlfing et al. [6]: the gradient $\partial E_c / \partial \phi_\iota = \omega_s \partial E_s / \partial \phi_\iota + \omega_p \partial E_p / \partial \phi_\iota$ of the cost function

(2) is computed, and next a simple line search (Van Wijngaarden–Dekker–Brent Method [11]) is performed along the direction of maximal descent. This procedure is repeated until the cost function cannot be improved any further, after which the algorithm continuous to a finer resolution (either by refining the deformation mesh or the image resolution).

Instead of using a finite-difference approximation to the derivative like in [6], we perform an analytical calculation of the derivative with respect to the transformation parameters Φ (see Thévenaz *et al.* [9] for more details). The derivative of the mutual information is given by

$$\frac{\partial E_s}{\partial \phi_\iota} = \frac{\partial I(R, F; \Phi)}{\partial \phi_\iota} = \sum_{r \in R} \sum_{f \in F} \frac{\partial p(r, f; \Phi)}{\partial \phi_\iota} \cdot \log \left(\frac{p(r, f; \Phi)}{p(f; \Phi)} \right). \quad (10)$$

using the fact that

$$\sum_{r \in R} \sum_{f \in F} \frac{\partial p(r, f; \Phi)}{\partial \phi_\iota} = \sum_{f \in F} \frac{\partial p(f; \Phi)}{\partial \phi_\iota} = 0 \quad (11)$$

The Frobenius norm of the matrix A is $\|A\|_F = \sqrt{\sum_{i,j}(A_{i,j})^2}$, such that the derivative of the penalty term with respect to a deformation parameter is given by

$$\frac{\partial E_p(\mathbf{T})}{\partial \phi_{\iota,\kappa}} = -\int_{R \cap F'} w(\mathbf{x}) \frac{\sum_{i,j} \left[J_\mathbf{T} J_\mathbf{T}^T - \mathbf{1} \right]_{ij} \left[\frac{\partial J_\mathbf{T}}{\partial \phi_{\iota,\kappa}} J_\mathbf{T}^T + J_\mathbf{T} \frac{\partial J_\mathbf{T}}{\partial \phi_{\iota,\kappa}}^T \right]_{ij}}{\left\| J_\mathbf{T} J_\mathbf{T}^T - \mathbf{1} \right\|_F} d\mathbf{x} \quad (12)$$

where

$$\frac{\partial J_\mathbf{T}}{\partial \phi_{\iota,\kappa}}^T = \begin{bmatrix} \frac{\partial^2 \mathbf{T}}{\partial \phi_{\iota,\kappa} \partial x} \\ \frac{\partial^2 \mathbf{T}}{\partial \phi_{\iota,\kappa} \partial y} \\ \frac{\partial^2 \mathbf{T}}{\partial \phi_{\iota,\kappa} \partial z} \end{bmatrix} = \begin{bmatrix} \frac{1}{\delta_x} \frac{dB_l^d(u)}{du} B_m^d(v) B_n^d(w) \\ \frac{1}{\delta_y} B_l^d(u) \frac{dB_m^d(v)}{dv} B_n^d(w) \\ \frac{1}{\delta_z} B_l^d(u) B_m^d(v) \frac{dB_n^d(w)}{dw} \end{bmatrix} \mathbf{e}_\kappa \quad (13)$$

for $\kappa = x, y, z$ and with $\mathbf{e}_\kappa$ the unit vector along coordinate axis κ. We see that the non-zero element of e.g. $\frac{\partial^2 \mathbf{T}}{\partial \phi_{\iota,\kappa} \partial x}$ is the same over all components of ϕ_ι and independent of its value, allowing for an efficient precalculation of its values.

3   Experiments

To indicate the feasibility and usefulness of the proposed approach, we applied it to three different data sets (figure 1). The first data set consists of artificial images, roughly depicting a vessel containing calcified regions. Although the vessel changes shape between the floating and the reference image, the shape of the calcified regions and bony structures is supposed to remain constant. Therefore, we chose a weight function $w(\mathbf{x}) = 1$ for high-intense regions and $w(\mathbf{x}) = 0$ otherwise. As can be seen from the results, the shape of the rigid structures is

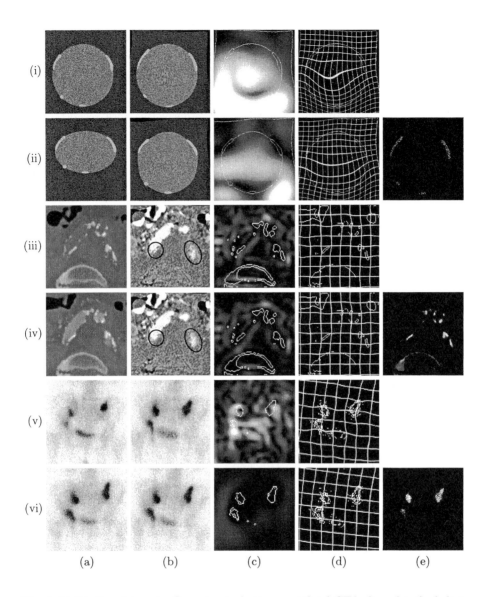

Fig. 1. Validation data sets. From top to bottom: artificial CTA slice, detail of clinical CTA slice, detail of clinical PET scan. Rows (i), (iii) and (v) display the reference images and the registration results without the penalty term, rows (ii), (iv) and (vi) display the floating images and the registration results with the penalty term. The columns contain (a) the reference and floating image, (b) the registered images (reference image subtracted from registered floating image in (iii) and (iv)) , (c) the unweighted penalty term, (d) the obtained deformation grid, and (e) the local weight function $w(\mathbf{x})$. The penalty term and deformation field images are overlaid with the edges of the registered image.

preserved better using the proposed penalty term then without. E.g., the bigger calcifications at the top of the image are more elongated, whereas the smaller calcifications at the bottom are slightly compressed. This is confirmed by the images in column (d), that show a high non-rigidity factor in the unconstrained case, and almost no deformation in the constrained case.

The second example (figure 1, rows (iii) and (iv)) shows a detail of a registered computed tomography angiography (CTA) slice. We chose a weight factor that increases linear with intensity in the high-intense regions, and is zero otherwise. As can be seen in column (c), an unconstrained registration causes local shape deformations in the calcified or bony regions. When we use the approach proposed in this article, the deformation is locally rigid in the selected structures. As expected, this has a positive influence on the artifacts in the difference images (column (b)).

The third data set we applied the algorithm to consists of full body PET images, acquired at different time points during treatment. As we want to study the evolution of the lesion over time, we do not want the non-rigid registration to locally deform it. The results of the registration are shown in figure 1, rows (v-vi). We used a weight function similar to the previous case, preventing the lesions to change shape. Close observation of column (b) shows that in the unconstrained case, the lower left region did slightly shrink while the lower middle lesion did grow.

4   Discussion

A new local rigidity penalty term for non-rigid image registration is proposed, modelling the weighted local rigidity of the transformation. This penalty term is useful for the registration of images where certain structures can not or should not change shape. Its applicability is shown on three example data sets.

The introduction of the local weight factor enables the deformation to preserve the shape in selected regions while still allowing the deformation to non-rigidly align both images. The determination of the weight factor necessitates some kind of segmentation, labelled or statistical, of at least one of the images. Several approaches for this segmentation are possible, ranging from simple intensity thresholding as in the samples shown here, over the use of a more advanced segmentation algorithm like e.g. level-set segmentation, to a joint segmentation/registration approach, where in each iteration the segmentation is updated based on the current registration and vice versa.

In future research, we will validate our registration method on different kinds of images in two and three dimensions, investigate the influence of the weight factors and compare the rigidity constraint with other constraints, especially the volume preserving constraint introduced by Rohlfing et al. [6]. However, because usually no ground truth exists giving the correct deformation field, the validation of nonrigid registration algorithms is difficult and an active area of research. A promising validation method was recently introduced by Schnabel et al. [12], using a biomechanical model to simulate non-rigid deformations.

Acknowledgements This work is part of K.U.Leuven/OF/GOA/1999/05, K.U.Leuven/OF/GOA/2004/05 and FWO G.0258.02.

References

1. West, J., Fitzpatrick, J.M., Wang, M.Y., Dawant, B.M., Maurer, Jr., C.R., Kessler, R.M., Maciunas, R.J., Barillot, C., Lemoine, D., Collignon, A., Maes, F., Suetens, P., Vandermeulen, D., van den Elsen, P.A., Napel, S., Sumanaweera, T.S., Harkness, B., Hemler, P.F., Hill, D.L.G., Hawkes, D.J., Studholme, C., Maintz, J.B.A., Viergever, M.A., Malandain, G., Pennec, X., Noz, M.E., Maguire, Jr., G.Q., Pollack, M., Pelizzari, C.A., Robb, R.A., Hanson, D., Woods, R.P.: Comparison and evaluation of retrospective intermodality brain image registration techniques. Journal of Computer Assisted Tomography **21** (1997) 554–566
2. Rueckert, D., Sonoda, L.I., Hayes, C., Hill, D.L.G., Leach, M.O., Hawkes, D.J.: Nonrigid registration using free-form deformations: Application to breast MR images. IEEE Trans. Med. Imag. **18** (1999) 712–721
3. Amit, Y., Grenander, U., Piccioni, M.: Structural image restoration through deformable templates. J. Amer. Statist. Assoc. **86** (1991) 376–387
4. Tanner, C., Schnabel, J.A., Chung, D., Clarkson, M.J., Rueckert, D., Hill, D.L.G., Hawkes, D.J.: Volume and shape preservation of enhancing lesions when applying non-rigid registration to a time series of contrast enhancing MR breast images. In Delp, S.L., DiGioia, A.M., Jaramaz, B., eds.: Medical Image Computing and Computer-Assisted Intervention (MICCAI 2000). Volume 1935 of Lecture Notes in Computer Science., Springer Verlag (2000) 327–337
5. Little, J.A., Hill, D.L.G., Hawkes, D.J.: Deformations incorporating rigid structures. Comput. Vis. Image Underst. **66** (1997) 223–232
6. Rohlfing, T., C.R. Maurer, J., Bluemke, D., Jacobs, M.: Volume-preserving nonrigid registration of MR breast images using free-form deformation with an incompressibility constraint. IEEE Trans. Med. Imag. **22** (2003) 730–741
7. Maes, F., Collignon, A., Vandermeulen, D., Marchal, G., Suetens, P.: Multimodality image registration by maximization of mutual information. IEEE Trans. Med. Imag. **16** (1997) 187–198
8. Viola, P., Wells, W.: Alignment by maximization of mutual information. International Journal of Computer Vision **24** (1997) 137–154
9. Thévenaz, P., Unser, M.: Optimization of mutual information for multiresolution image registration. IEEE Trans. Med. Imag. **9** (2000) 2083–2099
10. Unser, M.: Splines: A perfect fit for signal and image processing. IEEE Signal Processing Mag. **16** (1999) 22–38
11. Press, W.H., Teukolsky, S.A., Vetterling, W.T., Flannery, B.P.: Numerical Recipes in C: The Art of Scientific Computing. Cambridge University Press (1992)
12. Schnabel, J.A., Tanner, C., Castellano-Smith, A.D., Leach, M.O., Hayes, C., Degenhard, A., Hose, R., Hill, D.L.G., Hawkes, D.J.: Validation of non-rigid registration using finite element methods. In Insana, M.F., Leahy, R.M., eds.: XVIIth International Conference on Information Processing in Medical Imaging (IPMI'01). Volume 2082 of Lecture Notes in Computer Science., Springer Verlag (2001) 344–357

Fast Non-linear Elastic Registration in 2D Medical Image

Zhi-ying Long[1], Li Yao[2], and Dan-ling Peng[1]

[1] School of Psychology, Beijing Normal University, Beijing, P.R.China, 100088
{friskying@163.com}
[2] Department of Electronics, Beijing Normal University, Beijing, P.R.China, 100088
{yaoli@bnu.edu.cn}

Abstract. Non-linear image registration can match two images' local areas exactly. Linear elastic model that obeys the Navier-stokes equilibrium equations is especially fit for image registration with small deformation. Bro-Nielesen derived a linear elastic convolution filter from the eigenfunctions of the Navier-stokes differential operator. Based on the elastic filter, the elastic partial differential equation (PDE) is easy to be solved although the filter is mainly used in viscous PDE of fluid model at first. Gaussian filter used in the 'demon'-based registration method of Thrion could be regarded as an approximation to the elastic filter. Because of the complexity of the elastic filter and the poor performance of the gaussian filter, we propose a new simple filter, two-sided exponential filter, to approach the elastic filter. The results of experiments also show the new filter improves the algorithm's convergence speed and the precision greatly and its performance is superior to the other two filters.

1 Introduction

Image registration, which aims to match two images by searching a best transformation between them, has been widely used in many fields. Especially in medical image field, changes in different images of the same object over periods of time need to be observed, or the images between patient and normal personal need to be compared. So it is very important for the involved images to be matched in structure. Usually there exist two kinds of matching algorithm in medical image registration. They are linear and non-linear registration. Linear registration, such as rigid or affine transformation, is often applied to matching two images in global shape, while non-linear registration can match two images locally and finely. In most cases, non-linear matching algorithm also need initial linear alignment.

Non-linear registration usually transforms images in higher-dimensional anatomical mappings in order to match local variability across different anatomies. Physical continuum models can be used in non-linear registration because they allow extremely flexible deformations and the degrees of freedom can be as many as the number of the voxels in the images. Bajcsy et al. [2] were the first to construct the deforming image as 3D elastic solid and derived the body force from the gradient of the intensity cor

C. Barillot, D.R. Haynor, and P. Hellier (Eds.): MICCAI 2004, LNCS 3216, pp. 647–654, 2004.

relation. Because of the limitation of small deformation assumptions for liner elasticity model, Christensen [5] proposed a viscous fluid model to estimate large image deformations for keeping the non-linear topological behavior. In this model, internal restoring forces that exist in the linear elastic model disappear and large magnitude displacement can't be penalized any more by regularization methods based on linear elasticity. So the precise deformation can be achieved. However, because the viscous fluid PDE is sloved on a discrete lattice, the speed of the algorithm is too slow to be implemented on PC.

Based on the work of Christensen, Bro-Nielsen [3] derived a convolution filter for linear elasticity from the eigenfunctions of the Navier-stokes differential operator $L = \mu \nabla^2 + (\lambda + \mu)\nabla(\nabla\cdot)$. And the algorithm speed got an increase of several orders of magnitude. Although the elastic filter improved the algorithm, the time cost of producing the filter still increased exponentially with the size of the image. And it will be much more difficult to get the filter in the 3D images. Therefore, the more easily the filter can be got, the more efficient the algorithm will be. In fact Bro-Nielsen [3] also demonstrated that the 'demon'-based registration method of Thirion [11] colud be seen as using a gaussian filter to approach the elastic filter. Because big differences exist between the two filters, gaussian filter still has many disadvantages.

And because Navier-stokes differential operator can be extracted from elastic as well as fluid model, the linear elastic filter can be applied to the two models easily. Byviewing the global shape of the 2D elastic filter, we find it is more like the shape of two-sided exponential, especially in the middle areas acted by driving force. And because two-side exponential filter is also lowpass just like the elastic filter, we propose the new simple filter as an approximation of the elastic filter. In our work, MR images from two different subjects are matched in global shape initially then we mainly apply elastic registration by using the new two-side exponential filter. Comparing the three filters, the performance of the new filter is obviously better than the gaussian filter, its final precision can almost reach the same level as the elastic filter and its algorithm convergence speed is much faster than the elastic filter.

2   Theory

2.1 Image Registration Based on Elastic Models

We assume two images, an object image (O) and a template image (T), are to be registered. And a best smooth deformation field u (x) needs to be found, where x is the particles of O. When applying the transform u (x) to the coordinates of the particles in O, the transformed image should match the template image very well.

Considering the deformed image to be embed in elastic media, the displacement field u (x) resulting from internal deformation forces F (x), which is called body force, obeys the Navier-stokes equilibrium equations for linear elasticity [12].

$$\mu\nabla^2 u(x) + (\lambda + \mu)\nabla(\nabla^T \cdot u(x)) + F(x) = 0 \qquad \forall x \in R \qquad (1)$$

Here $\nabla^T \cdot u(x) = \sum \partial u_j / \partial x_j$, ∇^2 is the Laplacian operation. Lamé's coefficients λ and μ controls the elastic properties of the medium. Body force can be derived from the gradient of a cost function, such as intensity correlation.

2.2 Convolution Filters in the Solution of the Navier-Stokes Equation

From equation 1, we can see PDE must be solved in order to get deformation field. In order to simplify the solving of PDE, Bro-Nielesen developed the convolution filter to solve the linear PDE [3]. A Navier-stokes differential operator L can be extracted from equation 1.

$$L = \mu \nabla^2 + (\lambda + \mu) \nabla (\nabla \cdot) \tag{2}$$

When applying the linear operator L to the corresponding variable u (x), elastic models can be simplified like equation 3.

$$Lu(x) + F(x) = 0 \tag{3}$$

In fact, equation 3 describes a linear system with F (x) as the input and u (x) as the output. Based on the eigen-functions of the linear operator L, Bro-Nielsen derived the filter H as an approximation to the impulse response of an applied unit force in the middle of an image. A linear filter of size D×D for the x direction has the form of Equation 4.

$$H_1(x) = \frac{4}{\pi^2 \mu (2\mu + \lambda)} \sum_{i,j=0}^{D-1} \frac{p(c)}{(i^2 + j^2)^2 \Gamma) ij} \left[\begin{array}{c} -(i^2 \mu + (2\mu + \lambda) j^2) p(x) \\ (\mu + \lambda) ij q(x) \end{array} \right] \tag{4}$$

And detailed derivation can refer to Bro-Nielsen in [3]. However, time cost to create the filter increases rapidly with the size of image.

2.3 Properties of Linear Elastic Filter

As H_1 (x) is a vector field with a unit force acting in x direction, each point in the field is a vector that consists of two components in x and y dimensions separately. So H_1 (x) can be decomposed into two scalar fields, $H_x(x)$ along x direction and $H_y(x)$ along y direction. Fig. 1 shows displacement field of H_1 (x) with size 15×15. Force from x direction makes the $H_x(x)$ must be much larger than $H_y(x)$. Then $H_y(x)$ can also be ignored for simplicity.

Because a unit force acts on the center of the field, the center displacement around the force direction is much larger than the other areas. From fig. 1, we can see the scalar field $H_x(x)$ is almost symmetrical about x and y directions and the displacements of the five middle rows of x and y can nearly dominate the whole field. In order to study the property of the filter further, the middle five rows and columns of $H_x(x)$, corresponding to x and y direction separately, are extracted. And only three of them are drawn because of the field's symmetry.

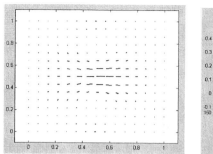 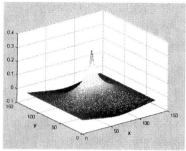

Fig. 1. Displacement vector field $H_1(x)$ (left) and the scalar field $H_x(x)$ of $H_1(x)$ shown in 3D space (right).

Fig. 2 shows those curves' shape along x and y directions are very similar. The main difference among them is that the curves' width along x direction is larger than that along y direction. That demonstrates the filter must be anisotropic.

In order to contrast gasussian filter with elastic filter, three middle rows in x and y direction of gaussian filter are also drawn in fig. 3. Comparing fig. 3 with fig. 2, we can see there are big differences between them.

2.4 2D Two-Sided Exponential Filter

Some problems may appear in the stability and precision of the deformation fields when applying the gaussian filter although the filter is very easy to be created. So the main work becomes whether we can find a new simple lowpass filter that is closer to the elastic filter than gaussian. When observing fig. 2 and 3 carefully, we can see that the curve's shape in fig. 2 is sharper and isn't like gaussian function at all, but more like two-sided exponential function in equation 5.

1D two-sided exponential filter:

$$H(x) = e^{(-\frac{|x|}{\alpha})} \tag{5}$$

2D two-sided exponential filter:

$$H_1(x, y) = e^{(-\frac{|x|}{\alpha_1} - \frac{|y|}{\alpha_2})} \qquad H_2(x, y) = e^{(-\frac{|x|}{\alpha_2} - \frac{|y|}{\alpha_1})} \tag{6}$$

Here the parameters α_1 and α_2 control the variation of data just like σ in gaussian function. If the two parameters are not identical, this filter is anisotropic too.

The subscript 1 and 2 of $H(x, y)$ denotes that the center unit force comes from x and y direction respectively.

Obviously two-sided exponential filter's shape (Fig. 4) is much more similar to linear elastic filter (Fig. 2) than that of Gaussian filter (Fig. 3). Therefore it can be inferred that the new filter must be superior to the Gaussian approximation and can also be created easily.

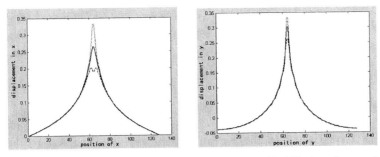

Fig. 2. Three middle rows of the scalar field $H_x(x)$ with 128×128 size along x (left) and y(right) direction. Row 62, 63 and 64 correspond to dashed, solid and dotted line.

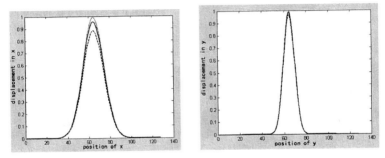

Fig. 3. Three middle rows of gaussian scalar field with 128×128 size along x (left) and y(right) direction. Row 62, 63 and 64 correspond to dashed, solid and dotted line.

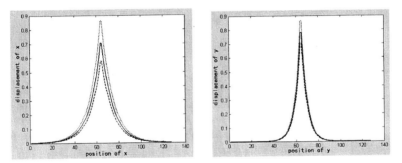

Fig. 4. Three middle rows of two-sided exponential scalar field with 128×128 size along x(left) and y(right) direction. Row 62, 63 and 64 correspond to dashed, solid and dotted line.

3   Experiments and Results

Two experiments based on elastic model are presented to demonstrate how the two-sided exponential filter is superior to the other two. And we focus on comparing the registration precision, convergence speed and time cost of the three filters under the same iterative times after the filters have been created. All programs were run in Matlab 6.1 software.

3.1 2D Square to Rectangular

In the first experiment, the object image was a square and the template was a rectangular (see fig. 5A). The dimension of the images is 128×128 pixels. Three filters, elastic, gaussian and two-sided exponential filters, were used to transform the square into the rectangular. Among three filters, two-sided exponential filter spent the least time, which is 4.7 seconds, with 120 iterative times, while elastic filter took 6.45 seconds and gaussian filter took 9.85 seconds. Fig. 5B shows that two-sided exponential filter got better precision than the other two filters. And from Fig. 5C, we can see that the convergence speed of two-sided exponential filter is also the fastest while the gaussian filter is the slowest among them.

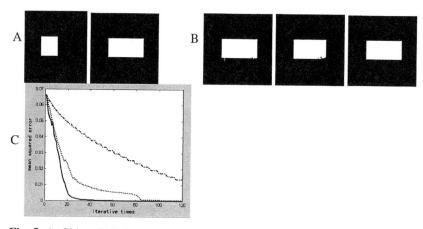

Fig. 5. A, Object (left) image and template (right) image. B, Transformed images after 120 iterative times using the linear elastic (left), Gaussian (middle) and two-sided exponential filter (right) respectively. And their corresponding mean squared errors are 4.20e-4, 0.0137 and 1.54e-7. C, Changes of mean squared error with iterative times, dotted line denotes elastic filter and the dashed line denotes gaussian filter.

3.2 2D MR Images of Human Brain

In medical field, medical images are often need to be matched so that some regional areas can be compared. In order to observe how the nonlinear transformation acted on image locally, we selected two 2D MR images from 3D MRI brain data of two subjects. The size of two images is 91×109 pixels. Only two-sided exponential filter and elastic filter are compared from the speed of convergence and the result precision.

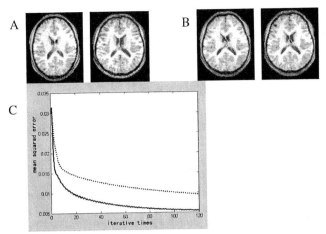

Fig. 6. A, Object (left) image and template (right) image. B, Transformed images after 120 iterative times using the linear elastic (left) and two-sided exponential filter (right). And their corresponding mean squared errors are 0.095 and 0.066. C, Changes of mean squared error with iterative times. The solid line denotes two-sided exponential filter and dotted line denotes elastic filter.

Fig. 6 shows that after nonlinear transformation, the original object image's global shape is almost consistent with the template and some local areas are also matched. Two-sided exponential filter get better result than elastic filter. And its convergence speed is also much faster.

4   Conclusion

Fast fluid registration based on the linear elastic filter has been a classical method for large displacement field. And because of the similarity between fluid and elastic model, the elastic filter can be used in the elastic model for small deformation. As the filter is based on the perfect physical model theory, it is also very robust for image registration in any cases. However, the creation speed of the linear elastic filter becomes slower and slower with the increase of the image size, which may increase the computation time cost greatly and reduce the algorithm's efficiency and practicability. When the new two-sided exponential filter is used in elastic model, the algorithm's time efficiency and result's precision are improved greatly because it has the following advantages. Firstly the filter's creation and the extension to 3D cases become much simpler than the elastic filter for images with any sizes. And that can make it very practicable especially for large size images. Secondly, the property of the new filter is much closer to the elastic filter than the Gaussian filter. So the result won't be worse than that of Gaussian filter and sometimes can even reach or overpass the elastic filter's precision. Lastly, its separable property, just like gaussian filter, improves the convolution speed greatly especially for 3D images with large sizes. It is all these attractive advantages that make the novel filter superior to the other filters in some aspects.

There are still some shortages in the two-sided exponential filter. Firstly, it is almost impossible for the two-sided exponential filter to have the same parameters in any cases. Specific images may correspond to specific parameters. And a bad parameter can degenerate deformation field greatly. So the parameters must be selected very carefully. Secondly, if we observe the two filters carefully in 3D space, we will find that the elastic filter's shape is much smoother than the two-sided exponential filter, which also makes its deformation field is smoother than the two-sided exponential filter. So the new filter may not be as robust as the elastic filter. And how to find a filter, which is smoother, more convenient and closer to the elastic filter than the two-sided exponential filter, is also worth studying further.

Acknowledgment. This work is supported by the National Natural Science Foundation of China. (60072003, 60271014).

References

1. Ashburner J. and Friston K.J., Nonlinear spatial normalization using basis functions, Hum. Brain Mapp., vol. 7, no. 4, (1999) 254-266.
2. Bajcsy R. and Kovacic S., Multiresolution elastic matching, Comput. Vision Graph. Image Process., vol. 46, (1989) 1-21.
3. Bro-Nielsen M. and Gramkow C., Fast fluid registration of medical images, Visualization in Biomedical Computing. Lecture Notes in Computer Science, vol. 1131. Springer-Verlag, Berlin Heidelberg New York (1996) 267-276.
4. Christensen G.E., Miller M.I. and Vannier M., A 3D deformable magnetic resonance textbook based on elasticity, in AAAI Spring Symposium Series: Applications of Computer Vision in Medical Image Processing, pp. 153-156, Stanford University, Mar. (1994).
5. Christensen G.E., Deformable shape models for anatomy, Washington University Ph.D. thesis, Aug. (1994).
6. Christensen G.E., Rabbitt R.D. and Miller M.I., Deformable templates using large deformation kinematics, IEEE Trans. Image Process., vol. 5, no. 10, Oct. (1996) 1435-1447.
7. Cachier P., Pennec X., and Ayache N., Fast non rigid matching by gradient descent: study and improvements of the "demons" algorithm. INRIA Technical Report RR-3707, June (1999).
8. Gramkow C. and Bro-Nielsen M., Comparison of three filters in the solution of the Navie-Stokes equation in registration, Proc. Scandinavian Conference on Image Analysis (1997) 795-802.
9. Miller M.I., Christensen G.E., Amit Y. and Grenander U., Mathematical textbook of deformable neuroanatomies, Proc. Natl. Acad. Sci. vol. 90, no. 24, (1993) 11944-11948.
10. Nielsen M., Florack L. and Deriche R., Regularization and scale space, INRIA Tech. Rep. RR-2352, Sep. (1994).
11. Thirion J.-P., Fast non-rigid matching of medical images, INRIA Internal Report 2547, Project Epidaure, INRIA, France, (1995)
12. Thompson P.M. and Toga A.W., A framework for computational anatomy, Comput. Visual. Sci., vol. 5, (2002) 13-34.

Multi-subject Registration for Unbiased Statistical Atlas Construction

Mathieu De Craene[1,2,3], Aloys du Bois d'Aische[1,2,3], Benoît Macq[1], and Simon K. Warfield[2,3]

[1] Communications and Remote Sensing Laboratory, Université catholique de Louvain, Louvain-la-Neuve, BELGIUM.
[2] Surgical Planning Laboratory
[3] Computational Radiology Laboratory, Brigham and Women's Hospital, Harvard Medical School, Boston MA, USA.

Abstract. This paper introduces a new similarity measure designed to bring a population of segmented subjects into alignment in a common coordinate system. Our metric aligns each subject with a hidden probabilistic model of the common spatial distribution of anatomical tissues, estimated using STAPLE. Our approach does not require the selection of a subject of the population as a "target subject", nor the identification of "stable" landmarks across subjects. Rather, the approach determines automatically from the data what the most consistent alignment of the joint data is, subject to the particular transformation family used to align the subjects. The computational cost of joint simultaneous registration of the population of subjects is small due to the use of an efficient gradient estimate used to solve the optimization transform aligning each subject. The efficacy of the approach in constructing an unbiased statistical atlas was demonstrated by carrying out joint alignment of 20 segmentations of MRI of healthy preterm infants, using an affine transformation model and a FEM volumetric tetrahedral mesh transformation model.

1 Introduction

Statistical atlases are an important representation for characterizing anatomy and anatomical variation. They have applications in characterizing normal anatomy, and in identifying structural differences between populations, such as between healthy newborn infants and infants with white matter injury. Furthermore, statistical atlases provide prior probability models useful to constrain segmentation and registration algorithms to ensure robust and rapid operation. For example, given prior information about the main modes of shape variation, a non-rigid registration algorithm may optimize initially upon these main modes of variation instead of considering all parameters of the deformation model simultaneously. The use of statistical atlases has also been investigated for improving the accuracy of automatic segmentations algorithms to extract data despite the noise and artifacts by capturing a priori information.

A statistical atlas is a model of the expected anatomy, usually represented as a probability of an anatomical structure or tissue being present at each voxel

C. Barillot, D.R. Haynor, and P. Hellier (Eds.): MICCAI 2004, LNCS 3216, pp. 655–662, 2004.

of a 3D lattice. Such an atlas may be constructed by sampling from a large population of subjects, identifying the anatomy or tissue present in each subject by segmentation and then projecting the segmentation into a common coordinate system. Previous approaches to do this have differed in the manner in which the appropriate alignment of the subjects is defined, and by the flexibility of the transformation aligning the subjects. For example, some have used manually selected landmarks [11] or intensity features [2] . As described in [2], a data-driven approach that avoids any bias introduced by selecting a set of landmarks is a desirable feature for next-generation statistical atlas construction algorithms. Furthermore, the bias introduced by selecting a particular subject (who has an anatomy of unknown typicality) and aligning further scans with that subject [4] is undesirable. Algorithms that attempt to undo this bias by removing an average transformation following the alignment to a single subject have been described (see [5] and [8]) but unfortunately require limiting assumptions regarding the accuracy of the individual subject-to-target alignment (see for example [8] note on page 1021) and in practice have generated statistical atlases that differ when different target subjects are selected.

We have previously investigated an approach to atlas construction that avoids the bias introduced by a single subject by carrying out simultaneous alignment of a collection of subjects [14]. This approach was built upon previous work in handwriting recognition by alignment [6]. This algorithm required the expensive construction of a large joint probability distribution. Bhatia[1] proposed to select one arbitrary image to act as an intensity reference, and then to add all pairs of intensities, comprising the voxel intensity in the reference and the corresponding intensity in each image, to the same joint histogram. We propose here a new algorithm, leveraging our recent work in the automated assessment of similarity of segmentations [14] to enable the construction of a statistical atlas by joint alignment of a collection of subjects. The new algorithm presented here is both efficient, in not requiring an unwieldy large joint probability distribution estimate, and avoids identifying any particular subject as a target and hence avoids any target bias. It does not require the identification of common and stable landmarks across subjects, but rather uses a data-driven approach to identify from the input data itself, the most consistent joint alignment of the subjects.

2   Algorithm Description

The purpose of the algorithm is to identify the best joint alignment of a collection of segmentations. This is done by solving for the set of transformations $\{T_j\}$ mapping each subject j into a common coordinate system. The common coordinate system is also estimated from the aligned data. To speed up the convergence, the set of $\{T_j\}$ is initialized to map the center of gravity of each subject to the center of the common coordinate system. The algorithm is a generalized Expectation-Maximization algorithm, where the subject segmentations are the observed data, and hidden data is the anatomical label of each voxel of the statistical atlas. The parameters to be estimated are the transform for each subject that aligns each subject best with the hidden statistical atlas, and parameters that describe the similarity of the subject labels with that of the hidden statistical atlas. The similarity parameters are estimated as in our earlier work on validation of image segmentation, and can be interpreted as, for each subject label, the probability that the subject label will match the atlas label at the same voxel under the current transformation. A closed form expression for these parameters is straightforward to solve, whereas the transformation parameters have no closed form solution and must be identified by an optimization procedure. Therefore, the implementation iterates between these two steps:

- Expectation step: A probabilistic estimate of the statistical atlas labels is made given the set of subjects $1 \ldots J$ and the set of current transformations $\{T_j\}$.
- Maximization step: For each subject j, the transformation T_j is updated to maximize the similarity of the subject with the probabilistic statistical atlas estimate computed in the first step. The parameters describing the consistency of each aligned subject to the probabilistic atlas are found by maximum likelihood estimation.

The entire procedure is then iterated to convergence, with the consistency parameter estimates being used to update the probabilistic atlas labels, which then allows new refined estimates of the simultaneous joint alignment of the subjects. As this constitutes a generalized Expectation-Maximization algorithm, convergence to a local optimum is guaranteed.

2.1   Probabilistic Atlas Estimation

In this step, a probability map for each label is computed over the whole atlas image domain using an iterative EM algorithm described in [13,14]. Rather than also updating estimates of the transformation parameters at each iteration, they are held fixed until the probabilistic atlas estimate is converged, and are only then updated. After convergence of the probabilistic atlas estimate, the probability to find the label s at the voxel i in the atlas can be written as

$$W_{si} = \frac{1}{\alpha} f(A_i = s) \prod_j f(D_{ij}|A_i = s, \hat{\Theta}, T_j) \tag{1}$$

$$= \frac{1}{\alpha} f(A_i = s) \prod_j \hat{\theta}^j_{D_{ij}s} \tag{2}$$

where α is a normalization constant to ensure $\sum_s W_{si} = 1$, $f(A_i = s)$ is a prior probability on the ground label A_i, D_{ij} is the value of the ith pixel in the jth subject. $\hat{\Theta}$ is the set of matrix of parameters describing the similarity of each subject with the probabilistic atlas. For a subject j, each element of the matrix is $\hat{\theta}^j_{s's}$, the probability for observing the label s' when the ground truth is s and can be computed from the set of W_{si} as:

$$\hat{\theta}^j_{s's} = \frac{1}{\beta} \sum_{i:D_{ij}=s'} W_{si} \tag{3}$$

where β is a normalization constant to get $\sum_{s'} \hat{\theta}^j_{s's} = 1$.

After convergence, the solutions of Equations 1 and 3 become stationary.

2.2   Subject to Probabilistic Atlas Registration

Once the probabilistic atlas W_{si} has been computed for each label s, at each position i of the atlas image domain, the set of transformations $\{T_j\}$ is updated for each subject by solving the transformation T_j maximizing the mean trace of the jth subject similarity matrix :

$$\frac{1}{N_s} \sum_s \hat{\theta}^j_{ss} \tag{4}$$

Since $\hat{\theta}^j_{ss}$ denotes the true positive fraction of the label s, this cost function seeks to align the subject j to have a spatial distribution of labels as similar as possible to that of the probabilistic atlas.

To illustrate the behavior of this metric around the optimum, the mean trace of the specifity matrix for one subject is plotted around the optimum as a function of translations and rotations parameters in Figure 1 for variations in a [-10,+10] interval.

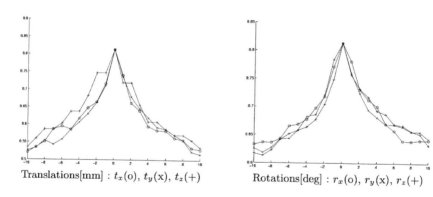

Translations[mm] : $t_x(\text{o})$, $t_y(\text{x})$, $t_z(+)$ Rotations[deg] : $r_x(\text{o})$, $r_y(\text{x})$, $r_z(+)$

Fig. 1. The cost function used for multi-subject registration is plotted for one subject around the optimum found by the algorithm as a function of the translations and rotations parameters.

3   Experiments

The 22 high resolution T1w, PDw and T2w MRI images of healthy preterm infants were segmented into tissue types (background, skin, sub-cortical and cortical gray matter, cerebrospinal fluid, myelinated white matter, unmyelinated white matter) using an intensity- and atlas- based optimal classifier as previously described and validated [12]. For this experiment, these labels have been gathered in four labels: background, unmyelinated white matter, basal ganglia and a class containing the remaining brain voxels.

The set of transformations mapping the atlas space on each subject was composed of a rigid and scale transformation followed by an FEM based non-rigid transformation. The process has been initialized by a set of translations sending the center of the atlas to the center of gravity of each subject using the itk::ImageMomentsCalculator class. This is done to improve the initialization and therefore reduce the computation time. The sum after bringing the center of the atlas to the center of gravity of each subject is plotted in Figure 3(a). The metric described in section 2.2 has been optimized using an iterative gradient ascent scheme. The gradient ascent is based on the Simultaneous Stochastic Perturbation Approximation (SPSA) of the gradient, firstly introduced by Spall [10]. The SPSA method incorporates two gains decreasing with the number of iterations shrinking the distance over which the finite differences are calculated as well as the learning rate. This method relies only on two measurements of the objective function to be optimized. The SPSA optimization routine has been integrated into the ITK[9] optimization framework.

3.1   Rigid and Scale Transformation Model

The algorithm described in Section 2 has been run using a transformation model allowing translations, rotations and three scale factors. After registration of each subject on the first estimate of the probabilistic atlas (to improve the consistency of each subject as described in Section 2.2) the probabilistic atlas (Ground Truth estimate) has been recomputed and plotted in Figure 2. The process is then iterated until convergence of the whole set of parameters (three iterations of probabilistic atlas estimation and registration parameters estimation were needed in this case). The sum of all subjects after rigid and scale alignment is plotted in Figure 3(b).

3.2   FEM Volumetric Tetrahedral Mesh Transformation Model

To refine the results obtained in the former section, a volumetric tetrahedral mesh has been used to extend the transformation model. The transformation is then parameterized by the displacements at each node of the mesh. The nodes displacements are propagated to any point of the common space of coordinates using the shape functions of the element containing this point.

$$u_l(x) = \sum_{n \in \text{Nodes}} v_l^n N^n(x) \tag{5}$$

where u_l stands for the lth component of the displacement field, x is the 3D position in the fixed image volume, v_l^n is the displacement of the nth node of the element and $N^n(x)$ is the shape function associated to the node n. In this experiment, a coarse mesh has been obtained from a $64 \times 64 \times 10$ voxels^3 BCC grid as described in [7]. To improve the convergence of the optimization process, we reduce the dimensionality of the space of parameters by selecting at each iteration a set of "active nodes". For this selection, a first derivative is computed by generating a large number of gradient estimates using stochastic perturbations on the whole set of nodes. The nodes where the norm of the derivative is above a fixed threshold are selected as active nodes. Active nodes displacements are propagated to other nodes by adding in the cost function a linear elastic regularization constrain as we describe in [3]. The sum of all subjects after FEM alignment of each subject on the probability map (starting from the results of section 3.1) is plotted in Figure 3 (c). The border of the brain has become more contrasted after FEM alignment. Figure 3 (d) plots a weighted sum of the four labels in all subjects after FEM alignment (the intensity at voxel i is equal to $\sum_j D_{ij} W_{D_{ij},s}$).

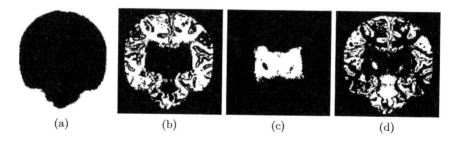

(a)   (b)   (c)   (d)

Fig. 2. The STAPLE ground truth probability for each label is plotted after 1 iteration of our algorithm for the background (a), the unmyelinated white matter (b), the basal ganglia(c) and the remaining brain voxels classified in a separate class (d). The steep rising from regions where the probability is 0 (black voxels) to regions where the probability is 1 results from the important weight give to consistent subjects in the W_{si} computation.

4   Conclusions and Future Work

This study, carried out on 22 preterm healthy infants, has demonstrated that the STAPLE estimate of a probability map for each label can be used to align a collection of subjects to a common space of coordinates. The use of volumetric adaptive FEM meshes could allow the refinement of the transformation model in specific areas, splitting elements where a significant variability is observed for the current alignment. Statistical analysis of the set of node displacements will allow to include prior information in non-rigid registration algorithms by seeking first to optimize the main deformations modes observed in the atlas.

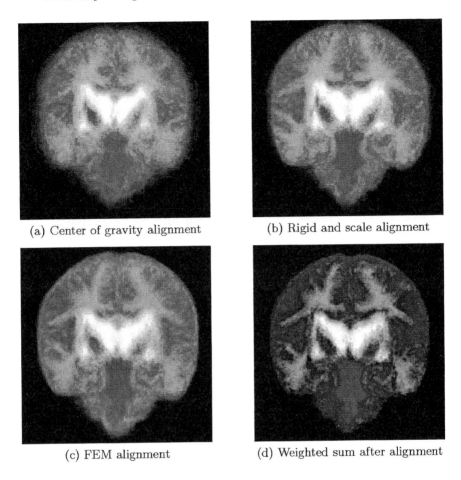

(a) Center of gravity alignment   (b) Rigid and scale alignment

(c) FEM alignment   (d) Weighted sum after alignment

Fig. 3. Sub-figure (a) plots the sum of all 22 pre-term healthy subjects after bringing the center of gravity of each subject to the center of the atlas image. Sub-figure (b) shows the sum of all subjects after alignment to the STAPLE probabilistic atlas (plotted in Figure 2) using translations, rotations around X, Y and Z axis, and 3 scale factors. A simple non-rigid transformation model using a regular FEM tetrahedral mesh has been used to improve the accuracy around the borders of the brain. The result is plotted in sub-figure (c). The FEM mesh has been built on a $64 \times 64 \times 10$ voxels^3 BCC regular grid. Sub-figure (d) plots a weighted - by the tissue probability in the statistical atlas - combination of labels for all subjects after FEM alignment.

Acknowledgments. Mathieu De Craene and Aloys du Bois d'Aische are working towards a Ph.D. degree with a grant from the Belgian FRIA. This investigation was supported in part by the Region Wallone Mercator project, NIH grants P41 RR13218, NIH P01 CA67165, NIH R01 RR11747 and NIH R01 AG19513 and by a research grant from the Whitaker Foundation. We thank Dr. Terrie Inder for the neonate MRI data used in this study.

References

1. K.K Bhatia, J.V. Hajnal, B.K. Puri, A.D. Edwards, and D. Rueckert. Consistent Groupwise Non-Rigid Registration for Atlas Construction. In *ISBI*, 2004.
2. D. L. Collins. *3D Model-based segmentation of individual brain structures from magnetic resonance imaging data.* PhD thesis, McGill University, Montreal, 1994.
3. Mathieu De Craene, Aloys du Bois d'Aische, Ion-Florin Talos, Matthieu Ferrant, Peter McL. Black, Ferenc Jolesz, Ron Kikinis, Benoit Macq, and Simon K. Warfield. Dense Deformation Field Estimation for Brain Intra-Operative Images Registration. In *SPIE Medical imaging : Image Processing*, 2004.
4. PF. D' Haese, V. Duay, B. Macq, T. Merchant, and Dawant B. Atlas-based segmentation of the brain for 3-dimensional treatment planning in children with infratentorial ependymoma. In *Sixth International Conference on Medical Image Computing and Computer-Assisted Intervention*. Springer-Verlag, 2003.
5. A. Guimond, J. Meunier, and J.-P. Thirion. Average brain models: A convergence study. *Computer Vision and Image Understanding*, 77(2):192–210, 1999.
6. Erik G. Miller. *Learning from One Example in Machine Vision by Sharing Densities.* PhD thesis, EECS, MIT, Boston, 2002.
7. N. Molino, R. Bridson, J. Teran, and R. Fedkiw. A crystalline, red green strategy for meshing highly deformable objects with tetrahedra. In *12th International Meshing Roundtable*, pages 103–114, Sandia National Laboratories, september 2003.
8. D. Rueckert, A. F. Frangi, and J. A. Schnabel. Automatic construction of 3-d statistical deformation models of the brain using nonrigid registration. *IEEE Trans Med Imaging*, 22(8):1014–25, 2003.
9. Luis Ibanez Will Schroeder. *The ITK Software Guide.* The Insight Consortium.
10. J. C. Spall. Overview of the simultaneous perturbation method for efficient optimization. *http://techdigest.jhuapl.edu/td/td1904/spall.pdf, Hopkins APL Technical Digest*, 19:482–492, 1998.
11. J. Talairach and P. Tournoux. Co-planar stereotaxic atlas of the human brain: 3-dimensional proportional system - an approach to cerebral imaging. *New York, NY: Thieme Medical Publishers*, 1998.
12. Simon K. Warfield, Michael Kaus, Ferenc A. Jolesz, and Ron Kikinis. Adaptive, Template Moderated, Spatially Varying Statistical Classification. *Med Image Anal*, 4(1):43–55, Mar 2000.
13. Simon K. Warfield, K. H. Zou, and III. W. M. Wells. Validation of image segmentation and expert quality with an expectation-maximization algorithm. In *Fifth International Conference on Medical Image Computing and Computer-Assisted Intervention*. Springer-Verlag, 2002.
14. Simon K. Warfield, K. H. Zou, and W. M. Wells. Simultaneous truth and performance level estimation (staple): An algorithm for the validation of image segmentation. *IEEE Trans Med Imag*, 2004. Accepted to appear.

Simultaneous Segmentation and Registration for Medical Image

Xiaohua Chen[1], Michael Brady[1], and Daniel Rueckert[2]

[1] Robotics Research Group, University of Oxford, Oxford, UK
{xchen, jmb}@robots.ox.ac.uk
[2] Department of Computing, Imperial College London, London, UK

Abstract. Although segmentation and registration are usually considered separately in medical image analysis, they can obviously benefit a great deal from each other. In this paper, we propose a novel scheme of simultaneously solving for segmentation and registration. This is achieved by a maximum a posteriori (MAP) model. The key idea is to introduce an additional hidden Markov random vector field into the model. Both rigid and non-rigid registration have been incorporated. We have used a B-spline based free-form deformation for non-rigid registration case. The method has been applied to the segmentation and registration of brain MR images.

1 Introduction

The large number of segmentation and registration methods found in the literature shows that these are two of the most studied topics in medical image analysis. However, most existing work considers them separately, even though they are closely related: the solution of one can greatly assist in the computation of the other. Using segmentation results can reduce the influence of noise on the original images and lead to improved registration. In the case that one image scan presents rather subtle information about the subject to be segmented, significant improvement may be obtained by combining information from images of the same subject acquired at different times or under different conditions. In order to use this information, images need to be perfectly aligned.

Until recently, little research has been done to simultaneously estimate the segmentation and registration problems in a single framework. Yezzi [2] proposed an active contour approach, but it is only suited to single object well-defined images with relatively large structures. Wyatt [4] used a method that applies Markov random fields in the solution of a MAP model of segmentation and registration. However, it is restricted to rigid registration, and its hard-assignment segmentation makes it vulnerable to noise.

In this paper, we present a novel MAP model for simultaneous segmentation and registration (SSR). We include a hidden Markov random vector field into the model to improve the performance of the segmentation method. We also incorporate B-spline based free-form deformation (FFD) to cope with the non-rigid registration.

C. Barillot, D.R. Haynor, and P. Hellier (Eds.): MICCAI 2004, LNCS 3216, pp. 663–670, 2004.
© Springer-Verlag Berlin Heidelberg 2004

2   Method

We have two images I and J, and we assume J corresponds to some unknown geometric transformation of reference image I. "Segmentation", or the labelling of each pixel to one tissue type can be regarded as a model of the underlying anatomy. I and J can be interpreted as a realization of a random process that corrupts the "Segmentation", e.g. by Gaussian noise. The problem can be formulated as follows: given image I and J, we wish to simultaneously estimate the label fields f of the images and recover the geometric transformation T that registers the two images. The MAP estimation is to find f and T to maximize $P(f, T | I, J)$.

2.1   Hidden Vector Field

We assume that there are M regions; discrete label $f(\boldsymbol{r})$ indicates to which region pixel $\boldsymbol{r} = (x_r, y_r)$ belongs. As noted above, the relationship between an image and its segmentation can be defined in terms of a Gaussian noise distribution:

$$P(I|f) = \prod_{\boldsymbol{r} \in \Omega_I} v_{f(\boldsymbol{r})}(\boldsymbol{r}) \, . \tag{1}$$

where Ω_I is the lattice of sites of I and each M-vector $\boldsymbol{v}(\boldsymbol{r})$ is defined by:

$$v_k(\boldsymbol{r}) = \sqrt{\frac{\gamma}{\pi}} \exp[-\gamma |I(\boldsymbol{r}) - \theta_k|^2] \, . \tag{2}$$

Here, γ and $\boldsymbol{\theta}$ are image parameters that depend on the noise variance and mean intensity value of each class. One can find the optional estimate for f by applying a classical MRF model and Bayesian MAP estimation [5].

Marroquin [3] proposed a different probabilistic model for the generation of label field to overcome the difficulties with classical MRF models like sensitive to noise and initialization. Instead of the conventional 1-step procedure, he proposed a 2-step probabilistic model, with an additional hidden Markov random vector field p: each vector $\boldsymbol{p}(\boldsymbol{r})$ indicates the probability the pixel $\boldsymbol{r}$ belongs to one of the regions given the intensity of that pixel, and it takes values on the M-vertex simplex S_M:

$$S_M = \{\boldsymbol{u} \in \mathcal{R}^M : \sum_{k=1}^{M} u_k = 1, u_k \geq 0, k = 1, ..., M\} \, . \tag{3}$$

Then, the optimal estimate for f can be calculated from p.

2.2   General Framework

We incorporate the Markov random vector field p into our framework. To obtain the optimal estimator f^* for the label field and T^* for transformation, we follow the steps:

1. Find the MAP estimators p^*, T^* for p, T: $p^*, T^* = \arg \max_{p \in S_M^N, T}$ $P(p, T | I, J)$
2. Determine $f^*(r) = \arg \max_{f(r)} P(f | p = p^*, I) = \arg \max_k p_k^*(r)$

The first step itself is a 2-step procedure, in which the best T is found given the current estimate for p, then the best estimate for p is found, given the current estimate for transformation T:

1. Find an initial estimate $\bar{p}$ for p by individual segmentation;
2. Repeat until convergence or often enough:
   (a): Set $\bar{T} = \arg \max_T P(T | \bar{p}, I, J)$
   (b): Set $\bar{p} = \arg \max_p P(p | \bar{T}, I, J)$

We now analyze step (a). We consider image I to be the reference image, transformation T to be a spatial mapping from I to J. Using Bayes' rule, we have:

$$P(T | \bar{p}, I, J) \propto P(I | \bar{p}) P(J | \bar{p}, T) P(T) . \tag{4}$$

In order to maintain spatial coherence and smoothness, the transformation $T(r)$ may be required to be similar to its value at the spatial neighbors. We assume a Gibbs distribution on the expected deformations: $P(T) = \exp(-E(T))$, where $E(T)$ is T in the form of an energy. The likelihood of the observations can be rewritten:

$$P(J | \bar{p}, T) = \prod_{r \in \Omega_I} P(J(T(r)) | \bar{p}) . \tag{5}$$

For a Gaussian noise distribution, we have:

$$p(J(T(r)) | \bar{p}) = \sum_{k=1}^{M} w_k(T(r)) \bar{p}_k(r) = w(T(r)) \cdot \bar{p}(r) . \tag{6}$$

where

$$w_k(T(r)) = \sqrt{\frac{\gamma}{\pi}} \exp[-\gamma | J(T(r)) - \theta_k)|^2] . \tag{7}$$

Finally we get:

$$P(T | \bar{p}, I, J) \propto \exp[-U(T)] . \tag{8}$$

where

$$U(T) = - \sum_{r \in \Omega_I} \log(w(T(r)) \cdot \bar{p}(r)) + E(T) . \tag{9}$$

Step (a) is equivalent to minimizing of $U(T)$.

For step (b):

$$P(p | \bar{T}, I, J) \propto P(I | p) P(J | p, \bar{T}) P(p) . \tag{10}$$

Since p is Markovian, $P(p)$ can be expressed as $P(p) = \exp(-V(p))$, where, for example,

$$V_{rs}(p(r), p(s)) = \lambda | p(r) - p(s) |^2 = \lambda \sum_{k=1}^{M} (p_k(r) - p_k(s))^2 . \tag{11}$$

where λ is a positive parameter, and $< r, s >$ are neighboring sites in Ω_I.

So, we get:

$$P(p|\bar{T}, I, J) \propto \exp[-U(p)] .\qquad(12)$$

with

$$U(p) = -\sum_{r \in \Omega_I} \log(v(r) \cdot p(r)) - \sum_{r \in \Omega_I} \log(w(\bar{T}(r)) \cdot p(r)) + \sum_C V_C(p) .\quad(13)$$

Step (b) is then equivalent to minimizing of energy $U(p)$. we use iterative gradient descent method for optimization of both T and p. Here, $p(r)$ must be projected back into S_M.

2.3   The Representation of Transformation

For the case where T is a rigid transformation, we represent it by a rotation matrix A and a translation vector c: $T(r) = Ar + c$. In two dimensions, the rotation matrix A depends upon a single angle α. Since for a rigid registration, all the pixels undergo the same transformation, it is sufficiently smooth for $E(T)$ to be dropped, so we can set it to zero. By minimizing $U(T)$, we get parameters α, c to represent $\bar{T}$.

For non-rigid transformation, we represent T using a combination of a global transformation and a local transformation:

$$T = T_{global} + T_{local} .\qquad(14)$$

The global transformation is represented by a rigid transformation, while for and the local transformation, we use a B-spline based FFD model [1]:

$$T_{local}(r) = \sum_{m=0}^{3} \sum_{n=0}^{3} B_m(u)B_n(v)\Phi_{i+m,j+n} .\qquad(15)$$

where Φ denotes lattice of control points, i, j denote the indices of the control points and u, v correspond to the relative positions of r in lattice coordinates. The lattice of control points is defined as a grid with uniform spacing which is placed on the underlying reference image.

For T_{global}, the $E(T)$ can be dropped, and for T_{local}, we may use a 5 pixels neighborhood clique C: $E(T) = \sum_C V_C(T)$ where

$$\sum_C V_C(T(r)) = 2(T(x_r, y_r+1) + T(x_r - 1, y_r) - T(x_r, y_r) - T(x_r - 1, y_r + 1))^2$$

$$+ (T(x_r - 1, y_r) + T(x_r + 1, y_r) - 2T(x_r, y_r))^2$$

$$+ (T(x_r, y_r - 1) + T(x_r, y_r + 1) - 2T(x_r, y_r))^2 .\qquad(16)$$

3   Experiments

In this section, we use brain MR images to illustrate the performance of our approach of simultaneous segmentation and registration presented above.

In order to compare the algorithms, we need to establish a performance index, which should be objective and quantitative. We propose the following performance index ξ:

$$\xi_k = \frac{2V_{GPk}}{V_{Pk} + V_{Gk}}$$

where V_{GPk} denotes the total number of pixels that were correctly assigned to class k by a given procedure; V_{Pk} is the total (correct + incorrect) number of pixels belonging to class k by this procedure and V_{Gk} denotes the total number of pixels belonging to class k in the ground truth. Higher performance index indicates better segmentation result here.

Our initial experiments are on brain MR images provided by Brainweb [6]. We segment the images into 3 tissue classes in the brain: cerebrospinal fluid (CSF), gray matter (GM), and white matter (WM). Our first experiment is on images with known rigid transformation between them. We make a transformation on zero noise brain image with 5.00 degree rotation and 11.0 pixels translations in both directions. Various amount of zero-mean Gaussian white noise are independently added to the original and transformed images to produce the observed images I and J. The test images, together with their single and SSR results are shown in Fig. 1. We compare these two results with our performance index: as can be seen from Table 1, in each tissue class, the performance index of SSR is always higher than that of the single segmentation. The recovered transformation is 5.03 degree and the translations in two direction are 10.7 and 10.4 pixels.

Our second experiment is on images with an unknown non-rigid transformation: we take two different slices of brain MRI as I and J; the image experimental results are shown in Fig. 2. We can see from the performance index in Table 2 that the SSR gives more correct classification for pixels in each class than the single segmentation. The recovered transformation is represented by transforming the floating image into the reference image domain, since no real transformation ground truth can be provided here, we can only get a visually qualitative impression of our registration result. We aim to study how to evaluate non-rigid registration methods later.

Table 1. Performance index comparison between single and SSR segmentation for experiment1

tissue class	CSF	GM	WM
single	0.893	0.869	0.930
SSR	0.894	0.874	0.937

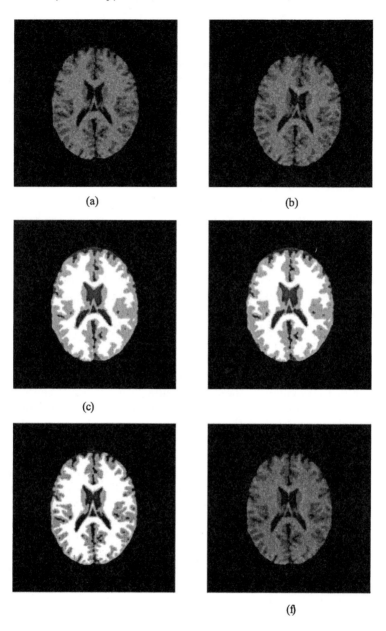

Fig. 1. Simultaneous segmentation and registration (SSR) experiment on rigid registration. (a)reference image I. (b)floating image J. (c)segmentation result of image I without SSR. (d)segmentation result with SSR. (e)segmentation ground truth in image I domain. (f)transformation of floating image to reference image using rigid registration.

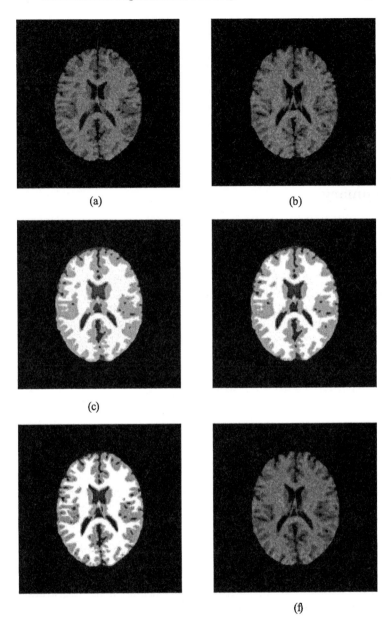

Fig. 2. Simultaneous segmentation and registration (SSR) on non-rigid registration. (a)reference image I. (b)floating image J. (c)segmentation result of image I without SSR.(d)segmentation result with SSR. (e)segmentation ground truth in image I domain. (f)transformation of floating image to reference image using non-rigid registration.

Table 2. Performance index comparison between single and SSR segmentation for experiment2

tissue class	CSF	GM	WM
single	0.882	0.888	0.939
SSR	0.890	0.892	0.942

4 Summary

In this paper, we have developed a framework to achieve simultaneously segmentation and registration to make the two problems' solutions facilitate each other. We use a hidden Markov measure vector field to make the interactions between these two problems possible. It is used for segmentation step to label each pixel with highest probability of certain tissue type and for registration step to act as a key element in similarity measure. For reason of space, we have only illustrated this framework to brain MR images for both rigid and non-rigid registration cases, with promising results for both segmentation and registration: the segmentation results achieved by fusion of the images performs better than the segmentation results got from single image, meanwhile, using the segmentation results also produces a good registration.

References

1. Rueckert, D., Sonoda, L.I., Hayes, C., Hill, D.L.G., Leach, M.O., Hawkes, D.J.: Nonrigid Registration Using Free-Form Deformations: Application to Breast MR Images. IEEE Trans. Medical Imaging, Vol. 18. Num. 8. (1999) 712–721
2. Yezzi, A., Zollei, L.: A Variational Framework for Integrating Segmentation and Registration Through Active Contours. Medical Image Analysis, Vol. 7. (2003) 171–185
3. Marroquin, J.L., Santana, E.A., Botello, S.: Hidden Markov Measure Field Models for Image Segmentation . IEEE Trans. Pattern Analysis and Machine Intelligence, Vol. 25. Num. 11. (2003) 1380–1387
4. Wyatt, P.P., Noble, J.A.: MAP MRF Joint Segmentation and Registration of Medical Images. Medical Image Analysis, Vol. 7. Num. 4. (2003) 539–552
5. Zhang, Y., Brady, M., Smith, S.: Segmentation of Brain MR Images Through a Hidden Markov Random Field Model and the Expectation Maximization Algorithm. IEEE Trans. Medical Imaging, Vol. 20. Num. 1. (2001) 45–57
6. Cocosco, C.A., Kollokian, V., Kwan, R., Evans, A.C.: BrainWeb: Onlie Interface to a 3D MRI Simulated Brain Database. Neuroimage, Vol. 5. Num. 4. (1997) 425

Mapping Template Heart Models to Patient Data Using Image Registration

Marcin Wierzbicki[1,2], Maria Drangova[1,2], Gerard Guiraudon[1,2,3], and Terry Peters[1,2]

[1] Imaging Research Laboratories, Robarts Research Institute,
London, Ontario, Canada, N6A 5K8
(mwierz,mdrangov,tpeters)@imaging.robarts.ca
[2] Department of Medical Biophysics, The University of Western Ontario,
London, Ontario, Canada, N6A 5C1
gguiraud@uwo.ca
[3] Canadian Surgical Technologies & Advanced Robotics (CSTAR),
London, Ontario, Canada, N6A 5A5

Abstract. Currently, minimally invasive cardiac surgery (MICS) faces several limitations, including inadequate training methods using non-realistic models, insufficient surgery planning using 2D images, and the lack of global, 3D guidance during the procedure. To address these issues we are developing the Virtual Cardiac Surgery Platform (VCSP) – a virtual reality model of the patient specific thorax, derived from pre-procedural images. Here we present an image registration-based method for customizing a geometrical template model of the heart to any given patient, and validate it using manual segmentation as the gold standard. On average, the process is accurate to within 3.3 ± 0.3 mm in MR images, and 2.4 ± 0.3 mm in CT images. These results include inaccuracies in the gold standard, which are on average 1.6 ± 0.2 and 0.9 ± 0.2 mm for MR and CT images respectively. We believe this method adequately prepares templates for use within VCSP, prior to and during MICS.

1   Introduction

Coronary artery disease (CAD) and atrial fibrillation (AF) are specific examples of heart disease – the most common cause of death in the developed world. Both conditions can be treated surgically, by strategic scarring of tissues in AF, and by coronary artery bypass grafting in CAD. Conventional surgery is performed via a median sternotomy on the arrested heart, requiring the use of cardiopulmonary bypass (CPB), aortic cross clamping, and myocardial preservation. The latter are the main causes of side effects that lead to increased patient recovery times and costs [1].

Unwanted side-effects, such as large incisions, CPB, or cardiac arrest can be reduced by performing cardiac surgery using an endoscope-aided, port-access approach described previously [2]. In practice however, operating on the beating heart without direct vision is extremely challenging. The first problem is the requirement to perform complex maneuvers, normally carried out in the open chest, inside the closed thoracic cavity. Several systems have been effective for such tasks when used by a trained practitioner [3]. The second and more prominent problem is the lack of proper

C. Barillot, D.R. Haynor, and P. Hellier (Eds.): MICCAI 2004, LNCS 3216, pp. 671–678, 2004.
© Springer-Verlag Berlin Heidelberg 2004

three-dimensional (3D) visualization during the training, planning, and guidance stages of surgery. Currently, only limited training is conducted, usually on unrealistic and expensive animal and cadaver models. Surgery planning of port locations is also inadequate, often based only on 2D images such as x-rays and angiograms. Finally, the current surgical guidance method is imperfect, due to the small field-of-view (FOV) of the endoscope, and the possibility that this view may become obstructed by blood, anatomy, moisture, etc. The lack of proper 3D surgery training, planning, and guidance can lead to improper patient selection, sub-optimal port placement, longer procedures, and increased risks to the patient [4, 5].

To address these issues, we continue to develop methods utilizing pre-operative images for 3D modeling of patient anatomy. These methods are combined and utilized in our Virtual Cardiac Surgery Planning (VCSP) platform [6], designed for training, planning, and guidance of minimally invasive cardiac surgeries. In this manuscript, we describe a method for generating patient-specific, geometric models of the heart and its components. Such models are essential in bringing VCSP closer to being an indispensable surgical support tool.

There are two main options for creating the necessary models from pre-operative images: direct segmentation and customization of a template. An example of the direct segmentation approach is the work by Sørensen *et al.* [7], who created a 3D geometric model of the entire heart from a specialized MR image acquired at end-diastole (ED). Clinical images are often noisy and of low resolution due to imaging time constraints (MR), dose limitations (CT), and unavailability of specialized imaging protocols, making direct segmentation of these images extremely challenging. In addition, it is difficult to use a single segmentation algorithm to detect the various heart structures in multi-modality images required for minimally invasive cardiac surgery. The more suitable method for our application is therefore the template customization approach. An example of this method is the work of Lorenzo-Valdéz, who build template myocardium, LV, and RV models from multiple MR images, and used voxel-based, elastic image registration for customization [8]. Voxel-based methods are well suited for our application, since the results are user independent and the time required per patient is minimal.

In this manuscript, we present our methods for building template models using manual segmentation and for customizing them to target images using a three-stage, image registration algorithm. We perform validation experiments on various MR and CT images, with manual segmentation of the target images acting as the gold standard. Following customization, any given model can be animated using the complete 4D data, as described in our previous work [9]. The final, patient-specific, dynamic model can then be easily integrated with VCSP.

2   Methods

In this section we outline our general methods for template-to-patient image mapping and specific methods for algorithm validation. Possible scanning protocols are discussed first, followed by a description of the template model extraction process, and a discussion of the template-to-patient image registration algorithm.

2.1   Image Acquisition

Both MR and CT imaging modalities were considered and tested with our template matching approach. The MR data, consisting of 4D images of six different human volunteers, were acquired with prospective ECG gating, using the 1.5 T, GE CVi scanner, with the fast cine SPGR pulse sequence, an image matrix of 256×128, eight views per segment, and a 20 degree flip angle. Five of the volunteers were imaged in a clinically practical manner, with two signal averages (NEX) and an average breath-hold duration of 23 sec ($1.5^2 \times 6$ mm^3 voxels). The sixth volunteer was imaged with four NEX, and a breath-hold duration of approximately 40 sec. (1.5^3 mm^3 voxels). The signal-to-noise ratio (SNR) in the higher resolution image was enhanced by registering the four adjacent image frames of the complete 4D data to the image at ED using the algorithm described in [9], and by averaging the resulting five images. This specialized image is a part of a separate project aimed at generating a dynamic cardiac MR dataset with high resolution and high SNR [10].

The CT data, consisting of four 4D images of canine subjects, were acquired using an eight-slice GE LightSpeed helical CT scanner, with retrospective ECG gating, and 120 kVp, 200 mA x-rays. The dogs were paralyzed and artificially ventilated during the 30 sec. scan time; one of the dogs was imaged on two different days. Prior to each scan, a bolus of iodine contrast agent (300 mg/mL) was injected intra-venously to enhance the image contrast inside the heart. The images were reconstructed with a voxel size of $0.35^2 \times 1.25$ mm^3.

2.2   Model Extraction

Model extraction is normally required once from the ED template image, however, for validation purposes, models of specific parts of the heart anatomy were extracted from *each* of the ED MR and CT images. A manual, paintbrush technique was used to generate binary data that were then smoothed using a spherical Gaussian filter to remove rough edges. The filtered data were then triangulated using the marching cubes algorithm [11], and finally decimated using a modified version of the algorithm of Schroeder *et al.* [12] to enable a reasonable rendering speed. For each MR image, the heart was divided into models of the left ventricular myocardium (LVM), right atrium and ventricle (RAV), left atrium and aorta (LAAo), and the epicardial surface (EH). We could only segment the epicardial surface in the canine CT images (EC) due to low contrast inside the heart. Figure 1 shows examples of the resulting models.

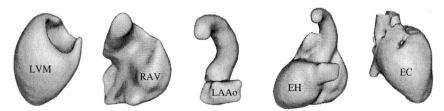

Fig. 1. Left ventricular myocardium (LVM), right atrium and ventricle (RAV), left atrium and aorta (LAAo), and the epicardium (EH) from the higher resolution, human MR image. Also shown is the epicardium obtained from one of the canine CT images (EC).

2.3   Registration Algorithm

For each customization task, the source and target images are selected from the complete 4D data sets so that both represent the heart at approximately the same time point in the cardiac cycle (ED according to the ECG). This reduces differences in morphology between the two hearts, thereby improving our ability to align them accurately. The chosen template image is then customized to the chosen target image using a three-stage registration approach. In the initial stage, the template image is roughly registered with the target image by aligning the two centroids. This is followed by a global registration using an affine transformation, representing translation, rotation, scaling, and shear operations. The 12-degree of freedom (DOF) transformation (T_G) can be parameterized in 3D using the variable a_{ij} as follows:

$$T_G(x, y, z) = \begin{pmatrix} a_{11} & a_{12} & a_{13} \\ a_{21} & a_{22} & a_{23} \\ a_{31} & a_{32} & a_{33} \end{pmatrix} \begin{pmatrix} x \\ y \\ z \end{pmatrix} + \begin{pmatrix} a_{14} \\ a_{24} \\ a_{34} \end{pmatrix}. \tag{1}$$

The solution is obtained by a downhill simplex optimization algorithm [13] that maximizes the normalized mutual information (NMI), a similarity metric often used for inter-subject registration [14]. NMI can be expressed as:

$$NMI(S, T) = \frac{E_S + E_T}{2 \cdot E_{ST}}, \tag{2}$$

where E_S and E_T are the marginal entropies of the source and target images, and E_{ST} is the join entropy. The division by 2 normalizes NMI to lie between 0.5 and 1.0.

Following affine registration, the algorithm begins the non-linear registration stage for local refinement of the template. This step is carried out in a free-form deformation (FFD) framework, where a mesh of control points (nodes) is placed on the template image and then assigned 3D vectors to indicate local deformation. The result at each node is found by minimizing the following cost function (C) using the downhill simplex method:

$$C(T_L^n) = -NMI\big(S(T_G T_L^n, V), T(V)\big) + \alpha \cdot BE(T_L^n), \tag{3}$$

where T_L^n is the translation vector at node n in the FFD grid, $S(T_G T_L^n, V)$ is the volume V of the source image surrounding n after the global transformation T_G and local translation T_L^i, $T(V)$ is the volume V of the target image surrounding n, and $BE(T_L^n)$ is the 3D thin plate spline bending energy attributed to T_L^i, included to ensure a smooth local transformation (weight controlled by α) [15]. To reduce the chance of the optimization procedure converging to a local minimum, the algorithm proceeds through three resolution levels of the FFD grid, with the V parameter progressing from ~ 7.5 to 5.0 to 2.5 cm^3. Larger V produces more accurate results since more samples are used to calculate NMI, while smaller V allows more local deformation to be extracted. The highly sampled version of T_L, required for application to images, is generated using linear interpolation.

3   Validation Experiments

Validation of our template customization algorithm was performed using a single observer, manual segmentation of the target image as the gold standard. Results and discussion are split into two sub-sections, based on the image set analyzed.

3.1   Human MR Images

The first task was to quantify the accuracy of the imperfect gold standard itself. For this purpose, an experienced observer manually segmented the LVM, RAV, LAAo, and EH, twice in each of the six images. The intra-observer variability was then quantified as the root mean square (RMS) of the Euclidian distance between a given pair of segmentation surfaces. Correspondence between the surfaces was established by searching for the closest points. Results are in Table 1 below.

Table 1. RMS Euclidian distance between pairs of manually segmented surfaces showing the intra-observer variability of the gold standard. Correspondence was established using nearest points. Image 6 is the high resolution image, not included in the calculation of the mean and standard deviation (SD).

Data Compared	RMS (mm) for:			
	LVM	**RAV**	**LAAo**	**EH**
1 vs. 1	1.85	1.97	1.95	1.71
2 vs. 2	1.36	1.39	1.69	1.39
3 vs. 3	1.50	1.35	1.46	1.49
4 vs. 4	2.06	2.14	1.74	1.53
5 vs. 5	1.37	1.56	1.11	1.16
Mean ± SD	1.6 ± 0.3	1.7 ± 0.4	1.6 ± 0.3	1.5 ± 0.2
6 vs. 6 (Hi-res)	1.35	0.79	1.22	0.95

Table 1 shows that the gold standard can be defined fairly precisely, with the mean RMS error at less than 2 mm. There is no dependence of precision on the anatomy of interest, indicating that inaccuracies arise mostly due to variability in segmenting a particular region, rather than deciding if that region should or should not be segmented. Finally and as expected, we found that the high-resolution image set (image 6 result) could be segmented significantly more precisely than the lower resolution images (mean result).

To determine the accuracy of the customization procedure, one of the two segmentations obtained above for each part of the heart anatomy was randomly selected for every volunteer image. The high-resolution image (6) was then chosen to form the template models, and was registered to each of the remaining images (1 through 5). The error in the customization process was then calculated as the RMS Euclidian distance between the template models, both before and after deformation, and the original target models (Table 2).

Overall, the algorithm was successful at customizing the template models to a given target image. On average 70% of the unregistered RMS distance was eliminated, with the best results seen in the LVM, due to the high contrast of this structure in MR images. Higher errors of 3.6 ± 0.4 mm for the RAV models and 3.5 ±

0.3 mm for the LAAo models are not unexpected due to the 1.5×1.5×6 mm^3 voxel size in the target images. Voxel size not only affects the accuracy of the registration, but also the creation of the imperfect "gold standard" model, as seen in Table 1. The errors presented in Table 2 therefore include components that are overestimated (errors calculated with imperfect gold standard) and underestimated (nearest neighbor surface correspondence method).

Table 2. RMS Euclidian distance between the template models before and after customization and the target models. Correspondence was established using nearest points. Unregistered (before customization) results were obtained with models after the centroid alignment stage of registration.

Data	Unregistered RMS (mm) for:				Registered RMS (mm) for:			
Compared	LVM	RAV	LAAo	EH	LVM	RAV	LAAo	EH
6 vs. 1	7.03	8.49	9.34	8.56	3.23	3.72	3.77	3.42
6 vs. 2	9.01	11.16	8.94	9.87	3.12	3.97	3.54	3.37
6 vs. 3	11.25	13.38	17.54	15.91	2.52	3.25	3.09	2.66
6 vs. 4	8.27	10.78	10.63	10.67	2.68	3.05	3.29	3.54
6 vs. 5	10.95	12.80	13.71	13.82	2.89	4.04	3.59	3.14
Mean±SD	9.3±1.8	11.3±1.9	12.0±3.6	11.8±3.0	2.9±0.3	3.6±0.4	3.5±0.3	3.2±0.4

3.2 Canine CT Images

As for the MR images, the intra-observer variability of the gold standard was quantified by manually segmenting each image twice, and by calculating the RMS Euclidian distance between model pairs. The results are shown in Table 3 below.

Table 3. RMS Euclidian distance between pairs of manually segmented surfaces showing the intra-observer variability of the gold standard. Correspondence was established using nearest points. Image 2 is from the same subject, obtained on two different days.

Data Compared	RMS (mm) for EC
1 vs. 1	0.68
2a vs. 2a	1.06
2b vs. 2b	0.91
3 vs. 3	0.98
Mean ± SD	0.9 ± 0.2

Data in Table 3 show a marked improvement in the intra-observer variability obtained with CT images compared to MR. This is most likely due to the almost 88 times increase in resolution of our CT images compared to our MR images, as well as the reduction in breathing motion artefacts achieved in the idealized canine images.

To determine the accuracy of the customization procedure, one of the two segmentations obtained above was randomly selected for each subject. One image was arbitrarily chosen to form the template model and was then registered to each of the remaining images. The error in the customization process was then calculated as the RMS Euclidian distance between the template models, both before and after deformation, and the original target models (Table 4).

Table 4. RMS Euclidian distance between the template models before and after customization and the target models. Correspondence was established using nearest points. Unregistered (before customization) results were obtained with models after the centroid alignment stage of registration.

Data Compared	Unregistered RMS (mm) for EC	Registered RMS (mm) for EC
1 vs. 2a	6.15	2.52
1 vs. 2b	6.06	2.62
1 vs. 3	6.84	2.07
Mean ± SD	6.3 ± 0.4	2.4 ± 0.3

The customization procedure with CT images yields models that are significantly more accurate than those obtained with the MR images. Again, note that the error in Table 4 contains components that are overestimated (calculated with imperfect gold standard) and underestimated (nearest neighbor surface correspondence method). The CT data yield better results than MR due to the increased resolution, ideal breath holding, and shorter scan duration.

4   Conclusions and Future Work

In this paper we have presented a registration algorithm for mapping template heart models to target images. Validation experiments on human and canine data showed that the method is sufficiently accurate (considering the imperfections in the gold standards) - customizing models with an error on the order of some of the smallest targets for minimally invasive cardiac surgery (coronary arteries). The method was especially successful with CT images, due to the improvement in resolution compared to MR, and the idealized scanning protocol used.

In the future we will use a more robust method of establishing correspondence between two surfaces when calculating registration error. While the nearest point method has been sufficient in this initial study, more sophisticated methods will be required for a thorough investigation. We also plan to perform validation studies on excised hearts, which can easily be segmented if scanned in air, and then surrounded by tissue-mimicking materials to model the heart surroundings in-vivo. Furthermore, we will combine this work and our previous approach [9] to investigate the effects of template registration error on model dynamics, to fully characterize the accuracy of our patient-specific, dynamic models of the heart.

Acknowledgements. The authors thank Aaron So and John Moore for the images, Rhonda Walcarius for MR acquisition, Atamai, Inc. for visualization software, and Ravi Gupta for help with code development. We also acknowledge funding from the Canadian Institutes of Health Research (MOP 14735), Canadian Heart and Stroke Foundation (NA 4755), Ontario Consortium for Image-guided Surgery and Therapy, National Science and Engineering Research Council of Canada, and the University of Western Ontario.

References

1. King, R.C., Reece, T.B., Hurst, J.L., Shockley, K.S., Tribble, C.G., Spotnitz, W.D., and Kron, I.L.: Minimally Invasive Coronary Artery Bypass Grafting Decreases Hospital Stay and Cost. Ann Surg 225(6) (1997) 805-811
2. Stevens, J.H., Burdin, T.A., Peters, W.S., Siegel, L.C., Pompili, M.F., Vierra, M.A., St.Goar, F.G., Ribakove, G.H., Mitchell, R.S., and Reitz, B.A.: Port-Access Coronary Artery Bypass Grafting: A Proposed Surgical Method. J Thorac Cardiovasc Surg 111(1996) 567-573
3. Pike, N. and Gundry, S.: Robotically Assisted Cardiac Surgery. J Cardiovasc Nurs 18(5) (2003) 382-388
4. Herzog, C., Dogan, S., Diebold, T., Khan, M.F., Ackermann, H., Schaller, S., Flohr, T.G., Wimmer-Greinecker, G., Moritz, A., and Vogl, T.J.: Multi-Detector Row CT versus Coronary Angiography: Preoperative Evaluation before Totally Endoscopic Coronary Artery Bypass Grafting. Radiology 229(2003) 200-208
5. Boyd, W.D., Desai, N.D., Kiaii, B., Rayman, R., Menkis, A.H., McKenzie, F.N., and Novick, R.J.: A Comparison of Robot-Assisted Versus Manually Constructed Endoscopic Coronary Anastomosis. Ann Thorac Surg 70(2000) 839-843
6. Chiu, A.M., Dey, D., Drangova, M., Boyd, W.D., and Peters, T.M.: 3-D Image Guidance for Minimally Invasive Robotic Coronary Artery Bypass. Heart Surg Forum 3(3) (2000) 224-231
7. Sørensen, T.S., Therkildsen, S., V, Knudsen, J.L., and Pedersen, E.M.: A New Virtual Reality Approach for Planning of Cardiac Intervention. Artif Intell Med 22(3) (2001) 193-214
8. Lorenzo-Valdés, M., Sanchez-Ortiz, G., I, Mohiaddin, R., and Ruckert, D.: Atlas-Based Segmentation and Tracking of 3D Cardiac MR Images Using Non-rigid Registration. MICCAI 2002, LNCS 2488(2002) 642-650
9. Wierzbicki, M. and Peters, T.M.: Determining Epicardial Surface Motion Using Elastic Registration: Towards Virtual Reality Guidance of Minimally Invasive Cardiac Interventions. MICCAI 2003, LNCS 2878(2003) 722-729
10. Moore, J., Drangova, M., Wierzbicki, M., Barron, J., and Peters, T.M.: A High Resolution Dynamic Heart Model Based on Averaged MRI Data. MICCAI 2003, LNCS 2878(2003) 549-555
11. Lorensen, W.E. and Cline, H.E.: Marching Cubes: A High Resolution 3D Surface Construction Algorithm. Comput Graph (ACM) 21(4) (1987) 163-169
12. Schroeder, W.J., Zarge, J.A., and Lorensen, W.E.: Decimation of Triangle Meshes. SIGGRAPH 92(26) (1992) 65-70
13. Nelder, J.A. and Mead, R.: A simplex method for function minimization. Computer Journal 7(1965) 308-313
14. Studholme, C., Hill, D.L.G., and Hawkes, D.J.: An overlap invariant entropy measure of 3D medical image alignment. Pattern Recognit 32(1) (1999) 71-86
15. Ruckert, D., Sonoda, L., I, Hayes, C., Hill, D.L.G., Leach, M.O., and Hawkes, D.J.: Nonrigid Registration Using Free-Form Deformations: Application to Breast MR Images. IEEE Trans Med Imaging 18(8) (1999) 712-721

A Framework for Detailed Objective Comparison of Non-rigid Registration Algorithms in Neuroimaging

William R. Crum[1], Daniel Rueckert[2], Mark Jenkinson[3], David Kennedy[4], and Stephen M. Smith[3]

[1] Computational Imaging Science Group, Division of Imaging Sciences, Thomas Guy House, Guy's Hospital, Kings College London, London SE1 9RT, UK, `bill.crum@kcl.ac.uk`
[2] Department of Computing, Imperial College, London SW7 2AZ, UK
[3] Oxford Centre for Functional Magnetic Resonance Imaging of the Brain, John Radcliffe Hospital, Headington, Oxford OX3 9DU, UK
[4] Center for Morphometric Analysis, Department of Neurology, MGH, 13th Street, Charlestown MA 02129, USA

Abstract. Non-rigid image registration is widely used in the analysis of brain images to the extent it is provided as a standard tool in common packages such as SPM. However the performance of algorithms in specific applications remains hard to measure. In this paper a detailed comparison of the performance of an affine, B-Spline control-point and viscous fluid registration algorithm in inter-subject brain registration is presented. The comparison makes use of highly detailed expert manual labellings of a range of structures distributed in scale and in location in the brain. The overall performance is B-Spline, fluid, affine (best first) with all algorithms struggling to improve the match of smaller structures. We discuss caveats, evaluation strategies for registration and implications for future registration-based neuroimaging studies.

1 Introduction

Image registration is now widely used in medical image analysis but detailed comparison of the performance and suitability of algorithms for specific applications remains difficult, especially in the non-rigid case. In brain image analysis a common task is to register an MRI brain scan of one subject to another or to a template image in standard anatomical space. This is challenging due to population variability in cortical anatomy and the poorly specified nature of anatomical versus functional correspondence [1]. Many registration algorithms exist which can attempt this task but one persistent problem is how to conduct a detailed evaluation of such algorithms under realistic conditions.

In this paper we describe an application-centric framework for comparison and use it to evaluate the relative success of applying an affine [2], B-Spline [3] and viscous fluid registration (e.g. [4]) to the problem of inter-subject brain registration. This comparison framework makes use of highly detailed expert labelling of neuro-anatomical structures on a set of test images [5], [6]. These labels allow two assessments to be made: (i) an assessment of the relative performance of the registration algorithms in aligning specific structures or tissue classes (ii) a generic assessment of

C. Barillot, D.R. Haynor, and P. Hellier (Eds.): MICCAI 2004, LNCS 3216, pp. 679–686, 2004.

which structures fail to be well registered by any algorithm. The latter case has important implications for the efficacy of large-scale neuroimaging studies where the identification of structural or functional differences relies on non-rigid registration. The evaluation is "application-centric" in that it tests the ability of each algorithm to bring a series of neuroanatomical structures into alignment, rather than testing the absolute correctness of the algorithms in recovering a known transformation between two data-sets. We put no conditions on how the registration algorithms were applied beyond suggesting that default or typical parameter settings should be used and that the registrations should be run once using these settings. We are assessing suitability for the task rather than performing a detailed technical comparison of algorithms.

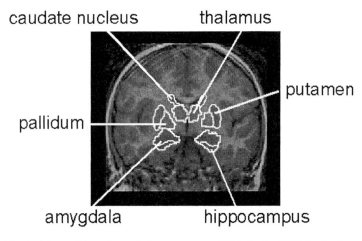

Fig. 1. A few of the sub-cortical structures available in the CMA brain data.

2   Method

2.1   Evaluation Data

We made use of eight labelled MR brain images obtained from the Centre of Morphometric Analysis at MGH (Boston). This centre has spent many years performing detailed reproducible manual labelling of MRI brain images [5], [6]. Each voxel has associated binary labels that identify it as a member of particular structures or tissue classes; there are 84 sub-cortical labels and 48 cortical labels. These brain images and a subset of the labels are available for use by the research community from the Internet Brain Segmentation Repository (http://www.cma.mgh.harvard.edu/ibsr/). For this work, the original labels have been grouped to produce a smaller hierarchy ranging from the entire brain and the primary lobes down to structures such as the hippocampus and the thalamus (see Table 1 for the full list of labels and Fig. 1 for some examples). The chosen groupings are arbitrary and can be defined to suit any specific application. In this paper we refer to the set of grouped labels as the test labels.

Table 1. The four groups of test labels used in the evaluation. The number of original anatomical labels used to create each test label is shown in brackets.

Major Structures	Major Lobes	Other Structures	Sub-Cortical
All (32)	Frontal (14)	Lat. Ventricle (2)	Thalamus (2)
Brain (25)	Occipital (8)	Cerebellum (4)	Caudate (2)
Cortex (6)	Parietal (7)	Brain Stem (3)	Putamen (2)
White Matter (2)	Temporal (16)	Sub-Cortex (10)	Pallidum (2)
CSF (7)			Hippocampus (2)
			Amygdala (2)

2.2 Evaluation Algorithms

Three non-rigid registration algorithms were evaluated. These were (a) an affine registration algorithm (FLIRT) available as part of the FSL image analysis toolkit (www.fmrib.ox.ac.uk/fsl) [2], [7] (b) a free-form deformation algorithm based on B-Splines [3], [8] and (c) a viscous fluid algorithm implemented following [4] and [9].

FLIRT: The affine registration method, FLIRT (FMRIB's Linear Registration Tool), was chosen as robust affine registration is widely used to register brain images and affine transformations are sufficient to successfully align many brain structures between individuals despite the relatively small number of degrees of freedom in the transformation model. It is designed to be highly robust to the initial alignment of the images by using a customised global optimisation method that runs over multiple scales (8, 4, 2 and 1mm); a large search space in rotation and scale is used at the 8mm resolution and many smaller perturbations on the best three candidate solutions used in the 4mm resolution. In addition, the cost functions are regularised such that they de-weight contributions near the edge of the overlapping field of view in order to produce a smoothly changing cost function. All of these factors combine to reduce the chance of the registration becoming "trapped" in a local minimum of the cost function. The correlation ratio is used to drive the registration.

B-SPLINE: Non-rigid registration based on free-form deformations and B-Splines is widely used in many registration applications including those involving inter-subject brain registration. The basic idea of FFDs is to deform an object by manipulating an underlying mesh of control points. The optimal control point locations are found by minimising a cost function which encompasses two competing goals: the first term represents the cost associated with the voxel-based similarity measure, in this case normalised mutual information, while the second term corresponds to a regularisation term which constrains the transformation to be smooth. The control-point spacing was set at 2.5mm for this study.

FLUID: The fluid methods have been used successfully for intra-subject brain registration [10] [11] and for registering structures from one brain to another [4]. They use a mathematical model of a compressible viscous fluid to model the transformation between images. They can accommodate large deformations but can be less robust than other methods without good initialisation. Therefore the fluid algorithm was initialised from a locally derived affine registration of each subject into a standard anatomical space. Additionally the registration was terminated after 5 regridding steps to reduce the influence of numerical error. The intensity cross correlation was used to drive the registration as in [9].

2.3 Evaluation Measures

We observe that for most applications of non-rigid registration in neuroimaging it is correspondence of brain structures on a variety of scales that is important as the absolute correctness of the transformation model cannot usually be determined; a corollary is that the amount of information contained in an MR brain image is insufficient to assess the point-accuracy of the registration but anatomical structures can be tested for correspondence post registration. Therefore the test labels that we have generated from the CMA data represent a natural means for evaluation of registration algorithms that is closely tied to their uses for neuroimaging research. Given pairs of test-labels, S and T, on registered brains a method for evaluating their overlap is required. There is considerable literature in this area, much of it applied to the assessment of segmentation algorithms (e.g. [12]). In this work we use P, the ratio of the number of overlapping voxels to the total number of voxels in the labelled structures.

$$P = \frac{N(S \cap T)}{N(S \cup T)} \tag{1}$$

This measure has been widely used but has the known disadvantage that errors in labelling small structures are magnified compared with larger structures.

2.4 Evaluation Framework

Each of the eight test subjects was registered to the other seven subjects using each of the three algorithms giving 56 inter-subject registrations for each algorithm. The registrations were run by the researchers most familiar with their operation; these researchers made any necessary parameter choices independently. After registration, each of the 19 test labels on each subject was transformed into the space of all the other subjects using the transformations determined by each registration algorithm. The binary labels were transformed using trilinear interpolation and then thresholded at 50% to produce transformed binary labels. The test-label overlap, P, was computed in all cases and this data was analysed to produce a mean and standard deviation fractional overlap for each test-label for each registration algorithm. The overlaps were also computed for all pairs of unregistered scans for comparison.

3 Results

The FLIRT registrations took approximately 5 minutes each to run on a contemporary desk-top Linux PC. Both the B-Spline and fluid registrations were run in a distributed fashion on a Linux condor cluster (one CPU per registration) and typically took be-

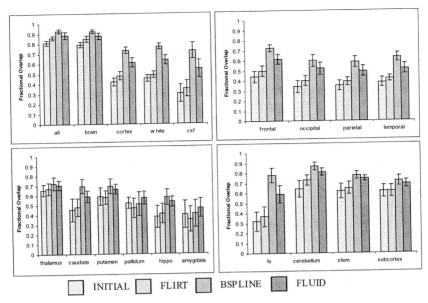

Fig. 2. The mean and standard deviation of the overlap measure for each structure registered by each registration algorithm. INITIAL refers to the original images.

tween 2 and 10 hours per registration. The results are summarised in Fig. 2. For each of the test labels, the mean fractional overlap is shown for each registration algorithm and the error bars show ±1 s.d. Some general observations can be made. In all cases all registration algorithms improved the mean label overlap except for the case of FLIRT applied to the pallidum and amygdala. We might expect that the potential accuracy of matching increases with the degrees of freedom available to the algorithms but that the potential for mis-registration also increases. In fact what we found is that for this study, the B-Spline method consistently performed well and was only outperformed by the fluid method for two structures (the pallidum and amygdala) where all methods struggled to improve the overlap. Conversely the B-Spline method proved far superior to all other methods for registering the larger tissue compartments (cortex, white, csf and lateral ventricle). There are some caveats associated with these results. The most obvious is that the sample-size of subject data is relatively small but another important point is that as part of the labelling process, the subject data was realigned and had already been interpolated prior to our analysis. This might have the largest impact on the alignment of small structures.

4   Discussion

We have assessed the ability of three registration algorithms to align a variety of brain structures between eight subjects and found overlaps ranging from ~0.3 (lateral ventricle) to ~0.9 (brain). The results enable us to distinguish the performance of the algorithms over different parts of the brain. Notable is that the B-Spline algorithm matches CSF and lateral ventricle particularly well, no algorithms match the major lobes better than ~0.7 and that there is less difference between the algorithms ability to match the sub-cortical structures than a consideration of the degrees of freedom of the transformation model used in each case might suggest. We would normally expect the largest increase in overlap to be achieved by the affine registration compared with no registration however due to the realignment applied to the images prior to manual segmentation the observed increases are relatively small. The fact that each algorithm used a different image similarity measure must impact on the results but reflects the current lack of consensus and deep understanding of the operation of such measures.

The most relevant recent work on registration evaluation is Hellier et al [13] where six registration algorithms were compared using a variety of measures including tissue overlap, correlation of differential characteristics and sulcal shape characteristics. They found that algorithms with higher degrees of freedom did not perform proportionately better at matching cortical sulci and that inter-subject cortical variability remains a severe challenge for voxel-based non-rigid algorithms. These findings are consistent with our experience. Their choice of a single reference subject could be a source of bias that we avoid by registering all permutations of the test subjects. Previously, Grachev et al [14] suggested using 128 carefully defined and manually placed landmarks per hemisphere to evaluate inter-subject registration accuracy. This approach, like ours, requires significant operator expertise to identify features. Landmarks enable a millimetre error to be computed but labels allow assessment that is more easily related to correspondence of the underlying neuroanatomy. Label-based evaluation approaches can also estimate the degree to which non-rigid registration can align anatomically and functionally important areas of the brain. This might prove important for establishing error bounds in studies using registration to compare groups of individuals. Another application is in serial scanning of individuals where labels defined on the first scan in a sequence may be propagated to subsequent scans using non-rigid registration.

Simple voxel-intensity driven algorithms will not on their own resolve the outstanding problem of cortical variability between subjects but are likely to remain useful for matching the locale of similar cortical structures. This degree of matching may be perfectly adequate for many applications especially where explicit allowance is made for uncertainty in structural matching e.g. in Voxel Based Morphometry [15]. For more specialised applications hybrid approaches may be required; for example cortical matching may be improved - or at least better controlled – by exploiting work done by Maudgil et al [16] where 24 points which were determined to be homologous between subjects were identified on the cortical surface. Such points can be incorporated into voxel-based registration algorithms [17].

There remain some questions as to the best way to define label overlaps. The measure we use in this paper is well known but does not account explicitly for inconsistency in the labelling process nor does it indicate the nature of the error in non-perfect overlaps. Crum et al [1] suggest the use of a tolerance parameter with overlap measures so that, for instance with the tolerance set to 1 voxel, the boundaries of two labels are regarded as completely overlapping if they are at most one voxel away from each other. A deeper consideration of overlap measures and the incorporation of labelling error is an urgent priority.

We plan to extend this study by including more registration algorithms and more labelled subjects in the evaluation. Future work will focus on a more detailed technical comparison of algorithms but this initial work has provided a benchmark for future performance in two ways. First, other registration techniques can be easily tested within the same framework for an operational comparison. Second, we can recognise that these algorithms are subject to many parameter choices that we have ignored in this study. We can optimise the parameter choice for each algorithm with respect to this well-defined task; this optimisation process may ultimately lead to new methods tuned to register structures of particular scale and intensity characteristics.

Acknowledgments. The authors are grateful for the intellectual and financial support of the Medical Images and Signals IRC (EPSRC and MRC GR/N14248/01). This work was made possible by the research environment created by this consortium. We also acknowledge valuable contributions from Professor David Hawkes and Dr Derek Hill.

References

1. Crum, W.R., Griffin, L.D., Hill, D.L.G. and Hawkes, D.J. : Zen and the Art of Medical Image Registration : Correspondence Homology and Quality. NeuroImage 20 (2003) 1425-1437
2. Jenkinson, M. and Smith, S.M. : A Global Optimisation Method for Robust Affine Registration of Brain Images. Medical Image Analysis 5(2) (2001) 143-156
3. Rueckert, D., Sonoda, L.I., Hayes, C., Hill, D.L.G., Leach, M.O. and Hawkes, D.J. : Non-Rigid Registration Using Free-Form Deformations: Application to Breast MR images. IEEE Transactions on Medical Imaging 18(8) (1999) 712-721
4. Christensen, G.E., Joshi S.C. and Miller, M.I. : Volumetric Transformation of Brain Anatomy. IEEE Transactions on Medical Imaging 16(6) (1997) 864-877
5. Kennedy, D.N., Fillipek, P.A. and Caviness, V.S. : Anatomic Segmentation and Volumetric Calculations in Nuclear Magnetic Resonance Imaging. IEEE Transactions on Medical Imaging 8 (1989) 1-7
6. Caviness, V.S., Meyer, J., Makris, N. and Kennedy, D.N. : MRI-based Topographic Parcellation of the Human Neocortex: an Anatomically Specified Method With Estimate of Reliability. Journal of Cognitive Neuroscience 8 (1996) 566-587
7. Jenkinson, M., Bannister, P., Brady, J.M. and Smith, S.M. : Improved Optimisation for the Robust and Accurate Linear Registration and Motion Correction of Brain Images. NeuroImage 17(2) (2002) 825-841
8. Rueckert, D., Frangi, A.F. and Schnabel, J.A. : Automatic Construction of 3D Statistical Deformation Models of the Brain using Non-Rigid Registration. IEEE Transactions on Medical Imaging 22(8) (2003) 1014-1025
9. Freeborough, P.A. and Fox, N.C. : Modeling Brain Deformations in Alzheimer Disease By Fluid Registration of Serial 3D MR Images. Journal of Computer Assisted Tomography 22(5) (1998) 838-843
10. Crum, W.R., Scahill, R.I., Fox, N.C. : Automated Hippocampal Segmentation by Regional Fluid Registration of Serial MRI : Validation and Application in Alzheimer's Disease. NeuroImage 13(5) (2001) 847-855
11. Fox, N.C., Crum, W.R., Scahill, R.I., Stevens, J.M., Janssen, J.C. and Rossor, M.N. : Imaging of Onset and Progression of Alzheimer's Disease with Voxel-Compression Mapping of Serial MRI. The Lancet 358 (2001) 201-205
12. Gerig, G., Jomier, M. and Chakos, M. : Valmet: A new validation tool for assessing and improving 3D object segmentation. In : Medical Image Computing and Computer-Assisted Intervention. Lecture Notes in Computer Science, Vol. 2208, Springer-Verlag, Berlin Heidelberg New York (2001) 516-528

13. Hellier, P., Barillot, I., Corouge, B., Gibaud, G., Le Goualher, G., Collins, D.L., Evans, A., Malandain, G., Ayache, N., Christensen, G.E. and Johnson H.J. : Retrospective Evaluation of Intersubject Brain Registration. IEEE Transactions on Medical Imaging, 22(9) (2003) 1120-1130

14. Grachev, I.D., Berdichevsky D., Rauch, S.L., Heckers, S., Kennedy, D.N., Caviness V.S. amd Alpert, N.M. : A Method For Assessing the Accuracy of Intersubject Registration of the Human Brain Using Anatomic Landmarks, NeuroImage 9 (1999) 250-268

15. Ashburner, J., and Friston, K.J. : Voxel-Based Morphometry – the Methods. NeuroImage 11 (2000) 805-821

16. Maudgil, D.D., Free, S.L., Sisodiya, S.M., Lemieux, L., Woermann, F.G., Fish, D.R., and Shorvon, S.D. : Identifying Homologous Anatomical Landmarks On Reconstructed Magnetic Resonance Images of the Human Cerebral Cortical Surface. Journal of Anatomy 193 (1998) 559-571

17. Hartkens, T., Hill, D.L.G., Castellano-Smith, A.D., Hawkes, D.J., Maurer, C.R., Martin, A.J., Hall, W.A., Liu, H. and Truwit, C.L. : Using Points and Surfaces to Improve Voxel-Based Non-Rigid Registration. in : Medical Image Computing and Computer-Assisted Intervention. Lecture Notes in Computer Science, Vol. 2489, Springer-Verlag, Berlin Heidelberg New York (2002) 565-572

Evaluation of Registration of Ictal SPECT/MRI Data Using Statistical Similarity Methods

Christophe Grova[1,2], Pierre Jannin[2], Irène Buvat[3], Habib Benali[3], and Bernard Gibaud[2]

[1] Montreal Neurological Institute, McGill University, Montreal
{christophe.grova}@mail.mcgill.ca
[2] Laboratoire IDM, Faculté de Médecine, Université de Rennes 1, France
{pierre.jannin,bernard.gibaud}@univ-rennes1.fr,
http://idm.univ-rennes1.fr
[3] INSERM U494, CHU Pitié Salpétrière, Paris
{irene.buvat,habib.benali}@imed.jussieu.fr

Abstract. In this study, we evaluated SPECT/MRI registration of ictal data, using similarity based registration methods. An absolute gold standard for registration evaluation was obtained by considering realistic normal and ictal SPECT simulations deduced from a high resolution T1-weighted MRI data set.

Those simulations were also used to study the impact of photon attenuation and Compton scatter corrections on registration accuracy. Evaluation of registration was also performed using inconsistency measurements for six patients with temporo-mesial epilepsy. For these data, as no Gold Standard was available, registration accuracy was assessed using inconsistency measurements involving a registration loop between inter-ictal SPECT, ictal SPECT and MRI data. Five registration methods based on statistical similarity measurements were compared, namely: mutual information (MI), normalized mutual information (NMI), L1 and L2 norm-based correlation ratios (CR) and correlation coefficient (CC). It was found that the simulation context had more influence on registration accuracy than the choice of the similarity criterion. Ictal SPECT as well as correction for uniform attenuation clearly decreased SPECT/MRI registration accuracy.

1 Introduction

Evaluation of SPECT/MRI registration methods is a difficult problem, especially when dealing with pathological data, such as ictal SPECT reflecting extreme perfusion changes occurring during an epileptic seizure. As ictal SPECT is currently the only imaging technique available to explore the ictal state in epilepsy with high sensitivity, achieving accurate registration with the anatomical MRI provides valuable information during the presurgical investigation. The purpose of this study is to perform a quantitative evaluation of SPECT/MRI statistical similarity-based registration methods, especially when dealing with ictal SPECT. Ictal SPECT usually shows large hyperperfusion that is likely

C. Barillot, D.R. Haynor, and P. Hellier (Eds.): MICCAI 2004, LNCS 3216, pp. 687–695, 2004.
© Springer-Verlag Berlin Heidelberg 2004

to occur during a seizure, whereas the anatomical MRI is generally considered as normal. Such situation creates intrinsic dissimilarities between SPECT and MRI data, that may affect registration methods based on statistical similarity measurements.

Quantitative evaluation of a registration method requires a reference geometrical transformation. When it refers to a ground truth, this reference transformation is called a Gold Standard. Although skin fiducial markers were used in some studies [1], the studies evaluating registration involving SPECT data generally lack any accurate gold standard. Evaluation on real data generally uses the result of one or several other registration methods as the reference transformation (e.g., [2]). Absolute gold standard may be obtained using physical phantom [3] or numerical simulations [2,4] of SPECT data. The effect of the dissimilarities introduced by ictal SPECT on registration accuracy has only been studied in the case of SPECT/SPECT registration [3]. The behaviour of registration methods in the presence of hypoperfused pathological areas has been studied under controlled conditions using numerical simulations [2,4]. When using numerical simulations, attention must be paid to the realism of the simulations, and validation bias may be introduced by the simulation method itself.

In the present study, we further investigate a validation methodology we first proposed in [5]. Attention was paid to a standardized description of our validation procedure [6]. Our registration evaluation method consisted in using realistic simulations of SPECT data, obtained from an anatomical MRI. We improved the accuracy of the perfusion model for SPECT simulations, using measurements performed on real data [7]. Pathological simulations mimicking ictal perfusion in temporal lobe epilepsy were added to normal SPECT simulations. Moreover, the simulations were used to assess the effect of attenuation and Compton scatter corrections on registration accuracy. Finally, our results were compared to those obtained on real data by measuring inconsistencies between the registrations of MRI, inter-ictal SPECT and ictal SPECT data of six subjects.

2   Material and Methods

2.1   Statistical Similarity-Based Registration Methods

We considered SPECT/MRI registration as rigid intra-patient registration. The purpose is to assess a rigid geometric T transformation defined by six parameters (three translations and three rotations). Let the reference image R be our SPECT data set and the floating image F our MRI data set. Statistical similarity-based registration methods assume that a similarity measurement $S(R, T(F))$ is optimal when the data sets are perfectly registered. Let us call f the theoretical function that relates intensities of both images, if it exists.

A first class of criteria are obtained by searching the optimal distance measurement on intensity values, given an *a priori* on the nature of f. The correlation coefficient (CC) is thus obtained under the assumption that f is linear. Assuming that there is a functional dependence between R and $T(F)$, without any assumption regarding the nature of f, Roche *et al.* [8] proposed to use the correlation ratio (CR). Two implementations of CR were studied here using the L1 and L2 norms as metrics in the intensity space. A second class of criteria assess similarity taking into account only information provided by intensity distributions of both images. Relying on entropy measurements, Mutual Information (MI)[9] measures a statistical dependence, making no assumptions regarding the nature of this dependence. Normalized Mutual Information (NMI) [10] is moreover invariant to the region overlapping between the two data sets.

Registration method implementation: All the similarity criteria were maximized according to the rigid transformation T, using Powell's multidimensional direction set method. $\hat{T}$ will denote the result of a registration method. 256-bin histograms and partial volume interpolation [9] were used to compute these similarity criteria. A two-level multiresolution strategy as described by [9] was applied to avoid the pitfall of local optima.

2.2   Validation Procedure

Characterization of the validation objective: We wanted to study the impact of ictal condition on SPECT/MRI registration. This study was performed in a fully controlled environment using simulated normal and ictal SPECT data as well as with real data for which no gold standard was available. The second objective of this study was to assess the impact of attenuation and scatter correction methods on registration accuracy.

Validation data sets: Validation data sets consisted of SPECT simulations generated from one MRI data set. The method to produce realistic SPECT simulations from MRI data was described in [7]. Simulations of SPECT data required an activity map representing the 3D spatial distribution of the radiotracer (^{99m}Tc-HMPAO) and the associated attenuation map describing the attenuation properties of the body. Monte Carlo simulations were used to model the response of a SPECT imaging system. Whereas Monte Carlo techniques are widely recognized to accurately model SPECT data [11], particular attention was paid to the realism of activity maps.

Generation of theoretical perfusion models: Theoretical normal and ictal perfusion models, i.e., activity maps, were deduced from measurements performed on anatomically standardized SPECT data. To perform perfusion measurements, we used Volumes of Interest (VOIs) deduced from an anatomically labelled T1-weighted MRI, Zubal phantom [12] (124 axial slices, matrix: 256×256, voxel size: $1.1 \times 1.1 \times 1.4$ mm^3). A theoretical map of photon attenuation coefficients was defined by assigning to each VOI a tissue type and an attenuation coefficient μ at $140keV$ for ^{99m}Tc. To define activity maps, an average model of normal perfusion was derived from the analysis of 27 normal SPECT data. Similarly, an average model of ictal perfusion was created from the analysis of 10 ictal SPECT data from patients showing a mesio-temporal epilepsy pattern. Several correction methods were taken into account to derive realistic activity values in the different compartments of our perfusion models. Assuming uniform attenuation in the head, first order Chang attenuation correction was performed. Scatter correction was only performed for the healthy subjects using the Jaszczak method. To derive a perfusion model as accurate as possible, perfusion measurements were corrected for partial volume effect (see [7] for a detailed description).

Monte Carlo SPECT simulations: Using attenuation and ^{99m}Tc-HMPAO activity maps, Monte Carlo simulations were performed using SimSET[1] [13]. Sixty-four projections over 360° (matrix: 128×128, pixel size: $4.51mm$) were simulated using a 20% energy window centred on 140 keV (126 - 154 keV) and a (111 - 125 keV) Compton window. All SPECT projections were then reconstructed by filtered backprojection using a ramp filter (Nyquist frequency cutoff) followed by 3D Gaussian filtering ($FWHM = 8mm$), leading to a spatial resolution of $FWHM = 12.2mm$ (see Figure 1). To assess the impact of several correction methods on registration accuracy, uniform attenuation correction (AC) and/or Jaszczak scatter correction (SC) methods were used. All simulated data will be referred to using a "simulation context" name (see Table 1).

Table 1. Simulation contexts explored by SPECT/MRI registration evaluation. Attenuation correction refers to first order Chang uniform correction, and scatter correction refers to Jaszczak window subtraction method.

Simulation context	Perfusion model	Correction methods
Normal none	average normal	none
Normal AC	average normal	attenuation correction
Normal SC	average normal	scatter correction
Normal SAC	average normal	attenuation + scatter correction
Ictal none	average ictal	none
Ictal AC	average ictal	attenuation correction
Ictal SC	average ictal	scatter correction
Ictal SAC	average ictal	attenuation + scatter correction

Clinical data for inconsistency measurements: Inconsistency measurements make it possible to study registration performance without any Gold Standard, when more than two data sets are available for each subject [2]. Among the 10 patients with mesio-temporal epilepsy, six subjects were selected, for whom inter-ictal and ictal SPECT, and anatomical MRI were available. Sampling rate, image dimensions and spatial resolution were similar to those used on simulated data.

Reference geometrical transformation:

Estimation of registration absolute errors: Simulated SPECT data being perfectly aligned with the MRI of Zubal phantom, our methodology provided us with an absolute Gold Standard for registration evaluation. $N_t = 50$ theoretical transformations T^* were generated by randomly sampling a 6 parameter vector

---

[1] Simulation System for Emission Tomography (SimSET) software package:
http://depts.washington.edu/~simset/html/simset_main.html

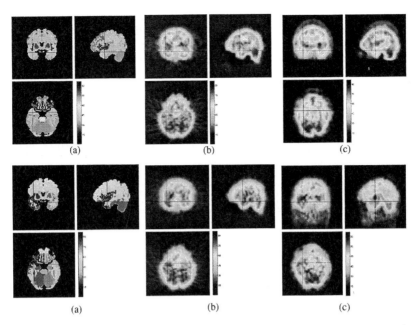

(a)   (b)   (c)

(a)   (b)   (c)

Fig. 1. Theoretical average perfusion model (a), corresponding SPECT simulation (b), and an example of a real SPECT data (c) for normal perfusion (top) and for ictal perfusion characteristic of mesio-temporal lobe epilepsy (bottom).

using a Gaussian distribution (Mean = 0, Standard Deviation = 10 mm or ^{o}). T^* was then applied to the MRI data and new unregistered MRIs were thus created using trilinear interpolation. Registrations were then sequentially performed using each pair of simulated SPECT and unregistered MRI. Let us call $\hat{T}$ the resulting computed geometric transformation.

Estimation of registration inconsistencies: As no Gold Standard was available for clinical data, registration loops allowed us to measure registration inconsistency (see for instance [2]). We assumed that inter-ictal SPECT → MRI transformation ($\hat{T}_{12}$) followed by MRI → ictal SPECT transformation ($\hat{T}_{23}$) should lead to the same transformation as the one provided by direct inter-ictal SPECT → ictal SPECT registration ($\hat{T}_{13}$). Those three registrations were performed using each method, on each of $N_t = 6$ subjects, and on SPECT data being corrected or not from uniform attenuation.

Validation criteria: Spatial registration errors or inconsistencies were estimated on $N_p = 1600$ points $\mathbf{x}_i$ uniformly distributed within the brain. For each registration test j, for each validation data set (cf. Table 1), and for each point $\mathbf{x}_i$ sampled within the brain, a local target registration error (TRE_{ij}) or a local inconsistency (INC_{ij}) was estimated as follows:

$$TRE_{ij} = \left\| \mathbf{x}_i - \hat{T}_j^{-1}\left(T_j^*(\mathbf{x}_i)\right) \right\| \ or \ INC_{ij} = \left\| \hat{T}_{13}^j(\mathbf{x}_i) - \hat{T}_{23}^j\left(\hat{T}_{12}^j(\mathbf{x}_i)\right) \right\| \quad (1)$$

Table 2. Validation criteria characterizing distributions of registration RMS_j (*Mean*, σ and $Q90$ in mm) for each similarity criterion. Top: SPECT/MRI registration in each simulation context (50 registrations tested in each case). Bottom : Inconsistencies measurement on clinical data using SPECT data with (AC) and without (none) attenuation correction (6 subjects). In each context, most accurate results are in bold.

Context	MI		NMI		CRL2		CRL1		CC	
	$Mean(\sigma)$	$Q90$	$Mean(\sigma)$	$Q90$	$Mean(\sigma)$	$Q90$	$Mean(\sigma)$	$Q90$	$Mean(\sigma)$	$Q90$
Normal none	2.71 (0.166)	2.90	2.72 (0.196)	2.95	**2.45** (0.221)	2.67	2.59 (0.251)	2.89	2.96 (0.229)	3.21
Normal SC	2.74 (0.180)	2.97	2.76 (0.158)	2.97	**2.38** (0.205)	2.59	2.52 (0.219)	2.71	2.65 (0.287)	3.06
Normal AC	3.10 (0.184)	3.28	3.10 (0.204)	3.33	2.98 (0.236)	3.28	**2.95** (0.233)	3.20	3.36 (0.249)	3.67
Normal SAC	3.19 (0.176)	3.46	3.13 (0.210)	3.42	**2.84** (0.199)	3.12	2.98 (0.215)	3.19	3.10 (0.229)	3.33
Ictal none	3.55 (0.189)	3.79	3.55 (0.229)	3.90	3.32 (0.177)	3.53	**3.29** (0.245)	3.51	4.06 (0.304)	4.50
Ictal SC	3.54 (0.235)	3.82	3.55 (0.182)	3.75	**3.22** (0.248)	3.50	3.37 (0.218)	3.55	3.59 (0.237)	3.85
Ictal AC	4.15 (0.212)	4.39	4.17 (0.197)	4.36	**4.05** (0.173)	4.27	4.09 (0.219)	4.29	4.57 (0.244)	4.80
Ictal SAC	4.11 (0.196)	4.30	4.13 (0.180)	4.32	**3.94** (0.157)	4.13	4.10 (0.227)	4.36	4.30 (0.168)	4.52
Correction	Registration inconsistencies on clinical data									
none	9.00 (3.68)	12.6	10.19 (4.55)	14.8	**7.21** (4.65)	11.7	8.03 (2.39)	10.1	11.12 (7.74)	17.6
AC	10.04 (5.33)	16.3	9.35 (5.14)	15.4	7.88 (4.51)	13.1	**7.67** (5.65)	14.8	11.87 (6.25)	17.4

with $i \in < 1, N_p >$ and $j \in < 1, N_t >$. $\| \ \|$ denotes the Euclidian norm in mm. To characterize the spatial distribution of TRE_{ij} or INC_{ij} within the brain, we estimated the root mean square (RMS_j) value of the local errors or local inconsistencies distribution:

$$RMS_j = \sqrt{\frac{1}{N_p} \sum_{i=1}^{N_p} TRE_{ij}^2} \ \text{ or } \ RMS_j = \sqrt{\frac{1}{N_p} \sum_{i=1}^{N_p} INC_{ij}^2} \qquad (2)$$

The validation criteria of a registration method were finally defined as global characteristics of registration errors or inconsistencies over the N_t registrations tested. Empirical mean (*Mean*) and the 90th quantile ($Q90$) of the RMS_j errors were computed to estimate registration accuracy, and standard deviation (σ) of the RMS_j errors was used to assess registration precision.

3 Results

3.1 Simulated SPECT/MRI Registration Errors

Distribution of registration errors RMS_j are summarized on Table 2. All statistical similarity-based registration methods were proved to be very accurate as all mean RMS errors were significantly lower than the SPECT voxel size of 4.51 mm (Student t-test, $pvalue < 0.001$). For each similarity criterion, analysis of variance proved a highly significant effect of the simulation context on registration accuracy (F-test: $pvalue < 0.001$ and adjusted determination coefficient $R^2_{ajust} > 0.86$). Registrations using normal SPECT simulations were more accurate than those involving ictal SPECT simulations, suggesting an effect of the pathology on registration accuracy. Moreover, attenuation correction seemed to decrease registration accuracy, whereas scatter correction slightly improved registration accuracy. Results showed that the effect of the registration method on accuracy is quantitatively lower than the effect of the simulation context, even if L1 and L2 norm-based correlation ratios (CRL1 and CRL2) were slightly more accurate than the other criteria for each context.

3.2 Registration Inconsistencies on Real Data

Inconsistency measurements are summarized on Table 2. Even if registration seems less accurate than when considering SPECT simulations, inconsistencies RMS_j were most often lower than the SPECT spatial resolution of 12.2 mm. Nevertheless, for non corrected data, few registrations failed and were excluded from the analysis (i.e., $RMS_j > 2 \times 12.2\ mm$): 2 subjects for CRL2, 1 for CRL1 and 3 for CC. CRL1 and CRL2 seemed to be the most accurate methods, whereas no effect of attenuation correction on registration accuracy was observed.

4   Discussion and Conclusion

Our results suggest that statistical similarity-based registration methods may achieve SPECT subvoxel accuracy in SPECT/MRI registration. We used realistic SPECT simulations to study the impact of ictal data, as well as attenuation and scatter corrections, on registration accuracy. To provide realistic SPECT simulations, attenuation, scatter and partial volume corrections were performed on real SPECT data to model realistic activity maps. When comparing simulated data to real data, relative quantification errors less than 20% were found in most anatomical structures, suggesting that our simulated data are quite realistic [7].

The simulation context strongly affected registration accuracy. Registration using normal simulations was more accurate than registration using ictal simulations, suggesting that pathological conditions significantly affected registration accuracy. Moreover, whereas scatter correction slightly improved registration accuracy, attenuation correction decreased registrations performances. Similar findings were observed by Kyme et al. [14] in the context of motion correction in SPECT. As Compton scatter has a smoothing effect, scatter correction increased the contrast, which should help the analysis of similarity between SPECT and MRI data. On the other hand, attenuation correction removes information related to the anatomy. Our hypothesis is that such information might be useful for SPECT/MRI registration based on statistical similarity, but this deserves further investigation. Statistical similarity criteria based either on mutual information (MI and NMI) or on correlation ratios (CRL1 and CRL2) seemed to be reliable for ictal SPECT/MRI registration. Even if only slight differences were shown among such methods, criteria based on the correlation ratios (CRL1 and CRL2) seemed to be slightly more accurate.

Using realistic simulations allowed us to study specifically the impact that each parameter may have on registration accuracy. As we did not model inter-individual variability, results might be too optimistic. On the other hand, inconsistency measurements allowed us to evaluate the registration of ictal and inter-ictal data on patients scans. As inconsistency measurements are obtained without any Gold Standard and as they result from the combination of three independent registration errors, they may over-estimate registration accuracy [2]. All registrations were pretty accurate, RMS_j being significantly lower than SPECT spatial resolution (12.2 mm), but always greater than SPECT voxel size (4.51 mm). Some registrations failed on this small patients group, suggesting that it is definitely not a trivial task to register ictal data. Registration based on the correlation ratios CRL1 and CRL2 seemed to be the most precise and accurate, whereas no effect of attenuation correction was observed. More subjects should be studied to confirm those tendencies.

Quantitative comparison of registration evaluation studies is a delicate task, notably because of the lack of standardization in validation procedures [6]. Our accuracy and precision measurements agree with previous results (e.g.,[1]). Thurjfell et al. [2] also simulated pathological data and found no significant effect of the pathological contexts on registration accuracy, but using analytical SPECT simulations. In our study, realistic Monte Carlo SPECT simulations showed an impact of the pathological context on registration accuracy. In [15], we proposed a method to explore functional variability on those data, such models may lead to even more realistic simulations reflecting the functional variability of a population of subjects.

References

1. L. Barnden, R. Kwiatek, Y. Lau, et al. Validation of fully automatic brain SPET to MR co-registration. Eur. J. Nucl. Med., 27(2):147–154, 2000.
2. L. Thurjfell, Y.H. Lau, J.L.R. Andersson, et al. Improved efficiency for MRI-SPET registration based on mutual information. Eur. J. Nucl. Med., 27(7):847–856, 2000.
3. B. Brinkmann, T. O'Brien, et al. Quantitative and clinical analysis of SPECT image registration for epilepsy studies. J. Nucl. Med., 40(7):1098–1105, 1999.
4. P. Radau, P. Slomka, et al. Evaluation of linear registration algorithms for brain SPECT and errors due to hypoperfusion lesions. Med. Phys., 28(8):1660–1668,2001.
5. C. Grova, A. Biraben, J.M. Scarabin, et al. A methodology to validate MRI/SPECT registration methods using realistic simulated SPECT data. In LNCS (MICCAI 2001, Utrecht), 2208:275–282, 2001.
6. P. Jannin, J.M. Fitzpatrick, D.J. Hawkes, et al. Editorial: Validation of medical image processing in image-guided therapy. IEEE TMI, 21(11):1445–1449, 2002.
7. C. Grova, P. Jannin, A. Biraben, et al. A methodology for generating normal and pathological brain perfusion SPECT images for evaluation of MRI/SPECT fusion methods: Application in epilepsy. Phys. Med. Biol., 48:4023–4043, 2003.
8. A. Roche, G. Malandain, et al. The correlation ratio as a new similarity measure for multimodal image registration. In LNCS (MICCAI'98), 1496: 1115–1124, 1998.
9. F. Maes, A. Collignon, D. Vandermeulen, et al. Multimodality image registration by maximization of mutual information. IEEE TMI, 16(2):187–198, 1997.
10. C. Studholme, D.L.G. Hill, and D.J. Hawkes. An overlap invariant entropy measure of 3D medical image alignment. Pattern Recognition, 32:71–86, 1999.
11. I. Buvat and I. Castiglioni. Monte carlo simulations in SPET and PET. Quarterly J. Nucl. Med., 46:48–59, 2002.
12. I.G. Zubal, C.R. Harrell, E.O. Smith, et al. Computerized three-dimensional segmented human anatomy. Medical Physics, 21(2):299–302, 1994.

13. R.L. Harrison, S.D. Vannoy, D.R. Haynor, *et al.* Preliminary experience with the photon history generator module of a public-domain simulation system for emission tomography. In *Conf. Rec. Nucl. Sci. Symp.*, vol. 2, p. 1154– 1158, 1993.

14. A.Z. Kyme, B.F. Hutton, R.L. Hatton, *et al.* Practical aspects of a data-driven motion correction approach for brain SPECT. *IEEE TMI*, 22(6):722–729, 2003.

15. C. Grova, P. Jannin, I. Buvat, *et al.* From anatomic standardization analysis of perfusion SPECT data to perfusion pattern modelling. In *LNCS (MICCAI 2003, Montreal)*, 2879(2):328–335, 2003.

Construction of a Brain Template from MR Images Using State-of-the-Art Registration and Segmentation Techniques

Dieter Seghers, Emiliano D'Agostino, Frederik Maes*, Dirk Vandermeulen, and Paul Suetens

Katholieke Universiteit Leuven, Faculties of Medicine and Engineering, Medical Image Computing (Radiology - ESAT/PSI), University Hospital Gasthuisberg, Herestraat 49, B-3000 Leuven, Belgium
dieter.seghers@uz.kuleuven.ac.be

Abstract. We propose a procedure for generating a brain atlas with mean morphology and mean intensity by state-of-the-art non-rigid registration of a database of MR images of normal brains. The new constructed atlas is much sharper that currently available linear atlases, as the residual inter-subject shape variability after both linear and subsequent non-linear normalization is retained. As a consequence, the resulting atlas is suited as a mean shape template for brain morphometry approaches that are based on non-rigid atlas-to-subject image registration.

1 Introduction

A brain atlas is an important tool in the processing of images of the brain. It contains prior knowledge about the human brain that is useful for the segmentation and registration of a new brain image. The construction of an atlas from a database of subject images consists of a spatial-normalization step and usually also an intensity-normalization step. The spatial normalization is needed to construct an averaged atlas image whith a mean morphology, while intensity normalization avoids that the intensities in the atlas image are dominated by a single subject image.

A widely used atlas of the human brain is the MNI atlas, that is the standard atlas template in SPM [1]. This atlas was constructed using spatial normalization by linear registration with 9 degrees of freedom. Linear registration does not comenpsate for local shape differences in the brain, which induces blurring, not only in the averaged MR template but also in the tissue distribution maps obtained by averaging segmentations of white matter (WM), gray matter (GM) and cerebrospinal fluid (CSF) over all subjects. This makes linear atlases not suited as a mean shape template for brain morphometry approaches that are

---

* Frederik Maes is Postdoctoral Fellow of the Fund for Scientific Research - Flanders (FWO-Vlaanderen, Belgium).

C. Barillot, D.R. Haynor, and P. Hellier (Eds.): MICCAI 2004, LNCS 3216, pp. 696–703, 2004.

based on non-rigid atlas-to-subject image registration. Hence, there is need for adequate brain atlases constructed by appropriate non-rigid spatial normalization.

In this paper we present a procedure for generating a brain atlas with mean morphology and mean intensity by state-of-the-art non-rigid registration of a database of MR images of normal brains. Similar to the approach of Guimond [2], all images in the database are aligned with a single template image. All images in the database are in turn selected as template image and subsequently deformed towards the mean shape of all other non-rigidly aligned images to eliminate bias in the atlas towards any of the original images in the database. Average segmentation maps for the distribution of WM, GM and CSF are also constructed from the intensity-based tissue classification maps of the original images. The resulting atlas is much sharper than currently available linear atlases, as only the residual inter-subject shape variability after both linear and subsequent nonlinear normalization is retained.

2   Materials and Methods

2.1   Image Database

The atlas is constructed from a database of MR images of normal brains. In this paper, a database of $N = 64$ images was used. The subjects were 41 males and 23 females, aged 22 to 40. All images were acquired using a 3D MPRAGE sequence with sagittal orientation. The images have dimensions $160 \times 256 \times 256$ with a voxelsize of $1 \times 1 \times 1$ mm^3.

2.2   Image Preprocessing

Segmentation and masking. A first step in the construction of the brain atlas is the masking of non-brain tissues in the images in the database. The images are therefore first segmented using the model-based tissue classification algorithm of Van Leemput et al [4] to obtain probabilistic WM, GM and CSF maps. A brain mask is created by summing these maps and thresholding at 50% probability. Figure 1 shows the result of this procedure for a particular brain.

Affine registration. Pose and size related differences in the position, orientation and scale of the brains in the images in the database are eliminated prior to atlas construction by transforming all images into the same space by a 12-parameter affine transformation. All images in the database are therefore affinely registered to the template MR image distributed with SPM99 [1] by maximization of mutual information [3].

2.3   Atlas Construction

Nonrigid registration. The key in the proposed procedure for atlas construction is non-rigid voxel-based image registration. Non-rigid registration finds the

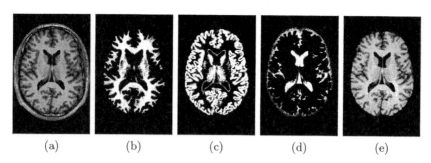

(a)   (b)   (c)   (d)   (e)

Fig. 1. The brain image is masked by first segmenting the image using the EMS algorithm of Van Leemput et al [4], which delivers probabilistic WM, GM and CSF maps. The sum of those maps serves as a mask to the brain image. From left to right: (a) the original image, its maps for (b) WM, (c) GM and (d) CSF and (e) the masked image.

deformation field $T(x, y, z) : \mathbb{R}^3 \to \mathbb{R}^3$ that maps coordinates (x,y,z) in the reference image R into coordinates (x', y', z') in the floating image F :

$$(x', y', z') = (x - T_x(x, y, z), y - T_y(x, y, z), z - T_z(x, y, z))$$

The warped image F' is computed as:

$$F'(x, y, z) = F(x - T_x(x, y, z), y - T_y(x, y, z), z - T_z(x, y, z)) \tag{1}$$

which requires interpolation to evaluate F at the non-integer positions (x', y', z') (in our case, trilinear interpolation is used). To simplify notation, equation (1) will be noted as $F' = T(F)$. The registration algorithm finds a transformation T that maximizes a similarity measure between the warped image F' and the reference image, subject to appropriate regularization constraints. The method used in this work is the algorithm proposed by D'Agostino et al [5] based on maximization of mutual information between the deformed floating image and the reference image. The deforming reference image is considered as a viscous fluid whose motion is governed by the Navier-Stokes equation of conservation of momentum. This algorithm is well suited to match one MR brain image to another because it allows large deformations. The mutual information criterium is chosen in order to cope with the intensity bias fields of the subject images.

Mean morphology. The aim of atlas construction is to recover the mean morphology of the brain from a database of images, assuming that the database is representative for the population of interest. To do so, we apply the following procedure (figure 2). Let A_0 denote any particular brain in the database. We want to transform A_0 in a new image A_1 with mean morphology as observed in the database. First, all database images $I_1, \ldots, I_N$ are registered to A_0 (A_0 is the floating image and the database images act as reference images), yielding deformations T_l $\forall l = 1, \ldots, N$. Consider an arbitrary point (i, j, k) at the same geometrical position in the space of each of the original images I_l (after affine registration as described above). This point corresponds to different anatomical locations in each image. These points are mapped by each T_l into the space of the selected template A_0:

$$(i_l, j_l, k_l) = (i, j, k) - (T_{l,x}(i, j, k), T_{l,y}(i, j, k), T_{l,z}(i, j, k)) \quad \forall l = 1, \ldots, N$$

We consider the point at the center of these projected points as the anatomical point that on average (for our database of images) matches the geometrical point (i, j, k). Hence, we define the mean morphology image A_1 as the image obtained from A_0 by the spatial transformation

$$A_1(i, j, k) = A_0(\overline{i}, \overline{j}, \overline{k}) \tag{2}$$

with

$$(\overline{i}, \overline{j}, \overline{k}) = \frac{1}{N} \sum_{l=1}^{N} (i_l, j_l, k_l) = (i - \overline{T}_x, j - \overline{T}_y, k - \overline{T}_z)$$

$\overline{T}_x, \overline{T}_y, \overline{T}_z$ represent the averaged sum of the deformation fields. Equation (2) becomes

$$A_1(i, j, k) = A_0(i - \overline{T}_x(i, j, k), j - \overline{T}_y(i, j, k), k - \overline{T}_z(i, j, k)) \tag{3}$$

which can be written as

$$A_1 = \overline{T}(A_0) \tag{4}$$

In words: the particular brain is warped to each of the individuals of the database, the mean deformation field is computed and this is applied to the particular brain.

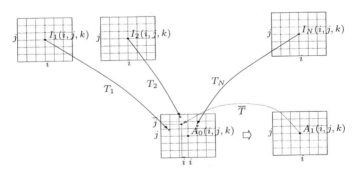

Fig. 2. A particular brain image A_0 is transformed into an image with mean morphology A_1 by the mean transformation $\overline{T}$ obtained by averaging all transformations T_l of A_0 to each of the images I_l in the database.

Mean intensities. The procedure described above does not result in a suitable atlas yet, because the computed image A_1 has only intensities originating from the particular brain A_0. Moreover the topology of image A_1 will be determined by the topology of the initial image A_0, while not every brain has the same topology. To overcome these limitations, we propose the scheme presented in figure 3. Each of the database images $I_1, I_2, ..., I_N$ is in turn selected as the template A_0 and transformed into images $\overline{I}_1, \overline{I}_2, ..., \overline{I}_N$ with mean morphology using the procedure described above. This requires $N(N-1)$ non-rigid registrations in total. These mean shape images are then averaged voxel-wise after appropriate intensity rescaling to compensate for global intensity differences between the images in the database. The need for this intensity rescaling is illustrated in figure 4. To match the intensities of two images $\overline{I}_i$ and $\overline{I}_j$, linear regression between the intensities of both images is performed and the intensities in one of the images are linearly rescaled to make the slope of the regression line equal to one and its intercept equal to zero.

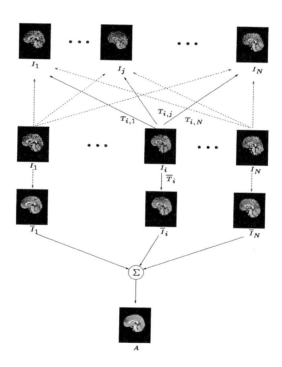

Fig. 3. Procedure to generate an atlas with mean morphology and mean intensities. Each of the images in the database is non-rigidly registered to all others and is subsequently transformed by the average deformation into a mean shape image. The mean shape images obtained for each database image are subsequently voxel-wise averaged after appropriate intensity rescaling to compensate for global intensity differences in the original images.

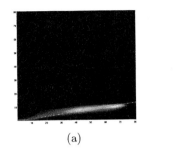
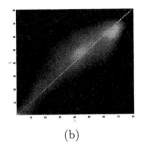

(a)   (b)

Fig. 4. (a) The joint histogram of two images $\overline{I}_i$ and $\overline{I}_j$. (b) The joint histogram of the images $\overline{I}_i$ and $\overline{I}_j$ after linear intensity rescaling to compensate for global intensity differences between both images.

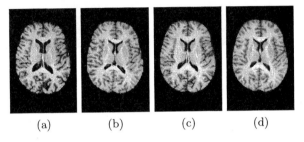

(a)   (b)   (c)   (d)

Fig. 5. Demonstration of the effect of the mean morphology transformation. (a) and (b): Two database images after preprocessing (masking and affine registration). (c) and (d): The same images but mapped into the mean morphology space. It is easy to remark that the shape of the ventricles has been normalized

Atlas with segmentation maps. Besides an atlas MR template with mean shape and gray values, we also construct the corresponding probability maps for WM, GM and CSF for use as spatially variant priors in atlas-driven intensity-based tissue classification. The segmentation maps obtained for each of the original images in the database are therefore first transformed into the mean morphology space using the already computed mean deformations $\overline{T}_i$ (figure 3). The projected probability maps are subsequently voxel-wise averaged.

3   Results

All results are computed using a database of $N = 64$ normal brains. The effect of the mean morphology transformation is illustrated in figure 5. The final atlas with mean morphology and mean intensities and its corresponding segmentation maps are shown in figure 6. In figure 7 the atlas is compared with the SPM-atlas. The new atlas is obviously less smooth then the SPM-atlas.

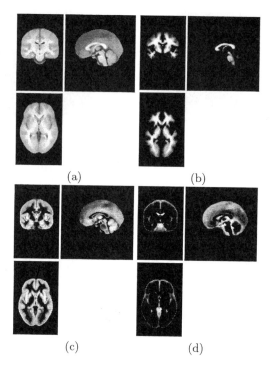

Fig. 6. Constructed atlas consisting of (a) a gray valued MR template with mean shape and intensity and corresponding probabilistic tissue distribution maps for (b) WM, (c) GM and (d) CSF.

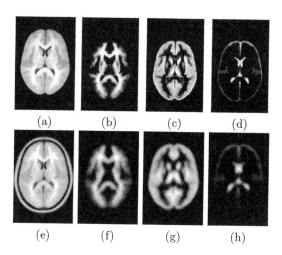

Fig. 7. Comparison of the new atlas ((a) gray values, (b) WM,(c) GM and (d) CSF) with the SPM-atlas ((e) gray values, (f) WM,(g) GM and (h) CSF). The new atlas is obviously less smooth than the SPM-atlas.

4   Discussion and Future Work

The resulting atlas is well suited for applications using non-rigid atlas-to-subject image registration, as blurring in the template image is avoided by compensating for local shape differences. The presented procedure also avoids the atlas to be dominated by any of the original images in the database. Instead of groupwise registration [6], each of the original subject images is deformed towards the mean shape of all other non-rigidly aligned images. If only one of the subject images would be taken as a target image, the atlas would be biased towards the chosen target image.

A possible improvement is the expansion of the atlas-generating procedure to multiple iterations. The original database is transformed to a database of mean morphology brains. This step can be repeated till a convergence criterium is reached.

In the future, this atlas has to be compared with other brain templates using non-linear spatial normalization. An other future step, is a statistical analysis of the deformation fields that transform the single subject templates to the mean shape. Hence, inter-subject local shape variability can be modeled.

Finally we need to mention the computational complexity. The number of registrations to be computed is $N(N - 1)$. All the computations were done with 2.6 GHz processors. One registration on one processor takes approximately one hour. The database consists of $N = 64$ images. The procedure would take 4096h (170 days) using only one processor. The computations were done using 18 processors simultaneously, which reduced the computation time to ± 10 days.

References

[1] Statistical Parameter Mapping. http://www.fil.ion.ucl.ac.uk/spm/spm99.html

[2] A. Guimond, J. Meunier and J-P. Thirion. Average brain models: a convergence study. Technical Report 3731, INRIA, 1999.

[3] F. Maes, A. Collignon, D. Vandermeulen, G. Marchal, and P. Suetens. Multimodality image registration by maximization of mutual information. *IEEE Trans. Medical Imaging*, 16(4):187–198, 1997.

[4] K. Van Leemput, F. Maes, D. Vandermeulen, P. Suetens. Automated model-based tissue classification of MR images of the brain. *IEEE Trans. Medical Imaging*, 18(10):897–908, 1999.

[5] E. D'Agostino, F. Maes, D. Vandermeulen, and P. Suetens. A viscous fluid model for multimodal non-rigid image registration using mutual information *Medical Image Analysis*, 7(4):565–575, 2003.

[6] C. Studholme. Simultaneous population based image alignment for template free spatial normalisation of brain anatomy. 2nd international workshop on biomedical image registration, June 2003, pp 81-90, LNCS 2717.

Non-rigid Atlas to Subject Registration with Pathologies for Conformal Brain Radiotherapy

Radu Stefanescu[1], Olivier Commowick[1,3], Grégoire Malandain[1],
Pierre-Yves Bondiau[1,2], Nicholas Ayache[1], and Xavier Pennec[1]

[1] INRIA Sophia - Epidaure team, BP 93, 06902 Sophia Antipolis Cedex, France
{Radu.Stefanescu, Olivier.Commowick}@sophia.inria.fr
[2] Centre Antoine Lacassagne, Département de Radiothérapie, 33 avenue de
Valombrose, 06 189 NICE Cedex 2, France
[3] DOSISoft S.A., 45-47 Avenue Carnot, 94 230 Cachan, France

Abstract. Warping a digital atlas toward a patient image allows the simultaneous segmentation of several structures. This may be of great interest for cerebral images, since the brain contains a large number of small but important structures (optical nerves, grey nuclei, etc.). One important application is the conformal radiotherapy of cerebral tumor, where a precise delineation of all these structures is required. However, in this case, the variability induced by the tumor or a surgical resection, that are not present in the digital atlas, prevents an accurate registration between the atlas and the patient images. Since our registration method allows to locally control the amount of regularization, we are able to explicitly introduce those areas in the warping process. For computational efficiency, we have created a parallel implementation that can be used from the clinical environment through a grid interface.

1 Introduction

The treatment of cerebral tumor may involve surgery, radiotherapy, or chemotherapy. Thanks to recent technological advances (on-line definition of the shape of the irradiation beam, irradiation intensity modulation during the treatment), conformal radiotherapy allows a high precision irradiation (homogeneous dose distribution within complex shapes), permitting an improvement of local control and the reduction of the complications.

This high precision radiotherapy is a powerful tool for the treatment of cerebral tumors, since the irradiation target may be close to critical structures (optical nerves, brain stem, etc.). In order to determine the best characteristics of the treatment planning, and to provide the patient follow-up, it is necessary to accurately locate all the structures of interest in the brain and the tumor. Currently, the segmentation of brain structures is manual and each structure must be delineated in each slice of a 3-D image (e.g. MRI). The treatment team spends a significant amount of time to delimit the various structures of interest with the precision requested for the conformal radiotherapy. An automatic segmentation algorithm of all the critical structures in a patient image is then an invaluable

C. Barillot, D.R. Haynor, and P. Hellier (Eds.): MICCAI 2004, LNCS 3216, pp. 704–711, 2004.

tool for radiotherapy, and its main requirement is a precise delineation of the structures of interest.

In order to extract all these structures in a specific patient's image, we chose to build a numerical reference atlas of all the structures we are interested in, and to use matching techniques to warp this atlas onto one patient's image. The atlas (Fig. 1b) was manually labeled from an artificial MR image (obtained from the Brainweb, see Fig. 1a). The first step is a rigid matching between atlas and the patient MRIs (usually T1, T2 and T1 injected). The recovered transformation is refined using non-rigid registration, and then applied to the atlas in order to obtain a segmentation of the patient image.

Due to its multi-subject nature, this registration problem is generally difficult. The topology of the brain, the shape of the ventricles, the number and shape of the sulci vary strongly from one individual to another. Thus, algorithms have to deal with the ambiguity of the structures to match, but they also have to take into account the large variability of the differences between the two brains.

A more important issue arises in our case with the presence of pathologies in the patient image, such as tumors or surgical resections. These structures have no equivalent in the atlas. They usually lead the non-rigid registration to important errors, especially around the pathology which is the area of interest for radiotherapy. Numerous methods and tools have been already devised to address non-rigid registration [1], but much fewer deal with pathological abnormalities.

Kyriacou et al. [2] used a biomechanical modeling of the brain and tumor based on non-linear elasticity. In the case of multi-subject patient/atlas registration, elastic models are of low relevancy, since the transformation to recover does not correspond to a physical deformation. Christensen [3] showed that in order to recover large deformations, such as the ones implied by multi-subject registration, a viscous component is needed.

Some methods [4,5] deal with the absence of pathology in the atlas by artificially introducing it. A first non-rigid registration between patient and atlas yields an initial deformation that is used to implant a "pathology seed" inside the atlas. This deformation is then refined by non-rigidly registering the subject image with the seeded atlas. The main problem consists in performing the first registration, which can easily fail, especially if the pathology is located closely to the brain border or the ventricles.

We have presented in [6] a non-rigid registration algorithm that uses anatomical information to locally adapt the regularization from fluid (for CSF) to visco-elastic-like (for grey/white matter). In this paper, we show how to take explicitly into account tumors and surgical resections in our framework. The first step, detailed in Section 2 consist in segmenting these areas in the patient image. Then, we recall in Section 3 the principle of the registration method, and show how the pathology is modeled as a non-informative area. Last but not least, we present in Section 4 comparative results that demonstrate the improvements brought by our method.

2   Segmentation of Tumors and Surgical Resections

In order to obtain a priori information on the tumor and the surgical resection to guide the atlas registration, we have to segment these regions in the patient's brain. Thereafter, we propose two different methods for automatically delineating respectively the surgical resection and the tumor.

2.1   Segmentation of a Surgical Resection

A surgical resection corresponds to an absence of matter in the considered region, filled with CSF, and possibly connected with the ventricles. Its shape is more spherical than the other structures of the CSF, and is composed of only one big connected component. These are the basic properties that we exploit for delineating the resection.

First, we extract all structures behaving like CSF in the joint MR T1 and T2 histogram (low signal in T1 and high signal in T2) by fitting a 2D Gaussian on the corresponding area of the histogram. Selecting all the voxels whose joint intensity is statistically compatible gives us an oversized segmentation of CSF which still contains structures like the eyes and the ventricles. The eyes are quite easy to remove since they appear as two isolated connected components. To select them, we robustly register an atlas with an affine transformation, and remove the connected components that have an intersection with the eyes of the atlas. To separate the ventricles from the surgical resection, we use a region labeling algorithm based on a skeletonization by influence zone (SKIZ) [7]. As this labeling is sensitive to narrowings in a connected component, it easily classifies the surgical resection and the ventricle as different regions. The regions that intersect the ventricles of the atlas are removed as above.

Finally, we have to select the surgical resection region among remaining structures. The sulci are relatively small with respect to a surgical resection and thus easy to remove. The main problem comes from the possible presence of a CSF component between the brain and the skull due to brain shift during the surgical operation. The volume of this component may be quite large, but its shape is mostly flat. Thus, we compute a distance map in each remaining CSF connected component, and select the one that has the largest inscribed ball radius.

2.2   Delineation of the Tumor

Delineating a tumor is a hard task due to the multiple forms it may take in the image. The tumor may generate an edema at its frontiers, and contain a necrotic center. The tumor tissues and the edema usually appear like partial volume (CSF and grey matter) intensities, while the necrosis resembles the CSF.

Traditional Expectation-Maximization algorithms [8] fail to provide good results because of the presence of these tissues. An alternative is to consider tumor intensities as outliers in this mixture of Gaussians, or to add some specific classes to model the tumor and edema intensities [9]. As this was often not sufficient, some anatomical knowledge was added, either by combining geometric priors given by the non-rigid registration of an atlas to a tissue classification [10], or by using Markov Random Fields [11]. Other methods include region growing from a region of interest delineated by one of the preceding methods using levelsets methods [12].

All these methods end up in very complex algorithm as attempt to segment all the tissues. In our case, we are only interested in the tumor segmentation, so that we could rely on a very simple mathematical morphology scheme as we developed in the previous section.

We fit this time the selected region of the joint T1 an T2 intensity histogram by a mixture of two Gaussians: one for the necrotic part of the tumor (which appear like CSF), and a second one for the tumor tissues and its edema (resembling partial volume CSF/grey matter). We obtain an oversized segmentation where we need to remove structures like the sulci or the ventricles without removing interesting parts. Indeed, we now have CSF and grey matter partial volume voxels, and the necrotic part of the tumor can be near a region containing CSF. The ventricles and the eyes are removed like before. Then the remaining part of the segmentation is labeled into SKIZ zones. Each region is then compared with an a priori statistical atlas of the CSF to compute the mean probability of belonging to the CSF. A threshold on this probability allows us to remove the CSF structures like the ventricles or the sulci. In each of these two steps we also compute a distance map to the CSF of the statistical atlas in each region to avoid removing regions containing voxels too far from the expected CSF.

3 A Grid-Powered Registration Algorithm

We developed in [6] an original registration method that appear particularly well fitted to our current problem. The algorithm models the transformation as a dense deformation field, which enables it to recover fine details. The degree of regularity imposed on the deformation is locally adapted in order to let the ventricles deform freely, while preserving the coherence of the brain. The user may locally tune the weight of matching versus regularization in the registration process. Finally, the resulting transformation is guaranteed to be invertible.

3.1 General Description of the Algorithm

Through this section, we consider J to be the source image, I the target image and $U = (U_1, U_2, U_3)$ the displacement field that transforms J into I, so that for each point p, the intensity of the transformed image $(J \circ U)(p) \triangleq J(p + U(p))$ matches the one of the image I at point p. The estimation of U is twofold: first a small correction $u = (u_1, u_2, u_3)$ is computed by optimizing a *similarity criterion*, and second it is composed with U before regularization.

Our registration problem is monomodal, thus the sum of squared differences is a sufficient (and adapted) measure to estimate the similarity between the images to be matched. Let the similarity criterion by $Sim(I, J) = \sum_p (I(p) - J(p))^2$. A gradient descent scheme allows to optimize $Sim(I, J \circ U \circ u)$, yielding a small correction u. However, this raw deformation field is usually noisy. This is particularly true in areas of the images where the intensity is uniform and the registration is mainly driven by noise. To filter out the unreliable "matches" from the raw deformation field, we use a method inspired by the image-guided anisotropic diffusion: once the gradient $u = \nabla Sim$ of the similarity criterion is computed, its values are filtered using a diffusion equation: $\frac{\partial u_i}{\partial t}(p) = (1 - k(p)) \cdot (\Delta u_i)(p)$, where $k(p) \in [0, 1]$. The parameter $k(p)$ measures the local degree of smoothing applied to u, or the *local confidence* that we have in the similarity criterion. For $k(p) = 1$, the local displacement $u_i(p)$ will be locally unaffected by this PDE, whereas the field is locally smoothed or even interpolated from neighboring values for $k(p)$ close to zero. For an intermediate value, this smoothing may be seen as an approximation of a viscous-elastic behavior. In practice, $k(p)$ is related to the image gradient, so that diffusion occurs in homogeneous regions.

The regularized small correction u being computed, we compose it with U (similarly to the regridding scheme proposed by [3]). This additionally allows for an invertible transformation U.

Let us now consider the regularization of U. Some authors used elasticity, but there are more evidences toward a visco-elastic behavior of brain material. Moreover, the resolution of these biomechanical models is quite slow. We chose a more heuristic approach that only approximates a biomechanical behavior, but which is much faster. We use the same diffusion equation than above, now with U, and with a *stiffness field* $D(p)$ (instead of $1 - k(p)$) that now depends on the local nature of the tissues, as in [6]. Thus, combined with the above regularization, this realizes a good approximation of a visco-elastic material.

For computational efficiency, the algorithm was implemented on an inexpensive and powerful parallel machine: a cluster of workstations. However, such a cluster is more easily located in a computing center than in a clinical environment. To provide the clinical user with a user friendly interface on a visualization workstation located in its own environment, we proposed in [13] a *grid service* running on a parallel computer outside the clinical environment which provides on demand the computing power needed to perform the registration.

3.2   Using A Priori Anatomical Information About the Patient

As for every registration algorithm, we explicitly assumes that the chosen similarity metric describes a meaningful correspondence between the two images. This assumption is of course violated when the patient image contains additional structures, such as tumors or resections. Since there is no correspondent in the atlas for voxels in the "pathological" region of the patient image, we remove the influence of these voxels from the similarity metric: we assigned a null confidence to all voxels inside a dilated mask of the pathology. The dilation is necessary in order to remove the influence of the gradient caused by the pathology. As a consequence, the correspondences in this area will be determined by interpolation from non-pathological neighboring voxels, for which correspondences can be reliably estimated. We assign the pathological region the same stiffness D as the surrounding tissues.

We use the methods described in Section 2 to estimate a binary mask of the patient pathology. When performing the confidence-weighted filtering of unreliable matches, we assign a null confidence to each voxel inside the pathology. Since we specify the confidence inside the source image, we use the patient image as the source. After registration, we inverse the transformation in order to resample the atlas labeling in the subject image.

4   Experimental Results

Our test dataset contains 22 T1-weighted MR images of different patients. After preliminary rigid registration, the images sizes are $256 \times 256 \times 60$.

The pathology segmentation takes between 1 and 3 minute, and the non-rigid registration takes about 4 minutes on a cluster of 15 personal computers (2GHz Pentium IV processors, 1GB/s network), which amounts to a total computation time of 5 to 10 minutes. The whole database has been processed. Results have been visually inspected by a radiotherapist, and appear satisfactory.

Figures 1a and 1b show, respectively, the atlas used for the registration, and its segmentation. The atlas has been registered with a patient image (Fig. 1c) presenting a large tumor. The pathology has been automatically segmented, and its segmentation has been introduced in the confidence field (Fig. 1d). If the tumor is not taken into account in the non-rigid registration, the displacement field is biased by the tumor. This results in a false segmentation of the right lenticular nucleus and lateral ventricle (Fig. 1e,g). Taking in consideration the pathology results in a interpolated displacement field in the tumor area. Therefore, the correspondences around the right lenticular nucleus and lateral ventricle are no longer biased, which leads to a better segmentation (Fig. 1f,h).

In Figure 2a, we present an example where the patient brain has a large surgical resection, that we segmented using the algorithm in Section 2. In the confidence, we assigned null values inside the resection area (see Fig. 2b). A simple non-rigid registration is not able to follow the contour of the cerebellum (see white arrow in Fig. 2c). If we use the resection segmentation in our algorithm, the segmentation is the cerebellum is largely improved (Fig. 2d).

5   Discussion

In this paper, we describe a non-rigid atlas to subject registration algorithm aimed at automating a brain image segmentation method for conformal radiotherapy. The main difficulty consists in the unpredictable and huge variability introduced either by the tumor or the surgical resection in the patient image, that has no correspondent in the digital atlas. These additional structures introduce false matches in the transformation, and result in a local failure of the registration around the pathology, that may also lead to errors because of the regularization. Our method is based on segmenting the pathology and reducing the weight of the voxels inside the pathology. In these regions, we locally increase the degree of regularity of the deformation field, which enables us to compute the

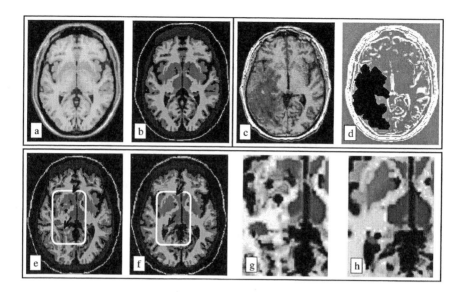

Fig. 1. Segmentation of a 3D patient image containing a large tumor. Top left: slice of atlas MRI (a) and segmentation (b). Top right: patient image (c), and confidence used for the registration (d). The confidence is 0 inside the tumor (in black on the image). Bottom line: transformation of the atlas segmentation into the patient geometry, by simple registration (e), or by taking into account the tumor (f). Fig. (g) and (h) present zooms on the same area of interest from figures (e) and (f).

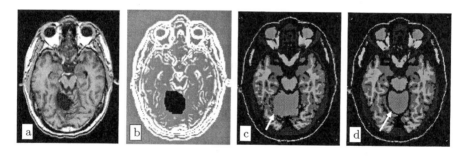

Fig. 2. Segmentation of a patient image containing a resection. (a) Patient image. (b) Confidence (resection is in black). (c) Result produced by a simple registration, un-aware of the resection. (d) Result produced by our algorithm, exhibiting a better segmentation of the cerebellum (see white arrows).

matches by interpolation. As we use a fuzzy segmentation of the pathology, the results of our algorithm gracefully degrade with the quality of the segmentation.

Results show an improvement of the segmentation in the pathology area. In the near future, we will validate this method by comparing segmentations produced by our algorithm to ones produced by clinical experts. Another future improvement is the use of our segmentation as an a priori for the pathology segmentation. We believe that iterating between registration and segmentation will result in future accuracy gains. In the future, we hope that automating the segmentation step will drastically reduce the time required by the conformal radiotherapy planning.

References

1. J.B.A. Maintz and M.A. Viergever. A survey of medical image registration. *Medical Image Analysis*, 2(1):1–36, 1998.
2. S.K. Kyriacou, C. Davatzikos, S.J. Zinreich, and R.N. Bryan. Nonlinear elastic registration of brain images with tumor pathology using a biomechanical model. *IEEE Trans. Med. Imaging*, 18(7):580–592, 1999.
3. G.E. Christensen, R. Rabitt, and M.I. Miller. Deformable templates using large deformation kinetics. *IEEE Trans. on Image Processing*, 5(10):1435–1447, 1996.
4. B.M. Dawant, S.L. Hartmann, Shiyan Pan, and S. Gadamsetty. Brain atlas deformation in the presence of small and large space-occupying tumors. *Computer Aided Surgery*, 7:1–10, 2002.
5. M. Bach Cuadra, J. Gomez, P. Hagmann, C. Pollo, J.-G. Villemure, B.M. Dawant, and J.-Ph. Thiran. Atlas-based segmentation of pathological brains using a model of tumor growth. In *Proc. of MICCAI'02*, volume 2488 of *LNCS*. Springer.
6. R. Stefanescu, X. Pennec, and N. Ayache. Grid enabled non-rigid registration with a dense transformation and a priori information. In *Proc. of MICCAI'03*, volume 2879 of *LNCS*, pages 804–811. Springer, 2003.
7. Pierre Soille. *Morphological image analysis : principles and applications*. Springer, 1999.
8. K. Van Leemput, F. Maes, D. Vandermeulen, and P. Suetens. Automated model-based tissue classification of MR images of the brain. *IEEE transactions on medical imaging*, 18(10):897–908, 1999.
9. N. Moon, K. van Leemput, E. Bullitt, and G. Gerig. Automatic brain and tumor segmentation. In *MICCAI*, pages 372–379, 2002.
10. Michael R. Kaus, Simon K. Warfield, Arya Nabavi, Peter M. Black, Ferenc A. Jolesz, and Ron Kikinis. Automated segmentation of mr images of brain tumors. *Radiology*, 218(2):586–591, 2001.
11. T. Kapur. *Model based three dimensional Medical Image Segmentation*. Ph.d thesis, Massachusetts Institute of Technology, May 1999.
12. S. Ho, E. Bullitt, and G. Gerig. Level set evolution with region competition: Automatic 3-d segmentation of brain tumors. In *Proc. 16th Int Conf on Pattern Recognition ICPR 2002*, pages 532–535, 2002.
13. R. Stefanescu, X. Pennec, and N. Ayache. A grid service for the interactive use of a parallel non-rigid registration algorithm. In *Proc. of HealthGrid'04*. European Commission, DG Information Society, 2004. To appear in Methods of Information in Medicine.

Ventricle Registration for Inter-subject White Matter Lesion Analysis

Cynthia Jongen, Jeroen van der Grond, and Josien P.W. Pluim

Image Sciences Institute, University Medical Center Utrecht, Heidelberglaan 100, E01.335,
Utrecht, The Netherlands
{cynthia, jeroen, josien}@isi.uu.nl

Abstract. A method is presented to non-rigidly register lateral ventricles to enable the automated analysis of peri-ventricular white matter lesions. A binary average image of the lateral ventricle system is used as a reference image for registration. To prevent false deformations of the lesions we non-rigidly register CSF segmentations to the average lateral ventricle image. The subvoxel accuracy achieved, allows accurate mapping of the peri-ventricular white matter lesions to the reference space of the average lateral ventricles. Application to patient data shows the feasibility of the presented approach.

1 Introduction

White matter lesions show as hyperintensities on T2-w and FLAIR MR images. These hyperintense white matter lesions are associated with age, vascular risk factors, such as hypertension and diabetes mellitus, and clinically silent stroke [1,2,3,4]. Analysis of white matter lesions has mainly focused on comparing lesion severity by grading the amount of lesion or volume measurements of segmented lesions. Analysis of differences in lesion location has been limited to distinguishing deep white matter lesions from peri-ventricular white matter lesions [4] and grading lesion severity for a small number of peri-ventricular areas [1,2].

The goal of this work is to analyze differences in lesion location between diabetes patients and controls on a voxel-by-voxel basis, without needing to classify lesions into a limited number of categories. To allow the analysis, MR images of different patients need to be matched. Since our interest is focused on peri-ventricular white matter lesions it is important that the ventricular system is correctly matched. Furthermore, matching should not actively deform the white matter lesions. Since the shape of the ventricular system has a high inter-subject variability, fine scale non-rigid deformations are necessary. If gray-value images are used, these fine scale deformations will also deform the lesions by matching lesion to lesion or lesion to healthy tissue. Of course this could be avoided by masking the lesions, but this approach will affect patients with different degrees of lesion severity differently. Therefore, we have chosen not to use the gray-value images for registration, but to match binary CSF segmentations of patients and controls to a binary reference lateral ventricle system image. Since peri-ventricular white matter lesions adjoin the lateral ventricles, any local inter-subject differences will be largely given by the differences between ventricular systems. So, deforming the ventricle systems to match with a

C. Barillot, D.R. Haynor, and P. Hellier (Eds.): MICCAI 2004, LNCS 3216, pp. 712–719, 2004.

reference lateral ventricle image will also register the peri-ventricular white matter lesions. We could also have included CSF around the cortex in our reference image, but the gyri and sulci pattern is highly variable between subjects. Therefore, mismatches of the CSF in different sulci are likely. This might adversely affect the registration of the lateral ventricles and thereby the peri-ventricular lesions. Even if a correct matching of CSF in the sulci is achieved, the beneficial effect on registration accuracy for the lesions will be small. No other structures that could easily be used for registration are present near the ventricles.

Thus, our approach of registering CSF segmentations to a binary average lateral ventricle image and applying these deformations to the lesions, allows us to place the lesions of different subjects in the same reference space. This enables us to compare the lesion pattern in patients to the lesion pattern in control subjects.

2   Methods

2.1   MR Imaging

Brain MR images were acquired on a Philips Gyroscan ACS-NT 15 whole body system operating at 1.5 Tesla (Philips Medical Systems, Best, The Netherlands). All patients were scanned using the same MR protocol consisting of T1-w, IR, T2-w, PD and FLAIR scans. All scans had a slice thickness of 4 mm, 38 continuous slices, a 230 x 230 mm field of view, and a 256 x 256 scan matrix. The scan parameters were: T1-w (FFE): 234/2 ms (repetition time (TR)/echo time (TE)); IR: 2919/410/22 ms (TR/inversion time (TI)/TE); T2-w: 2200/100 ms (TR/TE); PD: 2200/11 ms (TR/TE); and FLAIR: 6000/2000/100 ms (TR/TI/TE).

2.2   Image Preprocessing

The image preprocessing consisted of three steps. First, an automatic correction of shading artifacts in the T1-w, T2-w, PD, and FLAIR images was done. The intensity distortions were modeled with a multiplicative fourth order polynomial, as described by Likar et al. [5].

Second, for each patient and control the shading corrected T2-w, PD, FLAIR, and the IR images were registered to the shading corrected T1-w image using a normalized mutual information based registration algorithm [6] optimizing 9 parameters (translation, rotation, and scaling).

Third, CSF was extracted by k-means clustering of the 5 registered MR images into 8 clusters. Initialization of the cluster centers was done by clustering 10 random subsamples of 0.1% of all data using a random cluster center initialization and smoothing the result by clustering the centers found for the subsamples [7]. The CSF cluster was manually selected from the resulting clustered image. Making a distinction between lateral ventricle and other CSF structures would require much user interaction and the presence of non-ventricle structures was not expected to make a substantial difference to the registration results. Therefore, after interpolating the slices to isotropic voxels of 0.9 mm^3 using shape-based interpolation [8], the whole CSF cluster was used for registration to an average ventricle shape.

2.3 Construction of Average Ventricle

An average ventricle is needed as a template for inter-subject registration of CSF segmentations. Images of 24 patients with arterial vascular disease, who were not included in this study, were used. These patients are similar in age and in changes of the ventricle shape as the control and diabetics subjects. The lateral ventricles were segmented by thresholding and manual editing of their FLAIR scans (same protocol as used in this study). This resulted in 24 binary lateral ventricle segmentations. The slices of the segmentation images were interpolated to isotropic voxels using shape-based interpolation [8]. Eight segmented ventricles were registered together to determine their average ventricle position and size using a 12 parameter affine registration algorithm [9]. The eight ventricles were transformed to this position, summed, and thresholded. Then, this image was used as template for the affine registration of all 24 segmented ventricles. The 24 affinely registered images were summed. Next, a B-spline based non-rigid registration algorithm [9] was used with a control point spacing (CPS) of 32 voxels to register all 24 affinely registered ventricles to the sum image. A large CPS was chosen because we only want to correct for global differences in ventricle shape. The non-rigidly registered ventricles were summed and thresholded keeping the variation in ventricle shape that was present in at least a third of the ventricles. The resulting image was used as reference image for the affine and non-rigid registration of CSF segmentations of patients and controls.

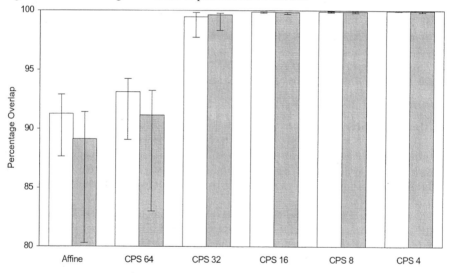

Fig. 1. Median percentage of average ventricle overlapped by CSF of diabetes patients (*white*) and control subjects (*gray*) after registration with an increasing degree of non-rigidity. Error bars indicate 25 and 75 percentiles

2.4 Registration

Registration of the CSF segmentations to the average ventricle shape was done using the method described by Rueckert et al. [9]. This method proceeds in two steps. First, a 15 parameter affine registration using normalized mutual information [6,10] was done to correct for global differences in position and size. Next, a free-form deformation using a B-spline based non-rigid registration algorithm with normalized mutual information as registration criterion was done. The spacing of the control points was decreased from 64 to 4 voxels by factors of 2.

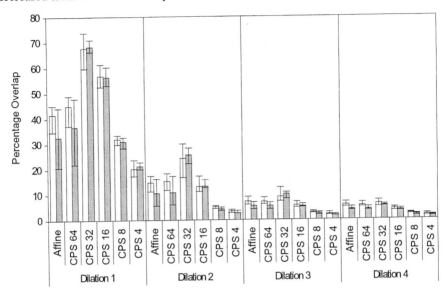

Fig. 2. Median percentage of overlap of rings of one voxel dilations around the average ventricle with CSF segmentations of diabetes patients (*white*) and control subjects (*gray*) after registration with an increasing degree of non-rigidity. Error bars indicate 25 and 75 percentiles

2.5 Statistical Analysis of White Matter Lesion Patterns

To illustrate the proposed method, we applied it to twenty-four diabetes mellitus patients and twelve control subjects matched for age. White matter lesion segmentations were made using the method described in [11]. All white matter lesion segmentations were transformed to the reference average ventricle shape by applying the transformations found for the CSF segmentation registration. Differences in white matter lesion patterns between diabetics and controls were analyzed using the non-parametric statistical analysis described by Holmes et al. [12]. This test is based on generating randomizations of the distribution of observations across the control and the diabetics group. The test statistics resulting from the randomizations were compared with the test statistic resulting from the experimental observation. Thus, the probability distribution of the test statistic was calculated based on the experimental data. This approach allowed us to calculate for each voxel the probability that the control and diabetics group were drawn from the same population.

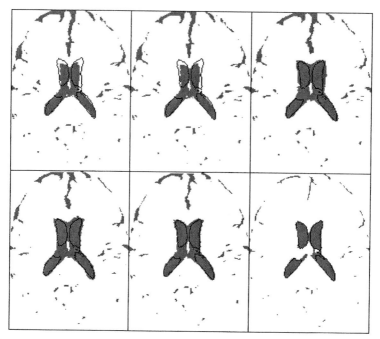

Fig. 3. Registration of the CSF segmentation of a subject (*gray*) to the average ventricle (*black lines*). The top row shows from left to right the result after registration using affine transformations, CPS 64 and CPS 32 non-rigid registration. The bottom row shows from left to right the result after non-rigid registration using CPS 16, CPS 8, and CPS 4

3   Results

3.1   Registration

Usually, the overlap between two segmentations is calculated as a measure of registration accuracy by taking two times the number of overlapping voxels divided by the sum of the total number of voxels in both segmentations. Since in this case one segmentation contains all CSF structures and the other only lateral ventricles, this would not yield relevant numbers. Therefore, we have constructed a one-voxel dilation around the average ventricles. Next, we constructed a one-voxel dilation around this first dilation, then around the second and around the third. So, we have four one voxel (0.9 mm) thick structures (referred to as dilation 1 (closest to the average ventricles) to 4 (farthest away)) and for each we counted the number of CSF segmentation voxels overlapping with this structure.

Figure 1 shows the percentage of average ventricle voxels that are overlapped by the CSF segmentation of diabetes patients and controls for the subsequent steps in the registration procedure. In Figure 2 the overlap of the CSF segmentation with the one-voxel dilations around the average ventricles is shown. Ideally, the overlap with the average ventricles is a hundred percent and the overlap with the dilations is zero.

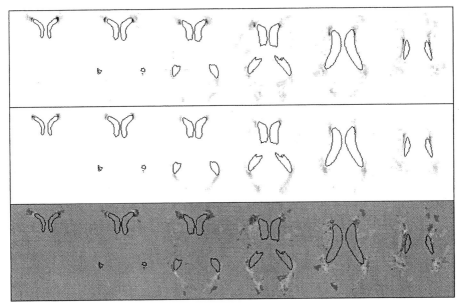

Fig. 4. Lesion pattern image for control subjects (*top row*) and diabetes patients (*middle row*). Darker gray indicates a higher prevalence of lesion. The bottom row shows the difference in lesion patterns with whiter areas indicating a higher lesion prevalence in diabetes patients and darker areas a higher prevalence in control subjects. The black lines show the outline of the average lateral ventricle.

After registration with a control point spacing of 32 voxels, almost all voxels of the average ventricle are overlapped by voxels of the CSF segmentations. However, this is at the expense of the overlap with the dilations, which is also increased. Thus, the CSF segmentation has deformed so that its ventricles have become somewhat larger than the average ventricles. Refinement of the control point grid decreases the overlap with the dilations while retaining and even slightly improving the overlap with the average ventricles.

For finer CPSs the overlap with the dilations is limited to the first dilation. The overlap in dilations two, three and four, especially for CPS eight and four, is caused by the presence of structures in the CSF segmentations other than lateral ventricles such as the third and fourth ventricle.

In Figure 3 the registration of a patient to the average ventricle is shown. Note that the CSF structures not present in the average ventricle image are subject to shrinkage. Inspection of the deformation fields reveals that this is only a local effect, which does not influence the deformations in the peri-ventricular areas.

3.2 White Matter Lesion Patterns

Figure 4 shows the lesion pattern in diabetes patients and control subjects, corrected for group size, and a subtraction image showing the differences between patients and controls. The lesion patterns did not differ significantly between diabetes patients and controls.

4 Discussion

We developed an automatic approach to inter-subject ventricle registration for the analysis of peri-ventricular white matter lesions. We constructed a binary average ventricle image as reference to match segmented CSF from different subjects. The registrations of the CSF to the lateral ventricles were accurate, mostly within one dilation of 0.9 mm. The approach of registering all CSF to only lateral ventricles did not lead to inaccuracies in the peri-ventricular regions.

The lesion patterns presented are preliminary and only intended to demonstrate the suitability of the presented method. The number of subjects is too small to have clinical implications. It is clear, however, that our approach provides a way to gain insight into the specifics of the lesion pattern of a patient group. In conclusion, the presented approach of registering CSF to an average ventricle is accurate, feasible, and well suited for the analysis of peri-ventricular white matter lesions.

Acknowledgements. The authors would like to thank the following people and laboratories for kindly supplying them with software and data:
- The Laboratory for Medical Imaging Research in Leuven for the software for mutual information-based registration
- B. Likar from the Department of Electrical Engineering of the University of Ljubljana for the software for MR intensity inhomogeneity correction
- D. Rueckert from the Computational Imaging Science Group, King's College London for the software for non-rigid registration using free-form deformations
- The Utrecht Diabetic Encephalopathy Study group of the University Medical Center Utrecht for the image data.

References

1. de Leeuw, F.E., de Groot, J.C., Achten, E., Oudkerk, M., Ramos, L.M., Heijboer, R., Hofman, A., Jolles, J., van Gijn, J., Breteler, M.M.: Prevalence of cerebral white matter lesions in elderly people: a population based magnetic resonance imaging study. The Rotterdam Scan Study. J. Neurol. Neurosurg. Psychiatry 70 (2001) 9-14
2. de Leeuw, F.E., de Groot, J.C., Oudkerk, M., Witteman, J.C., Hofman, A., van Gijn, J., Breteler, M.M.: Hypertension and cerebral white matter lesions in a prospective cohort study. Brain 125 (2002) 765-772
3. Longstreth, W.T., Jr., Manolio, T.A., Arnold, A., Burke, G.L., Bryan, N., Jungreis, C.A., Enright, P.L., O'Leary, D., Fried, L.: Clinical correlates of white matter findings on cranial magnetic resonance imaging of 3301 elderly people. The Cardiovascular Health Study. Stroke 27 (1996) 1274-1282
4. Taylor, W.D., MacFall, J.R., Provenzale, J.M., Payne, M.E. , McQuoid, D.R., Steffens, D.C., Krishnan, K.R.: Serial MR imaging of volumes of hyperintense white matter lesions in elderly patients: correlation with vascular risk factors. AJR Am. J. Roentgenol. 181 (2003) 571-576
5. Likar, B., Viergever, M.A., Pernus, F.: Retrospective correction of MR intensity inhomogeneity by information minimization. IEEE Trans Med Imaging 20 (2001) 1398-1410

6. Maes, F., Collignon, A., Vandermeulen, D., Marchal, G., Suetens, P.: Multimodality image registration by maximization of mutual information. IEEE Trans Med Imaging 16 (1997) 187- 198

7. Bradley, P.S., Fayyad, U.M.: Refining initial points for K-means clustering. International Conference on Machine Learning (1998) 91-99

8. Herman, G.T., Zheng, J.S., Bucholtz, C.A.: Shape-based interpolation. IEEE Computer Graphics and Applications 12 (1992) 69-79

9. Rueckert, D., Sonoda, L.I., Hayes, C., Hill, D.L.G., Leach, M.O., Hawkes, D.J.: Nonrigid registration using free-form deformations: application to breast MR images. IEEE Trans Med Imaging 18 (1999) 712-721

10. Studholme, C., Hill, D.L.G., Hawkes, D.J.: An overlap invariant entropy measure of 3D medical image alignment. Pattern Recognition 32 (1999) 71-86

11. Anbeek, P., Vincken, K.L., van Osch, M.J.P., Bisschops, R.H.C., van der Grond, J.: Probabilistic segmentation of white matter lesions in MR imaging. Neuroimage in press (2004)

12. Holmes, A.P., Blair, R.C., Watson, J.D.G., Ford, I.: Nonparametric analysis of statistic images from functional mapping experiments. J Cereb Blood Flow Metab 16 (1996) 7-22

Deformable Registration of Tumor-Diseased Brain Images

Tianming Liu, Dinggang Shen, and Christos Davatzikos

Section of Biomedical Image Analysis, Department of Radiology,
University of Pennsylvania, Philadelphia, PA 19104
{tliu, dgshen, christos}@rad.upenn.edu

Abstract. This paper presents an approach for deformable registration of a normal brain atlas to visible anatomic structures in a tumor-diseased brain image. We restrict our attention to cortical surfaces. First, a model surface in the atlas is warped to the tumor-diseased brain image via a HAMMER-based volumetric registration algorithm. However, the volumetric warping is generally inaccurate around the tumor region, due to the lack of reliable features to which the atlas can be matched. Therefore, the model structures for which no reliable matches are found are labeled by a Markov Random Field-Maximum A Posteriori approach. A statistically-based interpolation method is then used to correct/refine the volumetric warping for those structures. Finally, with the good initialization obtained by the above steps and the identification of the part of the model anatomy that can be recognized in the patient's image, the model surface is adaptively warped to its counterpart that is visible in the tumor-diseased brain image through a surface registration procedure. Preliminary results show good performance on both simulated and real tumor-diseased brain images.

1 Introduction

In neurosurgical planning, it is of interest to register a normal brain atlas to a patient's tumor-diseased brain image, in order to transfer the information available in the atlas to the patient's space for surgical guidance. In this paper, we propose an approach for deformable registration of a normal brain atlas to visible anatomic structures in a patient's brain image in the presence of tumor. We assume that only part of the patient's anatomy is visible, since some tissue might be severely distorted by the tumor and/or obscured by edema, and some tissue might have died during the tumor growth. Our long-term goal is to use the registered visible anatomy to estimate 1) the tumor location in a standardized atlas for the purpose of atlas construction from such patients and 2) the location of deformed and invisible structures for the purpose of neurosurgical planning. As an example, Figure 1 shows a normal atlas and a tumor-diseased brain image to be registered.

In general, the proposed approach extracts and exploits reliable information to drive the registration. There are four steps in our approach, as summarized in Figure 2. Firstly, a complete model surface (i.e., see Figure 1) in the atlas is warped to the space of a patient's brain by a HAMMER-based volumetric registration algorithm [6]. Secondly, a confidence level for the accuracy of volumetric warping for each model

C. Barillot, D.R. Haynor, and P. Hellier (Eds.): MICCAI 2004, LNCS 3216, pp. 720–728, 2004.
© Springer-Verlag Berlin Heidelberg 2004

surface vertex is determined by computing the possibility of this vertex has found its counterpart in the tumor-diseased brain. The degree of confidence will be low around the region where image features are missing due to the presence of tumor and/or edema. Based on the confidence map, we employ a Markov Random Field (MRF)-Maximum A Posteriori (MAP) approach to classify the model surface vertices into two groups, one roughly corresponding to the missing/invisible anatomy in the patient's brain, and the other roughly corresponding to the visible anatomy. Thirdly, a statistically-based interpolation method is used to correct/refine the deformation fields in the low confidence regions by those in the relatively high confidence regions. Finally, with the good initialization obtained by the first three steps and the identification of the part of the model anatomy that can be recognized in the patient's image, the model surface is adaptively warped to its counterpart visible in the patient's brain image by a surface registration procedure.

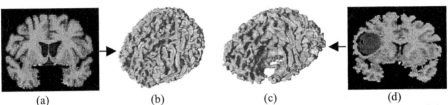

  (a)   (b)   (c)   (d)

Fig. 1. A normal atlas and a tumor-diseased brain image, to be registered. (a) A slice of the normal atlas. (b) The WM/GM surface reconstructed from the atlas. (c) The WM/GM surface reconstructed from a tumor-diseased brain image. (d) A typical slice of the tumor-diseased brain image (low grade glioma).

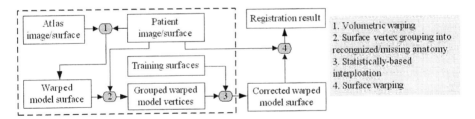

Fig. 2. The summary of our registration approach. The steps in the dashed block provide the initialization for the model surface in the atlas, to be adaptively deformed in step 4.

2 Method

2.1 Volumetric Warping

The HAMMER-based volumetric registration algorithm [6] is used to bring the model surface in the atlas close to its counterpart visible in the tumor-diseased brain image, in order to facilitate the subsequent steps. The registration accuracy is expected to be relatively high in normal brain regions [6]. However, the volumetric warping is expected to be less accurate around the tumor region, due to the lack of reliable features to which the atlas can be matched. To address this problem, a statistically-based interpolation method is used in Section 2.3 to correct/refine the volumetric warping around the tumor region, in order to provide better initialization for the model surface so that it can be registered with visible structures in the tumor-diseased brain through a surface registration described in Section 2.4.

2.2 Surface Vertex Grouping

To facilitate the statistically-based interpolation in Section 2.3, which requires hard grouping of the model surface vertices, the warped model vertices are classified into two groups. One group includes the vertices for which a good match can be found in the patient's brain after volumetric warping, and the opposite for the second group.

Firstly, we compute the confidence level of volumetric warping for each model surface vertex, in order to roughly measure the warping accuracy. The confidence level is defined as the similarity between this model surface vertex and its most likely counterpart in the surface of the tumor-diseased brain. Intuitively, if the similarity is higher for a model vertex, we can have more chance of detecting its correspondence in the registration procedure and thus have more confidence in the accuracy of the volumetric warping for this model vertex. The similarity between a model surface vertex s_i^{Mdl} and a surface vertex in the patient's brain s_j^{Ptn} is defined as:

$$f(s_i^{Mdl}, s_j^{Ptn}) = (n(s_i^{Mdl}) \bullet n(s_j^{Ptn})) \cdot C(s_i^{Mdl}, s_j^{Ptn}) \tag{1}$$

where $n(s_i^{Mdl})$ is a normal vector of the vertex s_i^{Mdl}, '$\bullet$' denotes the dot product of two vectors, and $C(s_i^{Mdl}, s_j^{Ptn})$ is the similarity of the surface curvatures of vertex s_i^{Mdl} and s_j^{Ptn}, which is defined next:

$$C(s_i^{Mdl}, s_j^{Ptn}) = 1 - \left\| c(s_i^{Mdl}) - c(s_j^{Ptn}) \right\| / (c(s_i^{Mdl}) + c(s_j^{Ptn})) \tag{2}$$

where $c(\bullet)$ is calculated as $\sqrt{(k_1^2 + k_2^2)/2}$, with k_1 and k_2 as two principle curvatures. For each model surface vertex s_i^{Mdl}, we look for a surface vertex in the patient's brain image with the largest degree of similarity. Here, $y_{s_i^{Mdl}}$ is used to denote the largest degree of similarity found for the model surface vertex s_i^{Mdl}. These computations create the confidence map, denoted by $Y = \{y_{s_i^{Mdl}}\}$.

To classify model surface vertices into two groups based on above confidence map, we employ a MRF-MAP method, because MRF theory provides an efficient and powerful framework for modeling spatial dependence and MAP estimation offers a mechanism for finding a desirable solution. Let $S^{Mdl} = \{s_i^{Mdl}\}$ denote the set of model vertices. For each vertex, a first-order neighborhood system, consisting of its immediate neighbors, is defined for the MRF. Let $\Lambda = \{0, 1\}$ be the label set, where 0 means recognized/matched vertex and 1 means unrecognized/missing vertex. Let $\omega = \{\omega_{s_i^{Mdl}}\}$ be the vertex grouping result, where $\omega_{s_i^{Mdl}}$ takes a value from Λ. Now, the objective of the grouping is to maximize the posteriori probability of $P(\omega|Y)$. According to the Bayes theory, the MAP-based vertex grouping is obtained by:

$$\omega^* = \arg\max_{\omega \in \Omega} (P(Y \mid \omega)P(\omega)) \qquad (3)$$

where Ω is the set of all possible grouping results. The term $P(Y \mid \omega)$ is modeled as an independent multivariate Gaussian distribution. According to the Hammersley-Clifford theorem [1], $P(\omega)$ has the Gibbs distribution, and its energy term is the sum of clique potentials over all possible cliques. Here, only cliques of a size up to two are considered, and the homogeneous multi-level logistic (MLL) distribution [1] is used to define the potential for two adjacent vertices. To solve Eq. (3), we use the local optimization method of Iterated Conditional Modes (ICM) [2].

Notably, we reconstruct anatomic surface in the patient's brain directly from the WM/GM volume in the tissue-classified image [4], without pre-segmentation of the tumor. This may introduce false WM/GM structures when performing the marching cubes algorithm to the possible extra WM/GM boundaries, produced during the tissue classification of the tumor-diseased brain image. However, those false structures have little effect on the surface vertex grouping and the following step of surface registration, since no structures of the model would match them.

2.3 Statistically-Based Interpolation

The general idea of the statistically-based interpolation is that we determine the deformation vectors of part of model surface by those of the remainder of the model surface using a statistical estimation method. In this paper, we use the statistically-based interpolation to correct/refine the volumetric warping in the low confidence regions.

More specifically, we discard the volumetric warping in the low confidence regions $\{s_i^{\text{Mdl}}, \omega_{s_i^{\text{Mdl}}}^* = 1\}$, and estimate it by that in the high confidence regions $\{s_i^{\text{Mdl}}, \omega_{s_i^{\text{Mdl}}}^* = 0\}$, using a statistical estimation method based on canonical correlation analysis in [5]. The statistical estimation is achieved by learning from a training set of deformation fields, which is obtained by warping a model surface in the atlas into individual normal brain images via the hybrid registration method in [3, 4].

It is worth noting that the statistically-based interpolation places the model structures much closer to their counterparts visible around the tumor region than the volumetric warping in Section 2.1, thus providing a good start for the next step of surface registration. In the future, we intend to take into account the statistics of the tumor mass effect, which can be obtained via a large number of tumor growth simulations at different brain locations [8, 9], in the statistically-based interpolation, thus leading to better initialization for the following step of surface warping.

2.4 Surface Warping

Based on the initialization obtained by the first three steps, the surface warping step is designed to adaptively deform the model surface $S^{\text{Mdl}} = \{s_i^{\text{Mdl}}\}$ to the surface in the patient's tumor-diseased brain image $S^{\text{Ptn}} = \{s_i^{\text{Ptn}}\}$, by using the above-collected confidence map and vertex grouping result as deformation adaptation knowledge to guide the surface registration. Notably, we allow only the model vertices with high confidence levels to search for their correspondences in the surface of the tumor-diseased brain image. For any model vertex s_i^{Mdl}, if that vertex finds its correspondence, then its surface patch $P(s_i^{\text{Mdl}}, r)$ within a geodesic distance r will be deformed to the patient's brain surface by a local transformation $T_{s_i^{\text{Mdl}}}$. Therefore, the whole transformation h for the warping of the model surface is decomposed into a number of local transformations $\{ T_{s_i^{\text{Mdl}}} \}$, i.e., $h = \{ T_{s_i^{\text{Mdl}}} \}$.

Mathematically, the surface warping can be formulated as a procedure of minimizing the energy function as defined next:

$$E\left(h = \{T_{s_i^{\text{Mdl}}}\}\right) = \sum_{s_i^{\text{Mdl}} \in S^{\text{Mdl}}, \omega_{s_i^{\text{Mdl}}} = 0} y_{s_i^{\text{Mdl}}} \left(w_{\text{Ext}} E_{s_i^{\text{Mdl}}}^{\text{Ext}}(T_{s_i^{\text{Mdl}}}) + w_{\text{Int}} E_{s_i^{\text{Mdl}}}^{\text{Int}}(T_{s_i^{\text{Mdl}}}) \right) \quad (4)$$

where $y_{s_i^{\text{Mdl}}}$ is the confidence level of s_i^{Mdl} and used to weight different model vertices differently. Only model vertices with high confidence levels, namely having $\omega_{s_i^{\text{Mdl}}} = 0$, are considered as viable to deform the model surface. w_{Ext} and w_{Int} are the weights for external and internal energies, respectively.

The external energy $E_{s_i^{\text{Mdl}}}^{\text{Ext}}(T_{s_i^{\text{Mdl}}})$ measures the similarity of the surface patches in the atlas and those in the patient, respectively. It requires that the curvature of the neighboring vertex s_j^{Mdl} in the model surface patch $P(s_i^{\text{Mdl}}, r)$ be similar to that of its counterpart in the patient, and also that the normal direction of vertex s_j^{Mdl} be close to that of its counterpart. The mathematical definition is given as:

$$E_{s_i^{\text{Mdl}}}^{\text{Ext}}(T_{s_i^{\text{Mdl}}}) = \sum_{s_j^{\text{Mdl}} \in P(s_i^{\text{Mdl}}, r)} \left(w_1 \left\| c(s_j^{\text{Mdl}}) - c\left(m\left(T_{s_i^{\text{Mdl}}}(s_j^{\text{Mdl}})\right)\right) \right\| + w_2 \left\| n(s_j^{\text{Mdl}}) - n\left(m\left(T_{s_i^{\text{Mdl}}}(s_j^{\text{Mdl}})\right)\right) \right\| \right) \quad (5)$$

where $c(\cdot)$ and $n(\cdot)$ denote the surface curvedness and the normal vector, respectively. $m(.)$ denotes a mapping of a vertex to the closest vertex in the patient's surface, since the transformed model vertex $T_{s_i^{\text{Mdl}}}(s_j^{\text{Mdl}})$ is not necessary on the patient's surface vertex. w_1 and w_2 are weighting parameters.

The internal energy term $E_{s_i^{\text{Mdl}}}^{\text{Int}}(T_{s_i^{\text{Mdl}}})$ is defined as the same as that in [3, 4], in order to preserve the shape of the model surface during deformation. To minimize the energy function, we use a greedy deformation algorithm. Similarly, we use the scheme in [4] to prevent self-intersection during deformation, and use the adaptive deformation strategy [4, 7] based on the confidence map to reduce the chances of being trapped of local minima. Notably, the confidence map and vertex grouping result are updated using the method in Section 2.2 after each iteration of the energy minimization process, since during the surface deformation procedure, some model structures might move outside the tumor, while other structures might move inside it.

So far, we have not used any tumor information in the registration. However, integrating tumor information, i.e., the location of tumor, into the registration procedure can potentially improve the registration accuracy.

3   Results

The performance of the proposed approach is tested by both simulated and real tumor-diseased brains. In these experiments, we register only WM/GM surfaces.

In this experiment using simulated tumor-diseased image, we compare the registration result obtained by our proposed approach with the ground-truth that is created as follows. We employ the method in [9] to grow a tumor in a normal brain image, and produce a tumor-induced deformation field. Then, the model WM/GM surface in the atlas is registered with its counterpart in the normal brain image [3, 4], and further deformed by the tumor-induced deformation field generated in the tumor simulation. The finally deformed model WM/GM surface is regarded as the ground-truth. Independently, we use the proposed approach to register the WM/GM surface reconstructed from the simulated tumor-diseased brain image. Figure 3 shows the histogram of registration errors of the proposed approach, compared to the ground-truth, after initialization and after final surface warping. The average registration error in the visible structures of the tumor-diseased brain drops from 1.4 mm to 1.1 mm, from initialization to final surface warping. As for the WM/GM surface around the tumor region, the average registration error drops from 2.5 mm to 1.8 mm. Figure 4 shows the overlay of a typical slice with the patient's WM/GM surface, the initialized model surface and the finally warped model surface. The registration result seems visually reasonable.

The performance of the proposed approach is also tested using real tumor-diseased brains obtained from the SPL brain tumor database [10]. Figure 5 shows the overlay of a typical slice with three surfaces, a patient's WM/GM surface, the initialized model surface and the finally warped model surface. It can be seen that the registration result is visually reasonable. For reference, the patient's WM/GM surface can be found in Figure 1. Since we do not know the true correspondences among the WM/GM surfaces in this experiment, we used the surface distance to measure the registration accuracy. By this measurement, the average distance is 0.3 mm from the finally warped model surface to the patient's surface, and is 0.46 mm from the patient's surface to the finally warped model surface. Here, only regions labeled high confidence are counted in the surface distance calculation. Notably, the average

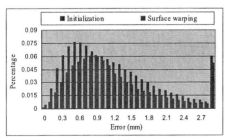 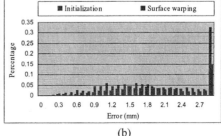

(a)   (b)

Fig. 3. Histogram of registration errors, after initialization and after final surface warping. The horizontal axis is the registration error, and the vertical axis is the percentage of the vertices on the model surface. (a) For all visible WM/GM structures. (b) Only for the visible WM/GM structures around the tumor.

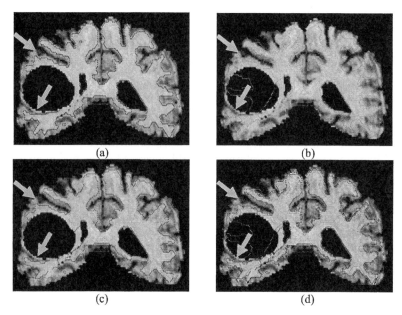

Fig. 4. Registration result for a simulated tumor-diseased brain. (a) Overlay of a typical slice and its own WM/GM surface. (b) The initialized model WM/GM surface. (c) The finally warped model WM/GM surface. (d) Overlay of all three surfaces. The arrows indicate the positions where the registration results were significantly improved by the surface warping.

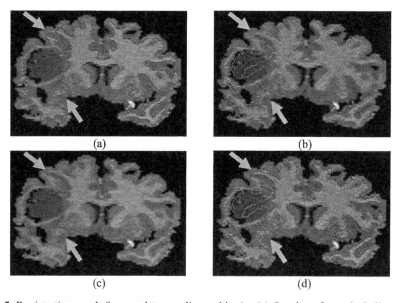

Fig. 5. Registration result for a real tumor-diseased brain. (a) Overlay of a typical slice and its own WM/GM surface. (b) The initialized model WM/GM surface. (c) The finally warped model WM/GM surface, shown only on visible WM/GM structures of tumor brain. (d) Overlay of all three surfaces.

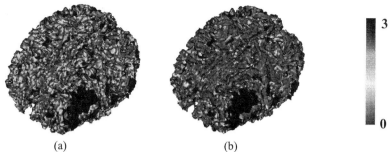

(a)   (b)

Fig. 6. Color-coded map of surface distance (mm), according to the color-bar at the right. (a) After initialization. (b) After final surface warping.

model-to-patient surface distance drops 57 percent after the surface warping. This can be confirmed by a color-coded map of distances of the warped model surface to the patient's surface in Figure 6.

4   Conclusion

We proposed an approach for deformable registration of a normal atlas to the visible anatomic structures in a tumor-diseased brain. Although we registered only WM/GM surface in this paper, our approach can be applied to register other surfaces in a tumor-diseased brain, including the GM/CSF surface. In the future, we intend to integrate into the registration approach the statistics of the mass effect of a tumor, which are determined via a large number of tumor growth simulations at different brain locations, and validate the approach using a larger number of patient brains.

Acknowledgement. The authors would like to thank Ashraf Mohamed for providing the simulated tumor-diseased brain and the SPL group of the Brigham and Women's Hospital for sharing the brain tumor database.

References

1.   Stan Z. Li, Markov random field modeling in image analysis, Springer-Verlag New York, Inc., Secaucus, NJ, 2001.
2.   J. Besag, "On the statistical analysis of dirty pictures," J. Roy. Statist. Soc. B 48(3), pp. 259-302, 1986.
3.   T. Liu, D. Shen, C. Davatzikos, "Deformable registration of cortical structures via hybrid volumetric and surface warping," MICCAI 2003, Canada, 2003.
4.   T. Liu, D. Shen, C. Davatzikos, "Deformable registration of cortical structures via hybrid volumetric and surface warping," submitted to NeuroImage.
5.   T. Liu, D. Shen, C. Davatzikos, "Predictive modeling of anatomic structures using canonical correlation analysis," To appear, ISBI 2004, April 15-18, Arlington, VA.
6.   D. Shen and C. Davatzikos, "HAMMER: hierarchical attribute matching mechanism for elastic registration," IEEE Transactions on Medical Imaging, 21(11): 1421-1439, 2002.

7. D. Shen, E. H. Herskovits, and C. Davatzikos, "An adaptive-focus statistical shape model for segmentation and shape modeling of 3D brain structures," IEEE Transactions on Medical Imaging, 20(4): 257-270, April 2001.
8. C. Davatzikos, D. Shen, A. Mohamed, and S. Kyriacou, "A framework for predictive modeling of anatomical deformations," IEEE TMI, 20 (8):836-843, 2001.
9. A. Mohamed and C. Davatzikos, "Finite element mesh generation and remeshing from segmented medical images," To appear, ISBI 2004, Arlington, VA, 2004.
10. M. Kaus, S. K. Warfield, A. Nabavi, P. M. Black, F. A. Jolesz, and R. Kikinis. "Automated segmentation of MRI of brain tumors," Radiology, 218:586-591, 2001.

Toward the Creation of an Electrophysiological Atlas for the Pre-operative Planning and Intra-operative Guidance of Deep Brain Stimulators (DBS) Implantation

Pierre-François D'Haese[1,2], Ebru Cetinkaya[1], Chris Kao[3],
J. Michael Fitzpatrick[1], Peter E. Konrad[3], and Benoit M. Dawant[1]

[1] Vanderbilt University, Nashville, TN, USA
{pierre-francois.dhaese, benoit.dawant}@vanderbilt.edu
http://www.vuse.vanderbilt.edu/~mip-web
[2] Université Catholique de Louvain, Louvain-la-Neuve, Belgique
[3] Department of Neurosurgery, Vanderbilt Medical Center, Nashville, TN, USA

Abstract. In current practice, optimal placement of deep brain stimulators (DBSs) is an iterative procedure. A target is chosen pre-operatively based on anatomical landmarks identified on MR images. This point is used as an initial position that is refined intra-operatively using both micro-electrode recordings and macro-stimulation. We hypothesize that boundaries of nuclei and sub-nuclei not visible in the anatomic images can be resolved in atlases that include electrophysiological information, thus improving both pre- and intra-operative guidance. In this work we report on our current progress toward creating such an atlas. We also present results we have obtained in creating an atlas of optimal target points that can be used for automatic pre-operative selection of the targets. We demonstrate that initial points selected with this atlas are closer to the final points than the initial points chosen manually.

1 Introduction

Since its first FDA approval in 1998 deep-brain stimulation (DBS) has gained significant popularity in the treatment of movement disorders [1,2]. The therapy has significant applications in the treatment of tremor, rigidity, and drug induced side effects in patients with Parkinson's disease and essential tremor. This procedure, which necessitates placing electrodes within targets ranging from 4-12 mm in diameter, requires stereotactic neurosurgical methodology. Typically, the process of implantation of a DBS electrode follows a step-wise progression of a) initial estimation of target localization based on imaged anatomical landmarks, b) intraoperative microanatomical mapping of key features associated with the intended target of interest, c) adjustment of the final target of implantation by appropriate shifts in three dimensional space, and d) implantation of a quadripolar electrode with contacts located surrounding the final desired target. These steps are required because the surgical targets of interest involve deep brain

C. Barillot, D.R. Haynor, and P. Hellier (Eds.): MICCAI 2004, LNCS 3216, pp. 729–736, 2004.

nuclei or subregions within the subthalamus or globus pallidus internus. These structures are not visible in any imaging modalities, such as magnetic resonance imaging (MRI), X-ray computed tomography (CT), or Positron Emission Tomography (PET). Pre-operatively, the location of these targets can thus only be inferred approximately from the position of adjacent structures that are visible in the images. Intra-operative adjustment of the target point is based on the surgical team's (at our institution, this team involves a neurosurgeon, a neurophysiologist, and a neurologist) interpretation of electrophysiological recordings and responses to stimulations. Anecdotal evidence based on conversations with the surgical team and observations of the procedure suggests that intra-operative electrode adjustment involves (1) matching a set of input data (e.g., loss of rigidity, firing rate, severity of side effects, stimulation voltage, etc.) with electrophysiological landmarks that can be related to the target of interest and (2) planning and execution of a displacement from the current position to the desired one. For instance, as a result of test stimulations applied through a trajectory, the clinical team may observe that unacceptable double vision occurs along with mild symptomatic relief of rigidity. The interpretation of this information would be that the trajectory is too medial. The difficult anatomical question at this point is: *in this particular patient* how far lateral does the trajectory need to be moved, e.g., 1, 2, or 3mm. Because of anatomical differences between patients, this question is difficult to answer. It could, however, be more easily answered if the current position could be mapped onto an atlas, the displacement determined in the atlas, and this displacement mapped back onto the patient. Doing so requires several key ingredients: (1) accurate algorithms to register patients and atlases, (2) populating the atlases with information that permits the labeling of structures and substructures based on their electrophysiological signatures, and (3) mapping electrophysiological signals to landmarks in the atlas. Others have proposed the creation of electrophysiological atlases [3] but these were populated with labels derived from intra-operative observations such as the type of side effect or its location. To the best of our knowledge we are the first to create an electrophysiological atlas directly from from the raw digitized signals. In the rest of the paper, we first present an extension of preliminary work presented earlier [4] that demonstrates the feasibility of using automatic nonrigid registration algorithms to create these atlases and to use them for preoperative planning. Then, we discuss the techniques we have developed for the creation of electrophysiological atlases. Finally, we present results we have obtained with recordings acquired on 8 patients.

2   Methods

2.1   Patients and Pre-operative Target Selection

All patients undergoing consideration for DBS implantation of the STN are first evaluated by a movement disorders neurologist and optimized on medications. If patients reach advanced parkinsonian symptoms (rigidity, bradykinesia, tremor, dyskinesias) despite optimal medical therapy, they are considered for surgical therapy by a multi-disciplinary group involving neurology, neurosurgery, neurophysiology, neuropsychiatry specialists. Target selection is decided upon by the team if no contraindications exist. A majority of patients with the above symptoms are recommended for STN (Sub Thalamic Nucleus) targeting of DBS therapy. Pre-operative target identification is performed by the functional neurosurgeon (P.E.K.) and is based on an identification of the AC-PC (anterior and posterior commissure) location and arriving at 4mm posterior, 12mm lateral, and 4mm inferior to the mid-commissural point for STN. Small adjustments to the target points can be made based on the width of the third ventricle and other anatomical asymmetries noted on the MRI scan, but these usually only consist of less than 1mm deviations from the initial intended target location.

2.2   Intraoperative Placement and Guidance System

Traditional methodology for carrying out the stepwise target localization procedure followed for DBS implantation requires an external, rigid fixture, called a "stereotactic frame" that encompasses the patient's head and upon which micro-manipulating equipment can be mounted and maneuvered with sub-millimetric precision. Recently, a market-cleared and CE-compliant miniature stereotactic positioner called a *microTargeting Platform* became clinically available (*microTargeting Drive System for Stereotactic Positioning, incorporating STarFix guidance*, FHC Inc., Bowdoinham, ME). This device, which is used at our institution presents several advantages: 1) Separation of the phase of the procedure that includes image acquisition and target planning from the actual day of the surgery. This allows for CT and MR images to be acquired under anesthesia and thereby reduce motion artifacts on the resultant images. 2) Patients are not tethered to the bed since the platform is small enough not to require stabilization thus reducing patient discomfort during the procedure. 3) The platform permits simultaneous bilateral implantation, which is not possible with traditional frames. Accuracy studies performed on this platform have also shown a placement accuracy at least good as the accuracy achievable with larger frames [5].

2.3   Data

A set of CT and MRI volumes are acquired pre-operatively for each patient. These are acquired with the patient anesthetized and head taped to the table to minimize motion. CT images are acquired at kvp = 120V, exposure = 350ms, 512x512 voxels ranging in size from 0.49 to 0.62 mm, slice thickness = 2 mm for one patient, 1.3 mm for 2 patients, 1mm for all others; MR images are 3D SPGR volumes, TR: 12.2, TE: 2.4, dimension 256x256x124 voxels, voxels dimensions 0.85X0.85X1.3mm3 except for subject 7 for which the voxels dimensions are 1X1X1.3mm3. Nineteen patients are included in the current study: 13 bilateral STN and 6 unilateral STN. For the 8 latest patients, micro-electrical signals have been recorded intra-operatively and saved using the dual channel LeadPoint system from Medtronic Neurological. These signals were recorded along the electrode path starting 10mm above the preoperative target point and ending 5mm below. Signals were recorded every .5mm for 10sec, and sampled at 22Khz. After the procedure, the digitized signals and the position at which these signals have been acquired are downloaded from the LeadPoint system and stored on file for further processing. At the time of writing, 850 signal epochs have been recorded.

2.4   Registration Algorithms

Two types of registrations algorithms are needed to process our data: rigid and non-rigid. The rigid registration algorithm is required to register MR and CT volumes of the same patient. This is necessary because the intra-operative positions of the recording and stimulating electrodes are given in CT coordinates. The algorithm we have used for this is an independent implementation of a standard MI-based algorithm [6]. Non-rigid registration is required to register patient data to an atlas and vice-versa. In this study, non-rigid registration is always performed on MR image volumes using an algorithm we have proposed recently [7]. Briefly, this algorithm computes a deformation field that is modeled as a linear combination of radial basis functions with finite support. The similarity measure we use is the Mutual Information between the images. We also compute two transformations (one from the atlas to the subject and the other from the subject to the atlas) that are inverse of each other.

3   Results

3.1   Registration Accuracy and Creation of an Atlas of Target Points

Validation of non-rigid registration algorithms is a notoriously difficult problem because of the lack of "gold standards". Fortunately, with a few assumptions, the nature of our problem allows us to assess in an indirect way the accuracy of our algorithms and their adequacy for our long term objectives. The STN is a very small structure (on the order of a few mm). Because of this and if one assumes that (1) the surgical team is able to place the electrode within the STN in each patient, (2) our intra-operative guidance system can provide us with the accurate position of the electrode in CT coordinates, and (3) our registration algorithms are accurate, then, mapping each and every target point selected intra-operatively onto the atlas should result in tight clusters of points in this atlas. In this work, we have chosen one of the subjects as the reference, which we call the atlas, and we have registered all the other volumes to it. We have then projected every final target point onto the atlas, thus creating two clouds of points (one for the left and the other for the right STNs). Figure 1 shows the results we have obtained and it demonstrates, at least qualitatively, our ability to cluster tightly the points selected intra-operatively onto the atlas. To quantify these results, we have computed the position of the centroid of each of these two clouds of points. We have then computed the distance between each point and its corresponding centroid, which we call Dc. Table 1 reports the results we have obtained.

Table 1. Position (mean and std) of the target points in the atlas and distance from centroids in mm

	Left				Right			
	X	Y	Z	Dc	X	Y	Z	Dc
Mean	121.6	106	50.2	2.8	97.5	106	49.2	2.8
Std	1.5	1.5	2.2	1.1	1.9	1.7	1.6	0.7

Table 2. Distances (in mm) between pre-operative target position and final intra-operative position.

	Pre-operative placement error			
	Left		Right	
	Auto	Man	Auto	Man
Mean	2.49	2.70	2.78	3.88
Std	1.31	1.98	0.76	2.04

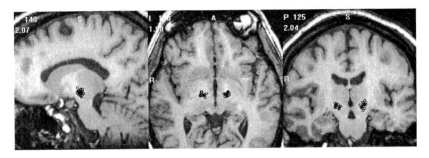

Fig. 1. DBS positions selected intra-operatively mapped onto the atlas.

3.2   Automatic Pre-operative Prediction of the Optimal Target Point

Rather than relying on a reference system based on the AC-PC line as it is done currently, the pre-operative target point could be predicted automatically by first selecting a standard target point in the atlas, registering the atlas to the patient image volume, and mapping the target point from the atlas to the patient volume. To evaluate this approach we have used the centroids introduced in the previous paragraph as our standard target points and we have mapped those onto the patient image volume to define the pre-operative position of the target point. To avoid both defining and evaluating the standard target point on the same data sets, we have used a leave-one-out strategy (i.e., the coordinates of the centroids have been computed using 17 volumes and projected on the 18th one; the process has been repeated 18 times). To compare the position of the pre-operative target point chosen manually using the current clinical procedure and the automatic technique we propose, we define the pre-operative placement error. This error is defined as the Euclidean distance between the final intra-operative position selected by the surgical team and the position chosen pre-operatively. It is thus the distance by which the surgical team adjusted the position of the electrode during the procedure. Table 2 reports both the manual and the automatic pre-operative placement errors. This table shows that the pre-operative target point selected automatically is closer to the final target point than the pre-operative target point chosen manually.

3.3   Electrophysiological Atlas Creation

An important component of our project is the development of a database that permits storage and access of all the pre-, intra-, and post-operative information pertaining to patients undergoing treatment at our institution. In this database, any spatially-dependent patient information can be related to a position in the atlas through registration. Albeit under construction, our current database already supports queries such as "return all the intra-operative recordings for patients with Parkinson we have in our database in a 5mm sphere centered at coordinates (x, y, z) in the atlas". This query returns a set of pointers to files that contain the digitized signals. These files can then be processed, features extracted, and these features associated with a point in the atlas. Intra-operative electrophysiological signals are often categorized in terms of firing rate (FR) that measures tonic activity and indices that measures phasic activity, including the burst index (BI), pause ratio (PR), pause index (PI), or interspike interval histogram (ISI) [8]. Figure 2 shows some of the results we have generated. From top to bottom the three

signals are epochs that have been recorded along an electrode path. The first row corresponds to a position above the STN, the middle one is in the middle of the STN, and the bottom one below the STN. The left panels show the raw signal as well as the spikes we have extracted from these signals (black spike trains on the bottom of the left panel). The right panel show the interspike interval histogram (ISI) as well

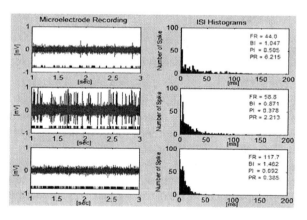

Fig. 2. Display of Electrophysiological signals and features extracted from these.

as the value for features commonly associated with these signals. Once features have been extracted, their values can be color-coded and displayed in the atlas. Figure 3 shows the mean value of the Burst Index in our current atlas. One can distinguish several regions with low, medium, and high values for this feature. Low values correspond to white matter, medium values to the STN, and high

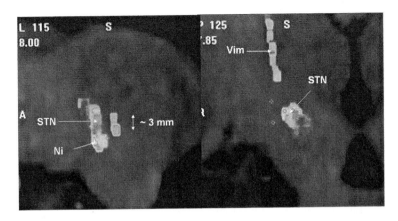

Fig. 3. Mean Burst Index in our electrophysiological atlas color-coded and superimposed on the MR images (Left, a sagital view; right a coronal view). Bright and dark pixels correspond to high and low values, respectively. Regions that correspond to various nuclei are shown with arrows.

values to structures such as the niagra and the ventralis intermedius (Vim) nucleus. Although the scarcity of data does not yet permit a precise localization of complete nuclei boundaries, the results we have obtained clearly show patterns in the data and clusters that correspond to known anatomical structures that are not visible in MR images.

4   Discussion and Conclusions

DBS placement requires selecting pre-operatively a candidate target point and adjusting this target point intra-operatively. In previously published work [4] we have demonstrated that automatic selection of the pre-operative target is not only feasible but better than the manual technique currently used. This conclusion was based on a limited data set (8 patients). Here we extend this study to 18 patients and we reach the same conclusion. With 18 patients, we have observed that the final target points, when mapped onto the atlas, form sub-clusters. This may be a discovery and an indication that the position of the optimal target point may be a function of parameters such as disease type or state. For example, patients who have prominent leg rigidity may benefit from an implant centered in a cluster more posterior and inferior in the STN than someone with arm rigidity whose ideal cluster may be more anterior and posterior. As the number of patients increases in our database, we will be able to confirm or disprove this finding. Results we have already obtained with the signals we have acquired indicate that features derived from these signals can be used to identify the STN and other nuclei, thus supporting the concept of an electrophysiological atlas that reveals the boundaries of structures and substructures not visible in current imaging modalities,which may be of value in target placement for other disorders, such as essential tremor [9]. Coupled with accurate registration algorithms, this atlas will not only permit the selection of preoperative target but also provide intra-operative guidance. This will be achieved by correlating intra-operative recordings with electrophysiological information contained in the atlas, which will permit the surgical team to identify the current location of the electrode, and plan and execute displacements from this position. The current difficulty with this concept is the intra-operative acquisition of signals that cover a region around the various targets of interest. Recording equipment used in current clinical practice only permit recording of one channel at a time. Thanks to a collaboration with FHC, Vanderbilt is the first site at which a device is used that permits recording along 5 parallel tracks on each side for a total of 10 simultaneous channels. At the time of writing one procedure has already been performed with this new device. This will allow us to rapidly expand our signal database which, in turn, will allow us to improve the localization of substructure boundaries based on electrophysiological signatures.

Acknowledgements. Pierre-François D'Haese is working towards a Ph.D. degree with awards from FRIA and FNRS (Belgian Science Foundation)(also supported by the Walloon Region by the MERCATOR grant). Supported in part by grant NIH/NCI 1R21 CA89657-01A2.

References

1. R. G. Deuschl, J. Volkmann, and P. Krack, "Deep brain stimulation for movement disorders," *Movement Disorders*, vol. 17, no. 3, pp. S1–S11, March/Arpil 2002.
2. B. Schrader, W. Hamel, D. Weinert, and H. M. Mehdorn, "Documentation of electrode localization." *Movement Disorders*, vol. 17, no. 3, pp. S167–S174, 2002.
3. K. Finnis, Y. P. Starreveld, A. G. Parrent, and T. M. Sadikot, A. F.and Peters, "Application of a population based electrophysiological database to the planning and guidance of deep brain stereotactic neurosurgery," *Medical Image Computing and Computer-Assisted Intervention - MICCAI 2002: 5th International Conference, Tokyo, Japan (T. Dohi, R. Kikinis (Eds))*, 2002.
4. B. Dawant, L. Rui, E. Cetinkaya, C. Kao, J. Fitzpatrick, and P. Konrad, "Computerized atlas-based positioning of deep brain stimulators:a feasibility study," *Second International Workshop, WBIR Philadelphia (James D. Gee, J.B. Antoine Maintz and Michael W.Vannier (Eds.))*, pp. 142–150, 2003.
5. C. Nickele, E. Cetinkaya, J. M. Fitzpatrick, and P. Konrad, "Method for placing deep-brain stimulators," *Proceedings of Medical Imaging, SPIE,* vol. 5029, 2003.
6. L. Rui, "Automatic placement of regions of interest in medical images using image registration," Master thesis in Electrical Engineering 2001.
7. G. K. Rohde, A. Aldroubi, and B. M. Dawant, "The adaptive bases algorithm for intensity based nonrigid image registration," *IEEE Transactions on Medical Imaging*, vol. 22, pp. 1470–1479, 2003.
8. J. Favre, J. Taha, T. Baumann, and K. J. Burchiel, "Computer analysis of the tonic, phasic, and kinesthetic activity of pallidal discharges in parkinson patient," *Surg Neurol*, vol. 16, no. 51, pp. 665–730, 1999.
9. E. Papavassiliou, G. Rau, S. Heath, A. Abosch, N. M. Barbaro, P. S. Larson, K. Lamborn, and P. A. Starr, "Thalamic deep brain stimulation for essential tremor: relation of lead location to outcome," *Neurosurgery*, vol. 54, pp. 1120–29, May 2004.

Detecting Regional Abnormal Cardiac Contraction in Short-Axis MR Images Using Independent Component Analysis*

A. Suinesiaputra[1], M. Üzümcü[1], A.F. Frangi[2,**], T.A.M. Kaandorp[1], J.H.C. Reiber[1], and B.P.F. Lelieveldt[1]

[1] Division of Image Processing, Department of Radiology, Leiden University Medical Center, Leiden, The Netherlands
[2] Computer Vision Group, Aragon Institute of Engineering, University of Zaragoza, Zaragoza, Spain

Abstract. Regional myocardial motion analysis is used in clinical routine to inspect cardiac contraction in myocardial diseases such as infarction or hypertrophy. Physicians/radiologists can recognize abnormal cardiac motion because they have knowledge about normal heart contraction. This paper explores the potential of Independent Component Analysis (ICA) to extract local myocardial contractility patterns and to use them for the automatic detection of regional abnormalities. A qualitative evaluation was performed using 42 healthy volunteers to train the ICA model and 6 infarct patients to test the detection and localization. This experiment shows that the evaluation results correlate very well to the clinical gold standard: delayed-enhancement MR images.

1 Introduction

Identification of reversible myocardial ischemic injury is a crucial assessment before coronary revascularization. Myocardial infarction is characterized by the presence of hypo-kinetic regions. MRI images have been used widely to diagnose myocardial infarction, especially recently with the delayed-enhancement MRI [1].

The effect of coronary artery occlusion is an abnormal myocardial contraction, particularly in the infarcted regions. Figure 1 shows two examples of MRI images from a healthy volunteer and an infarct patient, both at end-systole. Note that the inferior region (indicated by a white arrow) of the infarct heart does not contract, and has a reduced wall thickness.

The goal of this work is to automate the detection of abnormal cardiac motion from short-axis MRI images. This is achieved by deriving a statistical model of

* This work is supported by the Dutch Science Foundation (NWO), under an innovational research incentive grant, vernieuwingsimpuls 2001.
** A.F. Frangi is supported by a Ramón y Cajal Research Fellowship and grants TIC2002-04495-CO2 and ISCIII G03/185 from the Spanish Ministries of Science & Technology, and Health, respectively.

C. Barillot, D.R. Haynor, and P. Hellier (Eds.): MICCAI 2004, LNCS 3216, pp. 737–744, 2004.

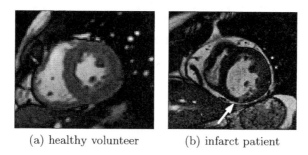

(a) healthy volunteer   (b) infarct patient

Fig. 1. MRI images of a healthy volunteer and an infarct patient at end-systole. The white arrow points to the infarcted tissue.

normal heart contraction and its local contractility patterns. In this paper, ICA is used to model the normal heart contraction and to detect and localize regions of the abnormal contraction in a patient. The contributions of this paper are threefold:

- We propose a geometry-based sorting method of independent components, providing an intuitive anatomical interpretation of the ICA modes.
- We demonstrate the potential of ICA in cardiac shape modeling to detect local contraction abnormalities.
- We present a qualitative evaluation of the detection and localization of my-ocardial infarctions. Results are compared with the corresponding "gold-standard" delayed-enhancement MRI images.

Section 2 describes shape modeling with ICA, the new sorting method for independent components and the method to detect local abnormalities. In Section 3, qualitative evaluation results are presented, followed by a discussion in Section 4.

2   Methodology

2.1   ICA Modeling of the Normal Cardiac Contraction

ICA is originally used for finding source signals from a mixture of unknown signals without prior knowledge other than the number of sources. In machine learning, ICA has been applied for feature extraction [2] and face recognition [3]. ICA can be applied to statistical shape modeling to extract independent components of the shape variation [4].

ICA is a linear generative model, where every training shape can be approximated by a linear combination of its components. Let $x = (x_1, y_1, \ldots, x_m, y_m)^T$ be a shape vector, consisting of m pairs of (x, y) coordinates of landmark points. The linear generative model is formulated as follows:

$$x \approx \bar{x} + \Phi b . \tag{1}$$

The matrix $\boldsymbol{\Phi} \in \mathbb{R}^{2m \times p}$ defines the independent components (ICs) and $\boldsymbol{b} \in \mathbb{R}^p$ is the weight coefficient vector. The mean shape, $\bar{x}$, is defined by

$$\bar{x} = \frac{1}{n} \sum_{i=1}^{n} x_i . \tag{2}$$

where n is the number of shapes and p is the number of retained components.

The goal of ICA is to find a matrix, $\boldsymbol{\Psi}$, such that

$$\boldsymbol{b} = \boldsymbol{\Psi} \left(x - \bar{x} \right) \tag{3}$$

with a constraint that columns of $\boldsymbol{\Psi}$ correspond to statistically independent directions. Thus the independent components are given by $\boldsymbol{\Phi} = \boldsymbol{\Psi}^{-1}$. The matrix $\boldsymbol{\Psi}$ is estimated by an optimisation algorithm (see [5] for survey of ICA).

Some pre-processing steps are necessarily performed before the ICA computation. The training shapes must be aligned, such that all shapes are invariant under Euclidean similarity transformations (rotation, translation and scaling). Procrustes analysis [6] is used for the shape alignment. Point correspondence between shapes is usually obtained by taking landmark points with the same anatomical interpretation. The resulting training shapes are zero mean, unit variance and all points are registered between shapes.

In this application, the observed data are left ventricular (LV) myocardial contours from short-axis cardiac MRI images at end-diastole (ED) and end-systole (ES) phases. To model the contractility pattern, contours for each subject are combined serially into one shape vector in the following order: endocardium contour at ED, epicardium contour at ED, endocardium contour at ES and epicardium contour at ES.

Figure 2(a) shows one example of an ICA derived shape variation mode. For comparison, the first mode of shape variation with PCA from the same data is shown in Fig. 2(b). ICA modes have a general shape of a local "bump", whereas the remainder of the shape is unaffected. This is an important property of ICA, which can be used to detect local shape anomalies. In contrast, PCA modes give global shape variations, distributed over the entire contour. A comparison study of ICA and PCA in cardiac shape modeling is given in [4].

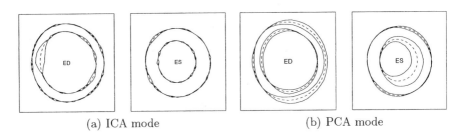

(a) ICA mode   (b) PCA mode

Fig. 2. Examples of modes from ICA and PCA models. The mean shape is drawn with a dashed line. The mode is drawn with a solid line. The shape variations are drawn with $\pm 3\sigma$ of the weight matrix distribution from the mean shape.

2.2   Geometry-Based Sorting of Independent Components

In our study, ICA is used to detect regional abnormalities, which are extracted from local shape variations. It would give a benefit in this case, if the position of each IC can be determined. Thus ICs are ordered based on their positions along the whole contour, giving an anatomically meaningful interpretation.

Let $\hat{\boldsymbol{x}}_i$ be a shape vector from the i-th component

$$\hat{\boldsymbol{x}}_i = \bar{\boldsymbol{x}} + \boldsymbol{\Phi a} \qquad (4)$$

where $1 \leq i \leq p$, $a_i = 1$ and $a_j = 0$ for $j \neq i$. A *displacement* vector $\boldsymbol{d}_i \in \mathbb{R}^m$ is defined as the distance of each element of $\hat{\boldsymbol{x}}_i$ to the mean shape

$$\boldsymbol{d}_i^{(j)} = \sqrt{\sum_{k=2j-1}^{2j} \left(\hat{\boldsymbol{x}}_i^{(k)} - \bar{\boldsymbol{x}}^{(k)} \right)^2} \qquad \text{where } j = 1, 2, \ldots, m \ . \qquad (5)$$

To determine the position of an independent component, a normalized circular cross-correlation is performed to each contour from the displacement vector with a bank of Gaussian filters. The parameter of the Gaussian filter giving the maximum response are stored for each component. The center of this filter defines the position of the component. Figure 3(a) shows an example of the cross-correlation response from a component.

There is an advantage of this sorting mechanism, that noise components can be detected. Noise components have a global wrinkled shape variation along the whole contour, which correlates best with the widest Gaussian filter. Figure 3(b) shows an example of the cross-correlation response for a noise component. Noise components are thus easily eliminated.

Figure 4 shows an example of the first four ICA modes after the geometry-based sorting mechanism. Note that the local shape variations are orderded clockwise.

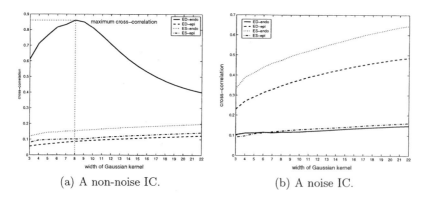

(a) A non-noise IC.   (b) A noise IC.

Fig. 3. Cross-correlation responses from two ICs.

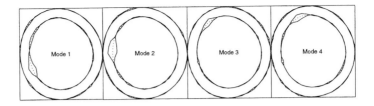

Fig. 4. The first four sorted ICA modes.

2.3   Determining the Number of Independent Components

One important parameter to determine is the number of independent components to estimate during the computation of ICA. Predicting this number with PCA may not always be a good idea, because PCA has a risk to eliminate "weak" ICs in the reduced data [7]. In shape modeling, this parameter affects appearance of the shape variations. As the number of computed ICs increases, the components represent more localized shape variations. If this parameter is too small, then the component gives global shape variation, much like PCA modes.

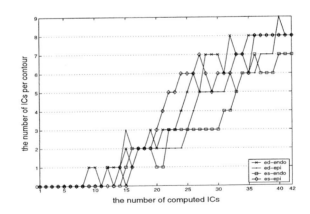

Fig. 5. A plot of the number of ICs per contour as a function of the number of computed ICs.

The determination of the optimal number of computed ICs is therefore task-specific. In this application to detect local abnormalities, we need sufficient regional segments. Too few segments will give an inaccurate localization. More segments will improve the detection resolution, but this is constrained by the computation time and the number of available shapes to avoid overlearning [8].

Figure 5 shows the number of segments as a function of the number of computed ICs from 42 shapes of normal hearts. From this, we took 40 as the number of computed ICs in our experiment, as it gives enough segments per contour.

2.4   Detection of Abnormal Contractility Patterns

Let $y \in \mathbb{R}^{2m}$ be a shape vector, fitted onto the mean shape of the model using the Procrustes fit [6]. The weight vector of the sample y is given by

$$b_y = \Phi^{-1} (y - \bar{x}) \tag{6}$$

which represents the parameters approximating the patient shape. Patient anomalies are estimated by elements in the weight vector that lie outside the distribution of parameters of the ICA model.

We have made a statistical test to test the gaussianity for the distribution of coefficient values for each component. We can assume that all components have normal distribution.

We define the anomaly at the i-th component $q_y^{(i)}$ as a value that falls beyond $\pm 3\sigma_i$ (99.7%), to make sure that the anomaly is an outlier. Thus the *anomaly vector* q_y is defined by taking the outlier components, normalized by their standard deviation. Each element of q_y is defined by

$$q_y^{(i)} = \begin{cases} 0 & \text{if } -3\sigma_i \le b_y^{(i)} \le 3\sigma_i \\ \dfrac{b_y^{(i)}}{\sigma_i} & \text{otherwise} \end{cases} \qquad \text{for } i = 1, \ldots, p \tag{7}$$

The anomaly vector (7) is mapped to a shape vector to facilitate a more intuitive regional interpretation. From the sorted ICs, the corresponding Gaussian filters giving the maximum responses for each IC are known. These Gaussian filters are generated to model the local bumps, resulting in a mixture of Gaussian functions. The regional sum of the Gaussian mixture gives a shape vector that indicates regional abnormal heart contraction of a patient.

3   Experimental Results

An ICA model was constructed from 42 healthy volunteers. The mid-ventricular level from short-axis MRI was taken from each subject. Contours were drawn manually and resampled to 40 landmarks defined by equi-angular sampling, starting from the intersection between left and right ventricle. The calculation of ICA was performed using the JADE algorithm [9], implemented in Matlab. The optimal number of computed ICs with minimum of 7 segments per contour is 40 (see Fig. 5).

To evaluate the infarct detection and localization of our method, MRI data of 6 patients with all necrotic infarcts were investigated. Mid-ventricular short-axis (SA) MRI images and the corresponding delayed-enhancement (DE) MRI images with the same orientation and the distance only < 1 mm were acquired. Regional abnormal contraction was compared visually with the corresponding DE-MRI. The myocardial infarct regions in the DE-MRI are demonstrated by signal hyperenhancement, corresponding to myocardial necrosis [1].

Six representative evaluation results are presented in Fig. 6. The anomaly vectors of patients were projected to the corresponding myocardial regions. The

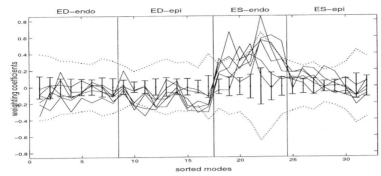

(a) Weight vectors (solid lines) of patients with the distribution of the ICA model (error bars). The dotted lines are the boundary of the normal contraction ($\pm 3\sigma_i$ for $i = 1, \ldots, p$).

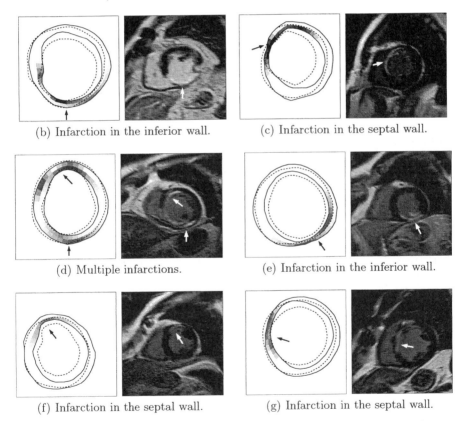

(b) Infarction in the inferior wall.

(c) Infarction in the septal wall.

(d) Multiple infarctions.

(e) Infarction in the inferior wall.

(f) Infarction in the septal wall.

(g) Infarction in the septal wall.

Fig. 6. Qualitative evaluation results. The top row figure shows projection of 6 patients to the ICA model of normal heart. Their abnormalities are shown below in the myocardial regions (ED=solid, ES=dashed). Dark areas have high abnormality value, whereas white areas are normal. The corresponding DE-MRI images are shown at the right side.

contraction patterns are also shown in the plot of ED contours (solid line) and ES contours (dashed line). It is clearly seen from Fig. 6, that the dark areas have a reduced contraction. The corresponding DE-MRI are given in the right side where the infarction regions are depicted by hyperintensity regions.

4   Discussion

This study shows the potential of ICA as an analysis tool for extracting local shape deformation. Using ICA to train a model of normal cardiac contraction, both global and regional motions are captured. To this end, we can automatically distinguish between abnormal and healthy cardiac motion.

An intuitive anatomical interpretation of the normal contraction model is achieved by ordering the ICs of the model geometrically along the whole contour. From this, anatomical shape information can be inferred, providing a method to localize the motion abnormalities.

In the qualitative comparison for 6 patients, the hypo-kinetic regions show an excellent correspondence to the hyperintensity regions of the "gold standard" DE-MRI. This demonstrates that the ICA-based infarct detection and localization from short-axis MRI images is a promising technique for computer aided infarct localization.

References

[1] Kim, R., Wu, E., Rafael, A., et. al.: The Use of Contrast-Enhanced Magnetic Resonance Imaging to Identify Reversible Myocardial Dysfunction. New England Journal of Medicine **343** (2000) 1445–1454

[2] Hoyer, P.O., Hyvärinen, A.: Independent Component Analysis Applied to Feature Extraction from Colour and Stereo Images. Network: Computation in Neural System **11** (2000) 191–210

[3] Bartlett, M.S., Movellan, J.R., Sejnowski, T.J.: Face Recognition by Independent Component Analysis. IEEE Trans. on Neural Networks **13** (2002) 1450–1464

[4] Üzümcü, M., Frangi, A.F., Reiber, J.H., Lelieveldt, B.P.: Independent Component Analysis in Statistical Shape Models. In Sonka, M., Fitzpatrick, J.M., eds.: Proc. of SPIE. Volume 5032. (2003) 375–383

[5] Hyvärinen, A.: Survey on Independent Component Analysis. Neural Computing Surveys **2** (1999) 94–128

[6] Dryden, I.L., Mardia, K.V.: Statistical Shape Analysis. John Wiley & Sons (2002)

[7] Nadal, J.P., Korutcheva, E., Aires, F.: Blind Source Separation in the Presence of Weak Sources. Neural Network **13** (2000) 589–596

[8] Hyvärinen, A., J.Särelä, Vígario, R.: Bumps and Spikes: Artifacts Generated by Independent Component Analysis with Insufficient Sample Size. In: Proc. Int. Workshop on ICA and BSS. (1999) 425–249

[9] Cardoso, J., Souloumiac, A.: Blind Beamforming for Non Gaussian Signals. IEEE Proceedings-F **140** (1993) 362–370

Non-rigid Atlas-to-Image Registration by Minimization of Class-Conditional Image Entropy

Emiliano D'Agostino, Frederik Maes*, Dirk Vandermeulen, and Paul Suetens

Katholieke Universiteit Leuven, Faculties of Medicine and Engineering, Medical
Image Computing (Radiology - ESAT/PSI), University Hospital Gasthuisberg,
Herestraat 49, B-3000 Leuven, Belgium
Emiliano.DAgostino@uz.kuleuven.ac.be

Abstract. We propose a new similarity measure for atlas-to-image matching in the context of atlas-driven intensity-based tissue classification of MR brain images. The new measure directly matches probabilistic tissue class labels to study image intensities, without need for an atlas MR template. Non-rigid warping of the atlas to the study image is achieved by free-form deformation using a viscous fluid regularizer such that mutual information (MI) between atlas class labels and study image intensities is maximized. The new registration measure is compared with the standard approach of maximization of MI between atlas and study images intensities. Our results show that the proposed registration scheme indeed improves segmentation quality, in the sense that the segmentations obtained using the atlas warped with the proposed non-rigid registration scheme better explain the study image data than the segmentations obtained with the atlas warped using standard intensity-based MI.

1   Introduction

An important problem in medical image analysis is the accurate and reliable extraction of brain tissue voxel maps for white matter (WM), grey matter (GM) and cerebrospinal fluid (CSF) from (possibly multispectral) MR brain images. Typical applications include the visualization of the cortex by volume or surface rendering, quantification of cortical thickness, quantification of intra-subject morphological changes over time and quantification of inter-subject morphological differences in relation to certain neurological or other conditions. While segmentation procedures that require some manual intervention (e.g. for initialization or supervised training) inevitably have to deal with some inter- and intra-observer variability and subjectivity, fully automated procedures for intensity-based tissue classification are more objective and potentially more robust and allow for efficient and consistent off-line processing of large series of data.

---

* Frederik Maes is Postdoctoral Fellow of the Fund for Scientific Research - Flanders
(FWO-Vlaanderen, Belgium).

C. Barillot, D.R. Haynor, and P. Hellier (Eds.): MICCAI 2004, LNCS 3216, pp. 745–753, 2004.

In previous work, we introduced a model-based approach for automated intensity-based tissue classification of MR brain images [4]. This method uses the Expectation-Maximization (EM) algorithm to iteratively estimate the parameters θ of a Gaussian mixture model (assuming the intensities of each tissue class to be normally distributed with unknown mean and variance, but corrupted by a spatially varying intensity inhomogenity or bias field) and simultaneously classify each voxel accordingly, such as to maximize the likelihood $p(I|\theta)$ of the intensity data I given the model. The method is initialized by providing initial tissue classification maps for WM, GM, CSF and OTHER derived from a digital brain atlas after appropriate spatial normalization of the atlas to the study images. However, the atlas is not only used to initialize the EM procedure, but also serves as a spatially varying prior that constrains the classification during parameter estimation and in the final classification step. The probabilistic tissue classification L is obtained as the a posteriori probability of tissue label given the observed image intensity and the estimated intensity parameters, which, assuming that all voxels are independent, is computed using Bayes' rule as $p(L_k = j|I_k, \theta) \propto p(I_k|L_k = j, \theta).p(L_k = j)$ with L_k the label assigned to voxel k, j the various tissue classes, I_k the intensity of voxel k, $p(I_k|L_k = j, \theta)$ the probability of the observed intensity given the specified class label as derived from the Gaussian mixture model and $p(L_k = j)$ the prior probability of voxel k to belong to class j, which is simply the atlas registered to the image I. Hence, the quality of the atlas-to-image registration has a direct impact on the segmentation result through the above relation and the impact of the atlas model $(p(L_k = j))$ is as important as that of the intensity data $(p(I_k|L_k = j, \theta))$ itself.

In the method described in [4], affine registration was used to align the brain tissue distribution maps provided with SPM [2] with the study image by maximization of mutual information of corresponding voxel intensities [3] of the study image and the MR template of the SPM atlas. But while affine registration provides an atlas-to-image registration that is globally satisfactory in most cases, it fails to compensate for local morphological differences between atlas and study images, for instance at the cortical surface or at the ventricular boundaries, especially in study images showing enlarged ventricles. Non-rigid image registration, using an appropriate similarity metric and regularization criterion, allows to locally adapt the morphology of the atlas to that of the image under study, such that a more specific prior model $p(L_k = j), \forall j$ is obtained, resulting in a more accurate segmentation that is more consistent with the image data. In this paper we derive a new similarity measure that matches the atlas class labels directly to the study image intensities, such that the likelihood of the data given the spatially deformed prior model is maximized. We show that the proposed scheme for atlas registration results in more optimal tissue segmentations that better explain the data than is the case with non-rigid atlas registration based on matching intensity images instead of class labels.

2   Method

2.1   Similarity Measure

Our aim is to apply non-rigid registration using an appropriate similarity measure to optimally align the prior tissue distribution maps of the atlas to the image under study, such that the a priori classification provided by the atlas best fits the image intensities. This is not necessarily guaranteed by matching the atlas MR template to the study image using an intensity-based similarity metric such as mutual information of corresponding voxels intensities, as is typically done [4]. Instead, what is needed is a measure that directly evaluates the correspondence between atlas tissue probabilities and study image intensities without having to rely on atlas intensity images. In this context, we propose the new information-theoretic similarity measure $I(Y, L)$ for voxel-based non-rigid image matching that measures the mutual information between study image intensities Y and atlas class label probabilities L. $I(Y, L)$ is defined as

$$I(Y, L) = \sum_k \sum_y p(k, y). \log \frac{p(k, y)}{p(k).p(y)} \tag{1}$$

with k indexing the different atlas class labels (WM,GM,CSF and OTHER), y the image intensity in the study image, $p(k, y)$ the joint probability distribution of class k and intensity y and $p(k)$ and $p(y)$ the corresponding marginal distributions for class label k and intensity y respectively. This measure is analogous to the traditional mutual information of voxel intensities similarity measure [3], but differs in the features used to estimate similarity and in the way the joint probability distribution $p(k, y)$ is computed. Samples i with intensity y_i at positions p_i in the image Y are transformed into the corresponding positions q_i in the atlas space using the transformation T_α with parameters α. The joint probability distributon $p(k, y)$ is constructed using partial volume distribution (PV) interpolation [3]:

$$p(k, y) = \frac{1}{N} \sum_{i=1}^{N} \sum_{j=1}^{8} w_{i,j} \delta(y - y_i).c_{i,j}(k) \tag{2}$$

with N the number of samples in the image, j indexing each of the 8 nearest neighbours on the grid of the atlas images of the transformed location q_i of sample i, $w_{i,j}$ the trilinear interpolation weight associated with neighbour j and $c_{i,j}(k)$ the probability for tissue class k at this grid point as given by the atlas. The marginal disributions $p(y)$ and $p(k)$ are derived by integration of $p(k, y)$ over k and over y respectively. $p(k, y)$ is a continuos and a.e. differentiable function of the registration parameters α through the weights $w_{i,j}$. Further on, we derive an expression for the derivative of $I(Y, L)$ with respect to local displacements of individual voxels to define a force field that drives the registration in order to maximize $I(Y, L)$.

$I(Y,L)$ can be interpreted as $I(Y,L) = H(Y) - H(Y|L)$ with $H(Y)$ the entropy of the image intensity data and $H(Y|L)$ the residual entropy (or uncertainty) of Y given the atlas classification L. Because $H(Y)$ is constant during registration (all samples of Y contribute always to the joint probability distribution $p(k,y)$), maximization of $I(Y,L)$ is equivalent to minimizing the class-conditional image intensity entropy $H(Y|L)$. The proposed method thus aims at aligning the atlas labels such that the atlas best explains the data, i.e. such that the intensities corresponding to each atlas class are optimally clustered.

2.2   Force Field Computation

To assess the effect of a displacement u_i of a particular voxel i on the similarity mesure $I(Y,L)$, we differentiate $I(Y,L)$ with respect to u_i, using a similar approach as in [5]:

$$\frac{\partial I(\boldsymbol{u} + \epsilon \boldsymbol{h})}{\partial u_i} = \sum_k \sum_y \frac{\partial}{\partial u_i} \left[p(k,y) \log \frac{p(k,y)}{p(y).p(k)} \right]$$

$$= \sum_k \sum_y \left[\log \frac{p(k,y)}{p(k)} \cdot \frac{\partial p(k,y)}{\partial u_i} \right] \tag{3}$$

using the fact that $\sum_k \sum_y \frac{\partial p(k,y)}{\partial u_i} = \sum_k \frac{\partial p(k)}{\partial u_i} = 0$. The derivative of $p(k,y)$ with respect to the displacement u_i of sample i is given by

$$\frac{\partial p(k,i)}{\partial u_i} = \frac{1}{N} \sum_{j=1}^{8} \frac{\partial w_{i,j}}{\partial u_i} \delta(y - y_i).c_{i,j}(k)$$

The derivative of the joint probability distribution is itself a joint probability constructed using the PV interpolation scheme, with weights that are the spatial derivatives of the weights of the original joint histogram. We can thus define the driving forces F_i in each voxel i as:

$$F_i = \frac{\partial I(Y,L)}{\partial \epsilon} = \frac{1}{N} \sum_k \log \frac{p(k,y_i)}{p(k)} \cdot \left(\sum_{j=1}^{8} \frac{\partial w_{i,j}}{\partial u_i} c_{i,j}(k) \right)$$

2.3   Viscous Fluid Regularization

We adopt the free-form registration approach of [5] and use the force field $\boldsymbol{F}(\boldsymbol{x}, \boldsymbol{u}) = F_i$ as defined above to drive a viscous fluid regularizer by iteratively solving its Navier-Stokes governing equation:

$$\nabla^2 \boldsymbol{v} + \nabla (\nabla.\boldsymbol{v}) + \boldsymbol{F}(\boldsymbol{x}, \boldsymbol{u}) = 0 \tag{4}$$

with $\boldsymbol{v}(\boldsymbol{x}, t)$ the deformation velocity experienced by a particle at position $\boldsymbol{x}$. An approximate solution of (4) is obtained by convolution with a Gaussian kernel

ψ and the deformation field $\boldsymbol{u}^{(m+1)}$ at iteration $(m+1)$ is found by integration over time:

$$\boldsymbol{v} = \psi \star \boldsymbol{F} \tag{5}$$

$$\boldsymbol{R}^{(m)} = \boldsymbol{v}^{(m)} - \sum_{i=1}^{3} v_i^{(m)} \left[\frac{\partial \boldsymbol{u}^{(m)}}{\partial x_i} \right] \tag{6}$$

$$\boldsymbol{u}^{(m+1)} = \boldsymbol{u}^{(m)} + \boldsymbol{R}^{(m)}.\Delta t \tag{7}$$

The time step Δt is constrained by $\Delta t \leq \max(\|\boldsymbol{R}\|).\Delta u$, with Δu the maximal voxel displacement that is allowed in one iteration. Regridding and template propagation are used as in [5] to preserve topology.

3   Results

The method presented above was implemented in Matlab. Image resampling, joint histogram construction and force field computation were coded in C. The maximal voxel displacement Δu at each iteration was set to 0.25 voxels and regridding was performed when the Jacobian of the deformation field became smaller than 0.5. Iterations were continued as long as negative $I(Y, L)$ decreased, with a maximal number of iterations of 180. The number of classes used for the template image was 4 (WM, GM, CSF and OTHER). After linear rescaling of the study image intensities to the range [0,127], the number of bins for the reference image was 128, such that the joint histogram size was 4×128.

Several experiments were conducted to evaluate the impact of the proposed registration measure on atlas-driven intensity-based tissue segmentation quality. In a first experiment the Brainweb MR brain template [1] was warped to 5 different high resolution MR images of normal brains. For each of these images, tissue maps for WM, GM and CSF were obtained independently using the method described in [4]. The atlas was first affinely aligned with the subject images using MI. Subsequently, three different non-rigid atlas-to-image registration schemes were compared: matching of atlas to subject image intensities using the MI measure as described in [5], matching of atlas to subject tissue class labels using the divergence measure as described in [6], and matching of atlas class labels to subject image intensities using the method proposed here. We refer to these methods as MI, D and HMI (hybrid mutual information) respectively. The performance of the different methods is compared by the overlap coefficient for WM, GM and CSF computed between the warped atlas tissue maps and the segmented tissue maps. All maps were hard segmented (after warping) to compute the overlap coefficients.

Table 1 shows the results. Non-rigid atlas warping using the HMI criterion proposed here generates, in all cases and for all tissue classes, tissue maps that are more similar to the intensity-based tissue segmentations itself than is the case with standard MI. The results obtained with measures HMI and D are comparable. However, the use of measure D, which matches atlas labels to subject class labels directly, requires availability of the subject segmentation maps, while the HMI measure proposed here does not. Moreover, matching atlas class labels to subject class labels using measure D does not consistently improve the registration quality compared to matching to subject intensities using the HMI measure.

In a second experiment an in-house constructed brain atlas, build from a database of 64 normal brain images by non-rigid warping, was warped to the same five subject images considered above. The atlas was first aligned with the subject images by affine registration and was subsequently non-rigidly warped to the subject images using the standard MI measure and the HMI measure proposed here (figure 1). The subject images were segmented with the method of [4] using a priori tissue probability maps derived from the affinely registered atlas and from the non-rigidly warped atlas using either of both methods.

Figure 2 shows the conditional probability $p(y|k)$ of intensities y in one of the subject images for the GM class before (i.e. only affine registration) and after non-rigid matching and, for both cases, before and after subsequent segmentation, i.e. using the warped a priori atlas GM classification or the computed a posteriori GM classification respectively. These graphs show the impact of the prior model and of the image data on the GM intensity model estimated during segmentation. It can be seen that non-rigid atlas registration (blue curve) clusters the GM intensities more than merely affine registration (black curve). HMI based warping (left) clusters the GM intensities more efficiently than standard MI (right). Subsequent intensity-based classification of the images using either the affinely or the non-rigidly warped atlas priors results in a class-conditional intensity distribution that is nearly Gaussian and that is fairly similar for segmentations obtained with both affinely and non-rigidly warped priors, especially with standard MI. Nevertheless, even if the intensity distribution within each tissue class might be more or less identical, the classification map itself can be quite different due to the impact of the prior model on the classification itself.

The effect of atlas warping on the segmentation quality can also be appreciated from the negative log-likelihood curves $-\log P(Y|\theta)$ of the data Y given the model parameters θ during iterative classification and parameter estimation [4]. As illustrated in figure 2 for one of the five subject images considered here, the negative log-likelihood associated with the segmentation based on priors warped using the HMI method presented here (red curve) is smaller than with the segmentation based on priors warped using standard MI (black curve). This confirms that the HMI warped prior better explains the image data than the standard MI warped prior.

Considering the tissue maps obtained independently using the affinely registered SPM atlas as ground truth (as in the first experiment), we can compute the overlap coefficients between this ground truth and the segmentations obtained with our atlas prior, after affine and after non-rigid warping using HMI and standard MI respectively. These results are summarized in table 2.

Table 1. Overlap coefficients (in %) for different tissue classes in 5 different subject images between the segmented tissue maps and atlas tissue maps warped to the study image using affine and subsequent non-rigid matching with three different registration schemes.

Case	Affine			MI			D			HMI		
	WM	GM	CSF	WM	GM	CSF	WM	GM	CSF	WM	GM	CSF
1	67.28	69.12	42.70	67.78	69.99	52.73	75.52	78.08	69.90	81.89	79.57	63.11
2	66.13	68.95	41.73	70.59	72.78	58.73	77.39	79.94	70.68	81.78	79.39	65.48
3	61.21	66.79	40.48	67.54	68.53	52.38	76.11	79.81	70.22	80.18	78.94	62.90
4	66.77	68.54	41.80	68.26	70.85	58.33	75.78	78.71	70.42	77.22	74.78	60.09
5	65.37	67.39	44.97	69.05	70.85	60.28	71.57	73.83	70.43	80.94	77.62	66.37

Table 2. Overlap coefficients (in %) for different tissue classes of tissue maps obtained with affinely registered and with non-rigidly warped atlas priors using HMI and standard MI, using an independent segmentation of the subject image as ground truth.

Case	Affine registration			HMI			MI		
	WM	GM	CSF	WM	GM	CSF	WM	GM	CSF
1	91.54	90.59	69.00	99.06	98.49	95.41	94.20	93.67	76.01
2	92.41	90.51	67.66	97.35	96.32	79.74	95.23	94.45	76.41
3	91.10	90.58	72.99	97.92	96.43	80.34	95.13	94.50	82.95
4	92.64	91.40	69.70	96.74	96.14	81.35	93.22	91.99	76.06
5	91.79	89.77	72.21	96.88	95.96	80.25	94.88	94.29	81.04

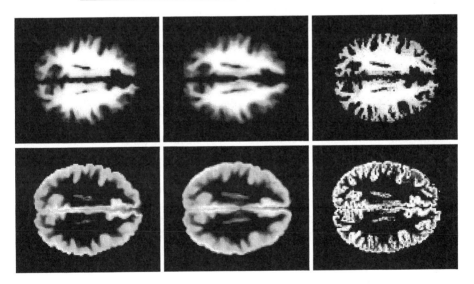

Fig. 1. WM (top) and GM (bottom) atlas priors warped to a particular subject brain using non-rigid registration with the proposed HMI measure (left column) and with standard MI (middle column). Right column: reference segmentation maps (ground truth).

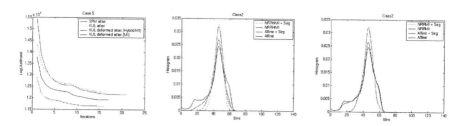

Fig. 2. Left: Negative log-likelihood $-P(Y|\theta)$ curves during iterative model-based tissue classification and parameter estimation for different segmentation strategies. Middle and right: conditional probabilties p(y—k) given one class (gray matter) before and after segmentation and/or non-rigid registration for one of the five cases. Middle: hybrid mutual information based non-rigid registration; Right: mutual information based non-rigid registration.

4   Discussion

In this paper we present a hybrid mutual information registration criterion for atlas-to-image matching that allows matching of atlas class probabilities to study image intensities. The new registration criterion measures how well the probabilistic atlas tissue distributions explain the intensities observed in the study image. A similar approach has been presented in [7]with the difference that in this paper the author uses mutual information between reference image intensities and binary labels in the floating image. Compared to the standard MI measure of corresponding voxel intensities, the proposed approach has the advantage that spatially varying tissue information is explicitly introduced in the registration criterion, which makes it more robust. On the other hand, in contrast with the divergence criterion introduced in [6] for matching atlas and study image class labels, no segmentation of the study image needs to be available for the method presented here.

The joint probability distribution $p(k, y)$ between atlas class labels k and study image intensities y from which the HMI measure $I(Y, L)$ is computed, is estimated during registration using PV interpolation [3], such that it varies smoothly with individual voxel displacements and can be analytically differentiated. A force field is thus obtained that acts to displace individual voxels such that the mutual information between atlas class labels and study image intensities is maximized. The approach presented here is completely discrete due to the PV interpolation scheme and, in contrast with the method of [5], the force field does not depend on spatial image intensity gradients.

Several experiments were performed to evaluate the impact of atlas warping using various registration schemes on atlas-driven intensity-based tissue segmentation, showing that the hybrid registration measure proposed here indeed performs better for this particular task than standard MI. Our further work will focus on merging atlas-driven labelling and label-based atlas matching in a single information-theoretic framework, whereby each process benefits from the output of the other.

References

[1] C.A. Cocosco and V. Kollokian and R.K.-S. Kwan and A.C. Evans. BrainWeb: Online Interface to a 3D MRI Simulated Brain Database. *Proceedings of 3-rd International Conference on Functional Mapping of the Human Brain*, 5(4), part 2/4, S425, 1997.

[2] The SPM package is available online at http://www.fil.ion.ucl.ac.uk/spm/

[3] F. Maes, A. Collignon, D. Vandermeulen, G. Marchal, and P. Suetens. Multimodality image registration by maximization of mutual information. *IEEE Trans. Medical Imaging*, 16(4):187–198, 1997.

[4] K. Van Leemput, F. Maes, D. Vandermeulen, P. Suetens. Automated model-based tissue classification of MR images of the brain. *IEEE Trans. Medical Imaging*, 18(10):897–908, 1999.

[5] E. D'Agostino, F. Maes, D. Vandermeulen, and P. Suetens. A viscous fluid model for multimodal non-rigid image registration using mutual information *Medical Image Analysis*, 7(4):565–575, 2003.

[6] E. D'Agostino, F. Maes, D. Vandermeulen, and P. Suetens. An information theoretic approach for non-rigid image registration using voxel class probabilities *MICCAI 2003*, Lectures Notes in Computer Science, vol 2878:812–820

[7] J. Kim, J. W. Fisher III, A. Jr. Yezzi, M. Cetin and A. S. Willsky. Nonparametric methods for image segmentation using information theory and curve evolution *IEEE ICIP 2002*, IEEE International Conference on Image Processing, vol. 3, pp. 797-800, Rochester, New York, September 2002.

Determination of Aortic Distensibility Using Non-rigid Registration of Cine MR Images

Maria Lorenzo-Valdés[1], Gerardo I. Sanchez-Ortiz[1], Hugo Bogren[2]*,
Raad Mohiaddin[2], and Daniel Rueckert[1]

[1] Visual Information Processing Group, Department of Computing,
Imperial College London, 180 Queen's Gate, London SW7 2BZ, United Kingdom
[2] Royal Brompton and Harefield NHS Trust, Sydney Street,
London, United Kingdom

Abstract. A novel method for the estimation of areas in 2D MR images of the aorta is presented. The method uses spatio-temporal non-rigid registration in order to obtain the 2D deformation fields of the vessels during the cardiac cycle. This is accomplished by aligning all time frames in the image sequence simultaneously to the first one. The determinant of the Jacobian of the 2D deformation fields are then computed to obtain the expansion (or contraction) at each time frame, with respect to the first time frame. By using 3D splines, the method exploits the relation between time frames in order to obtain continuous and smooth distensibility measurements throughout the cardiac cycle. Validation was carried out with MR images of the aorta. Experiments for the registration and estimation of areas in the aorta are presented in 60 data sets corresponding to three different sections of the aorta (proximal, mid and distal) in 20 different subjects, where each set consisted of 17 to 38 time frames. Manually estimated areas are compared to the areas estimated automatically in 8 data sets where the average error is 2.3% of the area manually obtained.

1 Introduction

The assessment of the elasticity of the great vessels is important in order to evaluate cardiovascular disease and performance since it reflects aging and atherosclerosis [1,2]. In addition, it can also be used to evaluate the results of plaque-reducing therapies. This elasticity assessment is usually accomplished by measuring compliance or distensibility, which are wall properties of great vessels. Arterial compliance reflects the buffering capacity of an artery and is defined as the absolute change in volume or cross-sectional area per unit of pulse pressure ($\triangle V / \triangle P$). Decrease in compliance increases cardiac after-load and the risk of cardiac hypertrophy. Arterial distensibility is defined as the relative change in volume or cross-sectional area per unit of pulse pressure ($[\triangle V/V]/ \triangle P$) and reflects mainly the elasticity of the wall.

---

* Hugo Bogren on sabbatical leave from the Department of Radiology, University of California Davis School of Medicine, California, USA

C. Barillot, D.R. Haynor, and P. Hellier (Eds.): MICCAI 2004, LNCS 3216, pp. 754–762, 2004.
© Springer-Verlag Berlin Heidelberg 2004

Two approaches for measuring compliance and distensibility are normally used. The first approach uses instantaneous pressure-dimension relations of single pulse waves at varying levels of distending pressures. A pulse wave travels with a speed of several metres/seconds from the aorta to the arterial branches. This velocity can be measured by recording the pressure pulse waves at two places with Doppler echo-probes [3], or using phase contrast MR [1,2]. The pulse wave velocity along the vessel of interest provides a measure of compliance C through the approximate relation $C = 1/(c^2\rho)$, where c is the pulse wave velocity and ρ is the blood mass density which can be considered to be constant. The second approach for obtaining compliance and distensibility uses measurements of area and pressure changes. While measuring pressure is simple to carry out for the recordings at end-systole and end-diastole using a sphygmomanometer, the measurement of volume changes is more difficult because there is no simple means of estimating regional changes in blood volume of a vessel. However, assuming that there is mainly radial and negligible axial vessel movement during pulse pressure, compliance and distensibility can be estimated as a change in radius, diameter, or cross-sectional area for a given change in pressure.

Manual delineation of the great vessels is usually performed in order to compute the area, however it is time consuming and there is a significant intra and inter-observer variability which make the results inconsistent. Deformable models have been previously proposed for the tracking and segmentation of the aorta [4]. However, this approach has not been applied on continuous measurements through a complete cardiac cycle.

This paper proposes a method to estimate the area changes of the aorta from MR images. We have successfully applied a similar approach for tracking cardiac MR image sequences [5]. First, each time frame of the image sequence is registered to the first frame using non-rigid registration to obtain the deformation fields of the aorta during the cardiac cycle. Subsequently, to calculate regional area changes the determinant of the Jacobian of the deformation field is integrated over the area of interest to quantify differences between registered images and the reference frame.

2   2D Registration of Cine MR Images

The purpose of image registration is to find the optimal correspondence between anatomical regions in two different images. Registration is a technique where the geometrical relation between two images is described by a transformation that maps points in one image to its corresponding point in another image [6]. Registration can be accomplished using different types of transformations that can be classified as rigid or non-rigid.

In our application non-rigid registrations are performed between a baseline (or reference) image at time $t = 0$ and all other images in the sequence to obtain transformations that can describe the deforming soft tissue such as the wall of the great vessels.

To model local deformations Rueckert $et\ al.$ [7] proposed a non-rigid transformation algorithm based on free-form deformations and B-splines. It manipulates control points allowing deformation of the shape of the 2D or 3D object producing a smooth and continuous transformation:

$$T_{local}(x,y) = \sum_{m=0}\sum_{n=0} B_m(u)B_n(v)\phi_{i+m,j+n} \tag{1}$$

where $i = \lfloor x/n_x \rfloor - 1, j = \lfloor y/n_y \rfloor - 1, u = x/n_x - \lfloor x/n_x \rfloor, v = y/n_y - \lfloor y/n_y \rfloor$ ($\lfloor$] means round down) and where B_m represents the m-th basis function of the B-spline described in [8].

To relate both images, a measurement of alignment is needed to find the correct transformation. If the images to be registered belong to the same image sequence, we can assume that the intensities in images A and B are closely related and Viola [9] demonstrated that in this case the correlation coefficient (CC) may be considered as the ideal similarity measure. For images A and B, the aim of the registration process is to find the transformation T which maximises:

$$CC = \frac{\sum_i (A(x_i) - \bar{A})(B(T(x_i)) - \bar{B}(T))}{\{\sum_i (A(x_i) - \bar{A})^2 \sum_i (B(T(x_i)) - \bar{B}(T))^2\}^{1/2}} \quad \forall i \in A \cap B \tag{2}$$

where $\bar{A}$ and $\bar{B}$ are the mean intensity values of voxels in image A and the transformed image B, respectively.

The resulting transformation maps each point of the image reference A to the corresponding point in the image B. After the optimal transformation has been obtained, the resulting deformation field can be analysed to identify areas which have expanded or contracted. This analysis requires the calculation of the determinant of the Jacobian matrix of the deformation field which defines the local volume change in the neighbourhood of a point $\mathbf{x}$.

3   3D Registration of Cine MR Images and Estimation of Area Changes in the Aorta

The idea of the proposed approach is to estimate the expansion or contraction of the aorta in different time frames with respect to a baseline image of the vessel. While the registration technique described in the previous section can be used to register all time frames in a sequence to their respective baseline image, it does not exploit the temporal coherence of the image sequence. In this section we propose a modified spatio-temporal registration which exploits the coherence of the image sequence.

Rather than considering each 2D cross-sectional image separately we use the 2D image sequence as a 3D (2D + time) image, where x, y describe the cross-sectional position and t the time during cardiac cycle. The goal of the spatio-temporal registration is to find the optimal transformation $T : (x, y, t) \mapsto (x, y, 0)$ which maps all points in the 3D image $I_{sequence}(x, y, t)$ to their corresponding anatomical location in the 2D baseline image $I_{baseline}(x, y)$.

Next, the image sequence $I_{sequence}$ is registered to the baseline image $I_{baseline}$ to find the optimal transformation T as presented in Fig 1. For this purpose we

$$I_{baseline} \qquad I_{sequence} \qquad I'_{sequence}$$

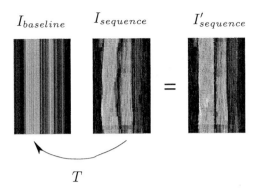

$$T$$

Fig. 1. Registration of the image sequence $I_{sequence}$ with the baseline image $I_{baseline}$.

modify eq. (1) to ensure a temporally smooth transformation:

$$\mathbf{T}_{I_0 I_N}(x,y,t) = \sum_{t=0}^{3}\sum_{m=0}^{3}\sum_{n=0}^{3} B_l(u)B_m(v)B_n(w)\phi_{i+l,j+m,k+n} \qquad (3)$$

Note that this transformation is a mapping from 3D (x, y, t) to 2D $(x, y, 0)$, i.e. the displacement of the control points is restricted to the x and y directions only. By optimising the location of all control points simultaneously we are able to simultaneously register all time frames of the image sequence to the baseline image. As a result we ensure a smooth deformation between time frames.

To calculate the change in area of a structure of interest we need to integrate the determinant of the Jacobian over the area of interest Ω in the baseline image that is on the region of the aorta. At any given point (x, y, t) the determinant of the Jacobian can be computed as

$$J(x,y,t) = \begin{bmatrix} \frac{\partial u_x}{\partial x} & \frac{\partial u_x}{\partial y} \\ \frac{\partial u_y}{\partial x} & \frac{\partial u_y}{\partial y} \end{bmatrix},$$

where $\frac{\partial u_i}{\partial j}$ is the rate of change of the i_{th} component of the displacement field u in the direction j. Note that this Jacobian only takes the spatial component of the transformation into account. The determinant of the Jacobian quantifies the expansion or contraction between the image sequence and the baseline image, for any given location in the baseline coordinate system. The resulting Jacobian values for frame t contained in the selected region Ω were averaged for each time frame.

$$\bar{J}_n = \frac{\int_\Omega J_{xy} dx dy}{\int_\Omega dx dy} = \frac{\sum_k J_{xy}(k)}{K} \quad \forall k \in T_{I(0)I(n)}(x,y) \cap \Omega \qquad (4)$$

where $\bar{J}_n$ is the average (or global) ratio of expansion or contraction of frame n, $J_{xy}(k)$ is the Jacobian of any transformed point found in the region Ω, and K is the total number of transformed points (or image voxels) in the region Ω. This would describe the global expansion or contraction ratio of the aorta at that particular time frame. The segmented area in the first time frame is then multiplied by this ratio to obtain the area in each time frame. In this way, not only the actual expansion ratio values but the absolute area changes of the vessel throughout a complete cardiac cycle can be visualised and used to estimate the elasticity of the vessel.

4   Experiments and Results

Images were acquired at Royal Brompton Hospital, London, UK, using a Siemens Sonata 1.5T scanner with a TrueFisp sequence. Images of the proximal, mid and distal parts of the ascending aorta were obtained from 20 different subjects with a resolution of 192×256 and pixel size around 0.6×0.6 mm with a slice thickness of 6 mm. The images were taken perpendicular to the aorta. For each subject between 17 and 38 time frames were acquired, at intervals of approximately 25-50msec. We divided the subjects in two age groups. The age of 10 subjects ranged between 23 and 34 years old and the age of the other 10 subjects ranged between 57 and 80 years old.

The proposed approach was applied to the 60 data sets from 20 subjects. First, the area change with respect to the first time frame image was computed with the proposed method. In five data sets the second or third time frame images were taken as the reference instead of the first time frame image because in those cases the first time frame image did not have good contrast and the boundaries of the aorta were not well defined. Therefore, frames with a better quality were chosen as the reference. Fig. 2 shows the expansion/contraction ratio of the cross-sectional area of the aorta in the three different sections (proximal, mid and distal) calculated with respect to the area of the first time frame. It presents the results for all the data sets of the younger and older subjects. The expansion of most of the older subjects do not exceed 120% of the area estimated in the first frame.

In order to evaluate our method, manual segmentations were performed by an expert observer in the complete time sequences of eight image sets where double determinations (i.e. two manual delineations) were averaged. The manually estimated area of the vessel was compared to those obtained with the proposed method. Fig. 3 presents the area manually estimated by the expert and by the proposed approach. Table 1 summarises the maximum difference between the manual and automatic estimates of the area. The maximum difference is 5.8% on average, while the average difference over all is 2.3%. For volunteer 6 the maximum difference between both areas is 9.9%, however, the source of this error is due to an inconsistent manual segmentation of the second time frame as can be seen in Fig. 3.

In order to visualise the results of the complete time sequence, using the transformation computed by the registration algorithm we have transformed the segmented image of the first time frame into the shape corresponding to the remaining time frames. This allows us to see the projected segmentation (or 2D delineation) of the vessels throughout the cardiac cycle. Figure 4 shows an

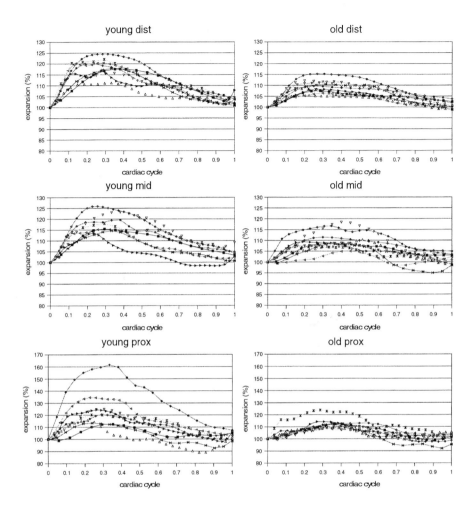

Fig. 2. Automatic estimation of the expansion/contraction ratio of the aorta with respect to the first time frame.

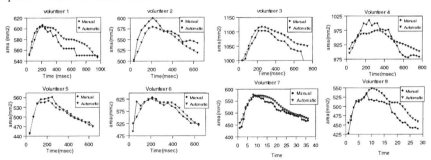

Fig. 3. Example of the manual and automatic estimation of the areas in a set of images. Notice the smooth time variations for the proposed method.

example of segmentation results on a cross-sectional image. Figure 5 illustrates the segmentation results on a 3D (2D + Time) representation.

Table 1. Differences between the area estimated manually and automatically for each curve of Fig. 3 divided by the area manually estimated.

Subject	1	2	3	4	5	6	7	8	Average
Maximum difference	4.4%	4.8%	5.5%	4.6%	3.6%	9.9%	5.1%	8.7%	5.8%
Average difference	2.0%	2.3%	2.0%	2.5%	1.1%	2.2%	2.0%	4.1%	2.3%

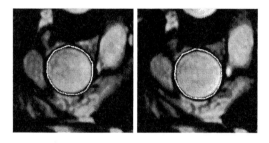

Fig. 4. Example of segmentation results shown on a cross section at (a) end-diastole and (b) end-systole. In order to help visualising results in this non-colour print, the continuous segmentation contour is shown as a dotted line.

5   Discussion

We have presented a procedure to estimate the transverse area in MR images of the aorta. The registration yields a deformation field from which the expansion or contraction ratio of the aorta could be accurately estimated. The 8 examples in Fig. 3 show that the area-time curve estimated by the proposed approach is smooth while the manual estimate of the area-time curve is noisy and has some abrupt changes due to the different criteria of the expert to segment the aorta in different time frames. The manual method was very time consuming with 60-100 measurements per section and took approximately one hour while the automatic method took 5 minutes once the program was set up. The automatic contours were consistent with no variation, contrary to the manual double determinations, and appeared more reliable. The method relates the images in time and the results are promising for physiological and clinical studies in the assessment of elasticity of the aorta as shown in Fig. 2 where the difference in elasticity between young and old subjects can be observed. The method is limited when the first time frame does not have a good contrast, however another time frame with better contrast can be chosen as a reference and the expansion/contraction ratio is calculated for that reference. At present only one time frame per sequence needs to be segmented manually. Future work will involve the automatic

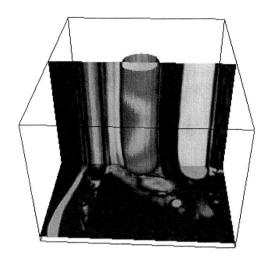

Fig. 5. Example of automatic segmentation results shown on a 3D (2D + Time) representation. The vertical axis (t) shows the time evolution of a section of the aorta. The colours on the segmentation surface show the magnitude of deformation in every region and at every time (blue is the minimum and red the maximum value).

segmentation of the first frame in order to make the approach fully automatic and measurements in the ascending and descending aorta, the aortic arch and the main, left and right pulmonary arteries will be performed.

References

1. R. H. Mohiaddin, S. R. Underwood, H. G. Bogren, D. N. Firmin, R. H. Klipstein, R. S. Rees, and D.B. Longmore. Regional aortic compliance studied by magnetic resonance imaging: The effects of age, training and coronary artery disease. *British Heart Journal*, 62:90–96, 1989.
2. H. G. Bogren, R. H. Mohiaddin, R. K. Klipstein, D. N. Firmin, R. S. Underwood, S. R. Rees, and D. B. Longmore. The function of the aorta in ischemic heart disease: a magnetic resonance and angiographic study of aortic compliance and blood flow patterns. *Am. Heart J.*, 118(2):234–247, 1989.
3. J. S. Wright, J. K. Cruickshank, S. Kontis, C. Dore, and R. G. Gosling. Aortic compliance measured by non-invasive doppler ultrasound: description of a method and its reproducibility. *Clinical Science*, 78:463–468, 1990.
4. D. Rueckert, P. Burger, S. M. Forbat, R. D. Mohiaddin, and G. Z. Yang. Automatic tracking of the aorta in cardiovascular MR images using deformable models. *IEEE Transactions on Medical Imaging*, 16(5):581–590, 1997.
5. M. Lorenzo-Valdes, G. I. Sanchez-Ortiz, R. Mohiaddin, and D. Rueckert. Atlas-based segmentation and tracking of 3D cardiac MR images using non-rigid registration. In *Fifth Int. Conf. on Medical Image Computing and Computer-Assisted Intervention (MICCAI '02)*, Lecture Notes in Computer Science, pages 642–650. Springer-Verlag, 2002.

6. J. M. Fitzpatrick, D. L. G. Hill, and C. R. Maurer, Jr. Image registration. In Milan Sonka and J. Michael Fitzpatrick, editors, *Handbook of Medical Imaging*, volume 2, pages 447–513. SPIE Press, 2000.
7. D. Rueckert, L.I. Sonoda, C. Hayes, D.L.G. Hill, M.O. Leach, and D.J. Hawkes. Nonrigid registration using free-form deformations: Application to breast MR images. *IEEE Transactions on Medical Imaging*, 18(8):712–721, 1999.
8. S. Lee, G. Wolberg, and S. Yong Shin. Scattered data interpolation with multilevel B-splines. *IEEE Transactions on Visualization and Computer Graphics*, 3(3):228–244, 1997.
9. P. Viola. *Alignment by Maximization of Mutual Information*. PhD thesis, Massachusetts Institute of Technology, 1995.

Integrated Intensity and Point-Feature Nonrigid Registration

Xenophon Papademetris[1,2], Andrea P. Jackowski[3], Robert T. Schultz[2,3], Lawrence H. Staib[1,2], and James S. Duncan[1,2]

[1] Departments of Biomedical Engineering, [2] Diag. Radiology, and [3] Child Study Center, Yale University New Haven, CT 06520-8042 papad@noodle.med.yale.edu

Abstract. In this work, we present a method for the integration of feature and intensity information for non rigid registration. Our method is based on a free-form deformation model, and uses a normalized mutual information intensity similarity metric to match intensities and the robust point matching framework to estimate feature (point) correspondences. The intensity and feature components of the registration are posed in a single energy functional with associated weights. We compare our method to both point-based and intensity-based registrations. In particular, we evaluate registration accuracy as measured by point landmark distances and image intensity similarity on a set of seventeen normal subjects. These results suggest that the integration of intensity and point-based registration is highly effective in yielding more accurate registrations.

1 Introduction

Non rigid image registration is a central task in medical image analysis. In the particular case of the brain, there are a number of important applications including comparing shape and function between individuals or groups, developing probabilistic models and atlases, measuring change within an individual and determining location with respect to a preacquired image during stereotactic surgery. The detailed comparison and nonrigid registration of brain images requires the determination of correspondence throughout the brain and the transformation of the image space according to this correspondence. In addition, a large number of other image analysis problems can in fact be posed as non rigid registration problems such as segmentation (via the use of an atlas), motion-tracking, etc.

There have been many approaches recently to nonrigid registration, with a particular emphasis on applications to brain imaging (see the collection [15]). Most commonly, non-linear registration methods use image intensities to compute the transformation (e.g. [2, 7, 14, 13, 8].) These techniques are potentially highly accurate but can be susceptible to local minima. In particular, the high anatomic variability of the cortex often results in intensity based methods yielding inaccurate results. Feature based and integrated feature-intensity methods

C. Barillot, D.R. Haynor, and P. Hellier (Eds.): MICCAI 2004, LNCS 3216, pp. 763–770, 2004.

have been developed to overcome such problems (e.g. [4, 6, 5, 11, 9, 1].) None of these methods, however, is able to handle outliers caused by large variations in sulcal anatomy, as well as irregular sulcal branching and discontinuity. We additionally note, that outliers can be present even in carefully manually segmented structures such as the ones used in this work. Brain structures are not always well defined and often part of their boundaries is set arbitrarily. For example, in the case of the amygdala typically manually traced on coronal slices, the selection of the posterior and the anterior extent is somewhat operator dependent. Hence a correspondence method that can explicitly handle outliers is important in this context.

In general, intensity-based methods are highly accurate in subcortical regions where the geometrical complexity is low. Feature-based registrations are often employed (typically with explicitly pre-segmented structures such as sulci) where accurate cortical registration is desired. In this paper we present a method which aim to integrate the strengths of both intensity and feature-based registration method. We test the results of these registrations one a set of 17 normal controls with manually extracted sulci and compare their performance to both point-based only and intensity-based only methods.

2   Methods

We first describe the components of our integrated method, namely the intensity-based registration module (section 2.1) and the robust point matching based-module (section 2.2). Then, the integrated method is presented in section 2.3.

2.1 Intensity-Based Module

We use a slightly modified form of the intensity-based non rigid registration method first described by Rueckert et al[13]. This method utilizes a free-form deformation transformation model based on tensor b-spline, and the normalized mutual information similarity metric. This metric can be expressed as:

$$d(A, B) = H(A, B)/(H(A) + H(B)) \qquad (1)$$

where A and B are the two images, and $H()$ is the image intensity entropy. This similarity metric is combined with a regularizing term to yield an optimization functional which is maximized in a multi-resolution framework. Our own implementation of this method which is used in the results section, first estimates a linear affine registration and then uses this as an input to estimate a full non-linear FFD transformation in a multiresolution manner. We modify the methodology in [13] in two ways: (a) we use a more efficient conjugate gradient optimization scheme, and (b) we implement an adaptive pre-processing scheme to better distribute the histogram bins over the intensity range in order to handle the often long tails at the upper end of the intensity of brain MRI images.

2.2   Robust-Point Based Matching Module

We present here a slightly modified form of the standard RPM methodology as can be found in Chui et al[3] and Papademetris et al[12]. The registration procedure consists of two alternative steps: (i) the correspondence estimation step and (ii) the transformation estimation step. In the following discussion we will label the reference point set as X and the transform point set as Y. The goal of the registration is to estimate the transformation $G : X \mapsto Y$. We will label G^k the estimate of G at the end of iteration k. G^0 is the starting transformation which can be the identity transformation.

Correspondence Estimation: Given the point sets X and Y we estimate the match matrix M, where M_{ij} is the distance metric between points $G^k(X_i)$ and Y_j. The standard distance metric is defined as:

$$M_{ij} = \frac{1}{\sqrt{2\pi T^2}} e^{\frac{-|G^k(X_i) - Y_j|^2}{2T^2}} \tag{2}$$

$$\forall i \quad \sum_j M_{ij} + C_i = 1, \quad \forall j \sum_i M_{ij} + R_j = 1$$

where $|X_i - Y_j|$ is the Euclidean distance between points X_i and Y_j and T is the temperature that controls the fuzziness of the correspondence. If the correspondence problem is to be thought of as a linear assignment problem, the rows and columns of M must sum to 1. The framework is further extended to handle outlier points by introducing an outlier column C and an outlier row R. C_i is a measure of the degree of 'outlierness' of a point in the reference point set X_i and R_j is the same for a point in the transform point set Y_j. C and R are initialized with constant values. The ability to model outliers allows this method to robustly match features of high variability such as cortical sulci. Once the normalization is completed we can compute the correspondence as follows. Let V_i be the corresponding point to X_i and w_i the confidence in the match. Then V_i is defined as a normalized weighted sum of the points Y_j where the weights are the elements of the match matrix M.

$$V_i = \frac{\sum_j M_{ij} Y_j}{\sum_j M_{ij}}, \quad \text{and } w_i = \left(\sum_j M_{ij}\right) = 1 - C_i \tag{3}$$

Note that a point that has a high value in the outlier column C will have low confidence and vice-versa. We note that in our integrated method (section 2.3) we simply use the correspondence piece of RPM.

Transformation Estimation: This is simply achieved by a regularized weighted least squares fit between X_i and V_i as follows:

$$G^k = \frac{\arg\min}{g} \sum_i w_i (g(X_i) - V_i)^2 + f(T)\mathcal{S}(g) \tag{4}$$

where $\mathcal{S}(g)$ is a regularization functional (e.g. bending energy function) weighted by a function of the temperature $f(T)$. This last weighting term is used to decrease the regularization as we approach convergence.

Deterministic Annealing Framework The alternating estimation of M and G is performed in a deterministic annealing framework. Starting with a high value of T corresponding to a rough estimate of the maximum mis-alignment distance we first estimate M, and then G. Then T is decreased by multiplying it with an annealing factor and the process is repeated until T becomes sufficiently small. In our implementation, first an affine transformation is estimated using $T = 15.0 \mapsto 2.0mm$ and then a non rigid FFD transformation is estimated using $T = 3.0 \mapsto 1.0$, with an annealing rate=0.93.

2.3   Integrated Method

Our method is closest in spirit to the work of Wang et al[16] and Harktens et al [9]. We first estimate an initial registration using the RPM method alone, to ensure that sulcal landmarks are correctly aligned. We then proceed to refine the estimate of the transformation by minimizing the following optimization functional which is a tradeoff between intensity similarity and adherence to point correspondence.

$$G = \underset{g}{\arg\max} \left(\underbrace{d(A,B)}_{\text{Intensity Similarity}} - \underbrace{\frac{\lambda}{N}\left(\sum_i w_i |g(X_i) - V_i|\right)}_{\text{Adherence to Point Correspondences}} \right)$$

(5)

where the first term is the intensity similarity distance (eqn. 1), the second is a measure of adherence to the corresponding points as estimated by RPM (eqn. 4) weighted by the constant λ (N is the number of points in the reference point-set). We note that during the optimization of this functional the correspondences maybe re-evaluated at each iteration at a constant temperature $T = 1.0mm$ which is equal to the minimum temperature used in the initial registration. In practice, however, keeping the correspondences fixed produced marginally better results. The transformation estimated has the exact same parameterization as the FFD transformation estimated by the RPM algorithm.

3   Results

In this section, we compare the performance of our new integrated algorithm to our previous point-based only method as well as a standard non-linear intensity-only based method. We evaluate the accuracy of the algorithms in matching cortical landmarks in a set of 17 normal controls.

   All images used in this work were high resolution ($1.2 \times 1.2 \times 1.2mm$) 3D SPGR images acquired using a GE 1.5 T scanner (2 NEX, TR= 24msec, TE

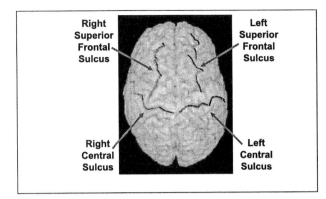

Fig. 1. Sulci used in the evaluation of the registration methods. Note that these are major sulci, hence the matching error of the intensity based method is smaller that what is reported by Hellier et al. [10]

= 5msec, flip = 45°). The scans were of excellent quality and without movement artifacts. The brains were next stripped and the following four sulci were manually traced (a) left central sulcus, (b) right central suclus, (c) left superior frontal sulcus and (d) right superior frontal sulcus, as shown in figure 1. For the purpose of both the integrated and the point-only based methods, labeled point sets for each subject were constructed using approximately 5000 points for the outer cortical surface and 250 points for each sulcus resulting in a total point set of approximately 6000 points/subject. All subjects were registered to a normal control reference subject, an example registration is shown in figure 2

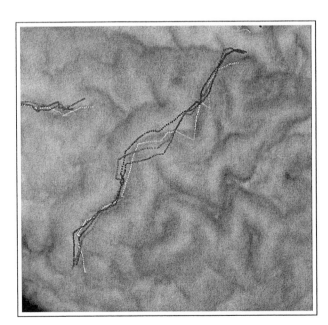

Fig. 2. Example registration result. In this close-up of the central sulcus overlaid on a volume rendered stripped brain, the target surface is shown in white. The warped template is shown for three different registrations RPM – red, Integrated ($\lambda = 0.1$) – blue and NMI – green.

For the purpose of comparison, the registrations were computed using (a) our point-based method RPM[12] and (b) our implementation of the non-linear

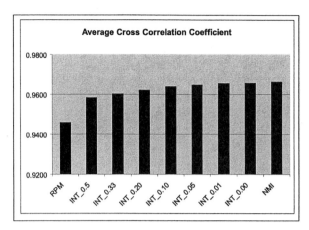

Fig. 3. Average intensity similarity for the point-based registration method (RPM), the new integrated algorithm (INT-λ) with seven different values of the weight of adherence to the point correspondences λ and the intensity only similarity algorithm (NMI) as computed from $N = 17$ normal controls.

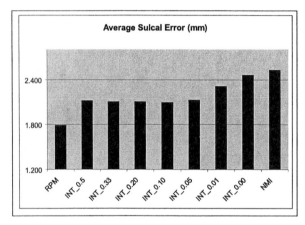

Fig. 4. Average sulcal matching error for the point-based registration method (RPM), the new integrated algorithm (INT-λ) as above and the intensity only similarity algorithm (NMI) as computed from $N = 17$ normal controls.

intensity (NMI) based method of Rueckert et al [13]. To test the effect of the tradeoff parameter λ, the integrated algorithm was applied using seven different values of λ (INT-λ). We used the following measures to evaluate the quality of the registration:

1. Cross-Correlation Coefficient (CC): This measures the degree of intensity similarity. We use this measure rather than NMI as it was not explicitly optimized by methods (ii) and (iii). In practice, though, there was found to be a monotonic relationship between CC and NMI. The values of CC for all registration methods are shown in figure 3.

2. Average Sulcal matching error: This was the mean distance of all points from the reference sulcus to the target sulcus using correspondences estimated by a nearest-neighbor matching method. The results for this are shown in figure 4.

We also report the total bending energy of the calculated transformations to give a sense of the extent of the deformation in each case. Note that the bending energy in RPM is very low as there are no sub-cortical features and hence the registration is very smooth away from the cortical surface and the sulci. The integrated algorithms with high values of λ also have low bending energy; the

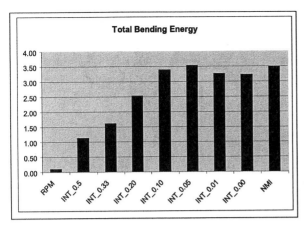

Fig. 5. Average bending energy for the registrations computed by the point-based registration method (RPM), the new integrated algorithm (INT-λ) and the intensity only similarity algorithm (NMI) as computed from $N = 17$ normal controls.

bending energy gradually increased and approaches that of the NMI method as λ goes to zero. The average total bending energy for all the registration methods is shown in the chart in figure 5.

The intensity similarity metric results shown in figure 3 indicate that the integrated method approaches the intensity-based method as the value of λ goes to zero as expected, especially for $\lambda < 0.05$. As expected the RPM algorithm is superior in terms of sulcal distance error point matching Note that in particular for $\lambda = 0.1$ or 0.05, the performance of the integrated algorithm the integrated method performs almost as well as the individual components (i.e. RPM and NMI) in their area of respective strengths, i.e. it produces an optimal tradeoff between sulcal matching error and intensity similarity.

4   Conclusions

In this work, we present a new method for the integration of intensity based and feature based registrations with encouraging results. In general, while feature based methods are highly accurate in specific areas, their accuracy decreases in regions away from the pre-extracted points. Intensity based methods, on the other hand are highly accurate in subcortical regions but their accuracy decreases in the cortex. Combining the two approaches offers the opportunity of an optimal tradeoff between localized feature-driven registration accuracy in the cortex and accurate intensity registration in the sub-cortex. We believe that this improvement would be more obvious in the case of variable sulci, as opposed to the major sulci that were available for this work. (Further, the brains used for all registrations were accurately pre-stripped hence improving the surface registration for the intensity-based method.)

We believe that such an integration is necessary for the computation of both morphometric differences between subjects, as well as composite activation maps from fMRI in cortical areas where intensity only methods are relatively inaccurate [10]. We are currently investigating reformulating our method in terms of two interacting modules to yield an EM-like algorithm.

References

1. P. Cachier, E. Bardinet, D. Dormont, X. Pennec, and N. Ayache. Iconic feature based nonrigid registration: the PASHA algorithm. *Computer Vision and Image Understanding*, 89:272–298, 2003.
2. G. E. Christensen, M. I. Miller, and M. W. Vannier. Individualizing neuroanatomical atlases using a massively parallel computer. *Computer*.
3. H. Chui, L. Win, R. T. Schultz, J. S. Duncan, and A. Rangarajan. A unified non-rigid feature registration method for brain mapping. *Medical Image Analysis*, 7(2):113–130, 2003.
4. D. L. Collins, G. Le Goualher, and A. C. Evans. Non-linear cerebral registration with sulcal constraints. In *Medical Image Computing and Computer Assisted Intervention*, pages 974–984. Springer, Berlin, 1998.
5. I. Corouge, C. Barillot, P. Hellier, P. Toulouse, and B. Gibaud. Non-linear local registration of functional data. In M.-A. Viergever, T. Dohi, and M. Vannier, editors, *Medical Image Computing and Computer Aided Intervention (MICCAI)*, pages 948–956, 2001.
6. C. Davatzikos. Spatial transformation and registration of brain images using elastically deformable models. *Comp. Vision and Image Understanding*, 66(2):207–222, 1997.
7. J. Feldmar, G. Malandain, J. Declerck, and N. Ayache. Extension of the ICP algorithm to non-rigid intensity-based registration of 3D volumes. In *Proc. Workshop Math. Meth. Biomed. Image Anal.*, pages 84–93, June 1996.
8. K.J. Friston, J. Ashburner, J.B. Poline, C.D. Frith, J.D. Heather, and R.S.J. Frackowiak. Spatial registration and normalization of images. *Human Brain Mapping*, 2:165–189, 1995.
9. T. Hartkens, D.L.G. Hill, A. D Castellano-Smith, D. J. Hawkes, C.R. Maurer Jr., A. J. Martin, W.A. Hall, H. Liu, and C.L. Truwit. Using points and surfaces to improve voxel-based non-rigid registration. In *Medical Image Computing and Computer Aided Intervention (MICCAI)*, pages 565–572, 2002.
10. P. Hellier, C. Barillot, I. Corouge, B. Gibaud, G. Le Goualher, D.L. Collins, A. Evans, G. Malandain, N. Ayache, G.E. Christensen, and H.J. Johnson. Retrospective evaluation of inter-subject brain registration. *IEEE Transactions on Medical Imaging*, 22(9):1120–1130, 2003.
11. T. Liu, D. Shen, and C. Davatzikos. Deformable registration of cortical structures via hybrid volumetric and surface warping. In *Medical Image Computing and Computer Aided Intervention (MICCAI) Part II LLNCS 2879*, pages 780–787. Springer-Verlag, 2003.
12. X. Papademetris, A. Jackowski, R. T. Schultz, L. H. Staib, and J. S. Duncan. Computing 3D non-rigid brain registration using extended robust point matching for composite multisubject fMRI analysis. In *Medical Image Computing and Computer Aided Intervention (MICCAI) Part II LLNCS 2879*, pages 788–795. Springer-Verlag, 2003.
13. D. Rueckert, L. I. Sonoda, C. Hayes, D. L. G. Hill, M.O. Leach, and D. J. Hawkes. Non-rigid registration using free-form deformations: Application to breast MR images. *IEEE Transactions on Medical Imaging*, 1999.
14. J. P. Thirion. Image matching as a diffusion process: An analogy with maxwell's demons. *Med. Image Anal.*, 2(3):243–260, 1998.
15. A. W. Toga. *Brain Warping*. Academic Press, San Diego, 1999.
16. Y. Wang and L. H. Staib. Physical model based non-rigid registration incorporating statistical shape information. *Med. Image Anal.*, 4:7–20, 2000.

Matching 3D Shapes Using 2D Conformal Representations

Xianfeng Gu[1] and Baba C. Vemuri[2]

Computer and Information Science and Engineering,
Gainesville, FL 32611-6120, USA
{gu,vemuri}@cise.ufl.edu

Abstract. Matching 3D shapes is a fundamental problem in Medical Imaging with many applications including, but not limited to, shape deformation analysis, tracking etc. Matching 3D shapes poses a computationally challenging task. The problem is especially hard when the transformation sought is diffeomorphic and non-rigid between the shapes being matched. In this paper, we propose a novel and computationally efficient matching technique which guarantees that the estimated non-rigid transformation between the two shapes being matched is a diffeomorphism.

Specifically, we propose to conformally map each of the two 3D shapes onto the canonical domain and then match these 2D representations over the class of diffeomorphisms. The representation consists of a two tuple (λ, H), where, λ is the conformal factor required to map the given 3D surface to the canonical domain (a sphere for genus zero surfaces) and H is the mean curvature of the 3D surface. Given this two tuple, it is possible to uniquely determine the corresponding 3D surface. This representation is one of the most salient features of the work presented here. The second salient feature is the fact that 3D non-rigid registration is achieved by matching the aforementioned 2D representations.

We present convincing results on real data with synthesized deformations and real data with real deformations.

1 Introduction

Matching 3D shapes is a fundamental problem in computer vision with several applications in medical imaging, archeology, augmented reality and many others. Several 2D and 3D shape matching techniques have been developed in the past couple of decades in the field of computer vision and some have been successfully applied to medical imaging, shape retrieval etc. Since our focus in this paper is 3D shape matching, in the following, we will restrict our literature review to matching 3D shapes and refer the reader to some recent works [1,2,3] and the references therein for 2D shape matching.

3D shape matching has a rich history in the field of Computer Vision specifically in object recognition applications. A key ingredient in shape matching has been the choice of the shape representation scheme. One of the first 3D shape

C. Barillot, D.R. Haynor, and P. Hellier (Eds.): MICCAI 2004, LNCS 3216, pp. 771–780, 2004.
© Springer-Verlag Berlin Heidelberg 2004

matching techniques involved the use of the curvature-based representations [4, 5], the modal based representations [6], harmonic images [7], spherical harmonic representation [8] and shape distributions [8], spline representations [9]. Very few of these representation along with the associated matching algorithms tackled non-rigid motions and when they did do so, the resulting motion was not a diffeomorphism. In some medical imaging applications, it is important to require that the estimated transformation be a diffeomorphism. Similar requirements are not uncommon in non-medical domains. More recently, there have been several techniques in literature [10] that yield a diffeomorphic mapping. These techniques however are relatively computationally expensive. In this paper, we propose a technique that is guaranteed to yield a diffeomorphic mapping in 3D and can be computed very efficiently via conformal matching of the corresponding 2D representation, described subsequently.

In [11], a technique for brain image warping was described and then applied to detect disease-specific patterns in [12]. In [13], yet another diffeomorphic warping scheme developed by Christensen [14] was used to study hippocampal morphometry. In [15] Twining et al. developed a method to construct diffeomorphic representations of non-rigid registrations of medical images. Automatic neuroanatomical segmentation based on warping of 3D models is addressed in [16]. More recently, conformal brain mappings have been studied in [17] and [18]. While some of these techniques yield diffeomorphic warps, they are however computationally expensive. In this paper, we present a technique that yields diffeomorphic warps which are easy to compute and relatively inexpensive.

The rest of the paper is organized as follows: Section 2 contains some mathematical preliminaries. This is followed by the description of the conformal representation in section 3. Section 4 contains the mathematical formulation of the matching problem and the optimization method to find the best Möbius transformation. Experimental results on both synthetic and real data cases is presented in section 5.

2   Mathematical Framework for the Proposed Model

We now present some definitions from differential geometry that are necessary to understand our shape representation.

Let $\phi : S_1 \to S_2$ be a smooth map between two manifolds, define the local coordinates for S_1 and S_2 by (x^1, x^2) and $\phi(x^1, x^2) = (\phi^1(x^1, x^2), \phi^2(x^1, x^2))$. The first fundamental forms of S_1 and S_2 are: $ds_1^2 = \sum_{ij} g_{ij} dx^i dx^j$ and $ds_2^2 = \sum_{ij} \tilde{g}_{ij} dx^i dx^j$. The pull back metric on S_1 induced by ϕ is then given by,

$$\phi^* ds_2^2 = \sum_{mn} \sum_{ij} \tilde{g}_{ij} \frac{\partial \phi^i}{\partial x_m} \frac{\partial \phi^j}{\partial x_n} dx^m dx^n. \tag{1}$$

If there exists a positive function $\lambda(x^1, x^2)$, such that $ds_1^2 = \lambda(x^1, x^2) \phi^* ds_2^2$, then we say ϕ is a *conformal map* between S_1 and S_2. Especially, if the map from S_1 to the local coordinate plane (x_1, x_2) is conformal, we say that (x_1, x_2) are the *conformal coordinates* of S_1. A 2-manifold S is a *Riemann surface*, if there exists an atlas, such that, (1) each local chart forms a conformal coordinate system on S and we treat each coordinate chart as an open set of the complex plane C. (2) The transition functions between charts are treated as complex functions, all of them being holomorphic. By the Riemann uniformization Theorem, all surfaces can be conformally embedded in a sphere, a plane or a hyperbolic space, wherein all the embeddings form special groups. The conformal parametrization continuously depends on the Riemannian metric tensor on the surface.

Surfaces can be represented as functions defined on their conformal coordinate systems. Thus, by using a conformal representation, the surface matching problems in 3D can be converted to matching of equivalent representations in 2D.

Suppose S_1 and S_2 are two surfaces we want to match and their conformal coordinate domains of S_1 and S_2 are D_1 and D_2 respectively. Let the conformal mapping from S_1 to D_1 be π_1, the one from S_2 to D_2 be π_2. Instead of finding the mapping ϕ from S_1 to S_2 directly, we want to find a map $\tilde{\phi} : D_1 \to D_2$, such that the diagram 2 is commutable i.e., $\pi_2^{-1} \circ \tilde{\phi} \circ \pi_1 = \phi$.

$$
\begin{array}{ccc}
S_1 & \xrightarrow{\ \phi\ } & S_2 \\
{\scriptstyle \pi_1}\Big\downarrow & & \Big\downarrow{\scriptstyle \pi_2} \\
D_1 & \xrightarrow[\ \tilde{\phi}\ ]{} & D_2
\end{array}
\qquad (2)
$$

Thus, finding a diffeomorphic ϕ between S_1 and S_2 can be achieved by finding a diffeomorphism $\tilde{\phi}$ from D_1 to D_2 and then using the commutative diagram.

3   The 2D Conformal Representation for Surfaces in 3D and Its Properties

In this section we will introduce the methods to represent surfaces using their *conformal coordinates*. This representation preserves all the geometric information of the surface and maps all surfaces to the canonical 2D domains. If two surfaces are close to each other under the Housdorff metric, the L^2 norm between their conformal representations are also close. Conversely, if two surfaces have similar conformal representations, then they also have similar shapes in R^3. The key advantage of our conformal representation is that it is complete in the sense that it allows us to reconstruct the original surface fully from the representation. Thus, there is no loss of information in this representation unlike most others e.g., shape distributions [8] and others.

Suppose surface S is mapped conformally to a canonical domain, such as the sphere. We can stereographically project the sphere to the complex plane, then use these conformal coordinates (u, v) to parameterize S. Then, We can compute the following two maps directly from the position vector $S(u, v)$. First, the *conformal factor map* or *stretch map* is the conformal factor function $\lambda(u, v)$

defined on (u, v), and conceptually represents the scaling factor at each point. Secondly, the *mean curvature function.*

$$\frac{\partial S}{\partial u} \times \frac{\partial S}{\partial v} = \lambda(u, v) n(u, v) \tag{3}$$

$$\Delta S(u, v) = H(u, v) n(u, v), \tag{4}$$

where Δ is the Laplace-Beltrami operator defined on S, $n(u, v)$ is the normal function, $H(u, v)$ is the mean curvature, $\lambda(u, v)$ conformal factor function. The tuple (λ, H) is the conformal representation of $S(u, v)$.

Theorem 1 Conformal Representation: *If a surface $S(u, v)$ is parameterized by some conformal parameter (u, v) on a domain D, then the conformal factor function $\lambda(u, v)$ and mean curvature function $H(u, v)$ defined on D satisfy the Gauss and Codazzi equation. If $\lambda(u, v)$ and $H(u, v)$ are given, along with the boundary condition $S(u, v)|_{\partial D}$, then $S(u, v)$ can be uniquely reconstructed.*

The conformal maps between two genus zero closed surfaces form the so called Möbius transformation group. If we map the sphere to the complex plane using stereo-graphic projection, then all Möbius transformations $\mu : S^2 \rightarrow S^2$ have the form

$$\mu(z) = \frac{az + b}{cz + d}, ad - bc = 1, a, b, c, d \in C. \tag{5}$$

Another important property of our representation is that it is *very stable.* If we slightly perturb a shape S, then its conformal representation $\lambda(u, v)$ will be perturbed only slightly. Hence, conformal representation is continuous and stable.

In summary, the conformal representation is intrinsic, continuous and stable, preserving all geometric information. It allows us to convert the problem of matching surfaces in 3D to the problem of matching the corresponding canonical 2D conformal representations.

4   3D Shape Matching Formulation

In this section, we present the mathematical formulation of the matching problem. Suppose we have two genus zero surfaces S_1 and S_2 embedded in R^3. Our goal is to find a diffeomorphism $\phi : S_1 \rightarrow S_2$, such that ϕ minimizes the following functional,

$$E(\phi) = \int_{D_1} ||S_1(u, v) - S_2(\phi(u, v))||^2 dudv. \tag{6}$$

If we want to find a conformal map ϕ between S_1 and S_2, we can restrict $\tilde{\phi}$ to be a Möbius transformation when D_1 and D_2 are spheres.

The position map/representation $S(u, v)$ is variant under rigid motion, and the conformal factor $\lambda(u, v)$ and mean curvature $H(u, v)$ are invariant under rigid motion. Therefore, it is most efficient to use $\lambda(u, v)$ and $H(u, v)$ for matching surfaces. The matching energy can therefore be defined as,

$$E(\tilde{\phi}) = \int_{D_1} ||\lambda_1(u, v) - \lambda_2(\tilde{\phi}(u, v))||^2 dudv + \int_{D_1} ||H_1(u, v) - H_2(\tilde{\phi}(u, v))||^2 dudv. \tag{7}$$

This energy is minimized numerically to obtain the optimal $\tilde{\phi}$ and then the corresponding ϕ is obtained from the commutative diagram shown earlier. There are many numerical optimization algorithms in literature that can be used to minimize the energy defined above for diffeomorphic matching of functions defined on the plane e.g., the gradient descent method with adaptive step size, the Gauss-Newton method or the quasi-Newton method. In this paper, we use the quasi-Newton method to compute the optimal diffeomorphism $\tilde{\phi}$.

During the matching, the boundary condition and geometric constraints should be considered. A general diffeomorphism may not guarantee that corresponding points between two instances of the same shape will map to each other however it is a necessary condition. Thus, in order to make sure that this constraint is satisfied, we may choose certain landmark points on S_1 which we want to map to predefined points on S_2. This leads to a constrained diffeomorphic matching.

For genus zero closed surface, in order to find a Möbius transformation, three landmarks are enough. Suppose three landmarks are given as $\{z_0, z_1, z_2\}$, corresponding to $\{\tilde{z}_0, \tilde{z}_1, \tilde{z}_2\}$, then a Möbius transformation $\tilde{\phi}$ which maps all the landmarks can be represented in a closed form, we use z_{ij} to denote $z_j - z_i$, and $\tilde{z}_{ij}$ for $\tilde{z}_j - \tilde{z}_i$,

$$\tilde{\phi}(z) = \frac{\tilde{z}_1(z - z_0)z_{12}\tilde{z}_{02} - (z - z_1)z_{02}\tilde{z}_{12}\tilde{z}_0}{(z - z_0)z_{12}\tilde{z}_{02} - (z - z_1)z_{02}\tilde{z}_{12}} \tag{8}$$

We match the landmarks first, then use that $\tilde{\phi}$ as the initial Möbius transformation , and optimize it to find the minimal matching energy.

5   Experimental Results

In order to test the performance of the matching algorithm, several experiments are carried out and described in this section. We use surfaces extracted from medical images for our testing. Their topologies are verified to be of genus zero. The shapes are represented by triangulated meshes in 3D which are subdivided using standard sub-division schemes in Computer Graphics to yield a smooth representation of the surfaces. These surfaces are conformally mapped to the canonical domain namely, the sphere, using the method introduced in [18] and these canonical mappings then form the input to our matching algorithm. We tested our algorithm with both synthetically generated deformations as well as real deformations. In the synthetic deformation cases, we applied known non-rigid deformations to a source shape to generate the target shape. The estimated deformation is then compared with the known ground truth deformation for several similarly generated data sets. The average and standard deviation of the error in estimated deformation was then computed over the entire source-target pairs of data. In the examples presented below, this error is quite small indicating the accuracy of our technique presented here.

5.1 Synthetic Deformations Applied to Real Surfaces

The deformation coefficients of ϕ are generated randomly using a Gaussian distribution. We used 20 sample deformations from the Guassian distribution of deformations to test our algorithm. As evident from the table 1, the mean and variance of the difference between ϕ and the reconstructed deformation $\hat{\phi}$ are very small indicating the accuracy of our algorithm.

In the next experiment, we present a cortical surface extracted from a human brain MRI image and represented using a triangular mesh as shown in 1. This cortical surface is then conformally mapped to a sphere as shown in (b) and (d). The conformal factor λ is color-encoded as depicted in (a) and (b), the mean curvature map is also color-encoded as shown in (c) and (d). The lowest values of λ and H are represented by the blue color and the highest by the red color. Values in between span the color spectrum.

We now define a non-rigid motion denoted by $\phi : R^3 \to R^3$ using affine maps and then apply it to the real anatomical surface extracted from the brain MRI scan. $\phi = (\phi^1, \phi^2, \phi^3)$ is represented as $\phi^k = \sum_i l_i^k x^i + t^k, i, j, k = 1, 2, 3$. All coefficients of ϕ are randomly drawn from a Gaussian distribution.

The anatomical surface S is deformed by a randomly generated ϕ, then we match S with $\phi(S)$ using the conformal representation. Using the algorithm described in the last section, we estimate ϕ and denoted it by $\hat{\phi}$. We computed the estimation error by comparing the original coefficients of ϕ and the estimated coefficients of $\hat{\phi}$. The results are depicted in the table 1. As evident, the estimates are very accurate. Figure 2 depicts one matching example. The deformation ϕ in 2 is

$$\phi(x, y, z) = \begin{pmatrix} 5.0 & 0.10 & 0.2 \\ 0.4 & 5.10 & 0.2 \\ 0.4 & 0.6 & 4.9 \end{pmatrix} \begin{pmatrix} x \\ y \\ z \end{pmatrix} + \begin{pmatrix} 5.0 \\ 10.0 \\ 15.0 \end{pmatrix}$$

Table 1. Mean and variance of the computed deformations between the source and target shapes.

# of Tests	$\mu_{l_i^k}$	$\sigma_{l_i^k}$	μ_{t^k}	σ_{t^k}	$\mu_{\hat{l}_i^k - l_i^k}$	$\sigma_{\hat{l}_i^k - l_i^k}$	$\mu_{\hat{t}^k - t^k}$	$\sigma_{\hat{t}_i - t_i}$
20	0.3	0.47	33.33	47.14	4.02e-4	0.538e-4	7.27e-4	4.69e-4
20	1.9	2.21	10.00	4.08	2.7333e-2	1.0607e-2	3.2645e-2	1.6135e-2
20	3.9	4.36	20.00	8.16	1.55339e-1	9.3372e-2	1.09864e-1	7.1456e-2
20	1.8	2.21	10.00	4.08	2.7333e-2	1.0607e-2	3.2645e-2	1.6135e-2
20	0.34	0.47	3.33e-3	4.714e-3	1.079e-3	9.83e-4	1.595e-4	3.05e-4

While the estimated deformation is,

$$\hat{\phi}(x,y,z) = \begin{pmatrix} 4.9562 & 0.1211 & 0.2492 \\ 0.3604 & 5.0734 & 0.2189 \\ 0.3729 & 0.5817 & 4.8887 \end{pmatrix} \begin{pmatrix} x \\ y \\ z \end{pmatrix} + \begin{pmatrix} 4.9897 \\ 10.0396 \\ 15.0480 \end{pmatrix}$$

The accuracy of the estimated deformation field is assessed by computing the standard deviation of the estimated deformation field for S. For each point, the displacement field on S is defined as $T_\phi(u,v) = \phi(S(u,v)) - S(u,v)$. The displacement field T_ϕ and the estimated displacement field $T_{\hat{\phi}}$ are color-encoded and illustrated in 2. We first normalize each channel, (x,y,z), of T_ϕ and $T_{\hat{\phi}}$ to be between 0 and 1. Then (x,y,z) are represented by (R,G,B) colors. Higher values of error in any of the 3 channels/directions will have a higher brightness in the corresponding color.

As evident, the estimated deformation is very accurate. The distortion of the conformal structure caused by ϕ in the above experiment is very large, for example, it changes an angle from 90° to 63° in the above experiment. Even with such big distortions of the conformal structure, our method is able to quite accurately recover this deformation. This illustrates the robustness of our algorithm.

5.2   Real Deformations Between Anatomical Surfaces

We also tested our algorithm on subcortical surfaces, specifically, the human hippocampus surface extracted from MR brain scans. We applied our algorithm to several distinct hippocampal surfaces to estimate the deformation between pairs of them. This deformation can be used in assessing the shape differences between them and assess the asymmetry between the left and right hippocampi for a subject with epilepsy or schizophrenia or other pathologies.

Figure 3 illustrates the conformal representation of a hippocampal surface. The matching results are illustrated in figure 4. We match the first hippocampal surface to other three. In order to illustrate the correspondence, we color encode the z value of the first surface and map the color to other surfaces by the matching deformation. Each surface has about 5000 faces, and it takes about 90 seconds to compute their conformal representation and 200 seconds (on a pentium 4) for estimating the 3D deformation.

6   Conclusions

In this paper, we introduced a novel method for 3D surface matching using conformal representations, which is based on Riemann surface theories. All orientable surfaces can be mapped conformally to canonical spaces and represented by conformal factor and mean curvature. The representation intrinsically and continuously depends on the geometry of the surface. Then, the 3D surface matching problem is converted to matching of 2D conformal representations.

In comparison to other matching methods, our new method is intrinsic and efficient. We presented several synthetic and real data examples depicting the

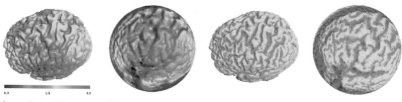

(a) conformal factor on (b)conformal factor (c) Mean curvature on (d)Mean curvature
   the brain surface.   on the sphere.   the brain surface.   on the sphere.

Fig. 1. Color encoding of the conformal factor on (a) the cortex, (b) on the canonical domain – the sphere; Color encoding of the Mean curvature on (c) the cortex and (d) the cortex conformally mapped to the sphere.

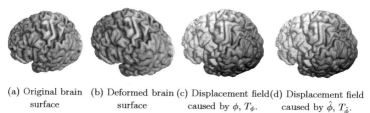

(a) Original brain (b) Deformed brain (c) Displacement field(d) Displacement field
      surface   surface   caused by ϕ, T_ϕ.   caused by $\hat{\phi}$, $T_{\hat{\phi}}$.

Fig. 2. Estimated deformation using the conformal representation. (a) Original cortical surface, (b) Synthetically deformed cortex. (c) and (d) depict color encoded deformation fields ϕ ((x, y, z) corresponding to (R, G, B)) and $\hat{\phi}$ applied to (a) respectively.

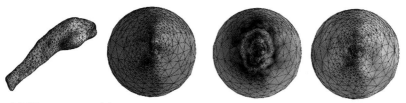

(a) Hippocampus (b) Conformal Mapping(c) Conformal Factor (d) Mean curvature
     surface

Fig. 3. Conformal factor and Mean curvature maps of the hippocampal surface. (a) Hippocampal surface, (b) Conformal mapping of (a) to a sphere, (c) & (d) color coded, conformal factor map and Mean curvature map respectively.

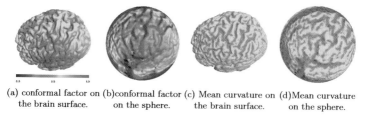

(a) conformal factor on (b)conformal factor (c) Mean curvature on (d)Mean curvature
   the brain surface.   on the sphere.   the brain surface.   on the sphere.

Fig. 4. Different hippocampal surfaces extracted from MRI images. The matching results are color encoded (see text for details). The regions of the same color exhibit the correspondence obtained from the matching algorithm.

accuracy of the estimated deformation between the source and target shapes. The achieved accuracy was quite high and comparable to those achieved by other methods reported in literature but at a much smaller computational expense. Our future work will focus on generalizing the conformal representations to surfaces with arbitrary genus.

Acknowledgements. This research was in part supported by the NIH grant RO1 NS42075 to BCV. Authors thank Professor C. M. Leonard of the UF-MBI for the hippocampal data.

References

1. H. D. Tagare. Shape-based nonrigid correspondence with application to heart motion analysis. In *IEEE Trans. Medical Imaging*, volume 18, pages 570–578, 1999.
2. B. B. Kimia C. M. Cyr, T. Sabestian. 2d to 3d registration based on shape matching. In *IEEE MMPIA*, 2000.
3. M. Frenkel and R. Basri. Curve matching using the fast marching method. In *EMMCVPR*, pages 35–51, 2003.
4. B. C. Vemuri, A. Mitiche, and J. K. Aggarwal. curvature-based representation of objects from range data. In *Image and Vision Computing*, volume 4, pages 107–114, may 1986.
5. Paul J. Besl and Ramesh C. Jain. Three-dimensional object recognition. In *ACM Computing Surveys*, volume 17, pages 75–145, 1985.
6. A. Pentland and S. Scalroff. Closed-form solutions for physically based shape modeling and recognition. In *IEEE Trans. on PAMI*, volume 13, pages 715–729, 1991.
7. Dongmei Zhang and Martial Hebert. Harmonic shape images: A representation for 3d free-form surfaces based on energy minimization. In *EMMCVPR*, pages 30–43, 1999.
8. Michael Kazhdan and Thomas Funkhouser. Harmonic 3d shape matching.
9. V. Camion and L. Younes. Geodesic interpolating splines. In *Proceedings of EMM-CVPR 2001*, pages 513–527, 2001.
10. A. Trouve. Diffeomorphisms groups and pattern matching in image analysis. In *International Journal of Computer Vision*, volume 28, pages 213–221, 1998.
11. P. Thompson and A. Toga. A surface-based technique for warping 3-dimensional images of the brain. In *IEEE Trans. Medical Images*, volume 15, pages 402–417, 1996.
12. P. M. Thompson, M. S. Mega, C. Vidal, J. L. Rapoport, and A. W. Toga. Detecting disease-specific patterns of brain structure using cortical pattern matching and a population-based probabilistic brain atlas. In *17th International Conference on Information Processing in Medical Imaging (IPMI2001)*, volume 18, pages 488–501, 2001.
13. Csernansky, J., Joshi, S., Wang, L., Haller, J., Gado, M., Miller, J., Grenander, U., Miller, and M. Hippocampal morphometry in schizophrenia via high dimensional brain mapping. In *Proceedings National Academy of Sciences*, pages 11406–11411, 1998.

14. G. E. Christensen, S. C. Joshi, and M. Miller. Volumetric transformation of brain anatomy. In *IEEE TMI*, volume 16, pages 864–877, 1997.

15. Carole Twining and Stephen Marsland. Constructing diffeomorphic representations of non-rigid registrations of medical images. In *18th International Conference on Information Processing in Medical Imaging (IPMI2003)*, volume 20, pages 413–425, 2003.

16. D. L. Collins, C. J. Holmes, T. M. Peters, and A. C. Evans. Automatic 3d model based neuroanatomical segmentation. In *Human Brain Mapping*, volume 3, pages 190–208, 1995.

17. S. Pentland, S. Angenent, A. Tannenbaum, R. Kikinis, G. Sapiro, and M. Halle. Conformal surface parameterization for texture mapping. In *IEEE Transaction on Visualization and Computer Graphics*, volume 6, pages 181–189, 2000.

18. X. Gu, Y. Wang, T.F. Chan, P.M. Thompson, and S.T. Yau. Genus zero surface conformal mapping and its application to brain surface mapping. In *IPMI2003*, pages 172–184.

Parallel Optimization Approaches for Medical Image Registration

Mark P. Wachowiak[1] and Terry M. Peters[1,2]

[1] Imaging Research Laboratories, Robarts Research Institute
[2] Department of Medical Biophysics, University of Western Ontario
London, ON N6A 5K8 Canada
{mwach, tpeters}@imaging.robarts.ca

Abstract. Optimization of a similarity metric is an essential component in most medical image registration approaches based on image intensities. The increasing availability of parallel computers makes parallelizing some registration tasks an attractive option. In this paper, two relatively new, deterministic, direct optimization algorithms are parallelized for distributed memory systems, and adapted for image registration. DIRECT is a global technique, and the multidirectional search is a recent local method. The performance of several variants are compared. Experimental results show that both methods are robust, accurate, and, in parallel implementations, can significantly reduce computation time.

1 Introduction

The robustness and performance of intensity-based image registration techniques depend on selecting an appropriate similarity metric suited to the particular application, choice of search space (linear, elastic, nonlinear), interpolation scheme, and the approach used to optimize the similarity metric. For the latter, the Nelder-Mead downhill simplex, Powell's method (line search), and methods requiring derivatives (conjugate gradient, Newton's method, Levenberg-Marquardt) have often been used [1,2]. If accurate first derivatives are available, then gradient descent methods are preferred [3]. However, these techniques are generally local, and are susceptible to premature convergence to local optima, and incorrect registration. Global optimization, usually having a stochastic component (e.g. [4,5,6]), has been shown to improve robustness, but at the cost of increased similarity metric evaluations and slower convergence. Faster processors and memory access have substantially reduced registration time, but parallel computing has the potential to further increase efficiency, and also to facilitate use of optimization techniques that were formerly considered too computationally expensive to be used for registration. Powell's method, while generally robust, is still prone to local minima entrapment for many similarity metrics [7], and is not easily parallelized. In gradient descent methods, gradients can be computed in parallel, but analytical expressions for the derivatives of many metrics (w.r.t. a transformation) are not available, or cannot be easily estimated.

C. Barillot, D.R. Haynor, and P. Hellier (Eds.): MICCAI 2004, LNCS 3216, pp. 781–788, 2004.

In the current work, two relatively new deterministic direct methods (not requiring evaluation of derivatives) are applied to medical image registration: DIRECT (for DIviding RECTangles) is a global technique that was designed for difficult optimization problems [8], and the multidirectional search (MDS) is a local method [3,9]. The inherent parallelism of both DIRECT and MDS can be easily exploited for improving registration performance. Other investigators have used DIRECT as a final, local step after stochastic optimization for registration [4], but in this paper, DIRECT is employed as a global strategy. In addition, a version of DIRECT with local bias is adapted for registration. To our knowledge, MDS has not previously been used in this application.

Other investigators have exploited parallelism to improve registration speed for clinical applications. In [10], resampling is multithreaded, and computation of similarity values, as well as segmentation and visualization, are parallelized on distributed memory clusters. In [11], vector field computations and resampling are performed in a hybrid distributed/shared memory environment. In the current paper, coarse-grained (high computation-to-communication ratio) parallelism is achieved by distributing the entire evaluation of the similarity metric, so that metrics for many transformations can be computed simultaneously. This technique is suitable for distributed, shared memory, and hybrid implementation, and is also extendible to include parallelization of other operations.

2   Dividing Rectangles (DIRECT)

DIRECT is a relatively recent algorithm for finding the global minimum of a multivariate function subject to linear bounds. It is essentially a Lipschitzian approach, but no Lipschitz constant needs to be specified [8]. DIRECT balances global search, which finds the "basin of attraction" of the minimum, with local search, which exploits this basin. In DIRECT, the search space is treated as an n-D rectangle with sides normalized to length 1, which is then recursively divided into smaller rectangles. Every rectangle i is centered at a point $\mathbf{x}_i$, and has a level $l = 0, 1, ...$ and stage p, $0 \leq p < n$. The rectangle has p short sides of length $3^{-(l+1)}$ and $n-p$ long sides of length 3^{-l}. Rectangles are grouped by their l_2 norm diameters, $d(l, p) = 3^l(n - 8p/9)^{1/2}$ [12]. The set of potentially optimal rectangles, or those that define the convex hull of a scatter plot of rectangle diameters versus $f(\mathbf{x}_i)$ for all rectangle centers $\mathbf{x}_i$, are identified, and are used as the centers for the next iteration. For each identified center, the $2n$ points $\mathbf{x}_i \pm 3^{(-l+1)}\mathbf{e}_j$, $j = 1, ..., n$, are evaluated. The rectangle is divided into thirds, first along the dimension with the smallest function value, and the resulting rectangles are then divided along the dimension with the next smallest value, and continuing until each new point is the center of a new rectangle. Division of an initial 2D rectangle with center $(\frac{1}{2}, \frac{1}{2})$ is shown in Fig. 1(a). Here, the initial normalized 2D rectangle is divided first along the y-axis, which is the side containing the smallest function value, $f(\frac{1}{2}, \frac{1}{2} - \frac{1}{3}) = 0.4$, and next along the x-axis, which is the side having the second smallest value, $f(\frac{1}{2} - \frac{1}{3}, \frac{1}{2}) = 0.8$.

A locally-biased form of the DIRECT algorithm has been developed for low-dimensional problems with few local minima [12]. The rectangles are grouped by the l_∞ norm, or maximum side length, given by: $d(l,p) = 3^{-l}$.

At each iteration, the number of function evaluations is $2n\times$ the number of points on the convex hull, and these can be performed in parallel. Several strategies exist, from simple master-slave models to load-balancing strategies [13]. The theoretical behavior of DIRECT has been explored, [8,12], and the algorithm has been adapted to engineering problems [12], and for local optimization in image registration [4]. Full descriptions of DIRECT are found in [8,12,13].

3   Multidirectional Search (MDS)

Like the Nelder-Mead method, MDS utilizes a simplex consisting of $n+1$ n-D vertices. A new simplex is generated at each iteration based on the current best point $\mathbf{x}_0$, i.e., the point attaining the lowest function value in the simplex. Initial vertices are usually chosen as $[\mathbf{I}_n - \mathbf{1}_{n\times1}]$ [9], where $\mathbf{I}_n$ is the $n \times n$ identity matrix, and $-\mathbf{1}_{n\times1}$ is a column vector of n -1's. The simplex changes by reflection, expansion, or contraction, as shown in Fig. 1 (b). In each iteration, the simplex is reflected and the new vertices are evaluated. If a new best vertex has been identified, an expansion step is computed. Otherwise, a contraction step is performed, and the new vertices are accepted. MDS has an outer loop that determines a new set of search directions by considering the best vertex, and an inner loop that determines the length of the steps to be taken [9]. These step lengths are determined by an expansion factor $\mu > 1$ and a contraction factor $\theta \in (0,1)$. MDS is a descent method, since for each iteration k, $f\left(\mathbf{x}_0^k\right) \leq f\left(\mathbf{x}_0^{k+1}\right)$. Furthermore, the simplex angles do not change, and thus, unlike the Nelder-Mead simplex, the search directions are guaranteed to be linearly independent. A full description of the MDS algorithm and its convergence properties is found in [9].

If P processors are available, then each CPU could evaluate about $3n/P$ vertices in parallel. However, if $P \geq 3n$, then each rotation, contraction, and expansion can be computed simultaneously, in a speculative manner[14].

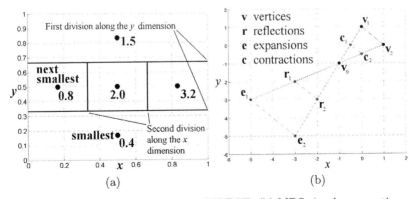

Fig. 1. (a) Division of rectangles in DIRECT. (b) MDS simplex operations.

4   Methods

Multiresolution rigid-body ($n = 6$) registration of 3D to 3D medical images was performed with global DIRECT (GD); locally-biased DIRECT (LD); GD at low resolution and LD at full resolution (GLD); MDS with $\mu = 2.0$ and $\theta = 0.5$; and Powell's (serial) method (P). Similarity metrics were mutual information (MI), normalized mutual information (NMI), entropy correlation coefficient (ECC), the correlation ratio (CR), and CR/NMI (CR at low and NMI at high resolutions). For MI, NMI, and ECC, histograms computed with trilinear partial volume interpolation [2] and 64 bins were found to give the best results.

The data were (Fig. 2): (1) Source volume: Simulated PD MRI brain volume (BrainWeb, Montreal Neurological Institute [15]) with multiple sclerosis lesions and 3% noise, with $181 \times 217 \times 35$ voxels, each voxel of size 1.0 mm^3. Target: Simulated normal T1 MRI volume with 9% noise $181 \times 217 \times 181$ 1 mm^3 voxels. (2) Same as (1), but with 9% noise in the source volume. (3) Source and target: porcine heart CT volumes, $143 \times 195 \times 168$ voxels of size 0.63 mm^3. The source and target were imaged with different CT parameters so that the target had very low contrast relative to the source. For all data, ground truth orientations were known. The source volumes were initially misregistered at random directions and with distances (d_0) of 5mm, 10mm, and 20mm from the target, and misrotated at $\pm10°$ about all three axes ($\pm30°$ for the heart volumes). For each d_0, 24 experiments were run. Convergence criteria were (1) a maximum budget of 2000 function evaluations, or (2) a tolerance of 0.005 between the best function values, or (3) for DIRECT, there are more than five iterations where the improved $\mathbf{x}$ is less than 0.1 mm and 0.01° from the previous best $\mathbf{x}$, with a tolerance of 0.005.

Performance was judged on: (1) The success rate (less than 2mm translation error and a maximum rotation error of $\pm2°$), (2) Translation and rotation accuracy for satisfactory registrations, and (3) Computation time. All experiments were run on a gigabit ethernet cluster of 900 MHz CPUs, each with 1 GB of memory, with MPI using MPICH libraries (www.mcs.anl.gov/mpi/mpich/).

5   Results

The success rates for the three volumes are shown in Table 1. The mean computation time and the ratio of computation time to number of similarity metric evaluations (T/E ratio) for the MRI registration trials are shown in Fig. 3, and in Fig. 4 for the CT heart trials. The mean translation and rotation errors, with minimum and maximum error values, are shown in Fig. 5. For the brain volumes, the DIRECT algorithms, especially LD, had the highest success rate. GD, GLD, and LD also outperformed MDS and P for $d_0 = 20$mm. MDS was successful for $d_0 = 5$mm and 10mm, but failed for $d_0 = 20$mm. GD, GLD, LD, and P performed best for MI, NMI, ECC, and CR/NMI (especially NMI), but MDS was most successful with MI. For the CT heart volumes, MDS had a low success rate (highest with MI). GD, GLD, LD, and P were successful for $d_0 = 5$mm and 10mm (with P the overall best for 10mm), but, as with the brain volumes, for $d_0 = 20$mm, the DIRECT methods had a high success rate while both P

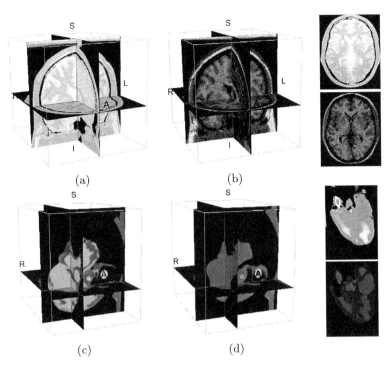

Fig. 2. (a) PD MRI brain, 3% noise. (b) T1 MRI brain, 9% noise. (c) Source CT heart volume. (d) Target CT heart volume.

and MDS performed poorly. All methods were accurate, with mean translation and rotation errors less than 1.5 mm and 2°, respectively. The parallel methods scaled well, with an almost linear decrease in time from 4 to 8 processors (DIRECT), and from 6 to 12 processors (MDS). The effect of similarity metric on timings was minimal. For "speculative" MDS, there was marginal improvement with $3n = 18$ CPUs. For the MR brain data, the mean computation time for Powell's method was 70.81, 138.22, 116.80, 72.79, and 86.90 sec. for NMI, MI, ECC, CR, and CR/NMI, respectively, and for the CT heart data, 217.3, 338.62, 339.44, 318.00 sec. for NMI, MI, ECC, CR, and CR/NMI, respectively, which were much higher than for DIRECT and MDS (except for LD with 4 CPUs). The T/E ratio was also generally higher with P. DIRECT has high overhead (rectangle division, finding the convex hull, etc.). Thus, T/E for these methods was high for 4 CPUs. MDS has low overhead, and had the best T/E for all trials.

6   Discussion and Conclusions

In this paper, optimization with parallel similarity metric computations was presented. These methods were applied to linear registration, an important global step prior to nonlinear matching. Many nonlinear methods compute deformation vectors from small blocks of voxels at different resolutions which are matched linearly [16], and therefore can also benefit from improved optimization.

Table 1. Ratio of successful registrations. (1) Brain MRI, PD-T1; MS lesions, 3% noise. (2) Brain MRI, PD-T1, MS lesions, 9% noise. (3) Heart CT.

Volume	Metric	5 mm					10 mm					20 mm				
		P	GD	GLD	LD	MDS	P	GD	GLD	LD	MDS	P	GD	GLD	LD	MDS
(1)	NMI	1.00	1.00	1.00	1.00	0.79	0.92	0.92	0.92	1.00	0.38	0.29	0.71	0.75	0.88	0.00
	MI	1.00	1.00	1.00	1.00	1.00	1.00	0.46	0.46	0.54	1.00	0.54	0.33	0.38	0.38	0.08
	ECC	1.00	1.00	1.00	1.00	1.00	1.00	0.54	0.54	0.54	1.00	0.29	0.33	0.42	0.38	0.12
	CR	1.00	0.88	0.92	0.96	1.00	1.00	0.29	0.38	0.38	0.83	0.25	0.21	0.21	0.29	0.00
	CR/NMI	1.00	0.96	0.92	0.96	1.00	1.00	0.33	0.38	0.71	0.75	0.17	0.29	0.21	0.67	0.00
(2)	NMI	1.00	1.00	1.00	1.00	0.12	1.00	0.71	0.62	0.83	0.12	0.08	0.75	0.71	0.88	0.00
	MI	1.00	1.00	1.00	1.00	1.00	1.00	0.58	0.46	0.58	0.88	0.17	0.29	0.42	0.38	0.00
	ECC	1.00	1.00	1.00	1.00	1.00	1.00	0.50	0.46	0.54	0.83	0.25	0.29	0.42	0.33	0.04
	CR	1.00	0.92	1.00	1.00	1.00	1.00	0.33	0.38	0.54	0.88	0.21	0.21	0.33	0.29	0.00
	CR/NMI	1.00	0.96	1.00	1.00	1.00	0.96	0.46	0.46	0.71	0.75	0.17	0.29	0.38	0.54	0.00
(3)	NMI	0.97	0.97	1.00	1.00	0.53	0.94	0.81	0.81	0.91	0.31	0.94	0.97	0.94	0.94	0.19
	MI	0.62	0.72	0.69	0.72	0.66	0.50	0.59	0.62	0.72	0.66	0.62	0.75	0.75	0.81	0.47
	CR/NMI	0.50	0.94	0.78	0.88	0.66	0.56	0.84	0.66	0.88	0.59	0.47	0.94	0.75	0.91	0.34

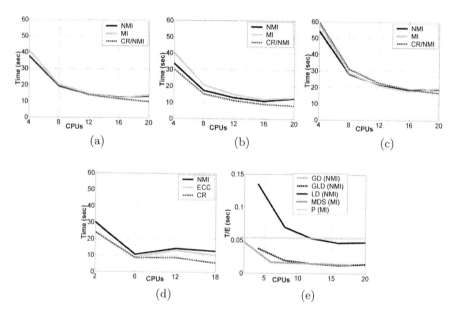

Fig. 3. Registration of brain volumes. Computation time for (a) GD (b) GLD (c) LD (d) MDS (e) Time per similarity metric evaluation.

Although Powell's method is robust and accurate, DIRECT and MDS easily exploit parallelism. DIRECT, especially LD, is also more robust for greater initial misregistrations (20mm). As a local method, MDS works well only for small capture ranges. Thus, MDS may be used as a local, high resolution search step after global optimization with DIRECT. DIRECT and MDS were also robust with respect to noise (e.g. 9% noise in the T1 MRI volume).

Because of the coarse granularity, the parallel methods scaled well. Function computation times are mostly consistent, and load balancing [13] is not expected to greatly increase speed. At least 8 CPUs for the DIRECT methods, and at

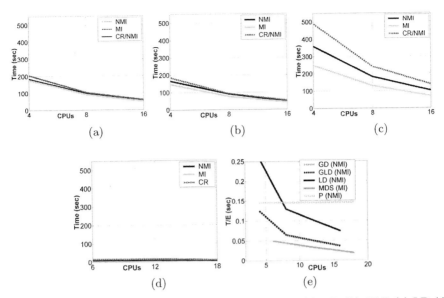

Fig. 4. Heart volume registration. Computation time for (a) GD (b) GLD (c) LD (d) MDS (efficient, but very low success rate) (e) Time per similarity metric evaluation.

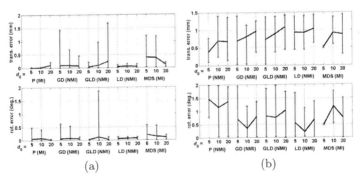

Fig. 5. Mean translation and rotation errors. (a) Brain volumes. (b) Heart volume.

least 12 for MDS, are required for speedup. Faster processors (> 2 GHz), shared memory, and optimized numerical libraries can also improve speed.

The robustness of DIRECT (and MDS for small capture ranges) and their scalability suggest that these methods should be considered as an alternative to Powell's method when many CPUs are available. However, on single or dual processor machines, the overhead in the DIRECT methods is prohibitive, and standard approaches should be used. The success of DIRECT and MDS for image registration merits further research into other non-stochastic parallel optimization approaches [17]. Future work includes implementation of these methods on shared-memory architectures, and on parallel methods in which other time consuming steps (resampling, joint histogram estimation) can also be parallelized.

Acknowledgments. The authors thank Hua Qian for heart CT data, Baolai Ge for technical assistance, Renata Smolíková-Wachowiak for helpful discussions, and the anonymous reviewers for constructive suggestions. This work was supported by SHARCNet, NSERC R3146-A02, CIHR 14735, and ORDCF.

References

1. Maes, F., Vandermeulen, D., Suetens, P: Comparative evaluation of multiresolution optimization strategies for multimodality image registration by maximization of mutual information Med. Image Anal. **3** (1999) 373–386.
2. Pluim, J. P. W., Maintz, J. B. A., Viergever, M. A.: Mutual-information-based registration of medical images: a survey. IEEE T. Med. Imag. **22** (2003) 986–1004.
3. Kolda, T. G., Lewis, R. M., Torczon, V.: Optimization by direct search: new perspectives on some classical and modern methods. SIAM Rev. **45** (2003) 385–482.
4. He, R., Narayana, P. A.: Global optimization of mutual information: application to three–dimensional retrospective registration of magnetic resonance images. Comput. Med. Imag. Graph. **26** (2002) 277-292.
5. Jenkinson, M., Smith, S.: A global optimization method for robust affine registration of brain images. Med. Image. Anal. **5** (2001) 143–156.
6. Matsopoulos, G. K., Mouravliansky, N. A., Delibasis, K. K., Nikita, K. S.: Automatic retinal image registration scheme using global optimization techniques. IEEE T. Inf. Technol. B. **3** (1999) 47–60.
7. Wachowiak, M. P., Smolíková, R., Peters, T. M.: Multiresolution biomedical image registration using generalized information measures. Proc. MICCAI 2003, LNCS 2879, Ellis, R. E., Peters, T. M., Eds., (2003) 846–853.
8. Jones, D. R., Perttunen, C. D., Stuckman, B. E.: Lipschitzian optimization without the Lipschitz constant. J. Optimiz. Theory App. **79** (1993) 157–181.
9. Torczon, V.: On the convergence of the multidirectional search algorithm. SIAM J. Optimiz. **1** (1991) 123–145.
10. Warfield, S. K., Jolesz, F. A., Kikinis, R: A high performance computing approach to the registration of medical imaging data. Parallel Comput. **24** (1998) 1345–1368.
11. Ourselin, S., Stefanescu, R., Pennec, X.: Robust registration of multi–modal images: Towards real-time clinical applications. Proc. MICCAI 2002, LNCS 2489, Dohi, T. and Kikinis, R. (Eds.) (2002) 140–147.
12. Gablonsky, J. M., Kelley, C. T.: A locally–biased form of the DIRECT algorithm. J. Global Optim. **21** (2001) 27–37.
13. Watson, L. T., Baker, C. A.: A fully-distributed parallel global search algorithm. Engineering Computation **18** (2001) 155-169.
14. Dennis, J. E., Torczon, V.: Direct search methods on parallel machines. SIAM J. Optimiz. **1** (1991) 448–474.
15. Kwan, R. K. , Evans, A. C., Pike, G. B.: MRI simulation-based evaluation of image processing and classification methods. IEEE T. Med. Imag. **18** (1999) 1085–1097.
16. Wierzbicki, M., Peters, T. M.: Determining epicardial surface motion using elastic registration. Proc. MICCAI 2003, LNCS 2878, Ellis, R. E., Peters, T. M., Eds., (2003) 722–729.
17. García-Palomares, U., Rodríguez, J.: New sequential and parallel derivative-free algorithms for unconstrained minimization. SIAM J. Optimiz. **13** (2002) 79–96.

Non-rigid Multimodal Image Registration Using Local Phase

Matthew Mellor* and Michael Brady

Medical Vision Laboratory, University of Oxford, UK
{matt,jmb}@robots.ox.ac.uk

Abstract. Non-rigid registration of multimodal images is a challenging problem. One approach, maximization of mutual information, has been shown to be effective for registering certain image modalities and is currently considered the standard against which all other techniques are measured. In this paper, we propose an alternative representation of an image based on local phases rather than intensities; we then show how mutual information can be extended to this representation. Local phase acts as a description of local image structure, enabling mutual phase information to detect complex image relationships that are hard or impossible to detect using mutual intensity information. Typical results are presented, comparing the performance of phase and intensity mutual information methods on simulated MR and ultrasound images.

1 Introduction

This paper illustrates the effectiveness of a representation of an image, based on local phase, which significantly enhances non-rigid registration of a wide variety of multimodal images. Since it has become the reference against which other measures and non-rigid registration algorithms are judged, the experiments in this paper use mutual information (MI) of local phases to maximise a *structural* relationship between images. It should be understood from the outset, however, that the statistical behaviour of phase is highly predictable and so it is theoretically possible to design multimodal non-rigid registration algorithms which employ substantially more prior information than is available to conventional intensity-based mutual information methods. Several methods for non-rigid registration of images based on mutual information of intensities have been introduced [1,2, 3]. These methods use the global intensity statistics to inform local alterations to the registration. Regardless of the specific method used, these methods are only able to register images for which the global intensity statistics are an accurate reflection of the local statistics. Unfortunately, but significantly, this is manifestly not the case for many modalities, potentially including some of those for which rigid registration using MI has been asserted to be feasible.

---

* Matthew Mellor is funded by the EPRSC as part of the MIAS-IRC. (GR/N14248)

C. Barillot, D.R. Haynor, and P. Hellier (Eds.): MICCAI 2004, LNCS 3216, pp. 789–796, 2004.

2   Local Phase and Energy

Local phase is a qualitative description of the shape of an image location. It may be thought of as an amplitude-weighted average phase of the (windowed) Fourier components at each point in the signal. At a locally anti-symmetric point in the signal, the Fourier components are also predominantly anti-symmetric (i.e. sine functions), whereas at locally symmetric, points they are predominantly symmetric (cosine functions). The local phase is often considered in conjunction with a second quantity, called the local energy. Local energy can be thought of as the combined energy, after interference, of the Fourier components and acts as a measure of local signal activity. Local phase has a number of important properties which make it a natural choice for image registration. First, the local variation of the phase is well approximated by the phase gradient, which has been shown to increase the accuracy of matching algorithms [4]. Second, the marginal distributions, the treatment of which distinguishes the various information theoretic methods (mutual information, joint entropy, normalised mutual information etc) are highly predictable for phase. Figure 1 shows typical intensity and phase distributions for an MR-T1 image. Whereas the phase statistics are relatively flat, the intensity statistics clearly show the presence of several different classes. In general, an intensity only has meaning when interpreted in the context of other pixels in the image. In contrast, phase is a fundamental property, requiring no context for interpretation and this is reflected in the marginal. From the perspective of mutual information, it may be argued that a phase marginal contains limited information, relative to a typical intensity marginal.

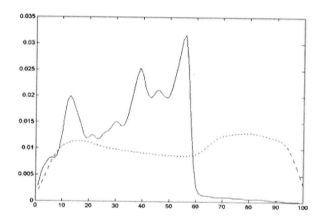

Fig. 1. Typical marginal distributions of an MR-T1 image: intensity (solid) is complex, while phase (dotted) is relatively flat

There is more than one way to extend the notion of phase to two dimensions. One possibility is to estimate the phase of the one dimensional signal in the direction of maximal local energy using steerable filters. For the results presented here, the local phase and energy have been estimated using the monogenic signal, described below. This choice was made in part for reasons of computational speed and simplicity, in part for mathematical elegance. However, in principle, there is no reason why the results presented here are particular to a method of phase estimation.

The monogenic signal [5] is a multi-dimensional extension to the analytic signal, which consists, at each image location, of three quantities: local energy, local phase, and local orientation. Space does not permit a detailed discussion of local energy and orientation, which can be found in [6]

The monogenic signal may be computed from the output of three filters. First, a rotationally symmetric, zero-mean filter is applied to the image, to give a bandpass image I_b: this constitutes the even component of the signal. The odd component is composed of the response of two anti-symmetric filters to the even part. These two filters, h_1 and h_2, are described in the Fourier domain by:

$$H_1(u, v) = \frac{u}{\sqrt{u^2 + v^2}}, H_2(u, v) = \frac{v}{\sqrt{u^2 + v^2}} \quad (1)$$

where u, v are the Fourier domain coordinates. Local phase, ϕ and local energy, E, can then be calculated from these filter responses and the bandpass image I_b as follows:

$$\phi(x, y) = \tan^{-1}\left(\frac{I_b}{\sqrt{(h_1 \otimes I_b)^2 + (h_2 \otimes I_b)^2}}\right) \quad (2)$$

$$E(x, y) = \sqrt{I_b^2 + (h_1 \otimes I)^2 + (h_2 \otimes I_b)^2} \quad (3)$$

$$(4)$$

3   Filter Choice

The measures of phase estimated using the method described above depend on the particular filters used to derive the bandpass image I_b. Criteria for the choice of bandpass filters for 1D signals have been studied extensively. However, the behaviour of a two dimensional filter to a two dimensional signal is more complex than the one dimensional case. For example, when a filter, such as a difference of Gaussians, is applied to a curved image structure, the blurring causes the phase contours to migrate from the feature towards the inside of the curve. This causes a problem for registration, since blurring by such filters is not affine invariant; this makes it difficult to predict phase after a local affine transform. To avoid this, we have developed filters which exhibit very little blurring:

$$f(r) = \frac{A}{r^{\alpha+\beta}} - \frac{B}{r^{\alpha-\beta}} \quad (5)$$

where r is the distance from the centre of the filter, α is a design parameter and β is a second parameter, which must be very small compared to α to avoid blurring. A and B are chosen to give zero mean and an appropriate amplitude.

The value of the filter is infinite for $r = 0$. To avoid having an infinite central value, the discrete versions of the filter must be calculated with the average of r over the pixel rather than the central value. For a more detailed discussion of these filters and their use see [6].

4   Algorithm

The results presented here are based on a method derived from that of Crum [2]. The algorithm deforms one image, the source, to match the second image, the target. At each iteration, the present estimate of the registration is applied to the source image and its local phase and energy are estimated using the monogenic signal, and using five different members of the filter family described in the previous section. These five filters are defined by $\alpha = [2.75, 3.25, 3.75, 4.25, 4.75]$ and $\beta = 0.25$ in each case. The joint distribution of the source image phases and target images phases for each filter is estimated. This proceeds by histogram binning with 100 bins per phase, followed by smoothing with a Gaussian of width $\sigma = 7$ bins. Only phase values with an energy greater than 5% of the maximum are binned, to reduce the effects of noise. Although the resolution of the joint distributions is quite low, because of the relatively small number of pixels typically available in 2D images, any increase in resolution decreased robustness. We anticipate that this effect will be less severe for 3D images. Once the joint distribution has been estimated, the mutual information forces are computed according to equation 6, for each of the phase images estimated with the five bandpass filters as follows:

$$F(x) = K(\log[P(\phi_1(x+1), \phi_2(x))/P(\phi_1(x+1))] - \log[P(\phi_1(x-1), \phi_2(x)/P(\phi_1(x-1))]) \tag{6}$$

where $\phi_1(x)$ is the local phase at position x in the source image, K is the timestep, and $\phi_2(x)$ is the phase in the target image. To regularise, the displacement field is convolved with a Gaussian ($\sigma = 4$) at each iteration.

For the purposes of comparing phase and intensity methods fairly, an intensity algorithm was designed, similar in as many respects as possible to the phase algorithm. The intensity is used directly, with no phase estimation. The time-step for each algorithm has been hand optimised such that both methods converge at, as near as possible, the same rate.

5   Results

The phase and intensity algorithms described above were applied to sets of synthetically generated two dimensional images. The first set consists of one MR-T2 image and thirty MR-T1 images to which were applied randomly generated warps. The second set consists of the same thirty MR-T1 images, but with the addition of a slowly varying, randomly generated, multiplicative bias field. The third set consists of thirty simulated ultrasound images. These were generated by using the randomly warped MR-T1 images as the scatter density field in a simple ultrasound simulation algorithm.

5.1   MR-T1 to MR-T2 Registration

The synthetic images from which the image pairs are generated were taken from the Brainweb simulated brain database [7]. Thirty deformed T1 images were generated by applying random warps to the original T1 image. The x and y components of the warps were each generated by convolving an IID normally distributed displacement field with a Gaussian of width $\sigma = 12$ pixels. The resulting warps were normalised such that the r.m.s displacement was three pixels. An example warped T1 image is shown in figure 2.

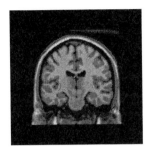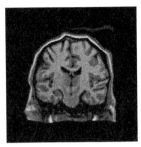

Fig. 2. T1-MR image before (left) and after (right) application of a randomly generated non-rigid deformation

Since the deformations are created using the same smoothing method as the regulariser, they should be very compatible with the registration algorithms: any failure should be due to the similarity measure and/or minimisation strategy, not the inability of the regulariser to produce the true deformation.

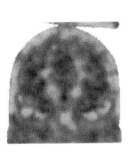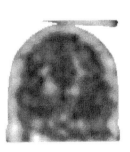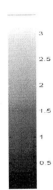

Fig. 3. mean displacement errors in pixels after registration with intensity (left) and phase (right)

The average performance of the two algorithms on the first synthetic data set is illustrated in figure 3. Both methods perform well on the brain, achieving sub-

Table 1. Average registration errors in pixels for the phase and intensity methods

		Phase	error	Intensity	error
		average	S.D.	average	S.D.
Brain & Skull	r.m.s	1.81	0.13	1.63	0.12
	mean	1.41	0.08	1.34	0.08
Brain Alone	r.m.s	1.39	0.15	1.45	0.13
	mean	1.11	0.11	1.21	0.09

Table 2. Average registration errors in pixels for both methods with bias field

		Phase	error	Intensity	error
		average	S.D.	average	S.D.
Brain & Skull	r.m.s	1.86	0.13	1.76	0.13
	mean	1.46	0.08	1.45	0.09
Brain Alone	r.m.s	1.42	0.15	1.66	0.13
	mean	1.14	0.11	1.38	0.12

pixel accuracy for a significant proportion, with the phase method performing better on average. The likely reason for this is the greater accuracy of linear interpolation for phase values [4]. In the region of the skull however, the intensity method outperforms phase. Since structures that are parallel in both images will create a mode in the phase joint histogram, it is difficult for phase based method to register them correctly, and this is the likely reason for the error in the skull region. The exact values for the average registration quality are given in table 1. The effects of bias field on the two registration schemes was assessed by introducing a synthetic bias field into the data set. The bias fields, like the deformations, were computed by convolving a Gaussian with a random field. Each bias field was scaled and shifted so that it had a mean of 1 and variation ± 0.2 and was then applied to one of the warped images of the previous data set by pixelwise multiplication. The experiment was then repeated on the bias corrupted images. Table 2 shows the overall performance of the two algorithms in the presence of bias field. A reduction in the performance of both algorithms is apparent. The phase method, however, is significantly less affected: the increase in mean error within the brain is only 3% for the phase method, while the mean error of the intensity method increases by 14%.

5.2 Ultrasound to MR Registration

The previous examples all involve images that are related by an intensity mapping. Phase mutual information algorithms are also able to register classes of images for which this is not the case. As a practically important example of this, a set of ultrasound (US) images were simulated from deformed MR-T1 images. The T1 intensity was used to determine tissue scatter density and the intensity gradient of the T1 image was used to determine ultrasound reflectivity. These were then used to generate US-like images. Since they are generated from deformed T1 images the registration between the US images and the generating

MR images is known. An example of a simulated US image is shown in figure 4. For more details of the model of US images and registration of US images see [6].

As for the previous two experiments, a set of thirty randomly deformed ultrasound images was generated. The two algorithms were then applied with very little alteration. The phase method had to be altered slightly to ignore phase estimate too close to the edge of the US image, since the phase at these points is dominated by the image edge rather than the image contents. The only other alteration was a re-optimisation of the time step for both algorithms and an increase in the width of the regularisation Gaussian.

Figure 5 shows the distribution of registration error for the phase and intensity methods applied to the synthetic ultrasound images. In both cases, the influence of the ventricles on the registration is clearly visible. In the case of intensity MI, the improvement is limited to the area within the ventricles, while the phase MI method correctly registers some of the tissue outside the ventricles. The probable reason for this is that intensity MI is unable to deal effectively with the reflections from the ventricle walls. Since the reflections are bright they appear more likely to belong to the outside of the ventricles than the inside, which biases the intensity algorithm in favor of enlarging the ventricles. The phase algorithm is able to interpret the reflections as the superpostion of an edge and a ridge and learn the correct relationship between this compound feature and the edge in the MR image.

6   Discussion

In this paper, we have described the initial development of a non-rigid registration algorithm based on local phase. To facilitate comparison with current techniques, we have analysed the extension of mutual information to use local phase. The primary motivation for this is to enable registration of certain classes of images for which intensity MI is unsuccessful. The ultrasound example (figure 5) shows that it succeeds to some extent in this.

This is not fortuitous, phase has intrinsic advantages over intensity, even for images which are well suited to registration with intensity MI. In particular,

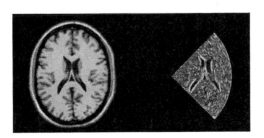

Fig. 4. An MR-T1 image and simulated (and deformed) ultrasound image

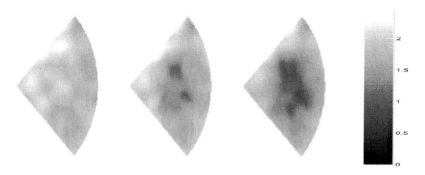

Fig. 5. Average registration error distribution for the synthetic ultrasound images (in pixels widths) prior to registration (left), after registration with intensity MI(centre) and after registration with phase MI (right)

the low information content of its marginal distribution greatly reduces the significance of the particular choice of information measure. It is also possible to make strong assumptions about the joint distributions of phase [6]; exploiting this prior knowledge in the registration scheme is a goal of our future research.

References

1. D. Rueckert; C. Hayes; C. Studholme; P. Summers; M. Leach; D.J. Hawkes. Non-rigid registration of breast MR images using mutual information. *Proc. MICCAI*, 1998.
2. W. Crum; D.L.G. Hill; D.J. Hawkes. Information theoretic similarity measures in non-rigid registration. *Proc. IPME*, 2003.
3. J.B.A. Maintz; E.H.W. Meijering; M.A. Viergever. General multimodal elastic registration based on mutual information. *Medical Imaging*, (3338):144–154, 1998.
4. D.J. Fleet. Disparity from local weighted phase-correlation. *IEEE International Conference on SMC*, pages 48–56, October 1994.
5. M. Felsberg; G. Sommer. A new extension of linear signal processing for estimating local properties and detecting features. *Proc. DAGM*, 2000.
6. Matthew Mellor. Phase methods for non-rigid medical image registration. *D.Phil Thesis, Oxford University*, 2004.
7. Brainweb: Simulated brain database. *http://www.bic.mni.mcgill.ca/brainweb/*.

Multi-channel Mutual Information Using Scale Space

Mark Holden[1], Lewis D. Griffin[1], Nadeem Saeed[2], and Derek L.G. Hill[1]

[1] CISG, Imaging Sciences, GKT School of Medicine, Guy's Hospital, King's College
London, UK
mark.holden@kcl.ac.uk
[2] GlaxoSmithKline, MRI Unit, The Frythe, Welwyn, UK

Abstract. We propose a new voxel similarity measure which utilises local image structure and intensity information. Gaussian scale space derivatives provide the structural information. Each derivative is assigned an information channel of N-D normalised mutual information. We illustrate the behaviour of the measure for a simulated signal and 2D medical brain images and demonstrate its potential for non-rigid, inter-subject registration of 3D thorax MR images as a proof of concept.

1 Introduction

Voxel intensity based image similarity measures, particularly mutual information, perform well for intramodality [1] and intermodality [2] rigid-body registration. However, non-rigid registration is a more difficult problem because the deformations that need to be recovered can be localised and have high frequency content which requires a high dimensional spatial transformation. As the dimensionality of the transformation increases so does the the likelihood of false optima of the similarity measure. Transformations with local support provide a useful model of tissue deformation, but as the dimensionality increases the number of voxels in the support region decreases which leads to a reduction in local information available for measuring similarity. False or local optima lead to ill-conditioning of the registration function which increases the possibility of a registration algorithm getting trapped in a local optima. There are approaches to reduce the likelihood of this by including additional constraints derived from modelling the physical tissue deformation or by regularising the transformation to reduce its dimensionality. The physical modelling approach has the disadvantage of requiring a labelled tissue model and the mechanical properties of the tissue which could vary between individuals and over time, for instance during disease progression or regression. Regularisation can restrict the solution space of transformations to satisfy certain mathematical constraints. This is definitely advantageous so long as the transformation adequately models the physical deformation. However, it cannot prevent the algorithm getting trapped in local optima. Here we investigate an approach aimed at improving the similarity measure by incorporating additional local structural image information.

C. Barillot, D.R. Haynor, and P. Hellier (Eds.): MICCAI 2004, LNCS 3216, pp. 797–804, 2004.

Related Work

Shen et al. [3] have designed a similarity measure that determines image similarity based on a attribute vector for each voxel at GM, WM and CSF interfaces. The attribute vector is derived from the voxel's edge type and geometric moment invariants calculated from voxel intensities in a spherical neighbourhood. This similarity measure is specifically designed for intra-modal, inter-subject MR brain image registration and requires a GM, WM and CSF segmentation.

In contrast, we aim for a general purpose registration algorithm that can be applied to intermodality data direct from the scanner without a pre-processing step. We start by establishing a set of desirable properties of the similarity measure and use these to devise a mutual information measure that utilises more structural image information than simple intensities. In this way we can retain the desirable intermodality property of mutual information. We use the derivatives of the Gaussian scale space expansion of the image to provide this local information. To assess the performance of the measure we present some simulations and results of inter-subject intramodality registration experiments.

2   Problem Analysis

Properties of Non-rigid Registration Similarity Measures

We require metrics that: (a) are suitable for intermodality data; (b) are translation and rotation invariant (invariance to non-rigid motion might also be desirable); (c) return values that are a smooth decreasing function of misregistration.

A problem often encountered in non-rigid registration arises when non-corresponding parts of the anatomy have similar MR signal intensities. When these regions overlap, voxel intensity based similarity measures can give a local optima (c.f. non-corresponding gyri [3]. Some authors have address this using additional information Cachier et al. [4]. To avoid this additional spatial information is required. Shen et al. [3] used geometrically invariant moments, Pluim [5] used intensity and first derivative, Butz [6] used a feature space. We want to use local image structure to provide this information. Ideally, we would like a small set of measures that unambiguously characterise each image voxel. To facilitate optimisation we desire measures that can be used in multi-resolution search, c.f. rigid-body registration [2].

Incorporating Local Image Structure in Mutual Information

Consider the Taylor series expansion of a 3D function $f(x, y, z)$ about (a, b, c):

$$f(x, y, z) = \sum_{l=0}^{\infty} \sum_{m=0}^{\infty} \sum_{n=0}^{\infty} \{\frac{\partial^{lmn} f(x, y, z)}{\partial x^l \partial x^m \partial x^n}\}_{a,b,c} \frac{(x - a)^l}{l!} \frac{(y - b)^m}{m!} \frac{(z - c)^n}{n!} \quad (1)$$

This equation describes how a continuous function $f(x, y, z)$ can be expanded in terms of its derivatives at (a, b, c). Since we are interested in discrete images we instead propose to use the analogous Gaussian scale space expansion [7].

$$I(x,y,z) = I_0(x,y,z,\sigma) + \sum_{i=x,y,z,\sigma} C_i I_i + \sum_{i,j=x,y,z,\sigma} C_{ij} I_{ij} + \dots \qquad (2)$$

Where I_0 denotes the image convolved with a Gaussian of standard deviation σ and $I_{ij}(x,y,z,\sigma)$ denotes the derivative of I_0 w.r.t. to the three Cartesian directions i,j and scale σ. It has been shown that such a representation maximally captures local image structure. The derivative terms are almost statistically independent. The small amount of dependence is not a problem.

We need a multivariate similarity measure that uses the derivative terms of the scale space expansion of the image. One way to do this is to consider each derivative term (I_{ij}) as a separate information channel. Then we can use multi-dimensional mutual information on the joint event $\{I_{ij}\}$. For two information channels, we get a 4D joint histogram and mutual information of the form:

$$MI(A,B,C,D) = H(A,B) + H(C,D) - H(A,B,C,D) \qquad (3)$$

$$NMI(A,B,C,D) = \frac{H(A,B) + H(C,D)}{H(A,B,C,D)} \qquad (4)$$

Where A, B and C, D refer to derivatives of the target and source respectively.

3   Materials and Methods

3.1   Implementation

Gaussian scale-space: In our experiments we consider only the luminance, first and second order derivative terms of the scale space expansion. These are reasonably invariant to rigid motion. Invariance to non-rigid motion could be achieved by recomputing them each time similarity is measured, however this would increase the computational overhead. The luminance image $I_0(\mathbf{x})$ is generated by convolving the image $I(\mathbf{x})$ with a Gaussian kernel $G(\mathbf{x})$ viz: $I_0(\mathbf{x}) = G(\mathbf{x}) \odot I(\mathbf{x})$ where $G(\mathbf{x}) = \frac{1}{2\pi\sigma^2}\exp(-|\mathbf{x}|^2/2\sigma^2)$. The gradient magnitude image $I_1(\mathbf{x}) = |\nabla(I_0)|$ and the Laplacian image $I_2(\mathbf{x}) = \nabla^2(I_0)$. In the experimental work we refer to these as luminance, GMOG (gradient magnitude of luminance) and LOG (Laplacian of luminance). The intensity of the LOG image was normalised by subtracting the minimum so that its minimum is zero. To avoid truncation during convolution, the image was reflected about each boundary by half the kernel width. Gaussian convolution and differentiation (central derivative) were implemented in matlab (Mathworks Inc, MA, USA) for 1D signals and 2D images and in C++ using vtk (Kitware, NY, USA) classes for 3D images. In all instances, the kernel radius was chosen to be three times larger than the standard deviation to avoid truncation effects.

Multi-dimensional mutual information: A major difficulty with this is that the dimensionality of the joint histogram array depends on the number of derivative terms (n). The array size grows as a power of n. This can lead to a sparsely populated array, also the memory required and access time grow as a power of n. Reducing the number of bins can help, but this only results in a linear reduction of size.

Image interpolation is generally the most computationally intensive part of voxel-based algorithms and grows linearly with n. A possible way of reducing the overhead could be to down-sample images. For 3D images, down-sampling by a factor of 2 reduces the number of voxels that need to be interpolated by a factor $2^3 = 8$. In summary, this approach seems viable for small n with down-sampling.

All similarity measures were implemented in both matlab (1D and 2D) and also in C++ for 3D images. For the non-rigid registration of 3D images a segmentation propagation algorithm based on method described in [8] and the 4D similarity measures were implemented in C++ and vtk by redesigning a number of classes of the CISG registration toolbox [9].

3.2   Simulation: Geometric Scaling of Synthetic Signal

A test signal was constructed by low-pass filtering a signal consisting of two rectangular pulses. We chose to model the imaging system using a unit width Gaussian low pass filter. The luminance, gradient magnitude of luminance GMOG and and Laplacian of luminance LOG signals were generated from the test signal using a Gaussian filter of standard deviation $\sigma = 6$ samples. To assess the behaviour of similarity measures as a function of misregistration (registration function) a copy of the test signal was geometrically scaled relative to the original signal. The similarity of these two signals was measured as a function of the scale factor $(s_x, 1 \leq s_x \leq 3)$, where $s_x = 1$ represents perfect registration.

Figure 2 shows the resulting graph for four similarity measures: standard normalised mutual information (NMI), NMI applied to luminance signal, 4D NMI using luminance and GMOG, 4D NMI using luminance and LOG.

For the standard form, there is a false maximum at $s_x \approx 1.6$ and the function is ill-conditioned for $s_x > 1.6$. Gaussian smoothing helps condition the registration function, but the function is flat around $s_x = 1.9$. For the 4D measures, both are well-conditioned and relatively easy to optimise.

3.3   Experiment: Translational Misregistration of a Brain Sub-image

This experiment was designed to evaluate the behaviour of our proposed similarity measure by taking two 2D images of the same anatomy and misregistering a small sub-image of one relative to the other. The data was acquired by scanning a volunteer's brain with a special T1W 3D gradient echo MR sequence with two interleaved readout lines. This data was reconstructed into two 3D spatial images separated by an interval of TR (a few milli-seconds). Essentially the difference between the two images is noise, but there is also a small difference in motion artefacts due to fast flowing blood. These images can be considered as a registration gold-standard, and the graphs of the registration function tell us how the similarity measure behaves as a function of misregistration for images with a noise difference. We took an axial slice through the lateral ventricles and

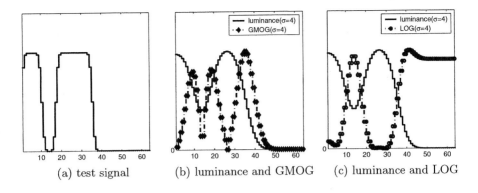

(a) test signal   (b) luminance and GMOG   (c) luminance and LOG

Fig. 1. (a)Test signal used for registration simulation experiments. (b) luminance signal, filtered with a Gaussian ($\sigma = 4$) and gradient magnitude of luminance (GMOG) ($\sigma = 4$). (c) luminance and Laplacian of luminance (LOG) ($\sigma = 4$).

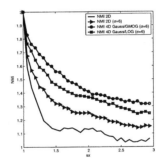

Fig. 2. Normalised mutual information (NMI) as a function of geometric scale change ($s_x, 1 \le s_x \le 3$). Comparison of standard form; standard form with Gaussian blurring $\sigma = 6$; 4D NMI with Gaussian and gradient magnitude of luminance (GMOG) input channels ($\sigma = 6$); 4D NMI with Gaussian and Laplacian of luminance (LOG) input channels ($\sigma = 6$).

extracted a 32×32 pixel sub-image. Then we misregistered the sub image relative to the other image by applying uniform scaling using a scale factor s_x in the range $1 \le s_x \le 3$ where $s_x = 1$ represents perfect registration.

Figure 3 shows the results of the experiment. The standard NMI flattens out for $s_x > 2$ making it difficult to optimise. For $\sigma = 1$ voxel (Figure 3 (a)), there is little difference between the other measures performance. However, for $\sigma = 8$ voxels there is a large difference. Standard 2D NMI applied to the luminance image has an optima around ($s_x = 1.8$) and is flat for ($s_x > 2.5$) whereas the 4D NMI measure based on the luminance and LOG has the least ill-conditioning and widest capture range. This behaviour could be important for multi-resolution optimisation, thought necessary for recovering large deformation.

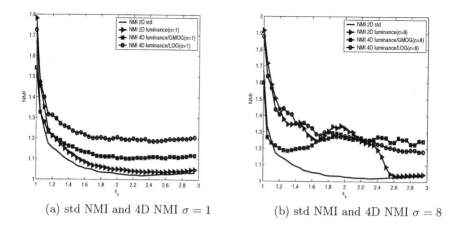

(a) std NMI and 4D NMI $\sigma = 1$ (b) std NMI and 4D NMI $\sigma = 8$

Fig. 3. Plots of the similarity as a function of geometrical scale misregistration of four similarity measures using different amounts of Gaussian blurring. (a) standard NMI (no blurring); standard NMI for Gaussian blurred (luminance) images ($\sigma = 1$); 4D NMI luminance and GMOG ($\sigma = 1$); luminance and LOG ($\sigma = 1$). (b) standard NMI; standard NMI applied to luminance images ($\sigma = 8$); 4D NMI luminance and GMOG ($\sigma = 8$); luminance and LOG ($\sigma = 8$).

3.4 Experiment: Non-rigid Intersubject Registration of the MR Lung

This experiment was designed to evaluate the accuracy of the similarity measures for a realistic 3D non-rigid registration problem involving large deformations. We used T1W 3D gradient echo MR scans of the thorax of seven murine subjects [1]. These images contained 128^3 isotropic voxels of dimension 0.234mm. The chest wall was manually segmented in each image by an expert with knowledge of the anatomy. We assigned one of these images as the atlas and registered this to the six other subjects using the segmentation propagation algorithm. We used the transformations to propagate the atlas segmentation into the space of the six other subjects. Because of the large difference in repositioning and subject size registration was initialised with a manually determined scaling transformation: six rigid-body plus three scale parameters. The registration strategy was based on a rigid-body stage followed by three B-Spline non-rigid stages with control point spacing of 5, 2.5 and 1.25 mm. To evaluate the accuracy of segmentation propagation we compared the propagated lungs with the manually defined segmentation using the overlap similarity index $S = \frac{2N(R1 \cap R2)}{N(R1) + N(R2)}$ as used in [8]. Where are $R1$ and $R2$ are the sets of voxels in the propagated and segmented regions and $N(.)$ refers to the number of voxels in a set. Table 1 shows similar performance of the 4D measure compared to the standard 2D one and indicates a similar accuracy for down-sampled and original resolution images.

---

[1] Animals were housed, maintained and experiments conducted, in accordance with the Home Office Animals (Scientific Procedures) Act 1986, UK.

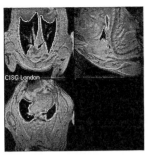 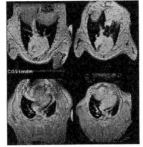 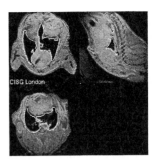

(a) lung segmentation   (b) initial misregistration   (c) resulting propagation

Fig. 4. (a) Manual segmentation of lungs. (b) Example of initial misregistration after manual alignment. (c) Example of a segmentation propagation.

Table 1. Overlap similarity index S after manual alignment (manual) and after rigid-body and non-rigid registration with B-spline control point spacing of 5mm, 2.5mm and 1.25mm. This table compares standard normalised mutual information and the 4D form using luminance and gradient magnitude of luminance GMOG and luminance and Laplacian of luminance (GLOG). The luminance image is created by filtering with Gaussian of $\sigma = 2$ and $\sigma = 4$. The three left hand columns refer to original resolution data and the three right hand ones to images down-sampled by a factor of 2.

target	manual	original resolution			down-sampled		
		NMI2D	GLOG	GMOG	2d	GMOG	GL
		$\sigma = 0$	$\sigma = 2$	$\sigma = 4$		$\sigma = 4$	
subject 1	0.36	0.82	0.76	0.75	0.79	0.72	0.73
subject 2	0.47	0.87	0.80	0.78	0.83	0.71	0.73
subject 3	0.41	0.87	0.81	0.80	0.83	0.74	0.76
subject 4	0.53	0.89	0.88	0.88	0.85	0.72	0.79
subject 5	0.26	0.87	0.86	0.86	0.84	0.78	0.81
subject 6	0.45	0.84	0.81	0.78	0.81	0.76	0.76

4   Discussion and Conclusions

We have established a set of properties of similarity measures for non-rigid inter-modality image registration. We used these to design a novel similarity measure based on Gaussian scale space derivatives. We demonstrated that this has a wider capture range than standard forms for large deformations with synthetically misregistered signals. We showed satisfactory performance for translating a sub-image of 2D brain slices. For non-rigid registration of 3D lung data there is similar performance with the standard measure for inter-subject registration accuracy, as assessed by comparing the overlap of propagations with manual segmentation. The lung images had little contrast between different tissues. This may be a reason why the 4D measure did not perform better than the standard one.

Acknowledgements. We are grateful to GlaxoSmithKline for funding this work.

References

1. M. Holden et al. Voxel similarity measures for 3D serial MR brain image registration. *IEEE Transactions on Medical Imaging*, 19(2):94–102, 2000.
2. C. Studholme, D. L. G. Hill, D. J. Hawkes. Automated 3-D registration of magnetic resonance and positron emission tomography brain images by multiresolution optimization of voxel similarity measures. *Medical Physics*, 24(1):25–35, 1997.
3. Dinggang Shen; Davatzikos, C.; Dinggang Shen; Davatzikos, C. HAMMER: hierarchical attribute matching mechanism for elastic registration. *IEEE Transactions on Medical Imaging*, 21(11):1421–1439, November 2002.
4. P. Cachier et al. Multisubject Non-Rigid Registration of Brain MRI using Intensity and Geometric Features. In *Medical Image Computing and Computer-Assisted Intervention (MICCAI '01)*, pages 734–742, Utrecht, Netherlands, 2001.
5. J. P. W. Pluim et al. Image registration by maximization of combined mutual information and gradient information. *IEEE TMI*, 19(8):809–814, 2000.
6. T. Butz et al. Affine registration with Feature Space Mutual Information. In *MICCAI '01*, pages 549–556, Utrecht, Netherlands, 2001.
7. L.M.J. Florack et al. Cartesian Differential Invariants in Scale-Space. *J. Math. Imaging Vision*, 3(4):327–348, 1993.
8. M. Holden, J. A. Schnabel, D. L. G. Hill. Quantification of small cerebral ventricular volume changes in treated growth hormone patients using non-rigid registration. *IEEE Transactions on Medical Imaging*, 21(10):1292–1301, 2002.
9. T. Hartkens et al. *VTK CISG Registration Toolkit*. CISG, Imaging Sciences, King's College London. http://www.imageregistration.com/.

Registration Using Segment Intensity Remapping and Mutual Information

Zeger F. Knops[1], J.B.A. Maintz[1], M.A. Viergever[1,2], and J.P.W. Pluim[2]

[1] Utrecht University, Department of Computer Science, PO Box 80089, NL-3508TB Utrecht, The Netherlands. {zeger,twan}@cs.uu.nl.
[2] University Medical Center Utrecht, Image Sciences Institute, PO Box 85500, NL-3508GA Utrecht, The Netherlands. {max,josien}@isi.uu.nl.

Abstract. A method for processing images prior to normalized mutual information based registration and an enhancement of the registration measure are presented. The method relies on k-means clustering of the intensity distribution and a gray-value remapping of spatially unconnected segments of similar intensity. Registration experiments using binary images from the MPEG-7 dataset and retinal images show our preprocessing to cause a significant reduction of the number of misregistrations without loss of accuracy or an increase in optimization steps.

1 Introduction

Image registration is a task required in many image processing applications where two or more similar images are involved. To exploit complementary information or express differences these images are often spatially aligned, i.e., registered.

Image content based registration uses the full intensity contents of the image or of a processed image. A measure of registration is defined and the images are assumed to be brought into registration by optimizing this measure. Well established measures include cross-correlation, mutual information and normalized mutual information.

Normalized mutual information (NMI) has proven to be a robust and accurate image registration measure for both mono- and multi-modality image registration [2,1,9,10,8]. During NMI-based registration an estimation of the image intensity distribution is necessary. The most common way to estimating an intensity distribution is by creating a histogram with equidistant binning. In this manner, the boundaries of the bins to be placed at arbitrary gray values rather than at locations meaningful to image structure. This could degrade the image alignment or registration process with respect to the number of misregistrations and speed [3,4]. In this paper we use an alternative binning method based on k-means clustering in order to compensate [3,4].

In an intensity histogram there is no distinction between multiple structures with similar intensities. They all fall into the same bin. This can negatively affect the registration process. We present a new technique, segment remapping,

C. Barillot, D.R. Haynor, and P. Hellier (Eds.): MICCAI 2004, LNCS 3216, pp. 805–812, 2004.
© Springer-Verlag Berlin Heidelberg 2004

in order to compensate for this effect: segments that are spatially unconnected but have equal intensity are each remapped to a new distinct intensity, e.g., in our "o" example the inside will be mapped to a new distinct intensity.

In section 2 we introduce our approach of combining NMI-based registration with both k-means clustering and segment remapping. We present the materials in section 3. In section 4 we discuss the results of registration with our new approach. Our conclusions are presented in section 5.

2   Methods

2.1   Normalized Mutual Information

The Shannon entropy H for image A with intensities a, n voxels and d distinct intensities is defined as

$$H(A) = -\sum_a p_A(a) \log p_A(a) = \log n - \frac{\sum_{x=1}^{d} f(a_x) \log f(a_x)}{n}, \qquad (1)$$

where $f(a)$ is the number of voxels with intensity a and $p_A(a)$ is the probability of intensity a in image A.

The Shannon entropy of of two images A and B is defined as

$$H(A,B) = -\sum_{a,b} p_{AB}(a,b) \log p_{AB}(a,b), \qquad (2)$$

where $p_{AB}(a,b)$ is the probability of intensity couple (a,b) of corresponding points in the overlapping part of A and B. A joint-histogam is generally used to compute the Shannon entropy for overlapping images. Note that increasing joint-histogram dispersion indicates a reduction in the registration quality.

A registration measure attuned to this effect is normalized mutual information, which is a well established registration measure [7,8,3,4] based on the Shannon entropy of the images:

$$\text{NMI}(A,B) = \frac{H(A) + H(B)}{H(A,B)}. \qquad (3)$$

2.2   Intensity Distribution Estimation

In order to compute the NMI of the overlapping part of two images their intensity distribution has to be estimated. Generally this is done by using a histogram with a fixed number of bins and a fixed number of gray values pooled in each bin. Gray values are converted to bin numbers in a rounded linear fashion. Remapping image intensities to bin numbers as described above could split segments over multiple bins, hence influencing the registration process with respect to the number of misregistrations and speed [3,4]. In this paper, we use k-means clustering based binning which takes the intensity distribution itself into account in order to reduce the splitting of segments. In previous work [3,4] we already have shown that adding k-means clustering based binning to NMI-based registration of 3D medical images (CT/MRI/SPECT) may greatly reduce the number of misregistrations and computational time of the process.

2.3   Segment Remapping

With equidistant binning spatially unconnected structures of similar gray value may be mapped to the same bin. This effect potentially degrades the registration process.

For example, consider an image where both the background and a large segment P have intensity a, and a corresponding image where the large segment P corresponds to a segment Q with intensity b. NMI uses the joint-histogram to determine the quality of the registration. As the overlap of segments P and Q increases so does the histogram entry (a, b) which indicates an increase of registration quality. On the other hand, overlapping segment Q with background, which clearly is not a good registration, also results in an increase of intensity couples (a, b) but not in an increase of registration quality.

We can compensate for this by remapping the intensities of spatially unconnected segments with equal intensity to distinct intensities. In our previous example we would, e.g., remap the intensity of the large segment P to c thus enabling NMI to distinguish between overlap of background and segment Q and overlap of segment P and Q.

2.4   Combining k-Means Clustering and Segment Remapping

A combination of both the standard NMI method and k-means clustering with segment remapping could enhance the registration with respect to the number of misregistrations and speed. We start by remapping the image intensities according to the pre-computed remapping function $k(i)$ where i is the intensity of voxel v. This function is based on the k-means clustering of the original intensity distribution of the image. See [3] and [4] for details of the computation of $k(i)$.

Next, a segment remapping of the image is done. First by determining the number of spatially unconnected segments and their respective size (using a 4-neighbor connectedness filter) for each bin. Second, by assigning a new distinct intensity to each segment. Note that the remapping function depends on the spatial location of the voxel v. Remapping starts with the largest segment. Remapping is stopped when a predetermined percentage of the image has been remapped. This avoids the creation of large numbers of spurious small segments for example, single voxel noise. We define the remapping function for voxel v as $r_v(i)$. Note that for a certain portion of the image the intensity is not affected by the segment remapping procedure.

2.5   Incorporating k-Means Clustering and Segment Remapping into the Standard NMI Framework

We include both the binned and the k-means clustered segment remapped image in the registration measure. We already noted that the regular binning method performs quite well in many circumstances, yet combining our method, $r_v(i)$, and the regular method could further enhance the registration process.

We first define the binning function $b(i)$. Next, we assign a vector s to each image voxel with intensity i according to:

$$s = (b, r) = (b(i), r_v(k(i))),\qquad(4)$$

where b is intensity i after applying the binning procedure.

Using the standard NMI approach an overlap of images A and B results in a joint-histogram with intensity couples (b_A, b_B). Our approach results in four distinct intensity couples for each corresponding voxel pair: (b_A, b_B), (b_A, r_B), (r_A, b_B) and (r_A, r_B), forming four distinct joint-histograms. For each of the images we define the entropy of the remapped intensities as $H(A_r)$ for image A and $H(B_r)$ for image B. We define four NMI equations based on (3):

$$NMI_{bb}(A, B) = \frac{H(A_b) + H(B_b)}{H(A_b, B_b)},\qquad(5)$$

$$NMI_{br}(A, B) = \frac{H(A_b) + H(B_r)}{H(A_b, B_r)},\qquad(6)$$

$$NMI_{rb}(A, B) = \frac{H(A_r) + H(B_b)}{H(A_r, B_b)},\qquad(7)$$

$$NMI_{rr}(A, B) = \frac{H(A_r) + H(B_r)}{H(A_r, B_r)},\qquad(8)$$

where subscripts b denote use of grey value employing the standard binning method and subscripts r indicate the use of clustered and remapped intensities.

Note that (5) is equal to the original NMI measure. Image registration can be performed using a combination of measures (5), (6), (7) and (8). Since each NMI measure contains image information that may be relevant to the registration process, we use the measure

$$NMI_s(A, B) = NMI_{bb}(A, B) + NMI_{br}(A, B) + NMI_{rb}(A, B) + NMI_{rr}(A, B),\qquad(9)$$

in our experiments.

3   Materials

Three 2D datasets have been used in this study, an artificial test image, the MPEG-7 dataset [5] and a medical retina dataset.

The artificial test image is a 1000 pixels square image, see figure 1(a), consisting of four distinct intensities $(1, 2, 3, 4)$ and eight spatially unconnected segments. This image was created so that some of the unconnected segments have equal intensity and are remapped by our method, see figure 1, in order to detect any changes in the parameter space for NMI_s(b) as compared to standard NMI.

The MPEG-7 data consists of a large number of test images, we randomly selected 50 images from the 'Regionn' part of the dataset. The complete 'Regionn' set is comprised of 3.628 images, however many of those images are made by applying a transformation to the same image, those were not used in our experiments. The data consists of binary images of 128 pixels square.

The retina data consists of 30 images of 768 by 527 pixels with a 8 bit pixel depth of the retina of a single healthy patient. The images were made in a single session during which a contrast agent was administered to the patient. The field of view was 40 by 25 degrees.

4   Experiments and Results

NMI_{bb} based registration, i.e., regular NMI-based registration was compared to NMI_s based registration. To optimize both measures as a function of 2D affine geometric transformations Powell's method was used [6]. The number of optimization steps needed to converge were used as a measure of computational speed. All images except the artificial image were registered to themselves by applying an offset transformation as initial starting position for the registration. The experiment using the artificial image is included only to demonstrate the added value of our new method, which is made clear by a parameter space cut.

4.1   Artificial Image

The artificial 2D image A consists of eight spatially unconnected segments but contains four distinct intensities $(1, 2, 3, 4)$. Intensities 2 and 4 both contain three unconnected segments. Applying our method results in a new image containing eight spatially unconnected segments and eight distinct intensities. The image is shown in figure 1.

A parameter space cut was made by registering the image to itself and applying a rotational offset T. Both the $NMI(A, T(A))$ and the $NMI_{rr}(A, T(A))$ were computed at 1440 equally spaced points comprising a full 360° rotation. To reduce the effects of varying overlap area, the background intensity was not used in the computation. The results can be seen in figure 2.

There is no difference between the two methods with respect to local and global maxima. However, there is a clear difference around the global optimum, whose base has a width of about 10 degrees using $NMI(A, A)$ and a width of about 80 degrees when using $NMI_{rr}(A, A)$. It is likely an optimization routine such as Powell or hill-climbing will use more optimization steps when using $NMI(A, A)$ instead of $NMI_{rr}(A, A)$.

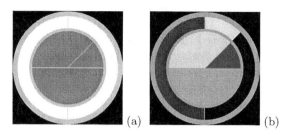

Fig. 1. The artificial image (1000 pixels square) has four distinct intensities (left) and eight spatially unconnected segments. On the right the same image is shown after remapping has been applied.

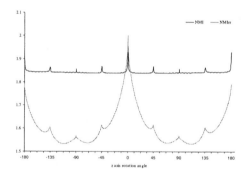

Fig. 2. $NMI(A, T(A))$ and $NMI_{rr}(A, T(A))$ of the artificial image (figure 1a) and a rotated version of the image, for rotation angles form -180 to 180 degrees.

4.2   MPEG-7 Data

Fifty binary were used in the experiment, which were clustered or binned using two bins and 100% binning. Each of the images was registered to itself with an initial null transform which corresponds to correct alignment. A rotation offset of -15, -30, 15 or 30 degrees, a translation offset of -10, -20, 10 or 20 pixels and a scaling of -10, -5, 5 or 10 percent was applied, resulting in 1024 registration starting positions for each image. For each of the registration measures $NMI(A, A)$ and $NMI_s(A, A)$ 51.200 registrations were done. The registration was considered a misregistration if the error was above 0.1 pixel. Some images used in this experiment are shown in figure 3.

Registering the images using both methods resulted in 58% misregistrations for $NMI(A, A)$ and 6% misregistrations for our NMI_s. There were no significant differences for both methods with respect to the number of optimization steps needed for a correct registration.

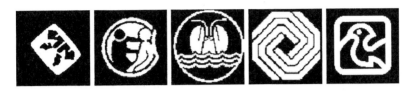

Fig. 3. Part of the MPEG-7 data used in our experiments.

4.3   Retina Data

Each retina image was registered to itself, using 32 bins for the $NMI(A, A)$ method. For $NMI_s(A, A)$ we used six to eight clusters and 80 to 90 percent segmentation depending on the images. The segmentation percentage was initially set to 80 and then increased until a remapping of large numbers of small segments occurred. Using these parameters resulted in 21 to 83 segments. An example image is shown in figure 4. Each image was registered to itself with an initial null transform which corresponds to correct alignment. A rotation offset of -20, -15, 15 or 20 degrees and a translation offset of -40, -20, 20 or 40 was applied, resulting in 64 starting positions for each image.

Ten images were registered using both methods resulting in 29% misregistrations for the $NMI(A, A)$ method and 9% misregistrations for $NMI_s(A, A)$. Registrations were considered a misregistration if the error was above 0.1 mm. There was no significant difference between the number of optimization steps used for both methods.

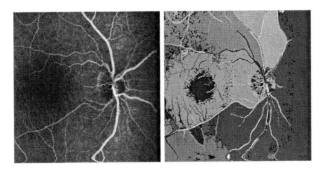

Fig. 4. A retina dataset after binning using 32 bins (left) and after applying our method using 6 clusters and adding 75 segments which comprised 90% of the image (right).

5   Conclusion and Discussion

In summary the combined use of k-means clustering and segment remapping improves the registration process with respect to the number of misregistrations when registering simple binary images or retina images. A parameter space cut made on an artificial image with four distinct intensities and eight spatially unconnected segments with equal intensity shows a significant improvement in the parameter space with respect to the standard NMI measure. Using our method on images with similar properties, i.e. several large spatially unconnected segments with equal intensity, could enhance the parameter space.

A drawback of our method is the presently manual selection of two parameters, the number of clusters and the percentage of the image to be segmented. However, this is a task that can in all likelihood be automated.

Future work will include the suggested automation and the investigation of the practical impact of the $NMI_s(A, A)$ measure on 2D and 3D medical image registration applications.

References

1. A. Collignon. *Multi-modality medical image registration by maximization of mutual information*. PhD thesis, Catholic University of Leuven, 1998.
2. A. Collignon, F. Maes, D. Delaere, D. Vandermeulen, P. Suetens, and G. Marchal. Automated multi-modality image registraction based on information theory. *Information Processing in Medical Imaging*, pages 263–274, 1995.
3. Z.F. Knops, J.B.A. Maintz, M.A. Viergever, and J.P.W. Pluim. Normalized mutual information based registration using K-means clustering based histogram binning. In M. Sonka and J.M. Fitzpatrick, editors, *SPIE Medical Imaging*, volume 5032, pages 1072–1080. SPIE press, 2003.
4. Z.F. Knops, J.B.A. Maintz, M.A. Viergever, and J.P.W. Pluim. Normalized mutual information based PET-MR registration using K-means clustering and shading correction. In J.C. Gee, J.B.A. Maintz, and M.W. Vannier, editors, *International Workshop on Biomedical Image Registration*, volume 2717 of *Lecture Notes in Computer Science*, pages 31–39. Springer, 2003.
5. MPEG-7 "Multimedia Content Description Interface" Documentation. WWW page, http://www.darmstadt.gmd.de/mobile/MPEG7, 1999.
6. W. H. Press, S.A. Teukolsky, W.T. Vetterling, and P.F. Brian. *Numerical recipes in C (2nd ed.): the art of scientific computing*. Cambridge University Press, 1992.
7. C. Studholme. *Measures of 3D medical image alignment*. PhD thesis, University of London, 1997.
8. C. Studholme, D.J. Hawkes, and D.L.G. Hill. An overlap invariant entropy measure of 3d medical image alignment. *Pattern Recognition*, 32(1):71–86, 1999.
9. P. Viola. *Alignment by maximization of mutual information*. PhD thesis, Massachusetts Institute of Technology, 1995.
10. W. M. Wells III, P. Viola, H. Atsumi, S. Nakajima, and R. Kikinis. Multi-modal volume registration by maximization of mutual information. *Medical Image Analysis*, 1(1):35–51, 1996.

Comparison of Different Global and Local Automatic Registration Schemes: An Application to Retinal Images

Evangelia Karali, Pantelis Asvestas, Konstantina S. Nikita, and
George K. Matsopoulos

National Technical University of Athens, School of Electrical and Computer Engineering,
Iroon Politechniou 9, Zografos 15780, Greece
ekarali@biosim.ntua.gr

Abstract. In this paper, different global and local automatic registration schemes are compared in terms of accuracy and efficiency. The accuracy of different optimization strategies based on a variety of similarity measures (cross-correlation, mutual information coefficient or chamfer distance) is assessed by means of statistical tests. Results from every optimization procedure are quantitatively evaluated with respect to the gold-standard (manual) registration. The comparison has shown that chamfer distance is a robust and fast similarity measure that can be successfully combined with common optimization techniques in retinal image registration applications.

1 Introduction

Retinal images are the common diagnostic tool in ophthalmology. Many eye diseases, like diabetic retinopathy, glaucoma, cataract and age-related macular degeneration can be detected in fundus images as well as many therapeutic techniques are planned and implemented according to eye vessels topography, as it is presented in ophthalmic images [1]. Comparison studies of ophthalmic images require thorough visual inspection because of their spatial misalignment, due to changes in the geometry between fundus camera and the retina or changes in retinal vessel topography because of pathological conditions, like glaucoma. Manual registration is the standard method used in clinical practice, however it depends on human knowledge and experience [2]. On the other hand, many automatic registration schemes that combine speed and accuracy have been applied to retinal images [1][3].

The most common ophthalmic imaging techniques are fluorescein angiography (FA) and indocyannine green angiography (ICG). FA images the fluorescence of a dye, fluoroscein, as it travels through retinal vessels because of blood circulation. Soon after intravenous injection to the patient of sodium fluoroscein 10% (usually after 5-7sec), FA images are obtained at a rate of 1 image/sec for the next 20sec. Prior to any examination, a Red-Free (RF) retinal image is acquired using a bandpass green filter, which cuts of the red light. In RF images, retinal blood vessels appear dark. Information from RF images in combination with FA and/or ICG data is used for the evaluation of disease progress [3].

C. Barillot, D.R. Haynor, and P. Hellier (Eds.): MICCAI 2004, LNCS 3216, pp. 813–820, 2004.
© Springer-Verlag Berlin Heidelberg 2004

In this work, automatic registration schemes based on various optimization techniques and on intrinsic image characteristics are compared in terms of accuracy and efficiency. In particular, three standard similarity measures, namely cross-correlation coefficient (C_{cc}), mutual information coefficient (MI) and chamfer distance (CD) have been used in combination with four different common optimization algorithms: Downhill Simplex (DSM), Powell's Method (PM), their combination (DSM-PM) and a combination of Simulated Annealing (SA) with PM (SA-PM). The accuracy of the different registration schemes has been assessed by means of statistical tests. Results from every optimization procedure have been quantitatively evaluated with respect to the gold-standard (manual) registration.

2 Materials and Methods

2.1 Image Acquisition

Retinal images were obtained using the IMAGEnet 1024 system, a fundus camera that provides 50% of coverage, 39mm working distance and specials filters for FA and acquired digital ophthalmic images 1024x1024 pixels in size. The automatic and manual registration techniques were applied to retinal images 512x512 pixels in size to increase optimization algorithm convergence speed.

2.2 Image Preprocessing

No preprocessing step was required for registration schemes based on C_{cc} or MI. Optimization techniques based on minimization of CD were applied to edge images of the retina, which were derived from the corresponding gray level images by applying first a canny edge detector with standard deviation $\sigma = 3$ and then the reconstruction opening operator that links edge fragments [4].

2.3 Registration Schemes

Every registration method is determined by the chosen transformation model, the similarity measure and the optimization strategy [5].

Transformation Model. The most suitable transformation model for registering retinal image pairs is a two dimensional (2D) affine transformation [5] that maps every pixel (x, y) of an image I to a pixel (x', y') of a reference image J according to the equation:

$$\begin{pmatrix} x' \\ y' \end{pmatrix} = \begin{pmatrix} a_1 & a_2 \\ a_3 & a_4 \end{pmatrix} \begin{pmatrix} x \\ y \end{pmatrix} + \begin{pmatrix} d_x \\ d_y \end{pmatrix}. \tag{1}$$

Similarity Measures. *Cross-correlation coefficient* (C_{cc}) is suitable for registering monomodal medical images [1]. The C_{cc} between two images I and J MxN pixels in size is mathematically expressed by:

$$C_{cc} = \frac{\sum_{x=1}^{M}\sum_{y=1}^{N}\left(I(x,y)-\bar{I}\right)\left(J(x,y)-\bar{J}\right)}{\sqrt{\sum_{x=1}^{M}\sum_{y=1}^{N}\left(I(x,y)-\bar{I}\right)^2 \sum_{x=1}^{M}\sum_{y=1}^{N}\left(J(x,y)-\bar{J}\right)^2}} \cdot \qquad (2)$$

where $\bar{I}$ and $\bar{J}$ are the mean gray values of I and J respectively and $C_{cc} \in [-1.1]$.

Mutual Information (MI) can be considered as a generalized non-linear correlation function. Considering two images I and J, which are geometrically associated by a transformation T, then if a and b are the gray values of $I(x,y)$ and $J(T(x,y))$ respectively, the coefficient of MI, $MI(I,J)$ can be mathematically expressed by:

$$MI(I,J) = \sum_{a,b} p_{IJ}(a,b)\ln\frac{p_{IJ}(a,b)}{p_I(a)p_J(b)} \cdot \qquad (3)$$

where $p_{IJ}(a,b)$ corresponds to the joint probability distribution of I and J and $p_I(a)$ and $p_J(b)$ are the marginal probabilities distributions of gray values α of image I and b of image J, respectively. A disadvantage of MI is that it usually presents many local extremes in which the optimization procedure may be trapped, which reduces registration efficiency and reliability. Furthermore MI based registration schemes are sensitive to the used interpolation method and their accuracy is limited due to the discrete nature of $MI(I,J)$ [1].

Chamfer Distance (CD): Two binary contour images are precisely aligned when the mean chamfer distance between them is minimum. 2D chamfer distance (CD) is computed by applying a suitable mask [6]. Usually the referenced contour distance map is computed prior to registration and used as a look-up table during the optimization procedure, in order to reduce execution time. Mean CD minimization is independent of the images gray level variances. However registration based on distance map is efficient when the image that contains the most contour information is assumed as the reference image [5].

Optimization Strategies

Downhill Simplex method (DSM), due to Nelder and Mead [7], is mostly recommended on applications that require execution speed. In this work, DSM was implemented as presented in [7]. The termination criterion was set equal to 10^{-6}, while the search space was restricted to [-0.1,+0.1] for scaling, [-6°,+6°] for rotation and [-150,+150] pixels for translation parameters around the initial specified position $P_{o=}(a_1,a_2,a_3,a_4,d_x,d_y)=(1,0,0,1,0,0)$ in each of the parameters directions separately.

Powell's direction set method (PM) finds the minimum of the similarity function in the N-dimensional parameter space, by iteratively minimizing the function in one direction along the set of N conjugate different directions. However PM may be trapped to a local and not the global minimum of the function. In the present work, PM was implemented as described in [7]. The initial set of directions was considered to be the basis vector in each dimension and the parameters were optimized in the order $(d_y,d_x,\alpha_4,\alpha_3,\alpha_2,\alpha_1)$. The search space and the termination criterion were determined as in DSM implementation.

Simulated Annealing method (SA) is commonly used in registration applications to extract similarity function's global minimum hidden among many local minima [5]. It has been successfully applied in retinal images in combination with correlation and mutual information [1][3]. The concept of the method relies on thermodynamics' laws and depends on the mathematical expression of the similarity function, the generation function of the random steps, the acceptance criterion and the annealing schedule [7]. In this work, the random steps were generated from a uniform function and were added to the function value. The used annealing schedule was defined by $T=T_o/1.25$, where $T_o=0.1$ and $k_{max}=100$, where T_o is the initial temperature and k the number of iterations. Because of its stochastic nature, SA algorithm was followed by PM, which provides more stable outputs.

3   Experimental Results

In this work the different registration schemes were assessed on 23 retinal image pairs, 18 temporal RF pairs and 5 FA-RF pairs. The temporal RF images were taken up to five years apart. The four common optimization techniques, DSM, PM, DSM-PM and SA-PM were combined with each of the three similarity measures; C_{cc}, MI and CD. PM was implemented after DSM or SA. Every registration algorithm was initialized so that a_1, $a_4 \in [-1.01,1.01]$, a_2, $a_3 \in [-0.1,0.1]$, and dx, $dy \in [-150,150]$ pixels. Bilinear interpolation was used and checkerboard images of the registration were produced to allow visual assessment of every method. As reference image was taken the one that had more edge information, including noise.

The mean value and the variance of every similarity function for every optimization method were calculated. For each similarity function, a pairwise comparison of the optimization methods was performed by means of Student's paired t-test. The null hypothesis was that the optimization methods under comparison did not differ as per the value of similarity function. Results are shown in Tables 1-3.

The registration schemes were also compared to the gold-standard (manual) registration, which was performed by an expert. From every image pair, six pairs of bifurcation points were chosen, according to which the affine transformation parameters were calculated using the Least-Squares method (LSM). This procedure was repeated three times. The best set of parameters was chosen as the one that corresponded to the smallest associated Root Mean Square Error (RMSE) value. The average RMSE of the LSM for all image pairs was 0.77 pixels, a rather low value that shows the good accuracy during pair points definition.

For the evaluation of the similarity measures, one thousand edge points of the image-to-be-transformed from each pair were randomly chosen. The mean Euclidean Distance (RMSE) between the manual and automatic registered points was computed. In Fig.1 the mean RMSE and in Table 4 the mean, medium and maximum RMSE [8] of C_{cc}, MI and CD for DSM, PM, SA-PM, DSM-PM are presented. Finally a pairwise comparison of the registration errors was performed by means of Student's paired t-test. The null hypothesis was that the similarity measures under comparison did not differ as per the value of RMS errors, namely present the same registration accuracy. Results are shown in Table 5.

Table 1. C_{cc} mean value and variance, p-value, execution time and mean number of iterations for DSM, PM, SA-PM, DSM-PM for the 18 temporal image pairs

	Mean	Variance	p-value				Time e (s)	Iterations
			DSM	PM	SA-PM	DSM-PM		
DSM	0.7775	0.1387	-	0.4918	0.4989	0.4993	29.9	396
PM	0.7785	0.1392	0.4918	-	0.4989	0.4996	119.9	1620
SA-PM	0.7786	0.1391	0.4907	0.4989	-	0.4993	92.2	1166
DSM-PM	0.7785	0.1391	0.4913	0.4996	0.4993	-	79.9	962

Table 2. MI mean value and variance, p-value, execution time and mean number of iterations for DSM, PM, SA-PM, DSM-PM for the 23 image pairs.

	Mean	Variance	p-value				Time (s)	Iterations
			DSM	PM	SA-PM	DSM-PM		
DSM	0.7887	0.3184	-	0.4589	0.4623	0.4571	45.3	354
PM	0.7549	0.3431	0.4589	-	0.4966	0.4982	186.0	1434
SA-PM	0.7976	0.3177	0.4623	0.4966	-	0.4948	171.8	1542
DSM-PM	0.7989	0.3161	0.4571	0.4982	0.4948	-	163.7	1289

Table 3. CD mean value and variance in pixels, p-value, execution time and mean number of iterations for DSM, PM, SA-PM, DSM-PM, for the 23 image pairs

	Mean	Variance	p-value				Time (s)	Iterations
			DSM	PM	SA-PM	DSM-PM		
DSM	8.0141	3.7033	-	0.4920	0.4832	0.4978	12.6	517
PM	7.9919	3.7270	0.4920	-	0.4754	0.4942	24.7	1580
SA-PM	8.0614	3.8782	0.4832	0.4754	-	0.4810	19.8	1336
DSM-PM	8.0079	3.7094	0.4978	0.4942	0.4810	-	14.1	1217

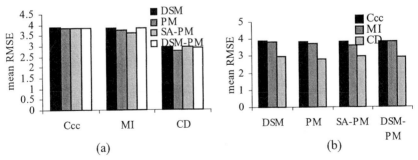

Fig. 1. (a) Mean RMSE of C_{cc}, MI and CD for DSM, PM, SA-PM, DSM-PM. (b) Mean RMSE of DSM, PM, SA-PM, DSM-PM for C_{cc}, MI and CD

According to Tables 1-3, and Fig. 1(a) no significant differences were observed (p-value>0.05, for all cases). All methods present the same registration accuracy. DSM is the fastest method and needs the lowest number of iterations. PM seems to be very slow because of the small steps it takes in the parameter space. DSM-PM presents an average performance of DSM and PM, as far as execution time and number of iterations are concerned. Almost all optimization techniques depend on the shape of the similarity measure. If it has many extremes, then the optimization algorithms must be initialized close to the best solution. PM showed the strongest dependence on the initial guess when it was combined with the MI, because of the deviation of this similarity function surface from quadratic form. SA-PM was almost independent from the initial guess, since it represents a global optimization technique.

Table 4. Mean , medium (med) and maximum (max) RMSE in pixels, for C_{cc}, MI, CD combined with DSM, PM, SA-PM, DSM-PM, for all image pairs

	C_{cc}			MI			CD		
	mean	med	max	mean	med	max	mean	med	max
DSM	3.897	1.777	19.57	3.837	2.857	17.52	2.968	1.823	11.45
PM	3.849	1.840	19.35	3.731	2.296	17.38	2.783	1.488	9.67
SA-PM	3.828	1.834	19.56	3.602	2.162	17.54	2.969	2.252	10.91
DSM-PM	3.864	1.777	19.57	3.829	2.291	17.52	2.899	1.823	9.87

Table 5. P-value for C_{cc}, MI, CD for all registration cases. The numbers in bold correspond to accepted p-value for the null hypothesis.

	p-value								
	mean			med			max		
	Ccc	MI	CD	Ccc	MI	CD	Ccc	MI	CD
Ccc	-	**0.07**	3×10^{-5}	-	**0.06**	4×10^{-4}	-	2×10^{-7}	10^{-4}
MI	**0.07**	-	10^{-5}	**0.06**	-	0.008	2×10^{-7}	-	2×10^{-4}
CD	3×10^{-5}	10^{-5}	-	4×10^{-4}	0.008	-	10^{-4}	2×10^{-4}	-

C_{cc}, seems to be very efficient combined with PM because it has a unique extreme. However C_{cc} did not succeed in registering FA-RF image pairs, due to the nonlinear dependence between the gray levels of the two images. Also C_{cc}, according to Fig.1 (b) and Tables 4 and 5 presents high registration errors in comparison with CD, due to small but existent deviation of the images gray levels dependence from linearity, probably because of noise.

MI coefficient presents many local extremes and has different shape with different values of the transformation parameters. An example is presented in Fig.3, which shows the dependence of MI on the affine model's parameters a_1 and a_4 for one of the examined image pairs, when the other parameters were kept constant. Only near the best solution presents MI a global extreme. According to Table 5 MI presents almost the same registration accuracy with C_{cc}. MI coefficient is well coupled with SA-PM, which does not present a strong dependence on the initial guess.

CD does not depend on the gray levels of the images. It seems to be a robust and fast similarity measure that, according to Fig.1 can be combined well with all optimi-

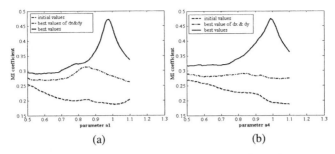

      (a)   (b)

Fig. 2. Dependence of MI coefficient on (a) a_4 and (b) a_1 transformation parameters, for a temporal RF image pair registration. Solid curves correspond to the best values of a_2, a_3, d_x, d_y and a_4 or a_1, dashdot curves to best values only of d_x and d_y, while in dashed curves the stable transformation parameters values were far from the best.

zation techniques, when contour extraction from images is possible. In Table 3 the required time includes the segmentation time interval as well. CD is the most accurate similarity measure. However CD depends strongly on translation parameters initial values. An example is shown in Fig. 4, that presents CD dependence on d_x and d_y parameters for another image pair.

For all the 23 examined cases, the error of the manual method was far and away smaller than those of the automatic techniques (mean RMSE=0.77, med RMSE=0.83 and max RMSE=1.14 pixels). Because of this and the fact that the placement of external markers in retinal image registration applications is not possible due to the great sensitivity of the human eye, manual registration was considered as a gold-standard procedure. In Table 4 the obtained errors of the automatic techniques include the error of the manual technique as well.

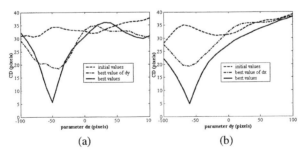

      (a)   (b)

Fig. 3. Dependence of CD on (a) dy and (b) dx transformation parameters, for a temporal RF image pair registartion. Solid curves correspond to the best values of a_1, a_2, a_3, a_4, and dx or dy, dashdot curves to best values only of dx or dy, while in dashed curves the stable transformation parameters values was far from the best.

Finally the affine model seems to be adequate for registering retinal images that are misaligned because of changes in the position between the camera and the patient. Deformable models could offer further improvements in the registration final result, especially in the case of glaucoma, where visual evaluation of vessels deformations in the area of the optic disk is essential.

Fig. 4 shows three different retinal image pairs, randomly chosen from the 23 pairs, registered with different schemes. As it can be seen from the images there is absolute continuity between vessels, something that shows the success of the registration schemes.

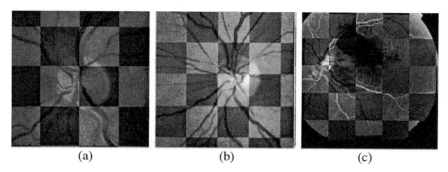

(a)   (b)   (c)

Fig. 4. (a) Chessboard image of a temporal RF image pair registered by PM combined with C_{cc}. (b) chessboard image of a temporal RF image pair registered by SA-PM coupled with MI. (c) chessboard image of an FA-RF image pair registered with DSM-PM combined with CD

4   Conclusion

In this work different global and local automatic registration schemes were applied to temporal RF and to FA-RF retina image pairs. The different techniques were compared on and evaluated against manual registration. The comparison showed that chamfer distance is an accurate and cost effective similarity measure that can be combined with common optimization techniques.

References

1. N. Ritter, et al "Registration of Stereo and Temporal Images of the Retina", IEEE Trans. on Medical Imaging, vol. 18, No. 5, May 1999.
2. F.Laliberte, L. Gagnon, "Registration and Fusion of Retinal Images-An Evaluation Study", IEEE Trans. on Medical Imaging, vol. 22, No. 5, May 2003.
3. G. Matsopoulos, N.A. Mouravliansky, K.K. Delibasis and K.S. Nikita, "Automatic Retinal Image Registration Scheme Using Global Optimization Techniques", IEEE Trans. on Inf. Tech. in Biomedicine, vol 3, No 1, March 1999.
4. L. Shaphiro, G Stockman: Computer Vision, Prentice Hall, New Jersey, 2001.
5. J. Mainz and M. Viergever, "A survey of medical image registration", Medical Image Analysis, vol.2, No 1, 1998.
6. G. Borgefors, "Distance Transformations in Arbitrary Dimensions", Com. Vision Graphics and Image Processing, vol. 27, 1984.
7. "Numerical Recipes in C: The Art of Scientific Computing", 1992 Cambridge University Press.
8. J. West, et al "Comparison and Evaluation of Retrospective Intermodality Brain Image Registration Techniques", J Comput Assist Tomogr, vol. 21, No 4, 1997.

Automatic Estimation of Error in Voxel-Based Registration

William R. Crum, Lewis D. Griffin, and David J. Hawkes

Division of Imaging Sciences, Thomas Guy House, Guy's Hospital, Kings College London,
London SE1 9RT, UK
{bill.crum, lewis.griffin, david.hawkes}@kcl.ac.uk

Abstract. Image registration driven by similarity measures that are simple functions of voxel intensities is now widely used in medical applications. Validation of registration in general remains an unsolved problem; measurement of registration error usually requires manual intervention. This paper presents a general framework for automatically estimating the scale of spatial registration error. The error is estimated from a statistical analysis of the scale-space of a residual image constructed with the same assumptions used to choose the image similarity measure. The analysis identifies the most significant scale of voxel clusters in the residual image for a coarse estimate of error. A partial volume correction is then applied to estimate finer and sub-voxel displacements. We describe the algorithm and present the results of an evaluation on rigid-body registrations where the ground-truth error is known. Automated measures may ultimately provide a useful estimate of the scale of registration error.

1 Introduction

Image registration is widely used in medical analysis with continuing efforts to improve, develop and validate existing algorithms [1]. A convenient distinction can be made between "manual" registration algorithms which use identified features and "automatic" algorithms that use voxel intensities. While the manual methods have some inherent error estimation through the identification of corresponding features, the automatic methods can only check that the voxel similarity measure is increasing and require further input (such as the laborious and error-prone identification of landmarks e.g. [2]) to measure registration error on a case-by-case basis. Where automatic registration algorithms are employed in large studies their behaviour is usually characterised on a representative subset of data.

In this paper we propose an approach for automatic estimation of error in voxel-based registration that combines statistical tests of significance on a residual image with a scale-selection process. The target application is retrospective estimation of registration error but it is also related to the problem of detection of change since image differences post-registration may represent biological changes of interest rather than error (e.g. lesion development in Multiple Sclerosis or contrast enhancement over time). In this latter case our approach will assign a spatial scale to such features and further interpretation will be required.

C. Barillot, D.R. Haynor, and P. Hellier (Eds.): MICCAI 2004, LNCS 3216, pp. 821–828, 2004.
© Springer-Verlag Berlin Heidelberg 2004

2   Method

A natural framework for examining image structures at different scales is provided by scale-space theory [3]. Images can be analysed at any scale desired by convolving them with a Gaussian filter of a specified standard deviation (s.d.). In image registration, it is common to examine a digital subtraction image (or more generally a residual image) post-registration to identify error or residual image differences. Our general approach is to identify the most significant scale associated with a structure in the residual image and interpret this as the scale of registration error. There are three required steps. First, a suitable residual image must be constructed, then scale selection must be applied to significant voxel clusters and finally these voxel intensities must be transformed into estimates of spatial displacement.

2.1   Constructing the Residual Image

The simplest case is mono-modal images assumed to differ only by additive Gaussian noise that are often registered by minimising their r.m.s. intensity difference. For multi-modal registration there is generally not a one-to-one relationship between the intensity at corresponding points in the two images. This can be dealt with by constructing a simulated difference image from the joint intensity probability distribution of the image pair (the target and source). For each voxel intensity in the source image, the most probable intensity in the target is selected and subtracted from the actual target voxel intensity. For true multi-modal images that do not have a one-to-one intensity relationship between source and target, the most probable intensity will not necessarily be the correct choice and will be a source of error.

2.2   Establishing Approximate Scale of Image Differences

Fig. 1(a) shows a 1D intensity profile of a displacing block edge, together with the 1D subtraction profile showing high signal over the region where the edge has displaced. Fig. 1(b) shows how the response of the difference profile to a Gaussian filter, once normalised by the noise response to the filter, exhibits a peak at a specific scale, σ. This suggests that by convolving the residual image with Gaussian filters of different scales to construct an isotropic scale-space and then normalising for noise, statistical tests on the intensity at each voxel can be used to find the most significant scale for features in the residual image.

In scale-space images there is substantial correlation between the intensities of neighbouring voxels introduced by the filtering process and the commonly used Bonferroni correction for large numbers of statistical tests is overly conservative. This problem has been addressed by Worsley *et al* [4] using the theory of Gaussian random fields to set the threshold for statistical significance from an estimate of the smoothness of the image and shape and extent of the search volume. The significance level sets the rate of false positive voxel clusters. We adopt this approach here assuming stationary Gaussian noise.

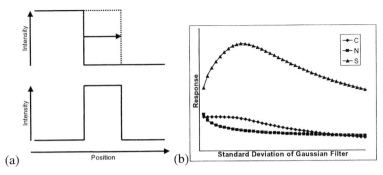

Fig. 1. 1D Edge Displacement. (a) Intensity profiles of a displacing edge and the difference between the displaced and the undisplaced edge. (b) Schematic showing the effect of convolving a Gaussian filter with the difference profile. C = Convolution of difference profile, N = Convolution of Gaussian noise, S = C/N is the normalised response of the difference profile

2.3 Measuring Sub-voxel Displacements

The method described in section 2.2 results in a relatively coarse assignment of scale that will be insensitive to sub-voxel edge-displacements. This is because tests are voxel-wise and a range of sub-voxel displacements may all be assigned the scale of the same applied Gaussian filter due to partial volume effects. To distinguish these displacements a single-voxel partial volume model of edge-displacement is used. In Fig. 2(a) an edge intensity profile is shown in different positions within the central voxel in the target (top) and source (bottom) images. The intensities of neighbouring voxels are presumed identical and equal to I_1 (right of centre) and I_2 (left of centre). The intensity of the central voxel in each image is related to the position of the edge (denoted by α and β) and given by:

$$T_C = \alpha I_2 + (1-\alpha)I_1 , \quad S_C = \beta I_2 + (1-\beta)I_1 \tag{1}$$

where T_C is the central intensity in the target image and S_C is the central intensity in the source image. In Fig. 2(b) the intensity profile in the subtraction image is shown together with the intensities of the voxels in the subtraction image. Then the central voxel intensity in the difference image, D_C, is given by:

$$D_C = T_C - S_C = (\alpha - \beta)(I_2 - I_1) \tag{2}$$

Writing $\Delta = -(\alpha - \beta)$ it can be seen that $\Delta = -D_C/(I_2 - I_1)$. Therefore the edge displacement can be estimated from the voxel intensity in the difference image normalised by the intensity gradient across the voxel in either the target or source image. In practice the target and residual images are resampled to the most significant scale so that the edge displacement can be modelled as within-voxel.

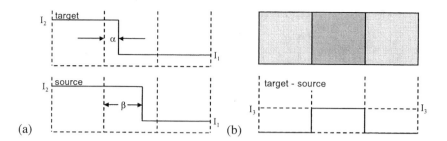

Fig. 2. The partial-volume model of a displacing edge. (b) The intensity profile of an edge within a voxel in two images. (b) The difference image and difference profile

3 Experiments

The algorithm was implemented in GNU C/C++ under Redhat Linux. Gaussian filtering was accomplished by multiplication in the frequency domain. Run times were < 5 minutes per case for the full algorithm applied to 2D images.

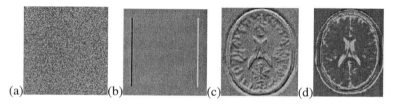

Fig. 3. Residual images used in the experiments (a) noise field (b) displaced square (c) T1-brain slices (d) T2 and T1 brain slices. (a)-(c) are difference images and (d) is a residual image computed from the joint intensity probability distribution. See text for further details

3.1 Rate of False-Positives

We need to check that the thresholds for significance are being set correctly so that only the expected number of false-positive significant voxel clusters are detected. Two independent 512x512 Gaussian noise images (Fig. 3(a)) were created and the number of significant voxel clusters determined over eleven scales in the range [0.8, 15] pixels and significance levels varying between [0.005, 0.5]. The experiment was repeated 1000 times for clusters detected as described in Section 2.1.

3.2 Detecting a Displacing Edge

Two copies of an image of a constant intensity square were created and one was displaced by varying amounts along the x-axis (one case is shown in Fig. 3(b)). Noise was added to each image and the displacement was estimated by (a) finding the mean most significant scale of difference and (b) the mean most significant scale after applying the partial volume correction. The experiment was run for 9 sub-voxel displacements in the range [0.1, 0.9] and 8 voxel displacements in the range [1, 10]. The experiment was repeated for 10 different levels of noise in the images in the range [1%, 10%]. Here and in the following experiments the significance level was set equal to 0.01 at all scales.

3.3 Detecting 2D Rigid-Body Motion from Subtraction Images

Two copies of a single slice of the MNI BrainWeb T1-weighted digital phantom were used [5], [6]. One copy was displaced by a random amount in the range $[0, 4\sqrt{2}]$ voxels (i.e. up to ±4 voxels in each of the x and y directions) and rotated by a random amount in the range ±2° forty times (Fig. 3(c)). Independent Gaussian noise of mean 3% was added to each image before analysis. The images were ranked for misregistration by computing the mean voxel-displacement in brain in each case. The mean displacement between the displaced image and the static image was then estimated as in 3.2 (b) for each of the forty cases.

3.4 Detecting 2D Rigid-Body Motion from Residual Images

Experiment 3.3 was repeated using the statistical residual image (Fig. 3(d)). In the first case the same pairs of T1-weighted images were used and in the second case the static image was replaced by a T2-weighted image.

4 Results

4.1 Rate of False Positives

Fig. 4 shows the total number of false positive significant voxel clusters detected over all scales compared with the expected number for the range of significance levels.

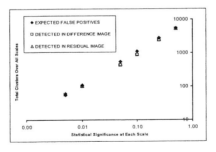

Fig. 4. The number of false positive voxel clusters detected in a Gaussian random noise field as a function of the statistical significance level

4.2 Detecting a Displacing Edge

Fig. 5 shows the most significant mean recovered scale of displacement as a function of the applied displacement for each noise level for (a) the simple approach and (b) the partial volume correction. Note that this mean is only computed over voxels that are significant in the residual image. There is a highly significant linear trend for all noise levels in the partial volume graph that extends to sub-voxel applied displacements.

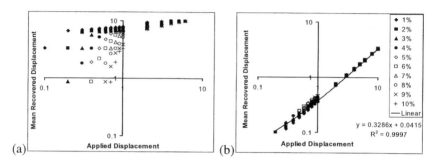

Fig. 5. The recovered mean displacement as a function of applied mean displacement for a translating square subject to 10 different noise levels (a) the most significant scale (b) with partial volume correction. The trend line is constructed for the 1% noise level

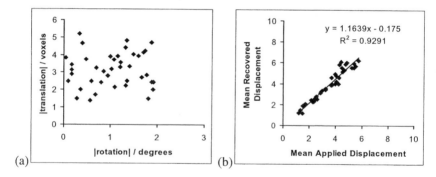

Fig. 6. (a) The distribution of 2D random translations and rotations applied to the example brain data. (b) The relationship between the mean applied voxel displacement and the mean recovered voxel displacement recovered the subtracted pairs of T1-weighted brain scans.

4.3 Detecting 2D Rigid Body Motion from Subtraction Images

Fig. 6 (a) shows the distribution of applied rotations and translations and (b) the relationship between the magnitude of the applied global displacement and the magnitude of the mean recovered displacement for the forty test cases.

4.4 Detecting 2D Rigid Body Motion from Residual Images

Fig. 7 shows the results for the same test cases as in figure 6 but with the displacement recovered from a statistical residual image rather than a difference image. The graphs show (a) T1-T1 displacement and (b) T2-T1 displacement.

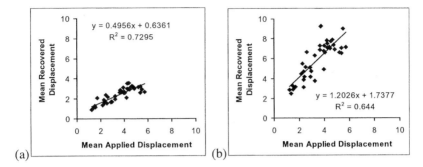

(a)　　　　　　　　　　　　　　　　　　(b)

Fig. 7. The relationship between mean applied and mean recovered voxel displacement for the cases shown in figure 6 calculated from (a) T1-T1 statistical residual image (b) T2-T1 statistical residual image

5 Discussion

We propose that registration error can be estimated from a post-registration residual image and have shown that rigid-body mis-registrations can be ranked by mean voxel displacement with a linear relationship between estimated and known mean voxel displacement. The techniques in this paper generalise immediately to 3D data. However, we have taken a simple approach to address a complex problem and a more general registration scenario will require further innovation. In particular, our attempt to treat the multi-modal case is simplistic and the results are data-dependent (Fig. 7). Spatial localisation of estimated error is the ultimate goal but will require a more thorough analysis. There is a deep relationship between the size and configuration of corresponding objects in the source and target images and the structures seen in residual images that should be explored and exploited. The displacement of objects that do not overlap will not be recovered with the current naïve approach.

There are other caveats. First, for simplicity we have applied the same statistical significance at all scales; this implies repeated tests at each voxel. Our experience is that the results are relatively insensitive to the significance level but note that previous work [9] suggests a more principled way of searching for significant structure within a scale-space. It may be more appropriate to specify the total significance across all scales and to weight the significance to favour smaller scale structures. Second, the structure in the residual image must be interpreted in light of the applied transformation model. A structure-less residual image may result from a highly non-physical transformation that does not reflect true correspondence. The particular transformation model will also affect spatial correlation of features in the residual image and this might be exploited to differentiate mis-registration from true change; for instance a rigid-body transformation will introduce correlated structures at opposing faces of a displaced object. In the future a scale-selective feature analysis of both the target image and the residual image may enable tighter bounds on error to be found.

These methods will not replace detailed evaluation studies (e.g. [7], [8]) but will complement them with estimates that can be obtained retrospectively or prospectively without special provision. The principle that an analysis of the residual image structure can be used to estimate the likely registration error or to automatically compare attempts at registration is a powerful one. With automatic voxel-based registration increasingly applied in large studies, novel methods to automatically monitor and estimate registration error are urgently required. Such methods will assist in validation and monitoring of existing techniques and ultimately may be used to initialise or to drive registration.

Acknowledgments. The authors are grateful for the intellectual and financial support of the Medical Images and Signals IRC (EPSRC and MRC GR/N14248/01).

References

1. Hajnal, J.V., Hill D.L.G. and Hawkes, D.J.: Medical Image Registration, CRC Press, Boca Raton, USA (2001)
2. Grachev, I.D., Berdichevsky D., Rauch, S.L., Heckers, S., Kennedy, D.N., Caviness V.S. amd Alpert, N.M.: A Method For Assessing the Accuracy of Intersubject Registration of the Human Brain Using Anatomic Landmarks, NeuroImage 9 (1999) 250-268
3. Koenderink, J.J.: The Structure of Images. Biological Cybernetics 50(5) (1984) 363-370
4. Worsley, K.J., Marrett, S. P., Neelin, Vandal, A.C., Friston, K.J. and Evans, A.C. : A Unified Statistical Approach for Determining Significant Signals in Images of Cerebral Activation. Human Brain Mapping 4 (1996) 58-73
5. Collins, D.L., Zijdenbos, A.P., Kollokian, V., Sled, J.G., Kabani, N.J., Holmes C.J. and Evans, A.C.: Design and Construction of a Realistic Digital Brain Phantom. IEEE Transactions on Medical Imaging 17(3) (1998) 463-468
6. Kwan, R.K.-S., Evans, A.C. and Pike, G.B.: MRI Simulation-Based Evaluation of Image Processing and Classification Methods. IEEE Transactions on Medical Imaging 18(11) (1999) 1085-1097
7. Hellier, P., Barillot, I., Corouge, B., Gibaud, G., Le Goualher, G., Collins, D.L., Evans, A., Malandain, G., Ayache, N., Christensen, G.E. and Johnson H.J.: Retrospective Evaluation of Intersubject Brain Registration. IEEE Transactions on Medical Imaging, 22(9) (2003) 1120-1130
8. Grachev, I.D., Berdichevsky D., Rauch, S.L., Heckers, S., Kennedy, D.N., Caviness V.S. amd Alpert, N.M.: A Method For Assessing the Accuracy of Intersubject Registration of the Human Brain Using Anatomic Landmarks, NeuroImage 9 (1999) 250-268
9. Worsley, K.J., Marrett, S., Neelin, P. and Evans, A.C.: Searching Scale Space for Activation in PET Images. Human Brain Mapping 4 (1996) 74-90

Rigid and Deformable Vasculature-to-Image Registration: A Hierarchical Approach

Julien Jomier and Stephen R. Aylward

Computer-Aided Diagnosis and Display Lab
The University of North Carolina at Chapel Hill, Department of Radiology
27510 Chapel Hill, USA
{jomier, aylward}@unc.edu

Abstract. Several recent studies demonstrate the potential of using tubular structures such as vessels as a basis for image registration. In this paper, we present a novel technique for the deformable registration of tubular structures. Our approach aligns tubular models, e.g. vessels of an organ, with an image by combining both rigid and non-rigid transformations in a hierarchical manner. The physical structure and properties of the vessels are taken into account to drive the registration process. Our model-to-image registration method shows sub-voxel accuracy as well as robustness to noise and a convergence time of less than one minute.

1 Introduction

Registration of vascular images has shown promising results compared to tissue based registration [3] and has been used to form vascular atlases [4] in order to diagnose cerebral malformations. Other extensions to this technique have also been applied to image-guided surgery.

Registration methods typically use mutual information [9,11] and related image-image metrics to register one image with another. Iterative closest point is also used to perform model-model registration of common features extracted from two images. A third type of registration is used in [1]: features from one image are registered directly with another image using a model-image match metric. However the extension of this method to deformable registration has not been shown.

A variety of deformation field estimation methods exist. Fluid based, image-image registration approaches [7] handle arbitrary deformations but do not take advantage of the object's geometry in images. Finite element modeling also shows excellent results [6] by deforming a mesh given image forces. On the other hand, model-to-model registration techniques may directly exploit the geometric correspondences have been developed. Our technique differs from these approaches by (1) combining both rigid and deformable transformations in a hierarchical manner, (2) combining geometry and intensity information and (3) persisting as an instance of model-to-image registration.

Our technique takes advantage of the typical tree structure of blood vessels and uses branch points to constrain the deformation field. We perform three

C. Barillot, D.R. Haynor, and P. Hellier (Eds.): MICCAI 2004, LNCS 3216, pp. 829–836, 2004.

distinct steps to achieve final registration of the model with the image: global rigid transformation, piece-wise rigid registration and deformable registration. The first stage deals with the global rigid body registration and has been shown to have sub-voxel accuracy, handle large initial mis-registrations and converge in 2-10 seconds [1]. Such rigid registration is a preliminary and necessary stage in order to be "close enough" to the deformed structure. The second stage uses the tree structure inherent in vascular network to perform a piece-wise rigid alignment. First, the root of the tree is aligned and then its children are registered, in order, from root to leaves. Branch points and physical parameters of the tubular structure have to be known to approximately constrain this task. Hierarchical local deformation is the concern of the third stage.

2   Method

Blood vessels in the human body are organized as a tree structure. For instance, in the liver, portal and hepatic vessels define two distinct trees; in the brain, vessels are divided into several trees, among them, right and left cerebral group. Formally, a tree is composed of at least one root, but vasculature trees can have multiple roots and can contain cycles. Our technique relies on this tree configuration to perform a global to local registration. First, a 3-dimensional model of the vasculature is formed using a ridge traversal technique [2]. Each extracted blood vessel is represented as a centerline with an associated radius at each point on the line. Next, we initiate our deformable registration strategy by solving for a global rigid transform.

2.1   Global Rigid Registration

Our rigid registration method maps a 3-dimensional vascular model into the target image using a tube-to-image technique developed by Aylward et al. [1]. This algorithm relies on blood vessels to have high intensity values in the target image. For each sample point of the model, the intensity is computed in the target image at a scale proportional to the radius of the vessel at that point. The sum of these intensities is the value of the match metric and the parameters of the transformation are optimized to maximize this metric. A unique additional property of this method is that it limits vessel to inducing registration updates in their normal directions. Furthermore, the iterative updates of the rigid transform are adjusted for the orientation bias of the vessels. The second step consists of a piece-wise rigid registration from root to leaves.

2.2   Piece-Wise Rigid Transformation via Propagation

A rigid registration is applied to each vessel in a hierarchical manner. As in our global rigid registration step, we align the model to match high intensity values in the target image. First the root of the tree is registered with the image using a rigid body transformation. Second, the branches of the tree are registered rigidly with the image one branch at a time using the parent-child hierarchy with anchor points at the branch points. That is during this step we solve for the rotation at each branch point using the parent-child hierarchy.

The magnitude of the rotation is given by the displacement vector v computed along each branch individually (sub-branches do not contribute). The evaluation of the rotation is done using a linear weighted factor $\lambda(i)$ along the child tube so that points close to the branch contribute more to the rotation. The image gradient is computed only at centerline points x at a scale σ proportional to the radius of the tube at that point. N represents the number of centerline points that compose the vessel. For each centerline point i the image gradient is projected onto its normal plane $n_i = (n_1, n_2)_i$.

$$v = \frac{1}{N} \sum_{i=1}^{N} \lambda(i) \nabla_x(\sigma) \cdot n_i \tag{1}$$

To translate a branch, the elastic property of the parent has to be taken into account. Specifically, the translation vector v of the child is projected onto the tangent direction t of its parent at the specified branch point x and the amount of translation T allowed is constrained by the elasticity γ of the parent tube multiplied by the initial distance d between the two consecutive points near the branch.

$$T = \max(v \cdot t, \gamma d - |x - x_0|) \cdot t \tag{2}$$

Once the branch point is moved, the points of the parent are updated to propagate the translation along the tube. We repeat the process until convergence before going to the next step: the deformable registration.

2.3   Deformable Registration

Non-rigid registration is also driven by derivative information from the target image. Our approach uses the image gradient computed at a scale proportional to the radius of the tube and projected onto the normal of the tube. Due to the potential complexity of the elastic deformations, i.e. folding, shrinking, expansion, etc., we add constraints to the registration process.

The first constraint is the elasticity coefficient γ of the tube which limits the movement of points along a tube. This is the same as 2.1 but now everypoint along a tube may move.

The second constraint is the rigidity coefficient which defines the bending factor of the tube. There are several ways to define such a coefficient. We define rigidity as the maximum angle between the initial tangent t_0 at rest and the actual tangent t. The rigidity coefficient can be different for each point along the structure or can be constant. Intuitively, the rigidity of a vessel is proportional to its radius and depends on its material and physical properties. In our implementation we choose to keep the rigidity constant and use a non-uniform sampling rate to accommodate the rigidity coefficient as the radius changes.

An iterative optimization process uses these two coefficients and the projected gradient at each point along a centerline to fit each centerline to the data. This continues until the full hierarchy has been fit to the data.

3   Results

In order to evaluate the accuracy of our registration algorithm we compared registered blood vessels with vessels that had been extracted from the target image. It is important to note that the extracted target image vessels are not used in the registration process, but only for validation purposes.

3.1   Simulated Data

First, we tested our algorithm on simulated data to perform noise sensitivity measurements. We created an artificial tree composed of a main trunk and two branches. The main trunk is a straight tube composed of 50 points while the branches are 20 points long. The three tubes have a constant radius of 2mm. Next, we deformed the tree and created a binary image of the deformed tree such that high intensity pixels fall inside the tubes. Finally, the image is blurred by a Gaussian filter ($\sigma = 5$) since blood vessel's cross section have a Gaussian profile in clinical data. Figure 1 shows a slice of the synthetic image.

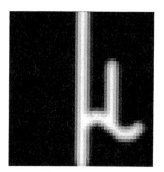 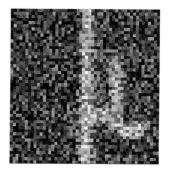

Fig. 1. Simulated image, with no noise(left) and with a noise range [0,255](right), used to test the robustness to noise of our algorithm.

Figure 2 shows the three consecutive steps of the algorithm, after rigid registration(left), after piece-wise rigid transformations(middle) and after non-rigid registration(left). Before and after the registration process we compute the cumulated measures of the percentile of points inside a given distance from the centerline using the closest point metric. Results are shown in Figure 3.

Next, we quantify the robustness to noise of our algorithm by adding uniform additive noise to the simulated image (Figure 1-right). Table 4 presents the results of the registration given different ranges of noise level. The accuracy of

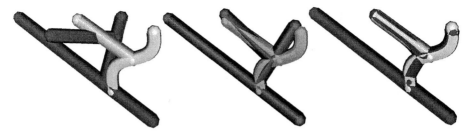

Fig. 2. Simulated tubes used to test the robustness of our algorithm. Original sets of tubes(left), After semi-rigid registration(middle) and after non-rigid registration(right). Only the light grey tubes are moving, they are being registered with the deformed image. The dark vessels are only being shown to illustrate "truth"

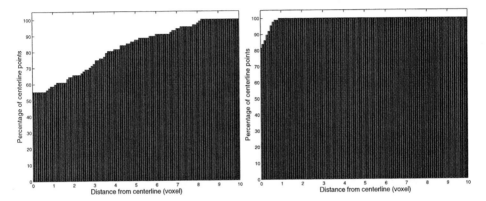

Fig. 3. Cumulative graphs representing the percentile of vascular points within a certain distance from the centerline of the true vasculature point, before registration(left) and after rigid and non-rigid transformations(right)

the registration process shows a fall-off of 3.5% only even when the noise pans the same range as the image. The summation of derivatives calculated using gaussians with standard deviation proportional to the size of the object is very robust to noise [8].

Noise level range	% of points $\leq$ 1 voxel	% of points $\leq$ 2 voxels	% of points > 2 voxels
[0,0]	100 %	100 %	0 %
[0,50]	100 %	100 %	0 %
[0,100]	97.7 %	100 %	0 %
[0,200]	96.8 %	99.7 %	0.3 %
[0,255]	96.5 %	99 %	1 %

Fig. 4. Influence of different additive white noise levels on the registration process

3.2   Pre-post-surgery Brain Data

We applied our algorithm on pre- and post-surgery brain Time-of-flight MRA data in which an arteriovenous malformation (AVM) had been embolized. The data volume sizes 256x256x104 and has been isotropically resampled to a spacing of 0.87. Approximately 100 vessels were extracted with an average of 150 points per vessel. An initial global rigid registration was performed using a sample factor of 10, i.e. approximately 15 points per vessel are used for registration. Fig.5-left shows the result. Next we applied 40 piece-wise rigid transformation iterations per branch, Fig.5-right. Fig.6 shows the final registration using both piece-wise rigid and non-rigid transformations.

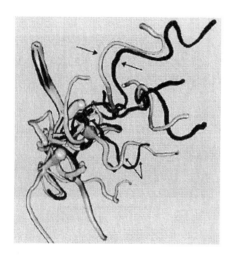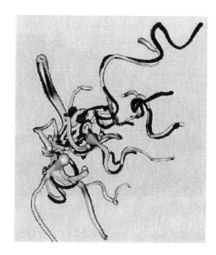

Fig. 5. Original set of tubes registered with a global rigid transformation(left) and the resulting set of tubes after the piece-wise rigid registration(right). Only the black vasculature is moving. The light grey vasculature is shown here as truth but is never used to drive the registration process. The data that produced the clinical MRA light grey tubes is actually driving the registration process

After each stage of the registration process we compute the percentile of centerline points inside a given distance from the centerlines of the vessels in the target image. Figure 7 shows the results. Both stages of the deformable registration requires less than 10 seconds to converge on a standard desktop PC Pentium 4 (2.4GHz) without any parallelization. Depending on the complexity of the vascular tree (number of branches, size of the tree) the computation time can be decreased significantly using parallel processing [1]. We are currently integrating our algorithm for Radio-Frequency Ablation (RFA) of liver tumors in the operating room and are pursuing parallelization and other speed improving enhancements.

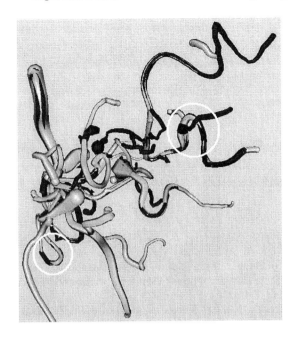

Fig. 6. Set of tubes after the deformable registration process. Non-rigid deformations are applied after the semi rigid registration. Again, the light grey vasculature is shown here as an illustration but is never used to drive the registration process. Circles highlight areas of larger non-rigid deformation

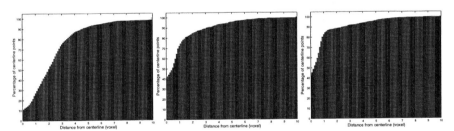

Fig. 7. Percentile of points inside a given distance from the centerlines of the vessels in the target image (cumulative graphs). Before registration(left), after semi-rigid registration(middle) and after semi-rigid plus deformable registration(right)

4   Discussion and Conclusions

We have developed a novel model to image registration technique that uses both rigid and deformable transformations in a hierarchical manner. The model, a set of blood vessels, is registered with the image by exploiting the parent-child hierarchy present in the vasculature. Furthermore, elasticity and rigidity coefficient of the vessels are taken into account during the registration process to constrain the deformation field. Our algorithm shows high accuracy and robustness to noise on simulated data and operate with $\approx 87\%$ of centerline points within 2 voxels on pre-to-post AVM embolization MRA registration. We are conscious that our definitions of elasticity and rigidity do not have "real" physical meaning and we are currently investigating the physical utility of incorporating the properties of blood vessels embedded in different tissues.

Acknowledgements. This work is funded in part by the Whitaker Foundation (RG-01-0341), the NIH-NIBIB (R01 EB000219), and the NIH-HLB (R01 HL69808).

References

1. Aylward, S., Jomier, J., Weeks, S., Bullitt, E.: Registration of Vascular Images International Journal of Computer Vision, November 2003, pages 15
2. Aylward, S., Bullitt, E.: Initialization, Noise, Singularities, and Scale in Height-Ridge Traversal for Tubular Object Centerline Extraction IEEE Transactions on Medical Imaging, Feb, 2002, Pages 61-75
3. Cool, D., Chillet, D., Kim, J., Foskey, M., Aylward, S.: Tissue-Based Affine Registration of Brain Images to form a Vascular Density Atlas MICCAI 2003, November 2003
4. Chillet, D., Jomier, J., Cool, D., Aylward, S.: Vascular Atlas Formation Using a Vessel-to-Image Affine Registration Method MICCAI 2003, November 2003
5. Danielsson, P.E.: Euclidean distance mapping Computer Graphics and Image Processing, 14, 1980, pp. 227-248.
6. Ferrant, M., Warfield, S., Guttmann, C., Mulkern, R., Jolesz, F., Kikinis, R.: 3D Image Matching Using a Finite Element Based Elastic Deformation Model MICCAI 1999,pp 202-209
7. Lorenzen, P. J., Joshi, S. C.: High-Dimensional Multi-modal Image Registration. WBIR 2003: 234-243
8. Lindeberg, T.: Linear Spatio-Temporal Scale-Space. Scale-Space 1997: 113-127
9. Maes, F., Collignon, A., Vandermeulen, D., Marchal, G., Suetens, P.: Multimodality image registration by maximization of mutual information IEEE Transactions on Medical Imaging, vol. 16, no. 2, pp. 187-198, April 1997.
10. Maintz, J.B.A., Viergever, M.A.: A Survey of medical image registration. In U. Spetzger, H.S. Stiehl, J.M. Gilsbach (Eds.), Navigated Brain Surgery (pp. 117-136). Aachen: Verlag Mainz.
11. Rueckert, D., Clarkson, M. J., Hill,D. L. G., Hawkes,D. J.: Non-Rigid Registration Using Higher-Order Mutual Information. Proc. SPIE Medical Imaging 2000: Image Processing, pp. 438-447
12. Wink, O., Niessen, W.J., Verdonck, B., Viergever, M.A.: Vessel Axis Determination Using Wave Front Propagation Analysis MICCAI 2001,LNCS 2208, pp. 845-853, 2001.

Rigid Registration of Freehand 3D Ultrasound and CT-Scan Kidney Images

Antoine Leroy[1], Pierre Mozer[1,2], Yohan Payan[1], and Jocelyne Troccaz[1]

[1] Laboratoire TIMC-GMCAO, Faculté de Médecine, Domaine de la Merci,
38700 La Tronche, France
Antoine.Leroy@imag.fr
[2] Service d'Urologie et de Transplantation Rénale. CHU Pitié-Salpêtrière. AP-HP,
75013 Paris, France

Abstract. This paper presents a method to register a preoperative CT volume to a sparse set of intraoperative US slices. In the context of percutaneous renal puncture, the aim is to transfer a planning information to an intraoperative co-ordinate system. The spatial position of the US slices is measured by localizing a calibrated probe. Our method consists in optimizing a rigid 6 degree of free-dom (DOF) transform by evaluating at each step the similarity between the set of US images and the CT volume. The images have been preprocessed in order to increase the relationship between CT and US pixels. Correlation Ratio turned out to be the most accurate and appropriate similarity measure to be used in a Powell-Brent minimization scheme. Results are compared to a standard rigid point-to-point registration involving segmentation, and discussed.

1 Introduction

Percutaneous Renal Puncture (PRP) is becoming a common surgical procedure, whose accuracy could benefit from computer assistance. The pre-operative imaging modality is CT, whereas either fluoroscopy or echography is used for intra-operative target visualization. A feasibility study on Computer-Assisted PRP has been carried out [3], in which the kidney surface, segmented from CT and localized US images, was registered using ICP. The study showed satisfying results; however it required a manual segmentation in both image modalities, which is not acceptable for a clinical use, especially intra-operatively.

We therefore investigated automatic CT/US registration. It was decided for the present study to propose and evaluate an automatic voxel-based registration algo-rithm, to avoid segmentation steps and to minimize user intervention.

Voxel-based registration methods have been deeply studied since 1995. Every method proposes a similarity measure and a cost minimization algorithm. Wells [12] first introduced Mutual Information (MI) combined with histogram windowing and a gradient descent algorithm. Maes [4] presented an interesting combination of MI and Powell-Brent (PB) search strategy. He also compared various search and multi-resolution strategies, and showed that PB was efficient with image subsampling [5]. Jenkinson [2], Studholme [11] and Sarrut [10] made a thorough comparison of differ-ent functional and statistical similarity measures.

C. Barillot, D.R. Haynor, and P. Hellier (Eds.): MICCAI 2004, LNCS 3216, pp. 837–844, 2004.
© Springer-Verlag Berlin Heidelberg 2004

Although those studies constitute the base of our research, none of them is applied to registering US images. We will therefore focus on the works of Roche [9], who registered 3D US of the brain with MRI, and Penney [6], who registered 2.5D US of the liver with MRI. The theoretical difficulty in registering CT and US is that the former gives information on tissues intensity, whereas the latter contains a speckled image of their boundaries. So a complex similarity measure and specific image preprocessing must be chosen.

This paper introduces a method to automatically register localized US images of the kidney onto a high-quality abdominal CT volume. The final algorithm uses image preprocessing in both modalities, Powell-Brent method as a search strategy, and Correlation Ratio (CR) as a similarity measure. Preliminary tests have been carried out on one data set, that allows us to draw the first conclusions on the method.

2 Image Preprocessing

2.1 CT Preprocessing

Penney [6] basically transformed the blurred MRI and US images of the liver into maps giving the probability of a pixel to be liver tissue or vessel lumen. However, as this process requires manual thresholding of the MRI, and as the segmentation of the kidney parenchyma is not a binary process, especially in the US images, we do not think that the technique can apply to our problem. Roche [9] proposed the combined use of the MRI image and its derivate, that we again decided not to use, because of the complexity of the bivariate correlation method and because of the observed chaotic correlation between CT gradient and US.

Our goal was to highlight the major boundaries in CT in order to increase the correlation with the US. The preprocessing of a CT slice consists in the superposition of a median blur and a bi-directional Sobel gradient from which we kept the largest connex components (fig. 1).

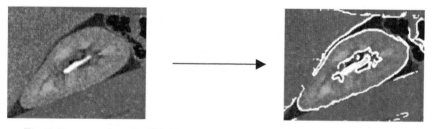

Fig. 1. Preprocessing of a CT oblique slice. The major boundaries are highlighted

2.2 US Preprocessing

Speckle Removal. US images are known to be low-quality gradient images, blurred by speckle noise. Still, the kidney, due to its small size and echogenic capsule, can be well and fully visualized through anterior access. The aim of preprocessing US images is to reduce the speckle, while preserving the boundaries of the organ. We applied the "sticks" filter proposed by Czerwinski [1], designed for that purpose.

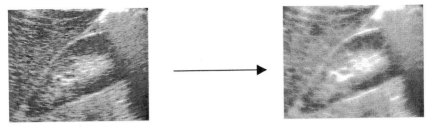

Fig. 2. Preprocessing of a US slice. Most speckle is removed while boundaries are preserved

Shadow Removal. Because they convey no relevant information for registration, acoustic shadows are removed in the US images, as proposed in [6]. The shadows are produced by large interfaces like the ribs or the colon that reflect quasi-totally the acoustic signal, the remaining waves decreasing in the distance in an exponential way. Shadow removal is based on the correlation between a US line profile and a heuristic exponential function. A shadow is detected when the correlation is higher than a given threshold, and when the maximum acoustic interface is close enough to the skin. Fig. 3 and 4 show the result of our automatic method on a sample slice.

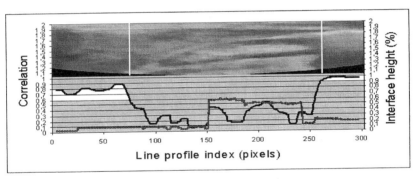

Fig. 3. Correlation profile (black curve) and height of shadow interface (grey curve) along the US fan. Left and right white areas correspond to shadow regions (high correlation, low height)

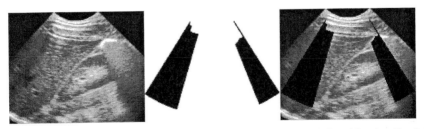

Fig. 4. US shadow removal. Left image shows the shadow profiles induced by the ribs (left) and the colon (right). Middle image shows the generated mask, superimposed on right image

3 Search Strategy: Powell-Brent Algorithm

PB algorithm [2][4] appears as a fairly efficient search strategy when the differentiation of the cost function is unknown [4]. Our implementation is based on [7]. We applied some changes since we found the method too slow and too sensitive to local minima, which are frequent in image registration.

3.1 Initial Attitude and Parameter Space

The minimization process consists in optimizing a 6D vector $(T_x, T_y, T_z, R_x, R_y, R_z)$. From the Arun-based Initial Attitude (IA) computation, we define the longitudinal axis of the CT kidney as the Z' axis of the new parameter space; this allows us to follow Maes' advice [5] to optimize the vector in the better-conditioned order $(T_{x'}, T_{y'}, R_{z'}, T_{z'}, R_{x'}, R_{y'})$.

3.2 Search Interval

Contrary to fundamental PB method, whose Brent 1D search interval, for each DOF, is defined by a time-consuming automatic bracketing, we chose an arbitrary interval length of $2*RMS_{ARUN}$ (20 to 30mm) around the IA.

Since PB tends to reach the solution very fast (only the first iteration makes a significant step), it was decided, for computation time improvement, to reduce the interval length at each Powell iteration.

3.3 1D Initial Search

As PB method tends to converge to local minima, and as the similarity between registered CT and US shows in most cases a non-ambiguous global minimum (fig. 6), we chose to perform before each Brent 1D optimization an initial search, with a step of 10% of the interval length, to find an approximate global minimum in that DOF. Then Brent method is applied around that minimum in a very restrained interval (fig. 5). This strategy does not significantly increase the computation time. Jenkinson [2] also proposed an initial search on the rotational DOF, previously to PB iterations, to make the solution "more reliable".

4 Similarity Measure: Correlation Ratio

4.1 Definition

Let X be the base image (CT), and Y the match image (US). CR is a functional similarity measure [2][8][10] based on conditional moments. It measures the functional relationship between the match pixels and the base pixels. Roche [8] writes:

$$\eta(Y|X) = 1 - \frac{1}{N\sigma^2} \sum_i N_i \sigma_i^2 \qquad (1)$$

where N is the number of overlapped pixels, and σ their variance in Y, where Ni is the number of overlapped pixels in X of value i, $σ_i$ their variance in Y.

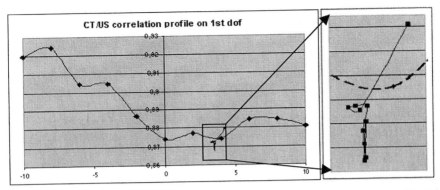

Fig. 5. CR profile along the search interval for T_x. The converging curve represents Brent iterations around the global minimum of the profile

4.2 Motivation

Theoretically, the functional relationship between an intensity CT image and a gradient US image is not obvious, thus a statistical similarity measure like normalized mutual information (NMI) should be more appropriate. However, although US images best enhance the boundaries between organs, they also convey an information on the tissues, as each of them diffuses the US waves its own way, in both intensity and frequency. So CR is somehow justified, especially with the preprocessing we presented above. We also chose CR against NMI for several reasons:

- CR looks more continuous than NMI (fig. 6); few local minima appear, even when subsampling: it is more precise, discriminative and robust [10].
- CR algorithm complexity is $O(N_x)$, where N_x is the number of overlapped grey levels in X, whereas NMI algorithm complexity is $O(N_xN_y)$ [8].
- CR continuous profile is particularly adapted to PB search algorithm, since Brent minimization is based on the fitting of a parabola onto the function curve [7].

4.3 2.5D Correlation Ratio

In the context of 2.5D US, the CR is computed as follows: for every rigid transform estimate, the CT volume is resliced in the plane of each US slice, using linear interpolation. Then the region of interest (ROI) defined in each US image is superimposed onto the corresponding CT slice. Finally, the CR is estimated on the set of pixels of the superimposed ROIs.

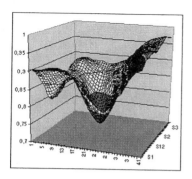 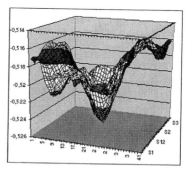

Fig. 6. CR (left) and NMI (right) profiles mapped along T_x and T_y while registering 2 images. Note the continuous aspect of CR and the unambiguous minimum

5 Preliminary Results and Discussion

5.1 Material and Methods

We worked on a single data set. The isotropic abdominal CT volume has 287x517x517 voxels, the voxel size being 0.6mm. Our experiments were carried out on a late acquisition CT, after iodine injection. Besides, for the use of our experiments, 100 US images (axial and longitudinal) of the right kidney were acquired with a localized calibrated echographic probe, through anterior access. Those images are then resized to match CT voxel size. In the final protocol, each registration will be carried out on only 5 slices of various orientations out of the whole set.

The accuracy study consists in performing 2 series of 10 registrations: on the one hand, by fixing the IA and changing the set of 5 US slices to match; on the other hand, by computing a new IA at each attempt, while keeping the same set of slices. Every IA is determined by the user from the choice of 4 points at the axial and lateral extremities of the kidney.

From our previous study [3] we have a "Bronze" Standard (BS) transform based on ICP matching, and segmented US and CT meshes. The quality of the solution is evaluated by the distance of the registered CT mesh to the BS CT mesh, and the difference between their gravity centers and their major axes inclinations.

5.2 Results

The registrations took on average 80s[1]. The algorithm appeared stable since a second matching pass kept the kidney in place. Table 1 shows matching statistics between the CT mesh transformed by our algorithm and the CT mesh obtained by the BS transform. *D(CT,BS)* (mm) shows the distance of the CT mesh to the BS mesh. *Δ Center* (mm) and *Δ Inclination* (°) are the differences between gravity centers and major axis inclinations. The choice of the criteria will be discussed later. Generally the IA sets the kidney at about 10mm in translation and 10° in inclination from the solution. For

---

[1] Tests performed on a Pentium IV 1.7GHz

example, with IA n°1 we obtained: 12.3mm±2.6 ; 9.6mm ; 9.0°. With 1mm to 6mm error we can say that every registration has succeeded, except n°13 and n°17 whose position and orientation hardly improved.

Table 1. Matching statistics when the IA is constant and when the set of slices is fixed

Constant IA				Constant set of slices			
Nb	D(CT,BS)	Δ Cent.	Δ Inclin.	Nb	D(CT,GS)	Δ Cent.	Δ Inclin.
1	5.6+/-2.1	2.7	4.1	11	3.7+/-1.3	1.3	4.3
2	6.8+/-2.0	3.2	6.7	12	3.2+/-0.8	2.9	1.5
3	5.2+/-1.5	3.2	1.3	13	8.8+/-2.5	5.7	10.5
4	6.2+/-1.8	4.0	5.3	14	5.7+/-2.0	4.0	5.3
5	5.8+/-1.8	2.3	9.5	15	6.7+/-2.6	5.1	8.2
6	6.0+/-2.0	4.3	4.7	16	6.0+/-1.3	5.8	3.2
7	4.1+/-1.1	2.7	5.5	17	11.9+/-4.8	8.1	6.4
8	5.1+/-1.1	3.4	5.2	18	6.5+/-2.1	5.0	7.6
9	5.1+/-1.9	3.0	5.4	19	6.2+/-1.6	5.6	6.0
10	3.7+/-0.9	2.1	2.9	20	5.4+/-0.9	4.1	4.3

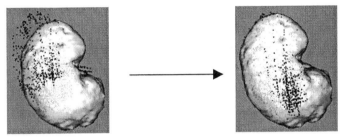

Fig. 7. Illustration of registration n°1 showing the US (black) and CT (white) meshes.

5.3 Discussion

We chose to compare homogeneous data, instead of computing the distance between the transformed CT mesh and the US cloud of points, as the bare information of an average distance between two sets of points does not appear relevant. To illustrate that, fig. 7 shows the result of matching n°1, which is visually very good. However, the distance of the US points to the IA-transformed CT mesh was 3.1mm±2.4 while the distance to the registered mesh was no smaller than 2.9mm±2.0. Furthermore, beside the quantitative evaluation of the solution, we also checked it visually, since the BS does not give an exact solution: in most cases the kidney position was acceptable for a further guiding procedure.

Although the results are satisfying in regard with accuracy, robustness and computation time, we must bear in mind that they highly depend on the choice of slices, the manual ROI, the manual IA and the search interval. The two failure cases were due to a bad IA. We expect to validate our method on other patient data sets in the following weeks. Anyway, the theoretical and practical difficulties in registering CT with US, particularly in terms of patient-dependent parameters settings, lead us to think that our method should be part of a higher-level algorithm that would also involve elastic registration, or the combination of rigid matching and deformable contour fitting, and certainly a minimal user intervention.

References

1. Czerwinski, R.N., Jones, D.L., and O'Brien, W.D., Detection of Lines and Boundaries in Speckle Images – Application to Medical Ultrasound, IEEE Transactions on Medical Imaging, 18(2):126-136, February 1999
2. Jenkinson, M., and Smith, S., A Global Optimization Method for Robust Affine Registration of Brain Images, Medical Image Analysis, 5(2):143-156, June 2001
3. Leroy, A., Mozer, P., Payan, Y., Richard, F., Chartier-Kastler, E., and Troccaz, J., Percutaneous Renal Puncture: Requirements and Preliminary Results, Surgetica'02, 303-309, 2002
4. Maes, F., Collignon, A., Vandermeulen, D., Marchal, G., and Suetens, P., Multimodality Image Registration by Maximization of Mutual Information, IEEE Transactions on Medical Imaging, 16(2):187-198
5. Maes, F., Vandermeulen, D., and Suetens, P., Comparative Evaluation of Multiresolution Optimization Strategies for Multimodality Registration by Maximization of Mutual Information, Medical Image Analysis, 3(4):373-386, 1999
6. Penney, G.P., Blackall, J.M., Hamady, M.S., Sabharwal, T., Adam, A., and Hawkes, D.J., Registration of Freehand 3D Ultrasound and Magnetic Resonance Liver Images, Medical Image Analysis, 8(1):81-91, January 2004
7. Press, W.H., Flannery, B.P., Teukolsky, S.A., and Vetterling, W.T., Numerical Recipes in C: The Art of Scientific Computing, Cambridge University Press, 1992
8. Roche, A., Malandain, G., Pennec, X., and Ayache, N., The Correlation Ratio as a New Similarity Measure for Multimodal Image Registration, MICCAI'98, 1115-1124, 1998
9. Roche, A., Pennec, X., Malandain, G., and Ayache, N., Rigid Registration of 3D Ultrasound with MR Images: a New Approach Combining Intensity and Gradient, IEEE Transactions on Medical Imaging, 20(10):1038-1049, October 2001
10. Sarrut, D. and Miguet, S. Similarity Measures for Image Registration, European Workshop on Content-Based Multimedia Indexing, p. 263-270. IHMPT-IRIT, Toulouse, France, 1999
11. Studholme, C., Hill, D.L.G., and Hawkes, D.J., Automated 3-D Registration of MR and CT Images of the Head, Medical Image Analysis, 1(2):163-175, 1996
12. Wells, W.M., Viola, P., Atsumi, H., Nakajima, S., and Kikinis, R., Multi-modal Volume Registration by Maximization of Mutual Information, Medical Image Analysis, 1(1):35-51, March 1996

Improved Non-rigid Registration of Prostate MRI

Aloys du Bois d'Aische[1,2,3], Mathieu De Craene[1,2,3], Steven Haker[2],
Neil Weisenfeld[2,3], Clare Tempany[2], Benoit Macq[1], and Simon K. Warfield[2,3]

[1] Communications and Remote Sensing Laboratory Université catholique de
Louvain, Louvain-la-Neuve, Belgium
[2] Surgical Planning Laboratory, Department of Radiology, Brigham and Women's
Hospital, Havard Medical School, Boston MA, USA
[3] Computational Radiology Laboratory, Children's Hospital, Brigham and Women's
Hospital, Harvard Medical School, Boston MA, USA

Abstract. This paper introduces a fast non-rigid registration method
for aligning pre-operative 1.5 T MR images to intra-operative 0.5 T MR
images for guidance in prostate biopsy.

After the acquisition of both pre-operative 1.5 T and intra-operative 0.5
T, an intensity correction method is applied to the pre-operative images
to reduce the significant artifacts in the signal intensities due to the
presence of an endo-rectal coil. A fast manual segmentation of prostate in
both modalities is carried out to enable conformal mapping of the surface
of the pre-operative data to the intra-operative data. A displacement
field is estimated with a linear elastic inhomogeneous material model
using the surface displacements established by the conformal mapping.
We then use this as an initialization for a mutual information based
non-rigid registration algorithm to match the internal structures of the
prostate. This non-rigid registration is based on a finite element method
discretization using the mutual information metric with a linear elastic
regularization constraint. The registration is accelerated while preserving
accuracy by using an adaptive mesh based on the body-centered cubic
lattice and a significantly improved registration is achieved.

1 Introduction

Prostate cancer is a leading cause of morbidity and mortality. This cancer is currently diagnosed by transrectal guided needle biopsy. In our institution, Magnetic Resonance Imaging (MRI) is used for intra-operative surgical navigation. MRI can clearly depict not only the prostate itself but also its substructure including the peripheral zone. However, the tumor foci can be better localized and identified on the pre-operative 1.5-T MRI than on the 0.5-T used for surgical navigation. Prostate shape changes appear between images caused by different patient positions before and during surgery. For this reason, the development of fast and accurate registration algorithms to fuse pre-operative and intra-operative data in the operating room is a challenging problem.

C. Barillot, D.R. Haynor, and P. Hellier (Eds.): MICCAI 2004, LNCS 3216, pp. 845–852, 2004.

Although rigid registration methods for the prostate have been presented [2,5], few non-rigid registration methods for this application are present in the literature. At our institution, we have used alternative methods in the past [3,8,7]. Bharatha et al.[3] presented an alignment strategy utilizing surface matching with an inhomogeneous material model. The surfaces of both segmented pre-operative and intra-operative MR images were registered using an active surface algorithm. Then the volumetric deformations were inferred from the surface deformations using a finite element model and applied to the pre-operative image. Later, the active surface step was replaced by a conformal mapping strategy [1]. More recently, we proposed a mutual information based deformation strategy to register multi-modality data [7].

Furthermore, the quality of tetrahedral meshes became an important issue to ensure a good convergence of FEM registration methods. Indeed, avoiding flat tetrahedrons so-called slivers can lead to better accuracy and stability of the numerical solutions. A broad range of strategies permits to refine adaptive tetrahedral meshes and to keep better shaped elements. The Laplacian smoothing technique is one of the most frequently applied. This method changes the positions of nodes by solving the Laplacian equation to move interior nodes with given positions of the boundary nodes. The smoothing is iteratively repeated until the movement of the nodes goes lower than a specified threshold. If the Laplacian smoothing technique increases the quality of the mesh in average, some elements may be more distorted. Other optimization methods have been proposed to optimize the element with respect to a specific cost function [4,9]. Recently, a body-centered cubic (BCC) based lattice offering a nice compromise between the density of the lattice and the number of nodes has been developped [14]. The elements composing this mesh may be divided into finer elements of same shape to adapt the object to mesh without moving nodes.

The new registration algorithm improves upon the surface to surface matching previously proposed by using an accelerated robust mutual information based volumetric registration. High speed and fidelity is achieved through an adaptive body-centered cubic lattice based meshing. Together, these methods enable a fast and accurate alignment of pre-operative and intra-operative MRI.

2   Registration Strategy

The mapping from the space of one image to another image is defined by a transformation model. We used a volumetric tetrahedral mesh to approximate the transformation which is parameterized by the displacements at each vertex of the mesh. The vertices displacements, derived from image based forces, are propagated to any point of the fixed image volume using the shape (basis) functions of the element containing this point. The finite element framework provides a broad family of elements and associated shape functions.

The registration strategy is divided into five steps. After the acquisition of both pre-operative and intra-operative images, an intensity correction has to be applied. After a manual segmentation of both images, the surface of the pre-operative prostate image is deformed to map onto the surface of the intra-operative data. The deformation field is then inferred into the whole volume. Finally, a mutual information based deformation method is applied to map the internal structures of the prostate.

2.1   Acquisition

Although 0.5 T T2-weighted images provide good visualization of the gland, 1.5 T imaging with endorectal coil provides better spatial resolutions and contrast. More precisely, the ability to visualize the substructure of the prostate is improved. Pre-treatement 1.5 T images provide detail, allowing accurate definition of the gland, its margins, and in most cases, the tumor, all of which are useful for complete treatment planning. It should be noted that of all modalities, MR imaging of the prostate provides the most optimal imaging not only of the gland and its adjacent structures, but importantly, of its substructure [3].

The 1.5 T fast spin echo MR-images were acquired using an endorectal coil with integrated pelvic phased multi-coil array. The intra-operative imaging was performed in the open-configuration 0.5 T MR Interventionnal Magnetic Resonance Therapy scanner. The typical acquisition times were 6 minutes.

2.2   Intensity Correction

Acquisition of pre-operative images using an endorectal coil resulted in significant intensity non-uniformity throughout the images acquired. Our experience has been that such an artifact can have a negative impact on the registration process [7]. In order to solve this problem, a retrospective correction method based on entropy minimization was employed. From the method described in [12] we developed an adaptive algorithm using a multi-resolution framework for speed and stability, to help accomodate the significant magnitude of the artifact in the images under study.

2.3   Transformation Model

We implemented the crystalline adaptive mesh based on the body-centered cubic lattice. The method was first proposed by [14]. The basic resolution of tetrahedrons is created by splitting two interlaced regular grids of hexahedrons. The mesh is then refined in specific regions of interest, as surfaces or specific organs, without loss of quality for the elements. The finer resolutions are obtained by dividing the principal tetrahedrons in eight children of same shape and quality. Specific patterns are then used to bind different resolutions. Our algorithm obeys the five following steps:

To obtain a new resolution, do at the current resolution:

Step-1. Find the neighbors of each tetrahedron by a search in the children of the neighbors of the father element at the previous resolution.

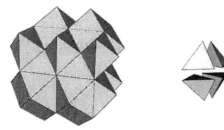

Fig. 1. The first resolution is based on a body-centered cubic lattice. The basic resolution of tetrahedrons is created by splitting two interlaced regular grids of hexahedrons.

Step-2. Search and mark which tetrahedrons have to be refined into 8 children (Figure 2-2) following a given criterion (curvature, edge, variance or other criterions).

Step-3. Complete the topology. Indeed if the neighboring tetrahedrons of the current one have to be split, mark that this current tetrahedron must be refined to avoid floating nodes.

Step-4. Bind the resolutions by labeling the tetrahedrons following patterns 3 to 5 (Figure 2) to avoid floating nodes. The father of these tetrahedrons should obey pattern 2 to keep a good quality ratio and avoid flat elements. Otherwise we return to the coarser resolutions to transform the ancestors of the current tetrahedrons into a pattern 2 and apply steps 2 to 4 again.

Step-5. Create the nodes and elements of the new resolution following the labels given during steps 2 to 4.

This mesh generation allows to fit the region of interest without loss of quality of the tetrahedrons. Furthermore, the choice of refinement criterion is free. Finally, we implemented the mesh generator within the ITK framework [11].

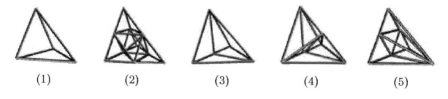

(1)	(2)	(3)	(4)	(5)

Fig. 2. The five possible patterns. A tetrahedron a one resolution (1) may be split into a pattern (2). The other patterns (3-5) bind the new resolution to the previous one.

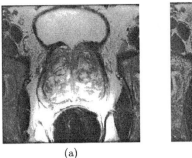
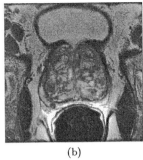

(a)   (b)

Fig. 3. Intensity correction results. The pre-operative image (a) was acquired using an endorectal coil resulting in significant intensity non-uniformity throughout the image. This image underwent an intensity correction based on entropy minimization (b).

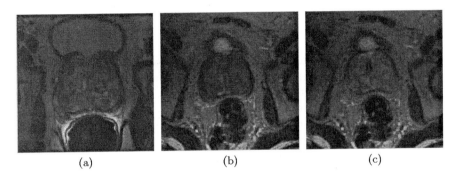

(a)   (b)   (c)

Fig. 4. Results of the surface based registration matching. The pre-operative image (a) has been manually segmented before the surgery and registered to the segmented intra-operative image (b). The result has been overlaid onto the intra-operative image for better visualization (c).

2.4   Registration Using Image Based Forces

First, an affine registration process has been applied to center the 0.5 T and 1.5 T segmented datasets and correct the scaling between images. Then a non-rigid registration driven by a conformal mapping technique [1] is applied to match the surface of the prostate from the pre-procedural image to the intra-procedural image. The volumetric displacement field is then inferred from the surface deformation field using the finite element method. The data scans are segmented using the 3D Slicer, a surgical simulation and navigation tool [10].

Finally, to refine the mapping between the internal structures of the prostate, we used a mutual information based [16,13] non-rigid registration method [6]. The finite element approximation of the transformation is regularized by the linear elastic energy

$$C(I_1, I_2) = MI(I_1, I_2) + \frac{\alpha}{2} \cdot u^t K u \tag{1}$$

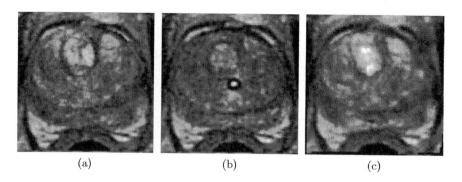

(a)   (b)   (c)

Fig. 5. Results of the mutual information based registration. The pre-operative image after surface registration (a) has then been registered to the intra-operative image (b) using our mutual information based registration method. We can observe in the resulting image (c) that the internal substructure aligns well with the intra-operative image.

where K is the stiffness matrix associated with the volumetric mesh [17], u the vector of vertex displacements and α is a weighting factor to balance the action of the mutual information term.

The optimization technique used is the Simultaneous Perturbation Stochastic Approximation (SPSA) firstly introduced by Spall [15]. SPSA has attracted considerable attention for solving optimization problems for which it is impossible or time consuming to directly obtain a gradient of the objective function with respect to the parameters being optimized. SPSA is based on a highly efficient gradient approximation that relies only on two evaluations of the objective function to be optimized regardless of the number of parameters being optimized and without requiring an explicit knowledge of the gradient of the objective function.

3   Results

Pre-operative 1.5 T endorectal coil images were acquired for the supine patient and intra-operative 0.5 T were acquired in the lithotomy position. The difference between positions let deformations appear. The images used were acquired in the Open Magnet System (Signa SP, GE Medical Systems, Milwaukee,WI).

The pre-operative prostate images were corrected in the gray-level domain. Figure 3 shows the prostate image before and after correction based on entropy minimization. The brightness artifact has been removed. The processing time is dependent of the machine and the size of the data. For a $256 \times 256 \times 60$ image, this process needs about 10 minutes but is made before surgery.

The following step is the segmentation and the surface registration of prostates in both modalities. The figure 4 presents a result for this step. The pre-operative prostate image (Figure 4-a) has been segmented to fit the segmented prostate of the intra-operative image (Figure 4-b). The result has been fused in the intra-operative image (Figure 4-c) for better visualization. This surface registration needs less than 90 seconds. While the pre-operative data can be segmented before the surgery, we need some more minutes to segment the prostate in the intra-operative images.

The last step is the mutual information based registration. Since we are mainly interested in capturing the deformations of the substructure inside the prostate, we use the segmentation of the intra-operative prostate as a mask to measure mutual information. Figure 5-a presents the pre-operative prostate after surface based registration, Figure 5-b the intra-operative image of the prostate and Figure 5-c the result after registration. This last step needs less than 2 minutes.

We placed a set of landmarks inside prostates. The minimum distance between landmarks after surface and after mutual information based registration is about 0.3 mm. The largest distance goes from 3.8 mm after surface registration to 2.5 after MI registration and the mean distance from 2.3 mm to 1.3mm for a voxel size of $0.9 \times 0.9 \times 2.5$mm.

4   Conclusions and Future Work

In the former section, our algorithm has been proven to estimate the deformation induced by different positions of the patient before and during prostate surgery. Prior information can be included in this registration strategy by using the adaptive mesh. This adaptation of the basis functions used to represent the dense deformation field is the main advantage of finite element meshes compared to radial basis functions. Pre-operative segmentations also enable to employ different material characteristics. Volumetric FEM meshes following the surfaces of the anatomical objects make possible the inclusion of statistical shape information in determined deformation patterns. Furthermore, other refinement strategies could be investigated. Refining only the mesh in elements with a high gradient of the mutual information would allow to improve the computation time.

Acknowledgments. Aloys du Bois d'Aische and Mathieu De Craene are working towards a Ph.D. degree with a grant from the Belgian FRIA. This investigation was also supported by the Region Wallone (MERCATOR grant), by a research grant from the Whitaker Foundation and by NIH grants R21 MH67054, R01 LM007861, P41 RR13218, R33 CA99015, P01 CA67165 and R01 AG 19513-03.

References

1. S. Angenent, S. Haker, A. Tannenbaum, and R. Kikinis. On the laplace-beltrami operator and brain surface flattening. *IEEE Trans Med Imaging*, 18:700–711, 1999.
2. R. Bansal, L. Staib, Z. Chen, A. Rangarajan, J. Knisely, R. Nath, and J.S. Duncan. Entropy-based, multiple-portal-to-3dct registration for prostate radiotherapy using iteratively estimate segmentation. In *MICCAI*, pages 567–578, September 1999.

3. A. Bharatha, M. Hirose, N. Hata, S. Warfield, M. Ferrant, K. Zou, E. Suarez-Santana, J. Ruiz-Azola, A. D'Amico, R. Cormack, F. Jolesz, and C. Tempany. Evaluation of three-dimensional finite element-based deformable registration of pre- and intra-operative prostate imaging. *Med. Phys.*, 2001.

4. J. Cabello, R. Lohner, and O.P. Jacquote. A variational method for the optimization of two- and three-dimensional unstructured meshes. Technical report, Technical Report AIAA-92-0450, 1992.

5. L. Court and L. Dong. Automatic registration of the prostate for computed-tomography-guided radiotherapy. *Med Phys.*, October 2003.

6. M. De Craene, A. du Bois d Aische, I. Talos, M. Ferrant, P. Black, F. Jolesz, R. Kikinis, B. Macq, and S. Warfield. Dense deformation field estimation for brain intra-operative images registration. In *SPIE Medical imaging*, 2004.

7. M. De Craene, A. du Bois d'Aische, N. Weisenfeld, S. Haker, B. Macq, and S. Warfield. Multi-modal non-rigid registration using a stochastic gradient approximation. In *ISBI*, 2004.

8. Matthieu Ferrant, Arya Nabavi, Benoit Macq, Peter McL. Black, Ferenc A. Jolesz, Ron Kikinis, and Simon K. Warfield. Serial Registration of Intraoperative MR Images of the Brain. *Med Image Anal*, 6(4):337–359, 2002.

9. L. Freitag, T. Leurent, P. Knupp, and D. Melander. Mesquite design: Issues in the development of a mesh quality improvement toolki. In *Proceedings of the 8th Intl. Conference on Numerical Grid Generation in Computational Field Simulation*, pages 159–168, 2002.

10. D. Gering, A. Nabavi, R. Kikinis, W.E.L Grimson, N. Hata, P. Everett, F. Jolesz, and W. Wells. An integrated visualization system for surgical planning and guidance using image fusion and interventional imaging. In *MICCAI*, 1999.

11. L. Ibanez, W. Schroeder, L. Ng, and Cates. *The ITK Software Guide*. the Insight Consortium, http://www.itk.org.

12. J.-F. Mangin. Entropy minimization for automatic correction of intensity non-uniformity. In *Mathematical Methods in Biomedical Image Analysis*, pages 162–169, Los Alamitos, California, 2000. IEEE Computer Society.

13. D. Mattes, D.R. Haynor, H. Vesselle, T.K. Lewellen, and W. Eubank. Pet-ct image registration in the chest using free-form deformations. *IEEE Transaction on Medical Imaging*, 22(1):120–128, January 2003.

14. N. Molino, R. Bridson, J. Teran, and R. Fedkiw. A crystalline, red green strategy for meshing highly deformable objects with tetrahedra. In *12th International Meshing Roundtable*, pages 103–114, Sandia National Laboratories, september 2003.

15. J. C. Spall. Overview of the simultaneous perturbation method for efficient optimization. *http://techdigest.jhuapl.edu/td/td1904/spall.pdf*, *Hopkins APL Technical Digest*, 19:482–492, 1998.

16. P. Viola and W.M. Wells III. Alignment by maximization of mutual information. In *Fifth Int. Conf. on Computer Vision*, pages 16–23, 1995.

17. O. C. Zienkiewicz and R. L. Taylor. *The Finite Element Method, Volume 1, Basic Formulation and Linear Problems*. McGraw-Hill, London, 4th edition, 1989.

Landmark-Guided Surface Matching and Volumetric Warping for Improved Prostate Biopsy Targeting and Guidance

Steven Haker, Simon K. Warfield, and Clare M.C. Tempany

Surgical Planning Laboratory
Harvard Medical School and Brigham and Women's Hospital
75 Francis St., Boston, MA 02115 USA
haker@bwh.harvard.edu

Abstract. We present a composite method for landmark-guided surface matching and volumetric non-rigid registration, with an application to prostate biopsy. The two-step method, based primarily on finite element and thin-plate spline techniques, consists of a boundary matching process, followed by a volumetric warping step. In practice, the boundary matching method allows for registration of anatomical surfaces, such as prostate gland capsules, in a way that is bijective, *i.e.* one-to-one and onto. The novelty of this approach is that it allows for the exact matching of pre-specified corresponding landmark points on the two surfaces to be matched. The second step, volumetric warping, is presented as an extension of our previous work in prostate registration, having been improved to address the problem of non-bijectivity (the "flipping" of tetrahedra) which can result from the linear-elastic modelling of the deformation. We discuss the use of our method for the registration of pre-operative magnetic resonance (MR) imaging for improved targeting and visualization during MR-guided prostate biopsy. Although presented within the context of prostate MR image registration, our composite surface matching and volumetric registration method has general applicability to other organs and imaging modalities such as CT and ultrasound.

1 Introduction

For the male population of the United States, prostate cancer (PC) is the most common non-cutaneous cancer, affecting one in six in his lifetime, and is the second most common cause of cancer death. Prostate cancer takes the life of nearly 40,000 men annually in the U.S., and the American Cancer Society predicted that 220 900 new cases would occur in the in 2003 [1]. In light of the generally aging populations of industrialized nations, prostate cancer will continue to be a major medical and socioeconomic problem.

Prostate cancer is commonly diagnosed by transrectal ultrasound-guided needle biopsy (TRUS), prompted by either an elevated prostate-specific serum antigen (PSA) level or a palpable nodule. TRUS does not target specific lesions, but rather uses a sextant approach, attempting to sample six representative locations

C. Barillot, D.R. Haynor, and P. Hellier (Eds.): MICCAI 2004, LNCS 3216, pp. 853–861, 2004.
© Springer-Verlag Berlin Heidelberg 2004

in the gland. Studies have shown that in more than 20% of cancers, at least two biopsy sessions were required to diagnose the tumor, and it is not yet clear how many samples (per session) are necessary to reach a diagnosis. Although increasing the number of random TRUS biopsy samples yields a marginal improvement in detection rate [16,9,18], only a very small fraction of the gland is sampled with even a dozen needle placements. Thus, it is unlikely that simply increasing the number of samples taken will solve the problem. Clearly, an imaging method capable of demarcating the regions of the gland most likely to harbor cancerous tissue could result in a diminished false negative rate of needle biopsy.

Standard MR imaging can clearly define the prostate and its sub-structures, as well as the rectum, neurovascular bundles and urethra. Endo-rectal coil MRI at 1.5 Tesla (1.5T), combined with a multi-coil array, is the method in routine clinical use for staging prostate cancer [17]. Further, several new MR imaging methods have recently shown promise in their ability to detect and characterize prostate cancer. These include MRSI (spectroscopy), T2maps, Line Scan Diffusion Imaging, and MR imaging with dynamic intravenous contrast enhancement (gadolinium). Indeed, we have performed a preliminary study, demonstrating the effectiveness of integration of multiple pre-operative MR image sets into a single image, which we call a summary statistical map [6], with validation based on the biopsy sample pathology.

The goal of this research is to increase the information content of images used by the physician during prostate biopsy, through registration of pre-operative MR imaging with intra-operative imaging. In this way, needle placement can be targeted specifically to those locations most likely to contain cancer. Although presented here in the context of MR-guided prostate biopsy, the methods presented are applicable to ultrasound-guided biopsy as well, and to other procedures, such as CT-guided radiation therapies.

2   Methods

Here we describe our method of prostate image registration. The prostate, being composed of soft tissue, can undergo significant shape changes between different imaging sessions. We have found, for example, that significant prostate shape changes occur between pre-operative 1.5T endorectal coil imaging, in which the patient is supine, and intra-operative 0.5T imaging, during which the patient is in the lithotomy position. This shape change is likely the result of changes in patient position and rectal filling necessitated by the procedures. We have performed a quantitative analysis of this deformation, reported in [14]. For this reason, we have pursued the development of non-rigid registration methods. We have performed [3] a preliminary study to develop and evaluate a finite element based non-rigid registration system. The method was an extension of an algorithm developed for brain registration [10]. The methods described here further extend, refine and improve upon this work.

The method involves the following steps general steps: 1.) A 3D tetrahedral model of the entire prostate is created from segmented pre-operative 1.5T images; 2.) the boundary surface of the prostate capsule is extracted from this tetrahedral mesh and is registered to a corresponding capsule surface obtained from segmented intra-operative images; 3.) the surface point matches from step 2 are used as boundary conditions when solving a finite element-based system of evolution equations which models the volumetric deformation within the gland; 4.) the final volumetric deformation field from step 3 step is used to interpolate pre-operative imaging data. We describe these steps in greater detail below.

2.1   Creation of a Tetrahedral Model of the Pre-operative Prostate

The starting point of our method is a segmentation of the prostate gland from high-quality pre-operative MR imaging. This segmentation may be obtained by contouring of the gland by hand, or by an automated segmentation method. The surface is extracted as a triangulated surface using the marching cubes algorithm. To create a tetrahedral mesh within this capsular surface, we register to it a high-quality meshing of the unit ball $\{(x, y, z) \mid x^2 + y^2 + z^2 \leq 1\}$. The procedure for this registration is the same as is used to register the pre-operative prostate to the intra-operative prostate, *i.e.* a surface matching procedure followed by a volumetric warp.

2.2   Boundary Surface Matching Using Landmark Points

Our original method for boundary matching [3,10] used an "active surface model." This method moved one surface toward the other through space, according to a specified attraction force between the surfaces, balanced by an internal energy force used to keep the moving surface smooth and topologically consistent. Difficulties arise from the need to balance these forces, the requirement of a bijective surface matching (a problem in practice), and from the desire for operating-room compatible speed.

We have now improved the speed and robustness of the algorithm by replacing with a direct approach based on our work in the theory of conformal (angle-preserving) mappings [12,2] of surfaces with spherical topology. In this method the surface of the prostate capsule is modeled as a thin elastic sheet which conforms to the altered shape of the capsule as given by the intra-operative imaging. Regardless of the degree of shape deformation, or changes from convexity to concavity, the method yields a one to one mapping of one surface onto another. Further, the method has several inherent advantages over our earlier methods which make it more suitable for use in the operating room. In particular, the core of the algorithm requires only the solution of a pair of sparse linear systems of equations, and thus can be made to run quickly enough to be practical. Indeed, this is the sense in which the method is direct, as the matching from pre-operative surface to inter-operative surface does not require the calculation of intermediate sets of points moving through space. The method also lends itself well to multi-processor parallelization, and standard parallel versions of linear solvers can be used to reduce the solution time significantly.

In order to find a conformal mapping u, we need to solve Laplace's equation,

$$\nabla^2 u = 0, \tag{1}$$

on the triangulated surface to be registered. Here ∇^2 is the Laplace-Beltrami operator, a generalization of the standard second-order Laplacian operator. The trick is to specify a condition, similar to a boundary condition, which results in a u which is conformal. See [12,2] for details. Although the conformal mapping method produces a matching of surfaces, it is not possible to use conformal mapping alone to match surfaces while, at the same time, requiring that the mapping take a general number of pre-specified landmark points on one surface to the corresponding points on the other. What we have now developed is a method which augments the conformal mapping with a simple thin-plate spline technique [4] to produce a mapping with the desired point-matching property. The use of this method allows for far more control over the final surface match. We typically use as landmark points the 6 points of intersection of the major axes of rotation of the prostate surface with the surface itself. See Fig. 1.

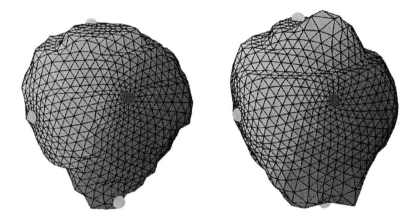

Fig. 1. Two prostate surfaces. The surfaces have been mapped to the sphere and re-triangulated in the same way to establish point correspondence. The small spheres represent landmark points which were matched during the registration process.

To see how this is done, let u_1 and u_2 be conformal mappings from two surfaces to the unit sphere, and let w_1 and w_2 be the corresponding conformal mappings to the plane obtained by composing u_1 and u_2 with stereographic projection, a standard map projection used in cartography. Let s be the standard 2D thin-plate spline mapping that takes a specified set of landmark points in the planar image of w_1 to the corresponding points in the image of w_2. Then $z := w_2^{-1} \circ s \circ w_1$ is a landmark-matching mapping from one surface to the other. Here $\circ$ represents composition of functions. In practice, the second surface is the usually the sphere itself, with phantom "landmark" points such as the poles, $(0, 0, \pm 1)$, etc. specified thereon. We can map any prostate surface to the sphere this way, and thus any prostate surface to any other, using compositions of mappings to the sphere and the inverses of these mappings, all the while matching corresponding landmark points. See Fig. 1.

When mapping to the sphere, we use the resulting z mapping as an initial condition for the geometric heat equation

$$\frac{\partial}{\partial t} z = \nabla^2 z, \tag{2}$$

while fixing the matched landmark points and re-projecting the evolving surface back to the sphere. This is iterated until near convergence, and helps to produce a smoother, harmonic mapping. Although [11] suggest the use of this type of *Jacobi relaxation* for finding conformal mappings to the sphere, it is in general too slow to be practical [15], and in fact global long-term solutions to (2) do not in general exist for arbitrary initial conditions and surfaces [19]. The reason it is practical for our use is that we have an initial condition that is already close to the final harmonic mapping, due to the use of our conformal mapping technique and perhaps to the intimate relation between thin plate splines and the bi-harmonic equation $\nabla^4 z = 0$.

We note, as an important caveat, that as with standard thin-plate spline methods, we have no guarantee that the final mapping produced will be bijective. We can report however, that in the more than 100 prostate cases that we have processed this way, we have not found the method to fail to produce a bijective mapping.

2.3   Background on Volumetric Warping

Given two prostate surfaces, obtained from segmentations of pre-operative and intra-operative images, we may map them to the sphere using the surface warping technique described above, while sending landmark points to pre-specified locations. By interpolating the resulting spherical maps at the vertices of a standard triangulation of the sphere, we can effectively re-triangulate the original prostate surfaces in a consistent manner, thereby providing a point-by-point registration of the surfaces. We use a spherical triangulation which is the boundary of the high-quality tetrahedral meshing of the unit ball, as mentioned in sub-section 2.1. See Fig. 1. We now describe how we use this surface matching to obtain a volumetric registration of the entire interior of the prostate gland.

As mentioned above, in previous work we have performed [3] a preliminary study to develop and evaluate a finite element based non-rigid registration system. The method was an extension of an algorithm developed for brain registration [10]. In this model, the prostate tissue is considered as a linear elastic material. The second-order partial differential equation governing the 3D deformation field p of the material under this model is

$$\nabla^2 p + \frac{1}{1 - 2\nu} \nabla \operatorname{div} p = 0 \tag{3}$$

subject to our specified boundary conditions. The use of the above equation has, of course, been the subject of investigations by several other research groups, see in particular the pioneering work [7] for an excellent discussion and application to medical image registration. Here *Poisson's ratio* ν is constant for a given tissue type, and governs the elastic properties of the deforming material. In [3] we reported that values of $\nu = 0.2$ kPa for the central gland and $\nu = 0.4$ kPa for the peripheral zone produced satisfactory results.

The tetrahedral mesh within the prostate surface defines the set of finite elements used to discretize a variational form of the partial differential equation above. The volumetric deformation field is found by solving for the displacement field that minimizes an associated energy. The finite element technique reduces the problem to the solution of a sparse system of linear equations that can be solved for the unknown displacements at each interior vertex.

2.4   Improving the Volumetric Warping

We have experienced some problems in practice using the basic method for volumetric warping described above. Specifically, we have found that tetrahedra can "flip" *i.e* turn inside out in certain cases, and thereby yield a non-bijective registration. This is especially true when some portion of the deforming surface goes from being convex to concave. This may well be the case in practice, as the prostate consists of soft tissue, and the the patient may be scanned using an endo-rectal coil in one imaging session, and with no such coil in another. The reason for this appears to be that the well-known assumption of small deformation required in order for equation (3) to be valid is not being satisfied. Large deformations also cast doubt on the validity of the solution even when no tetrahedra flip.

To address this problem, we have incorporated the following simple technique. Let us suppose we have found the surface mapping between prostate capsules obtained by the conformal mapping and thin plate spline technique described above. Using the surface point correspondence, we align the surfaces with a rigid transformation to minimize the sum-of-squares distance between them. Let $s_1 = s_1(x, y, z)$ be the resulting surface mapping between the prostate capsules after rigid registration. Introduce an artificial time parameter t and create a sequence of $N + 1$ surfaces $s(x, y, x, t) = (1 - t) \times (x, y, z) + t \times s_1(x, y, z)$, for $t = 0, 1/N, 2/N, ..., 1$. We can choose N large enough so that the pointwise change in s from one time to another is small with respect to the size of the tetrahedra in the mesh. At each time $t = 0, 1, ..., (N - 1)/N$, we compute the volumetric warping using the method described in the previous sub-section with boundary conditions specified by the steps in s, arriving in the end with a boundary which is the target capsule surface. We emphasize that it is essential here to re-compute, after each iteration, the matrix associated with the linear system of equations obtained from the finite-element discretization of equation (3). For our application, we have found a value of $N = 20$ to be sufficient.

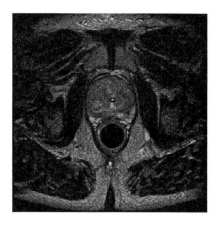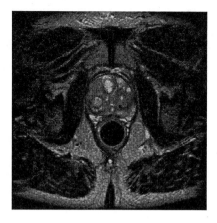

Fig. 2. On the left, an intra-operative 0.5T T2-weighted axial image of the prostate gland. On the right, within the gland, registered pre-operative 1.5T T2-weighted image data. Note the increased conspicuity of the prostate sub-structure; the urethra is not visible due to the absence of a Foley catheter.

In practice, we have found that the above technique eliminates the problem of tetrahedral flipping in all but the most extreme cases. The drawback, of course, is the increased computation time that is necessary.

2.5   Warping of Pre-operative Images

After the registration process is complete, we use the resulting mapping to interpolate the pre-operative MR image data into the space of the intra-operative images. Since our method only registers material inside the prostate capsule, we simply take as values outside the gland the data from the intra-operative images. See Fig. 2.

2.6   Rapid Solution of the System of Equations

In order for this strategy of obtaining a volumetric deformation field to be practical during surgery, we must be able to obtain the solution at a rate compatible with surgical decision making. Fortunately, since the heart of our algorithms involve the solution to linear systems of equations, there are many tools available within the scientific computing community which make this possible. In particular, we have investigated solving the system of linear equations on a set of parallel architectures. See [20] for details. We have recently experimented with both an inexpensive workstation, a Dell Precision 650n with dual 3.0 GHz Intel Xeon CPUs running Linux, and a cluster of such workstations connected by 100Mbps Fast Ethernet. This has enabled extremely rapid solution of the typical system of equations on inexpensive and widely available hardware, which holds out the possibility of widespread deployment of this technology. With such a set-up, we have found that the solution of (3) can be found in approximately 3 seconds, or $3 \times N$ seconds for the multi-step method of Subsection (2.4).

3   Results and Discussion

We regularly use the algorithm described in the above sections for registration of various MR prostate images, having done so on more than 100 cases to date. In particular, it is now run regularly as part of our MR-guided prostate biopsy procedure [13]. The mapping technique allows us to provide the physician with an integrated view of the intra-operative and high quality pre-operative imaging during the biopsy procedure. Fig. 2.

Although presented here for MR, the method has direct applicability to other less discriminating but widely used intra-operative imaging modalities such as CT and ultrasound, since the method does not require intensity information from within the target gland. We plan to test the algorithm's use for these modalities in the near future. Potential uses of the landmark-guided surface registration method include the registration of organs other than the prostate, and applications such as the creation of models of organ variability using principle component analysis. Finally, we mention that in the case where intra-operative images do contain information that might be useful for registration within the gland, we have experimented with using our method as an initial registration step to be improved through a mutual-information maximization process [8].

Acknowledgements. This work was funded by NIH grants R01 AG 19513-03 and P41 RR13218-06.

References

1. American Cancer Society. Cancer facts and figures. Atlanta GA, 2003.
2. Angenent S, Haker S, Tannenbaum A, Kikinis R. Laplace-Beltrami operator and brain surface flattening. IEEE Trans. On Medical Imaging, 1999; 18:700-711.
3. Bharatha A, Hirose M, Hata N, Warfield SK, Ferrant M, Zou KH, Suarez-Santana E, Ruiz-Alzola J, D'Amico A, Cormack R, Kikinis R, Jolesz FA, Tempany CM. Evaluation of three-dimensional finite element-based deformable registration of pre- and intra-operative prostate imaging. Med Phys 28: 2551-2560, 2001.
4. Bookstein FL. Size and shape spaces for landmark data in to dimensions (with discussion). Statist. Sci. 1 (1986), 181-242.
5. Brechbuhler C, Gerig G, Kubler O. Parametrization of closed surfaces for 3-D shape description. CVGIP: Image Under 61 (1995) 154-170.
6. Chan I, Wells W III, Mulkern RV, Haker S, Zhang J, Zou KH, Maier SE, Tempany CMC. Detection of prostate cancer by integration of line-scan diffusion, T2-mapping and T2-weighted MR imaging; a multi-channel statistical classifier Med Phys, 30 (9) September 2003, pp. 2390-2398.
7. Christensen, G. Deformable shape models for anatomy, Ph.D. thesis, University of Washington, 1994.
8. du Bois d'Aische A, De Craene M, Haker S, Weisenfeld N, Tempany CMC, Macq B, and Warfield SK. Improved nonrigid registration of prostate MRI, MICCAI 2004, submitted.
9. Epstein JI, Walsh PC, Sauvagerot J, et al. Use of repeat sextant and transition zone biopsies for assessing extent of prostate cancer. J Urol 158; 1886 1997.

10. Ferrant M, Nabavi A, Macq B, Jolesz FA, Kikinis R, and Warfield SK. 2001. Registration of 3-D intraoperative MR images of the brain using a finite-element biomechanical model. IEEE Trans Med Imaging 20 (12):1384-97.
11. Gu X, Wang Y, Chan T, Thompson P, Yau ST. Genus Zero Surface Conformal Mapping and Its Application to Brain Surface Mapping. IEEE Trans. Med. Image, vol. 23 (7), 2004.
12. Haker S, Angenent S, Tannenbaum A, Halle M, Kikinis R. Conformal surface parameterization for texture mappings. IEEE Trans. On Visualization and Computer Graphics, 2000 April-June.
13. Hata N, Jinzaki M, Kacher D, Cormack R, Gering D, Nabavi A, Silverman SG, D'Amico AV, Kikinis R, Jolesz FA, Tempany CMC. MRI-guided prostate biopsy using surgical navigation software: device validation and feasibility. Radiology, 220:263-268, 2001.
14. Hirose M, Bharatha A, Hata N, Zou K, Warfield S, Cormack R, D'Amico A, Kikinis R, Jolesz F, Tempany C. Quantitative MR imaging assessment of prostate gland deformation before and during MR imaging-guided brachytherapy, Acad. Rad., 9, 8, pp. 906-912. 2002.
15. Press W, Teukolsky S, Vetterling W and Flannery B. Numerical Recipes in C: The Art of Scientific Computing, 2nd Edition, Cambridge University Press, Cambridge U.K., 1992.
16. Rabbani R, Stroumbakis N, Kava BR, Incidence and clinical significance of false negative sextant prostate biopsies. J Urol 1998; 159: 1247.
17. Seltzer SE, Getty DJ, Tempany CMC, Pickett RM, Schnall MD, McNeil BJ, Swets JA. Staging Prostate cancer with MR imaging: A combined radiologist-computer system. Radiology 1997; 202: 219-226.
18. Stroumbakis N, Cookson MS, Reuter V. et al. Clinical significance of repeat sextant biopsies in prostate cancer patients. Urology Suppl 49; 113 1997.
19. Struwe M. On the evolution of harmonic mappings of Riemannian surfaces. Comment. Math. Helv. 60 (1985), no. 4, 558-581.
20. Warfield S K, Ferrant M, Gallez X, Nabavi A, Jolesz F, and Kikinis R. Real-Time Biomechanical Simulation of Volumetric Brain Deformation for Image Guided Neurosurgery. In SC 2000: High Performance Networking and Computing Conference; 2000 Nov 4-10; Dallas, USA.

Improved Regional Analysis of Oxygen-Enhanced Lung MR Imaging Using Image Registration

Josephine H. Naish[1], Geoffrey J.M. Parker[1], Paul C.Beatty[1], Alan Jackson[1], John C. Waterton[2], Simon S. Young[3], and Chris J. Taylor[1]

[1] Imaging Science and Biomedical Engineering, University of Manchester, Manchester, UK
[2] Global Sciences and Information, AstraZeneca, Alderley Park, Macclesfield,UK
[3] AstraZeneca R&D Charnwood, Bakewell Road, Loughborough, UK

Abstract. Oxygen enhanced MR imaging of the lung is a promising technique for monitoring a range of pulmonary diseases but regional analysis is hampered by lung motion and volume changes due to breathing. We have developed an image registration method to improve the quantitative regional analysis of both static and dynamic oxygen-enhanced pulmonary MRI. Images were acquired using a HASTE sequence at 1.5T for five normal volunteers alternately breathing air and 100% oxygen. Static images were used to calculate regional changes in relaxation rate between breathing air and oxygen which is directly related to the increase in the dissolved oxygen concentration. Dynamic scans were used to calculate regional maps of oxygen wash-in and wash-out time constants. The method provided significant improvements in the both the static and the dynamic analysis. This may provide improved information in the regional assessment of chronic obstructive lung diseases.

1   Introduction

Oxygen-enhanced MR imaging of the lung has been demonstrated in healthy volunteers and in patients with pulmonary diseases [1,2,3,4]. Molecular oxygen is paramagnetic and so acts as a contrast agent when dissolved in parenchymal plasma due to its effect on T_1. Breathing 100% oxygen results in an increase in the concentration of dissolved oxygen in the lung tissue producing a corresponding decrease in T_1 which can be detected as a regional signal intensity increase in a T_1-weighted image. Unlike hyperpolarized gas MRI, which visualizes directly the air spaces in the lung, oxygen-enhanced MRI provides an indirect assessment of lung ventilation that may also depend on available tissue surface area and oxygen clearance by the blood. The method has the advantage over hyperpolarized gas MRI of requiring little specialized equipment so being more straightforward to implement in a clinical setting.

While a number of studies have demonstrated regional ventilation using oxygen-enhanced MRI, a pixel-by-pixel analysis is made difficult by changes in size and shape of the lungs due to breathing. To date, little has been reported on characterizing regional time courses of oxygen wash-in and wash-out [5,6]. Breath-holding has been used in static ventilation studies [7,8] to overcome problems due to breathing motion but it can be uncomfortable for patients and it is difficult to perform in a reproducible manner. Various alternatives to breath-holding, designed to allow data acqisition during free

C. Barillot, D.R. Haynor, and P. Hellier (Eds.): MICCAI 2004, LNCS 3216, pp. 862–869, 2004.
© Springer-Verlag Berlin Heidelberg 2004

breathing, have also been suggested. These include time-averaging sets of images [2,5], retrospective respiratory gating by selecting images for which the diaphragm position matches [1,9], respiratory triggering [7,10] and correlation analysis [8,11]. In this study we have developed an image registration method to correct for breathing motion which leads to significant improvements in the determination of both regional oxygen induced changes in T_1 and in the time course of regional signal intensity change during oxygen wash-in and wash-out.

2   Methods

2.1   Imaging

Imaging was performed at 1.5T on five normal volunteers (non-smokers aged 30-39). A half Fourier single shot turbo spin-echo (HASTE) sequence was used with 68 phase encoding steps and inter-echo spacing of 4ms, 128 128 matrix, coronal section with slice thickness 10mm. Volunteers breathed air or 100% oxygen through an MR compatible Bain breathing system and tightly fitting face mask. Gas was supplied at 10l/min using a standard anaesthesia trolley.

Static T_1 measurements were performed using a saturation recovery HASTE sequence with nine saturation times (TS) between 100ms and 3.5s. Five images were collected for each saturation time to enable averaging over the cardiac cycle. Saturation recovery (SR) was chosen in preference to inversion recovery (IR) because of the shorter total imaging time (approximately 2.5min for the set of 45 images). Dynamic image acquisitions were performed using an IR HASTE sequence during oxygen wash-in and wash-out. An inversion time of 720ms was chosen to approximately null the signal while breathing air [3]. Dynamic images were acquired every 3.5s for a total of 200s and the gas supply was switched from medical air to 100% oxygen (or vice-versa) after the 10th image in the set.

2.2   Image Registration

During breathing the lung is deformed mainly in the longitudinal direction due to motion of the diaphragm and, to a lesser extent, expansion of the chest cage. The registration procedure that we have adopted is based on this observation and consists of two steps. The first step utilises an active shape model (ASM) [12] to allow an automated identification of the lung outline. An ASM combines a point distribution model (PDM) with an image search and enables the automatic detection of structures in a wide variety of both medical and non-medical images. In the second step the lung outline is registered to a reference using a 1D linear transformation.

The first ten images from a set of 116 dynamic scans (58 for oxygen wash-in and 58 for oxygen wash-out)were manually marked up to build the ASM. Ten points were manually marked along the diaphragm and a further twelve points were marked at landmarks around the lung outline; where possible these marked the intervertebral disks and the positions of the ribs. The ten points along the diaphragm were then re-sampled at equidistant points along the curve using an Akima spline interpolation [13]. The resulting set of 22 points for each of the ten images form the set of correspondences which are used to calculate the PDM. Over 99% of the variation in lung shape was described by the first two modes of variation of the PDM as illustrated in Fig. 1. The ASM search was used to locate the lung outline in the remaining 106 images in the dynamic set. An example search result is presented in Fig. 1.

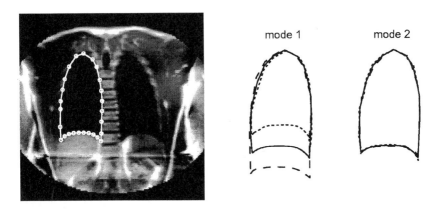

Fig. 1. An example image from a dynamic set showing the results of the active shape model search and the first two modes of variation of the active shape model. The solid line is the mean shape and the dashed and dotted lines are +2s.d and -2s.d respectively

The images were transformed onto a reference by re-sampling the lung outline at discrete horizontal pixel locations around the top edge of the lung and along the diaphragm and applying a simple linear transformation on each column of pixels. Signal intensity was sampled at off-pixel locations using linear interpolation and re-scaled according to the magnitude of the stretch to account for proton density variation during the breathing cycle.

The T_1 measurement SR HASTE images were registered by manually marking up all 45 images in each measurement set and transforming as described above. In this case it was not possible to build an ASM to minimize the user input because of the large variation in contrast between images with different TS.

2.3 Analysis

T_1 maps were produced from each set of 45 registered SR HASTE images by fitting on a pixel-by-pixel basis using an exponential of the form $S(TS) = A - B\exp(-TS/T_1)$ where $S(TS)$ is the pixel intensity at each TS and A and B are constants. Oxygen wash-in and wash-out times were calculated from the dynamic IR HASTE sets of images by fitting an exponential to the dynamic signal intensity both in regions of interest and on a pixel-by-pixel basis in a smoothed set of images.

3   Results

The ASM search successfully located the lung outline in all 116 dynamic images for three of the volunteers and in all but 3 of the 116 images for each of the other two volunteers. Virtually all of the shape variation is captured in the first mode, and this is mainly a simple linear stretch in the vertical direction as illustrated in Fig. 1.

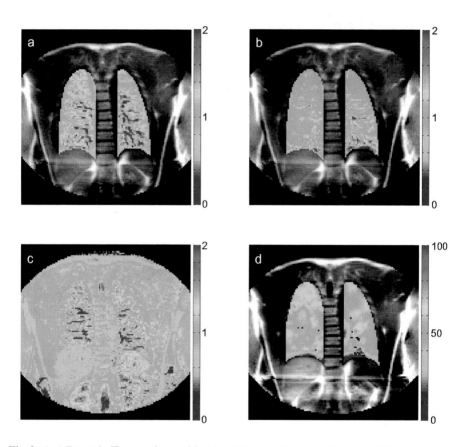

Fig. 2. a)-c) Example T_1 maps for a subject breathing medical air (a & c) and 100% oxygen (b). The maps in a & b are calculated using the full set of registered images and the map in c is calculated using a subset of images in which the right diaphragm position matches to ± 1 pixel (retrospective gating). d) Example regional uptake time map. The scales for all four maps are in units of s.

In Fig. 2a & b we present an example of matched T_1 maps for a volunteer breathing medical air and 100% oxygen. A reduction in T_1 on breathing oxygen is demonstrated across the whole of the lung. T_1 values averaged within the lung breathing air and oxygen are 1.27s and 1.08s respectively and are consistent with previously published values [2,14]. Figure 2c is a T_1 map calculated by selecting those images for which the

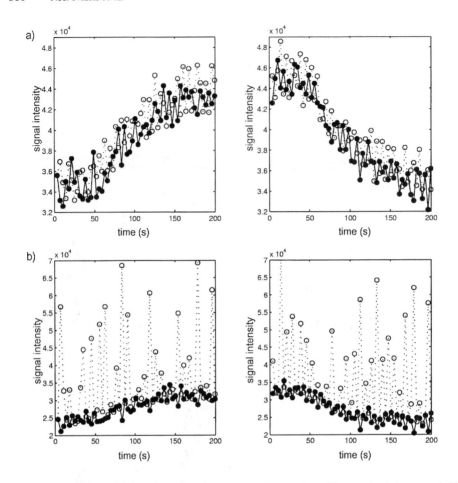

Fig. 3. Example dynamic wash-in and wash-out curves for a region of interest in a) the upper half of the right lung and b) the lower half of the right lung. The dotted lines (open symbols) are for raw images and the solid lines (filled symbols) are for registered images

right diaphragm matches to within 2 pixels (i.e. ± 1 pixel from the mean position in the subset of images), which effectively forms a retrospectively gated map. The T_1 map calculated from the registered set of images shows comparatively clearer structure and a reduction in breathing artefact. The contribution of dissolved oxygen to the relaxation rate depends linearly on its concentration [14]. The difference in relaxation rate between breathing air and 100% oxygen, $1/T_{1(\text{oxygen})} - 1/T_{1(\text{air})}$, is directly proportional to the additional dissolved oxygen on breathing 100% oxygen thus this technique allows a spatial mapping of the relative regional distribution of additional dissolved oxygen.

Signal intensity time courses are plotted in Fig. 3 for regions of interest defined in the upper and lower halves of the right lung. Registration leads to a small improvement in the upper ROI seen as a reduction in noise of the solid lines compared to the dotted lines. A more dramatic improvement can be seen for the lower ROI which is much more affected by the movement of the diaphragm during breathing. The results of fitting an exponential to the dynamic signal intensity in order to obtain oxygen wash-in and wash-out time constants for a ROI encompassing the whole of the left or the right lung are presented in Table 1 for the five volunteers. The mean wash-in times for the right and left lungs were 57 ± 5s and 46 ± 14s. The mean wash-out times for the right and left lungs were 38 ± 14s and 38 ± 13s. An example regional wash-in time map, found by fitting the smoothed images on a pixel-by-pixel basis, is presented in Fig. 2d.

Table 1. Average wash-in and wash-out times in seconds for the right and left lungs of five normal volunteers

subject	wash-in right	wash-in left	wash-out right	wash-out left
1	53.7	46.9	31.8	34.0
2	58.7	21.9	27.0	37.7
3	65.1	50.4	40.9	31.0
4	54.5	50.6	61.5	61.2
5	53.2	62.1	29.7	27.0
mean(s.d.)	57(5)	46(14)	38(14)	38(13)

4   Discussion

We have demonstrated an image registration method which results in significant improvements in the regional analysis of oxygen enhanced lung MR imaging. The increase in concentration of oxygen dissolved in the lung tissue as a result of breathing 100% oxygen leads to a shortening of the parenchymal T_1. A regional determination of change in relaxation rate directly corresponds to the regional increase in concentration of dissolved oxygen. The image registration method used therefore allows a pixel-by-pixel determination of relaxation rate change and hence the relative regional increase in dissolved oxygen.

Regional dynamic oxygen wash-in and wash-out analysis is also improved by the use of registration, particularly in the lower region of the lung which is most affected by diaphragm motion. There is some evidence that the wash-in is heterogeneous across the lung even in normal volunteers as indicated in Fig. 2d. Longer wash-in time constants seem to be present in the upper lobes which is consistent with what might be expected for a supine subject. The average time constants as presented in Table 1 are longer than those reported by Hatabu et al [5], possibly as a result of differences in the breathing apparatus used. In common with Hatabu et al, we observe shorter wash-out times compared to wash-in, probably due to dissolved oxygen being carried from the lungs in the blood and removed by tissues in other parts of the body.

During breathing, the majority of the movement and volume change observed in the lung is as a result of the diaphragm motion with an additional smaller effect due to the expansion of the chest wall. This observation is also confirmed by the modes of variation of the ASM and led to the selection of a 1D linear model to describe the deformation. A limitation of this model is that it does not take account of movement out of the coronal plane, although this is expected to be small compared to the in-plane motion, and of limited significance due to the relatively large (10mm) slice thickness used. In the present study we have investigated slices positioned posteriorly, further limiting out of plane motion. Another limitation of our study is that in rescaling the pixel signal intensity according to the magnitude of the stretch we are assuming that the total proton density within the lung remains constant over a breathing cycle. This may not be a valid assumption and in fact we observe a tendency to over-correct which may be due to an increase in blood volume in the lung at maximum inhalation. Methods which rely on some form of respiratory gating are less affected by out-of-plane movement and changes in proton density but suffer from remaining motion artefacts due to some remaining differences in diaphragm position. In the case of retrospective gating there is also a considerable loss of temporal resolution. An improvement to our method may be to combine it with respiratory triggering which would result in a relatively small loss of temporal resolution.

5   Conclusions

We have demonstrated that by using image registration we can improve the regional determination of both the change in relaxation rate on breathing 100% oxygen and the rate of change of signal intensity on switching from air to 100% oxygen. This results in an improved understanding of the regional change in oxygen concentration and the oxygen wash-in and wash-out rates which may be important in the regional evaluation of chronic obstructive pulmonary diseases.

References

1. Edelman RR, Hatabu H, Tadamura E, Li W, and Prasad PV. Noninvasive assessment of regional ventilation in the human lung using oxygen-enhanced magnetic resonance imaging. *Nat Med*, 2(11):1236–9, 1996.
2. Chen Q, Jakob PM, Griswold MA, Levin DL, Hatabu H, and Edelman RR. Oxygen enhanced mr ventilation imaging of the lung. *Magma*, 7(3):153–61, 1998.
3. Ohno Y, Hatabu H, Takenaka D, Adachi S, Van Cauteren M, and Sugimura K. Oxygen-enhanced MR ventilation imaging of the lung: preliminary clinical experience in 25 subjects. *AJR Am J Roentgenol*, 177(1):185–94, 2001.
4. Ohno Y, Hatabu H, Takenaka D, Van Cauteren M, Fujii M, and Sugimura K. Dynamic oxygen-enhanced MRI reflects diffusing capacity of the lung. *Magn Reson Med*, 47(6):1139–44, 2002.
5. Hatabu H, Tadamura E, Chen Q, Stock KW, Li W, Prasad PV, and Edelman RR. Pulmonary ventilation: dynamic MRI with inhalation of molecular oxygen. *Eur J Radiol*, 37(3):172–8, 2001.
6. Muller CJ, Schwaiblmair M, Scheidler J, Deimling M, Weber J, Loffler RB, and Reiser MF. Pulmonary diffusing capacity: assessment with oxygen-enhanced lung MR imaging preliminary findings. *Radiology*, 222(2):499–506, 2002.

7. Stock KW, Chen Q, Morrin M, Hatabu H, and Edelman RR. Oxygen-enhanced magnetic resonance ventilation imaging of the human lung at 0.2 and 1.5 t. *J Magn Reson Imaging*, 9(6):838–41, 1999.

8. Loffler R, Muller CJ, Peller M, Penzkofer H, Deimling M, Schwaiblmair M, Scheidler J, and Reiser M. Optimization and evaluation of the signal intensity change in multisection oxygen-enhanced MR lung imaging. *Magn Reson Med*, 43(6):860–6, 2000.

9. Mai VM, Liu B, Li W, Polzin J, Kurucay S, Chen Q, and Edelman RR. Influence of oxygen flow rate on signal and T(1) changes in oxygen-enhanced ventilation imaging. *J Magn Reson Imaging*, 16(1):37–41, 2002.

10. Vaninbroukx J, Bosmans H, Sunaert S, Demedts M, Delcroix M, Marchal G, and Verschakelen J. The use of ECG and respiratory triggering to improve the sensitivity of oxygen-enhanced proton MRI of lung ventilation. *Eur Radiol*, 13(6):1260–5, 2003.

11. Mai VM, Tutton S, Prasad PV, Chen Q, Li W, Chen C, Liu B, Polzin J, Kurucay S, and Edelman RR. Computing oxygen-enhanced ventilation maps using correlation analysis. *Magn Reson Med*, 49(3):591–4, 2003.

12. Cootes TF, Taylor CJ, Cooper DH, and Graham J. Active Shape Models- their training and application. *Comput Vis Image Underst*, 61(1):38–59, 1995.

13. Akima H. A new method of interpolation and smooth curve fitting based on local procedures. *J Acm*, 17(4):589, 1970.

14. Ohno Y, Chen Q, and Hatabu H. Oxygen-enhanced magnetic resonance ventilation imaging of lung. *Eur J Radiol*, 37(3):164–71, 2001.

An Uncertainty-Driven Hybrid of Intensity-Based and Feature-Based Registration with Application to Retinal and Lung CT Images*

Charles V. Stewart, Ying-Lin Lee, and Chia-Ling Tsai

Rensselaer Polytechnic Institute
Troy, NY 12180-3590 USA

Abstract. A new hybrid of feature-based and intensity-based registration is presented. The algorithm reflects a new understanding of the role of alignment error in the generation of registration constraints. This leads to an iterative process where distinctive image locations from the moving image are matched against the intensity structure of the fixed image. The search range of this matching process is controlled by both the uncertainty in the current transformation estimate and the properties of the image locations to be matched. The resulting hybrid algorithm is applied to retinal image registration by incorporating it as the main estimation engine within our recently published Dual-Bootstrap ICP algorithm. The hybrid algorithm is used to align serial and 4d CT images of the lung using a B-spline based deformation model.

1   Introduction

Feature-based and intensity-based registration algorithms differ considerably in the image-based features that drive the alignment process [4]. Intensity-based techniques use all image pixels and do not require explicit feature extraction. They tend to be more stable around minima of the objective function because they don't rely on uncertain feature locations or on correspondences which may fluctuate with slight changes in the transformation. On the other hand, feature-based techniques tend to be faster, have a wider capture range, and allow alignment to be focused on only selected subsets of the image data. These strengths and weaknesses are studied experimentally in [9].

A growing set of papers has begun to address the issue of combining feature-based and intensity-based registration. As examples, in [5] registration is driven both by intensity similarity error and by errors in the positions of matched features. In Feldmar et al. [7] intensity is treated as a 4th dimension for ICP matching, while Sharp et al. [13] combines ICP with invariant features. In a much

---

* The support of the GE Global Research Center and of the National Science Foundation through the Center for Subsurface Sensing and Imaging Systems is gratefully acknowledged.

C. Barillot, D.R. Haynor, and P. Hellier (Eds.): MICCAI 2004, LNCS 3216, pp. 870–877, 2004.

different approach, Aylward et al. [1] locate tubular structures in one image and then align images using gradient-descent of a "tubularness" measure evaluated at the transformed locations of these structures in the other image. Ourselin, et al. [10] use block-matching of intensities together with robust regression. Shum and Szeliski [15] use block matching of intensities to refine video mosaics. The PASHA algorithm [4] combines correspondence and deformation processes in a global objective function. In the HAMMER algorithm [14] registration is driven by the alignment of feature positions based on a hierarchical description of the surrounding intensity distribution.

This paper presents a new hybrid of intensity-based and feature-based registration and applies the resulting algorithm in two contexts: aligning low-overlap retina images and spline-based alignment of lung CT volumes. Feature points found in the moving image are matched against the intensity structure of the fixed image. Importantly, the search range for the match is dictated by both the properties of the feature and the uncertainty in the current transformation estimate. This differs from common intensity-based techniques where constraints are driven by local changes in the similarity measure. It also differs from correspondence-based methods like ICP [2] where matching is purely a nearest-point search.

This core algorithm is built into two different overall registration algorithms. The first is an extension of our recent Dual-Bootstrap ICP [17] algorithm for aligning retinal images. Replacing the feature-to-feature ICP algorithm with the new feature-to-intensity similarity matching increases the effectiveness for extremely different cases. The second overall algorithm is a new technique for non-rigid, B-spline alignment of lung CT volumes. Small regions with sufficient intensity variation in the moving image are matched against the fixed image. These matches control the estimate of hierarchical B-spline deformations. The algorithm is applied to effectively align serial CT volumes.

2   The Role of Uncertainty in Registration

We motivate the new hybrid algorithm by considering the importance of uncertainty in registration. Let $S(\mathbf{p}, \mathbf{q})$ measure the region-based similarity error between moving image I_m at location $\mathbf{p}$ and fixed (target) image I_f at location $\mathbf{q}$. Let $T(\mathbf{p}; \boldsymbol{\theta})$ be the transformation mapping $\mathbf{p}$ from I_m onto I_f based on the (to be estimated) parameter vector $\boldsymbol{\theta}$. Finally, let $\mathcal{P}$ be a set of locations in I_m where transformation constraints are applied.

Intensity-based algorithms search for the transformation minimizing the aggregate similarity error:

$$E(\boldsymbol{\theta}) = \sum_{\mathbf{p}_i \in \mathcal{P}} S(\mathbf{p}_i, T(\mathbf{p}_i, \boldsymbol{\theta})), \tag{1}$$

Regularizing constraints may be placed on $\boldsymbol{\theta}$, but we will ignore these for now. $E(\boldsymbol{\theta})$ is most frequently minimized through a gradient-descent technique [8]. The estimate, $\hat{\boldsymbol{\theta}}$, remains uncertain throughout the minimization process. This

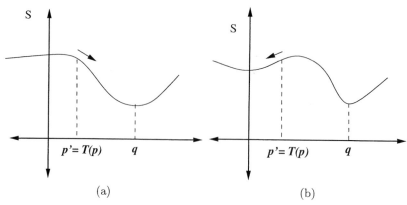

Fig. 1. Two examples of a one-dimensional cross-section of the similarity error function surface surrounding a transformed point $\mathbf{p}'$. The interval over which the function is plotted is the uncertainty region. The arrow shows the direction of gradient descent based on the point. The location q is the minimum of the similarity error function within the search region. In (a) the gradient descent direction is in the direction of the minimum, whereas in (b) the direction is away from the minimum.

in turn causes uncertainty in the location $T(\mathbf{p}_i, \hat{\boldsymbol{\theta}})$. We investigate the effect of this on the constraints used in registration.

Suppose we have a measure of the uncertainty on $\mathbf{p}'_i = T(\mathbf{p}_i, \hat{\boldsymbol{\theta}})$ and this can roughly be described in terms of a standard deviation σ. Consider a region of width $\pm c\sigma$ around $\mathbf{p}'_i$ in I_f. If the uncertainty model is reasonably accurate, this region will likely contain the true homologous point in image I_f to $\mathbf{p}_i$. Call this point $\mathbf{q}_i$. Moreover, if the similarity error function is correct, this point will also minimize $S(\mathbf{p}_i, \mathbf{q})$ for all $\mathbf{q}$ within this uncertainty region. If the gradient direction $\nabla S(\mathbf{p}_i, \mathbf{q})$ evaluated at $\mathbf{p}'_i$ points in the direction of $\mathbf{q}_i$, then the gradient descent direction computed for point i is consistent with the direction the estimate needs to move (based on the local constraints). This happens when the search region is convex, as illustrated in Figure 1(a). On the other hand, if the gradient points away from $\mathbf{q}_i$ then the constraint will pull the transformation estimate in the wrong direction (Figure 1(b)). This is likely to happen when the uncertainty region is large. When it happens at enough points, registration will descend into an incorrect local minimum. This problem can occur no matter at what resolution the images are represented. A similar problem occurs in ICP-like matching when the uncertainty region contains multiple points and the closer point drives registration in the wrong direction.

3   Iterative Most Similar Point (IMSP)

The natural alternative to gradient-based minimization is to search for the most similar location, $\mathbf{q}_i$, surrounding $\mathbf{p}'_i$. This leads to a conceptually straightforward registration algorithm: iteratively match the feature points by minimizing the similarity error and estimate the transformation based on the matches. The trick (and primary novelty) is using uncertainty to dictate the search region for minimizing the error. A summary outline of this "IMSP" procedure is presented below, followed by a sketch of important details:

1. Given are initial transformation estimate $\hat{\boldsymbol{\theta}}_0$, moving image I_m, fixed image I_f, and feature point set $\mathcal{P}$ from I_m.
2. Initialize $t = 1$.
3. For each $\mathbf{p}_i \in \mathcal{P}$,
    a) Use the properties of $\mathbf{p}_i$ and the uncertainty in the current estimate to determine a search region $N(\mathbf{p}'_i)$ surrounding $\mathbf{p}'_i = T(\mathbf{p}, \hat{\boldsymbol{\theta}}_{t-1})$ in I_f.
    b) Find the location $\mathbf{q}_i$ that minimizes $S(\mathbf{p}_i, \mathbf{q})$ over $N(\mathbf{p}'_i)$. Gather these image location pairs $(\mathbf{p}_i, \mathbf{q}_i)$ into a set of correspondences $\mathcal{C}_t$.
4. Estimate the new parameter set:

$$\hat{\boldsymbol{\theta}}_t = \underset{\boldsymbol{\theta}}{\operatorname{argmin}} \sum_{(\mathbf{p}_i, \mathbf{q}_i) \in \mathcal{C}_t} w_i D(T(\mathbf{p}_i, \boldsymbol{\theta}), \mathbf{q}_i)^2 \qquad (2)$$

Here $D(\cdot, \cdot)$ is an alignment error function, and w_i is a robust weight.
5. Compute the alignment error variance, σ_t^2, and the covariance of $\hat{\boldsymbol{\theta}}_t$.
6. $t = t + 1$
7. Repeat steps 3-6 until convergence.

3.1   Feature Points

Feature points may be extracted from I_m to form $\mathcal{P}$ in several ways. When aligning retinal fundus images, these are automatically-detected centerline points along the retinal vessels [6]. In the lung CT application, the volume is divided into small regions, and the gradient structure of each region is analyzed (eigen analysis) to determine if it is "landmark-like" (significant variation of intensity in all directions) "vessel-like" (significant variation in two directions), "face-like" (significant variation in one direction), or homogeneous. Matching of the feature points is restricted to the directions along which their intensity structure varies. For example, the search for a match for a face-like feature is only along the normal to the face after it has been (approximately) transformed into I_f based on the current transformation estimate. Alignment error constraints, $D(T(\mathbf{p}_i, \boldsymbol{\theta}), \mathbf{q}_i)$, are defined in the same way.

3.2   Uncertainties and Search Regions

The key to the new algorithm is calculating the uncertainty and the resulting search region, $N(\mathbf{p}'_i)$. The first issue is estimating the standard deviation of the alignment error, a difficult problem in robust estimation. We have found that a similarity-weighted average of the squared alignment errors (step 5 of the algorithm) is more effective than the usual robust estimation based on geometric distances. Intuitively, the reason is that the covariance-driven search already eliminates the possibility of gross outliers, making the similarity score a much better indication of match correctness. The weight for a correspondence[1] is

$$w_i = \frac{S''(\mathbf{p}_i, \mathbf{q}_i)}{1 + S(\mathbf{p}_i, \mathbf{q}_i)}.$$

This favors matches with lower overall similarity error and sharper local minima of the error. The similarity error used throughout the paper is normalized SSD. The scale estimate is $\sigma_t^2 = \sum w_i D(T(\mathbf{p}_i, \boldsymbol{\theta}), \mathbf{q}_i)^2 / \sum w_i$. For the first iteration of matching a prior estimate σ_0 must be used .

Once we have the scale there are two ways to use it in defining the search region. The first is to define an isotropic volume of radius $c\sigma$ around each transformed feature location, $\mathbf{p}_i'$, in I_f. The second is based on computing the covariance matrix $\Sigma_{\boldsymbol{\theta}}$ of the transformation parameters at each stage of the algorithm (see below). If we compute the Jacobian, $\mathbf{J}$, of the transformation function $T(\mathbf{p}_i, \boldsymbol{\theta})$ with respect to point location $\mathbf{p}_i$, then standard covariance propagation techniques show that the covariance matrix of $\mathbf{p}_i'$, the mapped point, is approximately $\mathbf{J}\Sigma_{\boldsymbol{\theta}}\mathbf{J}^T$. This covariance matrix defines a search volume (error ellipsoid) surrounding $\mathbf{p}_i'$ (in fact, the first way to define the search area approximates the covariance matrix as $\sigma^2\mathbf{I}$). Using either method, the final search region for each feature is then along the feature's search direction (mapped by the transformation estimation, as above) within this volume.

3.3   Robust Parameter Estimation

Parameter estimation in each iteration is based on weighted least-squares using the similarity weights above. Levenberg-Marquardt techniques are needed for estimating the spline parameters. The covariance matrix of the transformation parameters can be estimated approximately [11, Ch. 15] as $\Sigma_{\boldsymbol{\theta}} = \sigma_t^2 \mathbf{H}^{-1}(\hat{\boldsymbol{\theta}}_t)$, where $\mathbf{H}(\hat{\boldsymbol{\theta}}_t)$ is the Hessian matrix, evaluated at the parameter estimate. This explicit calculation is not practical for 3D B-spline deformation models. In ongoing work we are developing approximations.

4   Retinal Image Registration

The first application of the new IMSP algorithm is to use it in place of ICP within our Dual-Bootstrap ICP (DB-ICP) algorithm for retinal image registration [17]. DB-ICP generates a series of low-order initial transformation estimates based on automatic matching of small image regions. It then tests each initial transformation and associated region separately to see if it can be "grown" into an accurate, image-wide quadratic transformation (12 parameters). The growth process iteratively: (1) refines the transformation estimate, (2) expands the region, and (3) tests to see if a higher-order transformation model can be used, with steps (2) and (3) controlled by $\Sigma_{\boldsymbol{\theta}}$. IMSP can be used in place of ICP in

---

[1] See [16] for a different form of covariance-based weighting.

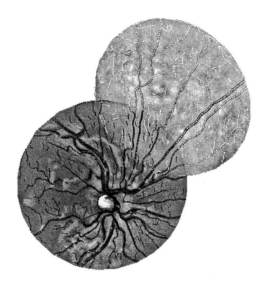

Fig. 2. An example retinal image alignment where DB-ICP failed but DB-IMSP succeeded. The small overlap region between the images contains little variation in the vessel contour directions, leading to instability in the feature-to-feature alignment but not in feature-to-intensity alignment.

step (1), matching vascular centerline points from the moving image against the intensities of the fixed image using normal distance constraints.

Although DB-ICP is extremely successful (100% success on image pairs that overlap by at least 35% and have at least a minima set of features), DB-IMSP is better. From our large data set we pulled 81 difficult image pairs having low image overlaps and poor contrast. DB-ICP aligned only 33% of these pairs (to a required average alignment error of less than 1.5 pixels on 1024x1024 images), whereas DB-IMSP aligned 86%. By not relying on consistency between extracted features in the two images, it was able to generate more constraints. An example is shown in Figure 2.

5   Spline-Based Lung CT Volume Registration

The second application of IMSP is in B-spline alignment [12] of lung CT volumes. As discussed above, feature set $\mathcal{P}$ is determined by analyzing the distribution of intensity gradients in regularly-spaced blocks in each image. In each iteration, the neighborhood search volume is isotropic, with radius $c\sigma_t$; due to the large number of transformation parameters, the covariance matrix is not explicitly computed. The algorithm proceeds in a coarse-to-fine manner, starting at 64x64 (within each slice) and ending at 256x256. The uniform B-splines are also estimated in a hierarchical fashion, with a knot spacing of 360 millimeters at the 64x64 resolution and 90 millimeters at the 256x256 resolution. For each combination of

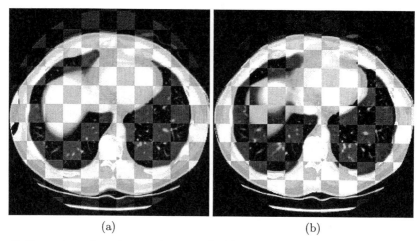

(a) (b)

Fig. 3. Example registration results using IMSP and a B-spline deformation on serial lung CT images. The left shows checkerboard results (alternating blocks from the two images) in a single slice following alignment. The right shows the affine alignment using the final IMSP correspondences from B-spline registration.

resolution and B-spline knot spacing, the algorithm proceeds as described above. The correspondence constraints are powerful enough, at least in this application, that no additional smoothness constraints must be placed on the B-spline.

In preliminary studies, this algorithm has been applied to align the individual volumes in a 4d CT sequence and serial, intra-patient 3d CT volumes taken 2 to 6 months apart. The 4d CT alignment was accurate to significantly less than a voxel. In the serial alignment problem, using images taken with GE Lightspeed 16 and GE Lightspeed Ultra scanners, the deformations were quite large. The final alignment error for 3 different patients (4 alignments — one patient had 3 volumes) we've studied averaged approximately 1.5mm as compared to an affine alignment error of 11.7mm (using the final B-spline correspondences). Therefore, unlike rigid registration [3], the deformable results are approaching the accuracy needed for serial CAD studies. An example side-by-side comparison of the B-spline results and the affine alignment for a single slice is shown in Figure 3.

6   Discussion and Conclusions

The results on retinal and lung CT registration show the promise of the new IMSP algorithm. The computation and use of uncertainty effectively controls the search range for feature-to-intensity matching. The algorithm produces accurate matches while relying less on consistency between feature locations in the two images. The results raise several interesting issues for on-going work. First is an effective combination of ICP-style feature-to-feature correspondences and IMSP-style feature-to-intensity correspondences to improve both reliability and efficiency. Second is using IMSP constraints to build a variable resolution

B-spline model, introducing higher resolutions where the deformations are more substantial and the constraint set richer. Third is using the resulting algorithm for serial registration of lung CT volumes in computer-aided diagnosis.

References

[1] S. Aylward, J. Jomier, S. Weeks, and E. Bullitt. Registration of vascular images. *IJCV*, 55(2-3):123–138, 2003.

[2] P. Besl and N. McKay. A method for registration of 3-d shapes. *IEEE T. Pattern Anal.*, 14(2):239–256, 1992.

[3] M. Betke, H. Hong, D. Thomas, C. Prince, and J. P. Ko. Landmark detection in the chest and registration of lung surfaces with an application to nodule registration. *Med. Image Anal.*, 7:265–281, 2003.

[4] P. Cachier, E. Bardinet, D. Dormont, X. Pennec, and N. Ayache. Iconic feature based nonrigid registration: the PASHA algorithm. *CVIU*, 89:272–298, 2003.

[5] P. Cachier, J.-F. Mangin, X. Pennec, D. Rivière, D. Papdopoulos-Orfanos, J. Régis, and N. Ayache. Multisubject non-rigid registration of brain MRI using intensity and geometric features. In *Proc. 4th MICCAI*, pages 734–742, 2001.

[6] A. Can, H. Shen, J. N. Turner, H. L. Tanenbaum, and B. Roysam. Rapid automated tracing and feature extraction from live high-resolution retinal fundus images using direct exploratory algorithms. *IEEE Trans. on Inf. Tech. in Biomedicine*, 3(2):125–138, 1999.

[7] J. Feldmar, J. Declerck, G. Malandain, and N. Ayache. Extension of the ICP algorithm to nonrigid intensity-based registration of 3d volumes. *CVIU*, 66(2):193–206, May 1997.

[8] L. Ibáñez, L. Ng, J. Gee, and S. Aylward. Registration patterns: the generic framework for image registration of the Insight Toolkit. In *IEEE Int. Symp. on Biomedical Imaging*, pages 345–348, Washington, DC, USA, 7–10July 2002.

[9] R. A. McLaughlin, J. Hipwell, G. P. Penney, K. Rhode, A. Chung, J. A. Noble, and D. J. Hawkes. Intensity-based registration versus feature-based registration for neurointerventions. In *Proc. Med. Image. Understanding Analysis*, 2001.

[10] S. Ourselin, A. Rocher, G. Subsol, X. Pennec, and N. Ayache. Reconstructing a 3D structure from serial histological sections. *IVC*, 19:25–31, 2000.

[11] W. H. Press, S. A. Teukolsky, W. T. Vetterling, and B. P. Flannery. *Numerical Recipes in C: The Art of Scientific Computing*. Cambridge University Press, 1992.

[12] D. Rueckert, I. Somoda, C. Hayes, D. Hill, M. Leach, and D. Hawkes. Nonrigid registration using free-form deformations: application to breast MR images. *IEEE Trans. Med. Imaging.*, 18:712–721, 1999.

[13] G. Sharp, S. Lee, and D. Wehe. ICP registration using invariant features. *IEEE T. Pattern Anal.*, 24(1):90–102, 2002.

[14] D. Shen and C. Davatzikos. Hammer: Hierarchical attribute matching mechanism for elastic registration. *IEEE Trans. Med. Imaging.*, 21(11):1421–1439, 2002.

[15] H. Shum and R. Szeliski. Construction of panoramic image mosaics with global and local alignment. *IJCV*, 36(2):101–130, 2000.

[16] A. Singh and P. Allen. Image-flow computation: An estimation-theoretic framework and a unified perspective. *CVGIP: Image Understanding*, 56(2):152–177, 1992.

[17] C. Stewart, C.-L. Tsai, and B. Roysam. The dual-bootstrap iterative closest point algorithm with application to retinal image registration. *IEEE Trans. Med. Imaging.*, 22(11):1379–1394, 2003.

Portal Vein Registration for the Follow-Up of Hepatic Tumours

Arnaud Charnoz, Vincent Agnus, and Luc Soler

IRCAD,
1, place de l'Hôpital - F67091 Strasbourg Cedex - France
Arnaud.Charnoz@ircad.u-strasbg.fr

Abstract. In this paper, we propose an original method which permits a follow-up of intra-patient evolution of tumours in the liver by using a registration of the portal vascular system.

First, several methods to segment the liver data structures (liver, vascular systems and tumours) on computed tomography scans are presented. Secondly, the skeleton of the vessels is computed and transformed into a graph representation. Then, the intra-patient graph registration is computed to determine an approximation of liver deformation. Finally, the deformation permits to match tumours to diagnose their evolution.

For each step, we present the methods we used and their results on CT-scan images.

1 Motivations

Liver surgery is a field in which computer-based surgery planning has great impact on selection of therapeutic strategy. In this paper, we focus on the follow-up of tumours from the same patient between two acquisitions. We propose an automatic method which permits to show how tumours evolve. The main purpose is to match tumours between two different moments.

Tumour matching provides an automatic framework to diagnose their evolutions. The comparison amongst matched tumours permits to see their evolutions by comparing their volumes. A tumour cannot be matched if it appeared or disappeared between the two acquisitions.

Tumour matching can not be accurately performed by using only their localization information. Indeed, between two acquisitions, their localization and shape can vary a lot. The shape deformation is due to disease development and the localization changes are due the deformation of liver.

The liver deformation gives an estimate of tumour displacement that helps to track them. The liver is lacking of reference points allow the estimation of its deformation, so its inner vascular system is preferred, particularly the portal system. On the CT-scan images, hepatic vessels are enhanced with a contrast medium. The vascular system gives a better reference point set in two respects: a) topologically, by providing junction points as reference points, b) geometrically, with diameter and orientation information of incident branches.

C. Barillot, D.R. Haynor, and P. Hellier (Eds.): MICCAI 2004, LNCS 3216, pp. 878–886, 2004.

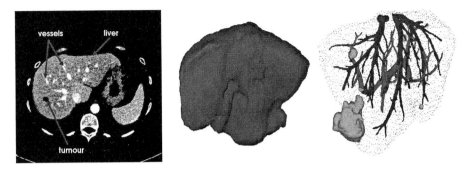

Fig. 1. Component extraction: [**left**] Slice obtained by CT-scan of a liver. The vascular systems are highly contrasted and tumours are poorly contrasted. [**center**] Liver surface obtained by robust segmentation of the CT-scans. [**right**] Visualization of different components of the liver (portal vein, hepatic vein and tumours).

To compute the deformation, the portal vein is modeled as a directed tree from the skeleton of segmented CT-scan images, then graph vertices are matched together. These matchings define a transformation which helps in tracking tumours. This method differs from traditional methods which generally work on grey level image registration [2,3]. Our approach is inspired by some methods employed to register airway tree [6,10] but whose purpose is to search for local liver deformations.

The remainder of this paper is organized as follows. Section 2 deals with the computation of the vascular graph from CT-scan images. Section 3 describes our graph registration algorithm. It also introduces energy functions used to measure resemblance between edges. Section 4 is dedicated to tumour registration. We finish with a discussion on future possible improvements.

2   Preprocessing: Segmentations and Thinning

Segmentation: Some methods are proposed in the literature to segment liver structures [4,8]. To extract them, we have used an automated algorithm [9] based on three segmentation steps. First, an approximation of the other structures allows to obtain a good localization of the liver in the image. A deformable model is used to segment the liver [5] (see fig. 1). Then, the method estimates the intensity distributions of three tissue classes: tumours, parenchyma and vessels, and classifies them. Finally, to separate hepatic and portal vascular systems, the skeleton of systems is computed and inconsistent links between graphs are removed to obtain two dissociated graphs.

Graph representation: The graph representing the portal system is constructed from a skeleton. The thining skeleton (see fig. 2) is obtained by iterative removing points (except end points) where removal preserves the topology

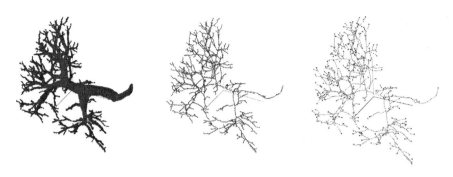

Fig. 2. Skeleton creation: [**left**] Voxel visualization representing the portal vascular system segmentation of a liver. [**center**] Thinning result of the portal vascular system. [**right**] 3D representation of the graph structure data obtained starting from previous skeleton.

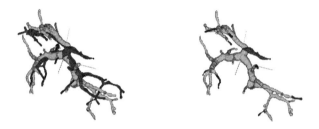

Fig. 3. Graph registration: [**left**] This figure shows the superimposition of two portal vascular systems created from two images of a same patient acquired at two different times. On this figure, only the node root has been registered. [**right**] This figure shows the good result of the registration graph (all nodes registered). Some differences appear between graphs, as some branches were detected in only one of the graphs.

(called simple points [1]). Then, the edges (resp. vertices) of graph are generated by branch voxels (resp. junction nodes). Furthermore, a few operations improve visualization and keep significant edges [4,8,9].

3   Graph Registration

Once the graph of the portal vascular system is created for both acquisitions of the same patient, we register their graphs. There are many approaches for graph matching in the graph theory, especially on the matching of hierarchical structures using weighted association graphs [7]. The algorithm proposed in this paper is simplified, faster and more specific although it strongly related to these concepts. Figure 3 shows the result of this registration.

3.1 Algorithm

The method is very fast (see alg. 1): a) roots are matched and registered, b) the first edge set is matched with the second set, c) local deformations are computed and d) we repeat this operation with child nodes. Figure 4 shows some steps of the iterative registration evolution.

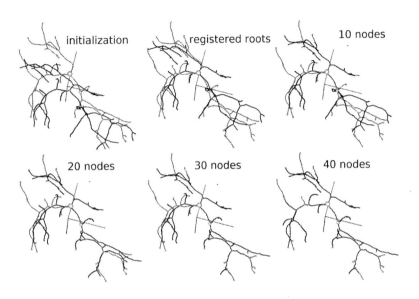

Fig. 4. Graph registration evolution: Images represent the evolution of graph registration (left → right, up → down) of a real patient case showed on fig. 3. Step by step, the graph matching evolves with a depth-first search.

3.2 Vessel Registration

The first step of the algorithm requires a matching of nodes in both graphs and tries to match the out-edges. This step is difficult because blood vessels are not always well segmented due to contrast medium propagation time. Two matched edges can have different lengths or can be slightly displaced in space. Sometimes edges have no match in the other graph.

To determine the best out-edges matching for a given node pair, the method minimizes an energy function. For this, an energy function f_g between two edges (see eq. 1 and fig. 5) is used and all possible one-to-one functions for the matching between $E_1 = \{e_1^1, e_1^2, ..., e_1^n\}$ first graph edge set and $E_2 = \{e_2^1, e_2^2, ..., e_2^m\}$ second graph edge set are tested. Finally, the function which minimizes the global matching energy is chosen (see eq. 2).

$$f_g(e_1, e_2) = f_1(e_1, e_2) \times f_2(e_1, e_2)$$

$$f_1(e_1, e_2) = \frac{1}{l_{min}} \times \sum_{i=1}^{l_{min}} \|p_1^i - p_2^i\|^2$$

$$f_2(e_1, e_2) = \sin(\frac{\hat{\theta}(e_1, e_2)}{2})^2 \times e^{\frac{l_{max} - l_{min}}{l_{max}} - 1}$$

(1)

where e_1, e_2 are edges (vessels) which are registered in their first node, l_{min} (resp. l_{max}) is the shortest (resp. longest) edge lenght beetween e_1 and e_2 and where p_k^i is the ith point of e_k.

$$F_g(E_1, E_2) = \min_{\sigma} \sum_{k=1}^{n} f_g(e_1^k, e_2^{\sigma(k)})$$

(2)

where $\sigma : [1...n] \to [1...m]$ is an injective function of correspondence and thus it is supposed that $n \leq m$. If this is not the case, E_1 and E_2 are permuted in equation.

The robustness of this method depends on the ability of the energy function to describe the matching between two edges. To improve this, the function f_2 is introduced in eq. 1 to influence small angles beetween edges with $\hat{\theta}(e_1, e_2)$ (the angle created by vectors $(p_1^1 p_1^{l_{min}}, p_2^1 p_2^{l_{min}})$) and the matching edge of same length with $e^{\frac{l_{max} - l_{min}}{l_{max}} - 1}$.

However, to improve matching quality, work on other energy functions is being study. These functions will focus on the matching impact on the subgraph or on the quality of the transformation to deform the edge.

Algorithm 1 Graph registration

{**Initialization**}
1/ Register graph roots which correspond to the entry of the portal vein.
2/ Compute their associated transformation.
3/ Push the common node in the process stack.

{**Principal loop**}
while all nodes are not registered (process stack is not empty) **do**
   Step 1/ Vessel registration (see sec. 3.2)
   From two already matched nodes, compute the best set of out-edge pairs (without parent edge) within both graphs. Some out-edges can have no match.
   Step 2/ Junction node registration (see sec. 3.3)
   If end points from edge pair do not match, a new artificial node has to be inserted in the graph at the longer edge. Go to step 1 and recompute with new edges.
   Step 3/ Local transformation (see sec. 3.4)
   A local transformation for each edge pair is computed to superimpose them and deform the edge subgraph.
   Step 4/ Push registered nodes of out-edges.
end while

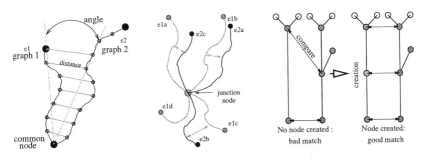

Fig. 5. Process registration visualization: [**left**] This figure shows how to compute the energy function f_g to know if two edges match (see eq 1). [**center**] This figure explains the problem of matching group for out-edges of a registered node and shows the problem of missed edges. For instance here, the best matching is: $((e_1^a, e_2^c)(e_1^b, e_2^a)(e_1^c, e_2^b))$, e_1^d has no correspondence. [**right**] Problem of junction node matching when edges and nodes miss.

3.3   Junction Node Registration

In this step, the best one-to-one function which matches the first edge set with the second edge set is found. However, some matched edges do not have the same length, due to squeeze pressure on the liver, methods used to compute the graph representation and injection time. If the end node of each edge match, they are registered together. It is also possible, that during the segmentation process, some edges are not segmented on one of the graphs. In this case, junction node does not appear in one of the graphs. This node will be inserted into it to preserve the efficiency of matching in the process continuation and to obtain in the end, a better registration (see fig. 5).

The difficulty is to distinguish between these two cases. Currently, the method is just a simple test on the relative length difference. But, in the future, criteria will take the impact of such a decision on the subgraph into account in terms of register costs.

3.4   Local Transformation Computation

At the begining of this step, pairs of edges match between themselves due to step 1 (see sec. 3.2) and edge endings (node ends) are equivalent due to step 2 (see sec. 3.3). It is now necessary to compute the local transformation T (translation, rotation, ...) to be applied to these edges to obtain the deformation that the subgraph of each edge will undergo.

$$T_{sol} = \min_T \sum_i \|p_1^i - T(p_2^i)\|^2 \tag{3}$$

Equation 3 shows the best local transformation which is chosen to minimize the euclidean distance error between edge points and the projection of associated points of the other graph. Currently, a translation is applied to register

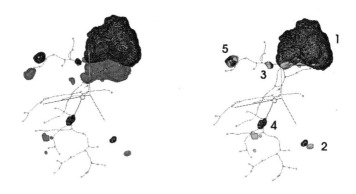

Fig. 6. Tumour registration: [**left**] This figure shows the tumours superimposition before tumour registration. The graph and tumours with the surface point represent the first acquisition. [**right**] This figure shows the tumour superimposition (associated with an id number) after tumour registration. All tumours have an improved matching (good correlation or reduction of the distance separation (see table 1)) but some of them did not overlap perfectly (2,4).

Table 1. Tumour registration results: This table shows some results on each tumour matching. Tumour numbers indicated in the table are shown in fig. 6. All measurements are in millimetres (excluding similarity) and are computed before and after registration.

Group id	Min $\min\limits_{a\in A,b\in B} d(a,b)$	Max $d_{Hausdorff}(A,B)$	Center $d(c_a,c_b)$	Similarity $\frac{2\times vol(A\cap B)}{vol(A)+vol(B)}$	Tumour to graph distance
1	0 → 0	35.5 → 16.5	27.7 → 9.5	12.1 → 58.0 %	11.6
2	14.8 → 2.5	22.1 → 10.7	21.6 → 10.4	0 → 0 %	22.6
3	14.8 → 0	22.5 → 4.0	22.1 → 2.4	0 → 48.2 %	7.7
4	25.4 → 7.6	37.8 → 19.6	35.8 → 16.7	0 → 0 %	6.1
5	9.5 → 0	25.1 → 2.4	25.4 → 0.9	0 → 81.8 %	1.8

node ends. In future works, this transformation will be approximated by a rigid transformation (rotation, translation). Finding the right 3D rotation is necessary to increase the robustness of the method with other patients.

4   Tumour Registration

In this part, lesion matching is evoked. From the local transformation computed in each node, a global transformation in the liver can be approximated. This transformation is applied to tumours in order to superimpose them.

Nowadays, the deformation applied to each tumour is only the local transformation of its graph closest node.

Figure 6 and table 1 show the result of tumour registration. The projection of tumours in the first patient acquisition is represented before and after registration. All tumour distance separations decrease with the matching. Groups 1, 3 and 5 have an efficient matching (good similarity).

However, groups 2 and 4 do not overlap, although the distance between them decreases. The worst matching can be explained for group 2 by a large separation between vessels (graph) and tumours, and for group 4 by a too simple deformation model. In a future work, it will be interesting to compute and merge sub-hepatic vascular system and liver surface deformations which will provide more information on liver deformation.

5   Discussion and Perspectives

We have presented a new method for tumour registration. It permits an automatic follow-up of tumour evolution. Our method works by registering the vascular system to approximate the liver deformation. The registration process is robust to topological changes within the vascular graph. Preliminary results promise an efficient approach.

However, this study must be tested on a larger database to be correctly evaluated. Future work will be directed towards defining a more complex local deformation model and improving the robustness of the energy function. We will also be able to introduce Kalman filtering to estimate a global deformation of the liver.

References

1. G. Bertrand and G. Malandain. A new characterization of three-dimensional simple points. *Pattern Recognition Letters*, 15(2):169–175, February 1994.
2. M. Bosc, F. Heitz, J.P. Armspach, I.J. Namer, D. Gounot, and L. Rumbach. Automatic change detection in multi-modal serial MRI: application to multiple sclerosis lesion evolution. *NeuroImage*, 20(2):643–656, 2003.
3. E. R. E. Denton, L. I. Sonoda, D. Rueckert, S. C. Rankin, C. Hayes, M. Leach, D. L. G. Hill, and D. J. Hawkes. Comparison and evaluation of rigid and non-rigid registration of breast MR images. *Journal of Computer Assisted Tomography*, 23:800–805, 1999.
4. P. Dokladal, C. Lohou, L. Perroton, and G. Bertrand. Liver blood vessels extraction by a 3-D topological approach. In *Medical Image Computing and Computer-Assisted Intervention*, volume 1679, 19 September 1999.
5. J. Montagnat and H. Delingette. Globally constrained deformable models for 3d object reconstruction. *Signal Processing*, 71(2):173–186, December 1998.
6. Y. Park. *Registration of linear structures in 3-D medical images*. PhD thesis, Osaka University, Japan. Departement of informatics and Mathematical Science, January 2002.
7. M. Pelillo, K. Siddiqi, and S.W. Zucker. Matching hierarchical structures using association graphs. *Pattern Analysis and Machine Intelligence*, 21:1105–1120, November 1999.
8. D. Selle, B Preim, and A. Schenk. Analysis of vasculature for liver surgery planning. *IEEE Transactions on Medical Imaging*, 21(11):1344–1357, November 2002.

9. L. Soler, H. Delingette, G. Malandain, J. Montagnat, N. Ayache, J.-M. Clément, C. Koehl, O. Dourthe, D. Mutter, and J. Marescaux. A fully automatic anatomical, pathological and fonctionnal segmentation from CT-scans for hepatic surgery. In *Medical Imaging 2000*, pages 246–255, February 2000.

10. J. Tschirren, K. Palágyi, J.M. Reinhardt, E.A. Hoffman, and M. Sonka. Segmentation, skeletonization, and branchpoint matching—A fully automated quantitative evaluation of human intrathoracic airway trees. In Takeyosihi Dohi and Ron Kikinis, editors, *Lecture Notes in Computer Science*, volume 2489, pages 12–19. Springer-Verlag, Utrecht, October 2002.

Fast Rigid 2D-2D Multimodal Registration

Ulrich Müller, Jürgen Hesser, and Reinhard Männer

Institute for Computational Medicine, Universities Mannheim and Heidelberg,
B6, 23, D-68131 Mannheim, Germany
ulrich.mueller@ti.uni-mannheim.de

Abstract. This paper solves the problem to assign optimal sample sizes to Viola's stochastic matching [1] and determines the best stochastic gradient optimizer to this sort of problems. It can be used for applications like X-ray based minimal invasive interventions or the control of patient motion during radiation therapy. The preprocessing for optimally estimating the parameters lies between 0.5-4.5 seconds and is only necessary once for a typical set of images to be matched. Matching itself is performed within 300-1300 milliseconds on an Athlon 800 MHz processor.

1 Introduction

Radiation therapy and many interventional techniques require real-time or at least sub-second control of patient motion. Often this information is obtained by point-pair matching with markers either attached on the skin surface or fixed in bone. In the case of X-ray fluoroscopy acquired images would already suffice to determine this motion. In order to achieve sub-second rates for image-based registration, however, matching algorithms have to be modified. L. Ng et al. [2] could increase matching speed by concentrating on shapes in a 2D image. A translation of 21.4 mm and 10 degrees was corrected in 0.954 seconds on a Pentium 4 with 2.4 GHz. A more complex case has been reported by Fei et al. [3]. They match a 2D slice against an MRI volume within 5 seconds on a 1.8 GHz Pentium 4 processor and achieve the short matching times by multiresolution, cross-correlation for the coarse levels, and mutual information for the fine-grained matching. Another option is based on graphics hardware acceleration. Strzodka et al. [6] demonstrated a monomodal non-rigid gradient flow registration for two 256^2 images in less than 2 seconds with the streaming architecture of the DX9 graphics hardware. Another result was reported from Soza et al. [8] for 3D-3D matching. He deformed medical data using Free-Form Deformation (FFD) based on three-dimensional Bezier functions. They accelerate the algorithm by computing the FFD only for a sparse grid and then propagate the deformation on the whole volume using trilinear interpolation done in graphics hardware.

Despite these results, most of the time is still consumed by processing all pixels of the image for evaluating the quality function. Therefore, a reduction of the number of image pixels required will have a high impact on the matching speed. Viola [1] suggested to use randomly chosen samples of the image, Parzen-window estimation of the bimodal histogram estimation, and a gradient based

C. Barillot, D.R. Haynor, and P. Hellier (Eds.): MICCAI 2004, LNCS 3216, pp. 887–894, 2004.

optimizer. The main cost, however, lies in the handling of the Parzen-windows that are essentially Gaussian functions. Meihe et al. [5] improve this algorithm by replacing the computations of exponentials by a precomputed index table.

Nevertheless, Viola's approach is still not able to provide sub-second matching times. Further, the sample set size and the parameters for the optimizers have to be hand-tuned; which may be difficult in practice. In this paper we concentrate on these two points. Firstly, we develop a method that allows to estimate the optimal sample size in less than a second for most image examples. Secondly, among the best available stochastic gradient optimizers we selected the one which performed best. Combining both approaches, we achieve sub-second matching times.

The subsequent paper is organized as follows: Firstly, we introduce concepts like mutual information, Viola's stochastic matching approach, and different stochastic gradient optimizers. Secondly, we derive the optimal sample size and show in the results section the sub-second matching performance of our approach using a dedicated stochastic gradient optimizer. A conclusion section finishes this paper.

2   Mutual Information

Let us consider the target image as random variable U and the model image as random variable $V(T)$ depending on a transformation T. The model image is pre-segmented to get a set L of "interesting" pixel positions. In each iteration step, a random sample set $a \subseteq L$ of S image points is chosen. The probability distribution of the variables is estimated by Parzen windows based on Gaussian kernels. In order to save computation time, look-up-tables are used [5]. For the sample point i in the target image, $u_i = U(i)$ is the grey value in image U and $v_i = V(T, i)$ is computed by transforming the model image V with T. The mutual information $I(U, V(T))$ is selected as similarity measure. We estimate the gradient by

$$\frac{dI}{dT} \approx \frac{1}{S \cdot (S-1)} \sum_{i \in a} \sum_{\substack{j \in a \\ j \neq i}} term(i, j) \frac{d}{dT}(v_i - v_j) \tag{1}$$

Hereby, the expression $term(i, j)$ is a shortcut for the Parzen estimates [1].

3   Stochastic Optimization

We determine the local gradient dv/dT by finite differences (FD)

$$\left(\frac{dv_i}{dT}\right)_k = \frac{v(T + c_k \cdot e_k, x_i) - v(T, x_i)}{c_k} \tag{2}$$

where k indexes the components of the gradient. Although Spall [4] states that in general, simultaneous perturbation (SP) requires the same amount of iterations as FD, we were not able to verify this. In our tests the overall cost of optimization for SP was higher. Probably our gain sequence tuning fitted better for FD than it did for SP. Among the different optimization techniques, gradient ascent, resilient backpropagation and conjugate gradient descent [7] we left out the latter in this paper since it performed worse compared to its other competitors.

3.1 Gradient Ascent

In each step of Gradient ascent the transformation T is updated, $T^{(i+1)} = T^{(i)} + \Delta T^{(i)}$; $\Delta T^{(i)} = a^{(i)} \frac{dI}{dT^{(i)}}$. Spall [4] proposes to choose $a^{(i)}$ as

$$a^{(i)} = \frac{a}{(i+1+A)^\alpha} \tag{3}$$

with $\alpha = 0.602$, $A > 0$ a stability constant, e.g. 10% of the iteration maximum, and a factor a such that $(a/(A+1)^{0.602}) \frac{dI}{dT^{(i)}}$ is approximately equal to the desired change magnitude in the early iterations. We give a rough estimation of a before the start and refine it after 25 iterations. The total number of iterations is fixed. Viola [1] uses a constant value for $a^{(i)}$ and reduces it after a fixed number of iterations. In our tests the Spall gain sequence had a better performance.

3.2 Resilient Backpropagation

Resilient Backpropagation (Rprop) uses only the signs of the gradient coordinates, not their absolute value.

$$\Delta T_j^{(i)} = \lambda_j^{(i)} \cdot sign\left(\frac{\partial I}{\partial T_j}(T^{(i)})\right) \tag{4}$$

The step size λ_j is changed for each coordinate j, using two constant factors $0 < \eta^- < 1 < \eta^+$ for decelerating/accelerating depending if the gradient of the last iteration pointed to the opposite or the same side. We used 0.9 and 1.1. The iteration stops when each $\lambda_j^{(i)}$ falls below a minimum learning rate.

4 Choosing the Sample Size

The optimal sample size for the optimization is as small as possible, while still providing sufficiently robust results. Given an image pair, i.e. given a set L of target image points and a model image, we want to compute the optimal sample size S. In order to overcome high initial cost for performing test runs to find an optimal parameter set, we propose a direct method described next.

4.1 Estimating Gradients

For a rigid 2D-2D transformation T (having three degrees of freedom), setting $S = L$ will produce a reference gradient. For each of the 3 coordinates of T we'll first estimate how many samples of that size will produce a gradient pointing into the same direction as the reference gradient.

Given a sample size S, let A be the set of all possible samples of S points in L. Then $\forall a \in A$ we define the gradient

$$\frac{dI}{dT}(a) = \frac{1}{S}\frac{1}{S-1}\sum_{i \in a}\sum_{\substack{j \in a \\ j \neq i}} term(i,j)\frac{d}{dT}(v_i - v_j) \qquad (5)$$

as a random variable, denoted as dI, depending on a sample set a of size S. We assume that dI is Gaussian distributed. Thus, if we know the mean and the variance of dI, we will be able to determine how many samples will lead to a gradient pointing into the same direction as the reference gradient. In our approximation of $\frac{dI}{dT}$ we replace the sample a by L; which is in good accordance to the expectation of the Gaussian and obtain:

$$\frac{dI}{dT}(L) = \frac{1}{L}\frac{1}{L-1}\sum_{i \in L}\sum_{\substack{j \in L \\ j \neq i}} term(i,j)\frac{d}{dT}(v_i - v_j). \qquad (6)$$

This is a measure for the quality of the gradient for both optimization methods straight gradient ascent and Rprop. Now for any given point pair $(i \neq j)$ the corresponding addend in the double sum does not depend on the sample any more. Hence the mean of dI is equal to the reference gradient because all point pairs $(i \neq j)$ have the same probability of being in sample a. Based on all possible point pairs in L the variance of dI can be computed at a cost of $O(L^3)$ which is too expensive. We rewrite the reference gradient as

$$\frac{dI}{dT}(L) = \frac{1}{L}\frac{1}{L-1}\sum_{i \in L}\sum_{\substack{j \in L \\ j \neq i}}(term(i,j) + term(j,i))\frac{d}{dT}(v_i). \qquad (7)$$

For each $i \in L$, only the term $d/dT(v_i)$ contains local information. $term(i,j)$ only contains terms of the form $u_i - u_j$ and $v_i - v_j$, i.e. it depends on the grey value pairs $(u_i, v_i), i \in L$. We estimate these addend terms for all possible grey value pair combinations, i.e. we consider a bihistogram generated from the model and the target image. Let G be the number of grey values, then the bihistogramm contains $G \times G$ entries. Processing all points in L we add all $(u_i, v_i), i \in L$ into the bihistogram. Since the grey values typically fall in-between the bins of the histogram, their weight is distributed among the four neighboring bins. Computing the bihistogram is therefore of $O(L + G^2)$. We also compute the single histograms for U and V.

In order to further reduce the complexity, G is split into C intervals. Given a grey value pair $(g_u, g_v) \in G \times G$ and $(c_1, c_2) \in C \times C$, we define

$$I(g_u, g_v, c_1, c_2) = \{(g_1, g_2) \in G \times G : |g_u - g_1| \in [c_1 \cdot G/C, (c_1 + 1) \cdot G/C - 1]$$
$$\wedge |g_u - g_1| \in [c_1 \cdot G/C, (c_1 + 1) \cdot G/C - 1]\}. \qquad (8)$$

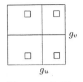

$I(g_u, g_v, 2, 3)$ inside
the bihistogram.

Any set $I(g_u, g_v, c_1, c_2)$ contains up to 4 rectangles. For each one of them the expectations $\mu(u_j)$ and $\mu(v_j)$ are computed. After that we replace $u_i - u_j$ by $g_u - \mu(u_j)$ and $v_i - v_j$ by $g_v - \mu(v_j)$ in equation (7). The computations inside the rectangles can be done in constant time by using summed area tables for precomputation.

Computing summed area tables [9] for the grey value expectations and for the bihistogram is of $O(G^2)$. Next, Parzen estimates $PE(g_u, g_v)$ are computed at $O(G^2 \cdot C^2)$. Again, we compute summed area tables of the Parzen estimates. This allows us to compute every possible addend of equation (8), $add(g_u, g_v)$. Finally, for every point $i \in L$, the corresponding 4 addends for the grey values are determined and form $add(i)$.

This way the whole estimation cost is $O(L + G^2 \cdot C^2)$. Having computed $add(i)$ for all points $i \in L$, we get

$$mean(dI) = dI(L) = \frac{1}{L} \sum_{i \in L} add(i). \qquad (9)$$

Then the variance can be computed as

$$\frac{1}{LS} \sum_{i \in L} (add(i))^2 + \frac{S-1}{L-1} \frac{1}{LS} \sum_{i \in L} \sum_{\substack{j \in L \\ j \neq i}} add(i) add(j) - mean(dI)^2$$

$$= \frac{1}{LS} \left(1 - \frac{S-1}{L-1} \right) \sum_{i \in L} (add(i))^2 + \left(\frac{S-1}{L-1} \frac{1}{LS} - \frac{1}{L^2} \right) \left(\sum_{i \in L} add(i) \right)^2 . \qquad (10)$$

Now we can use a lookup table containing the cumulative density function of the normal Gaussian to compute the desired percentage estimate.

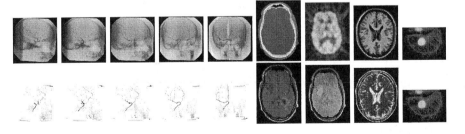

Fig. 1. Image pairs 1-5: CT images of a skull phantom and virtual X-ray projections of the 3D-volume reconstructed from 100 images. Pair 6: CT-MR scan of a brain slice [12]. Pair 7: PET-MR scan [12]. Pair 8: artificial MR slice obtained from [13] (T1-, T2-weighted). Pair 9: microscope image of a cell nucleus.

4.2 Verification

In order to verify the quality of this formula, we compared the estimations with real values based on a set of images in Fig.1. For each of the datasets we have applied our method to estimate mean gradients and percentages for sample sizes of 40-200 for 64 different poses and 3 parameter directions, denoted by k. Results are shown in table 3. For $G = 8$ and $C = 4$, this took 0.5-4.5 seconds, depending on L on an AMD Athlon, 800 MHz processor. We also computed the gradients dI/dT for 1000 random samples, computed the mean gradients and computed the percentage from the variance by the inverse Gaussian cdf. Some typical results are shown in Table 1.

For each sample size, all measured means and percentages are compared with the estimated ones (see table 2) showing good agreement between estimation and measurement.

Table 1. Data: Number of the data set, L: We presegmented the image into regions with high local gradient. Only these points are considered as relevant for matching. L denotes the number of pixels in the segmented regions. Sample: sample size, k: gradient coordinate, meas. %: measured percentage % , est. % estimated perc., meas. mean: measured mean, est. mean: estimated mean.

Data	L	sample	k	meas. %	est. %	meas. mean	est. mean
2	733	40	2	69.8	69.1	0.000728505	0.000720879
2	733	40	1	83.1	85.1	0.00145102	0.00151631
7	1819	100	0	86	86.9	0.00100356	0.00101309
7	1819	200	0	91.9	91.6	0.000677705	0.000687959

Table 2. Columns 4-6: mean of all 64 absolute differences of estimated and measured percentages for the three gradient coordinates k0-k2. Columns 7-9: normalized differences of estimated and observed means.

Data	L	sample	k0	k1	k2	k0	k1	k2
3	704	40	2.6875	2.0671	2.2546	0.3017	0.2568	0.3022
3	704	100	1.7296	1.3921	1.4156	0.09821	0.5366	0.05541
3	704	200	1.0265	0.875	0.9203	0.0322	0.0397	0.0349
7	1819	40	2.3781	1.9312	2.1968	2.4350	0.1093	0.1836
7	1819	100	1.0468	0.8734	0.8578	0.0986	0.0316	0.0306
7	1819	200	1.014	0.5765	0.6843	0.0838	0.0227	0.0289

5 Results

In table 3 we observe that for an estimated percentage of 75 the sample size is close to the optimum. For FD straight gradient ascent the optimal sample size is slightly greater. Table 3 shows two typical cases where we did not find a sample size that met our stability conditions. In these cases, even the deterministic approach of $S = L$ did not yield acceptable results. We conclude that

Table 3. Columns 3-11 show the mean over the $64 \cdot 3$ estimated percentages for each sample size 40-200. For some of the datasets we have chosen more than one segmentation, resulting in different values for L. The optimal sample sizes for Rprop are written bold.

Data	L	S=40	S=60	S=80	S=100	S=120	S=140	S=160	S=180	S=200
1	660	72.77	**76.78**	79.75	82.05	83.85	85.36	86.61	87.67	88.57
2	733	71.19	**75.02**	77.86	80.17	81.98	83.50	84.74	85.77	86.68
3	704	72.58	**76.44**	79.33	81.53	83.28	84.68	85.87	86.88	87.76
4	693	74.61	**78.83**	81.95	84.30	86.17	87.63	88.79	89.75	90.52
4	1518	70.51	**74.40**	77.34	79.71	81.68	83.34	84.72	85.92	86.94
4	265	72.42	76.40	79.46	82.01	84.25	86.20	87.95	89.55	91.07
5	647	70.26	73.91	**76.70**	78.88	80.69	82.21	83.50	84.62	85.59
6	1896	66.12	69.29	71.76	**73.78**	75.53	77.01	78.34	79.49	80.54
6	1073	68.21	71.63	74.24	76.39	78.13	79.60	80.91	82.02	83.00
7	1819	67.81	71.19	73.82	**75.98**	77.79	79.34	80.61	81.76	82.81
8	5743	68.69	**72.10**	74.74	76.86	78.60	80.03	81.30	82.37	83.30
8	3143	72.31	**76.18**	79.02	81.27	83.04	84.50	85.67	86.67	87.54
9	204	**78.18**	82.66	85.73	88.03	89.90	91.54	93.15	94.81	96.71

Table 4. Method: the stochastic optimization method, r_0, d_0: start angle in degrees, start translation in pixels for T. The resulting T gives an error rotation r_e in degrees and an error translation d_e in pixels. We consider the result as being good if $r_e < 1$ and $d_e < 1$. iter: average number of iterations, time: average time.

Data	method	r_0	d_0	good (%)	$r_e(deg)$	$d_e(pix)$	iter	time (ms)
1	Rrop	6	8	90	0.062	0.06	126	506
1	FD	6	8	89	0.192	0.177	150	682
1	Rrop	4	8	94	0.058	0.062	118	484
1	FD	4	8	92	0.175	0.168	150	682
1	Rrop(G)	6	8	92	0.068	0.076	132	460
9	Rrop(G)	14	28	100	0.072	0.065	99	314
7	Rrop	8	8	98	0.174	0.197	117	1229
7	Rrop	6	16	99	0.172	0.183	128	1271
8	Rrop	10	8	99	0.081	0.07	90	627
8	Rrop	6	12	87	0.078	0.076	108	850

if the alignment is not found for a 75%-sample size, a different segmentation is necessary that includes more information about the images.

For each row in table 4 we have run the experiments with 100 randomly chosen initial poses T, with a starting error angle of r_0 and a starting translation of d_0 pixels in a random direction. The optimal solution for all of them is $T = 0$. We use a two-stage multiresolution approach: The images are downsized two times, then a matching is performed, then the matching is done on the original size to improve the accuracy. In order to speed up our registration, we introduce a local method. We reduce the number of point pairs in equation (1) by laying a grid over the target image, thus splitting it into squares. For every point x_i, only the points x_j inside and in adjacent squares are taken into account. This approach, marked as (G), works for the datasets 1-5 and 9, but not for 6-8. In our experiments Rprop has been more accurate than FD while requiring less time. All testing was done on an AMD Athlon, 800 MHz processor.

6 Conclusion

As can be seen in table 3 the optimal sample size can be estimated in less than one second if $L < 800$. The estimation is, however, only valid if the point set L is large enough; otherwise the target function is ill-conditioned. Even choosing $L = S$ will then not yield satisfying results.

In all stochastic gradient-based optimization methods the choice of the gain sequences is crucial to the performance. We have found that Rprop is easier to handle than straight gradient ascent because less parameters have to be chosen to get good results. Depending on the images the local grid approach can speed up the registration by a factor of up to 4, especially for small motions.

Acknowledgment. This project was supported by BMBF-grant 01 EZ 0024.

References

1. P. Viola. Alignment by Maximization of Mutual Information. PhD-Thesis, Massachusetts Institute of Technology, 1995.
2. L. Ng, L. Ibanez. Narrow Band to Image Registration in the Insight Toolkit. WBIR'03, LNCS 2717, pp.271-280, Springer Verlag, 2003.
3. B. Fei, Z. Lee et al. Image Registration for Interventional MRI Guided Procedures: Interpolation methods, Similarity Measurements, and Applications to the Prostate. WBIR'03, LNCS 2717, pp.321-329, Springer Verlag, 2003.
4. J. Spall. Introduction to Stochastic Search and Optimization: Estimation, Simulation, and Control. Wiley, 2003.
5. Xu Meihe, R. Srinivasan, W.L. Nowinski. A Fast Mutual Information Method for Multi-modal Registration. IPMI'99, LNCS 1613, pp. 466-471, Springer Verlag, 1999.
6. R. Strzodka, M. Droske, M. Rumpf. Fast Image Registration in DX9 Graphics Hardware. Journal of Medical Informatics and Technologies, 6:43-49, Nov 2003.
7. N. Schraudolph, T. Graepel. Towards Stochastic Conjugate Gradient Methods. Proc. 9th Intl. Conf. Neural Information Processing, Singapore 2002
8. G. Soza, P. Hastreiter, M. Bauer et al. Non-rigid Registration with Use of Hardware-Based 3D Bezier Functions. MICCAI 2002, pp. 549-556
9. P. Lacroute. Fast Volume Rendering Using a Shear-Warp Factorization of the Viewing Transformation. PhD-Thesis, Stanford University, 1995.
10. J. Pluim, et al. Mutual-Information-Based Registration of Medical Images: A Survey. IEEE Transactions on Medical Imaging, Vol. 22, No. 8, Aug 2003.
11. U. Müller et al. Correction of C-arm Projection Matrices by 3D-2D Rigid Registration of CT-Images Using Mutual Information. WBIR'03, LNCS 2717, pp.161-170, Springer Verlag, 2003.
12. http://www.itk.org/HTML/MutualInfo.htm
13. http://www.bic.mni.mcgill.ca/brainweb/

Finite Deformation Guided Nonlinear Filtering for Multiframe Cardiac Motion Analysis

C.L. Ken Wong and Pengcheng Shi

Biomedical Research Laboratory
Department of Electrical and Electronic Engineering
Hong Kong University of Science and Technology
Clear Water Bay, Kowloon, Hong Kong
{eewclken, eeship}@ust.hk

Abstract. In order to obtain sensible estimates of myocardial kinematics based on biomechanics constraints, one must adopt appropriate material, deformation, and temporal models. Earlier efforts, although not concurrently adopted within the same framework, have shown that it is essential to carefully consider the fibrous structure of the myocardium, the large geometric deformation of the cardiac wall movement, the multiframe observations over the cardiac cycle, and the uncertainties in the system modeling and data measurements. With the meshfree particle method providing the platform to enforce the anisotropic material property derived from the myofiber architecture, we present the first effort to perform *multiframe* cardiac motion analysis under *finite deformation* conditions, posed as a nonlinear statistical filtering process. Total Lagrangian (TL) formulation is adopted to establish the myocardial system dynamics under finite deformation, which is then used to perform nonlinear state space prediction (of the tissue displacement and velocity) at each time frame, using the Newton-Raphson iteration scheme. The system matrices of the state space equation are then derived, and the optimal estimation of the kinematic state is achieved through TL-updated recursive filtering. Results from synthetic data with ground truth and canine cardiac image sequence are presented.

1 Introduction

In cardiac motion analysis, the imaging data typically only provide noisy measurements at some salient landmark points, such as the Lagrangian tag displacements from the MR tagging images and the Eulerian tissue velocities from the MR phase contrast data. In order to obtain the complete cardiac motion field, *a priori* material, deformation, and temporal constraints are required to obtain a unique solution in some optimal sense [3].

For successful and meaningful cardiac motion recovery using biomechanical models, the myocardial constitutive laws and the deformation properties need to be properly considered [4]. From experimental testings, it has been shown that the material properties along and cross the myofibers are substantially

C. Barillot, D.R. Haynor, and P. Hellier (Eds.): MICCAI 2004, LNCS 3216, pp. 895–902, 2004.
© Springer-Verlag Berlin Heidelberg 2004

different. Furthermore, it has long been observed that normal cardiac deformation (radial contraction) reaches at least 30% between end-diastole (ED) and end-systole (ES). Hence, spatial constraints with anisotropic properties and finite deformation models are required for realistic cardiac motion analysis. Sofar, however, with few recent exceptions [5,11], most of the efforts have been using the isotropic material model for computational simplicity [3]. Moreover, except our most recent work [12], no algorithm has undergone the essential finite deformation analysis. In addition, multiframe analysis is also of paramount importance for cardiac motion recovery. The temporal kinematics coherence plays key roles in achieving robust motion estimates, especially when there are uncertainties in system models and noises in input data [7,8,10]. Unfortunately, none of these multiframe works have employed the proper anisotropic and finite deformation constraints.

In our recent work, the importance of using anisotropic material and finite deformation models has been demonstrated for frame-to-frame analysis [12]. We have also shown the advantages of using the meshfree particle method (MPM) to deal with myofiber orientations, geometric and kinematics discontinuities, and representation refinements. In this paper, we extend that effort to perform multiframe analysis under finite deformation conditions as a nonlinear statistical filtering problem. Total Lagrangian (TL) formulation is adopted to establish the myocardial system dynamics under large deformation, which then relies on the Newton-Raphson scheme to perform nonlinear predictions of the displacement and velocity for the next time frame. The system matrices of the state space representation are then derived, and the optimal estimation of the kinematic state is achieved through TL-updated recursive filtering. Simulations on synthetic data have shown superior performance over existing strategies, and experiments with canine MR images have produced physiologically sensible outcomes.

2   Methodology

2.1   Meshfree Particle Representation of Myocardium

Using the meshfree particle method, the myocardium can be represented by a set of unstructured, adaptively sampled nodes, bounded by the segmented endo- and epi-cardial boundaries (see Fig. 2 for a MPM represented 2D LV slice). Let $u(\mathbf{x})$ be the displacement field of the myocardial tissue at point $\mathbf{x}$, the approximated displacement function $u^h(\mathbf{x})$ is then given by the moving least square (MLS) approximation: $u^h(\mathbf{x}) = \sum_{I=1}^{N} \phi_I(\mathbf{x}) u_I$, where $\phi_I(\mathbf{x})$ is the MLS shape function of node I, N is the total number of sampling nodes, and u_I is the nodal displacement value [8].

2.2   Anisotropic Composite Material Model

Realistic anisotropic material models are essential for the accurate recovery of cardiac movement. For elastic materials, both isotropic and anisotropic, the 2D stress-strain relationships obey the Hooke's Law:

$$\begin{bmatrix} S_{11} \\ S_{22} \\ S_{12} \end{bmatrix} = C \begin{bmatrix} \epsilon_{11} \\ \epsilon_{22} \\ \epsilon_{12} \end{bmatrix} \tag{1}$$

where ϵ_{ij} are the components of the Green-Lagrangian strain tensor, S_{ij} are the components of the second Piola-Kirchhoff (PKII) stress tensor, and C is the stiffness matrix. Let the 2D stiffness matrix of a point with 0° fiber orientation be C_o and of the form:

$$C_o = \begin{bmatrix} 1/E_f & -\nu/E_f & 0 \\ -\nu/E_f & 1/E_{cf} & 0 \\ 0 & 0 & 1/G \end{bmatrix}^{-1} \tag{2}$$

where E_{cf} and E_f are the cross-fiber and along-fiber Young's modulus respectively, ν is the Poisson ratio measuring the material compressibility, and $G \approx E_f/(2(1+v))$ describes the shearing properties. Then, the stiffness matrix at any point with fiber orientation θ can be calculated from C_o through $C_\theta = T^{-1}C_oRTR^{-1}$ [9], where T is the coordinate transformation matrix which is a function of θ, and R is a matrix responsible for the transformation between the strain tensor components and the engineering strain tensor components.

2.3   Myocardial System Dynamics under Finite Deformation

When the deformation is large, the strain calculated by directly using the linearized Green-Lagrangian strain calculation would not be accurate because the term $\frac{1}{2}u_{i,k}u_{j,k}$ in the full Green-Lagrangian strain calculation $\epsilon_{ij} = \frac{1}{2}(u_{i,j} + u_{j,i} + u_{k,i}u_{k,j})$ (where $u_{i,j} = \partial u_i/\partial x_j$) becomes large. Hence, to proper treat all kinematics nonlinear effects caused by large rotations, large displacements, and large strains, the dynamic equilibrium equation with linearized incremental Total Lagrangian (TL) formulation should be used [1].

Using the displacement field approximation derived at Section 2.1, the TL represents the equilibrium at time $t + \Delta t$ in the following form [1]:

$$({}_0^t\mathbf{K}_L + {}_0^t\mathbf{K}_{NL})\Delta\mathbf{U} = {}_0^t\tilde{\mathbf{K}}\Delta\mathbf{U} = {}^{t+\Delta t}\mathbf{R} - {}_0^t\mathbf{F} \tag{3}$$

where ${}_0^t\mathbf{K}_L$ and ${}_0^t\mathbf{K}_{NL}$ are the linear and nonlinear strain incremental stiffness matrices, respectively, ${}^{t+\Delta t}\mathbf{R}$ is the external force, ${}_0^t\mathbf{F}$ is the force related to the stress, and $\Delta\mathbf{U} = [\Delta u_1, \Delta u_2, ...\Delta u_N]^T$ is the incremental displacement vector caused by the force difference ${}^{t+\Delta t}\mathbf{R} - {}_0^t\mathbf{F}$.

Equation (3) is the complete governing equation for static finite deformation analysis. By considering the inertia of the system, it becomes the system governing equation for dynamic finite deformation analysis [1]:

$$ {}_0^t\mathbf{M}\,{}^{t+\Delta t}\ddot{\mathbf{U}} + {}_0^t\mathbf{C}\,{}^{t+\Delta t}\dot{\mathbf{U}} + {}_0^t\tilde{\mathbf{K}}\,\Delta\mathbf{U} = {}^{t+\Delta t}\mathbf{R} - {}_0^t\mathbf{F} \tag{4}$$

where ${}^{t+\Delta t}\ddot{\mathbf{U}}$ and ${}^{t+\Delta t}\dot{\mathbf{U}}$ are the acceleration and velocity at time $t+\Delta t$ respectively, ${}_0^t\mathbf{M}$ is the mass matrix, and ${}_0^t\mathbf{C}$ is the damping matrix.

---

[1] In all equations, the left subscript indicates the time at which the measurement is referred to, and the left superscript indicates the time at which the quantity is measured.

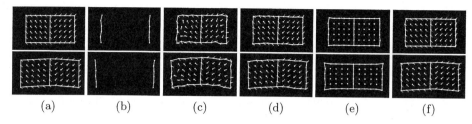

Fig. 1. Experiments on the synthetic data. (a): Two frames (#1 and #9, out of sixteen) of a deforming object which is composed of two materials. Generated by enforcing outward boundary displacements on the left and right edges, with frame #1 the original configuration. (b): Noisy displacement observations on the left and right edges (SNR= $2.919dB$), used as data inputs. (c)-(f): Recovered object geometry from the noisy data, using: frame-to-frame estimation with anisotropic material and finite deformation models (c); multiframe estimation with anisotropic material and infinitesimal deformation models (d); multiframe estimation with isotropic material and finite deformation models (e); and multiframe estimation with anisotropic material and finite deformation models (f).

2.4   Frame-to-Frame Nonlinear Kinematics Analysis

While solving for Equation (4), in order to reduce the error introduced by the linearization at any particular time instance, the Newton-Raphson iteration is employed [1]. Using the trapezoidal rules, i.e. ${}^{t+\Delta t}\dot{U} = {}^{t}\dot{U} + \frac{\Delta t}{2}({}^{t}\ddot{U} + {}^{t+\Delta t}\ddot{U})$ and ${}^{t+\Delta t}U = {}^{t}U + \frac{\Delta t}{2}({}^{t}\dot{U} + {}^{t+\Delta t}\dot{U})$, and the displacement update equation during the Newton-Raphson iteration ${}^{t+\Delta t}U^{k} = {}^{t+\Delta t}U^{k-1} + \Delta U^{k}$ where the right superscript k indicates the iteration and ${}^{t+\Delta t}U^{0} = {}^{t}U$, then we have

$$
{}^{t+\Delta t}\dot{U}^{k} = \frac{2}{\Delta t}({}^{t+\Delta t}U^{k-1} + \Delta U^{k} - {}^{t}U) - {}^{t}\dot{U} \tag{5}
$$

$$
{}^{t+\Delta t}\ddot{U}^{k} = \frac{4}{\Delta t^{2}}({}^{t+\Delta t}U^{k-1} + \Delta U^{k} - {}^{t}U) - \frac{4}{\Delta t}{}^{t}\dot{U} - {}^{t}\ddot{U} \tag{6}
$$

Substituting Equations (5) and (6) into Equation (4), after rearrangement, we obtain the governing iteration equation between time t and time $t + \Delta t$ as [2]:

$$
\hat{K}^{k-1}\Delta U^{k} = \Delta R^{k-1} - (\hat{K}^{k-1} - \tilde{K}^{k-1})U^{k-1} \tag{7}
$$

where

$$
\hat{K}^{k-1} = \frac{4}{\Delta t^{2}}M^{k-1} + \frac{2}{\Delta t}C^{k-1} + \tilde{K}^{k-1}
$$

$$
\Delta R^{k-1} = {}^{t+\Delta t}R - F^{k-1}
$$

$$
- M^{k-1}(-\frac{4}{\Delta t^{2}}{}^{t}U - \frac{4}{\Delta t}{}^{t}\dot{U} - {}^{t}\ddot{U}) - C^{k-1}(-\frac{2}{\Delta t}{}^{t}U - {}^{t}\dot{U})
$$

---

[2] In order to keep the equation simple to read, we assume that any parameter with right superscript k is measured at time $t + \Delta t$, thus we can omit the left scripts indicating the time.

Table 1. Positional differences between the ground truth and estimated nodal locations under different models.

temporal material deformation	frame-to-frame anisotropic finite	multi-frame anisotropic infinitesimal	multi-frame isotropic finite	multi-frame anisotropic finite
Frame #1	0.31170±0.25571	0.18633±0.09015	0.15672±0.12818	0.10805±0.10021
Frame #9	0.33567±0.20786	0.21138±0.12648	0.32348±0.19121	0.10881±0.10293

with $\mathbf{M}^0 = {}^t_0\mathbf{M}$, $\mathbf{C}^0 = {}^t_0\mathbf{C}$, $\mathbf{K}^0 = {}^t_0\mathbf{K}$, and $\mathbf{F}^0 = {}^t_0\mathbf{F}$. The governing iteration equation (7) would iterate until the unbalanced dynamic force $\Delta\mathbf{R}^{k-1} - (\hat{\mathbf{K}}^{k-1} - \tilde{\mathbf{K}}^{k-1})\mathbf{U}^{k-1}$ approaches zero.

Using Equation (7), the displacement update equation during the Newton-Raphson iteration becomes

$$\mathbf{U}^k = (\hat{\mathbf{K}}^{k-1})^{-1}\,\tilde{\mathbf{K}}^{k-1}\mathbf{U}^{k-1} + (\hat{\mathbf{K}}^{k-1})^{-1}\Delta\mathbf{R}^{k-1} \tag{8}$$

Let $\bar{k}$ be the iteration at which convergence occurs, and let $A^{k-1} = (\hat{\mathbf{K}}^{k-1})^{-1}\,\tilde{\mathbf{K}}^{k-1}$ and $B^{k-1} = (\hat{\mathbf{K}}^{k-1})^{-1}\Delta\mathbf{R}^{k-1}$. With Equation (8), the relation between $\mathbf{U}^{\bar{k}}$ and $\mathbf{U}^0$ is derived to be

$$\mathbf{U}^{\bar{k}} = (\prod_{i=0}^{\bar{k}-1} A^i)\mathbf{U}^0 + \sum_{i=1}^{\bar{k}-1}((\prod_{j=i}^{\bar{k}-1} A^j)B^{i-1}) + B^{\bar{k}-1} \tag{9}$$

Using this equation, Equation (5) can be written into

$$\dot{\mathbf{U}}^{\bar{k}} = \frac{2}{\Delta t}(\prod_{i=0}^{\bar{k}-1} A^i - \mathbf{I})\mathbf{U}^0 - \dot{\mathbf{U}}^0 + \frac{2}{\Delta t}(\sum_{i=1}^{\bar{k}-1}((\prod_{j=i}^{\bar{k}-1} A^j)B^{i-1}) + B^{\bar{k}-1}) \tag{10}$$

2.5 State Space Analysis of Nonlinear System Dynamics: Optimal Multiframe Kinematics Estimation

Since $\mathbf{U}^{\bar{k}} = {}^{t+\Delta t}\mathbf{U}$, $\mathbf{U}^0 = {}^t\mathbf{U}$, $\dot{\mathbf{U}}^{\bar{k}} = {}^{t+\Delta t}\dot{\mathbf{U}}$, and $\dot{\mathbf{U}}^0 = {}^t\dot{\mathbf{U}}$, Equations (9) and (10) can be combined in the form

$$x(t + \Delta t) = D(t + \Delta t)x(t) + w(t) \tag{11}$$

where

$$D(t + \Delta t) = \begin{bmatrix} \prod_{i=0}^{\bar{k}-1} A^i & 0 \\ \frac{2}{\Delta t}(\prod_{i=0}^{\bar{k}-1} A^i - \mathbf{I}) & -\mathbf{I} \end{bmatrix},$$

$$w(t) = \begin{bmatrix} \sum_{i=1}^{\bar{k}-1}((\prod_{j=i}^{\bar{k}-1} A^j)B^{i-1}) + B^{\bar{k}-1} \\ \frac{2}{\Delta t}(\sum_{i=1}^{\bar{k}-1}((\prod_{j=i}^{\bar{k}-1} A^j)B^{i-1}) + B^{\bar{k}-1}) \end{bmatrix},$$

$$x(t + \Delta t) = \begin{bmatrix} {}^{t+\Delta t}\mathbf{U} \\ {}^{t+\Delta t}\dot{\mathbf{U}} \end{bmatrix}, \quad \text{and} \quad x(t) = \begin{bmatrix} {}^t\mathbf{U} \\ {}^t\dot{\mathbf{U}} \end{bmatrix}.$$

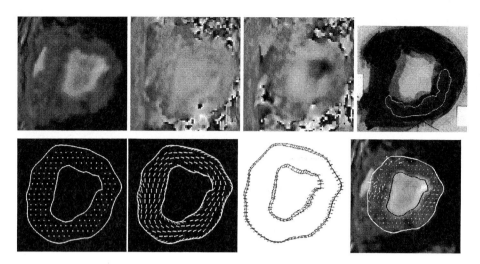

Fig. 2. Canine MRI phase contrast data. From left to right: MR intensity, x-velocity, y-velocity, and TTC-stained post mortem myocardium with infarcted tissue highlighted (top); meshfree representation of the slice, myofiber orientations, boundary displacement constraints, and phase contrast velocity field (bottom).

Including the zero-mean, additive, and white process noise $v(t)$ ($E[v(t)] = 0$, $E[v(t)v(s)'] = Q_v(t)\delta_{ts}$), Equation (11) becomes the TL-updated state-space equation which has performed nonlinear state prediction of tissue displacement and velocity using the Newton-Raphson iteration scheme:

$$x(t + \Delta t) = D(t + \Delta t)x(t) + w(t) + v(t) \tag{12}$$

Since the data observations $y(t + \Delta t)$ obtained from the imaging data are corrupted by noise $e(t)$ (once again, assuming zero-mean, additive, and white, with $E[e(t)] = 0$, $E[e(t)e(s)'] = R_e(t)\delta_{ts}$), the measurement equation thus is:

$$y(t + \Delta t) = Hx(t + \Delta t) + e(t + \Delta t), \tag{13}$$

where H is a known, user-specified measurement matrix.

With the discretized state space equations (12) and (13), the multiframe estimation of the cardiac kinematics over the cardiac cycle can be performed using standard recursive filtering procedures until convergence [6]:

1. Initialize state and error covariance estimates, $\hat{x}(t)$ and $P(t)$.
2. Prediction step: using the filter update equations to predict the state and error covariance at time $t + \Delta t$:

$$\hat{x}^-(t + \Delta t) = D(t + \Delta t)\hat{x}(t) + w(t) \tag{14}$$
$$P^-(t + \Delta t) = D(t + \Delta t)P(t)D^T(t + \Delta t) + Q_v(t) \tag{15}$$

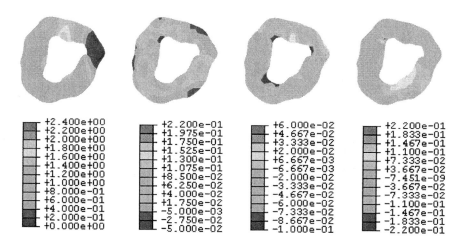

+2.400e+00	+2.200e-01	+6.000e-02	+2.200e-01
+2.200e+00	+1.975e-01	+4.667e-02	+1.833e-01
+2.000e+00	+1.750e-01	+3.333e-02	+1.467e-01
+1.800e+00	+1.525e-01	+2.000e-02	+1.100e-01
+1.600e+00	+1.300e-01	+6.667e-03	+7.333e-02
+1.400e+00	+1.075e-01	-6.667e-03	+3.667e-02
+1.200e+00	+8.500e-02	-2.000e-02	-7.451e-09
+1.000e+00	+6.250e-02	-3.333e-02	-3.667e-02
+8.000e-01	+4.000e-02	-4.667e-02	-7.333e-02
+6.000e-01	+1.750e-02	-6.000e-02	-1.100e-01
+4.000e-01	-5.000e-03	-7.333e-02	-1.467e-01
+2.000e-01	-2.750e-02	-8.667e-02	-1.833e-01
+0.000e+00	-5.000e-02	-1.000e-01	-2.200e-01

Fig. 3. Estimated displacement, and radial, circumferential, and RC shear strain maps for frame #9 (with respective to frame #1).

3. Correction step: with the use of filter gain $G(t + \Delta t)$, the predictions are updated using the measurements $y(t + \Delta t)$:

$$G(t + \Delta t) = P^-(t + \Delta t)H^T(HP^-(t + \Delta t)H^T + R_e(t + \Delta t))^{-1} \quad (16)$$

$$\hat{x}(t + \Delta t) = \hat{x}^-(t + \Delta t) + G(t + \Delta t)(y(t + \Delta t) - H\hat{x}^-(t + \Delta t)) \quad (17)$$

$$P(t + \Delta t) = (I - G(t + \Delta t)H)P^-(t + \Delta t) \quad (18)$$

3   Experiments

3.1   Synthetic Data

As shown in Fig. 1, experiments have been conducted on a synthetic image sequence (16 frames) with different material, deformation, and temporal models to verify the needs to adopt the proper model constraints. The importance of using multiframe filtering can be observed by comparing Fig. 1(c) to Fig. 1(d,e,f). From Fig. 1(d) and (f), it can be seen that Fig. 1(d) deviates comparatively more than Fig. 1(f). This is because when deformation is large, the error caused by linearized strain tensor would accumulate during the filtering loop, so the object gradually deforms away from the configuration at the previous loop and would not converge. The importance of using anisotropic material model is shown between Fig. 1(e) and (f). Similarly, it can be seen from Table. 1 that the deformed geometry using multiframe estimation with finite deformation and anisotropic material models deviates the least from the ground truth.

3.2   In Vivo Canine MRI Data

Experiments have also been performed using a canine cardiac phase contrast MRI sequence (Fig.2), which contains the cardiac anatomy and also the respective instantaneous velocities of the tissues. The myofiber orientations are mapped onto the particular image slice, based on the principal warps algorithm of the landmarks [2]. The heart boundaries and their shape-based displacements over the 16-frame cardiac cycle are estimated [13], along with the mid-wall phase contrast velocities (Fig.2). The recovered displacement and cardiac-specific strain maps are shown in Fig. 3. Compared to our earlier, frame-to-frame results [12], these outcomes are overall better correlated with the TTC stained tissue.

This work is supported, in part, by HKRGC CERG Grant HKUST6151/03E.

References

1. K.J. Bathe. *Finite Element Procedures*. Prentice Hall, 1996.
2. F.L. Bookstein. Principal warps: Thin-plate splines and the decomposition of deformations. *IEEE PAMI*, 11:567–585, 1989.
3. A.J. Frangi, W.J. Niessen, and M.A. Viergever. Three-dimensional modeling for functional analysis of cardiac images: A review. *IEEE TMI*, 20:2–25, 2001.
4. L. Glass, P. Hunter, and A. McCulloch, editors. *Theory of Heart*. Springer, 1991.
5. Z. Hu, D. Metaxas, and L. Axel. *In vivo* strain and stress estimation of the heart left and right ventricles from MRI images. *Medical Image Analysis*, 7:435–444, 2003.
6. E.W. Kamen and J.K. Su. *Introduction to Optimal Estimation*. Springer, 1999.
7. W.S. Kerwin and J.L. Prince. The kriging update model and recursive space-time function estimation. *IEEE TSP*, 47:2942–2952, 1999.
8. H. Liu and P. Shi. Meshfree representation and computation: applications to cardiac motion analysis. In *IPMI'03*, pages 560–572, 2003.
9. F.L. Matthews and R.D. Rawlings. *Composite Materials*. Chapman & Hall, 1994.
10. J.C. McEachen and J.S. Duncan. Multiframe temporal estimation of cardiac nonrigid motion. *IEEE TMI*, 16:270–283, 1997.
11. X. Papademetris, A.J. Sinusas, D.P. Dione, R.T. Constable, and J.S. Duncan. Estimation of 3D left ventricular deformation from medical images using biomechanical models. *IEEE TMI*, 21:786–799, 2002.
12. C.L. Wong, H. Liu, L.N. Wong, A.J. Sinusas, and P. Shi. Meshfree cardiac motion analysis framework using composite material model and total Lagrangian formulation. In *IEEE ISBI'04*, pages 464–467, 2004.
13. L.N. Wong, H. Liu, A. Sinusas, and P. Shi. Spatio-temporal active region model for simultaneous segmentation and motion estimation of the whole heart. In *IEEE VLSM'03*, pages 193–200, 2003.

Contrast-Invariant Registration of Cardiac and Renal MR Perfusion Images

Ying Sun[1], Marie-Pierre Jolly[2], and José M.F. Moura[1]

[1] Department of Electrical and Computer Engineering, Carnegie Mellon University,
Pittsburgh, PA 15213, USA
[2] Department of Imaging and Visualization, Siemens Corporate Research, Inc.
Princeton, NJ 08540, USA

Abstract. Automatic registration of dynamic MR perfusion images is a challenging task *due to the rapid changes of the image contrast caused by the wash-in and wash-out of the contrast agent.* In this paper we introduce a contrast-invariant similarity metric and propose a common framework to perform affine registration on both cardiac and renal MR perfusion images. First, large-scale translational motion is identified by tracking a selected region of interest with integer pixel shifts. Then, we estimate the affine transformation of the organ for each frame. We have tested the proposed algorithm on real cardiac and renal MR perfusion scans and obtained encouraging registration results.

1 Introduction

Dynamic perfusion magnetic resonance imaging (MRI) has demonstrated great potential for diagnosing cardiovascular and renovascular diseases [1] [2]. In dynamic perfusion MRI, the organ under study is scanned repeatedly and rapidly following a bolus injection of a contrast agent. Changes in pixel intensity corresponding to the same tissue across the image sequence provide valuable functional information about the organ being imaged. However, perfusion MR image sequences suffer from motion induced by patient breathing during acquisition. Therefore, registration must be performed on time-series images to ensure the correspondence of anatomical structures in different frames. Due to the vast amounts of data acquired in dynamic perfusion MRI studies (on average, over 100 images per scan), automatic registration is strongly desirable. This paper focuses on automatic registration of cardiac and renal MR perfusion images.

Goal: Given a sequence of perfusion MR images for the heart or the kidney, we want to solve the registration problem: establish the appropriate correspondence between every pixel in the region of interest in each frame of the sequence.

Difficulties: This is difficult and standard block matching techniques do not work because the intensity at the same physical location changes across the MR image sequence due to the wash-in and wash-out of the contrast agent. To the best of our knowledge, there has been limited work on image registration to address these difficulties. An image registration algorithm that utilizes the maximization of mutual information has recently been proposed for cardiac MR

C. Barillot, D.R. Haynor, and P. Hellier (Eds.): MICCAI 2004, LNCS 3216, pp. 903–910, 2004.

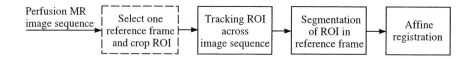

Fig. 1. The block diagram of the proposed registration algorithm

perfusion data [3]. Several methods have been developed for registration of renal MR perfusion images [4] [5] [6]. These methods all require manually drawn contours in one time frame to obtain a mask or a model; this model is then used to propagate the contours to other frames in the image sequence.

Our approach: We avoid manually drawn contours and only require the user to crop a rectangular region of interest (ROI). Since translation is the dominant motion caused by breathing, we divide the registration problem into two steps: large translation motion followed by affine transformation. The detailed sequence of steps is the following.

(1) Choose a reference frame and define a bounding box for the ROI;
(2) Compute the edge map in the bounding box of the reference frame and in the search window of other frames in the MR image sequence;
(3) Determine large-scale translation motion of the ROI by maximizing a contrast-invariant similarity metric between the current and the reference frames;
(4) Obtain the contours that delineate the boundaries of the organ in the reference frame through the segmentation of a difference image;
(5) Propagate the segmentation results to other frames by searching for the affine transformations that best match these frames to the reference frame.

Except for the first step, all other steps are automatic. The experimental results with real patient data show that by exploiting the invariance of the similarity metric our algorithm provides very good registration results.

2   Method

From the application point of view, it is reasonable to ask the user to select from the sequence of images one that has a good contrast and then crop an ROI in this selected frame. Fig. 1 illustrates the three main stages of the algorithm: tracking the ROI across the image sequence, segmentation of the ROI in the reference frame, and affine registration. Except for the segmentation block that is explained elsewhere, these stages are described in detail in the following sections with experiments on real MR perfusion patient datasets .

2.1   Tracking the ROI Across the Image Sequence

Given an ROI in one frame, the goal of this stage is to find the best match to the selected ROI in other frames. At this stage, we assume that the motion is reduced to translation with integer pixel shifts. Tracking the ROI is achieved by simple template matching. The key observation is that the orientation of the edges along tissue boundaries are always *parallel* across the image sequence, despite the fact that the relative intensities between tissues vary with time. Therefore, we choose the template defined by the orientation of the image gradient.

In our formulation, the image on which the ROI is manually cropped is called the *reference* frame. Let $\theta_r(x, y)$ and $M_r(x, y)$ stand for respectively the direction and the magnitude of the image gradient at pixel (x, y) in the reference frame; we obtain θ_r and M_r using a Sobel edge detector, [7]. We denote the set of pixels in the ROI as $\mathcal{R} = \{(x, y) | x_a \leq x \leq x_b, y_a \leq y \leq y_b\}$, where (x_a, y_a) and (x_b, y_b) are the two diagonal points that specify the bounding box of the ROI. Let $\theta_c(x, y)$ denote the edge orientation and $M_c(x, y)$ the edge magnitude at pixel (x, y) in the *current* frame. For each offset pair (dx, dy), we define the angle difference $\Delta\theta(x, y; dx, dy)$ and a weight function $w(x, y; dx, dy)$ by

$$\Delta\theta(x, y; dx, dy) = \theta_c(x + dx, y + dy) - \theta_r(x, y), \tag{1}$$

$$w(x, y; dx, dy) = \frac{M_c(x + dx, y + dy)M_r(x, y)}{\sum_{(x,y)\in\mathcal{R}} M_c(x + dx, y + dy)M_r(x, y)}. \tag{2}$$

We introduce a similarity metric:

$$S(dx, dy) = \sum_{(x,y)\in\mathcal{R}} w(x, y; dx, dy) \cos(2\Delta\theta(x, y; dx, dy)). \tag{3}$$

Note that $S(dx, dy)$ is the weighted average of the values of $\cos(2\Delta\theta)$ over the ROI, and its value lies in the interval of $[-1, 1]$. We use the cosine of the double angle to handle contrast inversions that commonly occur in perfusion studies. For instance, in a renal MR perfusion scan, see the first image in the bottom row in Fig. 2, the kidney is relatively darker compared to the surrounding tissues before the wash-in of the contrast agent; it becomes relatively brighter after the wash-in of the contrast agent as shown in the second image in the bottom row in Fig. 2. In addition, we choose the weight function as the normalized product of the edge magnitudes because it is desirable for the ROI to be attracted to strong edges in the current frame that are mostly parallel to the strong edges in the reference frame. The proposed similarity metric is invariant to rapidly changing image contrast, in the sense that its value is insensitive to changes in the contrast as long as the edge orientations are nearly parallel to those of the template. The integer shifts (dx^*, dy^*) that maximize S are determined by exploring all possible solutions (dx, dy) over a reasonable search space. It is important to point out that the value of $S(dx^*, dy^*)$ also plays a role as a confidence measure. To improve the robustness of the algorithm, we use both the *previous* frame and the *reference* frame as templates. The algorithm then chooses the match with maximum similarity metric.

We display in Fig. 2 selected frames from a renal (top row) and a cardiac (bottom row) MR perfusion scan, respectively. In cardiac perfusion, the contrast agent passes through the right ventricle to the left ventricle and then perfuses into the myocardium. Similarly, the intensity of the kidney increases as the contrast

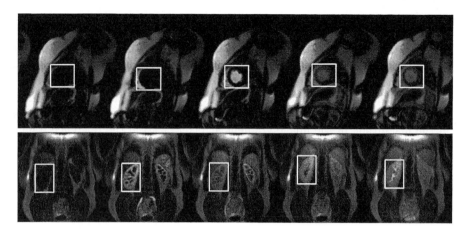

Fig. 2. Results obtained by tracking the ROI with integer pixel shifts on selected frames from a cardiac (top) and a renal (bottom) MR perfusion image sequence.

agent perfuses into the cortex, the medulla, and other structures of the kidney. To illustrate the performance of the proposed tracking algorithm, we shift the bounding box of the ROI to the best match location in each frame, see Fig. 2. Despite the rapidly changing image contrast and the fact that translational motion between two adjacent frames can be considerably large, the algorithm reliably tracks the selected ROI across the image sequence for both cardiac and renal perfusion studies, with minor tracking error in frames that lack strong edges. To further improve the accuracy of the registration results, we propose to estimate the local affine transformation of the heart or kidney by incorporating the knowledge of the contours delineating organ boundaries in the reference frame. This is considered in subsection 2.3.

2.2   Segmentation of the ROI

The purpose of this stage is to identify the boundaries of the organ in the reference frame, based on roughly registered ROI sequence resulting from the previous subsection. It has been demonstrated that myocardial boundaries can be detected by segmenting a subtraction image, in which the myocardium is accentuated [8]. Fig. 3(c) displays the image obtained by subtracting Fig. 3(a) from Fig. 3(b). Detecting the boundaries of the left ventricle becomes a less challenging problem, to which we can apply many available segmentation algorithms [8] [9] [10] [11]. We take an energy minimization approach and propose a customized energy functional to overcome some unique problems that arise in our particular application. To take into account the anatomical constraint that the distance between the endocardium and the epicardium is relatively constant, we borrow the idea of coupled propagation of two cardiac contours [9]. Since the emphasis of this paper is placed on registration, we will directly present the segmentation results with no further explanation. The detected endocardium and epicardium are delineated respectively using bright contours on top of the ref-

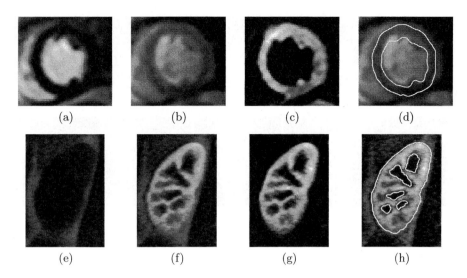

(a)   (b)   (c)   (d)

(e)   (f)   (g)   (h)

Fig. 3. Segmentation results of roughly registered images.

erence frame, see Fig. 3 (d). Although this is an approximate segmentation, it provides us with enough shape priors to refine the template for affine registration.

Similar to the case of cardiac MR perfusion data, the subtraction between Figs. 3(e) and (f) results in an enhanced image for the renal MR perfusion scan as shown in Fig. 3(g). We apply the level set method described in [11] to extract the renal cortex. This is an energy minimization based segmentation method. It assumes that the image is formed by two regions of approximatively piecewise constant intensities of distinct values [11]. It can be seen in Fig. 3(g) that the assumption is valid; the image contains a bright object to be detected in a dark background. The segmentation results are overlaid on top of the reference frame in Fig. 3(h). As shown, the outer boundary of the kidney is well delineated. These results demonstrate that the boundaries of the organ (heart or kidney) in the reference frame can be identified.

2.3   Affine registration

We have compensated for integer pixel shifts of the ROI and obtained the contours that delineate the boundaries of the organ in the reference frame. Next, we propagate the segmentation results to other frames by estimating the affine transformation of the organ in each frame.

The affine transformation includes translation, rotation, scaling and shearing. In 2D, the affine transformation between (x, y) and (x', y') is given by

$$\begin{bmatrix} x' \\ y' \end{bmatrix} = \mathbf{A} \begin{bmatrix} x \\ y \end{bmatrix} + \mathbf{t}, \tag{4}$$

where $\mathbf{A}$ is a 2×2 invertible matrix that defines rotation, shear, and scale, and $\mathbf{t}$ is a 2×1 translation vector.

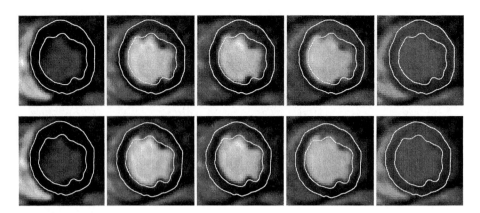

Fig. 4. Registration results for representative frames from a real patient cardiac MR perfusion scan. The top row shows the segmentation results obtained in Section 2.2 with the contours overlaid on the registered ROI. The bottom row shows the transformed contours after applying affine registration.

The segmentation results obtained in the previous step make it possible to refine the template by ignoring irrelevant edge information. Let $\mathcal{L} \subset \mathcal{R}$ denote the set of pixels in the ROI corresponding to pixels lying on the boundaries of the organ and their nearest neighbors under a second order neighborhood system. Let $\theta'_c(x, y; \mathbf{A}, \mathbf{t})$ and $M'_c(x, y; \mathbf{A}, \mathbf{t})$ denote the corresponding direction and magnitude of the image gradient in the current frame under the affine transformation defined by $\mathbf{A}$ and $\mathbf{t}$. The goal of the affine registration is to find the affine transformation $(\mathbf{A}, \mathbf{t})$ that maximizes the following similarity metric for the current image

$$S'(\mathbf{A}, \mathbf{t}) = \sum_{(x,y) \in \mathcal{L}} w'(x, y; \mathbf{A}, \mathbf{t}) \cos(2\Delta\theta'(x, y; \mathbf{A}, \mathbf{t})), \qquad (5)$$

where $\Delta\theta'(x, y; \mathbf{A}, \mathbf{t})$ and $w'(x, y; \mathbf{A}, \mathbf{t})$ are computed respectively by

$$\Delta\theta'(x, y; \mathbf{A}, \mathbf{t}) = \theta'_c(x, y; \mathbf{A}, \mathbf{t}) - \theta_r(x, y), \qquad (6)$$

$$w'(x, y; \mathbf{A}, \mathbf{t}) = \frac{M'_c(x, y; \mathbf{A}, \mathbf{t}) M_r(x, y)}{\sum_{(x,y) \in \mathcal{L}} M'_c(x, y; \mathbf{A}, \mathbf{t}) M_r(x, y)}. \qquad (7)$$

In the special case where the motion of the organ is highly constrained and approximately rigid, we can reduce the number of degrees of freedom in the affine transform by restricting the motion to rotation and translation. In our experiments, we adopt the following measures: (1) we keep the scaling fixed and let the rotation vary between -5 to 5 degrees in 1 degree steps; (2) the translation along either dimension is constrained between -2 to 2 pixels; (3) we construct a bank of templates for each combination of rotation and translation; and (4) we search for the best template that results in the largest similarity metric between the current frame and the reference frame, over the constrained parameter space. This algorithm is fast and insensitive to noise. Although not described here, the algorithm can be extended to maximizing $S'(\mathbf{A}, \mathbf{t})$ under affine transformation through a gradient descent method [12].

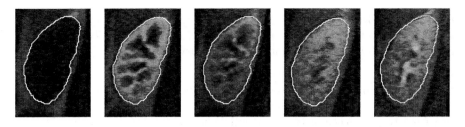

Fig. 5. Registration results for selected frames from a renal MR perfusion scan.

3   Results

Our algorithm has been tested on 15 cardiac and 12 renal MR perfusion datasets of real patients. Each dataset contains 3 or 4 slices. The images were acquired on Siemens Sonata MR scanners following bolus injection of Gd-DTPA contrast agent. In most cases, the image matrix is 256×256 pixels. The number of frames in each image sequence ranges from 50 to 350.

For all the data sets in our study, the registration results were qualitatively validated with visual analysis by displaying the registered image sequence in a movie mode. Using our ROI tracking algorithm, we are able to track the ROI reliably in all the sequences robustly, with a maximum tracking error less than 2 pixels in both directions. Furthermore, our experimental results show that affine registration helps improve the accuracy of the registration greatly. Fig. 4 compares the results obtained before and after applying affine registration for a real cardiac MR perfusion scan. As shown, the contours in the top row of images, before affine registration, do not lie exactly at the boundaries of the left ventricle. This is easily seen at the bottom left of each image where the edge information is relatively strong. On the other hand, the contours in the bottom row of images, after affine registration, delineate well the boundaries of the left ventricle. In particular, the accuracy of the estimated rotation can be visually validated by looking at the papillary muscle at the bottom of each image.

To illustrate the performance of the registration algorithm with renal MR perfusion data, we present the results for a real patient in Fig. 5. We have also validated the registration results quantitatively for a renal perfusion MR scan of 150 images, by comparing the estimated translation vector at each frame with a "gold standard," i.e., pixel shifts obtained manually. The error size is less than one pixel in each direction for more than 95% of the frames. These results strongly suggest that the motion caused by breathing can be successfully compensated using the registration algorithm presented here.

4   Conclusion

The paper presents a common framework for the registration of dynamic cardiac and renal MR perfusion images. The algorithm exploits image features that are invariant to a rapidly changing contrast and utilizes image segmentation results for the construction of templates. We have obtained encouraging registration results with real patient datasets. As future work, we plan to segment different anatomical structures within the ROI based on their distinct dynamics of the first-pass signal, i.e., the pixel intensity-time curve [13].

Acknowledgements. The authors would like to thank Niels Oesingmann from Siemens Medical Systems MR Division, Erlangen, Germany, and Stefan Schoenberg from the Institute of Clinical Radiology, Klinikum Grosshadern, Munich, Germany, for providing cardiac and renal MR perfusion data. The first and third authors acknowledge the support from NIH grants (P41EB001977 and R01EB/AI-00318) and from a Siemens research grant.

References

1. E. Nagel et al. Magnetic resonance perfusion measurements for the noninvasive detection of coronary artery disease. *Circulation*, 108(4):432-437, July, 2003.
2. S.J. Gandy et al. Dynamic MRI contrast enhancement of renal cortex: a functional assessment of renovascular disease in patients with renal artery stenosis. *J Magn Reson Imaging*, 18(4):461-6, Oct, 2003.
3. R. Bansal and G. Funka-Lea. Integrated image registration for cardiac MR perfusion data. *MICCAI*(1) 2002:659-666.
4. G. Gerig, R. Kikinis, W. Kuoni, G.K. van Schulthess, and O. Kübler. Semiautomated ROI analysis in dynamic MRI-studies: Part I: image analysis tools for automatic correction of organ displacements. *IEEE Trans. Image Processing*, 11(2):221-232, 1992.
5. E.L.W. Giele et al. Movement correction of the kidney in dynamic MRI scans using FFT phase difference movement detection. *J. Magn Reson Imaging*, 14:741-49, 2001.
6. P.J. Yim et al. Registration of time-series contrast enhanced magnetic resonance images for renography. *Proc. 14th IEEE Symp. Computer-Based Medical Systems*, pp. 516-520, 2001.
7. K.R. Castleman. *Digital Image Processing*. Prentice Hall, 1996.
8. L. Spreeuwers and M. Breeuwer. Automatic detection of myocardial boundaries in MR cardio perfusion images. *MICCAI* 2001:1228-1231.
9. N. Paragios. A variational approach for the segmentation of the left ventricle in MR cardiac images. *IEEE Workshop on Variational and Level Set Methods in Computer Vision*, Vancouver, Canada, pp.153-160, July 2001.
10. M.-P. Jolly. Combining edge, region, and shape information to segment the left ventricle in cardiac MR images. *Proc. Medical Image Computing and Computer-Assisted Intervention*, Utrecht, The Netherlands, pp.482-490, Oct 2001.
11. T. F. Chan and L. A. Vese. Active contours without edges. *IEEE Trans. Image Processing*, 10(2):266-77, 2001.
12. A. Yezzi, L. Zollei, and T. Kapur. A variational framework for joint segmentation and registration. *IEEE CVPR-MMBIA*, 2001.
13. Y. Sun, J. M. F. Moura, D. Yang, Q. Ye, and C. Ho. Kidney segmentation in MRI sequences using temporal dynamics. *Proc. 2002 IEEE Int. Symp. Biomedical Imaging*, pp.98-101, Washington, D.C., July 2002.

Spatio-temporal Free-Form Registration of Cardiac MR Image Sequences

Dimitrios Perperidis[1], Raad Mohiaddin[2], and Daniel Rueckert[1]

[1] Visual Information Processing Group, Department of Computing, Imperial College London,
180 Queen's Gate, London SW7 2AZ, United Kingdom
[2] Royal Brompton and Harefield NHS Trust, Sydney Street,
London, United Kingdom

Abstract. In this paper we develop a spatio-temporal registration algorithm for cardiac MR image sequences. The algorithm has the ability to correct any spatial misalignment between the images caused by global differences in the acquisition of the image sequences and by local shape differences. In addition it has the ability to correct temporal misalignment caused by differences in the length of the cardiac cycles and by differences in the dynamic properties of the hearts. The algorithm uses a 4D deformable transformation model which is separated into spatial and temporal components. The registration method was qualitatively evaluated by visual inspection and by measuring the overlap and surface distance of anatomical regions. The results demonstrate that a significant improvement in the alignment of the image sequences is achieved by the use of the deformable transformation model.

1 Introduction

Cardiovascular diseases are a very important cause of death in the developed world. Their early diagnosis and treatment is crucial in order to reduce mortality and to improve patients' quality of life. Recent advances in the development of non-invasive imaging modalities are enabling the high resolution imaging of the cardiovascular system. Among these modalities, magnetic imaging (MR) is playing an increasingly important role. MR imaging allows not only the acquisition of 3D images which describe the cardiac anatomy but also the acquisition of 4D cardiac image sequences which describe the cardiac anatomy as well as function.

The recent advantages in the development of cardiac imaging modalities have led to an increased need for cardiac registration methods (for recent reviews of cardiac image registration methods see [1] and [2] for a general review of image registration methods). In general, cardiac image registration is a very complex problem due to the complicated non-rigid motion of the heart and the thorax as well as the low resolution with which cardiac images are usually acquired. In the recent years cardiac image registration has emerged as an important tool for a large number of applications. It has a fundamental role in the construction of anatomical atlases of the heart [3,4]. It has also been used for the analysis of the myocardial motion [5] and for the segmentation of cardiac images [6]. Image registration has been also used for the fusion of information from a number of different modalities such as CT, MR, PET, and SPECT [7,8]. In addition, cardiac

C. Barillot, D.R. Haynor, and P. Hellier (Eds.): MICCAI 2004, LNCS 3216, pp. 911–919, 2004.

image registration is crucial for the comparison of images of the same subject, e.g. before and after pharmacological treatment or surgical intervention. Furthermore, inter-subject alignment of cardiac image sequences to the same coordinate space (anatomical reference) enables direct comparisons between the cardiac anatomy and function of different subjects to be made.

While a large number of registration techniques exist for cardiac images, most of these techniques focus on 3D images ignoring any temporal misalignment between the two image sequences. In this paper we extend a 4D cardiac MR image registration method based on voxel similarity measures which has been recently presented [9,10, 3]. This method will not only bring a number of sequences of cardiac images acquired from different subjects or the same subject (for example short and long axis cardiac image sequences) into the same spatial coordinate frame but also into the same temporal coordinate frame. This allows direct comparison between both the cardiac anatomy of different subjects and the cardiac function to be made. The aim of this contribution is to improve the accuracy of the cardiac MR image sequence registration algorithm by using a spatio-temporal free-form deformation model based on B-Splines. The registration method which has been previously presented [10] had the ability to correct spatial misalignment caused by both global and local differences of the shape of the heart as well as temporal misalignment due to differences in the temporal acquisition parameters but not temporal misalignment caused by different cardiac dynamics. This contribution will enable the correction of temporal misalignment not only caused by differences in the temporal acquisition parameters but also in the cardiac dynamics providing a spatio-temporal deformable registration method for cardiac MR image sequences.

2   Spatio-temporal Registration

Since the heart is undergoing a spatially and temporally varying degree motion during the cardiac cycle, 4D cardiac image registration algorithms are required when registering two cardiac MR image sequences. Spatial alignment of corresponding frames of the image sequences (e.g. the second frame of one image sequence with the second frame of the other) is not enough since these frames may not correspond to the same position in the cardiac cycle of the hearts. This is due to differences in the acquisition parameters (initial offset in the acquisition of the first frame and different frequency in the acquisition of consecutively frames), differences in the length of cardiac cycles (e.g. one cardiac cycle maybe longer than the other) and differences in the dynamic properties of the hearts (e.g. one heart may have longer contraction phase and shorter relaxation phase). Spatio-temporal alignment will enable comparison between corresponding anatomical positions and corresponding positions in the cardiac cycle of the hearts. It will also resolve spatial ambiguities which occur when there is not sufficient common appearance in the two 3D MR cardiac images. Furthermore, it can also improve the results of the registration because it is not restricted only to the alignment of existing frames but it can also use sub-frame information.

A 4D cardiac image sequence can be represented as sequence of n 3D images $I_k(x, y, z)$ with a fixed field of view Ω_I and an acquisition time t_k with $t_k < t_{k+1}$, in the temporal direction. The resulting image sequence can be viewed as 4D image

$I(x, y, z, t)$ defined on the spatio-temporal domain $\Omega_I \times [t_1, t_n]$. The goal of 4D image registration described in this paper is to relate each point of one image sequence to its corresponding point of the reference image sequence. In this case the transformation $\mathbf{T} : (x, y, z, t) \rightarrow (x', y', z', t')$ maps any point of one image sequence $I(x, y, z, t)$ into its corresponding point in the reference image sequence $I(x', y', z', t')$. The mapping used in this paper is of the following form:

$$\mathbf{T}(x, y, z, t) = (x'(x, y, z), y'(x, y, z), z'(x, y, z), t'(t)) \tag{1}$$

and can be of a subvoxel displacement in the spatial domain and of a sub-frame displacement in the temporal domain. The 4D mapping can be resolved into decoupled spatial and temporal components $\mathbf{T}_{spatial}$ and $\mathbf{T}_{temporal}$ respectively where

$$\mathbf{T}_{spatial}(x, y, z) = (x'(x, y, z), y'(x, y, z), z'(x, y, z)), \mathbf{T}_{temporal}(t) = t'(t)$$

each of which we choose to be one-to-one mappings. One consequence of this decoupling is that each temporal frame t in image sequence I will map to another temporal frame t' in image sequence I', ensuring causality and preventing different regions in a 3D image $I_t(x, y, z)$ from being warped differently in the temporal direction by $\mathbf{T}_{temporal}$.

2.1 Spatial Alignment

The aim of the spatial part of the transformation is to relate each spatial point of an image to a point of the reference image, i.e. $\mathbf{T}_{spatial} : (x, y, z) \rightarrow (x', y', z')$ maps any point (x, y, z) of a particular time frame t in one image sequence into its corresponding point (x', y', z') of another particular time frame t' of the reference image sequence. The transformation $\mathbf{T}_{spatial}$ consists of a global transformation and a local transformation:

$$\mathbf{T}_{spatial}(x, y, z) = \mathbf{T}_{spatial}^{global}(x, y, z) + \mathbf{T}_{spatial}^{local}(x, y, z) \tag{2}$$

The global transformation addresses differences in the size, orientation and alignment of the hearts while the local part addresses differences in the shape of the hearts. An affine transformation with 12 degrees of freedom utilizing scaling and shearing in addition to translation and rotation is used as $\mathbf{T}_{spatial}^{global}$.

A free-form deformation (FFD) model based on B-splines is used in order to describe the differences in the local shape of the hearts. To define a spline-based FFD we denote the spatial domain of the image volume as $\Omega_I = \{(x, y, z) \mid 0 \leq x < X, 0 \leq y < Y, 0 \leq z < Z\}$. Let Φ denote a $n_x \times n_y \times n_z$ mesh of control points $\phi_{i,j,k}$ with uniform spacing δ. Then, the FFD can be written as the 3D tensor product of the familiar 1D cubic B-splines [11]:

$$\mathbf{T}_{spatial}^{local}(x, y, z) = \sum_{l=0}^{3} \sum_{m=0}^{3} \sum_{n=0}^{3} B_l(u) B_m(v) B_n(w) \phi_{i+l, j+m, k+n} \tag{3}$$

where $i = \lfloor \frac{x}{n_x} \rfloor - 1, j = \lfloor \frac{y}{n_y} \rfloor - 1, k = \lfloor \frac{z}{n_z} \rfloor - 1, u = \frac{x}{n_x} - \lfloor \frac{x}{n_x} \rfloor, v = \frac{y}{n_y} - \lfloor \frac{y}{n_y} \rfloor, w = \frac{z}{n_z} - \lfloor \frac{z}{n_z} \rfloor$ and where B_l represents the l-th basis function of the B-spline. One advantage of B-Splines is that they are locally controlled which makes them computationally efficient even for a large number of control points. In particular, the basis functions of cubic B-Splines have a limited support, i.e. changing a control point affects the transformation only in the local neighborhood of that control point. This combined spatial deformation model has been introduced by Rueckert et al. [11].It has been used by a large number of approaches in cardiac MR imaging including for the analysis of the myocardial motion [5], and for the segmentation of the myocardium and the ventricles of cardiac MR image sequences [6].

2.2 Temporal Alignment

The temporal part of the transformation consists of a temporal global part, $\mathbf{T}^{global}_{temporal}$, and a temporal local part, $\mathbf{T}^{local}_{temporal}$:

$$\mathbf{T}_{temporal}(t) = \mathbf{T}^{global}_{temporal}(t') + \mathbf{T}^{local}_{temporal}(t')$$

$\mathbf{T}^{global}_{temporal}$ is an affine transformation which corrects for differences in the length of the cardiac cycles and differences in the acquisition parameters. $\mathbf{T}^{local}_{temporal}$ is modeled by a free-form deformation using a 1D B-spline and corrects for temporal misalignment caused by different cardiac dynamic properties (difference in the length of contraction and relaxation phases, different motion patterns, etc). To define a spline-based temporal free-form deformation we denote the temporal domain of the image sequence as $\Omega_t = \{(t) \mid 0 \le x < T\}$. Let Φ denote a set of n_t control points ϕ_t with a temporal spacing δ_t. Then, the temporal free-form deformation can be defined as a 1D cubic B-spline:

$$\mathbf{T}^{local}_{temporal}(t) = \sum_{l=0}^{3} B_l(u)\phi_{t_{i+l}} \qquad (4)$$

where $i = \lfloor \frac{t}{n_t} \rfloor - 1$, $u = \frac{t}{n_t} - \lfloor \frac{t}{n_t} \rfloor$ and B_l represents the l-th basis function of the B-spline.

$\mathbf{T}^{local}_{temporal}$ deforms the temporal characteristics of each image sequence in order to follow the same motion pattern with the reference image sequence. The combined 4D transformation model (equation 1) is the spatio-temporal free-form deformation (STFFD).

2.3 Voxel-Based Similarity of Image Sequences

The optimal transformation is found by maximising a voxel based similarity measure, the Normalised Mutual Information (NMI) [12] which is a very commonly used similarity measure in the field of medical image registration. The normalised mutual information of the two image sequences can be calculated directly from the joint intensity histogram of the two sequences over the spatio-temporal domain of overlap $\Omega_{I_A} \times [t_{A1}, t_{An}] \bigcap \mathbf{T}(\Omega_{I_B} \times [t_{B1}, t_{Bn}])$. During the optimisation new voxel values are generated in the temporal domain using linear interpolation and trilinear interpolation in the spatial domain. In the first part of the optimization procedure NMI is optimized as a function of $T^{global}_{spatial}$ and $T^{global}_{temporal}$ using an iterative downhill descent algorithm. In the second part, NMI is optimized as a a function of $T^{local}_{spatial}$ and $T^{local}_{temporal}$ using a simple iterative gradient descent method.

3   Results and Discussion

To evaluate the spatio-temporal deformable registration algorithm we have acquired fifteen cardiac MR image sequences from healthy volunteers. All image sequences used for our experiments were acquired on a Siemens Sonata 1.5 T scanner using TrueFisp pulse sequence. For the reference subject 32 different time frames were acquired (cardiac cycle of length 950msec). Each 3D image of the sequence had a resolution of 256 × 192 × 46 with a pixel size of $0.97mm × 0.97mm$ and a slice thickness of 3mm. Fourteen 4D cardiac MR images were registered to the reference subject. The length of the cardiac cycle of these images sequences varied from 300msec to 800msec. An initial estimate of the global spatial transformation was provided due to the large variety in the position and orientation of the hearts. Since all the image sequences contained almost entire cardiac cycles, the global temporal transformation was calculated in order to compensate the differences in length of the cardiac cycles of the subjects (by matching the first and the last frames of the image sequences). The spacing of the control points of the local transformation were 10mm in the spatial domain and 90msec in the temporal domain.

Figure 1 (a) shows the volume curves of the left ventricle after the optimization of the spatio-temporal global transformation, while 1 (b) shows the same volume curves and after the optimization of the spatio-temporal local transformation. The volume of the left ventricles were calculated using segmented images. The images were segmented using an EM-algorithm developed by Lorenzo-Valdés et al. [13]. We can clearly see that with the introduction of the deformable components the hearts are significantly better aligned in the temporal domain. All the hearts in 1,(b) follow a similar motion pattern.

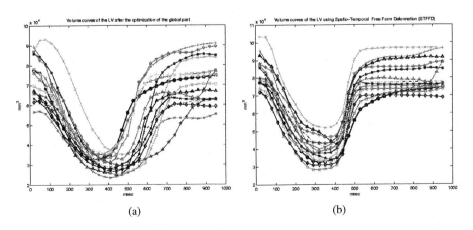

(a)   (b)

Fig. 1. The volume curves of the left ventricle for all subjects after optimisation of the global spatio spatio-temporal transformation (a) and the local spatio-temporal registration (b).

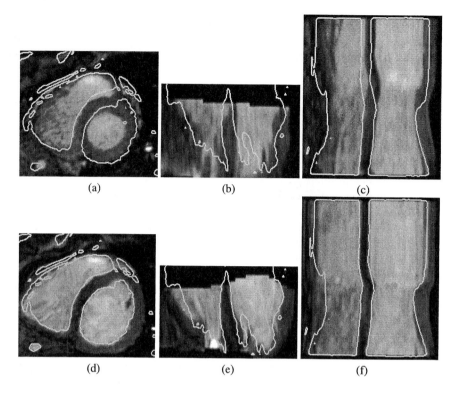

(a)   (b)   (c)

(d)   (e)   (f)

Fig. 2. Results of the 4D cardiac MR registration algorithm. (a-c) shows the short axis, the long axis and the temporal views after the affine alignment, (d-f) shows the corresponding short axis, long axis and temporal views after the spatio-temporal free-form registration. Animations of the registrations can be found at http://www.doc.ic.ac.uk/~dp1/Conferences/MICCAI04/

Figure 2 provides an example of the spatio-temporal free-form registration. The images in the top row (a-c) are the short axis, the long axis and the temporal views of a frame in the middle of the image sequence after the optimization of the global transformations (affine spatio-temporal registration). The lines in the images represent the contours of the reference image sequence. The images in the bottom row of figure 2 are the same images after spatio-temporal free-form registration. We can clearly see with the introduction of the deformable temporal and spatial transformation there is a significant improvement in the alignment of the image sequences both in the spatial and in the temporal domain. This enables comparisons between corresponding positions in the cardiac cycle to be performed. The blank areas in the long axis views are caused due to a smaller off-plane field of view in the current subject. The quality of the registration in the spatial domain was measured by calculating the volume overlap for the left and right ventricles as well as for the myocardium. The volume overlap for an object O is defined as:

$$\Delta(T, S) = \frac{2 \times |T \cap S|}{|T| + |S|} \times 100\%$$

(5)

Table 1. The mean volume overlap and surface distance after the affine 4D registration,after the deformable 3D and after spatio-temporal deformable registration.

	Volume Overlap			Surface Distance in mm		
Anatomical region	Affine 4D	Deformable 3D	Deformable 4D	Affine 4D	Deformable 3D	Deformable 4D
Left ventricle	76.15%	80.95%	85.76%	4.16	3.56	2.96
Right ventricle	77.39%	83.87%	84.86%	4.95	4.27	3.60
Myocardium	70.39%	71.64%	73.86%	4.77	3.87	4.16

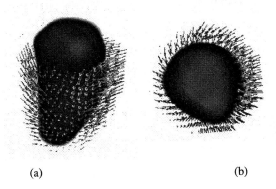

(a)   (b)

Fig. 3. Examples of the volume renderings of the probabilistic atlas of the left ventricle with the atlas of the myocardium's deformation [3]. Animations of the atlases can be found at `http://www.doc.ic.ac.uk/~dp1/Conferences/MICCAI04/`.

Here T denotes the voxels in the reference (target) image part of object O and S denotes the voxels in the other image part of object O. We have also calculated the mean surface distance of the above anatomical regions after the affine and the deformable 4D registration. In order to calculate the overlap of the anatomical structures and the surface distance we used segmented images. Table 1 shows the mean volume overlap and the mean surface distance (in mm) for each anatomical region after spatio-temporal affine registration, after 3D non-rigid registration of the first frames (by matching the first and the last time frames of the image sequences) and after the spatio-temporal deformable registration. The results indicate clearly that the use of the deformable spatial and temporal part provides a significant improvement in the quality of the registration compared to the other two methods.

4   Conclusions and Further Work

We have presented an extension to our earlier spatio-temporal registration method [9,10]. In this contribution we extended the registration method by introducing a spatio-temporal deformable transformation model. The proposed registration approach corrects temporal misalignment caused by different acquisition parameters, different length of cardiac cycles and different dynamic properties of the hearts. The approach also corrects spatial misalignment caused by global differences in the acquisition of the image sequences and local shape differences. There is a large range of applications for this spatio-temporal registration method. We are planning to use it for building a probabilistic atlas of the cardiac anatomy and function similar to the one we have recently presented [3]. In this case, image registration is used in order to map all the image sequences used for the atlas construction to the same spatio-temporal coordinate system. Then, the atlas can be constructed by averaging the transformed image sequences. Figure 3 provides an example of a 4D probabilistic atlas of the left ventricle with the average deformation of the myocardium [3]. Moreover, the method can be used anytime a comparison between image sequences from the same subject (before and after surgical intervention or pharmacological treatment) or from different subjects (comparison of different cardiac anatomies and functions, atlas based registration) is required. The method was evaluated using fifteen image sequences from healthy volunteers. The results indicate a significant improvement in the temporal and spatial registration of the image sequences with the use of the spatio-temporal deformable transformation model.

References

1. T. Mäkelä, P. Clarysse, N. Sipila, O.and Pauna, and Q. C. Pham. A review of cardiac image registration methods. *IEEE Transcactions on Medical Imaging*, 21(9), 2002.
2. B. Zitová and J. Flusser. Image registration methods: a survey. *Image and Vision Computing*, 21:977–1000, 2003.
3. D. Perperidis, M. Lorenzo-Valdés, R. Chandrashekara, A. Rao, R. Mohiaddin, G.I Sanchez-Ortiz, and D. Rueckert. Building a 4D atlas of the cardiac anatomy and motion using MR imaging. In *2004 IEEE International Symposium on Biomedical Imaging: From Nano to Macro*, 2004.
4. A.F. Frangi, D. Rueckert, J. A. Schnabel, and W.J. Niessen. Automatic construction of multiple-object three-dimensional statistical shape models: Application to cardiac modeling. *IEEE Transaction on Medical Imaging*, 21(9):1151–1165, 2002.
5. R. Chandrashekara, R. H. Mohiaddin, and D. Rueckert. Analysis of myocardial motion in tagged MR images using nonrigid image registration. In M. Sonka and J. Michael Fitzpatrick, editors, *Proceedings of the SPIE International Symposium on Medical Imaging*, pages 1168–1179, San Diego, California USA, 24–28 February 2002.
6. M. Lorenzo-Valdés, G.I. Sanchez-Ortiz, R. Mohiaddin, and D. Rueckert. Atlas based segmentation and tracking of 3D cardiac MR images using non rigid registration. In *Fith Int. Conf. on Medical Image Computing and Computer-Assisted Intervention (MICCAI'02)*, Lecture Notes in Computer Science, pages 642–650. Springer-Verlag, 2002.
7. M.C. Gilardi, G. Rizzo, A. Savi, C. Landoni, V. Bettinardi, C. Rosseti, G. Striano, and F. Fazio. Correlation of SPECT and PET cardiac images by a surface matching registration technique. *Computerized Medical Imaging and Graphics*, 22(5):391–398, 1998.
8. T. G. Turkington, T. R. DeGradom, M. W. Hanson, and E. R. Coleman. Alignment of dynamic cardiac PET images for correction of motion. *IEEE Transaction on Nuclear Science*, 44(2):235–242, 1997.
9. D. Perperidis, A. Rao, M. Lorenzo-Valdés, R. Mohiaddin, and D. Rueckert. Spatio-temporal alignment of 4D cardiac MR images. In *Lecture Notes in Computer Science: Functional Imaging and Modeling of the heart, FIMH'03*, Lyon, France, June 5-6, 2003. Springer.
10. D. Perperidis, A. Rao, R. Mohiaddin, and R. Rueckert. Non-rigid spatio temporal alignment of 4D cardiac MR images. In *Lecture Notes in Computer Science: Second International Workshop on Biomedical Image Registration (WBIR)*. Springer, 2003.

11. D. Rueckert, L. I. Sonoda, C. Hayes, D.L.G Hill, M.O. Leach, and D.J Hawkes. Non-rigid registration using free-form deformations: Application to breast MR images. *IEEE Transactions on Medical Imaging*, 18(8):712–721, 1999.

12. C. Studholme, D.L.G. Hill, and D.J. Hawkes. An overlap invariant entropy measure of 3D medical image alignment. *Pattern Recognition*, 32:71–86, 1999.

13. M. Lorenzo-Valdés, G. I. Sanchez-Ortiz, R. Mohiaddin, and D. Rueckert. Segmentation of 4D cardiac MR images using a probabilistic atlas and the EM algorithm. In *Sixth Int. Conf. on Medical Image Computing and Computer-Assisted Intervention (MICCAI'03)*, Lecture Notes in Computer Science. Springer-Verlag, 2003.

Author Index

Lecture Notes in Computer Science

For information about Vols. 1–3121

please contact your bookseller or Springer